EMERGENCY PROCEDURES FOR THE SMALL ANIMAL VETERINARIAN

Dedication

This edition is dedicated

— *to my family and to my very special friends, Michael Longoni, Melissa Manos, Diane Paster and Susan K. Wilkerson. Thank you for your continued loyalty, support, and encouragement.*

— *to Alie Amato, who I admire and respect for her devotion to the animals she rescues and to whom I am forever indebted for allowing me to enter her world, to meet people and to enjoy experiences I never would have imagined.*

— *to Stacey Hoffman, for her friendship, guidance, patience, and for having confidence in me. Thank you for standing up for what is right and not being afraid to speak up when something is wrong.*

— *and to Maureen McMichael, F. Tony Mann, Marie Kerl, Tim Hackett, Karl Jandrey, Jana Jones and all the specialists, residents and interns who helped me during my residency. I was very fortunate to spend a while with each of them. They each taught me so much more about life than just veterinary medicine.*

Content Strategist: Robert Edwards
Senior Content Development Specialist: Catherine Jackson
Senior Project Manager: Beula Christopher
Designer/Design Direction: Miles Hitchen/Christian J Bilbow
Illustration Manager: Jennifer Rose
Illustrator: Samantha Elmhurst

EMERGENCY PROCEDURES FOR THE SMALL ANIMAL VETERINARIAN

Signe J Plunkett DVM
Director, Urgent Care at Animal Health Services
Member, VECCS, Society of Critical Care Medicine,
Arizona Veterinary Medical Association,
and American Veterinary Medical Association
Cave Creek, Arizona

THIRD EDITION

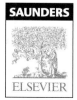

SAUNDERS

ELSEVIER

EDINBURGH   LONDON   NEW YORK   OXFORD   PHILADELPHIA   ST LOUIS
SYDNEY   TORONTO 2013

SAUNDERS
ELSEVIER

© 2013 Elsevier Ltd. All rights reserved.

First edition 1993
Second edition 2000
Third edition 2013

ISBN 978 0 7020 2768 0

British Library Cataloguing in Publication Data
A catalogue record for this book is available from the British Library

Library of Congress Cataloging in Publication Data
A catalog record for this book is available from the Library of Congress

Notices
Knowledge and best practice in this field are constantly changing. As new research and experience broaden our understanding, changes in research methods, professional practices, or medical treatment may become necessary.

Practitioners and researchers must always rely on their own experience and knowledge in evaluating and using any information, methods, compounds, or experiments described herein. In using such information or methods they should be mindful of their own safety and the safety of others, including parties for whom they have a professional responsibility.

With respect to any drug or pharmaceutical products identified, readers are advised to check the most current information provided (i) on procedures featured or (ii) by the manufacturer of each product to be administered, to verify the recommended dose or formula, the method and duration of administration, and contraindications. It is the responsibility of practitioners, relying on their own experience and knowledge of their patients, to make diagnoses, to determine dosages and the best treatment for each individual patient, and to take all appropriate safety precautions.

To the fullest extent of the law, neither the Publisher nor the authors, contributors, or editors, assume any liability for any injury and/or damage to persons or property as a matter of products liability, negligence or otherwise, or from any use or operation of any methods, products, instructions, or ideas contained in the material herein.

Printed in India

Last digit is the print number: 20 19 18 17

Contents

CONTENTS

Preface

Major changes have occurred since the publication of the second edition. I completed a residency in small animal emergency and critical care. I am also with a different practice.

During my residency, I spent time at the veterinary teaching hospitals of Texas A and M University, the University of California at Davis, Colorado State University, and the University of Missouri. I worked with, and learned from, several criticalists, emergency and critical care residents and interns, members of the other services in these hospitals, and numerous veterinary students. It was an incredible experience after being in private practice for 20 years. I learned so much from everyone who assisted me, and became a better emergency and critical care doctor as a result. At each location, I received thanks from many of the faculty members and residents for helping them make it through the emergency rotations of their internships and residencies by writing this book. I hope that this new edition continues to be helpful to those in internships, family practice veterinarians and veterinarians in emergency and critical care practices. I hope also that this new edition continues to be helpful when you need quick assistance with your emergency patient. This is not your reference for detailed information regarding pathophysiology or pharmacology, but hopefully you can quickly find the information you need to save a life when confronted with a seriously ill, injured, or poisoned patient.

This edition contains information on many more emergencies and additional toxicoses, including grapes and raisins, lilies, sago palm and xylitol. Chapters have been added to cover the basics of emergency care, including analgesia, fluid therapy, oxygen administration, supportive care and shock. Every section was updated and, hopefully, improved. Due to popular demand, the format has remained the same.

To enhance the quality, coauthors were brought in for three chapters. Sarah J. Deitschel DVM, DACVECC wrote the majority of the updates on respiratory emergencies. Elizabeth J. Thomovsky DVM, MS, DACVECC wrote the majority of the updates on urological emergencies and electrolyte disorders. Christoph Mans MED.VET rewrote the chapter on exotic emergencies, providing expert information for those of us who do not routinely work with these species.

We hope you find the third edition as helpful as, or more so than, the previous editions. Good luck in your efforts to make a difference in the lives of people by helping their friends with serious injuries or illnesses. Ours is not an easy task, but it is very rewarding.

Acknowledgments

I would like to acknowledge several people for their contributions to this project. Robert Edwards, Alison McMurdo, Catherine Jackson, Beula Christopher, and the entire staff of Elsevier were very helpful, providing encouragement, guidance and assistance in the preparation of this book. Several friends also helped complete this edition. I met Sarah J. Deitschel and Elizabeth J. Thomovsky at the University of Missouri, and they have continued to be wonderful friends. I was so lucky our paths crossed. Thank you to Dr. Christoph Mans for stepping in towards the end and assisting us with the completion of this project.

List of contributors

Sarah J Deitschel DVM, DACVECC
Criticalist
Pittsburgh Veterinary Specialty and Emergency Center
Pittsburgh, Pennsylvania

Christoph Mans MED. VET.
Clinical Instructor in Zoological Medicine
Department of Medical Sciences
School of Veterinary Medicine, University of Wisconsin
Madison, Wisconsin

Elizabeth J Thomovsky DVM, MS, DACVECC
Clinical Assistant Professor of Small Animal Emergency and Critical Care
Purdue University College of Veterinary Medicine
West Lafayette, Indiana

Supportive therapy

ACID–BASE DISTURBANCES

Evaluation of the blood pH, bicarbonate (HCO_3^-), P_{CO_2} and base excess may be very helpful in the assessment of a critically ill or injured animal. Arterial blood samples are necessary to evaluate the respiratory status and are the preferred sample, but venous blood samples are helpful to evaluate the status of the patient at the cellular level.

The normal arterial blood gas reference ranges for dogs and cats inspiring room air are listed in Table 1.1.

Evaluation of blood gas results is a process involving many steps

1. Determine whether the pH is normal.
2. Evaluate the partial pressure of carbon dioxide (P_{CO_2}) – the respiratory component.
3. Evaluate the bicarbonate concentration [HCO_3^-] – the nonrespiratory component.
4. What is the primary disorder? The direction of the expected changes are shown in Table 1.2.
5. Is the secondary or adaptive response as expected? The expected responses are shown in Table 1.3.
6. Which disease process(es) is(are) responsible for the acid–base disorder?

RESPIRATORY ACIDOSIS

Respiratory acidosis or primary hypercapnia indicates hypoventilation and hypoxemia. The blood pH is decreased, the Pa_{CO_2} is increased and, with compensation, the HCO_3^- increases.

Sympathetic activation, increased cardiac output and possibly tachyarrhythmias may occur in the presence of moderately elevated Pa_{CO_2}. As the Pa_{CO_2} increases, intracranial pressure and cerebral blood flow increase. Disorientation, narcosis, and coma may occur at extremely high Pa_{CO_2} levels (60–70 mm Hg).

Causes of respiratory acidosis include:

- Depression of the respiratory center
  - Associated with medications (inhalant anesthetics, opioids, barbiturates)

Table 1.1 *Typical reference ranges for normal arterial blood gas values for dogs and cats inspiring room air*

	Dog	**Cat**
pH	7.41 (7.35–7.46)	7.39 (7.31–7.46)
Pa_{CO_2} (mm Hg)	37 (31–43)	31 (25–37)
[HCO_3^-] (mEq/L)	22 (19–26)	18 (14–22)
P_{O_2} (mm Hg)	92 (81–103)	107 (95–118)

Table 1.2 *The changes in simple primary acid–base disorders*

Disorder	pH	P_{CO_2}	[HCO_3^-]
Respiratory acidosis	↓	↑	↑ or normal
Respiratory alkalosis	↑	↓	↓ or normal
Nonrespiratory (Metabolic) acidosis	↓	↓	↓
Nonrespiratory (Metabolic) alkalosis	↑	↑	↑

Table 1.3 *Expected compensatory response in simple acid–base disturbances in dogs and cats**

		Clinical guide for compensation	
Disturbance	**Primary change**	**Dogs**	**Cats[†]**
Metabolic acidosis	Each 1 mEq/L ↓ HCO_3^-	P_{CO_2} ↓ by 0.7 mm Hg	P_{CO_2} does not change
Metabolic alkalosis	Each 1 mEq/L ↑ HCO_3^-	P_{CO_2} ↑ by 0.7 mm Hg	P_{CO_2} ↑ by 0.7 mm Hg
Respiratory acidosis			
Acute	Each 1 mm Hg ↑ P_{CO_2}	HCO_3^- ↑ by 0.15 mEq/L	HCO_3^- ↑ by 0.15 mEq/L
Chronic	Each 1 mm Hg ↑ P_{CO_2}	HCO_3^- ↑ by 0.35 mEq/L	Unknown
Long-standing[‡]	Each 1 mm Hg ↑ P_{CO_2}	HCO_3^- ↑ by 0.55 mEq/L	Unknown
Respiratory alkalosis			
Acute	Each 1 mm Hg ↓ P_{CO_2}	HCO_3^- ↓ by 0.25 mEq/L	HCO_3^- ↓ by 0.25 mEq/L
Chronic	Each 1 mm Hg ↓ P_{CO_2}	HCO_3^- ↓ by 0.55 mEq/L	Similar to dogs[§]

*From DiBartola SP (ed), Fluid, Electrolyte, and Acid-Base Disorders in Small Animal Practice, 3rd edn, St Louis, Elsevier, 2006, p 298, reprinted with permission from Elsevier Ltd. Data in dogs from de Morais & DiBartola (1991). See DiBartola (2006) for reference in cats.

[†]Data from cats are derived from a very limited number of cats.

[‡]More than 30 days.

[§]Exact degree of compensation has not been determined, but in cats with chronic respiratory alkalosis maintain normal arterial pH.

- ○ Neurologic disease
  - – Cervical spinal cord lesion
  - – Brainstem lesion
- Neuromuscular disease
  - ○ Myasthenia gravis
  - ○ Botulism
  - ○ Tetanus
  - ○ Tick paralysis
  - ○ Severe hypokalemia
  - ○ Associated with medications or chemicals (organophosphates, aminoglycosides)
- Obstruction of large airways
  - ○ Aspiration
  - ○ Kinked or plugged endotracheal tube
  - ○ Tracheal collapse
  - ○ Brachycephalic syndrome
  - ○ Laryngeal paralysis
  - ○ Mass lesion (intraluminal or extraluminal)
  - ○ Infiltrative lower airway disease (chronic obstructive pulmonary disease (COPD), asthma).

Treatment of respiratory acidosis is aimed at treatment of the underlying disorder, discontinuation or reversal of possible pharmacologic causes, establishment of an airway if needed, ventilation, and oxygenation.

RESPIRATORY ALKALOSIS

Respiratory alkalosis or primary hypocapnia indicates hyperventilation. The blood pH is increased, the Pa_{CO_2} is decreased and, with compensation, the HCO_3^- decreases.

The P_{CO_2} can be falsely decreased by excessive dilution of the blood sample with heparin and by the presence of air bubbles in the sample. Arteriolar vasoconstriction occurs when Pa_{CO_2} decreases to less than 25 mm Hg and when arterial pH increases to 7.6. This results in a reduction in myocardial and cerebral blood flow.

Clinical signs are usually those of the underlying condition, although tachypnea may be noticed. Disorientation, seizures and cardiac arrhythmias may occur.

Causes of respiratory alkalosis include:

- Fear, excitement, anxiety, or pain
- Hyperventilation (either by the patient or by mechanical ventilation)
- Decreased inspired partial pressure of oxygen
- Pulmonary diseases such as pneumonia, pulmonary edema, pulmonary fibrosis, pulmonary thromboembolism
- Congestive heart failure
- Severe anemia
- Severe hypotension
- Central nervous system disease
- Stimulation of pulmonary stretch receptors or nociceptors

- Activation of central respiratory centers
- Medications such as xanthines (aminophylline), corticosteroids, salicylates
- Hepatic disease
- Hyperadrenocorticism
- Sepsis
- Heat stroke
- Exercise
- Following metabolic acidosis.

Treatment of respiratory alkalosis is aimed at the underlying disorder, decreasing fear or pain, decreasing mechanical ventilation, discontinuation of possible pharmacologic causes, and correcting hypoxemia.

NONRESPIRATORY ACIDOSIS (METABOLIC ACIDOSIS)

Nonrespiratory or metabolic acidosis is based on the presence of decreased blood pH, decreased HCO_3^-, decreased base excess (BE), and with compensation the P_{CO_2} decreases. The condition is considered severe if blood pH exceeds 7.1 or HCO_3^- is less than 8 mEq/L. Although depression can occur with severe nonrespiratory acidosis and tachypnea may be observed, the clinical signs are usually associated with the underlying cause. Treatment is directed at the underlying disorder.

Causes of nonrespiratory acidosis include:

- Strong ion difference (SID) acidosis
  - Organic acidosis
    - Toxicities such as ethylene glycol or salicylate
    - Lactic acidosis
    - Uremic acidosis
    - Diabetic ketoacidosis
  - Dilutional acidosis (increased free water, associated with hyponatremia)
    - Due to a gain of hypotonic fluid (hypervolemia)
      Congestive heart failure
      Severe hepatic failure
    - Due to a gain of water (normovolemia)
      Infusion of hypotonic fluids
      Psychogenic polydipsia
    - Due to a loss of hypertonic fluid (hypovolemia)
      Administration of diuretics
      Hypoadrenocorticism
  - Hyperchloremic acidosis
    - Renal failure
    - Total parenteral nutrition
    - Fluid therapy with 0.9% NaCl, 7.2% NaCl, or potassium chloride (KCl) supplemented fluids
    - Hypoadrenocorticism
    - Diarrhea

- Nonvolatile ion buffer acidosis
  - Hyperphosphatemic acidosis
    - Renal failure
    - Urethral obstruction
    - Uroabdomen
    - Intravenous phosphate supplementation
    - Administration of phosphate-containing enemas.

NONRESPIRATORY ALKALOSIS (METABOLIC ALKALOSIS)

Nonrespiratory or metabolic alkalosis is based on the presence of increased blood pH, increased HCO_3^-, increased base excess (BE), and with compensation the P_{CO_2} increases. The condition is considered severe if blood pH exceeds 7.6. The clinical signs of nonrespiratory alkalosis are associated with the underlying cause. Treatment is directed at the underlying disorder.

Causes of nonrespiratory alkalosis include:

- Strong ion difference (SID) alkalosis
  - Hypochloremic alkalosis
    - Vomiting of stomach contents
    - Administration of loop diuretics, thiazides, or sodium bicarbonate
  - Chloride-resistant alkalosis
    - Hyperaldosteronism
      Hyperadrenocorticism
  - Concentration alkalosis (from pure water loss, associated with hypernatremia)
    - Water deprivation
    - Vomiting or diarrhea
- Nonvolatile ion buffer alkalosis
  - Hypoalbuminemia
    - Protein-losing nephropathy
    - Protein-losing enteropathy
    - Hepatic failure.

Mixed disorders may occur and may involve combinations of two or three of any of the above disorders. If respiratory acidosis occurs simultaneously with nonrespiratory acidosis, the resulting pH tends to be much lower than with a solitary disorder. If respiratory acidosis occurs simultaneously with nonrespiratory alkalosis, the resulting pH may be within normal range.

STRONG ION APPROACH

According to this method of acid–base evaluation, three independent variables determine plasma pH.

1. P_{CO_2} – an increase causes respiratory acidosis; a decrease causes respiratory alkalosis.
2. Strong ion difference (SID) – the sum of the completely dissociated plasma anions does not equal the sum of the completely dissociated plasma cations. These strong ions act together as one positively charged unit (SID) to affect plasma pH. The strong ions of importance in plasma

Gamblegram

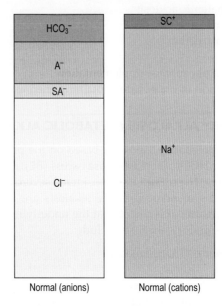

Normal (anions)   Normal (cations)

FIG 1.1   Gamblegram Normal plasma and change in ionic strength of anions secondary to increase (hyperchloremic acidosis) or decrease (hypochloremic alkalosis) in chloride. HCO_3^- = Bicarbonate, A^- = nonvolatile buffers, SA^- = strong anions, Cl^- = chloride, SC^+ = strong cations, Na^+ = sodium. *From DiBartola SP (ed), Fluid, Electrolyte, and Acid-Base Disorders in Small Animal Practice, 3rd edn, St Louis, Elsevier, 2006, p 315.*

are sodium (Na^+), potassium (K^+), calcium (Ca^{2+}), magnesium (Mg^{2+}), chloride (Cl^-), lactate, ketoacids (β-hydroxybutyrate, acetoacetate), and sulfate (SO_4^{2-}). An increase of the SID, caused by an increased [Na^+] or a decreased [Cl^-], results in strong ion or metabolic alkalosis. A decrease of the SID, caused by a decreased [Na^+] or an increased [Cl^-], [SO_4^{2-}], or organic anion concentration, results in strong ion or metabolic acidosis.

3. A_{TOT} – the effect of nonvolatile buffer ions, which act as weak acids at physiologic pH, are albumin, globulin, and inorganic phosphate. An increased A_{TOT} causes metabolic or nonvolatile ion buffer acidosis. A decreased A_{TOT} causes metabolic or nonvolatile ion buffer alkalosis.

A gamblegram is usually used to evaluate the strong ion approach (Fig. 1.1). There are six primary acid–base disturbances revealed by the strong ion approach:

1. Respiratory acidosis – increased P_{CO_2} as seen with hypoventilation
2. Respiratory alkalosis – decreased P_{CO_2} as seen with hyperventilation
3. Strong ion difference acidosis
   A. Dilutional acidosis (decreased [Na^+])
      I. Hypervolemia (congestive heart failure, nephrotic syndrome, severe hepatic disease)
      II. Normovolemia (administration of hypotonic fluids, psychogenic polydipsia)
      III. Hypovolemia (third space losses, administration of diuretics, hypoadrenocorticism, diarrhea, or vomiting)

B. Hyperchloremic acidosis (increased [Cl⁻])
   I. Excessive loss via diarrhea of sodium
   II. Gain of chloride (administration of total parenteral nutrition, fluid therapy with KCl, NaCl (0.9%, 3%, 5%, or 7.5%))
C. Retention of chloride (hypoadrenocorticism, renal failure)
D. Organic acidosis (uremia, diabetic ketoacidosis, lactic acidosis, and ethylene glycol or salicylate intoxication)
4. Strong ion difference alkalosis
   A. Concentrational alkalosis (increased [Na⁺])
      I. Hypotonic fluid loss (postobstructive diuresis, nonoliguric renal failure, vomiting)
      II. Pure water loss (diabetes insipidus, water deprivation)
   B. Hypochloremic alkalosis (decreased [Cl⁻])
      I. Excessive gain of sodium relative to chloride as with the administration of sodium bicarbonate
      II. Excessive loss of chloride relative to sodium (thiazide or loop diuretic administration or vomiting of stomach contents)
5. Nonvolatile buffer ion acidosis (increased [A_{TOT}])
   A. Hyperalbuminemia (dehydration, water deprivation)
   B. Hyperphosphatemia (tumor cell lysis, rhabdomyolysis or tissue trauma, administration of phosphate solutions or enemas, or decreased loss as occurs with renal failure, uroabdomen or urethral obstruction)
6. Nonvolatile buffer ion alkalosis (decreased [A_{TOT}] due to hypoalbuminemia)
   A. Excessive loss of albumin via protein-losing enteropathy or protein-losing neuropathy
   B. Sequestration of albumin into inflammatory effusions or into tissues via vasculitis
   C. Decreased albumin production due to malnutrition, starvation, chronic hepatic disease or the acute phase response of inflammation.

OXYGEN THERAPY

HYPOXEMIA

There are five causes of hypoxemia:

1. Hypoventilation
   A. Central nervous system disease (cervical spinal cord lesion above the fifth cervical vertebrae or a brainstem lesion)
   B. Neuromuscular disease (tetanus, botulism, tick paralysis, polyradiculoneuritis, myasthenia gravis, neuromuscular blocking agents)
   C. Medications that depress respiration (inhalant anesthetics, barbiturates, narcotics)
   D. Chest wall injury (fractured ribs, flail chest, pleural space disease, postoperative thoracotomy)
   E. Upper airway obstruction (aspiration, brachycephalic syndrome, tracheal collapse, laryngeal paralysis, mass, occluded endotracheal tube)

2. Decreased partial pressure of inspired oxygen (fraction of inspired oxygen (Fi_{O_2}))
   A. High altitude
   B. Faulty technique for inhalation anesthesia administration (inadequate minute ventilation, failure of the carbon dioxide filter or removal system)
3. Ventilation – perfusion mismatch (V/Q mismatch)
   A. Asthma
   B. Bronchitis
   C. Chronic obstructive pulmonary disease
   D. Pulmonary embolism
4. Diffusion impairment
   A. Diffuse pulmonary interstitial disease
   B. Vasculitis
   C. Emphysema
   D. Pneumonia
   E. Severe pulmonary edema
5. Right-to-left shunt
   A. Atelectasis
   B. Anatomic shunt with right-to-left blood flow (patent ductus arteriosus, ventricular septal defect, atrial septal defect, tetralogy of Fallot).

ASSESSMENT OF HYPOXEMIA

Along with adequate cardiac output, the oxygen content of arterial blood must be adequate to deliver sufficient oxygen to cells. Hypoxemia is the condition in which there is an inadequate oxygen level in the blood. Hemoglobin transports the majority of oxygen to cells. The normal hemoglobin level is 13–15 g/dL. Ideal oxygen delivery is thought to require a hemoglobin level of at least 10 g/dL, which corresponds to a packed cell volume (PCV) of about 30%, although 22–25% is usually adequate in healthy patients. One gram of hemoglobin (Hb) binds 1.34 mL of oxygen (98% of the oxygen content of blood) when it is fully saturated. Sa_{O_2} is the saturation of hemoglobin with oxygen; Pa_{O_2} is the partial pressure of oxygen dissolved in arterial plasma. The solubility coefficient of oxygen in plasma at body temperature = 0.003. By plugging these numbers in the following equation, the patient's arterial blood total oxygen content (Ca_{O_2}) can be calculated:

$$Ca_{O_2} = ([Hb] \times Sa_{O_2} \times 1.34) + (0.003 \times Pa_{O_2})$$

Pa_{O_2} can be measured by a blood gas analysis machine from an arterial blood sample obtained in an appropriate manner. Excessive heparin volume and air exposure to the sample should be avoided. Hypoxemia (inadequate oxygen level in blood) is a partial pressure of oxygen in arterial blood (Pa_{O_2}) less than 80 mm Hg. Visible cyanosis occurs at Pa_{O_2} levels of 40 mm Hg and requires an [Hb] of 5 g/dL of deoxygenated Hb.

The alveolar air equation allows assessment of the quantity of oxygen in the alveolus. The alveolar air equation is:

$$PA_{O_2} = (Fi_{O_2} \times [PB - P_{H_2O}]) - Pa_{CO_2}/RQ$$

PA_{O_2} = partial pressure of oxygen in alveolar air

Fi_{O_2} = fraction of inspired oxygen (21% [0.21] on room air)

PB = barometric pressure (about 760 mm Hg at sea level, decreases with increases in altitude)

P_{H_2O} = pressure of water vapor (about 50 mm Hg)

RQ = respiratory quotient = CO_2 production/oxygen consumption, usually 0.8 or 0.9

Pa_{O_2} = measured value which has a limited impact on Pa_{O_2} and will only cause hypoxemia in an animal breathing room air.

A–a gradient

Abnormalities of ventilation and perfusion can be assessed by determining the difference of the PO_2 of alveolar gas and arterial blood, known as the "A–a gradient". Pa_{O_2} should always be less than PA_{O_2}.

$$\text{Alveolar–arterial (A–a) gradient} = PA_{O_2} - Pa_{O_2}$$

<10–15 = normal

\>15 = impaired pulmonary oxygenation of blood

\>30 = severely impaired pulmonary gas exchange

Hypoxemia with a normal A–a gradient occurs with decreased Fi_{O_2} and hypoventilation. If a patient has hypoxemia due to hypoventilation, an increase of the Fi_{O_2} to 30% or more will usually remedy the situation. Hypoxemia with an increased A–a gradient occurs with conditions that cause diffusion impairment, V/Q mismatch, and shunts.

$Pa_{O_2} : Fi_{O_2}$ ratio (or P:F ratio)

Comparing the ratio of these values allows for a quick evaluation of oxygenation. Because Pa_{CO_2} is not measured, it is less accurate than the A–a gradient.

$Pa_{O_2} : Fi_{O_2}$ = 500 is normal

300–500 indicates mild disease

200–300 indicates moderate disease

<200 indicates severe disease

$Fi_{O2} \times 5$

A rapid estimation of pulmonary oxygenation ability can be made by multiplying the Fi_{O_2} by 5, which should approximate the Pa_{O_2} in a normal patient at sea level. Fi_{O_2} of 20% (room air) × 5 = Pa_{O_2} of 100 mm Hg; Fi_{O_2} of 100% (with 100% oxygen supplementation) × 5 = 500 mm Hg.

PULSE OXIMETRY

The saturation of hemoglobin with oxygen (Sa_{O_2}) is the main factor affecting the amount of oxygen presented to the tissues in a patient with normal cardiovascular function. Sa_{O_2} measured by a pulse oximeter is Sp_{O_2}. Two wavelengths of light are emitted by the probe, which differentiates oxygenated from deoxygenated hemoglobin. The measurement is inaccurate in the presence of hypoxemia, poor perfusion, hypothermia, vasoconstriction, cardiac arrhythmias, increased pigmentation, abnormal hemoglobin and movement. Jaundice has no significant effect on Sp_{O_2}.

An Sp_{O_2} of 98% corresponds to a Pa_{O_2} of 100–500 mm Hg.

An Sp_{O_2} of 95% corresponds to a Pa_{O_2} of 80 mm Hg and is mild hypoxemia.

An Sp_{O_2} of 90% corresponds to a Pa_{O_2} of 60 mm Hg and is severe hypoxemia.

Carboxyhemoglobin is read as oxyhemoglobin, resulting in a falsely high Sp_{O_2}.

Methemoglobin causes the Sp_{O_2} to read 85% regardless of the real Sp_{O_2}.

VENOUS P_{O_2}

Venous partial pressure of oxygen (Pv_{O_2}) can provide an approximation of tissue oxygenation. A Pv_{O_2} of <30 mm Hg in a sample obtained from a central vein indicates increased oxygen consumption or decreased oxygen deliver. An estimation of ventilatory status can be made from a venous P_{CO_2} (Pv_{CO_2}), which is usually 3–6 mm Hg higher than Pa_{CO_2}.

SUPPLEMENTAL OXYGEN THERAPY

Oxygen supplementation is needed if Pa_{O_2} is less than 60–80 mm Hg, Sp_{O_2} is less than 92% or the patient exhibits signs of hypoxemia. There are several methods to enrich the oxygen in the patient's environment. Some of the more common ways are listed. To avoid oxygen toxicity, an Fi_{O_2} of >60% should not be administered for more than 24–72 hours.

1. Flow-by
   A. By holding oxygen tubing within 2 cm of a patient's nostril or mouth, and running the oxygen at 2–3 L/min, the Fi_{O_2} can often be increased to 25–40%.
   B. Placing a loose plastic bag over the patient's head like a tent and positioning the oxygen tubing under the bag may improve patient compliance and provide similar results.
2. Mask
   A. An Fi_{O_2} of up to 60% can be obtained by applying a tight-fitting face-mask onto a patient's muzzle and an oxygen flow rate of 8–12 L/min.
   B. Carbon dioxide, humidity and temperature may increase within the mask to hazardous levels, requiring frequent venting of the closed system.
   C. Loose-fitting face-masks may require an oxygen flow rate of 2–5 L/min.
   D. Many conscious patients will not accept a face-mask, especially for prolonged periods. Struggling and patient resistance will compound hypoxemia and should be avoided.
3. Hood or Elizabethan collar (Fig. 1.2)
   A. An Elizabethan collar can be modified to allow supplemental administration of oxygen by covering the majority of the front of the collar with clear plastic wrap.

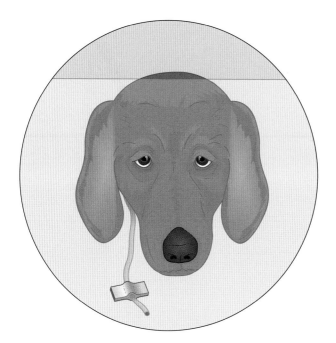

FIG 1.2 **Elizabethan collar hood oxygenation** Apply an Elizabethan collar that extends past the patient's nose about 1.5–2 inches (4–5 mm). Thread a 5–12 Fr. red rubber catheter into the collar. Secure the end of the catheter inside the Elizabethan collar with tape so that it lies near the patient's nose. Apply clear plastic food wrap over the front of the Elizabethan collar, leaving a 1.5–2 inch gap at the top to allow carbon dioxide to escape. A single strip of porous tape may be used to secure the top of the plastic wrap if desired. Secure the plastic wrap to the outside of the Elizabethan collar with tape. Attach an oxygen line to the outer end of the red rubber catheter and administer oxygen.

- B. It is important to leave a small space open in the front to allow carbon dioxide and moisture to escape.
- C. After the collar is applied to the patient, oxygen tubing is inserted from the back so that the tip of the tubing is near the nose and the tube is secured with tape.
- D. An Fi_{O_2} of 30–40% can be obtained with an oxygen flow rate of 0.5–1 L/min.
- E. Commercial hoods are also available.
- F. Most patients will tolerate hood oxygenation, especially if the collar is long enough to keep the plastic a comfortable distance from the nose.
4. Nasal (Figs 1.3, 1.4)
- A. Depending upon whether the patient is panting or mouth breathing, respiratory rate, and patient size, an oxygen flow rate of 50–150 mL/kg/min can provide an Fi_{O_2} of 30–60%.
- B. Nasal oxygen should be humidified to avoid excessive irritation to nasal tissues.
- C. Contraindications to nasal oxygenation include
  - I. Increased intracranial pressure or an intracranial mass lesion
  - II. Nasal or facial trauma

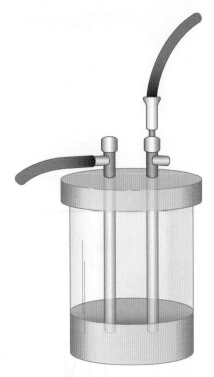

FIG 1.3   Equipment for administering nasal oxygen Intravenous tubing can be attached to an infusion bottle or other sterile bottle that is filled with sterile water. Oxygen is administered through water and IV tubing connected to the nasal catheter. An oxygen flow rate of 50–75 mL/kg will provide an oxygen concentration of 40–60%.

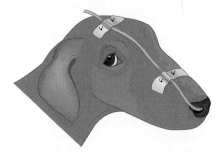

FIG 1.4   Placement of a nasal oxygen catheter Note that the tubing is brought up over the head between the eyes and sutured to the skin above the nose, on the forehead, and then draped behind the ears. The tubing is also secured with a 'Chinese fingerlock' suture.

     III. Epistaxis
     IV. Nasal mass
     V. Laryngeal obstruction
     VI. Coagulopathy.
   D. Methods of nasal oxygenation
     I. Human cannulas
       a. The small two-pronged nasal cannulas commonly used in human hospitals may be tolerated by many patients.

      b. Placement is easy and the supplemental oxygen provided via this route may be beneficial.

  II. Single nasal catheter

      a. A nasal catheter is quick and easy to place.

      b. Position the patient in either sternal or lateral recumbency.

      c. Instill several drops of dilute 2% lidocaine or proparacaine into the nostril while holding the patient's nose upward.

      d. A 5–10 Fr. red rubber or polypropylene catheter is commonly used.

      e. Measure the catheter by placing the tip of the catheter at the medical canthus of the eye then mark the length on the catheter with a permanent marker at the lateral aspect of the nostril.

      f. Lubricate the catheter tip with water-soluble lubricant.

      g. Hold the catheter as close to the tip as possible with one hand as close to the nostril as possible; hold the patient's nose with the other hand.

      h. Direct the catheter ventrally and medially into the nostril, to the mark on the catheter.

      i. Place a stay suture through the lateral aspect of the nares to secure the catheter.

      j. Place the catheter up the center of the muzzle between the eyes for dogs and to the side of the face for cats, avoiding the whiskers, and suture in place with 2–3 more sutures.

      k. Place an Elizabethan collar on the patient.

      l. Administer oxygen at flow rates of 50–100 mL/kg/minute.

      m. If additional oxygen is required, place another nasal catheter in the other nostril.

  III. Bilateral nasal catheters enable the F_{IO_2} to be increased to a higher level than at lower oxygen flow levels through a single nasal catheter.

5. Nasopharyngeal catheterization may enable the F_{IO_2} to be increased to a higher level than with nasal catheterization.

  A. The procedure for placement is the same as nasal catheterization, except the catheter is introduced to the level of the ramus of the mandible rather than the medial canthus of the eye.

  B. For placement of a nasopharyngeal catheter, it is helpful to pinch the dorsolateral portion of the external nares medially while pushing the nasal philtrum dorsally.

6. Endotracheal intubation

  A. Use a laryngoscope to perform the procedure as gently as possible and avoid inducing laryngeal trauma or a vagal response.

  B. Use a low-pressure high-volume cuffed endotracheal tube if possible.

  C. For cats, a small volume of lidocaine may be squirted onto the larynx to decrease laryngospasm.

  D. Secure the endotracheal tube in place. A section of IV line, a piece of gauze, rubber bands and other items have been used.

  E. Ensure proper placement of the endotracheal tube by palpation of a single tube in the neck, visualization of the tube entering the trachea through the oropharynx, or assessment of end tidal carbon dioxide.

F. The endotracheal tube should be connected to an oxygen source such as an anesthetic machine circuit and oxygen should be administered.

G. The cuff should be gently inflated until the airway exterior to the tube is occluded.

H. An Fi_{O_2} of 100% may be provided to the patient with a sealed system.

I. Maintenance of an endotracheal tube requires sedation to obliterate the gag reflex. If the patient requires continued intubation to maintain a patent airway, a tracheostomy may be indicated.

J. Complications of endotracheal intubation include:

    I. Airway obstruction from kinking or clogging of the tube resulting in hypoxemia

    II. Pressure-induced tracheal necrosis, which may lead to pneumomediastinum and subcutaneous emphysema

    III. Tracheal laceration, which may lead to pneumomediastinum and subcutaneous emphysema

    IV. Intubation of a mainstem bronchus rather than the trachea resulting in overinflation of one lung lobe, impaired gas exchange, and possible airway rupture

    V. Pressure necrosis of the gingiva, lips and tongue

    VI. Laryngeal trauma

    VII. Excessive lingual swelling

    VIII. Increased intracranial pressure

    IX. Increased intraocular pressure.

7. Tracheostomy tube placement (Fig. 1.5)

  A. Indications

    I. Severe upper airway obstruction

    II. Severe upper airway trauma

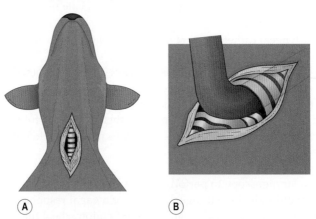

Ⓐ   Ⓑ

FIG 1.5 Procedure for performing an emergency tracheostomy (A) With the patient in dorsal recumbency, quickly clip and prep the neck just distal to the larynx. With a scalpel, make a 2–3 cm incision through the skin, subcutaneous tissue and fascia on the ventral midline. Separate the muscles with scissors and forceps to expose the trachea. (B) Make an incision between tracheal rings that is one-quarter to one-third the circumference of the trachea. With the scalpel handle, separate the tracheal rings and insert a tracheostomy or endotracheal tube, directed caudally down the trachea. Secure the tube in place with umbilical tape tied around the neck.

III. Laryngeal paralysis

IV. Long term positive pressure ventilation

B. Contraindications

  I. Tracheal injury

  II. Tracheal obstruction distal to the tracheostomy site

C. Procedure

  I. Ideal situations allow for general anesthesia and placement of an endotracheal tube.

  II. The patient should be positioned in dorsal recumbency with the neck extended and elevated from the table with a towel or other padding.

  III. The ventral cervical region is clipped and routine surgical preparation is performed, time allowing.

  IV. A ventral cervical midline incision is made from the cricoid cartilage toward the sternum for 2–5 cm in length.

  V. With lateral retraction and blunt dissection, the sternohyoid muscles are separated along midline.

  VI. A transverse incision less than 50% of the tracheal circumference is made in the annular ligament between the fourth and fifth or third and fourth tracheal rings.

  VII. A tracheostomy tube should be inserted through the incision into the trachea, with the end directed ventrally.

    a. A cuffed tracheostomy tube with an inner cannula is ideal, but an uncuffed tube, tube without an inner cannula, or a modified endotracheal tube may be used.

    b. The tube size can be estimated by measurement of the inner tracheal diameter on a lateral cervical radiograph.

  VIII. A long suture loop should be placed around a tracheal ring above and below the incision to facilitate future replacement of the tube.

  IX. The muscle and skin should be sutured to decrease the size of the incision.

  X. The tube should be secured by tying around the neck with umbilical tape or suturing the tube in place.

  XI. The patient may be provided with supplemental oxygen by either increasing the oxygen concentration of the surrounding air, as in an oxygen kennel, or anesthetic tubing may be connected directly to the tracheostomy tube.

  XII. Daily tracheostomy tube care is essential to maintain a functional tube.

8. Oxygen kennel

A. In addition to commercial oxygen kennels, which control humidity, temperature, and oxygen concentration, many other items can be substituted including a human pediatric incubator, a Plexiglas box, a Plexiglas door tightly fit onto a regular kennel, and, in the absence of any thing else in an emergency situation, a regular kennel door can be covered with plastic wrap and an oxygen line can be run into the kennel to increase the Fi_{O_2}.

    B. Depending upon the kennel, patient size, frequency of opening the kennel door, and oxygen flow rate, an Fi_{O_2} of 40–60% can be maintained.

    C. An oxygen kennel allows improvement of the Fi_{O_2} with minimal patient stress. When a dyspneic, distressed cat or small dog is brought in on emergency, it is often helpful to place the patient into an oxygen kennel, with oxygen supplementation, for several minutes to allow the patient to calm down, even if ultimately another method of oxygen supplementation will be provided to the patient.

    D. Problems associated with oxygen kennels include
      I. They are expensive to purchase and to maintain.
      II. They require more oxygen than other methods.
      III. Hyperthermia commonly occurs.
        a. Placement of ice packs in the kennel but not on the patient may be helpful.
        b. Ice packs may also be placed in or around the humidifier.
      IV. Respiratory sounds such as stridor or stertor are muffled to the outside observer.
      V. Hands-on assessment of the patient requires opening of the oxygen kennel door and subsequent decrease in Fi_{O_2}.

9. Hyperbaric oxygen
    A. The administration of hyperbaric oxygen requires a specialized commercial chamber and supra-atmospheric pressure (>760 mm Hg).
    B. The chamber generates an Fi_{O_2} of 100% and allows oxygen to diffuse readily into tissues.
    C. The indications for hyperbaric oxygen administration include:
      I. Osteomyelitis
      II. Burns
      III. Severe soft tissue infections.
    D. Hyperbaric chambers are usually not used in the treatment of patients with hypoxemia and are not often used in veterinary medicine.

FLUID THERAPY

There are many things to consider when evaluating the need and method of fluid therapy. Questions that should be answered include:

1. Does the animal require fluid therapy?
2. What type of fluid should be used?
3. Which route should be used?
4. How much should be given and over what period of time?
5. For how long should therapy continue?

Fluid therapy is beneficial for patients in shock or suffering from dehydration, or as a carrier for dilute intravenous medications. The signs of shock include:

1. Tachycardia
2. Pale oral mucous membranes
3. Weak or bounding peripheral pulses

Table 1.4 *Packed cell volumes and total solids in fluid losses*

PCV%	TS (g/dL)	Interpretation
Increased	Increased	Dehydration
Increased	Normal or decreased	Splenic contraction Polycythemia Dehydration with pre-existing hypoproteinemia
Normal	Increased	Normal hydration with hyperproteinemia Anemia with dehydration
Normal	Normal	Normal hydration Dehydration with pre-existing anemia and hypoproteinemia Acute hemorrhage Dehydration with secondary compartment shift
Decreased	Increased	Anemia with dehydration Anemia with pre-existing hyperproteinemia
Decreased	Normal	Non-blood-loss anemia with normal hydration
Decreased	Decreased	Blood loss Anemia with hypoproteinemia Overhydration

4. Prolonged capillary refill time
5. Altered mentation.

Dehydration occurs when fluid losses exceed fluid intake. The signs of dehydration include:

1. Decreased skin turgor – although subjective, this assessment provides a rough idea of fluid losses in the patient. The skin over the lumbar region is pinched into a fold and the time required for it to return to normal position is evaluated. Obese animals may appear well hydrated. Emaciated and older animals may appear more dehydrated.
2. Retraction of the eye
3. Dry or tacky oral mucous membranes
4. Urine specific gravity should be high (>1.045) in a dehydrated dog or cat with normal renal function.
5. Serial evaluation of body weight is the best indicator of hydration status.
   A. A loss of 1 kg of body weight = 1 liter fluid deficit.
   B. Fluid 'lost' to third spacing (ascites, pleural effusion) doesn't decrease body weight.
   C. Approximately 60% of total body weight in normal animals is fluid. This varies with age, metabolic status and the percentage of body fat:
      I. 10 kg dog = 6 kg of water
      II. 40 kg dog = 24 kg of water.

The packed cell volume and total solids (TS) increase with all types of fluid losses excluding hemorrhage (See Table 1.4.). The normal canine PCV = 38–55%, normal feline PCV = 29–45% and normal TS = 6.0–8.0 g/dL.

Table 1.5 *Crystalloid solutions*

Fluid	Osmolality (mOsm/L)	pH	Na	Cl	K	Ca	Mg	Glucose (g/L)	Buffer (mOsm/L)
Plasma	300	7.4	145	145	5	5	3		24 bicarbonate
5% Dextrose in water (D5W)	252	4.0	0	0	0	0	0	50	0
2.5% Dextrose in 0.45% NaCl	280	4.5	77	77	0	0	0	25	0
0.9% NaCl	308	5.0	154	154	0	0	0	0	0
LRS	272	6.5	130	109	4	3	0	0	28 lactate
Plasmalyte 148	294	5.5	140	98	5	0	3	0	27 acetate/ 23 gluconate
Normosol R	296	6.4	140	98	5	0	3	0	27 acetate/ 23 gluconate
Normosol M in D5W	364	5.5	40	40	13	0	3	50	16 acetate
3%NaCl	1026		513	513	0	0	0		0
5% NaCl	1712		855	855	0	0	0		0
7.2% NaCl	2400		1232	1232	0	0	0		0

FLUID TYPES

1. Crystalloids are water-based salt and/or sugar solutions with electrolytes added that resemble the extracellular fluid (ECF) compartment. Sodium ions [Na^+] are the major component. Within 30 minutes of administration, 75% of crystalloids leave intravascular space. Their primary effect is on the interstitial space, therefore they are recommended for replacing interstitial fluid losses (i.e. dehydration). Examples include lactated Ringer's solution (LRS), Normosol R or M, Plasmalyte, 0.9% NaCl (saline) and dextrose 5% in water (D5W). Maintenance solutions (Normosol M) have less sodium and more potassium than replacement (Normosol R) solutions (See Table 1.5.).

   Selection of the crystalloid fluid should be based on [Na^+] and [K^+], osmolality, and pH. Patients should be infused with fluids that match the volume and electrolyte composition of fluid that has been lost.

   A. Hypotonic fluids have an osmolality less than serum. Examples include 0.45% NaCl, 2.5% dextrose in 0.45% saline, and D5W. Since dextrose is rapidly oxidized to water and CO_2, giving 5% dextrose is equivalent to administering 'free water'.

Table 1.6 *Natural and synthetic colloids*

Colloid	MW (kDa)	Range (kDa)	Carrier	COP (mm Hg)
5% Albumin	69	66–69	–	20
25% Albumin	69	66–69	–	200
6% Dextran-70	70	20–200	0.9% NaCl	40
6% Hetastarch	480	30–2000	0.9% NaCl	32
10% Pentastarch	264	10–1000	0.9% NaCl	40
Oxyglobin	200	65–500	Modified LRS	43
Plasma	69			17–20

    I. These fluids should not be administered subcutaneously (could cause electrolyte imbalance).

    II. Caloric needs cannot be maintained with 5% dextrose except in very small animals, as 1 liter of 5% dextrose supplies only 200 kcal.

B. Isotonic fluids have an osmolality closest to serum (extracellular fluid), about 290–310 mOsm/L, so they do not change in cell volume. These fluids are recommended for maintenance needs and shock therapy. Examples: LRS, 0.9% NaCl, whole blood, synthetic colloids.

C. Hypertonic fluids have greater osmolality than extracellular fluid, and create a large osmotic gradient – they cause rapid movement of water into the vascular space. These fluids can be used to treat shock, since they draw fluid from the interstitial space, which then redistributes out of the ECF compartment just as quickly as other crystalloids.

    I. Hypertonic saline is available as NaCl 3%, 7.2%, 7.5% and 23%. The 23% solution should always be diluted prior to administration.

    II. The advantage is the small volume required to resuscitate, which allows rapid resuscitation.

    III. The recommended dose for the treatment of shock is hypertonic saline (7.2% NaCl), 3–5 mL/kg in dogs or 2–4 mL/kg in cats IV over 10 minutes in shock.

    IV. Rapid administration of hypertonic saline may cause vagal mediated hypotension and bradycardia.

    V. Hypertonic saline administration may provide rapid restoration of arterial blood pressure, higher blood pressure, a greater increase in cardiac contractility and cardiac output, improved blood flow and oxygen delivery to tissues. Hypertonic saline reduces endothelial swelling, microvascular permeability, and tumor necrosis factor levels. It also reduces intracranial pressure.

    VI. Hypertonic saline is recommended for the treatment of circulatory shock, head and spinal trauma.

    VII. Contraindications for hypertonic saline administration include dehydration, volume overload, hypernatremia, hyperosmolality, ventricular arrhythmias, and uncontrolled hemorrhage.

Supportive therapy

2. Colloids are fluids with large molecular weight particles that cannot readily cross capillary membranes, thus they are restricted to plasma, where they contribute to oncotic pressure and expand the intravascular volume. Colloids contain negatively charged molecules (anions), which, by electrostatic attraction, retain cations (positively charged sodium ions) within the intravascular space. Water molecules follow the sodium ions, which results in expanded intravascular volume. The osmotic pressure generated by plasma proteins or by colloids in solution is called the colloid oncotic pressure (COP). Osmotic pressure is proportional to the number of molecules present, rather than their size. RBCs, WBCs and platelets do not contribute to COP. Albumin makes up 60–70% of the COP with the remainder comprised of globulins and fibrinogen.

Natural colloids include: fresh whole blood, fresh frozen plasma (primarily contribute albumin).

Synthetic colloids include: Hetastarch, Pentastarch, Dextran 70, Oxyglobin (See Table 1.6.).

A. Albumin
   I. Albumin is the primary component in plasma responsible for maintaining intravascular oncotic pressure.
   II. Normal albumin values for the dog and cat are 2.9–4.3 g/dL.
   III. Hypoalbuminemia is a poor prognostic indicator in human medicine. If albumin values decrease below 1.5 g/dL, endothelial leakage of intravascular fluids occurs, resulting in peripheral edema and edema of multiple organs, which leads to organ dysfunction, respiratory distress, and death.
   IV. Other consequences of hypoalbuminemia include altered homeostasis, altered delivery and metabolism of drugs and endogenous products, coagulation disorders, and increased inflammation via many routes.
   V. Canine albumin has recently been introduced to the veterinary market in the USA.
   VI. One unit of canine plasma contains about 6–7.5 g of albumin, equal to about 25 mL of human serum albumin (HSA) 25%.
   VII. There are two human serum albumin concentrations commercially available: 5% and 25%. The 5% concentration has not been shown to be more beneficial than LRS. The use of the 25% HSA solution is controversial, has not been proven to improve survival, may increase mortality and may have the following beneficial effects:
      a. May increase intravascular volume by as much as 4–5 times the administered volume
      b. May improve oxygen delivery
      c. May improve organ function
      d. May reduce peripheral edema and the accumulation of pleural and peritoneal fluid
      e. May increase blood pressure when administered as a bolus followed by an IV continuous rate infusion (CRI) over 4 hours.
   VIII. The volume recommended for the treatment of hypotension in dogs is 4 mL/kg IV slow push or bolus followed by a CRI of

0.1–1.7 mL/kg/h. The maximum volume recommended for an individual dog is 25 mL/kg given over 72 hours.

IX. Although a vented delivery set is required for administration, a blood filter is not.

X. Adverse effects of human serum albumin administration include death from immediate or delayed immune responses, facial edema, polyarthritis, vasculitis, dermatitis, type III hypersensitivity reactions, and enteropathic polyarthritis. Normal dogs should not be given 25% HSA as there is increased morbidity and mortality in dogs with normal serum albumin levels.

XI. Because the administration of 25% HSA is controversial, and the complications can be severe, it is important to evaluate the risks versus the benefits for the individual patient and fully inform the owner of the potential risks.

B. Hetastarch

I. Hetastarch is a complex carbohydrate polymer made from amylopectin, a highly branched polysaccharide.

II. The molecular weight is 480 kilodaltons (kDa), with a COP of 32 mm Hg.

III. The administration of 20 mL/kg causes the intravascular volume to expand 70–200% of the volume administered.

IV. The total solids of Hetastarch = 4.5 g/dL.

V. The dosage is 10–20 mL/kg/day in the dog and 10–15 mL/kg/day in the cat. It is recommended to start with 5 mL/kg/day in the cat and carefully reassess to avoid volume overload. The bolus administration of 5 mL/kg is often called a shock bolus. After the initial IV dose has been administered, another daily dose may be administered as a slow IV as a CRI. It is recommended that one should avoid exceeding 40 mL/kg/day in dogs.

VI. Hetastarch may be associated with a dose related coagulopathy. The PTT may be prolonged, but there have been no clinical reports of excessive bleeding. There is no interference with platelet function.

VII. Hetastarch is recommended for colloidal support, hypovolemia, and hypotension due to hypovolemia or decreased systemic vascular resistance.

VIII. The hemodynamic benefits and colloidal support improve when Hetastarch is administered on successive days.

C. Pentastarch

I. Pentastarch is an analogue of Hetastarch and has similar qualities.

II. The COP is approximately 40 mm Hg and the molecular weight is 264 kDa.

III. The intravascular volume expands by 150% of the administered volume.

D. Dextran 70 is produced by bacteria from sucrose. The molecular weight is 70 kDa (similar to albumin).

      I. It expands intravascular volume by 80–100% of the administered volume.

     II. It causes a dose-related coagulopathy by coating platelets, decreasing von Willebrand's factor and factor VIII activity, precipitation and dilution of clotting factors, and increasing thrombolysis. It also can interfere with the cross matching of blood after it is absorbed onto red blood cell membranes.

   III. Another Dextran product, Dextran 40, causes acute renal failure and should not be used.

   IV. Dextran molecules <20 kDa are excreted by renal glomerular filtration. The larger molecules are degraded by the reticuloendothelial system.

    V. The dosage of Dextran 70 is 10–20 mL/kg/day.

   VI. The total solids of Dextran 70 are 4.5 g/dL.

E. Oxyglobin (no longer available at time of publication)

      I. Oxyglobin was a synthetic oxygen-carrying stroma-free hemoglobin solution that had colloidal and vasopressor properties. It was made from bovine red blood cells.

     II. Oxyglobin improved oxygen delivery to tissues by expanding intravascular volume, increasing arterial blood pressure, and carrying more oxygen per volume because it was less viscous than blood. It was better able to penetrate tissues that have low blood flow.

   III. Oxyglobin had a molecular weight of 200 kDa and provided expansion of intravascular volume. It could cause volume overload if cautious dosing and monitoring was not provided. The colloidal pull of Oxyglobin was greater than that of Hetastarch, which is greater than that of plasma.

   IV. Oxyglobin was an effective and useful vasopressor; it elevated arterial blood pressure.

    V. Oxyglobin had multiple species compatibility (ferrets, dogs, cats, etc.) and caused no immune reactions.

   VI. It had a long shelf life (2 years) but had to be used within 24 hours of opening.

   VII. No refrigeration was needed, no filtration was needed during administration, and no cross match was needed.

  VIII. Each 125 mL unit of Oxyglobin contained the same amount of hemoglobin as one 450 mL unit of fresh whole blood.

   IX. The recommended dosage for Oxyglobin in dogs was 5–30 mL/kg IV. In cats, the dose was 2–15 mL/kg IV. For cats, Oxyglobin needed to be administered slowly and the patient needed to be monitored very carefully for signs of volume overload.

    X. The effective half-life varied with the dosage, with a half-life of 30–40 hours when dosed at 30 mL/kg.

   XI. Administration of Oxyglobin could raise a patient's hemoglobin levels without raising the patient's PCV. The Oxyglobin dose of 30 mL/kg could increase hemoglobin as if PCV has increased 12%. A rough estimate of the PCV can be made by multiplying the hemoglobin by three.

XII. Disadvantages of Oxyglobin include:
   a. Limited availability (no longer manufactured)
   b. High cost
   c. The yellow orange discoloration of the patient's mucous membranes, sclera, skin, plasma and urine
   d. Interference with chemistry analysis.
F. Blood components
   I. Commonly available products include:
      a. Fresh whole blood
      b. Stored whole blood
      c. Packed red blood cells (packed RBCs or pRBCs)
      d. Fresh plasma: donor must be available, contains all plasma components including coagulation factors and albumin
      e. Fresh frozen plasma: rapidly frozen within 8 hours of collection, frozen less than 1 year, contains all plasma components including coagulation factors and albumin; the dose is 10–40 mL/kg
      f. Frozen plasma: plasma which was frozen more than 8 hours following collection or fresh frozen plasma that has been stored more than 1 year; maximum length of storage = 5 years; contains factors II, VII, IX, X and albumin
      g. Platelet-rich plasma or platelet concentrate: indicated for the treatment of thrombocytopenia in patients with life-threatening hemorrhage; dose = 1 unit/10 kg
      h. Cryoprecipitate: dose = 1 unit or more/10 kg
      i. Cryoprecipitate (Cryo)-poor plasma: contains albumin and decreased amounts of factors II, VII, IX and X.
   II. Dosages
      a. Standard formula:

$$\frac{\text{Body}}{\text{wt (kg)}} \times \frac{40 \text{ mL (dog) or}}{30 \text{ mL (cat)}} \times \left[\frac{\text{desired PCV} - \text{patient PCV}}{\text{PCV of donor blood}}\right] = \frac{\text{vol of blood (mL)}}{\text{to be administered}}$$

      b. Short cuts:
         i. 20 mL/kg fresh whole blood or 10 mL/kg packed RBCs will usually increase the PCV by 10%.
         ii. 1 mL/lb will usually increase the PCV by 1%.
         iii. Volume of whole blood (mL) to be administered $= \left[\begin{array}{c}\text{PCV \% increase} \\ \text{desired}\end{array} \times \begin{array}{c}\text{body} \\ \text{wt(kg)}\end{array}\right] \times 2$
   III. Administration
      a. All stored or frozen products should be gently brought to room temperature by use of immersion in a warm water bath prior to administration. If the patient is in urgent need of RBCs quicker than a unit can be warmed, 50–100 mL of warm sterile 0.9% NaCl can be added to the RBC unit and the IV line can be placed through a warm water bath or warming coil.
      b. A unit that has been thawed should be used within 24 hours.

      c. A unit should not be at room temperature longer than 4 hours. If the patient is small, the portion of the unit to be administered within 4 hours should be removed for administration and the remainder of the product should be returned to refrigerated storage.

      d. All blood component products should be administered through a blood filter. Depending upon the filter used, some filters require a new filter for each unit administered.

  IV. Anaphylactic or allergic reactions

      a. Monitor for transfusion reactions with blood components: urticaria, fever, vomiting, dyspnea, hemoglobinemia, hemoglobinuria, hematuria, restlessness, or pulmonary edema.

      b. Treatment of transfusion reactions

         i. Stop the transfusion.

        ii. Establish an airway, ensure adequate oxygenation.

       iii. Administer epinephrine, 0.01–0.02 mg/kg IV, IM, or SC.

       iv. Administer diphenhydramine, 0.5 mg/kg, IV or IM.

       v. Administer crystalloid IV fluids and treat for shock.

ROUTES OF FLUID THERAPY

1. Oral
    A. This route is the most physiologic and allows for administration of high-caloric-density and hypertonic solutions.
    B. The oral route is very safe, unless the patient struggles or displacement of a feeding tube occurs. Passing of a feeding tube can be very stressful.
    C. Contraindications to oral fluid administration include vomiting, diarrhea, other gastrointestinal dysfunction, and patients with acute or excessive losses of fluid or electrolytes.
2. Subcutaneous
    A. Useful in mild dehydration.
    B. Must use isotonic fluid. LRS is preferred as it is reported to sting the least.
    C. The flow rate is governed by patient comfort, may need to use multiple sites (usually administer 10–20 mL/kg per site).
    D. All of the fluids should be absorbed within 6–8 hours.
    E. Potassium chloride may be added in concentrations up to 35 mEq/L.
3. Interosseous
    A. This route is useful in pediatric and exotic patients in urgent situations and in adults when peripheral vascular access cannot be obtained.
    B. The most commonly used sites include:
        I. The medial surface of the proximal tibia (direct the needle slightly distally to avoid the proximal growth plate)
        II. The tibial tuberosity

III. The trochanteric fossa of the femur (with the hip joint rotated internally and in a neutral position, walk the needle off the medial aspect of the greater trochanter to avoid the sciatic nerve)
IV. The wing of the ilium
V. The ischium
VI. The greater tubercle of the humerus.
C. Aseptic preparation of the selected site is required.
D. Local anesthetic should be infiltrated into the area, especially into the periosteum.
E. A small skin incision should be made to facilitate passage of the needle.
F. Depending upon the patient size, an 18- to 30-gauge hypodermic needle, an 18- to 22-gauge spinal needle, bone marrow needle, or intraosseous infusion needle should be used. A commercial bone injection gun is also available.
G. Correct placement of the interosseous needle involves local palpation and the needle should move with the bone when the limb is moved, without being dislodged. When flushed with sterile saline, there should be no distension indicating leakage. Bone marrow may be aspirated from younger patients.
H. The needle entry site should be covered with antiseptic or antimicrobial cream or ointment.
I. A piece of tape may be placed in a butterfly fashion around the needle hub and sutured to the skin. Suture may also be secured directly to the needle hub with cyanoacrylate glue.
4. Intraperitoneal
A. Only warm isotonic fluids may be administered.
B. Patient discomfort may occur.
C. Peritonitis is a possible complication.
D. This route is not commonly used in practice.
5. Intravenous
A. For many patients, this is the preferred route of fluid administration, especially for those with acute or severe fluid loss.
B. Presence of an intravenous catheter also facilitates administration of intravenous medication, repeated blood sample collection, and provides vascular access for emergencies.
C. The most commonly used veins include the jugular, cephalic, femoral, and lateral saphenous veins.
D. Contraindications of jugular vein catheterization include:
I. Coagulopathies, thrombocytopenia, thrombocytopathia, vitamin K antagonist rodenticide intoxication
II. Hypercoagulable states as occur with hyperadrenocorticism, immune-mediated hemolytic anemia, protein-losing enteropathy and protein-losing neuropathy
III. Elevated intracranial pressure as with head trauma, intracranial mass lesions, and intractable seizures.
E. Complications of intravenous fluid therapy include phlebitis, thrombosis, embolism, electrolyte abnormalities from inappropriate therapy, volume overload, mechanical difficulties with fluid

administration including kinking of the catheter or fluid lines, localized infections, and sepsis.
F. Sterile procedure must be followed during placement of an intravenous catheter and while providing the daily maintenance care.
G. Explanation of various placement techniques and available intravenous catheters can be easily found in many of the references.

HOW MUCH FLUID?

1. Hydration deficit
   A. Usually replace hydration deficit over 8–24 hours with isotonic crystalloids.
   B. % dehydration × body weight in kilograms (BW kg) = fluid deficit (in liters). Example: an 11 kg dog that is 7% dehydrated needs 770 mL of fluid to replace deficit ($0.07 \times 11 = 0.77$).
2. Maintenance phase of fluid therapy begins once shock and/or dehydration has been corrected.
   A. $(30 \times BW \text{ kg}) + 70 = \text{mL}/24 \text{ h}$ for animals which weigh between 2 kg and 50 kg.
   B. For any dog or cat of any body weight, $70 \times BW \text{ kg}^{0.75} = \text{mL}/24 \text{ h}$.
   C. Traditionally, maintenance volumes are estimated at 60 mL/kg/day for adult patients.
   D. Neonatal patients (0–2 weeks of age) require 80–120 mL/kg/day for maintenance.
   E. Infants (2–6 weeks of age) and pediatric patients (6–12 weeks of age) require 120–200 mL/kg/day for maintenance.
   F. Shortcut version: multiply body weight (pounds) by 1.25 → hourly fluid rate (mL/h) or administer 1–2 mL/lb/h.
   G. 60 mL/kg/day for cats and small dogs; 40 mL/kg/day for large dogs.
   H. Depending upon the needs of the patient, it is common to administer 2–3 times the maintenance requirement and adjusting for losses as they occur.
   I. Fever will increase maintenance fluid requirements up to 15–20 mL/kg/day.
3. INS and OUTS
   A. It is important to monitor the volume of fluid administered or taken in by the patient (INS) in relationship to the amount of fluid lost by the patient (OUTS).
      I. If INS > OUTS, there is a risk of fluid overload.
      II. If INS < OUTS, there is a risk of dehydration.
   B. INS: fluids obtained by food and water intake, created during metabolism of carbohydrates and fats, includes intravenous fluids, blood products, liquid diets.
   C. OUTS: caused by sensible losses and insensible losses.
      I. Sensible losses include urine, feces, saliva, vomiting, 3rd space losses (losses into body cavities) = 27–40 mL/kg/day.

II. Insensible losses include evaporation, respiratory fluids, metabolic processes, sweat = about 12 mL/kg/day for cats and 20 mL/kg/day for dogs.

III. Normal body function losses = 40–60 mL/kg/day.

IV. Fever will increase maintenance fluid requirements up to 15–20 mL/kg/day.

V. Vomiting, diarrhea, polyuria, excessive salivation will increase fluid losses.

VI. May need to estimate OUTS or try to measure accurately if volume is critical using such methods as a closed urinary collection system and weighing soiled bedding (1 mL of urine = 1 gram).

D. Cannot start balancing INS and OUTS until initial dehydration deficit is corrected.

4. Administration

A. IV fluid infusion pumps are very helpful in assuring the desired volume of fluid is administered at the desired rate and within the desired time.

B. In the absence of an infusion pump, it is helpful to be able to determine the number of drops that need to be administered per minute.

I. Administration sets are either standard size (10 drops = 1 mL) or micro drip (60 drops = 1 mL).

II. Standard drip set;   mL/h × 1 h/60 min × 10 drops/mL or __ mL/h ÷ 6 = __ drops/min.

III. Micro drip set: __ mL/h × 1 h/60 min × 60 drops/mL or __ mL/h = __ drops/min.

IV. To determine drops per minute, calculate the total volume needed and divide by number of minutes. Example: patient needs 700 mL/24 h or 0.48 mL/min. If using a 60 drop/mL micro drip set, 0.48 mL/min = 29 drops/min or 1 drop/2 s.

C. Burette drip chambers can be used to control the total amount administered and can also be used to administer medications via a portion of the IV bag being infused.

5. Monitoring

A. Serial physical exams (increased respiratory rate, nasal discharge, chemosis, cough)

B. PCV/total solids

C. Body weight (evaluate every 12–24 hours)

D. Urine output and urine specific gravity

E. Central venous pressure

6. Cessation of fluid therapy

A. Resuscitate shock to end points.

B. Dehydration has been corrected.

C. The patient is stable, eating, and drinking.

D. The patient is not vomiting and has no or minimal diarrhea.

E. The BUN and creatinine are near normal and stable.

F. Also stop fluid therapy if fluid overload has occurred.

G. It is recommended to wean the patient off of IV fluid therapy over 12–24 hours.

Fluid rate during anesthesia

1. Fluids are administered during anesthesia to prevent hypotension, hypovolemia and to maintain perfusion of kidneys.
2. Basal rate is 5–10 mL/kg/h and for major exploratory surgery is 10–15 mL/kg/h.

BLOOD PRESSURE ASSESSMENT

Blood pressure is the force exerted by blood against any unit area of the blood vessel wall. It is usually measured in mm Hg, but may be measured in cm H_2O. To convert between units, 1 mm Hg = 1.36 cm H_2O. The ways to measure blood pressure include:

1. Direct arterial blood pressure measurement via an intravascular catheter that is connected to an electronic pressure transducer.
   A. The commonly used vessels include the metatarsal and dorsal pedal arteries. The femoral artery may be used in some cases.
   B. The site should be clipped and disinfected.
   C. A 21–23G indwelling venous or arterial catheter should be inserted via a small skin incision or percutaneously. The catheter is first introduced perpendicularly to the skin then advanced while being held flatly along the limb.
   D. Heparinized saline should be flushed through the catheter immediately upon placement and then intermittently via bolus fashion or via constant infusion.
   E. Specialized semirigid tubing is used.
   F. A bag of 0.9% NaCl with heparin 1 unit/mL added is connected to the tubing and pressurized to 300 mm Hg, monitored by a pressure transducer. The pressure transducer should be mounted level with the patient's heart.
   G. The pressure changes are converted into an electrical signal by the pressure transducer. The signal is carried by a transducer cable to a monitor where it is displayed as a pressure waveform.
   H. Common problems associated with direct blood pressure measurement include difficulty in placing an intra-arterial catheter, kinking of the catheter or tubing, the catheter positioned against the wall of the artery, clotting of the catheter or tubing, air bubbles in the catheter or tubing, and the use of compliant tubing. These problems tend to result in a dampened waveform.
   I. Complications of direct blood pressure measurement include hematoma formation, thrombosis, phlebitis, infection, and necrosis of distal tissues.
2. Indirect blood pressure measurement
   A. Doppler ultrasound – a sound frequency change (Doppler shift) is created by the re-entry of red blood cells into an occluded artery.
      I. A cuff that is connected to a manometer is applied around the limb. The cuff width should be about 38–40% of the circumference of the limb. The measurements will be falsely

low if the cuff is too wide and falsely high if the cuff is too narrow.

   a. Commonly used sites include the radial artery on the medial and proximal aspect of the carpus, the median caudal artery at the ventral base of the tail, the brachial artery on the upper forelimb of cats and small dogs, and the saphenous artery on the medial and proximal aspect of the tarsus.

   b. The limb should be level with the body.

II. An ultrasound transducer that is connected to an amplifier is placed distally to the cuff. The site must usually be clipped and conductive gel applied. The transducer should be held perpendicularly to the artery and should not be pressed too tightly against the artery.

III. The cuff is inflated until the artery is occluded then the air in the cuff is gradually released until the artery reopens.

IV. The systolic blood pressure corresponds to the sound made by the first pressure wave of blood passing through the artery.

V. The use of a headset may be helpful to avoid patient distress and to assist hearing.

VI. It is recommended to take 3–5 separate measurements, prior to performing a physical exam, in the least stressful environment, then average the measurements.

B. Oscillometry

   I. A pneumatic cuff that contains the sensor is placed at the same sites as used for the Doppler method. The same principles apply regarding the width of the cuff.

   II. The cuff is automatically inflated and deflated by the unit.

   III. Systolic blood pressure (SAP), diastolic blood pressure (DAP) and pulse rate are determined. Mean arterial pressure (MAP) is often also displayed.

   IV. Clipping of the measurement site is not necessary.

   V. Multiple measurements should be taken.

C. Plethysmography, either photo or pressure, is difficult to utilize in practice because of the interference of pigmentation and cuff size limitations.

D. Manual palpation

   I. Commonly used sites include the femoral, saphenous, radial and lingual arteries.

   II. The pulse pressure difference between systolic and diastolic pressure is what is palpable. A large difference in pressure results in a strong pulse and a small difference results in a weak pulse. It cannot be relied upon as an accurate measure of blood pressure.

   III. The lowest systolic blood pressure at which femoral artery pressure is usually palpable is about 80 mm Hg.

E. Pulse oximetry – does not measure blood pressure but when pulse waves are too small to detect or absent, or the systolic blood pressure is less than 70 mm Hg, a pulse oximeter may malfunction.

3. Central venous pressure corresponds to right atrial pressure in the absence of vascular obstruction.

A. A jugular catheter is advanced so that the tip of the catheter lies in the anterior portion of the vena cava.

B. A bag of IV fluids is connected to an IV line that is connected to a three-way stopcock. A water manometer is connected to a second port of the three-way stopcock, and another IV line is connected from the last port of the three-way stopcock to the jugular catheter.

C. The manometer is filled to above 20 cm H_2O with IV fluids, then the system is turned off to the fluid bag and opened between the patient and the manometer.

D. The zero point of the manometer should be level with the right atrium, which is the manubrium of the sternum when the patient is in lateral recumbency and the point of the shoulder if the patient is in sternal recumbency.

E. The fluid is allowed to equilibrate. The fluid level should move slightly along with respiration. The central venous pressure (CVP) is then read off of the manometer, the result being in mm H_2O.

F. The normal CVP = 0–5 cm H_2O. Monitoring of trends is more important than one individual reading.

G. A low CVP (less than 0 cm H_2O) indicates hypovolemia or vasodilation.

H. A high CVP (greater than 10 cm H_2O) indicates volume overload, pleural effusion, pericardial effusion and tamponade, restrictive pericarditis, right-sided myocardial failure or increased intrathoracic pressure as occurs with positive end-expiratory pressure (PEEP), during positive pressure ventilation, and in patients with pneumothorax.

I. A CVP greater than 16 cm H_2O is associated with the development of edema and effusions.

J. The contraindications to evaluation of CVP include coagulopathy, increased risk of thromboembolism, increased intracranial pressure, or infection at the catheter placement site.

4. Blood pressure abnormalities

A. Normal systolic arterial pressure (SAP) in dogs is 90–140 mm Hg; in cats is 80–140 mm Hg. Normal diastolic arterial pressure (DAP) in dogs is 50–80 mm Hg; in cats is 55–75 mm Hg. Mean arterial pressure (MAP) in dogs is 60–100 mm Hg; in cats is 60–100 mm Hg.

B. Hypotension is MAP <60 mm Hg.

I. Hypotension is caused by:

Hypovolemia	Poor diastolic or systolic cardiac
Myocardial fibrosis	function
Low venous return to the	Cardiomyopathy
heart	Ventricular arrhythmias
Positive pressure ventilation	Pericardial tamponade
Gastric distension	Patent ductus arteriosus
Tachycardia	Bradycardia
Outflow tract obstruction	Low systemic vascular resistance

Vasodilating effects of anesthetic or other drugs

Negative inotropic effects of anesthetic drugs, beta blockers, or calcium channel blockers.

II. The clinical signs of hypotension include tachycardia (cats usually have bradycardia), slow capillary refill time, pale mucous membranes, either weak or bounding peripheral pulses, hypothermia, cold extremities, decreased urine output, mental dullness, and weakness. Dogs with sepsis or SIRS may have injected mucous membranes rather than pallor.

III. The adverse effects of hypotension include acute renal failure, arrhythmias, mentation changes, coagulopathies, tachypnea, vomiting, and melena.

IV. Treatment is directed at identifying and remedying the underlying cause and aggressive fluid therapy for patients without cardiac disease as the primary etiology.

   a. Shock boluses (90 mL/kg in the dog and 60 mL/kg in the cat) and additional IV fluid therapy are administered as needed, with crystalloids and colloids.

   b. Inotropic support with β-adrenergic agonists, vasopressive support with α-agonists, or vasopressin may be needed in patients that fail to respond to adequate fluid therapy.

      i. β-adrenergic agonists are commonly used in patients with refractory hypotension, cardiogenic shock, congestive heart failure and oliguric renal failure and are usually the safest choice if poor cardiac contractility cannot be ruled out as the underlying cause. There is no one clear choice for therapy. Some studies recommend norepinephrine in the treatment of severe hypotension, with the second choice varying between dopamine and dobutamine.

         – Dopamine 5–10 μg/kg/min IV CRI increases cardiac contractility and heart rate along with causing a slight increase in systemic vascular resistance. Lower doses may cause splanchnic vasodilation and changes in renal and gastrointestinal blood flow. Higher doses may cause ischemia of the gastrointestinal tract, kidneys, or heart.

         – Dobutamine 2–20 μg/kg/min IV CRI in dogs (1–5 μg/kg/min IV CRI in cats) increases cardiac contractility but does not affect systemic vascular resistance or heart rate. Higher doses in cats may cause tremors or seizures.

         – Epinephrine 0.005–1 μg/kg/min IV CRI can cause an increase in systemic vascular resistance, cardiac contractility, and heart rate but also causes an increase in oxygen consumption. The use of epinephrine is reserved for patients with resistant hypotension or during cardiopulmonary resuscitation.

         – Isoproterenol 0.04–0.08 μg/kg/min IV CRI increases heart rate and contractility but may decrease systemic vascular resistance. It is usually reserved for the treatment of patients with third-degree heart block.

- Norepinephrine 0.05–2 µg/kg/min IV CRI increases systemic vascular resistance without causing much change in heart rate.
  ii. Vasopressin 0.5–2 mU/kg/min IV CRI in dogs has been shown to cause a significant increase in mean arterial blood pressure. The side effects are minimal although high doses can result in hypercoagulability and excessive coronary and splanchnic vasoconstriction.
  iii. Combinations of these medications are often utilized. It is recommended to start with a low dose, gradually titrate to a higher dose and if the desired response is not achieved, to add on an additional medication.
C. Hypertension is defined as >160/95 mm Hg. Hypertension may be primary or secondary to systemic illnesses or medications (glucocorticoids, erythropoietin) including:

Renal disease (renal failure, glomerulopathy)   Hyperthyroidism

Hyperadrenocorticism   Hyperaldosteronism
Pheochromocytoma   Diabetes mellitus
Hepatic disease   Polycythemia
Chronic anemia

  I. The adverse effects of hypertension include:
    a. Ocular changes associated with hypertension include retinal hemorrhage and/or detachment, hyphema, retinal vessel tortuosity, perivascular edema, papilledema, glaucoma, and acute blindness
    b. Cardiac changes associated with hypertension include left ventricular hypertrophy, gallop rhythm, and arrhythmias
    c. The neurological signs associated with hypertension include depression, stupor and seizures.
  II. The treatment of hypertension
    a. Treatment of secondary hypertension is directed at the underlying etiology. If the patient is exhibiting clinical signs of hypertension, additional therapy should be provided for hypertension.
    b. Hypertensive emergencies (SAP >200 mm Hg) require continuous blood monitoring and intensive care. It is recommended to decrease blood pressure less than 25% in the first hour and repeat in 2–6 hours if the patient remains stable. Recommended medications include:
      i. Fenoldopam 0.1–0.6 µg/kg/min IV CRI in dogs and cats
      ii. Enalaprilat 0.1–1 mg IV q6h in dogs
      iii. Sodium nitroprusside 1–3 µg/kg/min IV CRI in dogs and 1–2 µg/kg/min IV CRI in cats
      iv. Hydralazine 0.5–3 mg/kg PO q12h or 0.25–4 mg/kg IM or SC q8–12 h in dogs, or 0.1–0.2 mg/kg/h IV CRI in dogs; or 2.5 mg (total dose) titrated up to 10 mg (total dose) PO q12h in cats or 0.25–2 mg/kg IM or SC q8–12 h in cats

     v. Amlodipine 0.05–0.2 mg/kg PO or per rectum q24h in dogs or 0.625–1.25 mg PO or per rectum q24h in cats.

  c. Cats

     i. Amlodipine 0.625–1.25 mg PO or per rectum q24h is usually the drug of choice for hypertension secondary to renal disease in cats.

     ii. Benazepril 0.25–0.5 mg/kg PO q12–24 h in cats is often the second choice.

     iii. Enalapril 0.25–0.5 mg/kg PO q12–24 h is an alternative ACE inhibitor that is usually less effective in cats.

     iv. Prazosin 0.25–0.5 mg/cat PO q24h has been shown to be more useful to cause urethral smooth muscle relaxation in cats with micturition disorders in cats or pheochromocytoma in dogs.

  d. Dogs

     i. Amlodipine 0.05–0.2 mg/kg PO every 12–24 hours, adjusted up to 0.25 mg/kg as needed.

     ii. Enalapril 0.25–0.5 mg/kg PO q12–24 h, benazepril 0.25–0.5 mg/kg PO q12–24 h, lisinopril 0.75 mg/kg PO q24 h or other ACE inhibitors are often the first therapeutic agents recommended in the management of hypertension in dogs.

     iii. Prazosin 0.5–2 mg PO q8–12 h may be useful in the treatment of pheochromocytoma or to cause urethral smooth muscle relaxation in dogs with micturition disorders.

     iv. Propanolol 0.5–1 mg/kg PO q8–12 h may be used in dogs but should be avoided in asthmatic cats.

     v. Spironolactone 1–2 mg/kg PO q12h is useful in patients with hyperaldosteronism or in conjunction with other diuretics.

INTRA-ABDOMINAL PRESSURE

1. Values
   A. The normal intra-abdominal pressure for dogs is 0–5 cm H_2O. The normal intra-abdominal pressure following abdominal surgery in the dog is 0–15 cm H_2O. The normal values for cats have not been reported.
   B. 10–20 cm H_2O is mild intra-abdominal hypertension. The patient should be monitored, and fluid therapy should be reevaluated, often volume resuscitation will be beneficial.
   C. 20–35 cm H_2O is moderate to severe intra-abdominal hypertension. Attempt to identify the cause, provide volume resuscitation, and consider decompression.
   D. >35 cm H_2O is severe intra-abdominal hypertension and may cause abdominal compartment syndrome. Decompression is necessary.
2. Common causes of intra-abdominal hypertension include:
   A. Abdominal surgery

B. Abdominal effusion or fluid accumulation
   I. Hemoperitoneum / hemoretroperitoneum
   II. Peritonitis, including bile peritonitis
   III. Pancreatitis
   IV. Ruptured urinary bladder
C. Ileus or gastric distension
D. Pneumoperitoneum
E. Intra-abdominal mass
F. Urinary obstruction
G. Massive fluid resuscitation
H. Blunt or penetrating abdominal trauma
I. Pelvic fractures with retroperitoneal hemorrhage
J. Abdominal packing or management of an open abdomen
K. Mechanical ventilation.

3. Clinical signs include:
A. Short, shallow, rapid respiration
B. Tense abdomen
C. Decreased urine output
D. Vomiting
E. Obtundation, cranial nerve reflex deficits and seizures if increased intracranial pressure occurs.

4. Adverse effects
A. Decreased cardiac output
B. Decreased abdominal blood flow and visceral perfusion, increased blood lactate level
C. Decreased renal function, decreased glomerular filtration rate and urine output, azotemia
D. Decreased pulmonary compliance, increased pulmonary artery pressure and pulmonary capillary wedge pressure
E. Increased central venous pressure
F. Increased intracranial pressure.

5. Measurement
A. Position the patient in lateral recumbency.
B. A urethral catheter, preferably a Foley catheter, should be placed so that the tip is just inside the trigone of the urinary bladder.
C. Using two three-way stopcocks, a closed urinary collection system should be connected to the urethral catheter, a water manometer, and a bag or 60 mL syringe of sterile 0.9% NaCl.
D. After emptying the urinary bladder, 0.5–1 mL/kg of 0.9% NaCl should be instilled into the bladder.
E. The manometer system should be zeroed at the patient's midline at the symphysis pubis, then the manometer should be filled with 0.9% NaCl.
F. The stopcock to the fluids should be closed and the pressure in the system should be allowed to equilibrate. The meniscus will fluctuate with respiration.
G. The difference between the meniscus and the zero point is the intra-abdominal pressure.

6. Depending upon the situation, the following treatments have been utilized:
   A. Volume resuscitation including colloid administration if indicated
   B. Repositioning of the patient's body
   C. Sedation
   D. Neuromuscular blockade
   E. Abdominal paracentesis
   F. Rectal decompression via the administration of enemas, placement of a drainage catheter or tube
   G. Gastric decompression via nasogastric suction
   H. Surgical decompression
   I. Administration of prokinetic agents such as cisapride, metoclopramide, pantoprazole, erythromycin, domperidone, or prostigmin
   J. Administration of diuretics
   K. Venovenous hemofiltration or ultrafiltration.

NUTRITIONAL SUPPORT

ENTERAL NUTRITION

1 Oral intake
   A. Critically ill patients often have metabolic disturbances that put them into a catabolic state and predispose them to malnutrition. It is important for the patient to ingest sufficient calories and nutrients on a daily basis to meet its needs.
   B. Nausea, pain, and the anxiety associated with hospitalization often interfere with the appetite of veterinary patients.
   C. Many things may be tried to encourage ingestion of adequate nutrients, including:
      I. Offer a more palatable diet.
      II. Warm the food (but avoid overheating and potentially burning the patient's mouth).
      III. Gravies and taste enhancers are commercially available.
      IV. Offer the food by hand, rather than from a dish.
      V. Provide a quiet environment.
      VI. Have the owner hand-feed.
      VII. Appetite stimulants such as diazepam 0.2 mg/kg IV, oxazepam 2.5 mg/cat PO, or cyproheptadine 2 mg/cat PO two to three times a day may be tried, but are not often successful in emergency patients. Mirtazapine (Remeron ®) may be more successful. The dosage is 3.75 mg PO q72h in cats and 0.6 mg/kg PO q24h in dogs.
   D. If the patient will not ingest sufficient calories and nutrients on its own, supplemental nutritional support is needed. Force-feeding with a syringe is not recommended as it is very stressful.
   E. Utilize as much of the functional gastrointestinal tract as possible.

F. The benefits of enteral feeding include:
   I. Maintains gastrointestinal mucosal integrity
   II. Prevents intestinal villous atrophy
   III. Decreases risk of bacterial translocation
   IV. Maintains gastrointestinal immune function
   V. It is safer, cheaper and more physiologic than parenteral feeding.
G. The contraindications of enteral feeding include:
   I. Inability to protect the airway
   II. Uncontrolled vomiting
   III. Malabsorption or maldigestion
   IV. Gastrointestinal obstruction
   V. Ileus.
H. The daily water requirements of 50–100 mL/kg/day may be administered via the enteral feeding tube also. The amount of water used to dilute food for tube feeding and the amount of water used to flush the tubes should be subtracted from the daily water requirement, and the remaining amount should be given to the patient daily.

2. Nasoesophageal or nasogastric tubes (NE- or NG-tubes)
   A. Contraindications include those listed above plus facial trauma.
   B. Nasoesophageal tubes are preferred unless gastric suctioning is desired.
   C. Administer light sedation to the patient if desired or needed.
   D. Position the patient in sternal recumbency.
   E. Instill several drops of dilute 2% lidocaine or proparacaine into the nostril while holding the patient's nose upward.
   F. A 3.5–8 Fr. silicone or polypropylene catheter is commonly used.
   G. Premeasure the catheter by placing the tip of the catheter along the patient's side to the caudal edge of the scapula then mark the length on the catheter with the permanent marker.
   H. Lubricate the catheter tip with water-soluble lubricant.
   I. Hold the catheter as close to the tip as possible with one hand as close to the nostril as possible; hold the patient's nose with the other hand. Try to hold the head in a neutral position and avoid sticking the nose straight up. Lowering the nose makes it easier for the patient to swallow the tube.
   J. Direct the catheter ventrally and medially into the nostril. It may be helpful to push the nasal planum of the dog upward while initially directing the catheter. Advance the catheter to the mark on the catheter.
   K. Take a lateral thoracic radiograph to confirm proper placement within the thoracic segment of the esophagus. Do not pass the tip into the stomach as that increases the incidence of gastric reflux.
   L. Place a stay suture through the lateral aspect of the nares to secure the catheter.
   M. Place the catheter up the center of the muzzle between the eyes for dogs and to the side of the face for cats, avoiding the whiskers, and suture in place with 2–3 more sutures.
   N. Place an Elizabethan collar on the patient.

O. Only liquid diets may be administered via a nasoesophageal or nasogastric tube.
P. The complications of nasoesophageal or nasogastric tube feeding include sneezing, rhinitis, dacryocystitis, epistaxis, sinusitis, esophagitis, gastroesophageal reflux, misplacement of the tube or movement of the tube into the trachea, removal of the tube by the patient and obstruction of the tube.
3. Esophagostomy tubes (E-tubes)
A. Indications include:
    I. Inappetance
    II. Maxillofacial trauma
    III. Severe dental disease
    IV. Severe stomatitis secondary to infectious disease, ingestion of potpourri oil or ingestion of an alkali
    V. Orofacial or pharyngeal masses
    VI. Orofacial surgery.
B. Contraindications include:
    I. Vomiting or regurgitation
    II. Esophageal stricture or esophagitis
    III. Megaesophagus
    IV. Inability to protect the airway
    V. Severe cough
    VI. Pneumonia.
C. A 12–14 Fr. silicone feeding tube or red rubber catheter is usually used in cats. In dogs, depending upon the size of the patient, a tube up to 20 Fr. can be used.
D. General anesthesia is required.
E. The patient is positioned in lateral recumbency.
F. The tube should be premeasured by holding it alongside the patient and marking the distance on the tube with a permanent marker from the midcervical esophagus to just caudal to the caudal aspect of the scapula, about the 6th or 7th intercostal space. Avoid placement of the tip of the tube through the lower esophageal sphincter into the stomach to decrease the incidence of gastric reflux.
G. Placement of a mouth speculum facilitates oral manipulation but is not absolutely essential.
H. The tip of a long curved Carmalt forceps or Kelley hemostat is placed into the esophagus to the midcervical level. The curve of the instrument should follow the curve of the patient's neck.
I. The handle of the forceps is gently lowered towards the table so that the tip of the forceps causes the esophagus to tent up, making it readily apparent and differentiated from surrounding structures. The handle can be held in place by an assistant if needed.
J. Identify the location of the carotid artery and jugular vein, then avoid those and other vital structures and carefully incise through the skin over the tented esophagus with a number 15 scalpel blade. The incision should be extended through the skin and into the esophagus but should be as short as possible in length (1–2 cm) to allow passage of the tube.

K. The tips of the forceps should be advanced through the incision and the tip of the esophagostomy tube should be grasped by the forceps. The forceps is withdrawn into the mouth, carrying the tube with it.

L. Without pulling the tube entirely through the skin incision, the tip of the tube is looped around in the mouth then redirected down the esophagus.

M. The tube is pushed down the esophagus; once the tip has passed the incision, the tube will flip around so that the entire tube is directed down the esophagus.

N. The position of the tube in the esophagus should be confirmed with a lateral thoracic radiograph and the oropharynx should be evaluated to remove any excessive length of tube that may be remaining.

O. The esophagostomy tube should be sutured in place. If the incision was excessive, the skin may be partially closed. Caution must be used in the placement of a purse-string suture, to avoid skin necrosis. A simple interrupted suture may be sufficient to secure the tube to the neck. Then a Chinese-finger-trap knot may be placed to secure the tube to the suture in the neck and decrease sliding of the tube.

P. Antimicrobial ointment should be placed over the incision and then the tube should be bandaged to the neck.

Q. Feeding may commence immediately once the patient has recovered from anesthesia.

R. In addition to liquid diets, there are many commercial diets such as Hills a/d and Iams Max Cal that facilitate tube feeding. Also, most other canned food diets may be combined with water, liquidized in a blender, and filtered for tube feeding.

S. Complications include:
  I. Cellulitis at the stoma site
  II. Infection at the stoma site
  III. Displacement or removal of the tube by the patient
  IV. Gagging or vomiting of the tube
  V. Gastroesophageal reflux
  VI. Clogging of the tube.

4. Gastrostomy tubes (G-tubes)
  A. Indications include:
    I. Inappetance and the other indications for esophagostomy tube placement
    II. Esophageal stricture or dysfunction.
  B. There are various ways of placement of a gastrostomy tube, including surgical placement, endoscopy-guided placement, and a blind technique using a placement device.
  C. The procedure for tube placement is provided in detail in surgery texts and in DiBartola, *Fluid, Electrolyte and Acid–Base Disorders in Small Animal Practice,* 4th edition.
  D. Usually a 14–28 Fr. mushroom tipped feeding tube is used.
  E. General anesthesia is required for placement.
  F. The tube should not be used for the first 24 hours following placement.

G. The tube should not be removed for at least 10 days following placement.

H. Complications include:
   I. Peritonitis
   II. Dehiscence
   III. Cellulitis at the stoma site
   IV. Infection at the stoma site
   V. Damage to intra-abdominal organs
   VI. Pyloric outflow obstruction
   VII. Clogging of the tube.

I. Blender-liquidized diets and liquid diets can be fed through the tube.

J. Long-term maintenance of the tube is relatively easy. A T-shirt may be applied over the patient to distract the patient from the tube.

K. An Elizabethan collar should be applied to any patient that licks or chews at the tube.

5. Jejunostomy tubes (J-tubes)
   A. Indications include:
      I. Uncontrolled vomiting
      II. Pancreatitis
      III. Inability to protect the airway.
   B. The procedure for jejunostomy tube placement is provided in detail in surgery texts.
   C. A 5–8 Fr. feeding tube is placed directly into the proximal jejunum.
   D. General anesthesia is required for placement.
   E. The tube should not be used for the first 24 hours following placement.
   F. Only a liquid diet can be administered.
   G. Patient tolerance appears to be improved with constant infusion rather than bolus feeding.
   H. Complications include:
      I. Peritonitis
      II. Dehiscence
      III. Cellulitis at the stoma site
      IV. Infection at the stoma site
      V. Migration of the tube resulting in intestinal obstruction
      VI. Abdominal cramping
      VII. Clogging of the tube.
   I. A T-shirt may be applied over the patient to distract the patient from the tube.
   J. An Elizabethan collar should be applied at least initially to all patients.

6. Diet options
   A. The tube diameter will dictate the type of diet that may be fed, with NE-, NG-, and J-tubes requiring a liquid diet such as CliniCare®.
   B. The resting energy requirements (RER) should be fed. 'Illness factors' are no longer used. Obese patients should be fed based upon their optimal body weight.
      I. $(30 \times BW\ kg) + 70 = kcal/day$
      II. For animals that weigh <2 kg or >50 kg, $70 \times BW\ kg^{0.75} = kcal/day$

Protein requirements
  I. Cats require 6 or more grams of protein per 100 kcal; 25–35% of
      the total energy provided to cats should be in the form of protein.
  II. Dogs should be fed 4–6 grams of protein per 100 kcal; 15–25% of
      the total energy provided to dogs should be in the form of protein.
 D. CliniCare® Canine/Feline and CliniCare® RF feline renal solutions
     supply 1 kcal/mL. Hills Prescription Diet a/d supplies 1.3 kcal/mL.
     Iams® Veterinary Formula™Maximum-Calorie™ supplies
     1.5 kcal/mL.
 E. Divide the RER for the patient by the kcal supplied per mL in the
     chosen food, then divide this amount by 4 to determine the volume
     to be fed four times per day. For the first day of enteral feeding,
     administer ⅓ of the required volume (and about 33% of the RER),
     divided into four feedings. For the second day, increase to ⅔ of the
     required vol, divided into four feedings. For the third and subsequent
     days, feed the entire volume, divided into four feedings.
 F. The gastric volume of a pediatric patient = 50 mL/kg.
 G. Before feeding, evaluate the tube placement, flush the tube with
     3–5 mL of tap water, then slowly feed the patient warm or room
     temperature food. The patient should be sternal or sitting when fed
     to decrease aspiration.
 H. After feeding, flush the tube with 3–5 mL of tap water. Cap and
     replace the cover over the tube.
 I. Do not administer medications, especially crushed tablets, down a
     feeding tube.
7. Complications of enteral feeding
 A. Refeeding syndrome may occur in any patient after a period of
     prolonged anorexia. Rapid movement of electrolytes from the
     intravascular to the intracellular space causes severe hypokalemia,
     hypomagnesemia and hypophosphatemia. It is recommended to
     reintroduce susceptible patients to feeding conservatively with close
     monitoring, then gradually increase the amount being fed.
 B. Aspiration may occur.
 C. Inflammation and infection may occur around stromal sites. Basic
     hygiene and daily care of the tubes will usually minimize this
     complication.
 D. Vomiting, diarrhea, and ileus are signs of gastrointestinal intolerance.
     The administration of antiemetics or prokinetics or changing the diet
     may allow feeding to continue.
 E. If the tube becomes clogged, gently flushing repeatedly with warm
     water or cola may help to relieve the clog. The tube should be
     replaced if it is still needed and the tube cannot be unclogged.

PARENTERAL NUTRITION (PN)

1. Indications
 A. When nutritional support is necessary but the patient cannot tolerate
     enteral feeding
 B. Patients with intractable nausea and vomiting
 C. Patients unable to protect their airways

2. Requirements
  A. Vascular access must be able to be obtained and maintained aseptically. Either a dedicated venous catheter or a dedicated port of a multilumen catheter should be available.
    I. Blood sample collection should not be performed through this catheter or port.
    II. Other IV fluids or medications should not be administered through this catheter or port. Potentially fatal interactions between nutrients and medications may occur.
    III. Hemodynamic monitoring should not be performed using this catheter or port.
    IV. A catheter placed in a central vein is preferred and is essential for the administration of hyperosmolar total parenteral nutrition solutions.
  B. Nursing care must be available 24 hours a day, along with the ability to monitor basic serum chemistry results in house.
    I. Most of these patients require critical care monitoring for their illness.
    II. The central venous catheter needs close monitoring and daily care. Phlebitis is common.
    III. The preferred method of administration of PN is as a constant rate infusion.
    IV. The patient's albumin, glucose, blood urea nitrogen (BUN) and electrolytes usually need to be monitored at least once per day.
    V. The patient's hydration status should be assessed daily.
  C. The PN prescription must be able to be formulated and compounded.
    I. A sterile environment is essential to prevent microbial contamination.
    II. To avoid precipitation of nutrients, the solutions must be combined in the proper order.
3. Nutritional requirements (See Table 1.7 and Table 1.8)
  A. The resting energy requirements (RER) should be fed. 'Illness factors' are no longer used. Obese patients should be fed based upon their optimal body weight.
    I. RER (kcal/day) = $(30 \times BW\ kg) + 70$ = kcal/day (for animals which weigh 2–45 kg)
    II. RER (kcal/day) for animals which weigh <2 kg or >45 kg = $70 \times BW\ kg^{0.75}$
  B. Protein requirements
    I. Cats require 6 or more grams of protein per 100 kcal; 25–35% of the total energy provided to cats should be in the form of protein.
    II. Dogs should be fed 4–6 grams of protein per 100 kcal; 15–25% of the total energy provided to dogs should be in the form of protein.
    III. Animals with renal disease and cats with hepatic disease should be fed 50% of their normal protein requirements.
  C. On the first day of providing PN and once weekly thereafter, administer Vitamin K_1 SC.

Table 1.7 *Sample calculation of total parenteral nutrition for a 22 lb (10 kg) dog with pancreatitis*

Step	Equation
1. Calculate the BER	$30 \times (10\ kg) + 70 = 370$ kcal/day
2. Calculate the TER	In this case, the illness factor is 1.0 TER = 370 kcal/day
3. Determine the daily protein requirement	4 g/100 TER kcal/day $\times$ 370 kcal/day = 14.8 g of protein/day
4. Determine the volume of nutrient solutions required	
Dextrose	The patient will receive 60% of its daily energy requirement as dextrose 222 kcal/day $\div$ 1.7 kcal/mL of 50% dextrose
Lipids	The patient will receive 40% of its daily energy requirements as lipids $0.40 \times$ TER = 0.40×370 kcal/day = 148 kcal/day as lipids 148 kcal/day $\div$ 2 kcal/mL of 20% lipid solution = 74 mL/day of 20% lipid solution
Amino acids	14.8 g of protein/day $\div$ 85 mg/mL of 8.5% amino acid solution = 174.1 mL/day (rounded to 174 mL/day) of amino acids
5. Determine the total volume and hourly rate of TPN solution administration	131 mL + 74 mL + 174 mL = 379 mL/day of TPN solution 379 mL/day $\div$ 24 h = 15.8 mL/h of TPN solution
6. Determine the daily vitamin requirements	Vitamin K: 0.5 mg/kg $\times$ 10 kg = 5 mg SC once weekly, if needed. Supplementation with vitamin B may be necessary. For example: 370 kcal/day $\div$ 1 mL B complex/1000 kcal = 0.37 mL/day
7. Administer TPN	Day 1: Administer one-third of the calculated requirement. $\frac{1}{3} \times$ (379 mL/day + 0.37 mL/day of B vitamins) $\div$ 24 h = 5.3 mL/h Day 2: Administer two-thirds of the calculated requirement. $\frac{2}{3} \times$ (379 mL/day + 0.37 mL/day B vitamins) $\div$ 24 h = 10.5 mL/h Day 3 and on: Administer the full calculated requirement plus 0.37 mL/day B vitamins. 379 mL/day + 0.37 mL/day B vitamins $\div$ 24 h = 15.8 mL/h

From Thomovsky E, Backus R, Reniker A et al, Parenteral nutrition: formulation, monitoring, and complications, Compendium Continuing Education for Veterinarian, vol 29 (2), February 2007, p 90 and 91, with permission.

4. Complications
   A. Catheter complications include:
      I. Phlebitis
      II. Loss of vascular access due to malposition of the catheter
      III. Thrombosis
      IV. Catheter-related infections.
   B. Nutrient solution complications include:
      I. Microbial contamination

Table 1.8 *Total parenteral nutrition worksheet*

Step	Equation
1. Calculate the BER	30 × (_____ kg) + 70 = _____ kcal/day
2. Calculate the TER	TER = illness factor × BER = _____ kcal/day
3. Determine the daily protein requirement	Protein requirement × _____ kcal/day = _____ g/day of protein
4. Determine the volume of nutrient solutions required	
Dextrose	The patient will receive ____ % of its daily energy requirement as dextrose. ____% × TER = kcal/day as dextrose ____ kcal/day dextrose ÷ 1.7 kcal/mL of 50% dextrose = ____ mL/day of 50% dextrose
Lipids	The patient will receive (100–_____)% of its daily energy requirement as lipids. ____% × TER = ____ kcal/day as lipids ____ kcal/day ÷ 2 kcal/mL of 20% lipid solution = ____ mL/day of 20% lipid solution
Amino acids	____ g/day of protein ÷ 85 mg/mL of 8.5% amino acid solution = ____ mL/day of amino acids
5. Determine the total volume and hourly rate of TPN solution administration	____ mL of dextrose + ____ mL of lipids + ____ mL of amino acids = _____ mL /day of TPN solution ____ mL/day ÷ 24 h = ____ mL/h of TPN solution
6. Determine the daily vitamin requirements	Vitamin K: 0.5 mg/kg × ____kg = _____mg SC once weekly, if needed Supplementation with vitamin B may be necessary. For example: BER ÷ 1 mL of B complex/1000 kcal = ____ mL
7. Administer TPN	Day 1: Administer one-third of the calculated requirement. ⅓ × (____ mL/day + ____ mL/day of B vitamins) ÷ 24 h = ____ mL/h Day 2: Administer two-thirds of the calculated requirement. ⅔ × (____ mL/day + ___ mL/day of B vitamins) ÷ 24 h = ___ mL/h Day 3 and on: Administer the full calculated requirement plus ___ mL/day of B vitamins. ___ mL/day + ____ mL/day of B vitamins ÷ 24 h = ____ mL/h

From Thomovsky E, Backus R, Reniker A et al, Parenteral nutrition: formulation, monitoring, and complications, Compendium Continuing Education for Veterinarian, vol 29 (2), February 2007, p 90 and 91, with permission.

    II. Drug–nutrient interactions
    III. Precipitation of nutritional components such as separation or layering of the lipid emulsion
    IV. Fat embolism.
  C. Metabolic complications
    I. Refeeding syndrome may occur (see description under Enteral nutrition).

II. Persistent hyperglycemia may occur and may require the administration of regular insulin 0.1 U/kg IV, IM, or SC, or CRI IV.

III. Signs of hepatic encephalopathy may develop in patients with hepatic insufficiency.

5. If total PN is not available or the cost is prohibitive, partial PN may be used to meet some of the energy requirements. There are several commercial nutritional combinations that are various combinations of amino acids and dextrose. A commonly used product is ProcalAmine®.

A. ProcalAmine has an osmolality of 735 mOsm/L and provides 246 kcal/L.

B. ProcalAmine may be administered through a peripheral venous catheter but the vein should be monitored for phlebitis.

C. A maintenance fluid rate of 66 mL/kg/day for dogs and 50 mL/kg/day for cats is recommended as a 24-hour CRI. At this dose, 30–40% of the patient's energy requirements, 100% of a dog's protein requirements, and most of a cat's protein requirements are met.

ANALGESIA

Many of the patients encountered in emergency veterinary practice will be suffering from pain. In human medicine, pain is now considered the fifth vital sign. Stress and anxiety can also affect the emergency patient. There are many differences between dogs and cats, and between breeds of dogs, regarding their response to pain, stress and anxiety. When possible, anticipation of pain and the administration of pre-emptive analgesics should be provided. Analgesia improves the speed and quality of recovery. For dosages, see Table 1.9.

Table 1.9 *Analgesics*

Analgesic class	Analgesic	Canine dosage	Feline dosage
Opioid	Buprenorphine	0.005–0.02 mg/kg q4–8 h IV, IM 5–20 µg/kg IV, IM q4–8 h 2–4 µg/kg/h IV 120 µg/kg OTM 0.12 mg/kg OTM	0.005–0.01 mg/kg q4–8 h IV, IM 5–10 µg/kg IV, IM q4–8 h 1–3 µg/kg/h IV CRI 20 µg/kg OTM 0.02 mg/kg OTM* q6–8 h
	Butorphanol	0.1–0.4 mg/kg IV, IM, SC q1–2 h 0.05–0.2 mg/kg/h IV CRI	
	Codeine	0.5–2 mg/kg PO q6–8 h	0.5–1 mg/kg PO q12h
	Fentanyl	2–10 µg/kg IV to effect 1–10 + µg/kg/h IV CRI 0.001–0.01 mg/kg/h IV CRI	1–5 µg/kg IV to effect 1–5 µg/kg/h IV CRI 0.001–0.005 mg/kg/h IV CRI
		Or transdermally as follows: *Body weight*	*Patch size*
		<5 kg	Fold back the liner to expose ⅓–½ of a 25 µg/h patch
		>5 kg	Fold back the liner to expose ⅔ of a 25 µg/h patch or use the full patch

Table 1.9 *Analgesics—cont'd*

Analgesic class	Analgesic	Canine dosage	Feline dosage
		<10 kg (20 lb) 10–25 kg (20–50 lb)	25 µg/h 50 µg/h
		25–40 kg (50–88 lb) >40 kg (>88 lb)	75 µg/h 100 µg/h
	Hydromorphone	0.05–0.2 mg/kg IV, IM or SC q2–6 h premed 0.1 mg/kg with acepromazine, 0.02–0.05 mg/kg IM	0.0125–0.05 mg/kg/h IV CRI 0.02–0.1 mg/kg IV, IM or SC q2–6h (C) and 0.0125–0.03 mg/kg/h IV CRI (C)
	Morphine	0.5–1 mg/kg IM, SC 0.1–0.05 mg/kg IV q2–4 h 0.05–0.5 mg/kg/h 0.1–0.3 mg/kg epidural q4–12 h	0.05–0.2 mg/kg IM, SC
	Oxymorphone	0.02–0.2 mg/kg/h IV q2–4 h 0.05–0.2 mg/kg IM, SC q2–6 h 0.05–0.3 mg/kg/h epidural	0.02–0.1 mg/kg IV 0.05–0.1 mg/kg IM, SC q2–4 h
	Tramadol	2–8 mg/kg q8–12 h PO	2–5 mg/kg q12h PO
NSAIDs	Aspirin	10–20 mg/kg q8–12 h PO	1–25 mg/kg q72h PO
	Carprofen	4.4 mg/kg q24h 2.2 mg/kg q12h PO	4 mg/kg SC or IV once
	Deracoxib	3–4 mg/kg q24h PO	
	Etodolac	10–15 mg/kg q24h PO	
	Firocoxib	5 mg/kg q24h PO	0.75–3 mg/kg PO once
	Flunixin meglumine	1 g/kg PO or IM once	
	Ketoprofen	2 mg/kg IM, IV, SC q24h for maximum 3 days Or 1 mg/kg PO q24h for 3–5 days	2 mg/kg IV, IM, SC once Or 1 mg/kg PO q24h for a maximum of 5 days
	Meloxicam	0.2 mg/kg initial dose then 0.1 mg/kg q24h PO	0.1 mg/kg SC or PO once
	Naproxen	5 mg/kg initial dose then 2 mg/kg q48h PO	
	Piroxicam	0.3 mg/kg q24–48 h PO	
	Robenacoxib	1–2 mg/kg or PO q24h or 2 mg/kg SC once	1–2 mg/kg PO q24h up to 6 days or 2 mg/kg SC once
	Tepoxalin	20 mg/kg initial dose then 10 mg/kg q24h PO	
	Tolfenamic Acid	4 mg/kg IM, SC once then PO q24h	4 mg/kg IM, SC once, or PO q24h for 3 days
NMDA antagonists	Ketamine	0.2–0.6 mg/kg/h 2–10 µg/kg/min CRI IV	
	Amantadine	3–5 mg/kg PO q24h	
α_2-adrenergic agonists	Dexmedetomidine	0.1–1.5 µg/kg/h	0.1–1 µg/kg/h
	Medetomidine	1–3 µg/kg/h	0.5–2 µg/kg/h
Miscellaneous	Gabapentin	3–10 mg/kg PO q8–12 h	
	Lidocaine	2–4 mg/kg/h	

*OTM = oral transmucosal.

1. Physiologic signs of pain
   A. Salivation
   B. Increased respiratory rate
   C. Dilated pupils
   D. Increased heart rate with or without arrhythmias
   E. Increased temperature
2. Behavioral signs of pain
   A. Increased aggression or timidity
   B. Restlessness or agitation to depression and inactivity
   C. Trembling
   D. Licking or chewing at the painful area and resisting handling of the painful area
   E. Alterations in gait
   F. Abnormal posturing or reluctance to lie down
   G. Fixed facial expression (staring or squinting)
   H. Vocalization
   I. Failure to groom or to use the litter box (cats)
   J. Increased or decreased urination
   K. Insomnia or inappetance
3. There are multiple classes of medications, administrative routes, and techniques for administration. It is recommended that the practitioners become familiar with the indications, contraindications and administration of medications of many different classes.
4. General information about each class
   A. Opioids
      I. Indications – include the treatment of acute and chronic pain and for sedation. They take effect quickly, and can be maintained for long periods. The pure agonists (morphine, hydromorphone, oxymorphone, fentanyl) can be reversed with an antagonist such as naloxone.
      II. Contraindications – they can cause gastroparesis and ileus, vomiting, stimulation of pancreatic secretions, respiratory depression and bradycardia. They should be used with caution in neonatal, geriatric or severely debilitated patients and those with adrenocortical insufficiency, hypothyroidism, severe renal insufficiency, head injuries, acute abdominal conditions, severe respiratory dysfunction or receiving monoamine oxidase inhibitors (MAOIs). Dose reduction should be considered in these patients. They should be avoided in those patients with hypersensitivity to opioid medications.
      III. Specific information – partial agonists and mixed agonist–antagonists have a ceiling effect, but the pure μ-receptor agonists do not, so they are beneficial in the treatment of severe pain. The potency, in order from weakest to strongest with morphine being the standard at 1, is:
      meperidine (0.1),
      morphine (1),
      oxymorphone (10),
      hydromorphone (10–15),

buprenorphine (25),
fentanyl (100), and
sufentanil (1000).

Opioids can be administered safely to cats to provide analgesia. They should be titrated slowly to effect. The onset of mydriasis indicates adequate analgesia in cats, additional opioid medication may result in agitation or hyperexcitability. Opioids can be combined with various other analgesics to lessen the side effects and provide analgesia.

B. Nonsteroidal anti-inflammatory drugs (NSAIDs)

I. Indications – anti-inflammatory, antipyretic, analgesia, acute pain (surgically induced or traumatic), chronic pain.

II. Contraindications – hepatic dysfunction, renal insufficiency, shock, dehydration, hypotension, coagulopathy, in the presence of gastrointestinal disease or pregnancy, trauma, pulmonary disease. They should not be used in combination with other NSAIDs or with corticosteroids. They should be used with caution in cats, geriatric patients and those with chronic illnesses. They should be used with caution during the perioperative period due to detrimental dysfunction of platelets.

III. Specific information

a. Meloxicam is labeled for one single dose for cats.

b. Many NSAIDs are administered once daily owing to their extended duration of activity.

c. NSAIDs can cause detrimental interactions with several other medications.

d. Regular monitoring of physical exam, complete blood count (CBC), complete blood count (UA), and serum chemistry panel (including hepatic and renal function tests) are recommended.

C. NMDA (N-methyl-D-aspartate) antagonists (ketamine, amantadine)

I. Indications – NMDA receptor antagonists are used in the treatment of acute and chronic pain. They are adjunctive analgesics, used in combination with other analgesics such as opioids. They are useful in the treatment of neuropathic pain, in the prevention of wind-up, to decreased opioid tolerance, allowing lower doses of opioids to be effective, and cause less dysphoria. Ketamine causes minimal cardiovascular depression and less respiratory depression than opioids. Tremors and sedation are side effects. Amantadine is used in the treatment of neuropathic pain. It is used to prevent wind-up pain, opioid tolerance and allodynia.

II. Contraindications – ketamine should not be administered as a sole agent for sedation or analgesia. It is contraindicated in patients with head trauma and those in which increased CSF or intraocular pressure would be detrimental. Ketamine is also contraindicated in patients with heart failure, hepatic or renal insufficiency, severe hypertension, or seizures.

III. Specific information
   a. Loud noises and minimal handling help to decrease the incidence of emergence reactions.
   b. Cats keep their eyes open following ketamine administration and therefore require lubrication with an ophthalmic lubricant such as Puralube®.
   c. Amantadine appears to have a narrow margin of safety. It may cause agitation, diarrhea, and flatulence in dogs.

D. Alpha$_2$-adrenergic agonists – these medications bind to receptors in the CNS and cause sedation, analgesia, bradycardia, diuresis, peripheral vasoconstriction, muscle relaxation, and respiratory depression.
   I. Indications – they can be administered in conjunction with opioids to produce synergistic analgesia and increase the duration of analgesia. They can provide sedation for short procedures in the stable patient and are reversible.
   II. Contraindications include cardiac disease, shock, severe debilitation, hepatic or renal disease, and respiratory disease.
   III. Specific information
      a. Treatment of alpha$_2$-adrenergic-agonist-induced bradycardia with atropine or glycopyrrolate is not recommended.
      b. Atipamezole is the preferred reversal agent.
      c. Adverse effects include urination, vomiting, altered gastrointestinal (GI) muscle tone, hyperglycemia, hypothermia, bradycardia, A-V blocks, depressed respiration or apnea, paradoxical excitation, and death from circulatory failure.

E. Lidocaine
   I. Indications – local anesthetic and antiarrhythmic agent, useful as an adjunctive analgesic agent when combined with an opioid and also in opioid–ketamine combinations as a CRI IV.
   II. Contraindications – heart block or severe bradycardia, hypersensitivity to lidocaine, shock, hypovolemia, respiratory depression, hepatic disease, congestive heart failure, patients susceptible to malignant hyperthermia.
   III. Specific information
      a. Must be used cautiously in cats.
      b. Drowsiness, depression, nystagmus, ataxia, muscle tremors, and seizures are signs of overdose, which improve rapidly when lidocaine is discontinued.

F. Gabapentin
   I. Indications – treatment of chronic pain, allodynia, hyperalgesia, and refractive or complex partial seizures.
   II. Contraindications include renal insufficiency and patients with known hypersensitivity.
   III. Specific information
      a. The oral liquid usually contains xylitol so it should not be administered to dogs.
      b. Start at a low dose and gradually increase, and then gradually wean off when discontinuing to avoid seizures.

ACID–BASE DISTURBANCES

Bateman, S.W., 2008. Making sense of blood gas results, advances in fluid, electrolyte, and acid-base disorders. In: de Morais, H.A., DiBartola, S.P. (Eds.), Veterinary Clinics: Small Animal Practice, vol 38, no 3. Elsevier, St Louis, pp. 543–558.

de Morais, H.A., 2008. Metabolic acidosis, advances in fluid, electrolyte, and acid-base disorders. In: de Morais, H.A., DiBartola, S.P. (Eds.), Veterinary Clinics: Small Animal Practice, vol 38, no 3. Elsevier, St Louis, pp. 439–442.

de Morais, H.A., Bach, J.F., DiBartola, S.P., 2008. Metabolic acid-base disorders in the critical care unit, advances in fluid, electrolyte, and acid-base disorders. In: de Morais, H.A., DiBartola, S.P. (Eds.), Veterinary Clinics: Small Animal Practice, vol 38, no 3. Elsevier, St Louis, pp. 559–574.

de Morais, H.A., Constable, P.D., 2006. Strong ion approach to acid base disorders. In: DiBartola, S.P. (Ed.), Fluid, Electrolyte, and Acid-Base Disorders in Small Animal Practice, third ed. Elsevier, St Louis, pp. 310–321.

de Morais, H.A., DiBartola, S., 1991. Ventilatory and metabolic compensation in dogs with acid-base disturbances. Journal of Veterinary Emergency and Critical Care 1 (2), 39–49.

de Morais, H.A., Leisewitz, A.L., 2006. Mixed acid-base disorders. In: DiBartola, S.P. (Ed.), Fluid, Electrolyte, and Acid-Base Disorders in Small Animal Practice, third ed. Elsevier, St Louis, pp. 296–309.

DiBartola, S.P. (Ed.), 2006. Fluid, Electrolyte, and Acid-Base Disorders in Small Animal Practice, third ed. Elsevier, St Louis, pp. 229–283.

Foy, D., de Morais, H.A., 2008. Metabolic alkalosis, advances in fluid, electrolyte, and acid-base Disorders. In: de Morais, H.A., DiBartola, S.P. (Eds.), Veterinary Clinics: Small Animal Practice, vol 38, no 3. Elsevier, St Louis, pp. 435–438.

Haskins, S.C., 1977. An overview of acid-base physiology. Journal of the American Veterinary Medical Association, 170, 423–428.

Johnson, R.A., 2008. Respiratory alkalosis, advances in fluid, electrolyte, and acid-base disorders. In: de Morais, H.A., DiBartola, S.P. (Eds.), Veterinary Clinics: Small Animal Practice, vol 38, no 3. Elsevier, St Louis, pp. 427–430, 431–434.

Johnson, R.A., de Morais, H.A., 2006. Respiratory acid-base disorders. In: DiBartola, S.P. (Ed.), Fluid, Electrolyte, and Acid-Base Disorders in Small Animal Practice, third ed. Elsevier, St Louis, pp. 283–296.

Kaae, J., de Morais, H.A., 2008. Anion gap and strong ion gap, advances in fluid, electrolyte, and acid-base disorders. In: de Morais, H.A., DiBartola, S.P. (Eds.), Veterinary Clinics: Small Animal Practice, vol 38, no 3. Elsevier, St Louis, pp. 443–448.

Kovacic, J.P., 2009. Acid-base disturbances. In: Silverstein, D.C., Hopper, K. (Eds.), Small Animal Critical Care Medicine. Elsevier, St Louis, pp. 249–254.

Sorrell-Raschi, L., 2009. Blood gas and oximetry monitoring. In: Silverstein, D.C., Hopper, K. (Eds.), Small Animal Critical Care Medicine. Elsevier, St Louis, pp. 878–882.

Whitehair, K.J., Haskins, S.C., Whitehair, J.G., et al., 1995. Clinical applications of quantitative acid-base chemistry. Journal of Veterinary Internal Medicine 9 (1), 1–11.

Wingfield, W.E., Van Pelt, D.R., Hackett, T.B., et al., 1994. Usefulness of venous blood in estimating acid-base status of the seriously ill dog. Journal of Veterinary Emergency and Critical Care 4 (1), 23–27.

OXYGEN THERAPY

Bach, J.F., 2008. Hypoxemia, advances in fluid, electrolyte, and acid-base disorders. In: de Morais, H.A., DiBartola, S.P. (Eds.), Veterinary Clinics: Small Animal Practice, vol 38, no 3. Elsevier, St Louis, pp. 423–426.

Callahan, J.M., 2008. Pulse oximetry in emergency medicine. Emergency Medicine Clinics of North America. vol 26, Elsevier, St Louis, pp. 869–879.

Fudge, M., 2009. Tracheostomy. In: Silverstein, D.C., Hopper, K. (Eds.), Small Animal Critical Care Medicine. Elsevier, St Louis, pp. 75–77.

Hackett, T.B., 2009. Tachypnea and hypoxemia. In: Silverstein, D.C.,

Hopper, K. (Eds.), Small Animal Critical Care Medicine. Elsevier, St Louis, pp. 37–40.

Hopper, K., Haskins, S.C., Kass, P.H., et al., 2007. Indications, management, and outcome of long-term positive-pressure ventilation in dogs and cats: 148 cases (1990–2001). Journal of the American Veterinary Medical Association 230, 64–75.

Lee, J.A., Drobatz, K.J., Koch, M.W., et al., 2005. Indications for and outcome of positive-pressure ventilation in cats: 53 cases (1993–2002). Journal of the American Veterinary Medical Association 226, 924–931.

Mazzaferro, E.M., 2009. Oxygen therapy. In: Silverstein, D.C., Hopper, K. (Eds.), Small Animal Critical Care Medicine. Elsevier, St Louis, pp. 78–81.

Van Pelt, D.R., Wingfield, W.E., Hackett, T.B., et al., 1993. Respiratory mechanics and hypoxemia. Journal of Veterinary Emergency and Critical Care 3 (2), 63–70.

Van Pelt, D.R., Wingfield, W.E., Hackett, T.B., et al., 1993. Airway pressure therapy. Journal of Veterinary Emergency and Critical Care 3 (2), 71–81.

FLUID THERAPY

Aldrich, J., 2009. Shock fluids and fluid challenge. In: Silverstein, D.C., Hopper, K. (Eds.), Small Animal Critical Care Medicine. Elsevier, St Louis, pp. 276–280.

Chan, D.L., 2008. Colloids: current recommendations, advances in fluid, electrolyte, and acid-base disorders. In: de Morais, H.A., DiBartola, S.P. (Eds.), Veterinary Clinics: Small Animal Practice, vol 38, no 3. Elsevier, St Louis, pp. 587–594.

DiBartola, S.P., Bateman, S., 2006. Introduction to fluid therapy. In: DiBartola, S.P. (Ed.), Fluid, Electrolyte, and Acid-Base Disorders in Small Animal Practice, third ed. Elsevier, St Louis, pp. 325–344.

Giger, U., 2009. Transfusion medicine. In: Silverstein, D.C., Hopper, K. (Eds.), Small Animal Critical Care Medicine. Elsevier, St Louis, pp. 281–286.

Hohenhaus, A., 2006. Blood transfusion and blood substitutes. In: DiBartola, S.P. (Ed.), Fluid, Electrolyte, and Acid-Base Disorders in Small Animal Practice, third ed. Elsevier, St Louis, pp. 367–583.

Hughes, D., Boag, A.K., 2006. Fluid therapy with macromolecular plasma volume expanders. In: DiBartola, S.P. (Ed.), Fluid, Electrolyte, and Acid-Base Disorders in Small Animal Practice, third ed. Elsevier, St Louis, pp. 621–634.

Macintire, D.K., 2008. Pediatric fluid therapy, advances in fluid, electrolyte, and acid-base disorders. In: de Morais, H.A., DiBartola, S.P. (Eds.), Veterinary Clinics: Small Animal Practice, vol 38, no 3. Elsevier, St Louis, pp. 621–628.

Mazzaferro, E.M., 2008. Complications of fluid therapy, advances in fluid, electrolyte, and acid-base disorders. In: de Morais, H.A., DiBartola, S.P. (Eds.), Veterinary Clinics: Small Animal Practice, vol 38, no 3. Elsevier, St Louis, pp. 607–620.

Mensack, S., 2008. Fluid therapy: options and rational administration, advances in fluid, electrolyte, acid-base disorders. In: de Morais, H.A., DiBartola, S.P. (Eds.), Veterinary Clinics: Small Animal Practice, vol 38, no 3. Elsevier, St Louis, pp. 575–586.

Prittie, J., 2006. Optimal endpoints of resuscitation and early goal-directed therapy. Journal of Veterinary Emergency and Critical Care 16 (4), 329–339.

Rozanski, E., Rondeau, M., 2002. Choosing fluids in traumatic hypovolemic shock: the role of crystalloids, colloids, hypertonic saline. Journal of the American Animal Hospital Association 38, 499–501.

Silverstein, D.C., 2009. Daily intravenous fluid therapy. In: Silverstein, D.C., Hopper, K. (Eds.), Small Animal Critical Care Medicine. Elsevier, St Louis, pp. 271–275.

BLOOD PRESSURE ASSESSMENT

Bond, B.R., 2009. Nitroglycerin. In: Silverstein, D.C., Hopper, K. (Eds.), Small Animal Critical Care Medicine. Elsevier, St Louis, pp. 768–770.

Brown, S., 2009. Hypertensive crisis. In: Silverstein, D.C., Hopper, K. (Eds.), Small Animal Critical Care Medicine. Elsevier, St Louis, pp. 176–179.

Hansen, B., 2006. Technical aspects of fluid therapy. In: DiBartola, S.P. (Ed.), Fluid, Electrolyte, and Acid-Base Disorders in Small Animal Practice, third ed. Elsevier, St Louis, pp. 371–374.

Labato, M.A., 2009. Antihypertensives. In: Silverstein, D.C., Hopper, K. (Eds.),

Small Animal Critical Care Medicine. Elsevier, St Louis, pp. 763–767.

Silverstein, D.C., 2009. Vasopressin. In: Silverstein, D.C., Hopper, K. (Eds.), Small Animal Critical Care Medicine. Elsevier, St Louis, pp. 759–762.

Simmon, H.P., Wohl, J.S., 2009. Hypotension. In: Silverstein, D.C., Hopper, K. (Eds.), Small Animal Critical Care Medicine. Elsevier, St Louis, pp. 27–30.

Simmons, J.P., Wohl, J.S., 2009. Vasoactive catecholamines. In: Silverstein, D.C., Hopper, K. (Eds.), Small Animal Critical Care Medicine. Elsevier, St Louis, pp. 756–758.

Waddell, L.S., Brown, A.J., 2009. Hemodynamic monitoring. In: Silverstein, D.C., Hopper, K. (Eds.), Small Animal Critical Care Medicine. Elsevier, St Louis, pp. 859–864.

Wohl, J.S., Clark, T.P., 2000. Pressor therapy in critically ill patients. Journal of Veterinary Emergency and Critical Care 10 (1), 19–33.

INTRA-ABDOMINAL PRESSURE

An, G., West, M.A., 2008. Abdominal compartment syndrome: a concise clinical review. Critical Care Medicine 36, 1304–1310.

Drellich, S., 2009. Intraabdominal pressure. In: Silverstein, D.C., Hopper, K. (Eds.), Small Animal Critical Care Medicine. Elsevier, St Louis, pp. 872–874.

Vidal, M.G., Weisser, J.R., Gonzalez, F., et al., 2008. Incidence and clinical effects of intra-abdominal hypertension in critically ill patients. Critical Care Medicine 36, 1823–1831.

NUTRITIONAL SUPPORT

Abood, S.K., McLoughlin, M.A., Buffington, C.A., 2006. Enteral nutrition. In: DiBartola, S.P. (Ed.), Fluid, Electrolyte, and Acid-Base Disorders in Small Animal Practice, third ed. Elsevier, St. Louis, pp. 601–620.

Cavanaugh, R.P., Kovak, J.R., Fischetti, A.J., et al., 2008. Evaluation of surgically placed gastrojejunostomy feeding tubes in critically ill dogs. Journal of American Veterinary Medical Association 232, 380–388.

Chandler, M.L., Guilford, W.G., Payne-James, J., 2000. Use of peripheral parenteral nutritional support in dogs and cats. Journal of the American

Veterinary Medical Association 216 (5), 669–673.

Crabb, S.E., Freeman, L.M., Chan, D.L., et al., 2006. Retrospective evaluation of total parenteral nutrition in cats: 40 cases (1991–2003). Journal of Veterinary Emergency and Critical Care 16 (2) suppl 1, S21–S26.

Elliott, D.A., 2009. Nutritional assessment. In: Silverstein, D.C., Hopper, K. (Eds.), Small Animal Critical Care Medicine. Elsevier, St Louis, pp. 856–859.

Elliott, D.A., Riel, D.L., Rogers, Q.R., 2000. Complications and outcomes associated with use of gastrostomy tubes for nutritional management of dogs with renal failure: 56 cases (1994–1999). Journal of the American Veterinary Medical Association 217, 1337–1342.

Freeman, L.M., Chan, D.L., 2006. Total parenteral nutrition. In: DiBartola, S.P. (Ed.), Fluid, Electrolyte, and Acid-Base Disorders in Small Animal Practice, third ed. Elsevier, St Louis, pp. 584–601.

Mazzaferro, E.M., 2001. Esophagostomy tubes: don't underutilize them! Journal of Veterinary Emergency and Critical Care 11 (2), 153–156.

Mohr, A.J., Leisewitz, A.L., Jacobson, L.S., et al., 2003. Effect of early nutrition on intestinal permeability, intestinal protein loss, and outcome in dogs with severe parvoviral enteritis. Journal of Veterinary Internal Medicine 17, 791–798.

Thomovsky, E., Reniker, A., Backus, R., et al., 2007. Parenteral nutrition: uses, indications, and compounding. Compendium on Continuing Education for the Practicing Veterinarian 76–85.

Thomovsky, E., Backus, R., Reniker, A., et al., 2007. Parenteral nutrition: formulation, monitoring, and complications. Compendium on Continuing Education for the Practicing Veterinarian, 88–103.

Wortinger, A., 2006. Care and use of feeding tubes in dogs and cats. Journal of the American Animal Hospital Association 42, 401–406.

Yagil-Kelmer, E., Wagner-Mann, C., Mann, F.A., 2006. Postoperative complications associated with jejunostomy tube placement using the interlocking box technique compared with other jejunopexy methods in dogs and cats: 76 cases (1999–2003). Journal of Veterinary

Emergency and Critical Care 16 (2) Suppl 1, S14–S20.

ANALGESIA

Abbo, L.A., Ko, L.C.H., Maxwell, L.K., et al., 2008. Pharmacokinetics of buprenorphine following intravenous and oral transmucosal administration in dogs. Veterinary Therapeutics, 9 (2), 83–93.

Bergh, M.S., Budsberg, S.C., 2005. The Coxib NSAIDs: potential clinical and pharmacologic importance in veterinary medicine. Journal of Veterinary Internal Medicine 19, 633–643.

Dyson, D.H., 2008. Analgesia and chemical restraint for the emergent veterinary patient. Veterinary Clinics Small Animal 38, 1329–1352.

Hansen, B., 2008. Analgesia for the critically ill dog or cat : an update. Veterinary Clinics Small Animal 38, 1353–1363.

Harvey, R.C., 2009. Narcotic agonists and antagonists. In: Silverstein, D.C., Hopper, K. (Eds.), Small Animal Critical Care Medicine. Elsevier, St Louis, pp. 784–789.

ISFM and AAFP consensus guidelines, long-term use of NSAIDs in cat 2010. Journal of Feline Medicine and Surgery 12, 521–538.

Krotscheck, U., Boothe, D.M., Little, A.A., 2008. Pharmacokinetics of buprenorphine following intravenous administration in dogs. American Journal of Veterinary Research 69, 722–727.

Lamont, L.A., 2008. Multimodal pain management in veterinary medicine: the physiologic basis of pharmacologic therapies. Veterinary Clinics Small Animal 38, 1173–1186.

Lamont, L.A., 2008. Adjunctive analgesic therapy in veterinary medicine. Veterinary Clinics Small Animal 38, 1187–1203.

Luna, S.P.L., Basílio, A.C., Steagall, P.V.M., et al., 2007. Evaluation of adverse effects of long-term oral administration of carprofen, etodolac, flunixin meglumine, ketoprofen, and meloxicam in dogs. American Journal of Veterinary Research 68, 258–264.

Mathews, K.A., 2005. Analgesia for the pregnant, lactating and neonatal to pediatric cat and dog. Journal of Veterinary Emergency and Critical Care 15 (4), 273–284.

Mathews, K.A., 2008. Neuropathic pain in dogs and cats: if only they could tell us if they hurt, Veterinary Clinics Small Animal 38, 1365–1414.

Papich, M.G., 2008. An update on nonsteroidal anti-inflammatory drugs (NSAIDs) in small animals. Veterinary Clinics Small Animal 38, 1243–1266.

Perkowski, S.Z., 2009. Pain and sedation assessment. In: Silverstein, D.C., Hopper, K. (Eds.), Small Animal Critical Care Medicine. Elsevier, St Louis, pp. 696–699.

Quandt, J., Lee, J.A., 2009. Analgesia and constant rate infusions. In: Silverstein, D.C., Hopper, K. (Eds.), Small Animal Critical Care Medicine. Elsevier, St Louis, pp. 710–716.

Robertson, S.A., 2005. Assessment and management of acute pain in cats. Journal of Veterinary Emergency and Critical Care 15 (4), 261–272.

Sparkes, A.H., Heiene, R., Lascelles, B.D.X., et al., 2010. ISFM and AAFP consensus guidelines: long-term use of NSAIDs in cats. Journal of Feline Medicine and Surgery 12, 521–538.

Shock

INTRODUCTION

There are many definitions for shock, but the most basic is the condition in which oxygen demand exceeds oxygen delivery, resulting in inadequate production of cellular energy. Shock usually occurs following a severe decrease in the delivery of oxygen (D_{O_2}) to tissues and the consumption of oxygen (V_{O_2}) by tissues, as commonly occurs in states of poor tissue perfusion. There are three general mechanisms that commonly result in a decreased D_{O_2}: cardiac pump failure (cardiogenic shock), vascular volume maldistribution (distributive shock), and intravascular volume loss (hypovolemic shock). In addition, conditions of failure of cellular metabolism can result in metabolic shock and conditions that decrease arterial blood oxygen content can cause hypoxemic shock.

CAUSES AND TYPES OF SHOCK

Hypovolemic or circulatory
  Dehydration (severe)
  Hemorrhage (internal or external)
  Trauma
Cardiogenic
  Cardiac arrhythmias
  Cardiac tamponade
  Congestive heart failure
  Drug overdose (β-blockers, calcium channel blockers, anesthetics, etc.)
Distributive
  Anaphylaxis
  Obstruction (thrombosis, thromboembolism, heartworm disease, etc.)
  Sepsis
Hypoxemic
  Anemia
  Carbon monoxide toxicity
  Methemoglobinemia
  Pulmonary disease

Metabolic
  Cyanide intoxication
  Cytopathic hypoxia of sepsis
  Hypoglycemia
  Mitochondrial abnormality

HYPOVOLEMIC OR CIRCULATORY SHOCK

Diagnosis

History—There may be a history of trauma, with or without hemorrhage and with or without head trauma; there may be a history of severe or prolonged fluid losses such as severe vomiting and diarrhea, which occurs in canine Parvovirus gastroenteritis; or the history may be unknown.

Clinical signs—There are various different classifications of shock and the clinical signs depend upon the phase.

1. Hyperdynamic or compensatory phase (in dogs)
   A. Heart rate may be increased or normal.
   B. Respiratory rate may be increased or normal.
   C. Oral mucous membranes are usually injected or hyperemic.
   D. Capillary refill time is usually more rapid (<1 second).
   E. Peripheral pulses may be bounding or normal.
   F. Mentation is usually normal to mild obtundation.
   G. Blood pressure is normal to increased.
2. The hyperdynamic phase of shock is rarely seen in cats. The common signs of shock in cats are:
   A. Pale mucous membranes
   B. Hypothermia, with cold extremities
   C. Mental obtundation
   D. Generalized weakness or collapse
   E. Respiratory distress
   F. Tachycardia or bradycardia.
3. Hypodynamic or early decompensatory phase
   A. Hypothermia
   B. Poor peripheral pulse quality
   C. Blood pressure is normal to decreased
   D. Pale oral mucous membranes
   E. Prolonged capillary refill time
   F. Tachycardia
   G. Dull mentation
   H. Oliguria
4. Terminal phase or late decompensatory phase of shock
   A. Stupor or coma
   B. Hypothermia
   C. Bradycardia
   D. Weak or absent peripheral pulses
   E. Pale or cyanotic mucous membranes
   F. Prolonged capillary refill time

G. Severe hypotension

H. Oliguria or anuria

Laboratory findings—

1. Venous or arterial blood gas evaluation – metabolic acidosis is common in shock

2. Base deficit (BD) – normal = 0 +/– 2; reflects metabolic acid–base disturbances and directly correlates with the severity of perfusion and oxygenation deficits. Whereas arterial BD may be the best predictor of blood volume changes, venous BD is a reliable indicator of physiologic status during shock and resuscitation

3. Blood lactate level – normal is <2.5 mmol/L; lactate levels >7 mmol/L are considered severely elevated and indicate poor tissue perfusion, tissue hypoxia, anaerobic metabolism

3. CBC

4. Serum chemistry panel

5. Coagulation panel

6. Urinalysis

Diagnostic imaging—The following tests may be beneficial based upon history and clinical signs:

1. Thoracic and abdominal radiographs

2. Abdominal ultrasound

3. Echocardiography.

Additional monitoring techniques—

1. Blood pressure measurement – maintain mean arterial pressure (MAP) above 65 mm Hg:

$$MAP = 3 \times \frac{\text{systolic arterial pressure} - \text{diastolic arterial pressure}}{\text{diastolic arterial pressure}}$$

2. ECG monitoring

3. Pulse oximetry – should be greater than 98% on room air

4. Urine output measurement – minimum urine output should be above 1–2 mL/kg/h

5. Central venous pressure measurement – minimum of 0–2 cm H_2O if ongoing hemorrhage, 2–5 cm H_2O if head trauma, and 8–10 cm H_2O if shock was due to hypovolemia or trauma without ongoing hemorrhage; for cats, the CVP should be 2–5 cm H_2O

6. Body temperature monitoring

7. Monitoring of heart rate, respiratory character and rate, mental attitude, mucous membrane color, capillary refill time, warmth of extremities and other physical parameters

Advanced monitoring procedures—

1. Placement of a pulmonary artery catheter (Swan-Ganz catheter) allows for the measurement of pulmonary capillary wedge pressure (PCWP), cardiac output, mixed venous blood gases (Pv_{O_2} and Sv_{O_2}), central venous pressure, and pulmonary artery pressure.

2. Central venous oxygen saturation (Scv_{O_2}) can also be measured from a central venous catheter that extends into the cranial vena cava; Sv_{O_2} is usually lower than Scv_{O_2}, which should be maintained above 70%.

Prognosis

The prognosis varies with the cause, duration, and extent of shock.

Treatment

The goal is to recognize the disorder rapidly and to stabilize the cardiovascular system to return the delivery of oxygen to tissues to normal levels. For all forms of shock except cardiogenic shock, the first priority of treatment is rapid restoration of the effective circulating volume and tissue perfusion by the administration of intravenous fluids.

1. Inform the client of the diagnosis, prognosis, and the cost of treatment.
2. Establish and maintain a patient airway.
3. Administer oxygen and ventilate if necessary.
4. Resuscitate to end points with early goal-directed therapy:
   A. MAP = 60–80 mm Hg
   B. Normal heart rate, temperature
   C. Urine output should be at least 1–2 mL/kg/hr
   D. Stroke index (heart rate/systolic blood pressure) >0.9
   E. Blood lactate concentration (surrogate marker of tissue oxygenation) = less than 2.5 normally
   F. Base deficit (BD): mild = 2 to –5, moderate = –6 to –14, severe = <–15.
5. Place a short, large bore IV catheter into a central or peripheral vein as quickly as possible. Perform a cut-down or place an intraosseous catheter if it is not possible to secure venous access owing to cardiovascular collapse.
6. Administer intravenous fluids rapidly.
   A. Isotonic crystalloid fluids such as Normosol R or Lactated Ringer's solution are usually recommended.
   B. The recommended dosage of crystalloid IV fluids is 90 mL/kg for dogs and 40–60 mL/kg for cats. It is often beneficial to administer this volume of fluid in aliquots of ¼ to ½ the dosage (30–40 mL/kg), and re-evaluate the patient, titrating fluid therapy to the patient's needs and desired end points.
7. The administration of synthetic colloids such as Hetastarch, Dextran 70 or Pentastarch may help to retain fluid in the intravascular space more effectively than crystalloids and cause a greater increase of intravascular volume.
   A. Initially colloids may be administered in 5–10 mL/kg IV increments followed by patient reassessment. It is usually not recommended to exceed bolus administration of 20 mL/kg.
   B. An IV CRI of 20 mL/kg for the first 24 hours may follow the initial shock boluses.
8. The administration of 3.5%, 7%, or 7.5% sodium chloride (hypertonic saline), 2–4 mL/kg IV in cats, 2–5 mL/kg IV dogs

A. Avoid in patients with pre-existing hypernatremia.

B. Administer slowly over 5–10 minutes.

9. Blood component therapy

A. Plasma should be administered only if the patient has a coagulopathy, not for volume.

B. Red blood cells or blood should be administered only to those patients with severe anemia.

10. Hemoglobin-based oxygen carrier solutions, such as Oxyglobin

A. A shock dose of 5 mL/kg IV may be beneficial in some shock patients.

B. The maximum dose is 30 mL/kg IV in dogs and 15 mL/kg IV in cats.

11. Vasopressors

A. Dopamine 5–10 µg/kg/min IV CRI increases cardiac contractility and heart rate along with causing a slight increase in systemic vascular resistance. Lower doses may cause splanchnic vasodilation and changes in renal and gastrointestinal blood flow. Higher doses may cause ischemia of the gastrointestinal tract, kidneys, or heart.

B. Norepinephrine 0.05–2 µg/kg/min IV CRI increases systemic vascular resistance without causing much change in heart rate.

C. Epinephrine 0.005–1 µg/kg/min IV CRI can cause an increase in systemic vascular resistance, cardiac contractility, and heart rate but also causes an increase in oxygen consumption. The use of epinephrine is reserved for patients with resistant hypotension or during cardiopulmonary cerebral resuscitation.

D. Phenylephrine 0.15 mg/kg IV.

E. Vasopressin 0.5–2 mU/kg/min IV CRI in dogs has been shown to cause a significant increase in mean arterial blood pressure. The side effects are minimal although high doses can result in hypercoagulability and excessive coronary and splanchnic vasoconstriction.

F. Glucagon 0.15 mg/kg IV bolus followed by CRI of 0.05–0.1 mg/kg IV.

CARDIOGENIC SHOCK

Causes of cardiogenic shock include congestive heart failure and cardiomyopathy. Patients in cardiogenic shock may have different clinical signs, including:

1. Respiratory distress
2. Tachycardia
3. Hypothermia and possibly cold extremities
4. Cardiac murmur
5. Gallop heart rhythm
6. Jugular venous distension may be present.

Cardiogenic shock causes decreased blood pressure, decreased stroke volume, decreased cardiac output, increased heart rate, increased peripheral vascular resistance, increased right atrial pressure, increased pulmonary arterial pressure, and increased pulmonary capillary wedge pressure. The result is decreased tissue perfusion, pulmonary edema, and dyspnea. A cardiac murmur or gallop rhythm and pulmonary crackles may be heard on thoracic auscultation. Cats with heart failure usually have hypothermia, which may be a key to differentiating heart failure from other causes of acute respiratory distress. A cat with heart failure may also present with signs of thromboembolic disease. For further discussion please see the section under congestive heart failure in Chapter 3.

DISTRIBUTIVE SHOCK

ANAPHYLACTIC SHOCK AND ACUTE ALLERGIC REACTIONS

Allergic reactions are the result of the release of histamines, leukotrienes and other chemical mediators from mast cells and basophils. A type I hypersensitivity occurs, resulting in various clinical signs. Urticaria is a superficial systemic allergic reaction that produces wheals on the skin. Angioedema is a deeper systemic allergic reaction that affects blood vessels resulting in edema, causing localized swelling. Anaphylaxis is a severe, acute immunologic reaction that occurs within 30 minutes of exposure. The target tissues for the chemical mediators of anaphylaxis are the blood vessels and smooth muscles.

> *In dogs*—The liver is the main 'shock organ' in anaphylaxis. Signs include excitability, vomiting, defecation, urination, respiratory depression, collapse, and peracute death.
>
> *In cats*—The respiratory and gastrointestinal tracts are the main 'shock organs' in anaphylaxis. Signs include pruritus (around the face and head), hypersalivation, ataxia, dyspnea, vomiting, diarrhea, collapse, and peracute death.

> Massive envenomation from large numbers of stings, as with Africanized bee attacks, may result in severe systemic toxic reactions, including cytotoxic, hepatotoxic, nephrotoxic, and neurotoxic effects.

Sources

Several families of insects within the order Hymenoptera commonly cause allergic reactions in dogs and cats, including *Apidae* (bees), *Formicidae* (ants) and *Vespidae* (hornets, wasps, and yellow jackets). *Apis mellifera scutellata* (Africanized or killer bees) are more aggressive than other bees, resulting in multiple stings, and systemic toxic reactions.

Vaccinations, drug allergies (including penicillin, sulfa, BNP ophthalmic ointment in some cats, etc.), food allergies, contact allergies, etc. manifest in similar ways to insect bite reactions.

Diagnosis

> *History*—The patient may have a history of food allergies, ingestion of spoiled protein material, insect bites, contact allergies, blood transfusions, or vaccinations. The owner may notice facial swelling, including puffiness around the eyes, lips, and ears. He or she may notice

hives, vomiting, or diarrhea. The patient may have become restless and may have been rubbing its face or pawing at its face. Dogs may become victims of multiple *Hymenoptera* stings owing to their curious nature.

Clinical signs—An acute allergic reaction is often characterized by swelling of the soft tissues of the head, especially around the eyes, ears, and mouth. The patient may be pruritic. Urticaria, localized angioedema, marked pruritus, erythema and wheals are seen if the skin is involved in localized anaphylaxis. Vomiting, diarrhea and tenesmus may be observed if the reaction is localized to the gastrointestinal tract. Local inflammation and pain may be evident at the site of an insect sting or bite. Hepatic and / or renal failure may occur.

Signs may develop within 30 minutes after contact with the allergen. Signs may progress to systemic anaphylaxis. Patients should be observed for 12–24 hours.

A patient in anaphylactic shock may have collapsed and may be comatose, with pale mucous membranes, weak and thready femoral pulses, tachycardia, no facial swelling or urticaria, cold extremities, and oliguria or anuria. These patients can develop symptoms of disseminated intravascular coagulopathy (DIC).

Laboratory findings—
1. The PCV is often elevated.
2. The serum lactate level is usually elevated.
3. An inflammatory leukogram may be observed.
4. A serum biochemical profile may reveal elevations of alanine aminotransferase (ALT), total bilirubin and alkaline phosphatase (ALP).
5. If the patient develops DIC, anemia, thrombocytopenia, increased prothrombin time (PT), increased partial thromboplastin time (PTT), increased activated clotting time (ACT) and increased levels of D-dimers may be observed.
6. If acute tubular nephrosis leads to acute renal failure, the BUN and creatinine may be elevated. Granular casts may be observed by urinalysis.

Prognosis

The prognosis is usually favorable but may be guarded to grave if the patient exhibits signs of DIC.

Treatment

1. Inform the client of the diagnosis, prognosis, and the cost of treatment.
2. Establish and maintain a patient airway. Monitor for severe laryngeal edema and occlusion.
3. Administer oxygen, via mask, cage, flow-by, nasal catheter, or hood (with an Elizabethan collar). Provide assisted ventilation if needed.
4. Place an intravenous catheter.

Shock

5. Administer a balanced electrolyte crystalloid replacement fluid such as lactated Ringer's solution (LRS), Plasma-Lyte or Normosol®-R IV.
   A. Dogs may require a shock dose of fluids (90 mL/kg) IV, which should be administered in boluses of 20–45 mL/kg the first 1–2 hours IV, with evaluation during and following each bolus.
   B. Cats may require a shock dose of fluids (40–60 mL/kg) IV, which should be administered in boluses of 10–15 mL/kg the first 1–2 hours, with evaluation during and following each bolus.
   C. After the first 1–2 hours, re-evaluate the patient's cardiovascular status. Generally decrease the rate to 20–40 mL/kg/h in dogs and 20–30 mL/kg/h in cats until the patient is stabilized. Continue at 10–20 mL/kg/h to maintain perfusion. Fluid rate requirements may range from 2 to 7 times normal maintenance rates.
   D. Monitor for fluid overload or continued hypotension.
6. Consider the administration of Hetastarch:
   A. Dogs – administer a 5–10 mL/kg IV bolus, which can be repeated then followed by an IV CRI for a total of 1–2 mL/kg/day if needed.
   B. Cats – administer a 3–5 mL/kg IV bolus, which can be repeated then followed by an IV CRI for a total of 15 mL/kg/day if needed.
   C. Reduce the crystalloid fluid volume administered by 40–60%.
7. Administer epinephrine (1:10000) if the patient is in anaphylaxis.
   A. Administer 0.5–1 mL slowly IV while monitoring the patient's pulse rate, blood pressure, and cardiac rhythm.
   B. Recommended epinephrine dosages include 2.5–5 µg/kg IV, 10 µg/kg IM, and 0.05 µg/kg/min IV via CRI.
8. Administer rapidly acting glucocorticoids: dexamethasone sodium phosphate 0.25–0.5 mg/kg IV or prednisolone sodium succinate, 2 mg/kg slow IV.
   A. For treatment of anaphylaxis or allergic reactions in a Shar Pei, do **not** give dexamethasone; instead administer prednisolone sodium succinate. Although not published, several veterinarians have commented that dexamethasone causes the wrinkles to disappear, potentially permanently.
   B. Glucocorticoids may cause allergic reactions and anaphylaxis so it is recommended to obtain a brief history from the client of any medication allergies, prior to their administration.
9. Administer diphenhydramine, 1–2 mg/kg slow IV, IM, or PO.
10. Administer famotidine 0.5–1 mg/kg IV, SC, or PO.
11. Measure and monitor the patient's PCV/TS.
    A. PCV >60% is common; >70% is not unusual.
    B. Administer balanced electrolyte crystalloid fluids IV as necessary, depending on clinical signs and PCV/TS.
    C. IV fluid therapy is recommended if PCV ≥55% (>60% if the patient is a dachshund or greyhound), the patient is vomiting excessively, has severe diarrhea, or presents in a state of shock
12. Remove the irritating substance, by scraping off the bee stinger rather than grasping it with tweezers or a hemostat, administering an enema, performing gastric lavage or bathing the patient, if indicated.

13. A cool water bath or application of a baking soda paste may decrease skin irritation.
14. Monitor blood pressure. Maintain systolic pressure above 90 mm Hg and mean arterial pressure above 60 mm Hg.
    A. Monitor central venous pressure (maintain between 8 and 10 cm H_2O).
    B. Monitor urine output (minimum should be 1–2 mL/kg/h).
15. For the patient with dyspnea administer oxygen and aminophylline 4–8 mg/kg IM or slow IV in dogs, 2–4 mg/kg IM or slow IV in cats. If bronchospasms persist, administer terbutaline, 0.01 mg/kg SC in dogs and cats.
16. Monitor hepatic and renal function and coagulation parameters. Anticipate complications such as systemic inflammatory response syndrome, sepsis, DIC and multiple organ failure. Treat aggressively.
17. Monitor for the occurrence of severe laryngeal edema.
18. Patients having an allergic reaction that is manifested by moderate to severe swelling of the neck may or may not be dyspneic upon entry.
    A. These patients should be hospitalized for observation until the external visible swelling has decreased.
    B. A tracheostomy may be necessary.
    C. Consider the administration of furosemide to reduce edema.
19. Victims of massive envenomation, such as occurs from an Africanized (killer) bee attack, may exhibit a toxic reaction (additional information is available in the Toxicology chapter).
    A. There may be an absence of urticaria or edema.
    B. The patient may appear depressed, febrile, with vomiting of brownish fluid, hematochezia, hematuria or myoglobinuria, ataxia, facial paralysis, seizures, or death.
    C. The clinical signs may occur acutely or be delayed by several days.
    D. Treatment includes aggressive intravenous fluid therapy and supportive care. Systemic inflammatory response syndrome (SIRS) and DIC are common sequelae and necessitate monitoring of the patient's cardiovascular, respiratory, hematologic, and urinary system functions.
20. Upon discharge
    A. Dispense prednisone, 0.5–1 mg/kg PO q12–24 h for 1–2 days.
    B. Recommend restriction of activity for 24 hours.

SEPTIC SHOCK AND SYSTEMIC INFLAMMATORY RESPONSE SYNDROME (SIRS)

Etiology

Any infection in any part of the body can lead to septic shock and systemic inflammatory response syndrome (SIRS). Other causes of SIRS include heat stroke, trauma, snake envenomation, bite wounds, neoplasia, and pancreatitis. Various cytokines are produced and released in response to an inciting stimulus. These cytokines are the mediators of SIRS. The clinical syndrome is similar, regardless of the inciting stimulus.

Table 2.1   Criteria for SIRS in Dogs and Cats

Criteria	Dogs	Cats
Heart rate (beats per minute)	>120	<140 or >225
Respiratory rate (breaths per minute)	>20	>40
Body temperature	<100.6 or >102.6	<100 or >104
WBC ($\times 10^3$) or % bands	<6 or >16; >3%	<5 or >19

Diagnosis

The diagnosis of SIRS is dependent on the presence of at least two of the criteria in Table 2.1 in dogs and at least three of the criteria in cats.

Septic shock is a combination of cardiogenic, hypovolemic, and distributive shock. It is characterized by two of the above physical findings, plus hypotension (systolic blood pressure <90 mm Hg), despite appropriate fluid therapy. In addition, perfusion abnormalities such as alteration of mental status, oliguria, or lactic acidosis are present.

History—The patient may have a history of receiving immunosuppressive medications or chemotherapy. There may be a history of previous trauma, wounds, infection, or recent dental procedure.

The patient may have an underlying predisposing disease such as advanced age, diabetes, hyperadrenocorticism, malnutrition, hypoproteinemia, burns, trauma, leukopenia, or viral infection.

If the patient is an intact female, inquire as to recent delivery of puppies or kittens, and the time lapse since the last heat cycle.

Inquire as to the use of the animal and its home environment, including whether it roams off the owner's property, if there is exposure to wild animals, whether it lives in a rural area or is confined to an apartment or home.

In addition, invasive procedures performed in the hospital, such as the use of long term intravascular catheters, indwelling urinary catheters, peritoneal lavage, total parenteral nutrition, and organ biopsies, may predispose a patient to sepsis.

Physical exam—
1. Initially, the dog in the early phase of septic shock may present with:
   A. Injected, 'brick' red mucous membranes
   B. Capillary refill time <1 second
   C. Tachycardia
   D. Tachypnea
   E. Fever
   F. Bounding pulses
   G. Depression or agitation
   H. The patient is usually warm to the touch.
2. A cat in septic shock typically presents with:
   A. Relative bradycardia
   B. Hypotension

C. Pale mucous membranes
D. Prolonged capillary refill
E. Poor pulse quality
F. Hypothermia.
3. As septic shock continues:
    A. The mucous membranes appear cyanotic, muddy pink to gray or pale.
    B. The capillary refill time prolongs to >2 seconds.
    C. Pulses become weak and difficult to palpate.
    D. The extremities become cool to the touch.
4. Examine the entire body for signs of a septic focus:
    A. Look for swelling, heat and pain, even when there are no visible wounds.
    B. Auscultate the heart. An abnormal heart rate, rhythm or a murmur may indicate endocarditis. Muffled heart and lung sounds may indicate the presence of a pyothorax.
    C. Patients with pneumonia may cough and may have auscultable crackles and wheezes.
    D. Thoroughly palpate all areas of the abdomen and look carefully for signs of penetrating wounds.
    E. Palpate all four limbs and the muscles of the thorax, abdomen and pelvis for fasciitis, myositis, or cellulitis.
    F. Carefully examine the cervical region and the entire spine. Meningitis patients will often exhibit cervical pain and a decreased range of motion. Pain along the spine may indicate discospondylitis.
5. The major sites for septic foci include the:
    A. Abdominal cavity (septic peritonitis)
    B. Gastrointestinal tract (bacteremia secondary to bacterial gastrointestinal disease, translocation)
    C. Reproductive tract (pyometra, prostatitis)
    D. Urinary tract (pyelonephritis)
    E. Respiratory tract (pneumonia)
    F. Thoracic cavity (pyothorax)
    G. Heart valves (endocarditis)
    H. Teeth and periodontal tissues (periodontitis, oral abscess)
    I. Skin (bite wounds, cellulitis)
    J. Bones, joints (osteomyelitis, septic arthritis).
6. As septic shock and systemic inflammatory response syndrome progresses, the patient develops multiple organ dysfunction syndrome (MODS) or failure of several body organ systems.
7. Death soon follows.

Laboratory evaluation—
1. For initial rapid evaluation of the critical patient, obtain a PCV, TS, blood glucose screen, BUN (azostick), ACT, or PT and PTT and urinalysis on urine collected by cystocentesis.
2. Obtain a CBC, complete serum biochemical profile including electrolytes, coagulation panel and blood gases.

Shock

    A. Initially, neutropenia and thrombocytopenia are observed. As the disease continues, neutrophilia with a left shift is expected.

    B. Hemoconcentration is common in dogs but anemia is more common in cats.

    C. Blood glucose concentration may vary.

    D. Hypoalbuminemia is common.

    E. Hyperbilirubinemia and icterus are common.

    F. Serum ALP may be increased in dogs but is usually normal in cats.

3. Measure magnesium levels. If serum magnesium is <0.7 mmol/L then supplementation is indicated.

4. Submit urine for culture and sensitivity testing. Obtain samples by performing sterile cystocentesis.

5. Measure arterial and central venous blood pressure.

6. Submit samples of abdominal and / or pleural effusion or aspirates from abscesses or suspected septic focal sites for cytologic analysis and culture and sensitivity.

    A. Measure the glucose level of the peritoneal fluid and compare it with the patient's blood glucose level. If the peritoneal fluid glucose level is >20 mg/dL lower than the blood glucose level, septic peritonitis is strongly suspected.

    B. In dogs, comparison of the lactate level of the peritoneal fluid with the serum lactate level may be helpful. If the peritoneal lactate level is higher than the serum lactate level, septic peritonitis is strongly suspected.

7. If the septic focal site is suspected to be intra-abdominal, but results of abdominocentesis are not forthcoming, perform diagnostic peritoneal lavage or perform a FAST ultrasound assessment and aspirate fluid if possible.

8. In patients with suspected bacterial pneumonia, bronchoalveolar lavage or tracheal wash may be beneficial.

9. Aspiration of joints (arthrocentesis) should be performed if lameness, fever, pain, joint effusion, or swelling are found.

10. After surgically preparing sites on two different veins, collect blood for blood cultures using sterile technique. Collect two samples no less than 1 hour apart within a 24-hour period. Two collection bottles should be obtained at each collection period. Vent one bottle, for aerobic culture, by inserting a sterile needle through the rubber stopper. Leave the second bottle sealed for anaerobic culture.

    The sample size is 10 mL of whole blood, inserted into 100 mL of culture broth medium.

    The most commonly cultured pathogens include gram-positive cocci (coagulase-positive *Staphylococcus aureus* and β-hemolytic streptococcus), enteric gram-negative bacteria (*Escherichia coli* and *Klebsiella, Enterobacter, Proteus,* and *Serratia* spp.), *Enterococcus* spp. and *Pseudomonas* spp. Other organisms cultured that are clinically significant include *Bacteroides* spp., *Clostridium* spp., *Fusobacterium* spp., *Erysipelothrix* spp. and *Corynebacterium* spp.

    If the patient has been on prior antibiotic therapy, the growth of organisms may be delayed past the normal 7-day period when 95%

of the bacteria can be detected. Hold the cultures for 14 days in these patients, to allow detection of delayed or slow-growing organisms.
11. Perform a CSF tap if meningitis or discospondylitis is suspected.
12. Perform a prostatic wash if prostatic disease is suspected.
13. If the patient has had an indwelling intravascular or urinary catheter, remove the catheter and submit the tip for culture.
14. Obtain additional samples and perform further testing based on the patient's history and physical exam.

ECG—Evaluate cardiac rate, rhythm, and appearance of the complexes.
Ultrasound—Evaluation of the abdomen and thorax may be beneficial in locating the septic focus.

Differential diagnosis

Patients with heat stroke, hypovolemic shock, cardiogenic shock, and several toxicities can exhibit similar signs.

Prognosis

The prognosis varies with the condition of the patient on presentation, the location of the septic focus, and the response to therapy. In general:

1. The patient that presents with the early signs of sepsis (injected mucous membranes, tachycardia, bounding pulses) has a fair to guarded prognosis.
2. The patient that presents with signs of septic shock (the mucous membranes acquire a cyanotic, muddy pink to gray or pale appearance, capillary refill time is prolonged and pulses are weak) has a guarded to poor prognosis.
3. The patient that presents with multiple organ dysfunction syndrome has a poor to grave prognosis.

Treatment

1. Inform the client of the underlying etiologies, diagnosis, prognosis and cost of the treatment.
2. Attempt to find and treat the underlying condition causing sepsis.
3. Anticipation of complications, not reaction to clinical signs, is necessary for patient survival.
4. Rebecca Kirby, DVM, DACVECCS, DACVIM, has developed a 'Rule of 20' checklist of 20 clinical parameters to evaluate twice daily in every patient with SIRS (Box 2.1).
5. Administer oxygen supplementation.
6. Place an intravenous catheter and obtain blood and urine samples.
7. Administer high-volume intravenous fluid therapy with a balanced electrolyte solution such as LRS, PlasmaLyte or Normosol-R to prevent stasis and organ ischemia.
   A. Dogs: 90–100 mL/kg for the first 1–2 hours IV, then re-evaluate.
   B. Cats: 45–60 mL/kg for the first 1–2 hours.

BOX 2.1 'Rule of 20' checklist	
1. Fluid balance	11. RBC/hemoglobin
2. Blood pressure/perfusion	12. Renal function
3. Cardiac function/rhythm	13. Immune state/WBC/antibiotic +
4. Albumin	14. GI motility/integrity
5. Oncotic pull	15. Drug metabolism/dosages
6. Oxygenation/ventilation	16. Nutrition
7. Glucose	17. Pain control
8. Electrolytes/acid–base balance	18. Nursing mobility/catheter care
9. Mentation/intracranial pressure	19. Bandage/wound care
10. Coagulation	20. Tender loving care

From Kirby, R., Crowe, D.T. (Eds.), Small Animal Practice, Emergency Medicine, 1994, vol 24, no 6 ©Elsevier, The Veterinary Clinics of North America, with permission of WB Saunders Co.

   C. After the first 1–2 hours, re-evaluate the patient's cardiovascular status. Generally decrease the rate to 20–40 mL/kg/h in dogs and 20–30 mL/kg/h to maintain perfusion. Fluid rate requirements may range from 2 to 7 times normal maintenance rates.

   D. Monitor for fluid overload or continued hypotension.

      I. Monitor blood pressure. Maintain systolic pressure above 90 mm Hg and mean arterial pressure above 60 mm Hg.

      II. Monitor central venous pressure (maintain between 8 and 10 cm of water).

      III. Monitor urine output (minimum should be 1–2 mL/kg/h).

8. Administration of 7.5% hypertonic saline, 4 mL/kg, will help to achieve peracute volume resuscitation, but should be followed by or accompanied by either crystalloid fluid therapy or crystalloid and colloid fluid therapy.

9. Administer colloid therapy to improve perfusion and expansion of the vascular space while avoiding peripheral edema.

   A. Hetastarch

      I. Dogs: administer a 20 mL/kg IV bolus, followed by an additional 20 mL/kg IV over 4–6 hours daily for at least 3 days.

      II. Cats: administer a 10–15 mL/kg IV bolus, followed by an additional 10–15 mL/kg IV over 4–6 hours daily as needed.

      III. Reduce the crystalloid fluid volume administered by 40–60%.

   B. Dextran 70 (avoid in patients with thrombocytopenia or coagulopathy)

      I. Dogs: administer 14–20 mL/kg IV.

      II. Cats: administer 10–15 mL/kg IV.

   C. Plasma: administer when the serum albumin level is less than 2.0 g/dL.

10. Administer antibiotic therapy as indicated by the suspected potential pathogens responsible for the septic condition and also prophylactically for gastrointestinal and hepatic translocation.

   A. When the source of infection is unknown or a mixed population of bacteria is suspected.

I. Administer clindamycin, 10–12 mg/kg q8–12 h IV, and enrofloxacin, 5–10 mg/kg q12h IV or 5–20 mg/kg q24H IV in dogs. Do not exceed the dosage of 5 mg/kg/day for enrofloxacin in cats.
   a. Administer enrofloxacin at the dose of 15–20 mg/kg only twice, then decrease the dose, as seizures may occur with high doses.
   b. Avoid the use of enrofloxacin in all puppies under 8 months of age and in giant breed puppies under 18 months of age.
II. Administer a combination of ampicillin (20–40 mg/kg q8h IV), or a first-generation cephalosporin (cefazolin (20 mg/kg q8h IV) or cephalothin (20–30 mg/kg q6h IV)), with a fluoroquinolone (enrofloxacin, ciprofloxacin), ciprofloxacin dose = 5–15 mg/kg PO q12h or 10–20 mg/kg PO q24h, an aminoglycoside [amikacin (3.5–5 mg/kg q8h IV or 10–15 mg/kg q24h IV), gentamicin (6–9 mg/kg/24 h IV or 2–3 mg/kg q8h IV), or tobramycin (2–4 mg/kg q8h IV)], or a third-generation cephalosporin (ceftizoxime 25–50 mg/kg IV, IM, SC q6–8h)) or cefotaxime (20–80 mg/kg IV, IM q6–8h).
   a. The penicillins have been combined with a β-lactamase inhibitor (ticarcillin-clavulanate (Timentin®, dose = 30–50 mg/kg IV q6–8h), ampicillin-sulbactam (Unasyn®, dose = 50 mg/kg IV, q6–8h), and piperacillin-tazobactam (Zosyn® dose = 50 mg/kg IV, IM, q4–6h) for increased efficacy.
   b. Aminoglycosides should be avoided in the presence of dehydration or azotemia as they may cause renal failure.
   c. If furosemide is utilized, aminoglycosides should be discontinued, as the combination increases the risk of inducing iatrogenic renal failure.
   d. When the patient is on aminoglycosides, urine sediment should be evaluated at least daily for casts and cellular debris.
   e. If an anaerobic infection is suspected, add either metronidazole (10 mg/kg IV CRI over 1 h q8h), clindamycin, cefoxitin (40 mg/kg IV initially and continued at 20 mg/kg IV q6–8h in the dog and q8h in the cat), or penicillin G aqueous (20 000–100 000 μ/kg q4–6h IV, IM, SC) to the above combinations.
III. Administer imipenem, 2–5 mg/kg IV CRI over 1 h, q8h.
   a. Imipenem may cause seizures in young animals.
   b. Nausea, diarrhea, and allergic reactions may occur.
B. For translocation and hepatic or gastrointestinal infections, administer cefoxitin, 40 mg/kg IV, initially and continued at 20 mg/kg IV q6–8h in the dog and q8h in the cat.
C. For gram-positive infections, except streptococcal infections, administer cefazolin, 20 mg/kg IV q6h, or trimethoprim-sulfa, 15 mg/kg q12h IM.
D. For streptococcal infections, administer clindamycin, 10 mg/kg q12h IV.

E. For gram-negative rods, administer enrofloxacin, amikacin, gentamicin, tobramycin, or trimethoprim-sulfa.

F. If *Pseudomonas* is suspected, administer enrofloxacin, tobramycin or piperacillin-tazobactam.

G. If the patient is receiving chemotherapy, is immunosuppressed, or neutropenic, administer imipenem.

H. If an anaerobic infection is suspected, administer metronidazole, 10 mg/kg IV CRI over 1 h, q8h.

I. If septic shock has occurred after a dental procedure, administer clindamycin, ampicillin, or ticarcillin-clavulanate.

J. If Ehrlichiosis or a rickettsial infection is suspected, administer doxycycline 5–10 mg/kg PO, IV q12h, or imidocarb, 5 mg/kg IM, once.

K. For suspected fungal infections, administer itraconazole, 5–10 mg/kg PO q12h or fluconazole 2.5–5 mg/kg PO q12h.

11. If there is no improvement in the patient's status, fever, white blood cell (WBC) count or band count after 36–48 hours, consider changing the antibiotic therapy. Reassess the patient and review the history and diagnostic data.

12. Administer vasopressor and positive inotropic agents if the cardiovascular status is still compromised following volume replacement:

A. Dobutamine, 5–10 µg/kg/min IV CRI in dogs, and 2.5–5 µg/kg/min IV CRI in cats

B. Dopamine, 1–3 µg/kg/min IV CRI

C. Norepinephrine, 0.01–0.4 µg/kg/min IV CRI.

13. If the patient has pressor-refractory hypotension, consider the presence of critical illness-related corticosteroid insufficiency (CIRCI). Administer hydrocortisone 0.5 mg/kg IV q6h (2 mg/kg/day), prednisone 0.5 mg/kg/day, or dexamethasone 0.07 mg/kg/day.

14. Monitor PCV, maintain at a minimum of 21%. Administer red blood cells or whole blood if necessary.

15. Monitor serum glucose levels and maintain between 80 and 140 mg/dL.

16. Monitor blood gases and optimize the patient's pH.

17. Monitor serum electrolytes q2–4h initially, as rapid changes occur.

18. Monitor serum magnesium levels and serum potassium levels, as magnesium reduces the loss of potassium.

A. If serum magnesium is <0.7 mmol/L, supplementation is indicated.

B. Administer magnesium intravenously at the rate of 30 mg/kg over 4 hours as a CRI IV.

C. Supplementation can be repeated as needed up to three times in a 24-hour period.

D. The maximum amount of magnesium that should be administered is 125 mg/kg/day.

19. Monitor coagulation parameters for DIC, which should be expected to occur.

A. Recheck the platelet count and PTT or ACT daily.

B. Trends should be followed, rather than one test in a point in time.

C. Treat DIC as discussed in that chapter with fluid therapy, oxygenation, treatment of the underlying disorder, plasma administration and possibly heparin therapy.

20. Antiemetic therapy may be indicated.
    A. Ondansetron (Zofran®), 0.1–0.18 mg/kg IV q6–8h.
    B. Dolasetron (Anzemet®), 0.6–1 mg/kg IV, SC, PO q24h.
    C. Maropitant (Cerenia®), 1 mg/kg SC q24h or 2 mg/kg PO q24h.
    D. Chlorpromazine, 0.05–0.1 mg/kg slowly IV q4h in dogs, and 0.01–0.025 mg/kg slowly IV q4h in cats, if the patient has been adequately fluid volume replaced.
    E. Prochlorperazine, 0.13 mg/kg IM or SC q6h.
    F. Metoclopramide, 1–2 mg/kg q24h as a CRI IV 0.1–0.5 mg/kg IV, IM, PO q8–12h, may be used if a gastrointestinal obstruction has been ruled out.
    G. Butorphanol, 0.2–0.4 mg/kg q2–4 h IV, provides some antiemetic benefit.
    H. Auscult and palpate the abdomen 2–3 times a day.

21. Gastric protection should be provided by treating prophylactically with:
    A. Famotidine (Pepcid®), 0.5–1 mg/kg IV, IM, PO q12–24h
    B. Omeprazole (Prilosec®), 0.7–1 mg/kg PO q24h
    C. Ranitidine (Zantac®), 2–5 mg/kg IV, IM, PO q8–12h in dogs, 2.5 mg/kg IV q12h or 3.5 mg/kg PO q12h in cats
    D. Sucralfate, 250 mg for a cat PO q8h, 250–500 mg for a dog <20 kg PO q6–8h, and 1 g PO q6–8h for a dog >20 kg.

22. Administer analgesics as indicated by the individual patient's needs:
    A. Fentanyl
       I. Dog: 2–10 μg/kg IV to effect, followed by 1–10 μg/kg/h IV CRI
       II. Cat: 1–5 μg/kg/hr to effect, followed by 1–5 μg/kg/h IV CRI
    B. Hydromorphone
       I. Dog: 0.05–0.2 mg/kg IV, IM, or SC q2–6h; 0.0125–0.05 mg/kg/h IV CRI
       II. Cat: 0.05–0.2 mg/kg IV, IM, or SC q2–6h
    C. Buprenorphine
       I. Dog: 0.005–0.02 mg/kg IV, IM q4–8h; 2–4 μg/kg/h IV CRI; 0.12 mg/kg OTM
       II. Cat: 0.005–0.01 mg/kg IV, IM q4–8h; 1–3 μg/kg/h IV CRI; 0.02 mg/kg OTM
    D. Butorphanol, 0.1–0.4 mg/kg IV, IM, SC q1-2h, 0.05–0.2 mg/kg/hr IV CRI (dog and cat)
    E. Oxymorphone, 0.05–0.1 mg/kg q3–4h.
    F. Morphine
       I. Dog: 0.5–1 mg/kg IM, SC; 0.05–0.1 mg/kg IV
       II. Cat: 0.005–0.2 mg/kg IM, SC

23. If the patient develops oliguria:
    A. Review fluid therapy and provide adequate fluid volume replacement.
    B. Measure CVP and MAP. Maintain CVP between 8 and 10 cm of water and MAP above 60 mm Hg.
    C. Administer dopamine, 1–3 μg/kg/min CRI IV.

D. Administer mannitol, 0.1–1 g/kg IV, and furosemide, 1 mg/kg/h CRI IV for 4 hours if the patient is not volume overloaded. Use mannitol carefully in SIRS because in the presence of vasculitis mannitol can leak into interstitial tissues and worsen interstitial edema.

24. Nutritional support should be initiated within 12 h of presentation.
    A. Provide a minimum of 25% of the patient's protein and energy requirements within the first 12 hours.
    B. Provide a minimum of 75% of the patient's protein and energy requirements within 72–96 hours.
    C. After the patient has been rehydrated, administer a 3.5% amino acid solution with glycerine (Procalamine®). The amino acid solution should make up ¼–½ of the patient's maintenance fluid needs and can be administered through a peripheral vein, 'piggy-backed' on the maintenance fluid line. The usual dose is 45 mL/kg/day IV.
    D. The patient can then be eased onto an enteral nutrition program, with electrolytes, glucose, and glutamine supplementation, as available in commercial products, including Resorb® and Vivonex TEN®.
       I. For dogs and cats, the package of Vivonex, TEN® should be diluted with double the amount of fluid recommended on the package for human consumption.
       II. The dose is 45 mL/kg/day.
       III. The first day, administer 33% of the recommended dose, in divided feedings given every 1–2 hours.
       IV. The second day, administer 66% of the recommended dose, in divided feedings given every 1–2 hours.
       V. The third day, administer the recommended dose, in divided feedings given every 1–2 hours.
    E. If vomiting does not occur, a bland diet can be given.
       I. It may be beneficial to administer a liquid diet, such as CliniCare®, first to see if the patient can tolerate oral feeding.
       II. CliniCare® should initially be diluted to a 50% solution to decrease the incidence of osmotic diarrhea.
       III. Hills i/d®, or a/d®, or Eukanuba recovery formula® are examples of diets that may be considered.
    F. Patients that have anorexia, pancreatitis or gastroduodenal pathology can receive nutritional supplementation via various feeding tubes:
       I. Nasogastric tube
       II. Esophagostomy tube
       III. Gastrotomy tube
       IV. Jejunostomy tube – the preferred method for patients with pancreatitis.
    G. Total parenteral nutrition can be utilized as an adjunct, but the benefits are greater and the risks are reduced by utilizing enteral nutrition if at all possible.

25. Consider the administration of a daily dose of physiologic glucocorticoids to patients with relative adrenocortical insufficiency:

A. Prednisone 0.2–0.3 mg/kg/day (dog and cat)
B. Dexamethasone 0.02–0.1 mg/kg/day (dog and cat).

26. Monitor the patient's mentation status. If the patient becomes depressed, check the serum osmolality and glucose levels. Provide appropriate nursing care, including elevation of the head, prevention of aspiration, lubrication of the eyes, turn the patient every 4 hours, etc.
27. Provide comfort and general nursing care.
   A. Turn the recumbent animal over from one side to the other every 4 hours.
   B. Keep the patient clean and dry.
   C. Provide padding, towels, pillows, etc. to provide comfort.
   D. Check the intravenous catheter site frequently.
   E. Provide kind words and affection.
   F. Allow the patient to rest, when possible, by decreasing the light and noise levels.

REFERENCES/FURTHER READING

Allen, S.E., Holm, J.L., 2008. Lactate: physiology and clinical utility. Journal of Veterinary Emergency and Critical Care 18 (2), 123–132.

Day, T.K., Bateman, S., 2006. Shock syndromes. In: diBartola, S.P. (Ed.), Fluid, Electrolyte, and Acid-Base Disorders in Small Animal Practice, third ed. Elsevier, St Louis, pp. 541–564.

De Backer, D., Biston, P., Devriendt, J., et al., for the SOAP II investigators, 2010. Comparison of dopamine and norepinephrine in the treatment of shock. New England Journal of Medicine 362, 779–789.

Ellender, T.J., Skinner, J.C., 2008. The Use of vasopressors and inotropes in the emergency medical treatment of shock. Emergency Medical Clinics of North America 26, 759–786.

Prittie, J., 2006. Optimal endpoints of resuscitation and early goal-directed therapy. Journal of Veterinary Emergency and Critical Care 16 (4), 329–339.

Silverstein, D.C., Waddell, L.S., Drobatz, K.J., et al., 2007. Vasopressin therapy in dogs with dopamine resistant hypotension and vasodilatory shock. Journal of Veterinary Emergency and Critical Care 17 (4), 399–408.

HYPOVOLEMIC OR CIRCULATORY SHOCK

deLaforcade, A.M., 2009. Shock. In: Silverstein, D.C., Hopper, K. (Eds.), Small Animal Critical Care Medicine. Elsevier, St Louis, pp. 41–45.

Pachtinger, G.E., Drobatz, K., 2008. Assessment and treatment of hypovolemic states, advances in fluid, electrolyte, and acid-base disorders. In: deMorais, H.A., DiBartola, S.P. (Eds.), Veterinary Clinics: Small Animal Practice, vol 38, no 3. Elsevier, St Louis, pp. 629–645.

Rudloff, E., Kirby, R., 2008. Fluid resuscitation and the trauma patient, advances in fluid, electrolyte, and acid-base disorders. In: deMorais, H.A., DiBartola, S.P. (Eds.), Veterinary Clinics: Small Animal Practice, vol 38, no 3. Elsevier, St Louis, pp. 645–652.

CARDIOGENIC SHOCK

Atkins, C., Bonagura, J., Ettinger, S., et al., 2009. Guidelines for the diagnosis and treatment of canine chronic valvular heart disease. Journal of Veterinary Internal Medicine 23, 1142–1150.

Brown, A.J., Mandell, D.C., 2009. Cardiogenic shock. In: Silverstein, D.C., Hopper, K. (Eds.), Small Animal Critical Care Medicine. Elsevier, St Louis, pp. 146–149.

DeFrancesco, T.C., 2008. Maintaining fluid and electrolyte balance in heart failure, advances in fluid, electrolyte, and acid-base disorders. In: deMorais, H.A., DiBartola, S.P. (Eds.), Veterinary Clinics: Small Animal Practice, vol 38, no 3. Elsevier, St Louis, pp. 727–746.

Topalian, S. , Ginsberg, F., Parrillo, J., 2008. Cardiogenic shock. Critical Care Medicine 36 (suppl), S66-S74.

DISTRIBUTIVE SHOCK

ANAPHYLACTIC SHOCK AND ALLERGIC REACTIONS

Dowling, P.M., 2009. Anaphylaxis. In: Silverstein, D.C., Hopper, K. (Eds.), Small Animal Critical Care Medicine. Elsevier, St Louis, pp. 727–729.

Plunkett, S.J., 2000. Anaphylaxis to ophthalmic medication in a cat. Journal of Veterinary Emergency and Critical Care September 10 (3), 169–171.

Schaer, M., Ginn, P.E., Hanel, R.M., 2005. A case of fatal anaphylaxis in a dog associated with a dexamethasone suppression test. Journal of Veterinary Emergency and Critical Care 15 (3), 213–216.

SEPTIC SHOCK AND SIRS

Bentley, A.M., Otto, C.M., Shofer, F.S., 2007. Comparison of dogs with septic peritonitis: 1988–1993 versus 1999–2003. Journal of Veterinary Emergency and Critical Care 17 (4), 391–398.

Boller, E.M., Otto, C.M., 2009. Sepsis. In: Silverstein, D.C., Hopper, K. (Eds.), Small Animal Critical Care Medicine. Elsevier, St Louis, pp. 454–458.

Boller, E.M., Otto, C.M., 2009. Septic shock. In: Silverstein, D.C., Hopper, K. (Eds.), Small Animal Critical Care Medicine. Elsevier, St Louis, pp. 459–463.

Burkitt, J.M., Haskins, S.C., Nelson, R.W., et al., 2007. Relative adrenal insufficiency in dogs with sepsis. Journal of Veterinary Internal Medicine 21, 226–231.

Costello, M.F., Drobatz, K.J., Aronson, L.R., et al., 2004. Underlying cause, pathophysiologic abnormalities, and response to treatment in cats with septic peritonitis: 51 cases (1990–2001). Journal of the American Veterinary Medical Association 225, 897–902.

deLaforcade, A.M., 2009. Systemic inflammatory response syndrome. In: Silverstein, D.C., Hopper, K. (Eds.), Small Animal Critical Care Medicine. Elsevier, St Louis, pp. 46–48.

de Laforcade, A.M., Freeman, L.M., Shaw, S.P., et al., 2003. Hemostatic changes in dogs with naturally occurring sepsis. Journal of Veterinary Internal Medicine 17, 674–679.

Dellinger, R.P., Levy, M.M., Carlet, J.M., et al., for the International Surviving Sepsis Campaign Guidelines Committee, 2008. Surviving Sepsis Campaign: International guidelines for management of severe sepsis and septic shock: 2008. Critical Care Medicine 36, 296–327.

Johnson, V., Gaynor, A., Chan, D.L., et al., 2004. Multiple organ dysfunction syndrome in humans and dogs. Journal of Veterinary Emergency and Critical Care 14 (3), 158–166.

Kenney, E.M., Rozanski, E.A., Rush, J.E., et al., 2010. Association between outcome and organ system dysfunction in dogs with sepsis: 114 cases (2003–2007). Journal of the American Veterinary Medical Association 236, 83–87.

Levin, G.M., Bonczynski, J.J., Ludwig, L.L., et al., 2004. Lactate as a diagnostic test for septic peritoneal effusions in dogs and cats. Journal of the American Animal Hospital Association 40, 364–371.

Cardiovascular emergencies

3

CARDIOPULMONARY RESUSCITATION (CPR)

There have been many recent changes in the recommendations for CPR in dogs and cats based upon the guidelines from the 2010 review of CPR conducted by the International Liaison Committee on Resuscitation (ILCOR) and published by the American Heart Association. The key recommendations are to provide continuous uninterrupted chest compressions, to minimize both the frequency and duration of interruptions and to avoid excessively rapid ventilator rates. The following recommendations are based on these updated published guidelines.

When possible, before CPR occurs, have a discussion with the client regarding the likelihood of cardiac arrest and their desire for CPR. The success rate for CPR in dogs is 5–6%, and for cats it is 6–9%. About 10% of these patients leave the hospital alive. Place all hospitalized patients in one of three categories: (1) no CPR, (2) closed-chest CPR, or (3) open-chest CPR.

The most successful CPR is also the one avoided. In small animal practice, there are many predisposing causes for cardiopulmonary arrest (CPA), including sepsis, cardiac failure, pulmonary disease, neoplasia, coagulopathies, anesthesia, toxicities, multisystem trauma, traumatic brain injury and systemic inflammatory response syndrome. Anticipation of CPA and vigilant monitoring for deterioration in critical patients are essential. If the patient is in a kennel, place the head facing out to improve access for monitoring. Frequent re-evaluation and repetition of critical diagnostic tests and procedures may be necessary.

Before CPA occurs, several changes may be observed, including obtundation, hypothermia, bradycardia, hypotension and dilated, unresponsive pupils. Changes in respiratory depth, rate or rhythm may occur, progressing to gasping and finally agonal breaths at death. Mucous membrane color and capillary refill time should not be used to assess the patient for CPA because they may remain normal for several minutes after arrest. The definitive clinical signs of CPA include loss of consciousness, absence of spontaneous ventilation, absence of heart sounds on auscultation, and absence of palpable pulses.

When cardiac arrest occurs, if the patient is receiving inhalation anesthesia, stop the administration of the inhalant but continue the administration of oxygen. It the patient has received an anesthetic or analgesic with a reversal agent, administer the reversal agent. Immediately start chest compressions then proceed with the following 'ABCs' of basic life support CPR.

BASIC LIFE SUPPORT

A = airway

1. Check the patient for a patent airway. If the patient is apneic and total airway obstruction is suspected:
   A. Extend the patient's neck, open the mouth and pull the tongue out and down, then look for an obstruction and perform a rapid finger sweep of the pharynx.
   B. Give the patient two or three abdominal thrusts, similar to the Heimlich maneuver.
   C. Repeat the finger sweep, then ventilate the patient.
   D. Turn the patient on its side and give blows to the patient's back.
   E. Repeat if needed, but only two or three times.
   F. If the patient's airway is still obstructed, perform a tracheostomy (see Fig. 1.5 p. 14).
   G. While performing a tracheostomy, place a large bore needle or IV catheter percutaneously into the trachea, in between the tracheal rings, caudal to the tracheostomy site. Attach an oxygen line and administer oxygen to the patient at the rate of 0.2–0.5 L/min whilst performing the tracheostomy. This will provide oxygen to the patient.
2. If there is no airway obstruction, place an endotracheal tube.
   A. Use a laryngoscope to perform the procedure as gently as possible and avoid inducing laryngeal trauma or a vagal response.
   B. Use a low-pressure, high-volume cuffed endotracheal tube if possible, or any other hollow tube of the appropriate size for the patient.
   C. Secure the endotracheal tube in place.
   D. Proper placement should be confirmed by visualization, appropriate chest wall excursions during ventilation, and palpation of the tube in the trachea rather than palpation of 'two tracheas,' which indicates the endotracheal tube is in the esophagus.
3. End-tidal carbon dioxide ($ETCO_2$) monitoring has been helpful to confirm endotracheal tube placement in anesthetized animals. A positive reading for exhaled CO_2 is usually a reliable indicator of proper tube placement within the trachea in animals with normal circulation. However, in the patient with CPA, $ETCO_2$ initially may read near zero because of lack of perfusion and therefore may not be a reliable indicator of proper tube placement in these patients.

B = breathing

1. 100% oxygen administration.
2. Positive-pressure ventilation:
   A. Give 2 initial breaths of 1–2-second duration, then re-evaluate the patient.

B. If spontaneous ventilation does not return, ventilations are begun at a rate of 15–20 breaths per minute (bpm) at airway pressures of ≤20 cm H_2O.

C. Avoid providing an excessive ventilatory rate. Excessive ventilatory rates adversely affect the outcome of CPR by causing decreased coronary perfusion pressure, decreased cardiac preload, decreased cardiac output, decreased right ventricular function, increased intrathoracic pressure and decreased venous return to the heart.

D. All breaths should be given over 1 second with sufficient volume to cause a visual rise in the chest wall, and then normal relaxation of the chest wall is allowed.

E. The ventilations delivered to the patient should be neither too large nor too forcefully administered, otherwise barotrauma of the lungs may occur.

F. An ambu bag or rebreathing bag on an anesthetic machine with the inhalant anesthetic turned off should be used.

G. In patients with pre-existing hypoxia or severe pulmonary disease, higher ventilation rates, 20–25 or higher bpm, may be beneficial.

3. Acupuncture of the Jen Chung (GV26) point should be considered. This technique is performed by twirling a 25-G, ⅝-inch needle inserted to the bone in the nasal philtrum at the ventral aspect of the nares. This technique has been effective at increasing the ventilation rate in dogs.

4. Reversal agents should be administered for medications that may cause apnea, including opioids (naloxone), benzodiazepines (flumazenil), and $alpha_2$ antagonists (atipamezole or yohimbine):

A. Yohimbine or atipamezole, 0.1–0.2 mg/kg IV slowly

B. Flumazenil, 0.01–0.02 mg/kg IV

C. Naloxone, 0.02–0.04 mg/kg IV

D. The administration of inhalation anesthetics should be stopped and the breathing circuit should be evaluated before cardiopulmonary resuscitation (CPR) is initiated.

5. Doxapram administration is contraindicated because it decreases cerebral blood flow and increases cerebral oxygen consumption and requirement.

C = cardiac massage

The most important finding in the 2010 American Heart Association guidelines for CPR is that providing continuous, uninterrupted chest compressions is the more important aspect of CPR. For by-stander CPR in humans, mouth-to-mouth resuscitation is no longer recommended. The emphasis of chest compression only CPR has proven to be beneficial at saving lives.

1. Provide external chest compressions continuously until return of spontaneous circulation (ROSC) occurs.
   A. Avoid interruptions; stop only when absolutely necessary, such as when administering a defibrillatory shock.
   B. Minimize interruptions to less than 10 seconds.

2. Place the patient on a firm surface in right lateral recumbency, with the head and chest lower than the rest of the body. Avoid moving the patient. For a patient with a round or barrel chest, such as a bull dog,

consider placing the patient in dorsal recumbency and performing sternal chest compressions.

3. The patient should be lower than the person providing chest compressions (the compressor).
4. The compressor should stand behind the patient's back.
5. Perform chest compressions on the animal's left side at the 4th–6th intercostal spaces. Place one hand on top of the other hand, with the palm fully against the chest wall. Avoid using fingertips.
   A. In patients weighing >15 kg, the compressor's hands should be placed flatly over the widest part of the chest and one hand should be placed on top of the other hand with the hands parallel, applying even pressure to the chest wall with the palm of the hand.
   B. In patients weighing <15 kg, the compressor should place his or her hands directly over the apex of the heart, which lies at or slightly dorsal to the costochondral junction.
   C. For smaller dogs (<7 kg) and cats, the fingers of one hand should be placed on one side of the chest and the thumb on the other side. Compressions with the fingertips should be avoided.
6. Perform 100–120 chest compressions per minute. The timing of chest and cardiac compressions may be synchronized with the beat in the song 'Stayin' Alive' performed by the Bee Gees or 'Another One Bites the Dust' performed by Queen, in dogs. For cats, the chest compressions may be synchronized with the beat in the songs 'Footloose' performed by Kenny Loggins or 'Livin' La Vida Loca' performed by Ricky Martin.
7. Compress the chest in a 'cough-like manner', using 1–2 lb (0.5–1 kg) of compression force per pound (0.5 kg) of the patient's body weight to cause a 25–30% displacement of the chest wall, then allow the chest wall to completely recoil; otherwise, decreased coronary and cerebral perfusion and increased intrathoracic pressure occur, leading to decreased survival to discharge from the hospital.
8. The compression duration should be 50% of the total cycle time, allowing equal time for chest wall re-expansion.
9. The person performing the chest compressions should change with another every 2 minutes if possible to maintain adequate force and rate. Avoid cessation of compressions while switching people and utilize this time to quickly puncture a vein for placement of an intravenous catheter or to assess the ECG.
10. Monitor the effectiveness of chest compressions by monitoring end-tidal carbon dioxide ($ETCO_2$).
11. Delivery of a precordial thump is no longer recommended and may result in asystole.
12. Interposed abdominal compression when performed by those with advanced training may increase venous return to the heart, but no survival benefit has been shown. Evidence for or against the use of interposed abdominal compression is lacking in the new CPR guidelines. Because it can be traumatic, at this time interposed abdominal compression is not recommended.
13. The goal of CPR is ROSC as indicated by a palpable pulse.

Future possibilities

1. Compression assist devices
   A. There are several compression assist devices available for CPR in humans.
   B. The theory of the active compression–decompression device is that venous return to the heart can be increased during decompression by expanding the chest cavity and decreasing intrathoracic pressure.
   C. Such a device may be difficult to use in most veterinary patients because of the hair coat.
2. Impedance threshold devices (ITD)
   A. An ITD is a valve that limits air entry into the lungs during chest recoil between chest compressions to improve venous return to the heart by increasing negative intrathoracic pressure during the decompression phase of CPR without affecting exhalation.
   B. In animal models, the ITD can improve hemodynamic parameters, increase cerebral perfusion by lowering intracranial pressure, improve myocardial perfusion when intrathoracic pressure becomes increasingly negative, and improve ROSC when used as an adjunct to CPR in intubated cardiac arrest patients.
   C. Although ITDs have been used successfully in research animals, their use in small animal practice had not yet been reported at the time of publication of this text.

Internal cardiac massage (ICM)

1. ICM is an invasive procedure with a chance of causing infections, excessive bleeding, and damage to the lungs, heart, and major vessels. It has been shown to be superior to external chest compressions in maintaining blood pressure, arterial and perfusion pressures, and cardiac output. The following are the current recommendations and procedure.
2. ICM indications
   A. ICM should be instituted immediately in dogs >20 kg.
   B. Initiate ICM within 2–5 minutes of unsuccessful external chest compressions in any size animal.
   C. Penetrating chest wounds
   D. Thoracic trauma with rib fractures
   E. Pleural space disease:
      I. Pneumothorax
      II. Hemothorax
      III. Chylothorax
      IV. Pyothorax
      V. Hydrothorax
   F. Diaphragmatic hernia
   G. Pericardial effusion
   H. Hemothorax
   I. Severe obesity
   J. Intraoperative sudden cardiac arrest while under anesthesia

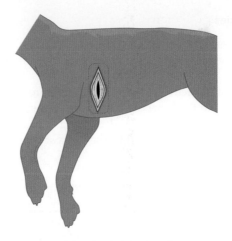

FIG 3.1 **Thoracotomy site for performing internal cardiac massage.** On the left side of the chest, between the 5th and 6th intercostal spaces, incise the skin and underlying muscles from the origin of the rib dorsally to the sternum ventrally. The technique for performing internal cardiac massage is described in the text.

3. Procedure
   A. Right-sided thoracotomy, 5th–6th intercostal space (ICS) from just below the origin of the rib dorsally to the sternum ventrally. For rapid identification, this ICS is usually just caudal to the scapula (Fig. 3.1).
   B. Rapid sterile preparation of the chest wall should be performed: minimal shaving of the incision site, disinfection, and sterile drape.
   C. Incise the skin with a no.10 scalpel blade.
   D. Between positive-pressure ventilations, penetrate the pleural space carefully with the tips of a curved Mayo scissors, hemostat, or the fingers.
   E. Open the scissors slightly, then slide them along the cranial edge of the caudal rib to enlarge the opening. A self-retaining retractor is helpful.
   F. Avoid the internal thoracic artery, which lies about 1 cm lateral to the sternum and runs the length of the chest.
   G. Perform a pericardiectomy – by sliding the left hand down the cranial and ventral aspect of the thoracotomy incision along the thoracic wall, hooking the left index finger through the pericardial–diaphragmatic ligament and incising through it with Mayo scissors. Enlarge the opening and peel the sac from the heart.
   H. In the larger patient, place the left hand underneath the heart so that the base lies in the palm of the hand and the fingers encircle the apex. Do not displace or rotate the heart or damage the myocardium with fingertips. Begin cardiac compressions by pressing down on the heart with the right hand, compressing from the apex to the base.
   I. In the smaller patient, gently cup the heart within the right hand so that the base lies in the palm of the hand and the fingers encircle the apex. Do not displace or rotate the heart or damage the myocardium with fingertips. Begin cardiac compressions by pressing down on the heart with the right hand, in a flowing motion starting with the fingers, which are grouped together and flat and ending with compression by the palm.

J. The rate of cardiac compressions should be about 100–120 compressions per minute, dictated by the rate of ventricular filling.
K. Place a cross-clamp around the descending aorta, caudal to the heart, to increase coronary and cerebral blood flow. Only utilize the cross-clamp tourniquet for <10 minutes and release it slowly.

Arrhythmias

1. Although rhythm analysis is important and ECG assessment should occur early in CPA, it should be carried out as briefly as possible to avoid impeding chest compressions.
2. There are only four rhythms that can cause a pulseless cardiac arrest: asystole, ventricular tachycardia, ventricular fibrillation, and pulseless electrical activity (PEA).
   A. Asystole is the most common arrest rhythm in dogs and cats.
      I. In humans, the survival rate from cardiac arrest with asystole is very low.
      II. Causes of asystole include numerous serious disease processes, trauma, and increased vagal tone.
      III. Evaluation of all leads of an ECG is important, because fine ventricular fibrillation can mimic asystole.
      IV. Administration of a defibrillation shock to a patient in asystole may prove detrimental to survival.
      V. Resuscitation efforts should be directed at performing high-quality CPR with minimal interruptions and to identify and treat reversible causes or complicating factors. No medications have been shown to be effective in the treatment of asystole. The administration of epinephrine or vasopressin and atropine should be tried.
   B. Ventricular tachycardia results from repetitive firing of an ectopic focus or foci in the ventricular myocardium or Purkinje system and can precipitate ventricular fibrillation.
      I. Causes of ventricular tachycardia include hypoxia, pain, ischemia, sepsis, electrolyte changes, trauma, pancreatitis, gastric dilatation and volvulus, primary cardiac disease, and other conditions.
      II. Treatment of the underlying cause should be addressed.
      III. Treatment options include the administration of amiodarone, lidocaine, or a defibrillatory shock.
   C. Ventricular fibrillation is unorganized ventricular excitation resulting in poorly synchronized and inadequate myocardial contractions that cause cardiac pump failure. Sudden loss of cardiac output leads to global tissue ischemia, the brain and myocardium being most susceptible.
      I. Ventricular fibrillation may be either fine, with lower amplitude and complete lack of organization, or coarse, with higher amplitude and more orderly appearance.
      II. Orthogonal leads (lead I and aVF, lead II and aVL) should be checked to verify fine ventricular fibrillation, which can mimic

asystole on the ECG. Fine ventricular fibrillation may be more difficult to convert to sinus rhythm than coarse ventricular fibrillation.

   III. Treatment is the administration of a defibrillatory shock.

D. Pulseless electrical activity is the condition in which, despite a normal heart rate and rhythm on ECG, there is an absence of myocardial contractility.

   I. Pulseless electrical activity was referred to previously as 'electrical mechanical dissociation' and has been combined with asystole under the new 2010 guidelines for humans. Under the new guidelines, many rhythms are grouped in the PEA category, including idioventricular rhythms and ventricular escape rhythms.

   II. No medications have proven effective in the treatment of PEA (i.e. defibrillation is not beneficial), and resuscitation should focus on performing consistent chest compressions and treatment of reversible causes or complicating factors. The administration of epinephrine or vasopressin and atropine should be tried.

   III. The prognosis is poor for successful resuscitation.

3. Another arrhythmia of importance is sinus bradycardia (a heart rate <40–60 bpm in dogs and <120–140 bpm in cats with a normal sinus rhythm on ECG).

A. Increased vagal tone, hypothermia, increased intracranial pressure, and medications can cause sinus bradycardia.

B. Treatment of sinus bradycardia includes atropine 0.04 mg/kg IV or 0.08 mg/kg intratracheal or glycopyrrolate, 0.005–0.01 mg/kg IV.

Defibrillation

Defibrillation is termination of ventricular fibrillation for at least 5 seconds after delivery of an electric shock that depolarizes myocardial cells and eliminates ventricular fibrillation. There are two types of defibrillators – monophasic and biphasic – referring to the type of current used. Newer defibrillators are usually biphasic and are effective at terminating ventricular fibrillation in humans at lower energy levels (120–200 J) than are monophasic defibrillators (360 J). It is important to know the type of defibrillator available and the energy level proven by the manufacturer to be effective at terminating ventricular fibrillation.

Defibrillation procedure—

1. Chest compressions should be performed while the defibrillator is being connected and charged.
2. Alcohol, ultrasound gel, or other nonconductive gels should not be used on electrode paddles. Conductive paste should be applied liberally to the paddles or self-adhesive pads should be used.
3. The largest electrode paddles or pad that will fit on the patient's chest should be used because small electrodes may cause myocardial necrosis.
4. The patient should be placed in dorsal recumbency and the paddles should be placed with pressure on opposite sides of the chest.

5. All electrical equipment that has not been certified by the manufacturer to be protected from defibrillatory shocks should be disconnected from the patient.
6. When the defibrillator is charged, the word 'clear' should be shouted to warn personnel to cease contact with the patient and anything connected to the patient, and then one shock should be administered as quickly as possible.
7. The person administering the shock must avoid contact with the patient's limbs, the table, the ECG leads, and everything connected to the patient. Doing so can be difficult with the patient in dorsal recumbency.

   Alternatively, the patient can remain in right lateral recumbency, a flat paddle can be placed under the patient's chest on the down side, and a standard paddle can be used on the upper side of the chest.
8. The initial counter-shock energy for external defibrillation is 2–5 J/kg.
9. For internal defibrillation, saline-soaked sponges should be placed between the paddles and the heart. The energy of the counter-shock for internal defibrillation is $\frac{1}{10}$ of the dosage used for external defibrillation (0.2–0.5 J/kg).
10. Under the 2010 guidelines, to minimize the interruption in chest compressions, one shock should be administered rather than the three successive shocks recommended previously.
11. Chest compressions should immediately be resumed for 1.5–2 minutes before reassessing the cardiac rhythm and administration of an additional shock.
12. After successful defibrillation, a short period of a nonperfusing rhythm, either asystole or pulseless electrical activity, is common before returning to normal sinus rhythm.

ADVANCED LIFE SUPPORT

D = drug therapy (See Table 3.1)

1. Route of administration
   A. The ideal route for drug administration during CPR is through a central venous catheter, but one is rarely in place and there is no time to place one during CPR.
   B. The other routes, in order of preference, include through a peripheral IV catheter, intratracheal (via an endotracheal tube) and interosseous.
   C. The intratracheal (IT) route is preferred by some as it is often the first available route and the easiest to obtain.
      I. The medications that are safe to administer IT are epinephrine, vasopressin, atropine, lidocaine, and naloxone.
      II. All medications which are administered IT should be administered at double the IV dosage except for epinephrine, which should be administered at triple the dosage.
      III. Medications administered IT should be diluted with 3–10 mL of sterile water, or sterile saline if sterile water is not available.

Table 3.1 *Medications and shock energy doses used in CPCR*

Medication	Canine	Feline	Details
Amiodarone	5.0 mg/kg IV, IO over 10 minutes Repeat dose 2.5 mg/kg IV, IO over 10 minutes	Same	Only repeat 1 dose, after 3–5 minutes, is recommended Do not administer IT
Atropine	0.04 mg/kg IV, IO 0.08–0.1 mg/kg IT*	Same	Can repeat every 3–5 minutes for a maximum of 3 doses
Calcium gluconate	10% 0.5–1.5 mL/kg IV slowly	Same	Do not administer IT
Epinephrine	0.01 mg/kg IV, IO 0.03–0.1 mg/kg IT* Repeat dose 0.1 mg/kg IV, IO, IT*	Same	Initial dose Repeat doses should be administered every 3–5 minutes
Lidocaine	2.0–4.0 mg/kg IV, IO 4.0–10 mg/kg IT*	0.2 mg/kg IV, IO, IT	Use cautiously in cats
Magnesium sulfate	0.15–0.3 mEq/kg IV slowly over 10 minutes	Same	Can repeat to a maximum of 0.75 mEq/kg Do not administer IT
Naloxone	0.02–0.04 mg/kg IV 0.04–0.10 mg/kg IT*	Same	Opioid reversal agent
Sodium bicarbonate	0.5 mEq/kg IV, IO 0.08 × BW (kg) × base deficit = no. of mEq to administer	Same	Do not administer IT Administer cautiously after 10–15 minutes of CPA; can repeat every 10 minutes
Vasopressin	0.2–0.8 U/kg IV, IO 0.4–1.2 U/kg IT*	Same	Repeat every 3–5 minutes or alternate with epinephrine
External defibrillation shock energy (J)	2–5 J/kg	Same	
Internal defibrillation shock energy (J)	0.2–0.5 J/kg	Same	

IO, intraosseous; IT, intratracheal; CPCR, cardiopulmonary cerebral resuscitation.

*All medications administered IT should be diluted in 5–10 mL of sterile water.

IV. It is helpful to administer IT medications through a long urinary catheter passed through the endotracheal tube to the level of the tracheal bifurcation.
D. Place an IV catheter.
E. If an IV catheter cannot be placed, either surgically cut down to a vein to place the catheter or place an intraosseous catheter in the femoral trochanteric fossa, proximal humerus, or the tibial crest.
2. Intravenous fluid therapy
   A. In the euvolemic CPA patient, the recommended dosage for crystalloid IV fluids is a 20 mL/kg bolus for dogs and a 10 mL/kg bolus for cats, as rapidly as possible.
   B. IV fluids should not be administered at shock dosages (90 mL/kg for dogs and 45 mL/kg for cats) unless the patient was hypovolemic before CPA. The administration of excessive volumes of IV fluids to

euvolemic patients during CPR in animal studies decreased coronary perfusion pressure and adversely affected survival.

C. If colloids are necessary, the IV dosage of Hetastarch or plasma is 20 mL/kg/day for dogs and 5–10 mL/kg/day for cats. Hetastarch may be administered as an IV bolus during CPR at a dosage of 5 mL/kg for dogs and 2–3 mL/kg for cats.

D. Hypertonic saline (3%, 5%, 7.2%) has been shown to improve survival from ventricular fibrillation when compared with 0.9% NaCl in animal studies. The recommended dosage in dogs is 4–5 mL/kg and in cats is 2–4 mL/kg IV, given slowly over 5 minutes to avoid vagal-induced bradycardia and hypotension.

3. Epinephrine hydrochloride

A. Epinephrine is a mixed adrenergic agonist, acting on alpha- and beta-receptors.

B. Epinephrine is administered during CPR mainly for its alpha$_2$-adrenergic receptor-stimulating effects, including peripheral arteriolar vasoconstriction, which leads to increased coronary and cerebral perfusion pressure.

C. The optimal dosage of epinephrine is not known. In veterinary patients, epinephrine (1:1000) should be administered initially at 0.01 mg/kg IV, unless it is being administered IT, in which case the dosage is 0.03–0.1 mg/kg.

D. Epinephrine administration should be repeated every 3–5 minutes if indicated or may be interchanged with the administration of vasopressin.

E. If repeated doses are not successful, vasopressin can be administered instead or the epinephrine dosage can be increased to 0.1 mg/kg IV.

4. Vasopressin

A. Vasopressin is a nonadrenergic endogenous pressor peptide that causes peripheral, coronary and renal vasoconstriction.

B. At a dosage of 0.2–0.8 U/kg IV or 0.4–1.2 U/kg IT, vasopressin stimulates specific V1A receptors in the smooth muscle of the vasculature, leading to nonadrenergic vasoconstriction.

C. Vasopressin may improve cerebral perfusion by causing dilatation of cerebral vasculature. It causes less constriction in coronary and renal blood vessels than in peripheral tissue, resulting in preferential shunting of blood to the central nervous system and heart.

D. Vasopressin can be used with or instead of epinephrine in the treatment of ventricular fibrillation, ventricular tachycardia and PEA.

E. Vasopressin is also indicated in the treatment of asystole, where some clinical studies in people have shown it was superior to epinephrine in survival to discharge from the hospital.

F. The responses of the V1A receptors remain intact in an acidotic environment, as encountered in cardiac arrest, allowing vasopressin to function, whereas epinephrine and other catecholamines lose much of their vasopressor effects in hypoxic and acidotic environments.

G. The initial dosage of vasopressin can be repeated every 3–5 minutes, or vasopressin can be alternated with epinephrine every 3–5 minutes.

5. Atropine sulfate
   A. Atropine is an anticholinergic parasympatholytic that is effective at muscarinic receptors.
   B. Atropine reverses cholinergic-mediated responses and parasympathetic stimulation and acts to increase heart rate, control hypotension, and increase systemic vascular resistance. It is most effective in the treatment of vagal induced asystole.
   C. Although there are no prospective controlled studies supporting the use of atropine in asystole or PEA cardiac arrest, the 2010 guidelines recommend atropine in these instances.
   D. The recommended dosage for atropine during CPR in dogs and cats is 0.04 mg/kg IV.
   E. If there is no effect, the dose can be repeated every 3–5 minutes for a maximum of 3 doses.
6. Amiodarone
   A. Amiodarone is a class III antiarrhythmic agent with several effects, including prolongation of myocardial cell action potential duration and refractory period by affecting sodium, potassium, and calcium channels, and noncompetitive alpha- and beta-adrenergic inhibition.
   B. It is the medication of choice for treatment of refractory ventricular fibrillation after defibrillation and if defibrillation is anticipated.
   C. Amiodarone is indicated for the treatment of atrial fibrillation, narrow-complex superventricular tachycardia, ventricular tachycardia, wide-complex tachycardia of uncertain origin, and refractory ventricular fibrillation that is unresponsive to compressions, defibrillation, and vasopressor administration.
   D. The dosage of amiodarone is 5.0 mg/kg IV or IO over 10 minutes.
   E. One repeated dose of amiodarone, at a dosage of 2.5 mg/kg IV, may be administered after 3–5 minutes.
7. Lidocaine
   A. Lidocaine is a class Ib antiarrhythmic agent that stabilizes cell membranes by sodium channel blockade and also acts as a local anesthetic.
   B. In clinical trials, in comparison with amiodarone, lidocaine resulted in decreased ROSC and increased incidence of asystole after defibrillation.
   C. Because it has no proven efficacy in cardiac arrest, the 2010 guidelines state that lidocaine should be considered an alternative treatment to amiodarone.
   D. Lidocaine is not recommended for treatment of ventricular fibrillation if defibrillation is planned, because it may make electrical defibrillation more difficult by increasing the defibrillation threshold and decreasing myocardial automaticity.
   E. For ventricular arrhythmias after resuscitation, lidocaine may be beneficial and should be considered if amiodarone is not available.
   F. The dosage of lidocaine in dogs is 2.0–4.0 mg/kg IV or IO.

G. For IT administration in dogs, the lidocaine dosage is increased 2–2.5 times and it is diluted in sterile water.

H. Lidocaine should be used cautiously, if at all, in cats at a dosage of 0.2 mg/kg IV, IO, or IT.

8. Magnesium sulfate

A. The administration of magnesium sulfate may be beneficial in the treatment of refractory ventricular arrhythmias, including ventricular fibrillation and torsades de pointes (a life-threatening, polymorphic form of ventricular tachycardia).

B. The dosage of magnesium sulfate during cardiac arrest is 0.15–0.3 mEq/kg administered slowly IV over 10 minutes, repeated to a maximum dosage of magnesium sulfate of 0.75 mEq/kg/day.

9. Dextrose

A. Check blood glucose levels.

B. Administer IV dextrose only if the patient is hypoglycemic.

C. Hyperglycemia has been shown to be detrimental to outcome.

10. Sodium bicarbonate

A. Sodium bicarbonate is recommended only in the treatment of tricyclic antidepressant overdose, severe pre-existing metabolic acidosis, and severe hyperkalemia.

B. For these conditions, sodium bicarbonate may be administered at a dosage of 0.5 mEq/kg IV.

C. The best treatment for the respiratory acidosis and nonrespiratory (metabolic) acidosis that occur during CPA is to maximize ventilation and perfusion.

D. Sodium bicarbonate may inactivate catecholamines that are administered simultaneously and can cause hypernatremia, hyperosmolality, extracellular alkalosis, decreased systemic vascular resistance, left shift of the oxyhemoglobin curve, and decreased release of oxygen from hemoglobin.

11. Calcium is currently recommended for the treatment of calcium channel blocker toxicity, hyperkalemia, and documented ionized hypocalcemia, rather than routine use during CPR.

A. When indicated, the dosage of 10% calcium gluconate is 0.5–1.5 mL/kg slowly IV.

B. In critically ill patients, serum total calcium concentration is an inadequate reflection of serum ionized calcium concentration, which is affected by interactions of serum pH, individual serum protein-binding capacity and affinity, and serum protein concentration.

E = evaluate status

1. End-tidal carbon dioxide ($ETCO_2$) level should be monitored as an indication of perfusion.

A. If ventilation during CPCR is relatively constant, changes in cardiac output are reflected by changes in $ETCO_2$ levels.

B. In studies of humans, patients who could not be resuscitated had significantly lower $ETCO_2$ levels than did those who were successfully resuscitated.

2. Assessment of blood flow
   A. The presence of a palpable carotid or femoral pulse may not be a reliable indicator of successful CPR.
   B. Venous pulses may be felt in the absence of adequate arterial blood flow during CPR due to the backflow of blood from the caudal vena cava.
   C. Assessment of cerebral blood flow can be performed by placement of a Doppler ultrasound transducer on the lubricated cornea.
3. Assessment of oxygenation
   A. During CPR, monitoring of central venous blood gases from a pulmonary artery catheter sample allows assessment of oxygenation at the tissue level.
   B. Evaluation of central venous blood gases provides a more accurate assessment of tissue acid–base status during CPR because it takes into consideration the effects of low peripheral blood flow and the resulting tissue hypoxia, hypercarbia and acidosis that occur during CPA.
   C. Studies have shown that evaluation of arterial blood gases during CPR does not adequately reflect the effectiveness of ventilation, or the severity of tissue acidosis or tissue hypoxemia.
   D. Pulse oximetry is not helpful because peripheral pulsatile blood flow is inadequate.

CARE OF THE PATIENT POST-RESUSCITATION

1. Respiratory or CPA commonly recurs after successful CPR in veterinary patients.
2. A 'sepsis-like syndrome' characterized by coagulopathy, immunologic dysfunction and multiple organ failure has been documented after successful resuscitation in people because of the presence of global ischemia and reperfusion injury.
3. Monitor the following parameters: pulse rate, rhythm and character, mental status, ECG, pulse oximetry, body temperature, lung sounds, mucous membrane color, capillary refill time, urine output, electrolytes, blood gases, PCV and total solids, blood glucose concentration, serum lactate concentration, central venous pressure, neurologic function and patient comfort.
4. Oxygen supplementation
   A. Supplemental oxygen should be provided via ventilatory support if inadequacies in spontaneous ventilation are present, or via a nasal catheter, a hood or an oxygen kennel.
   B. Initially, the patient should be ventilated with 100% oxygen, but the oxygen concentration should be decreased to <60% as quickly as possible to avoid oxygen toxicity.
   C. If continued ventilation is required, arterial blood gases and direct arterial blood pressure or indirect systolic blood pressure should be monitored continuously.

5. Permissive hypothermia
   A. If the animal has mild hypothermia or becomes hypothermic during CPR, permissive hypothermia should be allowed.
   B. Permissive hypothermia is the term used when hypothermia is allowed to continue without taking steps to rewarm the patient to a normal body temperature. This term differs from induced hypothermia, in which the human patient is manipulated via medical treatment and external devices to a body temperature of 32–34°C (90–93°F) and maintained at this low body temperature for 12–24 hours.
   C. Although induced hypothermia may be useful in human patients, it requires advanced monitoring and medical devices not typically available in veterinary practice.
   D. Complications of hypothermia include arrhythmias and coagulopathy.
   E. The target temperature for dogs and cats is 33–34°C (90–93°F).
   F. Permissive hypothermia diminishes the oxygen demands of tissues, reduces neurologic impairment after CPA, and may increase the success rate from CPCR.
6. Fluid therapy
   A. IV fluid therapy should be administered cautiously.
   B. Crystalloids should not be administered at shock fluid dosages unless the patient was hypovolemic before CPA.
   C. To improve peripheral perfusion and cardiac output, it may be beneficial to administer an IV bolus of a colloid such as Hetastarch (5–10 mL/kg IV for dogs and 2–3 mL/kg IV slowly over 15 minutes for cats).
   D. If the colloid bolus does not improve cardiac output, blood pressure, and peripheral perfusion, it may be beneficial to administer a positive inotrope or vasopressor.
7. Positive inotropes
   A. After an adequate IV fluid bolus, if the patient is normotensive, with decreased perfusion and decreased cardiac contractility as evaluated by echocardiography, administration of a positive inotrope (e.g. dobutamine or dopamine) may be indicated.
   B. Peripheral perfusion can be evaluated by assessing serum lactate concentration, urine output, capillary refill time, and rectal and peripheral temperatures.
   C. Dobutamine is usually the drug of choice to improve cardiac output without causing excessive vasoconstriction. The dosage of dobutamine for infusion is 2.0–20.0 µg/kg/min IV as a constant rate infusion (CRI) titrated to effect.
   D. Dopamine administration may be beneficial if dobutamine does not produce the desired response.
      I. Dopamine has a greater impact on systemic arterial blood pressure but may cause excessive vasoconstriction without an additional increase in cardiac output.
      II. The dosage of dopamine to produce a positive inotropic effect is 5–15 µg/kg/min IV as a CRI titrated to effect.

E. The following formula may be used to calculate a dobutamine or dopamine CRI:

$6 \times$ body weight in kilograms = the number of milligrams of dobutamine or dopamine added to a total volume of 100 mL 0.9% NaCl.

   I. When this preparation is delivered at 1.0 mL/h IV, 1.0 µg/kg/min is administered.

   II. The CRI solution should be protected from light.

8. Vasopressors

A. After an adequate IV fluid bolus, if the patient is hypotensive, with normal cardiac contractility as evaluated by echocardiography, the administration of a vasopressor (e.g. epinephrine, vasopressin or norepinephrine) IV as a CRI titrated to effect may be beneficial to increase systemic arterial blood pressure and cardiac output, but cautious administration is necessary because excessive vasoconstriction may occur.

B. Epinephrine

   I. The dosage of epinephrine (1:1000) for infusion is 0.1–1.0 µg/kg/min IV as a CRI titrated to effect.

   II. The following formula may be useful to calculate an epinephrine CRI:

$0.6 \times$ body weight in kilograms = the number of milligrams of epinephrine added to a total volume of 100 mL 0.9% NaCl.

   III. When this preparation is delivered at 1.0 mL/h IV, 0.1 µg/kg/min is administered.

   IV. The CRI solution should be protected from light.

C. Vasopressin

   I. The dosage of vasopressin for infusion is 0.01–0.04 U/min IV as a CRI titrated to effect.

   II. Vasopressin may be particularly beneficial for patients in septic shock.

D. Norepinephrine

   I. Norepinephrine is a potent vasoconstrictor and inotropic agent with mixed alpha- and beta-adrenergic receptor actions that may be indicated in the patient who remains hypotensive despite adequate volume replacement and treatment with other, less potent, inotropes such as dopamine.

   II. Cardiac contractility, cardiac oxygen demand, heart rate, and stroke volume increase after the administration of norepinephrine.

   III. Renal, splanchnic and pulmonary vasoconstriction also occurs.

   IV. Norepinephrine is available in two forms. Norepinephrine, 1 mg, is equivalent to 2 mg of norepinephrine bitartrate.

      a. Norepinephrine 4 mg, or 8 mg of norepinephrine bitartrate, should be diluted in 250 mL of 5% dextrose in water or 5% dextrose in normal saline before administration.

b. The dosage of norepinephrine is 0.5–1.0 µg/kg/min IV as a CRI, titrated to effect.
9. Neurologic dysfunction occurs commonly after CPCR.
   A. Often, the clinical abnormalities resolve over 24–48 hours.
   B. The patient should be allowed a minimum of 48 hours before a prognosis is made regarding neurologic abnormalities.
   C. To avoid increasing the brain's oxygen requirements, hyperthermia should be avoided and antiepileptic treatment should be administered to a patient with seizures.
   D. Situations that cause increased intracranial pressure such as sneezing caused by nasal oxygen cannulas and neck wraps for jugular catheters or esophagostomy tubes should be avoided.
   E. Place a board or other flat support underneath the patient's head and neck then elevate the end of the board near the nose as shown in Figure 3.2 to slightly elevate the head. Position the nose in a normal resting position, careful to avoid kinking the neck either ventrally or to either side.
   F. If the patient is placed in a kennel, have the head pointing out for easy access and evaluation.
   G. Glucocorticoid administration is contraindicated in these patients and may worsen neurologic injury secondary to ischemia by causing hyperglycemia.
   H. The administration of hypertonic saline or mannitol (0.5–1 g/kg IV over 20 minutes) may be beneficial for patients with cerebral edema.
10. Nutritional support should be instituted as soon as possible depending on the patient's mentation after resuscitation, original disease process, and underlying clinical status. If oral enteral nutritional support is not possible, placement of a feeding tube or parenteral nutritional support should be considered.
11. Studies in humans identified four clinical signs that correlate with poor neurologic outcome when observed 24 hours after resuscitation:
    A. Absent corneal reflex
    B. Absent pupillary response
    C. Absent withdrawal response to pain
    D. Absent motor response.

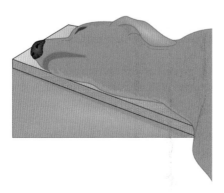

FIG 3.2 Proper positioning of patient's head post-resuscitation. Note the head is elevated and the neck is extended.

12. Common complications that can be seen after CPCR include cerebral edema, hypoxemia, reperfusion injury, abnormal hemostasis, acute renal failure, sepsis, multiple organ dysfunction syndrome, and recurrent CPA.
13. In addition, treatment is needed to address the underlying disease process that resulted in the initial CPA.

CONGESTIVE HEART FAILURE

Diagnosis

History—The patient may or may not have a history of a previous problem. The patient may or may not be on medication. The patient may have a dry and harsh cough, especially at night, in the early morning or after exercise. The patient may be restless at night, or have orthopnea, exercise intolerance, syncope or respiratory distress. Loss of appetite and weight loss are often noted. Small breed dogs, including Cavalier King Charles Spaniels, Dachshunds, and Miniature and Toy Poodles, have a higher predisposition for development of heart failure. Large breed dogs, such as Doberman Pinscher and Boxer, have a higher predisposition for development of cardiomyopathy, which leads to heart failure.
Clinical signs—Left-sided heart failure: heart murmur, dyspnea, tachypnea, tachycardia, coughing, cyanosis, hemoptysis, arrhythmia, cardiac cachexia, cardiogenic shock, pulmonary edema, fever.

Right-sided heart failure: possibly pleural effusion, muffled heart sounds, pericardial effusion, ascites, distended jugular veins with visible pulsations, pallor, syncope.
Laboratory tests—CBC, electrolytes, serum biochemistry profile, lactate, serum *N*-terminal pro-B-type naturetic peptide (BNP) concentration, cardiac troponin I, serum thyroxin levels, heartworm microfilaria or immunologic tests, and urinalysis. A minimum of hematocrit, total protein concentration, creatinine and urinalysis is indicated in all patients. Cystocentesis should be avoided in patients in distress. Do not withhold therapy while waiting for urination.
Thoracic radiographs—With left-sided heart failure, one may see dorsal displacement of the trachea, prominent pulmonary veins, and pulmonary edema. With right-sided heart failure, one may see pleural effusion, enlarged caudal vena cava, and hepatomegaly. Assessment of the vertebral heart score (VHS) may help assess cardiomegaly, which is increased in heart failure.
1. Using a lateral thoracic radiograph, the VHS is obtained by measuring both the long axis and short axis of the heart, in terms of vertebral body length.
2. The long axis (L) is measured from the ventral border of the left mainstem bronchus to the most ventral aspect of the apex of the heart.
3. The short axis (S) is measured at the area of maximum cardiac width, perpendicular to the L.
4. The sum of the L and S measurements is compared with the thoracic vertebrae, starting at the cranial edge of T4, estimated to the nearest 0.1 vertebrae.

5. The normal VHS for most dogs is between 8.5 and 10.5, although there are variations with some breeds.
6. The normal VHS for most cats is between 6.7 and 8.0, with a mean VHS of 7.5.

Echocardiography—May see mitral or tricuspid regurgitation, dilated cardiac chambers, thickened ventricular walls, pericardial effusion, or dilated pulmonary vessels.

Prognosis

The prognosis is fair to grave depending upon the severity of clinical signs on presentation.

Treatment

1. Inform the client of the diagnosis, prognosis and cost of the treatment.
2. Hospitalize the patient for observation.
3. Provide supplemental oxygen as needed. The goal is a Sp_{O_2} >95% on room air.
4. Place an intravenous catheter.
5. Depending upon the severity of clinical signs, administer furosemide as needed. The recommended initial dosage is 1–4 mg/kg IV.
   A. In dogs, if the pulmonary edema is severe, administer furosemide, 2–4 mg/kg IV; repeat every 1–4 hours as needed until respiratory rate and effort decrease.
   B. In cats with severe pulmonary edema, administer furosemide 1–2 mg/kg IV or IM; repeat every 1–4 hours as needed until respiratory rate and effort decrease.
   C. Furosemide can also be administered as a CRI in refractory patients, 1 mg/kg/h IV for a maximum of 4 hours. It is recommended to dilute the veterinary formulation to 5 or 10 mg/mL in D5W, sterile water, LRS, or 0.9% NaCl and to administer via syringe pump if possible, minimizing the volume of IV fluids administered until the pulmonary edema resolves.
   D. Some patients may require higher or lower dosages of furosemide.
   E. After diuresis has started, offer free access to water.
   F. Decrease furosemide to 1–4 mg/kg q6–12h in dogs and 1–2 mg/kg q6–12h in cats.
   G. *Caution:* Monitoring of serum potassium levels and creatinine is necessary as hypokalemia, azotemia, and dehydration may result.
6. Pimobendan, 0.25–0.3 mg/kg PO q12h (if the condition is severe, an additional 0.3 mg/kg dose may be administered with owner consent).
7. Administration of an ACEI (angiotensin-converting enzyme inhibitor) such as enalapril 0.5 mg/kg PO q12h, or benazepril 0.5 mg/kg PO q24h is useful for patients with left atrial enlargement.
8. If severe pulmonary edema is present, an afterload reducer may be combined with the above medications. Blood pressure should be monitored closely with these medications.
   A. Hydralazine 0.5–2 mg/kg PO

B. Amlodipine 0.05–0.1 mg/kg PO
C. Nitroglycerine 2% ointment, approximately 0.25 inch (0.65 cm) per 5 kg body weight transdermally q6–8h for 24–36 hours. Apply the ointment to a clipped area on the thorax or on the abdomen. Wear gloves during application, use a tongue depressor to apply and cover the area with nonporous tape. Avoid contact with the applicator's skin. The dose for cats is 0.25–0.5 inch (0.65–1.3 cm) transdermally q6–8h, with a 12-hour dose-free interval.
D. Sodium nitroprusside, starting at 0.5–1 µg/kg/min IV. Increase the dosage every 15–30 minutes as needed to a maximum of 10 µg/kg/min for up to 48 hours. The solution must be protected from light.

9. If inotropic support is needed for the hypotensive patient, administer dobutamine, 0.5–1 µg/kg/min IV. Increase the dosage every 15–30 minutes as needed to a maximum of 10 µg/kg/min for up to 48 hours. Blood pressure and ECG should be monitored continuously. The solution must be protected from light.

10. Control anxiety.
    A. Butorphanol 0.2–0.25 mg/kg IM or IV
    B. Buprenorphine 0.0075–0.01 mg/kg combined with acepromazine (acetylpromazine) 0.01–0.03 mg/kg IV, IM, SC
    C. Morphine 0.2 mg/kg SC or IM
    D. Hydromorphone 0.05–0.1 mg/kg IV, IM, SC

11. Administer antiarrhythmic therapy as needed.

12. The administration of a bronchodilator may be beneficial, but the inotropic and chronotropic effects may be detrimental in a patient with severe tachycardia or a tachyarrhythmia.
    A. Aminophylline, 5–10 mg/kg IV, IM or PO q8h
    B. Theophylline (extended release), 10 mg/kg PO q12h
    C. Terbutaline, 0.01 mg/kg SC q4h, or 1.25–5.0 mg PO q8–12h.

13. Thoracocentesis and/or abdominal paracentesis may be beneficial for some patients.

14. Mechanical ventilatory assistance may be beneficial for some patients.

15. Some cardiologists recommend the administration of spironolactone 0.25–2.0 mg/kg PO q12–24h after the patient has stabilized, for chronic therapy.

16. Intravenous fluids are contraindicated in the treatment of congestive heart failure. If severe electrolyte abnormalities or severe dehydration develops, cautious therapy may be initiated.
    A. Although D5W or 2.5% dextrose in 0.45% NaCl are usually recommended owing to their lower sodium content, these fluids supply free water and may actually increase cellular edema.
    B. CVP monitoring should be performed if possible.
    C. Monitor the patient's body weight, mucous membrane color, pulse rate and quality, respiratory rate and effort, and repeat thoracic auscultation several times a day to monitor fluid therapy.
    D. Also evaluate urine output, blood gas analysis, serum urea nitrogen, serum creatinine, ECG and thoracic radiographs.

3

I. DILATED FORM (DCM)

The dilated form is the most common form. It occurs in large breed dogs, such as Doberman Pinschers, Boxers, Scottish Deerhounds, Irish Wolfhounds, Great Danes, German Shepherds, and English and American Cocker Spaniels. It occurs most often in middle-aged to older dogs; however a juvenile-onset form occurs in Portuguese Water Dogs under 6 months of age. The clinical signs are often more severe in male dogs.

Diagnosis

History—Lethargy, exercise intolerance, anorexia, weight loss, cough, dyspnea, tachypnea, abdominal distension, syncope, or sudden death may be seen.

Physical exam—Poor peripheral pulses and possible pulse deficits, dull mentation, cool extremities, decreased rectal temperature, prolonged capillary refill, harsh lung sounds, dyspnea, tachypnea, cough, tachycardia, systolic murmur over left cardiac apex, arrhythmias, S_3 gallop rhythm, jugular pulsation, hepatojugular reflux (positive abdominojugular test) which is a more noticeable jugular pulse caused by pressure applied to the cranial abdomen, cyanosis, ascites, and cardiac cachexia may be seen.

Thoracic radiographs—Generalized cardiomegaly or enlargement of the left ventricle or left atrium or biventricular enlargement, an alveolar, interstitial or mixed pulmonary parenchymal pattern most commonly in the caudodorsal or perihilar areas consistent with pulmonary edema (may have an atypical pattern also), pulmonary venous distention, compression of the left mainstem bronchus, caudal vena caval enlargement, pleural effusion, ascites, and hepatomegaly may be observed.

Assessment of the vertebral heart score (VHS) may help assess cardiomegaly, which is increased in with DCM.

1. Using a lateral thoracic radiograph, the VHS is obtained by measuring both the long axis and short axis of the heart, in terms of vertebral body length.
2. The long axis (L) is measured from the ventral border of the left mainstem bronchus to the most ventral aspect of the apex of the heart.
3. The short axis (S) is measured at the area of maximum cardiac width, perpendicular to the L.
4. The sum of the L and S measurements is compared with the thoracic vertebrae, starting at the cranial edge of T4, estimated to the nearest 0.1 vertebrae.
5. The normal VHS for most dogs is between 8.5 and 10.5, although there are variations with some breeds.

Echocardiography—One may see left atrial enlargement, left ventricular or biventricular hypertrophy (the left ventricular wall thickness may be normal or decreased with chamber size increase), mitral regurgitation, increased left ventricular internal dimension (>49 mm in Doberman

Cardiovascular emergencies

Pinschers), increased left ventricular end systolic dimension (>42 mm in Doberman Pinschers), diastolic dysfunction or relaxation abnormalities and evidence of systolic dysfunction. Fractional shortening (FS) is usually decreased to <15% (normal FS for most dogs is <25% but some large and giant breed dogs normally have an FS = 20 to 25%).

ECG—Tachycardia is common. Many arrhythmias may be seen including atrial premature contractions, atrial fibrillation and ventricular tachycardia. Increased P-wave duration or amplitude, as with left or right atrial enlargement, and increased R-wave amplitude, as with left ventricular hypertrophy, may be seen in lead II.

Blood pressure—SAP and MAP are usually decreased.

Laboratory abnormalities—

1. The patient may have a stress leukogram.
2. Arterial blood gas analysis may show metabolic acidosis.
3. Pa_{CO_2} is usually decreased.
4. Pa_{O_2} is usually decreased.
5. Sp_{O_2} is usually decreased.
6. The serum lactate level is usually elevated.
7. Azotemia is seen, with an increased creatinine and BUN.
8. Hyponatremia and hypokalemia may be present.
9. ALT, ALP, and AST (aspartate aminotransferase) may be elevated.
10. Abdominal or pleural effusion analysis usually reveals a modified or pure transudate.
11. Plasma taurine level should be evaluated.

Differential diagnosis

1. Cardiomyopathy due to taurine deficiency
2. Chronic degenerative atrioventricular valve disease
3. Inflammatory or infectious myocarditis or cardiomyopathy
4. Pericardial effusion
5. Heartworm disease (especially if right-sided cardiac enlargement is present)
6. Arrhythmogenic right ventricular cardiomyopathy in Boxers

Prognosis

The prognosis is guarded to poor. The average life span after diagnosis is 6 months to 2 years. The prognosis is more favorable for those patients with subclinical or occult DCM. Warn the owners about the possibility of sudden cardiac death.

Treatment

1. Inform the client of the diagnosis, prognosis and cost of the treatment.
2. If the patient presents with occult DCM consider the following:
   A. ACE inhibitor such as enalapril (0.5 mg/kg PO q12h) or benazepril (0.5 mg/kg PO q24h)

B. Beta blocker such as carvedilol (Coreg®) 0.2 mg/kg PO q12h, atenolol (Tenormin®) 0.25–1 mg/kg PO q12h, or metoprolol (Dutoprol®) 0.2 mg/kg PO q12h.
C. Spironolactone, 1–2 mg/kg PO q12h.

3. If the patient presents in congestive heart failure, treat as previously discussed.
   A. Place an IV catheter.
   B. Provide supplemental oxygen as needed until $Sp_{O_2} > 95\%$ on room air.
   C. Administer furosemide, 2–4 mg/kg IV q8h.
   D. Administer pimobendan, 0.2–0.3 mg/kg PO q12h.
   E. Administer an ACE inhibitor such as enalapril (0.5 mg/kg PO q12h) or benazepril (0.25–0.5 mg/kg PO q12–24h).
   F. If there is no improvement, administer dobutamine, nitroprusside, or hydralazine as needed.
      I. Dobutamine 2.5–20 µg/kg/min IV infusion:
         a. (Wt in kg) × (no. of µg/kg/min) = no. of mg to add to 250 mL D5W at a drip rate of 15 ml/h.
         b. You must protect the solution from light.
         c. Usually an effect is seen within 3–5 minutes.
      II. Nitroprusside, 1–3 µg/kg/min IV CRI in dogs. Start at 1–2 µg/kg/min, increase every 3–5 minutes until patient improves, maximum 8–10 µg/kg/min, can maintain for 12–48 hours then wean off.
      III. Hydralazine, 0.5–3 mg/kg PO q12h
   G. Digoxin (0.005 mg/kg PO q12h) may be beneficial if the patient is in systolic failure.
   H. Administer taurine and L-carnitine supplements until a normal taurine level is confirmed:
      I. Taurine, if <25 kg 0.5–1.0 g PO q12h; if 25–40 kg 1–2 g PO q8–12h
      II. L-carnitine, if <25 kg 1 g PO q8h; if 25–40 kg 2 g PO q8h.
   I. For patients with atrial fibrillation or other supraventricular tachycardias (>160 bpm), administer esmolol, atenolol or sotalol (Class II antiarrhythmic, beta blockers) or diltiazem (Class IV, calcium channel blocker). Once stabilized they may be maintained on digoxin, atenolol, propranolol, diltiazem or diltiazem extended release.
      I. Esmolol, 200–500 µg/kg IV over 1 minute then 25–200 µg/kg/min CRI IV
      II. Atenolol, 0.2–1 mg/kg PO q12–24 h.
      III. Sotalol (also has Class III properties) 1.0–5.0 mg/kg PO q12h
      IV. Diltiazem, 0.05–0.25 mg/kg IV over 2 minutes, repeat as needed, or 0.5 mg/kg PO followed by 0.25 mg/kg PO q1h until conversion or maximum total dose of 1.5 mg/kg has been administered
      V. Diltiazem extended release
      VI. Digoxin, 0.0025 mg/kg PO q12h
      VII. Propanolol, 0.1–0.2 mg/kg PO q8h or 0.02 mg/kg IV

J. For patients with ventricular tachycardia, administer lidocaine (Class Ib), procainamide (Class Ia), sotalol or amiodarone (Classes I–IV). Once stabilized, the patient may be maintained on mexiletine (Class Ib), procainamide, sotalol or amiodarone as needed.

   I. Lidocaine, 1–2 mg/kg IV, repeat to a maximum total of 8 mg/kg for conversion, 25–75 μg/kg/min CRI IV for maintenance

   II. Procainamide, 2–4 mg/kg IV slowly over 2 minutes, up to 12–20 mg/kg until conversion, 10–40 μg/kg/min CRI IV for maintenance

   III. Amiodarone, 5.0 mg/kg IV or IO over 10 minutes

   IV. Mexiletine, 4–10 mg/kg PO q8h

K. If the patient has intractable coughing, hydrocodone (0.25 mg/kg PO q6–24 h) or butorphanol tartrate (0.5 mg/kg PO q12h) may be administered as needed.

4. Treat anxiety if needed.

   A. Butorphanol 0.2–0.25 mg/kg IM or IV

   B. Buprenorphine 0.0075–0.01 mg/kg transmucosal, IV, IM, SC

   C. Morphine 0.2 mg/kg SC or IM

   D. Hydromorphone 0.05–0.1 mg/kg IV, IM, SC

5. Auscultate lungs and monitor respiratory rate and effort regularly. Keep in mind that severe respiratory fatigue or clinical improvement may cause decreased respiratory effort or rate. Provide mechanical ventilatory support if respiratory fatigue occurs.

6. Monitor blood pressure.

7. Monitor renal parameters, electrolytes and hydration status at least q12h when providing aggressive diuretic therapy.

8. Therapeutic thoracocentesis or abdominocentesis may be indicated if the patient has respiratory distress.

9. A mild sodium-restricted diet may be beneficial.

10. Conservative intravenous fluid administration is recommended in CHF patients only if electrolyte depletion of severe dehydration occurs. In these instances, 0.45% sodium chloride or D5W is usually recommended.

II. HYPERTROPHIC FORM (HCM)

Diagnosis

History—This form of cardiomyopathy is very rare in dogs. Syncope or signs of left-sided heart failure may be seen, although most patients are asymptomatic until sudden death.

Physical exam—In the small number of symptomatic dogs, dyspnea, moist rales, a systolic murmur and a gallop rhythm may be observed.

ECG—Possible atrial or ventricular arrhythmias, ST-segment or T-wave abnormalities.

Blood pressure —Is usually normal.

Thoracic radiographs—May be normal. Pulmonary edema and left atrial or left ventricular enlargement may be present.

Echocardiography—Left atrial enlargement, thickening of the interventricular septum and / or left ventricular free wall.

Prognosis

The prognosis is guarded to grave.

Treatment

1. Inform the client of the diagnosis, prognosis and cost of the treatment.
2. Treatment is provided for symptomatic patients.
3. Administer oxygen as needed.
4. Place an intravenous catheter.
5. Administer furosemide.
6. Administer an ACE inhibitor.
7. Potent arteriolar dilators should be avoided.
8. The administration of a beta blocker or calcium channel blocker is controversial.
9. Restrict exercise, excitement and stress.

FELINE CARDIOMYOPATHY

Differentiation of disease types by physical findings.

HYPERTROPHIC FORM (HCM)

This is the most common form. It usually occurs in male cats with a mean age of 4–7 years at the time of diagnosis, but has been reported in cats from 3 months to 17 years of age. Domestic Shorthair cats, Maine Coon cats, Persians, Ragdolls, and American Shorthair cats are the most commonly affected breeds. Genetic mutation has been shown to be the cause in the Maine Coon cat and Ragdoll. The cause is unknown in other cats.

Diagnosis

History—Affected cats may be asymptomatic, have signs of heart failure and / or thromboembolism, or they may die suddenly. Acute onset of dyspnea, tachypnea, lethargy, anorexia, syncope, lameness, paresis, vocalization, or sudden death.

Clinical signs—Dyspnea, tachypnea, possibly cyanosis, hypothermia, harsh lung sounds with rales in patients with pulmonary edema, diminished lung sounds in patients with pleural effusion, poor body condition score. Cats with heart failure do not commonly cough. A gallop rhythm (diastolic S4 sound) or premature beats may be auscultated. A systolic murmur may best be heard in the parasternal region. Jugular vein distention and pulsations may be visible. Thromboembolism may cause absent or poor quality femoral pulses, paresis or paralysis, usually of one or both hindlimbs, cyanosis of the affected limb(s) and cooler limb(s).

Thoracic radiographs—Generalized cardiomegaly or biatrial enlargement, pulmonary venous dilation, pulmonary arterial enlargement, pulmonary edema and, possibly, pleural effusion. The heart may appear normal in size or may have the classic 'valentine' shape. Assessment of the vertebral heart score (VHS) may help assess cardiomegaly, which is increased in DCM:

1. Using a lateral thoracic radiograph, the VHS is obtained by measuring both the long axis and short axis of the heart, in terms of vertebral body length.
2. The long axis (L) is measured from the ventral border of the left mainstem bronchus to the most ventral aspect of the apex of the heart.
3. The short axis (S) is measured at the area of maximum cardiac width, perpendicular to the L.
4. The sum of the L and S measurements are compared with the thoracic vertebrae, starting at the cranial edge of T4, estimated to the nearest 0.1 vertebrae.
5. The normal VHS for most cats is between 6.7 and 8.0, with a mean VHS of 7.5.

ECG—May be normal or may have prolonged P-wave duration or increased P-wave amplitude and a prolonged QRS interval in lead II, possible arrhythmias and occasional left axis deviation in the frontal plane.
Echocardiography—Left atrial enlargement, thickening of the interventricular septum and / or left ventricular free wall, and papillary muscle hypertrophy.
Laboratory findings—CBC, electrolytes, serum biochemistry profile, lactate, serum N-terminal pro-B-type naturetic peptide (BNP) concentration, cardiac troponin I, serum thyroxin levels, heartworm microfilaria or immunologic tests, urinalysis. A minimum of hematocrit, total protein concentration, creatinine and urinalysis is indicated in all patients. Cystocentesis should be avoided in patients in distress. Do not withhold therapy while waiting for urination.

1. Prerenal azotemia may be present or may occur with diuretic therapy.
2. Hyperthyroidism is an underlying cause.
3. Analysis of pleural or abdominal effusion may reveal a modified or pure transudate or chylous effusion.

Blood pressure—Blood pressure measurement may reveal systemic hypertension (SAP >180 mm Hg) or hypotension (SAP <80 mm Hg) in cardiac failure.

Prognosis

The prognosis is fair to guarded as some cats will survive for as long as 3 years following the diagnosis.

Treatment

1. Inform the client of the diagnosis, prognosis and cost of the treatment.
2. Provide oxygen supplementation, preferably with an oxygen cage to decrease stress. The goal Sp_{O_2} is >95% on room air.
3. If the cat is highly stressed and difficult to manage, very low doses of butorphanol (0.2 mg/kg IV or 0.055–0.11 mg/kg SC or IM) have been

used to facilitate a diagnostic work-up. Avoid the administration of ketamine.

4. Place an intravenous catheter.
5. Administer furosemide, 1–2 mg/kg IV or IM, repeat every 1–4 hours as needed until respiratory rate and effort decrease.
   A. Furosemide can also be administered as a CRI in refractory patients, 1 mg/kg/h IV for a maximum of 4 hours. It is recommended to dilute the veterinary formulation to 5 or 10 mg/mL in D5W, sterile water, LRS or 0.9% NaCl and to administer via syringe pump if possible, minimizing the volume of IV fluids administered until the pulmonary edema resolves.
   B. Some patients may require higher or lower dosages of furosemide.
   C. After diuresis has started, offer free access to water.
   D. Decrease furosemide to 1–2 mg/kg q6–12h in cats.
   E. *Caution:* Must monitor serum potassium levels and creatinine as hypokalemia, azotemia, and dehydration may result.
6. If pulmonary edema is present, also consider nitroglycerin ointment 2% transdermally 0.25–0.5 inch (0.65–1.3 cm) on the skin of the thorax or abdomen (then cover the skin with nonporous tape) q6–8h with a 12-hour dose-free interval.
7. Provide external heat support if indicated.
8. Administer an ACE inhibitor such as enalapril 0.25–0.5 mg/kg PO q12–24h, or benazepril 0.25–0.5 mg/kg PO q24h.
9. Perform pleurocentesis if needed to decrease respiratory distress in patients with pleural effusion.
10. Monitor femoral pulses bilaterally for possible thromboembolism.
11. The administration of diltiazem is controversial and has not proven to be beneficial. The dosage of diltiazem is 7.5 mg/cat PO q8–12h. The dosage of extended release diltiazem is 10–30 mg/cat PO q12–24h. It may be useful by decreasing myocardial oxygen consumption, left ventricular end-diastolic pressure, ischemia, and outflow obstruction. It should not be administered to a patient in CHF.
12. Another controversial medication that has also not proven to be beneficial is atenolol. The dosage is 6.25–12.5 mg/cat PO q12–24h. It may decrease myocardial oxygen demand and left ventricular outflow obstruction, and slow heart rate. The dose should be slowly titrated to a goal heart rate of 140–160 bpm.
13. Thromboprophylaxis should be initiated in patients with moderate to severe left atrial enlargement, a visible thrombus or spontaneous contrast on echocardiography and in those patients that have had a thromboembolic event.
    A. Aspirin 5–81 mg PO q72h
    B. Clopidogrel 18.75 mg PO q24h
14. If thromboembolism occurs, see that section for therapy.

DILATED FORM

Occurs in middle-aged to older males, often in Siamese, Burmese or Abyssinians.

Diagnosis

History—Anorexia, lethargy, weakness, dyspnea, tachypnea, occasionally vomiting.

Signs—Hypothermia, weakness, prolonged capillary refill, poor femoral pulse quality, dyspnea, tachypnea, muffled lung sounds in patients with pleural effusion, crackles in patients with pulmonary edema. Tachycardia, bradycardia or a normal heart rate may be present. A systolic mitral murmur, arrhythmia or gallop rhythm may be auscultated. Aortic thromboembolism may occur.

Thoracic radiographs—Generalized cardiomegaly, pleural effusion, pulmonary edema, or the heart may appear normal.

Echocardiography—Left atrial enlargement, thin ventricular walls, enlarged left ventricular end-systolic and end-diastolic dimensions, and low fractional shortening.

ECG—May be normal; arrhythmias, or left atrial or ventricular enlargement patterns may be present.

Laboratory findings—CBC and serum biochemistry profile, urinalysis and thyroid panel. Abnormalities are similar to cats with the hypertrophic form.
1. Hyperthyroidism may be an underlying cause.
2. The plasma taurine level may be <40 nmol/L or the whole blood taurine level may be <250 nmol/L which are below normal.
3. Prerenal azotemia may be present or may occur with diuretic therapy.
4. Analysis of pleural or abdominal effusion may reveal a modified or pure transudate or chylous effusion.

Blood pressure—Blood pressure measurement may reveal systemic hypertension (SAP >180 mm Hg) or hypotension (SAP <80 mm Hg) in cardiac failure.

Prognosis

The prognosis is guarded to poor, as most cats are unresponsive to therapy.

Treatment

1. Inform the client of the diagnosis, prognosis and cost of the treatment.
2. Provide oxygen supplementation, usually by placing the cat in an oxygen cage to decrease stress.
3. Avoid stress.
4. Sedation – if the cat is highly stressed and difficult to manage, administer butorphanol 0.2 mg/kg IM or IV. Avoid ketamine.
5. Place an intravenous catheter.
6. Perform pleurocentesis if indicated.
7. Administer furosemide, 1–3 mg/kg IM or IV, then 0.5–1 mg/kg q8–12h.
8. Administer nitroglycerin ointment 2% 0.25–0.5 inch (0.65–1.3 cm) transdermally q4–6h as needed with a 12-hour dose-free interval.
9. Administer enalapril 0.25–0.5 mg/kg PO q24h.
10. Consider the administration of pimobendan 0.1–0.3 mg/kg PO q12h. Pimobendan is not currently licensed for use in cats.
11. Initiate thromboprophylaxis therapy.

12. Treat aortic thromboembolism if present.
13. Digoxin is optional
14. Treat arrhythmias as indicated.
15. Beta blockers and calcium channel blockers are controversial.
16. Administer taurine 250 mg PO q12h until the patient fails to respond.

ARTERIAL THROMBOSIS OR THROMBOEMBOLISM

A thrombus is an aggregation of platelets and other elements that forms locally (a clot) and partially or completely occludes a blood vessel in the heart or a vessel. An embolus is a clot that breaks away from the site of origin and is carried to a smaller vessel where it lodges, causing partial or complete occlusion of blood flow. Both can occur in the same patient.

The presence of three abnormalities referred to as Virchow's triad (static or slowed blood flow, endothelial structure or function abnormalities, and a hypercoagulable state due to increased procoagulant substances or decreased fibrinolytic or anticoagulant substances) predisposes the patient to the development of thromboembolism (TE).

In cats, thrombosis most commonly occurs as TE associated with hypertrophic cardiomyopathy.

In dogs, thrombosis is rarely associated with cardiac disease. The most common causes are:

Protein-losing nephropathy (PLN) (25% of PLN patients at necropsy
   have TE)
Protein-losing enteropathy (PLE)
Pulmonary thromboembolism (PTE)
Immune-mediated hemolytic anemia (IMHA) (80% of IMHA patients at
   necropsy have PTE)
Hyperadrenocorticism
Neoplasia
Major surgery such as hip replacement (82% of hip replacement patients
   have PTE)
Disseminated intravascular coagulation (DIC)
Diabetes mellitus, which may increase the incidence of occurrence.

Other disease conditions associated with TE formation include:

Sepsis / SIRS	Injection of an irritant substance
Heartworm disease	Endocarditis
Massive trauma	Congestive heart failure (CHF)
Shock	Cardiomyopathy
Reperfusion injury	Glucocorticoid therapy
Prolonged recumbency	Hypoviscosity (anemia)
Aneurysm	Pancreatitis
AV fistula	Fungal disease
Gastric dilatation volvulus (GDV)	Hyperviscosity (polycythemia,
Intravenous catheterization	hyperglobulinemia, leukemia).

In PLN, increased platelet adhesion and loss of antithrombin contribute to a hypercoagulable state that cannot be detected with PT and PTT. In

IMHA, TE is thought to be due to hypoviscosity and systemic inflammation (immune mediated). Hyperadrenocorticism is associated with elevation of procoagulant factors, decreased fibrinolysis and increased platelet activator inhibitor (PAI) activity. Diabetes mellitus causes hypofibrinolysis and increased platelet aggregation. Cats with myocardial disease, especially those with marked left atrial enlargement, develop turbulent blood flow, altered coagulability and local tissue injury. A thrombus commonly forms in the left atrium and emboli shower the body.

Clinical signs

1. The signs are referred to as the 'five P's':
   A. Pain
   B. Paresis
   C. Pallor
   D. Pulselessness
   E. Poikilothermy.
2. A thrombus can lodge anywhere in the body with corresponding clinical signs:
   A. Lungs – respiratory distress
   B. Brain – CNS disorder
   C. Kidney – acute renal failure
   D. Gastrointestinal tract – bowel ischemia
   E. Brachial artery – foreleg paresis and pain
   F. Caudal aorta (saddle thrombus) – most common in cats, paraparesis of the hind limbs and pain
3. Vocalization due to pain and distress
4. Acute limb paresis – possible monoparesis, posterior paresis, + / – intermittent claudication (pain, weakness and lameness that develops during exercise, becomes intensely painful, then disappears with rest, associated with peripheral occlusive vascular disease)
5. The affected limb may be painful and cool with pale footpads, cyanotic nail beds and an absent arterial pulse. Contracture of the affected muscles may occur.
6. Tachypnea or dyspnea due to pain or CHF
7. Hypothermia
8. Signs of cardiac disease or congestive heart failure may be present.
9. TE to the renal, mesenteric or pulmonary circulation may result in failure of the affected organs and death.
10. Coronary artery TE may be associated with ventricular tachyarrhythmias, AV blocks or other arrhythmias, along with ST-segment and T-wave changes on ECG.
11. Animals with PTE may have tachypnea, dyspnea, increased lung sounds and hypoxia due to a ventilation / perfusion (V / Q) mismatch.

Diagnostic procedures

Thoracic radiography (three views)—To assess for metastasis and to evaluate heart, pleural effusion, appearance of pulmonary lobar vessels

and pulmonary alveolar infiltrates. Radiographs may be particularly beneficial in evaluation of the feline patient where, if TE is accompanying heart failure, there may be generalized cardiomegaly or biatrial enlargement, pulmonary venous dilation, pulmonary arterial enlargement, pulmonary edema and, possibly, pleural effusion. The heart may appear normal in size or enlarged with the classic 'valentine' shape.
Coagulation profile including assessment of D-dimer and fibrinogen concentrations—To check baseline coagulation status and assess possible hypercoagulability or disseminated intravascular coagulation.
Abnormalities may include:
1. Azotemia (prerenal or renal)
2. Increased creatine phosphokinase (CK or CPK) activity
3. Assessment of systemic blood lactate levels in comparison with the lactate level from blood obtained from the affected limb (the limb lactate level would be higher)
4. Hyperglycemia (stress)
5. Lymphopenia (stress)
6. Thrombocytopenia, prolonged PT and PTT (DIC).

Thyroid panel—In cats with cardiac disease, a thyroid panel should be evaluated because hyperthyroidism is a common underlying cause.
Assessment of blood pressure via Doppler ultrasonography—To establish presence of blood flow in the distal portion of the affected limbs and to evaluate for systemic hypertension.
Echocardiography—To evaluate for endocarditis, heartworms, cardiac thrombi, left atrial enlargement, contractility, etc. With feline hypertrophic cardiomyopathy, you may see intracardiac thrombi, left atrial enlargement, thickening of the interventricular septum and / or left ventricular free wall, and papillary muscle hypertrophy.
Abdominal ultrasonography—To evaluate for aortic thrombus or neoplasia.
Assessment of urine protein-to-creatinine ratio—To evaluate for primary protein-losing nephropathy (i.e. predisposition to a hypercoagulable state).
Thromboelastography (TEG)—Can detect a hypercoagulable state and assist in patient selection for therapy and monitoring of treatment. Compatible changes of the TEG include a decreased R (reaction time), decreased K (clotting time), increased α (angle) and MA (maximum amplitude).

Evaluation of arterial blood gases and calculation of the alveolar–arterial (A–a) gradient is indicated if respiratory distress is persistent or severe.

Radiographs of the affected limb may help to rule out trauma, including a fracture.

Angiography, nuclear scintigraphy, CT or MR angiography may be helpful in diagnosing TE disease.

Prognosis

The prognosis is guarded to poor. Treatment with thrombolytic agents is often cost prohibitive and associated with complications. Permanent paralysis or limb dysfunction and gangrene are possible. Recurrence is also possible,

Cardiovascular emergencies

especially if the underlying metabolic diseases are not controlled. Additional thrombi may develop at distant sites.

Therapeutic plan

1. Inform the client of the diagnosis, prognosis and cost of the treatment.
2. Analgesic therapy
   A. Buprenorphine 0.01–0.03 mg/kg IV, IM, transmucosal, or 1–3 µg/kg/h CRI IV
   B. Fentanyl 1–5 µg/kg IV to effect, then 1–5 µg/kg/h IV CRI
   C. Hydromorphone 0.05–0.1 mg/kg IV, IM, SC or 1–5 µg/kg/h CRI IV
   D. Morphine 0.05–0.2 mg/kg IM or SC q4–6h
   E. If the cat is highly stressed and difficult to manage, the administration of butorphanol (0.2 mg/kg IV or 0.055–0.11 mg/kg SC or IM) or buprenorphine has been used to facilitate a diagnostic work-up
   F. Avoid ketamine
3. Supportive care
   A. Supplemental oxygen as needed based on clinical signs, Sp_{O_2}, arterial blood gas evaluation
   B. IV fluids as indicated (not with CHF)
   C. Management of CHF if present
   D. Correct azotemia and electrolyte imbalances
   E. Nutritional support if needed
   F. External warming if needed
   G. Keep the affected limbs warm and dry
4. Surgical thrombectomy is best performed within 6 hours of clot formation and has a guarded to poor prognosis, with common recurrence.
5. Treatment of any underlying disease that could predispose the patient to a hypercoagulable state is also recommended.
6. Antiplatelet therapy
   A. Aspirin
      I. Dog: 0.5 mg/kg PO q12–24h
      II. Cat: 5 mg/cat every 72 hours
   B. Clopidogrel (Plavix®)
      I. Dog: 75 mg PO q24h
      II. Cat: 18.75 mg/cat PO q24h
   C. Abciximab (ReoPro®) platelet integrin glycoprotein IIb/IIIa-receptor blocker
      I. Dog: 0.25 mg/kg IV bolus followed by 0.125 µg/kg/min IV CRI (experimental)
      II. Cat: unknown
7. Anticoagulant therapy
   A. Unfractionated heparin (sodium heparin, UH) – monitor aPTT (target is 1.5–2.5 × baseline) or anti-Xa (target is 0.35–0.7 U/mL)
      I. Dog: 250 U/kg IV or SC q6h, or 18 U/kg/h CRI IV
      II. Cat: 175–475 U/kg SC or IV q6–8h, or 18 U/kg/h CRI IV
      III. If an overdose or excessive hemorrhage occurs, heparin activity may be immediately neutralized by protamine sulfate,

administered slowly IV at the dose of 0.5–1 mg of protamine per 100 U heparin, if within 1 hour of the heparin administration. If greater than 1 hour has elapsed since the last heparin dose, decrease the protamine dose by half. If 2 hours have elapsed, 0.12–0.25 mg of protamine per 100 U heparin should be administered. (**Note: Excessive administration of protamine may result in a hemorrhagic condition for which there is no known therapy.**)

   B. Low molecular weight heparin (LMWH) – increased affinity for factor Xa. Minimal ability to inhibit thrombin, less likely to cause bleeding
      I. Dalteparin sodium: 100–150 U/kg SC q4h in cats, q8h in dogs
      II. Enoxaparin: 1.5 mg/kg SC q6h in cats, 0.8 mg/kg SC q6h in dogs
   C. Warfarin – monitor aPT (target is 1.5–2.5 × baseline). Because warfarin has a very narrow therapeutic index and there is constant risk of severe life-threatening hemorrhage, it is not commonly used in clinical practice.
      I. Dog: 0.2 mg/kg then 0.05–0.1 mg/kg PO q24h
      II. Cat: 0.1–0.2 mg/kg PO q24h
8. Thrombolytic therapy
   A. Streptokinase – no longer available
      I. Dog: 90,000 IU infused over 20–30 minutes, then 45,000 IU/h CRI IV for 6–12 hours
      II. Cat: same
   B. t-PA (tissue plasminogen activator)
      I. Dog: 0.4–1 mg/kg bolus IV q1h for 10 doses over 2 days
      II. Cat: 0.25–1 mg/kg/h (up to a total of 1–10 mg/kg) IV CRI
9. Monitor for reperfusion injury, necrosis and gangrene.

PERICARDIAL EFFUSION

Etiology

1. Neoplasia of the heart, heart base, or pericardium
   A. Right atrial hemangiosarcoma.
   B. Chemodectoma.
   C. Metastatic adenocarcinoma.
   D. Lymphoma.
   E. Thymoma.
   F. Undifferentiated carcinoma.
2. Idiopathic pericardial hemorrhage
3. Congestive heart failure
4. Peritoneopericardial diaphragmatic hernia
5. Pericardial cysts
6. Infectious pericarditis
   A. Bacterial (*Actinomyces* and *Nocardia* spp.)
   B. Fungal (coccidioidomycosis)
   C. Viral
   D. Trypanosomal

7. Noninfectious pericarditis (uremia)
8. Cardiac rupture
9. External chest trauma
10. Foreign bodies (foxtails, grass awns, etc.)
11. Hypoalbuminemia
12. Anticoagulant rodenticide toxicity
13. Other coagulopathies

Diagnosis

History—The most common cause of pericardial effusion in dogs is right atrial hemangiosarcoma, which most commonly occurs in large breed dogs, particularly the German Shepherd and Golden Retriever, 5 years of age or older. Lymphoma and feline infectious peritonitis are the most common causes in cats. Weakness, exercise intolerance, lethargy, dyspnea and abdominal distention are common client complaints.

Physical exam—
1. Weakness
2. Dyspnea
3. Ascites and / or pleural effusion
4. Weak and thready femoral pulses
5. Muffled heart sounds and muffled respiratory sounds
6. Jugular pulse and peripheral venous distension
7. Sinus tachycardia
8. May have hepatomegaly
9. Cachexia

Thoracic radiographs—Pleural effusion, hepatomegaly and ascites may be seen. If there is significant fluid accumulation in the pericardium, an enlarged globoid or round heart shadow may be seen. Tracheal elevation may be observed, especially if a heart base neoplastic mass is present. Distention of the caudal vena cava and underperfusion of the pulmonary vasculature may also be observed.

ECG—Sinus tachycardia, decreased R-wave amplitude with electrical alternans (a change in the size and shape of the QRS complexes and ST segment from beat to beat).

CVP—The patient's CVP is often >12 cm H_2O.

Echocardiography—A fluid-filled space is visible surrounding the heart, between the parietal pericardium and the epicardium. In severe cases of cardiac tamponade, the right atrium and ventricle may appear collapsed. Masses may be observed, as well as cardiac disorders.

Laboratory findings—Routine CBC and serum biochemical profile is usually nonspecific, but may show hypoproteinemia, anemia, leukocytosis, possibly elevated hepatic enzymes due to congestion or mild azotemia if there is impairment of renal perfusion. PT and PTT may be prolonged in patients with coagulopathy. Serum titers for FIP, coccidioidomycosis, ehrlichiosis and other infectious diseases could be measured. Thrombocytopenia, coagulation disorders, and erythrocyte abnormalities may be seen with hemangiosarcoma.

Prognosis

The prognosis is guarded to poor, depending upon the underlying etiology. The average survival of patients with hemangiosarcoma, with chemotherapy, is about 3 months. The long-term survival of these patients is 3–5 months.

Treatment

1. Inform the client of the diagnosis, prognosis and cost of the treatment.
2. Place an intravenous catheter; administer intravenous fluids if in shock.
3. Perform pericardiocentesis if serious cardiac tamponade exists.
   A. Position the patient in either left lateral or sternal recumbency.
   B. Clip and surgically prepare the right 5th or 6th intercostal space just above the costochondral junction.
   C. Attach ECG leads to the patient.
   D. Administer a lidocaine local anesthetic block.
   E. Make a small skin incision.
   F. Use an intravenous catheter of sufficient length and diameter (8-French, 9 cm) to penetrate the pericardial sac.
   G. Perform pericardiocentesis by carefully advancing the catheter through the intercostal space and into the pericardial sac, directed towards the opposite shoulder.
   H Monitor the ECG continuously.
   I. Once pericardial fluid is obtained, advance the catheter over the stylet, attach extension tubing, a three-way stopcock, and a 6 mL syringe. Initially place a small volume of fluid into a red-topped tube. Monitor the red-topped tube for clot formation. If a blood clot forms, the fluid sample may reflect acute pericardial hemorrhage or may have come directly from the heart and the catheter should be repositioned. Once proper placement of the catheter is confirmed, connect a larger 35–60 mL syringe to the stopcock and continue fluid aspiration.
   J. Apply gentle suction and remove as much fluid as possible without causing patient distress. Removal of a small volume of fluid may improve patient comfort so it is not necessary to drain all of the fluid from the pericardial sac.
   K. Place fluid samples in a red-topped and a lavender-topped blood tube. Save and submit the samples for lab analysis.
4. If the patient has an anticoagulant rodenticide intoxication, administer vitamin K_1 and plasma.
5. Treat heart failure if that is the underlying etiology.
6. Avoid the use of diuretics, unless indicated in the treatment of heart failure. Diuretic administration may lead to hypotension, weakness and azotemia.
7. Afterload- and preload-reducing agents (including ACE inhibitors) should be avoided.
8. Surgical exploratory of the thorax and pericardiectomy will allow for detection of small masses, the collection of biopsy specimens, and avoidance of cardiac tamponade.

9. Treat infectious pericardial disease with the appropriate antimicrobial agent:
   A. *Actinomyces* spp. – penicillins
   B. *Nocardia* spp. – potentiated sulfonamides
   C. Coccidioidomycosis – fluconazole, itraconazole, or amphotericin B.
10. Treatment of neoplastic pericardial disease with the appropriate chemotherapeutic agents can be directed based on the biopsy results.

HYPERTENSIVE CRISIS

History

Hypertension is defined as arterial blood pressure (systolic/diastolic) >150/95 mm Hg. Hypertension may be primary or secondary to systemic illnesses or medications (glucocorticoids, erythropoietin) including:

Renal disease (renal failure, glomerulopathy)
Hyperadrenocorticism
Pheochromocytoma
Hepatic disease
Chronic anemia
Obesity
Pregnancy
Renin-secreting tumors

Hyperthyroidism
Hyperaldosteronism
Diabetes mellitus
Polycythemia
Intracranial lesions
Acromegaly
Hyperviscosity / polycythemia
Patients with pheochromocytoma

Clinical signs

The clinical signs will vary with the underlying disease. Signs of end-organ damage may occur. The most common signs are ocular signs, especially sudden blindness due to retinal detachment or hemorrhage. Hemorrhage into the anterior or vitreal chamber, closed-angle glaucoma, perivasculitis and papilledema may also occur. Polyuria and polydipsia also occur owing to pressure diuresis, renal disease, hyperadrenocorticism in dogs and hyperthyroidism in cats. Epistaxis may occur. Paresis, ataxia, collapse, behavioral changes, vocalization, seizures and other neurologic signs can result from hypertensive encephalopathy. A soft systolic murmur or gallop sound may be heard on cardiac auscultation.

Intracranial disease that raises intracranial pressure can cause an increase in systemic blood pressure, which then results in a compensatory drop in heart rate. This is referred to as the Cushing's reflex.

Laboratory tests

A CBC, serum biochemistry profile and urinalysis should be performed on all hypertensive patients. Additional tests that may be useful, depending upon the underlying cause, include endocrine function tests, ECG, urine electrolytes, etc.

Diagnostic imaging

Depending upon the underlying cause, thoracic radiography, abdominal and thoracic ultrasonography, echocardiography, CT or MRI may be indicated.

Other diagnostics

There are various other diagnostic tests available for which the patient should probably be referred to an internal medicine specialist.

Prognosis

The prognosis varies with the underlying etiology. Surgical therapy of a pheochromocytoma can be complicated and has a mortality rate of about 50%.

Treatment

1. Inform the client of the diagnosis.
2. Hypertensive emergencies require continuous blood pressure monitoring and intensive care. It is recommended to decrease blood pressure less than 25% in the first hour and repeat in 2–6 hours if the patient remains stable.
   A. Fenoldopam (dopamine agonist) 0.1–0.6 µg/kg/min IV CRI in dogs and cats
   B. Enalaprilat (ACE inhibitor) 0.1–1 mg IV q6h in dogs.
   C. Sodium nitroprusside (vasodilator) 1–3 µg/kg/min IV CRI in dogs and 1–2 µg/kg/min IV CRI in cats.
   D. Hydralazine (vasodilator) 0.5–3 mg/kg PO q12h or 0.25–4 mg/kg IM or SC q8–12h in dogs, or 0.1–0.2 mg/kg/h IV CRI in dogs; or 2.5 mg (total dose) titrated up to 10 mg (total dose) PO q12h in cats or 0.25–2 mg/kg IM or SC q8–12h in cats.
   E. Amlodipine besylate (calcium channel blocker) 0.05–0.2 mg/kg PO or per rectum q24h in dogs or 0.625–1.25 mg PO or per rectum q24h in cats.
   F. Esmolol (beta blocker) 200–500 µg/kg IV over 1 minute then 25–200 µg/kg/min CRI IV.
   G. Phentolamine (alpha blocker) 0.02–1 mg/kg IV bolus then CRI IV to effect.
   H. Acepromazine (phenothiazine) 0.05–1 mg/kg up to 3 mg total IV
3. Treatment of hypertension in cats
   A. Amlodipine besylate 0.625–1.25 mg PO or per rectum q24h is usually the drug of choice for hypertension secondary to renal disease in cats.
   B. Benazepril (ACE inhibitor) 0.25–0.5 mg/kg PO q12–24h in cats is often the second choice.
   C. Enalapril (ACE inhibitor) 0.25–0.5 mg/kg PO q12–24h is an alternative ACE inhibitor that is usually less effective in cats.
   D. Prazosin (alpha-adrenergic antagonist) 0.25–0.5 mg/cat PO q24h has been shown to be more useful to cause urethral smooth muscle relaxation in cats with micturition disorders in cats or pheochromocytoma in dogs.

4. Treatment of hypertension in dogs
    A. Enalapril 0.25–0.5 mg/kg PO q12–24h, benazepril 0.25–0.5 mg/kg PO q12–24h, lisinopril 0.75 mg/kg PO q24h, or another ACE inhibitor, is often the first therapeutic agent recommended in the management of hypertension in dogs.
    B. Amlodipine besylate 0.05–0.2 mg/kg PO every 12–24 hours, adjusted up to 0.25 mg/kg as needed.
    C. Prazosin 0.5–2 mg PO q8–12h may be useful in the treatment of pheochromocytoma or to cause urethral smooth muscle relaxation in dogs with micturition disorders.
    D. Phenoxybenzamine (alpha-adrenergic antagonist) 0.2–1.5 mg/kg PO q8–12h is often used in dogs with pheochromocytoma.
    E. Propanolol (beta blocker, used in conjunction with phenoxybenzamine or prazosin) 0.5–1 mg/kg PO q8–12h may be used in dogs but should be avoided in asthmatic cats.
    F. Atenolol (beta blocker, used in conjunction with phenoxybenzamine or prazosin) 0.2–1 mg/kg PO q12–24h.
    G. Spironolactone (aldosterone antagonist) 1–2 mg/kg PO q12h is useful in patients with hyperaldosteronism or in conjunction with other diuretics.
5. Treatment of pheochromocytoma
    A. Phentolamine mesylate (alpha-adrenergic antagonist) 0.02–0.1 mg/kg IV bolus followed by CRI IV to effect
    B. An alpha-adrenergic antagonist, such as phenoxybenzamine or prazosin, should be started then a beta blocker such as atenolol or propanolol can be added. Beta blockers should not be used alone.

CAVAL SYNDROME OF HEARTWORM DISEASE

Caval syndrome is an acute life-threatening complication of heartworm disease that occurs in 16–20% of dogs with heartworm disease. It is characterized by hemolytic anemia, impaired hemodynamics and multisystemic dysfunction. Caval syndrome occurs most often in large, male, sporting breed dogs and only rarely in cats. It usually occurs in the spring and early summer.

Diagnosis

History—Sudden onset of anorexia, weakness, and depression. Some patients present with dyspnea, coughing, hemoglobinuria, jaundice and occasionally hemoptysis.
Physical exam—Weakness, mucous membrane pallor, prolonged capillary refill time, weak peripheral pulses, jugular vein distention and jugular pulses, increased lung sounds, dyspnea, a right apical systolic murmur of tricuspid insufficiency, a gallop rhythm, hepatosplenomegaly, ascites, and jaundice.
Thoracic radiographs—Distention of the caudal vena cava, right atrial enlargement, an enlarged main pulmonary artery segment, and tortuous pulmonary arteries. Some patients have pleural effusion and right ventricular enlargement.

ECG—Signs of right-sided heart disease, including a right deviation of the mean electrical axis, sinus tachycardia.

Echocardiography—May show massive worm infestation that moves from the right atrium into the right ventricle during diastole. Right ventricular lumen enlargement, paradoxical septal motion, and a decreased diastolic diameter of the left ventricle may also be observed.

Laboratory findings—

1. The CBC often reveals moderate regenerative anemia, hemoglobinemia, microfilaremia, leukocytosis with eosinophilia, neutrophilia and a left shift.
2. DIC is indicated by thrombocytopenia, prolonged coagulation parameters and decreased fibrinogen concentration.
3. Serum chemical abnormalities include increases in aspartate aminotransferase, alanine aminotransferase, total and direct serum bilirubin, and lactic dehydrogenase, elevated BUN, and hypoalbuminemia with hyperglobulinemia.
4. Urinalysis often reveals hemoglobinuria.
5. The *Dirofilaria immitis* adult antigen test is positive.

Central venous pressure should be monitored as it is increased in 80–90% of patients.

Prognosis

The prognosis is guarded to grave.

Treatment

1. Inform the client of the diagnosis, prognosis and cost of the treatment.
2. Monitor central venous pressure.
3. Monitor arterial and venous blood gases.
4. Place an intravenous catheter and administer intravenous fluids at a rate dictated by the central venous pressure. The intravenous fluid of choice is either D5W or 2.5% dextrose in 0.45% NaCl.
5. Strict confinement to a hospital cage.
6. Administer aspirin, 5 mg/kg/day in dogs.
7. Monitor and treat for sepsis and DIC as indicated.
8. As soon as possible, perform surgical removal of the adult heartworms.
   A. With the patient under light sedation or without sedation in a severely compromised patient, place the patient in left lateral recumbency.
   B. Clip and prepare the ventral cervical region.
   C. Instill local anesthesia.
   D. Isolate the right jugular vein and place a ligature cranially.
   E. Make a small incision into the right jugular vein caudal to the ligature.
   F. Insert 20–40 cm straight alligator forceps into the right jugular vein and carefully guide them down the vein to the level of the 4th or 5th intercostal space.

G. Open the jaws of the forceps, grasp the worms, then close the forceps and retract them from the vein. Often 35–50 or more adult worms can be removed.

H. Repeat the extraction until 5–6 repeated attempts fail to produce worms.

I. Ligate the jugular vein and close the incision.

9. Monitor for and treat right-sided heart failure as indicated.

10. After 2–3 weeks of stabilization, adulticide therapy can be initiated.

SYNCOPE

Syncope is defined as a brief and temporary period of unconsciousness due to a disturbance in cerebral function, often as a result of diminished cerebral blood flow secondary to reduced cardiac output, a cerebral vascular accident, or from hypoxemia or hypoglycemia.

Etiology

1. Cardiovascular causes include:
   A. Dysrhythmias such as sinus bradycardia, atrioventricular blocks, atrial standstill, atrial fibrillation, supraventricular tachycardia and ventricular tachyarrhythmias
   B. Congenital cardiac diseases such as tetralogy of Fallot, pulmonary stenosis and subvalvular aortic stenosis
   C. Acquired cardiac disease such as chronic valvular disease, cardiomyopathy, cardiac tamponade, myocardial infarction, thromboembolic disease and heartworm disease
   D. Cerebral vascular disease secondary to thromboemboli, coagulopathies, hyperproteinemia, atherosclerotic disease, trauma and neoplasia
   E. Severe acute blood loss
   F. Hypotension.

2. Pulmonary causes include:
   A. Tracheal collapse
   B. Chronic bronchitis
   C. Violent coughing ('cough drop' syncope)
   D. Pulmonary hypertension
   E. Pulmonary emboli.

3. Neurogenic causes include:
   A. Glossopharyngeal neuralgia
   B. Peripheral or neurogenic dysfunction
   C. Vasovagal stimulation
   D. Postural hypotension
   E. Hyperventilation
   F. Carotid sinus sensitivity
   G. Thromboembolic disease
   H. Neoplasia.

4. Miscellaneous causes include:
   A. Anemia
   B. Hypoglycemia (insulin-secreting tumors, insulin overdose, glycogen storage diseases)
   C. Medications such as acepromazine, digitalis, diuretics and vasodilators
   D. Starvation.

Differential diagnosis

1. Seizure disorders – with syncope, there are no pre-ictal or post-ictal behavior changes. Syncope is usually very short and is often associated with vigorous activity. Opisthotonos, crying, urination and transient forelimb rigidity may be observed during both a seizure and a syncopal episode. Hypersalivation and facial chomping are rare in syncope.
2. Systemic disorders that result in profound weakness, such as hypoadrenocorticism, hypokalemia, bleeding intrathoracic or intra-abdominal hemangiosarcoma, and neuromuscular diseases, may cause collapse, but rarely cause a loss of consciousness or are as sudden in onset as a syncopal episode.
3. Narcolepsy.
4 Catalepsy.

Diagnosis

History—Certain breeds have genetic predispositions to specific cardiovascular or pulmonary diseases, such as Boxer cardiomyopathy and obstructive airway disease in brachycephalic dog breeds.

Listen carefully to the events immediately prior to the syncopal episode (exertion or coughing). Determine whether the patient is receiving medication such as insulin, vasodilators or tranquilizers.

Often the owner will describe generalized muscle weakness that progresses rapidly to ataxia, followed by collapse and a brief period of unconsciousness. The animal may initially be relaxed but then may develop jerking motion of the muscles that may resemble seizure activity. Involuntary urination and / or defecation may occur. The animal may cry out.

The episode usually lasts from a few seconds to a few minutes, with a rapid recovery.

Physical exam—Carefully auscultate the heart for the presence of murmurs, arrhythmias and gallop rhythms. Palpate peripheral pulses. Examine the nares and pharynx. Palpate and percuss the chest. Listen carefully for abnormal lung sounds or muffled lung sounds. Examine mucous membranes for color and capillary refill time. Measure blood pressure. Perform a thorough neurologic examination. Provide exercise and stimulation, and monitor the patient's response.

Thoracic radiographs—May reveal cardiac disease, pulmonary disease or pleural effusion.

ECG—May reveal a dysrhythmia or signs of cardiac chamber enlargement. Run a lead II rhythm strip for at least 2 minutes. Consider the use of continuous ECG monitoring during hospitalization.

Echocardiography—May reveal abnormal cardiac structure or function.

Laboratory findings—Perform a CBC and serum chemistry profile, with particular emphasis on PCV, TS, glucose, cholesterol and electrolytes. Measure acid–base balance, blood ammonia levels, serum thyroxine levels, and test for heartworm microfilaria.

Prognosis

The prognosis depends on the underlying etiology.

Treatment

1. Inform the client of the diagnosis, prognosis and cost of the treatment.
2. Place an intravenous catheter.
3. Correct the underlying etiology if possible.
4. Treat any dysrhythmia accordingly.
5. Provide volume replacement with intravenous fluids if the patient is hypotensive or has acute blood loss.
6. Provide oxygen for pulmonary disorders and treat the underlying specific disorder.
7. For Boxers with cardiomyopathy, antiarrhythmic therapy is crucial as these dogs are prone to sudden death.
   A. Sotalol (Betapace®), at a dose of 1.0–5.0 mg/kg PO q12h, is recommended as a ventricular antiarrhythmic unless there are clinical signs of congestive heart failure or advanced systolic dysfunction. Sotalol appears to cause fewer lethal pro-arrhythmic effects than quinidine, procainamide and mexitiline in dogs with serious structural cardiac disease.
   B. Procainamide, 250–500 mg PO q8–12h, may be used in combination with propranolol, 20–40 mg PO q8h, for sustained or paroxysmal ventricular tachyarrhythmias.
   C. Metoprolol, 12.5–25 mg PO q12h, may be administered for vasovagal syncope related to bradycardia.
   D. Bradycardia-induced syncope can also be prevented by using either propantheline bromide, 15 mg PO q8h, or isopropamide, 2.5–5 mg PO q8–12h.
   E. Administration of atropine sulfate, 0.01–0.02 mg/kg IV or IM, may be beneficial in a crisis situation.
   F. Supplementation with L-carnitine, 1–2 g q8–12h PO, may be beneficial.
8. Administer antitussive therapy for animals with 'cough drop' syncope.

CARDIOPULMONARY RESUSCITATION

Barton, L., Crowe, D.T., 2000. Open chest resuscitation. In: Bonagura, J. (Ed.), Kirk's Current Veterinary Therapy XIII. WB Saunders, Philadelphia, pp. 147–149.

Cabrini, L., Beccaria, P., Landoni, G., et al., 2008. Impact of impedance threshold devices on cardiopulmonary resuscitation: A systematic review and meta-analysis of randomized controlled studies. Critical Care Medicine 36, 1625–1632.

Cammarata, G., Weil, M.H., Csapoczi, P., et al., 2006. Challenging the rationale of three sequential shocks for defibrillation. Resuscitation 69, 23–27.

Cole, S.G., 2009. Cardiopulmonary resuscitation. In: Silverstein, D.C., Hopper, K. (Eds.), Small Animal Critical Care Medicine. Elsevier, St Louis, pp. 14–21.

Cole, S.G., 2009. Cardioversion and defibrillation. In: Silverstein, D.C., Hopper, K. (Eds.), Small Animal Critical Care Medicine. Elsevier, St Louis, pp. 220–232.

Cole, S.G., Otto, C.M., Hughes, D., 2002. Cardiopulmonary cerebral resuscitation in small animals – A clinical practice review (part I). Journal of Veterinary Emergency and Critical Care 12, 261–267.

Cole, S.G., Otto, C.M., Hughes, D., 2003. Cardiopulmonary cerebral resuscitation in small animals – A clinical practice review (part II). Journal of Veterinary Emergency and Critical Care 13, 13–23.

Crowe, D.T., 1988. Cardiopulmonary resuscitation in the dog: A review and proposed new guidelines (part I). Seminars in Veterinary Medicine and Surgery (Small Animal) 3, 321–327.

Crowe, D.T., 1988. Cardiopulmonary resuscitation in the dog: A review and proposed new guidelines (part II). Seminars in Veterinary Medicine and Surgery (Small Animal) 3, 328–348.

Crowe, D.T., 1992. Triage and trauma management. In: Murtaugh, R.J., Kaplan, P.M. (Eds.), Veterinary Emergency and Critical Care. Mosby-Year Book, St Louis, pp. 77–121.

Crowe, D.T., Fox, P.R., Devey, J.J., et al., 1999. Cardiopulmonary and cerebral resuscitation. In: Fox, P.R., Sisson, D., Moisse, N. (Eds.), Textbook of Canine and Feline Cardiology, Principles and Clinical Practice, second ed. WB Saunders, Philadelphia, pp. 427–445.

Davies, A., Janse, J., Reynolds, G.W., 1984. Acupuncture in the relief of respiratory arrest. New Zealand Veterinary Journal 32, 109–110.

Ditchey, R.V., Lindenfeld, J., 1988. Failure of epinephrine to improve the balance between myocardial oxygen supply and demand during closed-chest resuscitation in dogs. Circulation 78, 382–389.

ECC Committee, Subcommittees and Task Force of the American Heart Association, 2005. American Heart Association guidelines for cardiopulmonary resuscitation and emergency cardiovascular care. Circulation 112, IV1–IV203.

Gilroy, B.A., Dunlop, B.J., Shapiro, H.M., 1987. Outcome from cardiopulmonary resuscitation: Laboratory and clinical experience. Journal of the American Animal Hospital Association 23, 133–139.

Hackett, T.B., Van Pelt, D.R., 1995. Cardiopulmonary resuscitation. In: Bonagura, J. (Ed.), Kirk's Current Veterinary Therapy XII. WB Saunders, Philadelphia, pp. 167–175.

Hahnel, J.H., Lindner, K.H., Schurmann, C., et al., 1990. What is the optimal volume of administration for endobronchial drugs? American Journal of Emergency Medicine 8, 504–508.

Haldane, S., Marks, S.L., 2004. Cardiopulmonary cerebral resuscitation: Techniques (part I) Compendium on Continuing Education for the Practicing Veterinarian 26, 780–790.

Haldane, S., Marks, S.L., 2004. Resuscitation: Emergency drugs and postresuscitation care (part 2). Compendium on Continuing Education for the Practicing Veterinarian 26, 791–799.

Haskins, S.C., 1992. Internal cardiac compression. Journal of the American Veterinary Medical Association 200 (12), 1945–1946.

Haskins, S.C., 2000. Therapy for shock. In: Bonagura, J. (Ed.), Kirk's Current Veterinary Therapy XIII. WB Saunders, Philadelphia, pp. 140–147.

Henik, R.A., 1992. Basic life support, and external cardiac compression in dogs and cats. Journal of the American Veterinary Medical Association 200 (12), 1925–1931.

Hilwig, R.W., Kern, K.B., Berg, R.A., et al., 2000. Catecholamines in cardiac arrest: Role of alpha agonists, beta- adrenergic blockers and high-dose epinephrine. Resuscitation 47, 203–208.

Hofmeister, E.H., Brainard, B.M., Egger, C.M., et al., 2009. Prognostic indicators for dogs and cats with cardiopulmonary arrest treated by cardiopulmonary cerebral resuscitation at a university teaching hospital. Journal of the American Veterinary Medical Association 235, 50–57.

Kass, P.H., Haskins, S.C., 1991. Survival following cardiopulmonary resuscitation in dogs and cats. Journal of Veterinary Emergency and Critical Care 2 (2), 57–65.

Kern, K.B., Hilwig, R.W., Berg, R.A., et al., 2002. Importance of continuous chest compressions during cardiopulmonary resuscitation: Improved outcome during a simulated single lay-rescuer scenario. Circulation 105, 645–649.

Kern, K.B., Sanders, A.B., Voorhees, W.D., et al., 1989. Changes in expired end-tidal carbon dioxide during cardiopulmonary resuscitation in dogs: A prognostic guide for resuscitation efforts Journal of the American College of Cardiology 13, 1184–1189.

Kruse-Elliott, K.T., 2001. Cardiopulmonary resuscitation: Strategies for maximizing success. Veterinary Medicine 16, 51–58.

Macintire, D.K., 1995. The practical use of constant-rate infusions. In: Bonagura, J., Kirk, R. (Eds.), Kirk's Current Veterinary Therapy XII. WB Saunders, Philadelphia, pp. 184–188.

Naganobu, K., Hasebe, Y., Uchiyama, Y., et al., 2000. A comparison of distilled water and normal saline as diluents for endobronchial administration of epinephrine in the dog. Anesthesia and Analgesia 91, 317–321.

Paradis, N.A., Wenzel, V., Southall, J., 2002. Pressor drugs in the treatment of cardiac arrest. Cardiology Clinics 20, 61–78, viii.

Paret, G., Vaknin, Z., Ezra, D., et al., 1997. Epinephrine pharmacokinetics and pharmacodynamics following endotracheal administration in dogs: The role of volume of diluent. Resuscitation 35, 77–82.

Plunkett, S.J., McMichael, M., 2008. Cardiopulmonary resuscitation in small animal medicine: An update. Journal of Veterinary Internal Medicine 22, 9–25.

Rea, R.S., Kane-Gill, S.L., Rudis, M.I., et al., 2006. Comparing intravenous amiodarone or lidocaine, or both, outcomes for inpatients with pulseless ventricular arrhythmias. Critical Care Medicine 34, 1617–1623.

Rieser, T.M., 2000. Cardiopulmonary resuscitation. Clinical Techniques in Small Animal Practice 15, 76–81.

Rush, J.E., Wingfield, W.E., 1992. Recognition and frequency of dysrhythmias during cardiopulmonary arrest. Journal of the American Veterinary Medical Association 200 (12), 1932–1937.

Schmittinger, C.A., Astner, S., Astner, L., et al., 2005. Cardiopulmonary resuscitation with vasopressin in a dog. Veterinary Anaesthesia and Analgesia 32, 112–114.

Silverstein, D.C., 2009. Vasopressin. In: Silverstein, D.C., Hopper, K. (Eds.), Small Animal Critical Care Medicine. Elsevier, St Louis, pp. 759–804.

Simmons, J.P., Wohl, J.S., 2009. Vasoactive catecholamines. In: Silverstein, D.C., Hopper, K. (Eds.), Small Animal Critical Care Medicine. Elsevier, St Louis, pp. 756–804.

Valenzuela, T.D., Kern, K.B., Clark, L.L., et al., 2005. Interruptions of chest compressions during emergency medical systems resuscitation. Circulation 112, 1259–1265.

van Pelt, D.R., Wingfield, W.E., 1992. Controversial issues in drug therapy during cardiopulmonary resuscitation. Journal of the American Veterinary Medical Association 200 (12), 1938–1944.

Waldrop, J.E., Rozanski, E.A., Swank, E.D., et al., 2004. Causes of cardiopulmonary arrest, resuscitation management, and functional outcome in dogs and cats surviving cardiopulmonary arrest. Journal of Veterinary Emergency and Critical Care 14, 22–29.

Weihui, L., Kohl, P., Trayanova, N., 2006. Myocardial ischemia lowers precordial thump efficacy: An inquiry into mechanisms using three-dimensional simulations. Heart Rhythm 3, 179–186.

Wenzel, V., Lindner, K.H., 2006. Vasopressin combined with epinephrine during cardiac resuscitation: A solution for the future? Critical Care 10, 125.

Wingfield, W.E., 2002. Cardiopulmonary arrest. In: Wingfield, W.E., Raffe, M.R. (Eds.), The Veterinary ICU Book. Elsevier, Jackson Hole, Teton New Media, pp. 421–452.

Wingfield, W.E., Van Pelt, D.R., 1992. Respiratory and cardiopulmonary arrest in dogs and cats: 265 cases (1986–1991). Journal of the American Veterinary Medical Association 200, 1993–1996.

Wittnich, C., Belanger, M.P., Saberno, T.A., et al., 1991. External vs internal cardiac massage. Compendium on Continuing Education for the Practicing Veterinarian 13, 50–59.

Wright, K.N., 2009. Antiarrhythmic agents. In: Silverstein, D.C., Hopper, K. (Eds.), Small Animal Critical Care Medicine. St Louis, pp. 807–804.

Zhong, J.Q., Dorian, P., 2005. Epinephrine and vasopressin during cardiopulmonary resuscitation. Resuscitation 66, 263–269.

CONGESTIVE HEART FAILURE

Atkins, C., Bonagura, J., Ettinger, S., et al., 2009. ACVIM consensus statement. Guidelines for the Diagnosis and Treatment of Canine Chronic Valvular Heart Disease. Journal of Veterinary Internal Medicine 23, 1142–1150.

Bond, B.R., 2009. Nitroglycerin. In: Silverstein, D.C., Hopper, K. (Eds.), Small Animal Critical Care Medicine. Elsevier, St Louis, pp. 768–804.

Chetboul, V., Serres, F., Tissier, R., et al., 2009. Association of plasma N-terminal pro-B-type natriuretic peptide concentration with mitral regurgitation severity and outcome in dogs with asymptomatic degenerative mitral valve disease. Journal of Veterinary Internal Medicine 23, 984–994.

Francey, T., 2009. Diuretics. In: Silverstein, D.C., Hopper, K. (Eds.), Small Animal Critical Care Medicine. Elsevier, St Louis, pp. 801–804.

Goutal, C.M., Keir, I., Kenney, S., et al., 2010. Evaluation of acute congestive heart failure in dogs and cats: 145 cases (2007–2008). Journal of Veterinary Emergency and Critical Care 20 (3), 330–337.

Lee, J.A., Herndon, W.E., Rishniw, M., 2011. The effect of noncardiac disease on plasma brain natriuretic peptide concentration in dogs. Journal of Veterinary Emergency and Critical Care 21 (1), 5–12.

Lombard, C.W., Jöns, O., Bussadori, C.M., 2006. Clinical efficacy of pimobendan versus benazepril for the treatment of acquired atrioventricular valvular disease in dogs. Journal of the American Animal Hospital Association 42, 249–261.

Oyama, M.A., Fox, P.R., Rush, J.E., et al., 2008. Clinical utility of serum N-terminal pro-B-type natriuretic peptide concentration for identifying cardiac disease in dogs and assessing disease severity. Journal of the Am Vet Med Assoc 232, 1496–1503.

Ware, W.A., 2007. Cardiovascular Disease in Small Animal Medicine. Manson, London, pp. 34–46, 164–193, 263–272.

Wey, A.C., 2009. Valvular heart disease. In: Silverstein, D.C., Hopper, K. (Eds.), Small Animal Critical Care Medicine Elsevier, St Louis, pp. 165–170.

CANINE CARDIOMYOPATHY

Borgarelli, M., Tarducci, A., Tidholm, A., et al., 2001. Canine idiopathic dilated cardiomyopathy. Part II: Pathophysiology and therapy. The Veterinary Journal 162, 182–195.

Burkett, D.E., 2009. Bradyarrhythmias and conduction abnormalities. In: Silverstein, D.C., Hopper, K. (Eds.), Small Animal Critical Care Medicine. Elsevier, St Louis, pp. 189–194.

Gordon, S.G., Miller, M.W., Saunders, A.B., 2006. Pimobendan in heart failure therapy – a silver bullet? Journal of the American Animal Hospital Association 42, 90–93.

Kirk, R.W., Bonagura, J.D. (Eds.), 1992, Current Veterinary Therapy XI. WB Saunders, Philadelphia, pp. 773–779.

Pariaut, R., 2009. Ventricular tachyarrhythmias. In: Silverstein, D.C., Hopper, K. (Eds.), Small Animal Critical Care Medicine. Elsevier, St Louis, pp. 200–202.

Prošek, R., 2009. Canine cardiomyopathy. In: Silverstein, D.C., Hopper, K. (Eds.), Small Animal Critical Care Medicine. Elsevier, St Louis, pp. 160–165.

Tidholm, A., Häggström, J., Borgarelli, M., et al., 2001. Canine idiopathic dilated cardiomyopathy. Part I: Aetiology, clinical characteristics, epidemiology and pathology. The Veterinary Journal 162, 92–107.

Ware, W.A., 2007. Cardiovascular Disease in Small Animal Medicine. Manson, London, pp. 280–299.

Wright, K.N., 2009. Supraventricular tachyarrhythmias. In: Silverstein, D.C., Hopper, K. (Eds.), Small Animal Critical Care Medicine. Elsevier, St Louis, pp. 195–199.

FELINE CARDIOMYOPATHY

Abbott, J.A., 2009. Feline cardiomyopathy. In: Silverstein, D.C., Hopper, K. (Eds.), Small Animal Critical Care Medicine. Elsevier, St Louis, pp. 154–159.

Birchard, S.J., Sherding, R.G., 1994. Saunders Manual of Small Animal Practice. WB Saunders, Philadelphia, pp. 464–473.

Bonagura, J.D., Kirk, R.W. (Eds.), 1995. Current Veterinary Therapy XII. WB Saunders, Philadelphia, pp. 854–862.

Litster, A.L., Buchanan, J.W., 2000. Vertebral scale system to measure heart size in radiographs of cats Journal of the American Veterinary Medical Association 216, 210–214.

Mathews, K.A., 1996. Veterinary Emergency and Critical Care Manual. Lifelearn, Ontario, pp. 9–1 to 9–4.

Miller, M.S., Tilley, L.P., 1995. Manual of Canine and Feline Cardiology, second ed. WB Saunders, Philadelphia, pp. 367–369.

Murtaugh, R.J., Kaplan, P.M., 1992. Veterinary Emergency and Critical Care Medicine. Mosby, St Louis, pp. 242–246.

Schober, K.E., Maerz, I., Ludewig, E., et al., 2007. Diagnostic accuracy of electrocardiography and thoracic radiography in the assessment of left atrial size in cats: Comparison with transthoracic 2-dimensional echocardiography. Journal of Veterinary Internal Medicine 21, 709–718.

Ware, W.A., 2007. Cardiovascular Disease in Small Animal Medicine. Manson, London, pp. 300–319.

ARTERIAL THROMBOEMBOLISM

Birchard, S.J., Sherding, R.G., 1994. Saunders Manual of Small Animal Practice. WB Saunders, Philadelphia, pp. 473–475.

Hogan, D.F., 2009. Thrombolytic agents. In: Silverstein, D.C., Hopper, K. (Eds.), Small Animal Critical Care Medicine. Elsevier, St Louis, pp. 801–804.

Lunsford, K.V., Mackin, A.J., Langston, V.C., et al., 2009. Pharmacokinetics of subcutaneous low molecular weight heparin (enoxaparin) in dogs. Journal of the American Animal Hospital Association 45, 261–267.

Mathews, K.A., 1996. Veterinary Emergency, and Critical Care Manual. Lifelearn, Ontario, pp. 9–1 to 9–4.

Moore, K.E., Morris, N., Dhupa, N., et al., 2000. Retrospective study of streptokinase administration in 46 cats with arterial thromboembolism. Journal of Veterinary Emergency and Critical Care 10, 245–257.

Murtaugh, R.J., Kaplan, P.M., 1992. Veterinary Emergency and Critical Care Medicine. Mosby, St Louis, pp. 242–246.

Stokol, T., Brooks, M., Rush, J.E., et al., 2008. Hypercoagulability in cats with cardiomyopathy. Journal of Veterinary Internal Medicine 22, 546–552.

Van De Wiele, C.M., Hogan, D.F., Green, H.W., et al., 2010. Antithrombotic effect of enoxaparin in clinically healthy cats: A venous stasis model. Journal of Veterinary Internal Medicine 24, 185–191.

Ware, W.A., 2007. Cardiovascular Disease in Small Animal Medicine. Manson, London, pp. 145–163.

PERICARDIAL EFFUSION

Davidson, B.J., Paling, A.C., Lahmers, S.L., et al., 2008. Disease association and clinical assessment of feline pericardial effusion. Journal of the American Animal Hospital Association 44, 5–9.

Hall, D.J., Shofer, F., Meier, C.K., et al., 2007. Pericardial effusion in cats: A retrospective study of clinical findings and outcome in 146 cats. Journal of Veterinary Internal Medicine 21, 1002–1007.

Hoit, B.D., 2007. Pericardial disease and pericardial tamponade. Critical Care Medicine 35 (suppl), S355-S364.

Laste, N.J., 2009. Pericardial diseases. In: Silverstein, D.C., Hopper, K. (Eds.), Small Animal Critical Care Medicine. Elsevier, St Louis, pp. 184–188.

Shaw, S.P., Rush, J.E., 2007a. Canine pericardial effusion: Pathophysiology and cause. Compendium on Continuing

Education for the Practicing Veterinarian 29 (7), 400–403.

Shaw, S.P., Rush, J.E., 2007b. Canine pericardial effusion: Diagnosis, treatment, and prognosis. Compendium on Continuing Education for the Practicing Veterinarian; 29 (7), 405–411.

Shubitz, L.F., Matz, M.E., Noon, T.H., et al., 2001. Constrictive pericarditis secondary to *Coccidioides immitis* infection in a dog. Journal of the American Veterinary Medical Association 218 (4), 537–540.

Ware, W.A., 2007. Cardiovascular Disease in Small Animal Medicine. Manson, London, pp. 320–339.

HYPERTENSIVE CRISIS

Brown, C.A., Munday, J.S., Mathur, S., et al., 2005. Hypertensive encephalopathy in cats with reduced renal function. Veterinary Pathology 42, 642–649.

Brown, S., 2009. Hypertensive crisis. In: Silverstein, D.C., Hopper, K. (Eds.), Small Animal Critical Care Medicine. Elsevier, St Louis, pp. 176–179.

Labato, M.A., 2009. Antihypertensives. In: Silverstein, D.C., Hopper, K. (Eds.), Small Animal Critical Care Medicine. Elsevier, St Louis, pp. 763–804.

Tissier, R., Perrot, S., Enriquez, B., 2005. Amlodipine: One of the main anti-hypertensive drugs in veterinary therapeutics. Journal of Veterinary Cardiology 7, 53–58.

CAVAL SYNDROME OF HEARTWORM DISEASE

Kirk, R.W., Bonagura, J.D. (Eds.), 1992. Current Veterinary Therapy XI. WB Saunders, Philadelphia, pp. 721–725.

Murtaugh, R.J., Kaplan, P.M., 1992. Veterinary Emergency and Critical Care Medicine. Mosby, St Louis, pp. 238–241.

Ware, W.A., 2007. Cardiovascular Disease in Small Animal Medicine. Manson, London, pp. 351–371.

SYNCOPE

Barnett, L., Martin, M.W.S., Todd, J., et al., 2011. A retrospective study of 153 cases of undiagnosed collapse, syncope or exercise intolerance: the outcomes. Journal of Small Animal Practice 52, 26–31.

Ettinger, S.J. (Ed.), 1989. The Textbook of Veterinary Internal Medicine, Diseases of the Dog and Cat, third ed. WB Saunders, Philadelphia, pp. 82–87.

Nelson, R.W.C., Guillermo, C., 1998. Small Animal Internal Medicine, second ed. Mosby, St Louis, pp. 58, 109–110.

Ware, W.A., 2007. Cardiovascular Disease in Small Animal Medicine. Manson, London, pp. 139–144.

Cardiovascular emergencies

Respiratory emergencies
Sarah J Deitschel DVM, DACVECC and Signe J Plunkett DVM

UPPER AIRWAY OBSTRUCTION (CHOKING)

LARYNGEAL OBSTRUCTIONS

Diagnosis

History—Sudden onset of respiratory distress, a history of chewing on a bone, ball, or a toy just prior to the onset of problems, or having been found with a collar, leash, rope or other object causing strangulation. Mildly or chronically affected animals may have a slow onset of clinical signs such as stridor, sterdor, coughing, or change in voice.
Physical exam—Inspiratory stridor, inspiratory dyspnea, ptyalism, cyanosis, tachypnea, pawing at the face or mouth, anxiety and distress. May be able to visualize or palpate a foreign body in the larynx.
Radiographs—Should not be taken unless resuscitative treatment is started and the patient is stable, or they are felt to be absolutely necessary.

Differential diagnosis

Laryngeal foreign body, laryngeal neoplasia, laryngeal edema, laryngeal paralysis, laryngeal trauma, brachyocephalic syndrome in brachyocephalic breeds, nasopharyngeal polyps, laryngeal polyps, chronic proliferative laryngitis, cervical mass (neoplasia, abscess, lymphadenopathy, rattlesnake envenomation).

Prognosis

The prognosis is good to grave, depending upon etiology, severity and duration of the obstruction.

Treatment

1. Inform the client of the diagnosis, prognosis and cost of the treatment. If the situation is critical, quickly obtain the owner's permission for sedation, an attempt at foreign-body removal, or tracheostomy tube placement.

2. Provide oxygen without causing additional stress to the animal and obtain venous access if the patient can tolerate restraint.

3. These patients have the ability to decompensate quickly. This is partially due to stress, which increases the respiratory rate and demand for oxygen. Anxiolysis can be life saving. Acepromazine, 0.05 mg/kg IV/IM, may be administered if the patient is hemodynamically stable because acepromazine can cause venodilation and hypotension. Butorphanol 0.1–0.6 mg/kg IV/IM may be given alone or in combination with acepromazine for anxiolysis.

4. Hyperthermia occurs commonly in cases of airway obstruction. External methods of cooling should begin along with other stabilization methods.

5. Oral intubation (if possible) or tracheostomy is indicated if the patient has significant respiratory distress despite the above measures, is hypoxic, or respiratory fatigue is imminent. Propofol given to effect at 1–6 mg/kg IV may be used to accomplish intubation or foreign body removal. Propofol causes vasodilation and myocardial depression and should be used with caution in a critical patient. Diazepam (0.1–0.5 mg/kg IV) in combination with ketamine (5–10 mg/kg IV) may also be used. Opioids can be used for induction in critical patients.

6. A tracheostomy may be needed if the foreign body is not easily removed or a mass is causing the obstruction. While performing a tracheostomy (see Fig. 1.5, p. 14), place a large bore needle percutaneously into the trachea, in between the tracheal rings, caudal to the tracheostomy site. Attach an oxygen line and administer oxygen to the patient while performing the tracheostomy. Aspiration should be performed if a mass is causing the obstruction. An abscess or cyst may be drained to alleviate obstruction; special care must be taken to protect the airway.

7. Administration of short-acting corticosteroids, dexamethasone sodium phosphate 0.2–0.4 mg/kg IV/IM may be recommended to reduce laryngeal or tracheal inflammation. Steroids should be avoided if neoplasia is suspected as the underlying cause because administration complicates interpretation of diagnostics.

8. Thoracic radiographs are indicated once the patient is stable, particularly to monitor for signs of aspiration pneumonia or noncardiogenic pulmonary edema.

9. Administer broad-spectrum antibiotics if an abscess or an infectious process is suspected. Obtain culture and susceptibility if possible before administration of antibiotics.

10. Diuretics are usually not beneficial and may be detrimental.

TRACHEAL AND TRACHEOBRONCHIAL OBSTRUCTIONS

Diagnosis

History—Sudden onset of respiratory distress, a history of chewing on a bone, ball or a toy just prior to the onset of problems, or having been found with a collar, leash, rope or other object causing strangulation.

Mildly or chronically affected animals may have a slow onset of clinical signs such as stridor, sterdor, coughing or change in voice.

Physical exam—Inspiratory stridor, inspiratory dyspnea, ptyalism, cyanosis, tachypnea, pawing at the face or mouth, anxiety and distress. May be able to palpate a swelling in the cervical portion of the trachea. Auscultate the lungs carefully and monitor for pulmonary edema. Vomiting or regurgitation may also occur.

Radiographs—Should not be taken unless resuscitative treatment is started and the patient is stable, or they are felt to be absolutely necessary.

Bronchoscopy—Bronchoscopy is often needed to confirm a diagnosis of a tracheal or bronchial obstruction. The patient must be stabilized prior to this diagnostic step.

Differential diagnosis

Tracheal intraluminal foreign body, intraluminal neoplasia, tracheal stenosis and / or collapse, tracheal trauma; cervical, intrathoracic, heart base or mediastinal mass (neoplasia, abscess, hemorrhage, edema), lymphadenopathy.

Prognosis

The prognosis is good to grave, depending upon etiology, severity and duration of the obstruction.

Treatment

1. Inform the client of the diagnosis, prognosis and cost of the treatment. If the situation is critical, quickly obtain the owner's permission for sedation, an attempt at foreign-body removal, or tracheostomy tube placement.
2. Provide oxygen without causing additional stress to the animal and obtain venous access if the patient can tolerate restraint.
3. These patients have the ability to decompensate quickly. This is partially due to stress, which increases the respiratory rate and demand for oxygen. Anxiolysis can be life saving. Acepromazine, 0.05 mg/kg IV/IM may be administered if the patient is hemodynamically stable because acepromazine can cause venodilation and hypotension. Butorphanol 0.1–0.6 mg/kg IV/IM may be given alone or in combination with acepromazine for anxiolysis.
4. Hyperthermia occurs commonly in cases of airway obstruction. External methods of cooling should begin along with other stabilization methods.
5. Oral intubation (if possible) or tracheostomy is indicated if the patient has significant respiratory distress despite above measures, is hypoxic or respiratory fatigue is imminent. Propofol given to effect at 1–6 mg/kg IV may be used to accomplish intubation or foreign body removal. Propofol causes vasodilation and myocardial depression and should be used with caution in a critical patient. Diazepam (0.1–0.5 mg/kg IV) in

combination with ketamine (5–10 mg/kg IV) may also be used. Opioids can be used for induction in critical patients.

6. A tracheostomy may be needed if the foreign body is not easily removed or a mass is causing the obstruction. While performing a tracheostomy (see Fig. 1.5, p. 14), place a large bore needle percutaneously into the trachea, in between the tracheal rings, caudal to the tracheostomy site. Attach an oxygen line and administer oxygen to the patient while performing the tracheostomy. Aspiration should be performed if a mass is causing the obstruction. An abscess or cyst may be drained to alleviate obstruction; special care must be taken to protect the airway.

7. Administration of short-acting corticosteroids, dexamethasone sodium phosphate 0.2–0.4 mg/kg IV/IM may be recommended to reduce laryngeal or tracheal inflammation. Steroids should be avoided if neoplasia is suspected as the underlying cause because administration complicates interpretation of diagnostics.

8. Thoracic radiographs are indicated once the patient is stable, particularly to monitor for signs of aspiration pneumonia or noncardiogenic pulmonary edema.

9. Administer broad-spectrum antibiotics if an abscess or an infectious process is suspected. Obtain culture and susceptibility if possible before administration of antibiotics.

10. Diuretics are usually not beneficial and may be detrimental

LARYNGEAL PARALYSIS

Laryngeal paralysis occurs most commonly in large breed, older dogs, though it can occur in cats. The recurrent laryngeal nerve innervates the cricoarytenoideus dorsalis muscle. Denervation of the recurrent laryngeal nerve causes atrophy of this muscle. Subsequently, the arytenoid cartilages are unable to abduct and cause narrowing / obstruction of the glottis.

Etiology

1. Idiopathic laryngeal paralysis is the most common cause of laryngeal paralysis and is commonly observed in medium to giant breed dogs. Labrador Retrievers, Golden Retrievers, Saint Bernards, Siberian Huskies and Irish Setters, of 7 years of age or older, are commonly affected. Males appear more predisposed than females. Although the etiology is unknown, it is likely the result of a peripheral neuropathy.

2. Congenital laryngeal paralysis occurs in English Bulldogs, Bouvier des Flandres, Siberian Huskies, Malamute and, possibly, in Bull Terriers. They usually present with respiratory distress between 4 and 18 months of age.

3. Acquired laryngeal paralysis can result from trauma or iatrogenic injuries to the recurrent laryngeal nerve such as surgery. Compression and / or inflammation of the recurrent laryngeal nerve can result from intra- or extrathoracic neoplasia, abscess, lymphadenopathy or parasitic infiltration.

4. Diffuse neuromuscular diseases such as myasthenia gravis, polyneuropathy, polymyopathy and hypothyroidism can also cause laryngeal paralysis.

Diagnosis

History—Exercise intolerance, increased respiratory effort (especially with exercise or excitement), stridor, change of voice, gagging, coughing, dysphagia or collapse.

Physical exam—Respiratory distress, inspiratory stridor, hyperthermia, cyanosis or ptyalism may be present. Pulmonary edema may occur.

Radiographs—Radiographs of the laryngeal area are rarely useful. Thoracic radiographs are indicated once the animal has been stabilized, particularly in animals with dyspnea. Aspiration pneumonia, megaesophagus and pulmonary edema may occur.

Laryngoscopic examination—Examine laryngeal function under light sedation or anesthesia for several respiratory cycles. Oxygen should be provided by flow-by methods and pulse oximetry should be closely monitored and remain greater than 95%. Failure of the arytenoid cartilages to abduct during inspiration is diagnostic of laryngeal paralysis. Doxapram 1 mg/kg IV may aid in diagnosis in animals that are not breathing well after induction. An assistant may also be helpful, to call out when inspiration and expiration are occurring. Endoscopic transnasal laryngeal exam may also be utilized to diagnose laryngeal paralysis.

Differential diagnosis

Laryngeal or tracheobronchial foreign body, laryngeal or tracheobronchial mass, and pulmonary disease (pulmonary edema, aspiration pneumonia, pulmonary thromboembolism).

Prognosis

Medical management consists of managing stress, temperature and weight. Medical management is typically effective in mildly affected or unilaterally affected animals. Most animals will progress to a more serious form. Surgery is the only definitive treatment. Unilateral arytenoid lateralization has been associated with the best outcome and fewest complications. Post-operative complications are still reported in 10–28% of dogs post-operatively. The most common complications are aspiration pneumonia, coughing, laryngeal edema, surgical failure and sudden death.

Treatment

1. Inform the client of the diagnosis, prognosis and cost of the treatment. If the situation is critical, quickly obtain the owner's permission for sedation and intubation.
2. Provide oxygen without causing additional stress to the animal and obtain venous access if the patient can tolerate restraint.

3. These patients have the ability to decompensate quickly. This is partially due to stress, which increases the respiratory rate and demand for oxygen. Anxiolysis can be life saving. Acepromazine, 0.05 mg/kg IV/IM, may be administered if the patient is hemodynamically stable because acepromazine can cause venodilation and hypotension. Butorphanol 0.1–0.6 mg/kg IV/IM may be given alone or in combination with acepromazine for anxiolysis.

4. Hyperthermia occurs commonly in cases of laryngeal paralysis. External methods of cooling should begin along with other stabilization methods.

5. Oral intubation is indicated if the patient has significant respiratory distress despite above measures, is hypoxic or respiratory fatigue is imminent. Propofol given to effect at 1–6 mg/kg IV may be used to accomplish intubation. Propofol causes vasodilation and myocardial depression and should be used with caution in a critical patient. Diazepam (0.1–0.5 mg/kg IV) in combination with ketamine (5–10 mg/kg IV) may also be used. Opioids can be used for induction in critical patients.

6. A tracheostomy may be needed if intubation is required for more than several hours. The patient should be orally intubated and pulse oximetry and end-tidal carbon dioxide should be closely monitored while performing a tracheostomy (see Fig. 1.5, p. 14).

7. Administration of short-acting corticosteroids, dexamethasone or sodium phosphate 0.2–0.4 mg/kg IV/IM may be recommended to reduce laryngeal or tracheal inflammation. Steroids should be avoided if neoplasia is suspected as the underlying cause because administration complicates interpretation of diagnostics.

8. Thoracic radiographs are indicated once the patient is stable, particularly to monitor for signs of aspiration pneumonia or noncardiogenic pulmonary edema.

9. Diuretics are usually not beneficial and may be detrimental.

10. Keep the patient calm and cool until surgical correction is performed.

TRACHEAL COLLAPSE

Tracheal collapse is a condition that occurs most commonly in toy breed dogs, the Yorkshire Terrier being the most commonly affected. It is rare in cats. The underlying cause is unknown, but several mechanisms have been proposed such as congenital malformation, hypocellular tracheal cartilages, chronic lower airway disease, extratracheal masses and trauma. The weakened tracheal cartilages result in laxity of dorsoventral membranes causing partial or complete obstruction of the trachea. Collapses may be cervical, thoracic, or both.

Diagnosis

History—An intermittent cough that worsens with excitement, stress or exercise. It is commonly described as a 'goose honk' due to vibrations in the collapsing segment of the trachea. Cyanosis or collapse may be observed.

Physical exam—Patients may appear clinically normal at presentation or have severe respiratory distress. They may be wheezing, coughing, or have stertor, cyanosis, hyperthermia or collapse. Many patients with a collapsing trachea are obese. A cough can often be induced upon tracheal palpation. Careful thoracic and tracheal auscultation may reveal wheezing, referred upper airway sounds, or an end-expiratory 'pop.' Concurrent pulmonary disease such as noncardiogenic edema can also exist.

Thoracic radiographs—The patient should be treated as necessary and be stable prior to radiographs. Thoracic and lateral cervical radiographs are most often used to diagnose collapsing trachea. Inspiratory and expiratory films are often needed to diagnose collapsing; however, some cases cannot be diagnosed with radiographs alone.

Fluoroscopy—Dynamic images of the trachea are sometimes necessary to diagnose collapsing trachea. Fluoroscopy allows for real time evaluation of the trachea and mainstem bronchi.

Bronchoscopy—Bronchoscopy allows for visualization of the trachea and mainstem bronchi in order to characterize the severity of the collapse or evidence of concurrent infection. It is often considered the 'gold standard' of diagnosis and establishes the grade of collapse (I–IV). This allows the clinician to perform a bronchoalveolar lavage (BAL) for cytologic exam and culture and susceptibility. Careful laryngeal exam should be performed at the time of bronchoscopy. Careful anesthetic monitoring during the procedure and after recovery are vital as these patients can decompensate.

Differential diagnosis

Laryngeal paralysis, tracheobronchial obstruction, tracheobronchitis, hypoplastic trachea, tracheal stenosis, tracheal neoplasia, bronchitis, pulmonary disease and cardiac disease.

Prognosis

Medical management typically provides long-term success (greater than 12 months) in 70% of dogs. However, long-term prognosis remains guarded depending on the severity and on whether concurrent diseases are present. Medical management is recommended prior to attempting more invasive treatment. Surgical options are considered if medical management fails or the collapse is severe. Surgical options include tracheal ring chondrotomy, dorsal tracheal membrane plication, tracheal resection and anastomosis. Extraluminal ring prostheses and intraluminal wall stents are the most commonly used surgical options. These procedures are associated with a high risk of complications including laryngeal paralysis, continued clinical signs and stent migration.

Emergency treatment

1. Inform the client of the diagnosis, prognosis and cost of the treatment. If the situation is critical, quickly obtain the owner's permission for sedation in intubation.

2. Provide oxygen without causing additional stress to the animal and obtain venous access if the patient can tolerate restraint; administer fluids as needed for hemodynamic stability and hydration.
3. These patients have the ability to decompensate quickly. This is partially due to stress, which increases the respiratory rate and demand for oxygen. Anxiolysis can be life saving. Butorphanol may be particularly useful in patients with collapsing trachea because, in addition to providing sedation, it is an antitussive. Butorphanol 0.1–0.6 mg/kg IV/IM may be given alone or in combination with acepromazine. Acepromazine 0.05 mg/kg IV/IM may be administered if the patient is hemodynamically stable because acepromazine can cause venodilation and hypotension.
4. Hyperthermia occurs commonly in cases of airway obstruction. External methods of cooling should begin along with other stabilization methods.
5. Endotracheal intubation is indicated if the patient has significant respiratory distress despite above measures, is hypoxic or respiratory fatigue is imminent. Propofol given to effect at 1–6 mg/kg IV may be used to accomplish intubation. Propofol causes vasodilation and myocardial depression and should be used with caution in a critical patient. Diazepam (0.1–0.5 mg/kg IV) in combination with ketamine (5–10 mg/kg IV) may also be used. Opioids can be used for induction in critical patients. Intubation may not fully alleviate clinical signs if the animal has severe collapse of the thoracic trachea or mainstem bronchi.
6. A tracheostomy is typically not recommended as collapsing trachea usually involves more than just the upper airway.
7. Administration of short-acting corticosteroids, dexamethasone sodium phosphate 0.2–0.4 mg/kg IV/IM may be recommended to reduce laryngeal or tracheal inflammation.
8. Thoracic radiographs are indicated once the patient is stable, particularly to monitor for signs of aspiration pneumonia or noncardiogenic pulmonary edema.
9. The use of bronchodilators is controversial. They will not increase the diameter or the trachea, but potentially decrease intrathoracic pressure and tendency to narrow during expiration through dilator effects on the pulmonary airways. Some bronchodilators may provide anti-inflammatory properties: aminophylline 5–10 mg/kg IV q8–12h, terbutaline 0.1 mg/kg IV/IM.

Medical management

1. Environmental changes: restrict activity in heat/humidity, change to harness from collar, and weight loss.
2. Anti-inflammatory therapy: prednisone 0.5–1.0 mg/kg PO q24h
3. Antitussive therapy: butorphanol 0.5–1 mg/kg PO q6–12h, hydrocodone 0.22 mg/kg PO q6–12h
4. Bronchodilator therapy (controversial): aminophylline 10 mg/kg PO q8–12h, theophylline 10 mg/kg PO q12h, terbutaline 1.25–5 mg PO q8–12h
5. Sedation if needed: acepromazine 0.5–2 mg PO q8–12h
6. Glucosamine/chondroitin, 13–15 mg/kg of the chondroitin portion, PO q24h, may improve tracheal cartilage health.

INFECTIOUS TRACHEOBRONCHITIS

Infectious tracheobronchitis, ITB, is commonly referred to as 'kennel cough.' It most commonly affects young dogs with an unknown vaccination status, though recently vaccinated dogs may be affected in settings where there is a high population density such as pet shops, shelters, boarding facilities, breeding kennels and animal hospitals. The viral agents most commonly associated with ITB are canine parainfluenza virus, canine adenovirus-2, canine distemper virus, and canine herpesvirus. The bacterial agents most commonly associated with ITB are *Bordetella bronchiseptica*, *Mycoplasma* and *Streptococcus* spp. Transmission usually occurs by aerosolized droplets. Incubation is typically 3–10 days with viral shedding occurring for 6–8 days after infection.

Diagnosis

History—The animal may present with an unremarkable history aside from an acute onset of paroxysmal cough and retching. The owner may confuse a productive cough with vomiting. However, dogs that are more severely affected with concurrent bacterial infections may present with a history of lethargy, anorexia, tachypnea, mucopurulent nasal and ocular discharge, and cough. A recent exposure to other dogs is also typical such as occurs in pet shops, shelters, boarding facilities, breeding kennels, and animal hospitals.

Physical exam—Findings vary depending upon the severity of disease. Patients with uncomplicated ITB typically have no abnormal physical exam findings other than a cough. Severely affected patients may be dehydrated, febrile, or have tachypnea or mucopurulent nasal / ocular discharge. Some patients may have significant respiratory distress that requires immediate therapy.

Laboratory tests—A CBC and chemistry profile will not diagnose ITB, but provide more information about the overall health status of the patient. The CBC may show a stress leukogram. In patients with concurrent pneumonia a neutrophilia with a left shift may be present and in severely affected animals leukopenia may be present.

Radiographs—Thoracic radiographs are typically unremarkable in dogs with uncomplicated ITB. However, patients with concurrent pneumonia may show evidence of bronchopulmonary infiltration.

Other diagnostics—Transtracheal wash or bronchoalveolar lavage may be helpful in patients that have been previously been treated with antimicrobials or have failed to respond to medical therapy. Oral or nasal swabs are typically contaminated with normal microflora and offer little diagnostic or therapeutic utility. Patients can quickly decompensate after these diagnostics are performed; therefore, special attention must be made in regards to patient selection and monitoring.

Prognosis

The prognosis is good to poor depending upon whether ITB is complicated by secondary bacterial infection and pneumonia.

Treatment – uncomplicated

1. Inform the client of the diagnosis, prognosis and cost of the treatment.
2. Isolation protocols should be used to limit the possibility of spread to other patients.
3. Antimicrobial therapy: doxycycline 5 mg/kg PO q12h × 7–10 days.
4. Antitussive therapy: butorphanol 0.5–1 mg/kg PO q6–12h, hydrocodone 0.22 mg/kg PO q6–12h.
5. Address the patient's hydration status as needed with IV or subcutaneous fluids.

Treatment – complicated

1. Inform the client of the diagnosis, prognosis and cost of the treatment. If the situation is critical, quickly obtain the owner's permission for sedation in intubation if severe dyspnea or hypoxia is present.
2. Provide oxygen without causing additional stress to the animal and obtain venous access if the patient can tolerate restraint; administer fluids as needed for hemodynamic stability and hydration.
3. Isolation protocols should be used to limit the possibility of spread to other patients.
4. Thoracic radiographs are indicated once the patient is stable.
5. Antimicrobial therapy with broad-spectrum antibiotics. These patients will likely require parenteral antimicrobials. Doxycycline 5 mg/kg IV, PO q12h for 7–10 days should still be utilized in addition to other antimicrobials.
6. Nebulization with saline and coupage may be beneficial in the management of tracheal and bronchial secretions. Antimicrobials may also be nebulized if indicated by culture and susceptibility, or in severe cases that are unresponsive to therapy.
7. Careful monitoring of pulse oximetry, respiratory rate and character are warranted.
8. Nutritional support should be provided as appropriate.
9. The use of bronchodilators is controversial and often not recommended. Some bronchodilators may provide anti-inflammatory properties: aminophylline 5–10 mg/kg IV q8–12h.

ASPIRATION PNEUMONITIS AND PNEUMONIA

Aspiration pneumonitis is defined as acute lung injury due to the inhalation of irritants such as gastric acid, hydrocarbons or water. Aspiration pneumonia occurs when bacteria colonize the injured lungs or contaminated materials were aspirated. There are several disorders that predispose patients to aspiration. This discussion will focus on aspiration pneumonia.

Etiology

Aspiration pneumonia rarely occurs in normal animals. It is usually secondary to other pathology. Aspiration pneumonia is uncommon in cats.

1. Altered level of consciousness – central nervous system disease, head trauma, seizures, general anesthesia / sedation.
2. Esophageal disorders – megaesophagus, esophageal foreign bodies or strictures, lower esophageal sphincter dysfunction, nasoesophageal or nasogastric feeding tubes, esophageal dysmotility, esophageal reflux.
3. Intrinsic volume or fluid – gastric outflow obstruction, delayed gastric emptying, gastric motility disorders, obesity, pregnancy, ileus, gastric motility disorders, opioids.
4. Persistent vomiting of any etiology.
5. Iatrogenic / other – inadvertent administration of activated charcoal, mineral oil, tablets, capsules, barium, etc. into the patient's trachea rather than the esophagus, force-feeding, cleft palate, weakness or paralysis.

Diagnosis

History—Often the inciting cause (aspiration pneumonitis) is not witnessed. Coughing, tachypnea and dyspnea may be observed 6–8 hours later. The patient will often have a history of an underlying etiology such as those listed above or drowning.

Physical exam—Food particles or fluid may be observed in the oropharynx, tachypnea, dyspnea, orthopnea, wheezing, coughing, gagging, cyanosis, shock, hypotension, fever, malaise, mucopurulent nasal or oropharyngeal secretions.

Thoracic radiographs—A patchy or focal pattern of alveolar pattern most commonly affecting the right middle lung lobe or the ventral portions of other lung lobes. However, the pattern can be dorsal or lateralized depending upon the position of patient when aspiration occurred. Megaesophagus may be observed.

Laboratory findings—Leukocytosis with or without a left shift may be present. A transtracheal wash or bronchoalveolar lavage is indicated for cytology and culture and susceptibility. Arterial blood gas is useful for characterizing the severity of respiratory impairment. Hypoxia, hypocapnea or hypercapnea may be present. If megaesophagus is detected, an acetylcholine receptor antibody titer should be run to test for myasthenia gravis.

Differential diagnosis

Pulmonary edema, acute respiratory distress syndrome, bronchopneumonia, hematogenous pneumonia.

Prognosis

Aspiration causes serious morbidity and mortality. The prognosis can range from good to grave. The number of lung lobes affected appears to be correlated with outcome. One affected lung lobe typically results in a good outcome with appropriate care. Patients with hypoxia despite oxygen therapy, respiratory fatigue or ARDS may require mechanical ventilation and have a poor to grave prognosis.

Treatment

1. Inform the client of the diagnosis, prognosis and cost of the treatment.
2. If the aspiration event is witnessed, remove all foreign material from the mouth, oropharynx and esophagus. Endotracheal intubation may be needed to accomplish this and suction of the oropharynx or esophagus may be needed.
3. Administer oxygen.
4. Place an intravenous catheter (if not already in place). Judicious use of IV fluid is warranted. It is important to keep the patient well hydrated in order to keep bronchial secretions moist.
5. Transtracheal wash or bronchoalveolar lavage using sterile saline as indicated by patient status.
6. Antibiotics are not indicated in the early stages of aspiration pneumonitis, but are indicated in aspiration pneumonia.
7. Treat or remove cause of aspiration if possible; i.e. prevent vomiting.
8. The use of bronchodilators is controversial and may be helpful immediately after aspiration occurs:
   A. Aminophylline: 6–10 mg/kg PO, IM or IV, q6–8h in dogs or 4–8 mg/kg IM, SC, PO q12h in cats
   B. Terbutaline:
      I. Dogs: 1.25–5 mg PO q8–12h or 0.01 mg/kg SC q4h
      II. Cats: 0.625 mg PO q8h or 0.01 mg/kg SC q4h.
9. Perform nebulization with saline and thoracic coupage q4–6h. It is unclear if this treatment is beneficial.
10. Corticosteroid administration is not recommended.
11. Monitor arterial blood gas and / or pulse oximetry serially.
12. Prevention is the most effective method of treating aspiration pneumonia.
    A. Fast patients prior to anesthesia or sedation if feasible.
    B. Gastroprotectants (H_2 receptor antagonists or proton pump inhibitors) may help.
    C. Prokinetic medications such as metoclopramide in patients at risk or undergoing surgery without being fasted.
    D. Confirming proper placement of any feeding tube prior to use.
    E. Vigilant nursing care for down animals.

PULMONARY THROMBOEMBOLISM

Pulmonary thromboembolism (PTE) is the occlusion of one or more pulmonary vessels by a blood clot, septic emboli, fats, neoplastic metastasis or parasites.

Etiology

Most cases of PTE result from other systemic disease. Disorders commonly associated with PTE include: immune-mediated hemolytic anemia, sepsis, protein losing enteropathy (PLE) and nephropathy (PLN), neoplasia, cardiac disease, trauma, central catheter use, major orthopedic surgery or injury, and hyperadrenocorticism.

Diagnosis

Definitive diagnosis of PTE requires selective pulmonary angiography and / or ventilation perfusion scans. Diagnosis is usually made based upon clinical suspicion and the below diagnostics. PTE is likely underdiagnosed because advanced imaging is not always available or practical and because emboli are difficult to find or have already broken down on post-mortem exam.

History—Usually acute onset of tachypnea or dyspnea. Patients may also present with altered mental status as a result of hypoxia. Coughing, hemoptysis or collapse may also be seen. The patient may have a history of one of the above conditions.

Physical exam—Patients may be tachypneic or dyspneic. Crackles or wheezes may be auscultated. Pleural effusions can be present resulting in dull heart and bronchovesicular sounds. Patients with underlying cardiac disease may have a heart murmur.

Thoracic radiographs—May be normal or may show hyperlucent lung regions, alveolar infiltrates, loss of definition of the pulmonary artery, or cardiomegaly.

Laboratory findings—CBC and chemistry are not diagnostic for PTE but may reveal underlying disease. Urinalysis is recommended as routine health screening and to rule out PLN.

Coagulation profiles—Routine coagulation profiles such as ACT, PT and PTT are not diagnostic for PTE. These values may be abnormal owing to concurrent disease associated with PTE. D-dimers may be helpful in conjunction with other clinical data. Patients with a large pulmonary embolus are likely to have a positive D-dimer. However, D-dimers can also be positive because of concurrent systemic disease. A negative D-dimer does not rule out PTE. Thromboelastography (TEG) may be beneficial in assessing a hypercoagulable state.

Arterial blood gas—ABG will typically reveal hypoxia and hypocapnea. This is the result of ventilation perfusion mismatch. The A–a gradient can be utilized to assess the extent and possible causes of hypoxia:

$$(A-a) = PA_{O_2} - Pa_{O_2}$$

$$PA_{O_2} = [Fi_{O_2}(Pb - P_{H_2O}) - Pa_{CO_2}/RQ]$$

Fi_{O_2} = fraction of inspired oxygen
Pb = barometric pressure (760 mm Hg at sea level)
P_{H_2O} = water vapor pressure (47 mm Hg)
RQ = respiratory quotient (0.8–1.0)
Normal A–a is less than 10–15 mm Hg on room air (inaccurate on supplemental O_2).

Responsiveness to oxygen therapy can be monitored using the P:F ratio, or the $Pa_{O_2}:Fi_{O_2}$ ratio. This is accomplished by dividing the Pa_{O_2} by the Fi_{O_2}. The normal P:F ration should be 450 mm Hg or greater.

Differential diagnosis

Aspiration pneumonia, pulmonary edema, acute heart failure, bronchopneumonia, airway obstruction.

Prognosis

The prognosis is guarded to poor and is dependent upon the underlying cause and whether or not it can be eliminated. Prognosis is poor if the underlying disease cannot be corrected because the patient is likely to continue forming emboli.

Treatment

Treatment is primarily supportive with removal of the underlying cause if possible.

1. Administer oxygen.
2. Inform the client of the diagnosis, prognosis and cost of the treatment.
3. Place an intravenous catheter (if not already in place). Judicious use of IV fluid is warranted.
4. Correct any underlying disorder if possible.
5. Thrombolysis can be achieved with streptokinase and tissue plasminogen activator. These medications are rarely used owing to their risks of serious side effects and expense. They are also time sensitive and definitive diagnosis of PTE is rarely made in veterinary medicine.
6. Anticoagulation will not resolve the PTE, but may prevent additional PTE from forming. Careful monitoring is required to prevent serious side effects. Unfractionated heparin therapy, 200–400 U/kg SC q6h to prolong activated partial thromboplastin by 3–4 fold. An alternative monitoring test is the ACT, which should be prolonged by 15–20 seconds over baseline values. Low molecular weight heparin can also be used. Warfarin therapy has also been used, but can be more difficult to regulate. Platelet inhibitors such as aspirin and clopidogrel are also utilized.
7. Prophylaxis for patients considered at risk is important and may prevent PTE. The efficacy and appropriate dosage of low dose aspirin in cats and dogs remains controversial.
   A. Heparin 75–100 units SC q8h
   B. Aspirin 0.5 mg/kg PO q12h (dogs)
   C. Aspirin 81 mg/cat q72h (cats)
   D. Clopidogrel 18.75–37.5 mg/day (cats)

NONCARDIOGENIC PULMONARY EDEMA

Etiology

Noncardiogenic pulmonary edema is caused by increased pulmonary vascular permeability. Increased vascular permeability occurs when the pulmonary microvascular endothelium separating the pulmonary interstices becomes injured. This causes protein-rich fluid to leak into the pulmonary interstices. Noncardiogenic pulmonary edema occurs as a consequence of primary lung injury such as drowning, electrocution, smoke inhalation, aspiration of gastric contents, oxygen toxicity or blunt trauma. Edema may result from secondary pulmonary injury. This occurs most commonly in systemic illness that causes inflammation such as sepsis, pancreatitis, uremia and polytrauma.

Diagnosis

History—Acute onset of respiratory distress following one of the events listed under etiology above.

Physical exam—Tachypnea, dyspnea, cyanosis, orthopnea and coughing may occur. Pulmonary crackles may be auscultated.

Thoracic radiographs—Radiographs are vital for the diagnosis, but should not be obtained until the patient is stable. Noncardiogenic edema typically has an interstitial or a mixed intestinal to alveolar pattern. It is most often located bilaterally in a caudodorsal location.

Laboratory findings—CBC, chemistry and urinalysis should be performed to evaluate concurrent disease but are not diagnostic for noncardiogenic pulmonary edema.

Arterial blood gas—ABG will typically reveal hypoxia and hypocapnea. This is the result of ventilation perfusion mismatch. The A–a gradient can be utilized to assess the extent and possible causes of hypoxia:

$$(A-a) = PA_{O_2} - Pa_{O_2}$$

$$PA_{O_2} = [Fi_{O_2}(Pb - P_{H_2O}) - Pa_{CO_2}/RQ]$$

Fi_{O_2} = fraction of inspired oxygen
Pb = barometric pressure (760 mm Hg at sea level)
P_{H_2O} = water vapor pressure (47 mm Hg)
RQ = respiratory quotient (0.8–1.0)
Normal A–a is less than 10–15 mm Hg on room air (inaccurate on supplemental O_2).

Responsiveness to oxygen therapy can be monitored using the $P : F$ ratio, or the $Pa_{O_2} : Fi_{O_2}$ ratio. This is accomplished by dividing the Pa_{O_2} by the Fi_{O_2}. The normal $P : F$ ration should be 450 mm Hg or greater.

Prognosis

This is always guarded but depends upon the underlying etiology. It is usually more difficult to treat than cardiogenic pulmonary edema because the edema fluid is rich in protein and typically does not respond to diuretics. Patients with Pa_{O_2} 60 mm Hg or less despite oxygen therapy require mechanical ventilation and have poor prognosis. Increased work of breathing and risk of respiratory failure (hypercapnea Pa_{CO_2} of 60 mm Hg or greater) are also indications for mechanical ventilation.

Treatment

1. Administer oxygen.
   A. Place the animal in an oxygen cage.
   B. Place a nasal catheter and administer nasal oxygen.
   C. Sedate, intubate and provide mechanical ventilation.
2. Inform the client of the diagnosis, prognosis and cost of the treatment.
3. Place an intravenous catheter (if not already in place). Judicious use of IV fluid is warranted.
4. Treat or remove the underlying cause if possible.

5. Administration of diuretic is controversial. It may be beneficial by reducing pulmonary hydrostatic pressure, but is generally ineffective at clearing protein-rich edema fluid. Administer furosemide, 2 mg/kg IV initially, then repeat the same dose every 6–8 hours. Alternatively, a furosemide CRI can be use at 0.1 mg/kg/h after the initial dose. Careful monitoring of hydration is required.

6. Vasopressor administration may be needed to maintain normotension in certain circumstances.

7. Decrease stress, provide sedation if needed with butorphanol 0.1–0.6 mg/kg IV q6–12h. A full mu agonist should be used if the patient has noncardiogenic pulmonary edema as a result of a painful process such as trauma.

8. Perform transtracheal wash or bronchoalveolar lavage using sterile saline as indicated by patient status. Cytology and culture and susceptibility may help determine etiology and whether antibiotics are needed.

9. Administration of a β_2-agonist such as terbutaline may increase alveolar water absorption. However, this is unproven and should be used with caution, particularly in cats that may have restrictive cardiomyopathy or hyperthyroidism. The dosage of terbutaline is:
   A. Dogs: 1.25–5 mg PO q8–12h or 0.01 mg/kg SC q4h
   B. Cats: 0.625 mg PO q8h or 0.01 mg/kg SC q4h.

10. Antibiotic therapy is not required in all cases of noncardiogenic pulmonary edema depending on the underlying cause. Antibiotics should be used when the cause is from infection such as sepsis, but cases of sterile inflammation do not require antibiotics.

11. Monitor respiratory rate and effort, arterial blood gases and / or pulse oximetry serially.

12. Positive-pressure ventilation may be required if the patient remains hypoxic, has increased work or breath, or is at risk of going into respiratory failure.

ACUTE LUNG INJURY AND RESPIRATORY DISTRESS SYNDROME

Acute lung injury, ALI, and acute respiratory distress syndrome, ARDS, are potentially life-threatening consequences of critical illness that result in pulmonary edema. The difference in the degree of hypoxia is the key component in defining the difference between ALI and ARDS, with ARDS being more severe. A ratio of arterial oxygen tension to fraction of inspired oxygen, called the PF ratio or the $Pa_{O_2}:Fi_{O_2}$ ratio (see below in arterial blood gas), is used to differentiate between the two.

Etiology

ALI and ARDS result from the increased vascular permeability that occurs when inflammatory cells and inflammatory mediators injure the pulmonary microvascular endothelium separating the pulmonary interstices. This causes protein-rich edema fluid to leak into the pulmonary interstices. ALI and ARDS can occur from primary lung injury such as drowning, electrocution, smoke inhalation, aspiration of gastric contents, oxygen toxicity or blunt trauma. Edema may result from secondary pulmonary injury that occurs with systemic illness such as sepsis, shock, heat stroke, bee envenomation, pancreatitis, uremia and polytrauma. The proposed criteria for the identification of ALI and ARDS in dogs are as follows:

- Pre-existing severe critical illness or injury
- Increased respiratory rate and effort
- Bilateral pulmonary infiltrates on thoracic radiographs
- Severe hypoxia defined by the PF ratio:
  ○ ALI:PF ratio of 200–300 mm Hg
  ○ ARDS:PF ratio less than 200 mm Hg
    (Normal PF ratio is 450 mm Hg and greater.)
- No evidence of left atrial hypertension (based on echocardiogram or pulmonary artery catheter).

Diagnosis

History—Acute onset of dyspnea with one of the predisposing factors above.

Physical exam—Tachypnea and various degrees of dyspnea present. Harsh lung sounds and crackles may auscultate. The patient may be using accessory respiratory muscles to breathe and may be orthopneic. In severe cases the patient may cough pink frothy fluid. It is important to perform a thorough physical exam to look for concurrent disease.

Thoracic radiographs—Bilateral caudodorsal infiltrates. The pattern may be more diffuse in serious cases.

Laboratory findings—CBC, chemistry and urinalysis are important in the evaluation of underlying health and concurrent disease, but are not diagnostic for ALI or ARDS. The patients are prone to developing multiple organ dysfunction or failure and serial CBC, chemistry and urinalysis are often indicated.

Arterial blood gas—ABG will typically reveal hypoxia and hypocapnea, although hypercapnea may be present in ventilatory failure or severe ALI and ARDS. This is the result of ventilation perfusion mismatch. The A–a gradient can be utilized to assess the extent and possible causes of hypoxia:

$$(A-a) = PA_{O_2} - Pa_{O_2}$$

$$PA_{O_2} = [Fi_{O_2}(Pb - P_{H_2O}) - Pa_{CO_2}/RQ]$$

Fi_{O_2} = fraction of inspired oxygen
Pb = barometric pressure (760 mm Hg at sea level)
P_{H_2O} = water vapor pressure (47 mm Hg)
RQ = respiratory quotient (0.8–1.0)
Normal A–a is less than 10–15 mm Hg on room air (inaccurate on supplemental O_2).
Responsiveness to oxygen therapy can be monitored using the P:F ratio, or the Pa_{O_2}:Fi_{O_2} ratio. This is accomplished by dividing the Pa_{O_2} by the Fi_{O_2}. The normal P:F ration should be 450 mm Hg or greater.

Echocardiography—May be useful to rule out cardiogenic edema.

Differential diagnosis

Cardiac failure with pulmonary edema, noncardiogenic pulmonary edema, fungal pneumonia, diffuse pulmonary primary or metastatic neoplasia.

Prognosis

The prognosis varies from fair to grave, depending on the underlying etiology and whether or not it can be treated quickly. Patients with a Pa_{O_2} 60 mm Hg or less despite oxygen therapy require mechanical ventilation and have poor prognosis. Increased work of breathing and risk of respiratory failure (hypercapnea Pa_{CO_2} of 60 mm Hg or greater) are also indications for mechanical ventilation.

Treatment

1. Administer oxygen, often by sedation and mechanical ventilation with positive end-expiratory pressure.
2. Obtain venous access and use IV fluids judiciously to maintain hemodynamic status and hydration.
3. Inform the client of the diagnosis, prognosis and cost of the treatment.
4. Pursue the underlying etiology and treat appropriately.
5. Provide nutritional support early in the course of the disease.
6. Administration of diuretics is controversial. It may be beneficial by reducing pulmonary hydrostatic pressure but is generally ineffective at clearing protein-rich edema fluid. Administer furosemide, 2 mg/kg IV initially, then repeat the same dose every 6–8 hours. Alternatively, a furosemide CRI can be used at 0.1 mg/kg/h after the initial dose. Hydration status must be carefully monitored.
7. Vasopressor administration may be needed to maintain normotension in certain circumstances.
8. Decrease stress, provide sedation if needed with butorphanol 0.1–0.6 mg/kg IVq6–12h. A full mu agonist should be used if the patient has noncardiogenic pulmonary edema as a result of a painful process such as trauma.
9. Perform transtracheal wash or bronchoalveolar lavage using sterile saline as indicated by patient status. Regular sampling is often indicated in mechanically ventilated patients if they show signs of infection (fever, leukocytosis, left shift) as ventilator-associated pneumonia is a common complication. Cytology and culture and susceptibility may help determine etiology and whether antibiotics are needed.
10. Antibiotic therapy is not required in all cases of ALI and ARDS (though the need may develop later) depending on the underlying cause. Antibiotics should be used when the cause is from infection such as sepsis.
11. Monitor respiratory rate and effort, arterial blood gases and / or pulse oximetry serially.

FELINE CHRONIC BRONCHIAL DISEASE (FELINE ASTHMA)

Chronic bronchial disease in cats has been referred to by many names including feline lower airway disease, allergic bronchitis and asthma. It results in hyperresponsiveness of the lower airways to inhaled allergens and ultimately results in increased bronchial secretions and bronchospasm. Cats presenting in respiratory distress are fragile and can decompensate quickly. It is important to treat them appropriately prior to diagnostics.

Diagnosis

History—There may be a history of coughing, wheezing or tachypnea, which may or may not be associated with dyspnea. The client may report a history of anxiety, open-mouthed breathing and possibly cyanosis. Exposure to allergens such as dust from cat litter, smoke, household dust particles, perfume, pollen or other may be described.
Physical exam—The patient will exhibit expiratory dyspnea with increased abdominal effort. The patient may also present with open-mouthed breathing, cyanosis, orthopnea, anxiety, increased bronchovesicular lung sounds, wheezing and coughing.
Thoracic radiographs—Radiographs may be normal or show increased interstitial densities and peribronchial markings, overinflation, straightening of the diaphragm, hyperlucency of the lungs and possibly aerophagia. Pneumothorax has been observed in some patients, particularly after bronchoscopy.
Laboratory findings—The CBC and serum chemistry profile are not diagnostic but are useful in determining other causes of respiratory distress. Peripheral eosinophilia may be present but is often absent. Fecal exam should be performed in addition to heartworm antigen and antibody tests.
Bronchoscopy—Bronchoscopy may reveal increased amounts of mucus in erythematous, narrowed airways. BAL should be performed for cytologic evaluation and culture susceptibility testing. Cytology is not pathognomonic, but is helpful in conjunction with other diagnostics.

Differential diagnosis

Cardiac disease, acute or chronic bronchitis, infectious pneumonia, pulmonary neoplasia.

Prognosis

The prognosis is guarded to fair depending upon the duration, severity and response to therapy. The prognosis is better in cats that have an identifiable and treatable underlying cause.

Treatment (acute)

1. Inform the client of the diagnosis, prognosis and cost of the treatment. If the situation is critical, quickly obtain the owner's permission for sedation and possible intubation.

EMERGENCY PROCEDURES FOR THE SMALL ANIMAL VETERINARIAN

2. Provide oxygen without causing additional stress to the animal and obtain venous access if the patient can tolerate restraint.
3. These patients have the ability to decompensate quickly. This is partially due to stress, which increases the respiratory rate and demand for oxygen. Anxiolysis can be life saving. Butorphanol 0.1–0.6 mg/kg IV/IM may be given alone or in combination with acepromazine for anxiolysis. Butorphanol is also an antitussive. Acepromazine, 0.05 mg/kg IV/IM, may be administered if the patient is hemodynamically stable because acepromazine can cause venodilation and hypotension.
4. Administration of short-acting corticosteroids, dexamethasone sodium phosphate 0.2–1.0 mg/kg IV/IM to reduce inflammation is recommended. However, it is important to verify that dyspnea is related to asthma as glucocorticoids will exacerbate other causes such as heart failure and infectious disease.
5. Administer bronchodilators (caution in patients with cardiac disease). Albuterol inhaler: 108 µg q30–60min until severe dyspnea resolves or terbutaline 0.01 mg/kg IM/SC up to q4h until severe dyspnea resolves.
6. Intubation is indicated if the patient has significant respiratory distress despite the above measures, is hypoxic or respiratory fatigue is imminent. Propofol given to effect at 1–6 mg/kg IV may be used to accomplish intubation. Propofol causes vasodilation and myocardial depression and should be used with caution in a critical patient. Diazepam (0.1–0.5 mg/kg IV) in combination with ketamine (5–10 mg/kg IV) may also be used. Opioids can be used for induction in critical patients.
7. Consider the administration of maropitant (Cerenia), 1 mg/kg SC, which has been reported to decrease bronchoconstriction and ease respiratory distress.

Treatment (maintenance)

1. Terbutaline sulfate 0.312–1.25 mg (total dose/cat) PO q24h
2. Albuterol sulfate 108 µg inhaled as needed
3. Prednisolone 1–2 mg/kg PO per day
4. Theophylline extended release 25 mg/kg PO q24h
5. Theophylline 6–8 mg/kg PO bid
6. Fluticasone propionate 44–220 µg inhaled bid

PLEURAL EFFUSION

The pleural space is a potential space formed by the visceral and parietal pleura. This space normally contains minimal amounts of fluid to facilitate lung movement. Pleural effusion is the abnormal accumulation of fluid in this space and can be caused by a multitude of disease processes.

Diagnosis

History—A wide variety of clinical signs are possible. The owner may notice clinical signs ranging from lethargy, anorexia, weight loss, fever or tachypnea to an acute onset of severe dyspnea.

Physical exam—Tachypnea, orthopnea, cyanosis, open-mouthed breathing. Respiratory movements will be short, shallow and rapid, and there may be paradoxical movement. The patient may be very distressed. Upon auscultation, cardiac and pulmonary sounds may appear muffled and a murmur may be heard. Ascites and distention and pulsation of the jugular vein may be observed. The patient may have a fever.

Thoracic radiographs—If severe effusion is suspected, do not take radiographs without first performing thoracocentesis; portable ultrasound may be utilized in thoracocentesis.

Note: Radiographs are not therapeutic. The patient must be stabilized first, including thoracocentesis, otherwise taking radiographs may become a terminal procedure. Lateral and DV (provides additional information about the dorsal lung field and may be better tolerated by the patient) views reveal a loss of cardiac silhouette in severe cases, scalloping of fluid around the lung lobes, rounded lung lobe edges, pleural fissure lines, and retraction of lung lobes from the thoracic wall. Other lesions to look for include cardiomegaly, intrapulmonary masses or infiltrates, diaphragmatic hernia, lung lobe torsion, mediastinal masses, and concurrent ascites. Subcutaneous emphysema or fractures of the vertebrae, ribs or sternebrae may be observed in the trauma patient. Pre- and post-thoracocentesis radiographs may elucidate other pathologic changes.

ECG—Evaluate for signs of cardiomyopathy, dysrhythmias and pericardial effusion.

Echocardiography and thoracic ultrasonography—Evaluate cardiac function; look for pericardial effusion, valvular lesions, congenital cardiac defects, and cardiac and mediastinal masses. Ultrasonography is more rewarding if performed prior to thoracocentesis, if the patient is stable.

Laboratory findings—

1. Pleural effusion analysis – Place any sample obtained by thoracocentesis into purple topped (2 mL) and sterile red topped (2–3 mL) blood collection tubes. Submit the samples for laboratory analysis, including cytology, culture and susceptibility.
2. Perform a CBC, chemistry and urinalysis to evaluate overall health and to identify potential disease processes.
3. Perform serum tests for infectious diseases such as heartworm, fungal infections, feline infectious peritonitis, feline leukemia virus and feline immunodeficiency virus.

Differential diagnosis

1. Transudate to modified transudate (hydrothorax) – hypoproteinemia (hepatic disease, renal disease, protein-losing enteropathy), heart failure, fluid overload, neoplasia, pulmonary thromboembolism, diaphragmatic hernia.
2. Nonseptic exudate – neoplasia, lung lobe torsion, diaphragmatic hernia, renal disease, pancreatitis, feline infectious peritonitis, feline leukemia virus infection.
3. Purulent exudate (pyothorax) – septic pleuritis (bacterial, fungal, viral), foreign body penetration.

4. Chylous effusion (chylothorax) – ruptured thoracic duct, obstructed thoracic duct, neoplasia (lymphosarcoma), heart failure, heartworm disease, idiopathic.
5. Hemorrhagic exudate (hemothorax) – neoplasia (heart base, heart, pericardium, intrathoracic vessels), trauma, coagulation abnormalities.

Prognosis

The prognosis is guarded to fair depending on the underlying cause, concurrent disease and severity.

Treatment

1. Provide oxygen without causing additional stress to the animal and obtain venous access if the patient can tolerate restraint.
2. Administer IV fluids as needed for hemodynamic stability and to maintain hydration.
3. Inform the client of the diagnosis, prognosis and cost of the treatment.
4. Have material ready for CPR prior to commencement of thoracocentesis. Open-chest CPR is indicated with any pleural space disease.
5. Sedate with butorphanol (0.2–0.6 mg/kg IV) or a full mu agonist such as fentanyl.
6. Perform bilateral thoracocentesis (Fig. 4.1), and assess the character of the pleural effusion, save a specimen for submission to the diagnostic lab. Use sterile technique (clip and scrub the site, wear sterile gloves, use sterile equipment). Place 2 mL of the pleural effusion into an EDTA tube and 2–3 mL of the pleural effusion into a sterile red-top tube.
7. Obtain blood samples for CBC, serum chemistries and infectious disease screens as listed above. Perform a CBC, BUN and blood glucose screens immediately, in house if possible.
8. It is usually recommended to perform thoracocentesis 2–3 times before placing a thoracotomy tube, unless the patient has pyothorax.
9. Placement of a thoracostomy tube:
   A. The patient should be preoxygenated before the procedure.
   B. Thoracocentesis should be performed prior to placement of a thoracostomy tube.
   C. Intubation under heavy sedation or general anesthesia is recommended.
   D. The animal is placed in lateral recumbency and the area caudal to the shoulder blade to the last rib is clipped and surgically prepared. Strict aseptic technique is used.
   E. Local anesthetic nerve block.
   F. Incise the skin with a scalpel blade creating an incision slightly larger than the thoracostomy tube at the 10th intercostal space.
   G. Undermine the skin with the trocar thoracotomy tube, hold it perpendicular and point it slightly ventral.
   H. Advance the thoracotomy tube three intercostal spaces from the cranial border of the rib. Avoid the caudal border of the rib to prevent traumatizing the intercostal vessels and nerve.

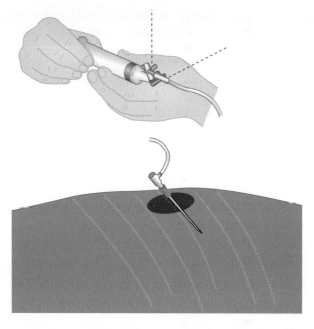

FIG. 4.1 **Performing thoracocentesis.** The patient can lie in either sternal or lateral recumbency, whichever causes the least distress. Utilizing sterile technique, clip and prep the area between the 6th and 8th intercostal spaces bilaterally. Insert the needle at the level of the costochondral junction to aspirate fluid (more dorsally to aspirate air). Insert the needle off the cranial edge of the rib, to avoid the intercostal vessels. Insert the needle into the chest wall at a 30° angle to avoid pulmonary trauma.

I. Position the thoracostomy tube perpendicular to the chest wall with one hand holding the tube securely at the entry point. Vigorously thrust the trocar into the chest with a sudden, short blow while maintaining control with the other hand to prevent overpenetration. Tell the assistant to hold the patient's breath during this portion if the patient is being manually ventilated.

J. Retract the trocar after penetration to avoid injury to the lungs and advance the tube toward the elbow.

K. Clamp the thoracostomy tube with hemostats as the trocar is being removed in order to prevent iatrogenic pneumothorax. An extension set, three-way stopcock, or continuous suction may be connected to the tube.

L. Secure the tube using a finger trap or friction sutures.

M. Evacuate the tube until negative pressure is achieved.

Alternative method:

A. Prepare the patient as above.

B. Place a local anesthetic nerve block.

C. Have an assistant pull the skin cranially and incise the skin with a scalpel blade creating an incision just larger than the thoracostomy tube at the 7th intercostal space.

D. Bluntly dissect through the subcutaneous tissue and musculature with hemostats.

E. Tell the assistant to hold the patient's breath if the patient is being manually ventilated. A finger is placed closed to the edge of the tip of the hemostat to prevent overpenetration. The pleura is penetrating by placing firm pressure on the hemostat. Once the pleura is penetrated, the thoracostomy tube is place over the site and the trochar is retracted. The tips of the hemostat are opened and the tube is introduced into the chest and guided cranially towards the elbow.

F. Attach and secure as above.

G. Good nursing care is essential. Keep the thoracostomy tube clean and bandage at the insertion site.

10. Exploratory thoracotomy is indicated in trauma and recommended in canine pyothorax. Feline pyothorax is typically managed medically.

11. Thoracostomy tubes are painful and all patients should be treated appropriately with opioid analgesics. Bupivacaine can be administered through the chest tube to provide additional analgesia. The recommended dosage is 0.5 mg/kg/tube q6h, diluted with sterile saline and allow to sit in the thorax for 15 minutes.

12. Administration of antibiotics may be required depending upon the underlying cause of pleural effusion.

13. Some patients may produce a tremendous amount of fluid through the thoracostomy tube. Careful attention to fluid balance is paramount.

14. The patient's respiratory rate, effort, arterial blood gas and pulse oximetry should be monitored serially.

15. Repeated cytologic exam of pleural effusion may help determine whether disease is resolving or other complications have occurred, such as infection.

16. Remove the thoracotomy tube when less than 2 mL/kg of fluid are aspirated from the tube per day.

REFERENCES/FURTHER READING

UPPER AIRWAY OBSTRUCTION (CHOKING)

Bonagura, J.D., Twedt, D.C. (Eds.), 2009. Kirk's Current Veterinary Therapy XIV. Elsevier, St Louis, pp. 627–630.

Millard, R.P., Tobias, K.M., 2009. Laryngeal paralysis in dogs. Compendium on Continuing Education 31 (5), 212–219.

Payne, J.D., Mehler, S.J., Weisse, C., 2006. Tracheal collapse. Compendium on Continuing Education 28 (5), 373–382.

Silverstein, D.C., Hopper, K. (Eds.), 2009. Small Animal Critical Care Medicine. Elsevier, St Louis, pp. 67–72.

LARYNGEAL PARALYSIS

Bonagura, J.D., Twedt, D.C. (Eds.), 2009. Kirk's Current Veterinary Therapy XIV. Elsevier, St Louis, pp. 627–630.

Millard, R.P., Tobias, K.M., 2009. Laryngeal paralysis in dogs. Compendium on Continuing Education 31 (5), 212–219.

Silverstein, D.C., Hopper, K. (Eds.), 2009. Small Animal Critical Care Medicine. Elsevier, St Louis, pp. 67–72.

TRACHEAL COLLAPSE

Bonagura, J.D., Twedt, D.C. (Eds.), 2009. Kirk's Current Veterinary Therapy XIV. Elsevier, St Louis, pp. 630–635, 635–641.

Payne, J.D., Mehler, S.J., Weisse, C., 2006. Tracheal collapse. Compendium on Continuing Education 28 (5), 373–382.

Silverstein, D.C., Hopper, K. (Eds.), 2009. Small Animal Critical Care Medicine. Elsevier, St Louis, pp. 67–72.

INFECTIOUS TRACHEOBRONCHITIS

Bonagura, J.D., Twedt, D.C. (Eds.), 2009. Kirk's Current Veterinary Therapy XIV. Elsevier, St Louis, pp. 646–649.

Datz, C., 2003. Bordetella infection in dogs and cats: pathogenesis, clinical signs and diagnosis. Compendium on Continuing Education 25 (12), 896–901.

Datz, C., 2003. Bordetella infection in dogs and cats: treatment and prevention. Compendium on Continuing Education 25 (12), 902–914.

Greene, C.E. (Ed.), 2006. Infectious Diseases of the Dog and Cat. Elsevier, St Louis, pp. 54–61.

ASPIRATION PNEUMONIA

Bonagura, J.D., Twedt, D.C. (Eds.), 2009. Kirk's Current Veterinary Therapy XIV. Elsevier, St Louis, pp. 658–662.

Silverstein, D.C., Hopper, K. (Eds.), 2009. Small Animal Critical Care Medicine. Elsevier, St Louis, pp. 91–97, 97–101.

Tart, K.M., Babski, D.M., Lee, J.A., 2010. Potential risks, prognostic indicators, and diagnostic and treatment modalities affecting survival in dogs with presumptive aspiration pneumonia: 125 cases (2005-2008). Journal of Veterinary and Emergency Critical Care 20 (3), 319–329.

PULMONARY THROMBOEMBOLISM

Bonagura, J.D., Twedt, D.C. (Eds.), 2009. Kirk's Current Veterinary Therapy XIV. Elsevier, St Louis, pp. 689–696.

Goggs, R., Benigni, L., Fuentes, V.L., et al., 2009. Pulmonary thromboembolism. Journal of Veterinary Emergency and Critical Care 19 (1), 30–52.

Silverstein, D.C., Hopper, K. (Eds.), 2009. Small Animal Critical Care Medicine. Elsevier, St Louis, pp. 114–117.

NONCARDIOGENIC PULMONARY EDEMA

Bonagura, J.D., Twedt, D.C. (Eds.), 2009. Kirk's Current Veterinary Therapy XIV. Elsevier, St Louis, pp. 663–665.

Myers, III, NC, Wall, R.E., 1995. Pathophysiologic mechanisms of noncardiogenic edema. Journal of the American Medical Association 206 (11), 1732–1736.

Silverstein, D.C., Hopper, K. (Eds.), 2009. Small Animal Critical Care Medicine. Elsevier, St Louis, pp. 86–90.

ACUTE LUNG INJURY AND ACUTE RESPIRATORY DISTRESS SYNDROME

DeClue, A.E., Cohn, L.A., 2007. Acute respiratory distress syndrome in dogs and cats: A review of clinical finds and pathophysiology. Journal of Veterinary and Emergency Critical Care 17 (4), 376–385.

Silverstein, D.C., Hopper, K. (Eds.), 2009. Small Animal Critical Care Medicine. Elsevier, St Louis, pp. 102–104.

Wilkins, P.A., Otto, C.M., Baumgardner, J.E., 2007. Acute lung injury and acute respiratory distress syndromes in veterinary medicine: consensus definitions: The Dorothy Russell Havemeyer Working Group on ALI and ARDS in Veterinary Medicine. Journal of Veterinary and Emergency Critical Care 17 (4), 339–339.

FELINE CHRONIC BRONCHIAL DISEASE (FELINE ASTHMA)

Bonagura, J.D., Twedt, D.C. (Eds.), 2009. Kirk's Current Veterinary Therapy XIV. Elsevier, St Louis, pp. 650–658.

Byers, C.G., Dhupa, N., 2005. Feline bronchial asthma: pathophysiology and diagnosis. Compendium on Continuing Education 27 (6), 418–425.

Byers, C.G., Dhupa, N., 2005. Feline bronchial asthma: treatment. Compendium on Continuing Education 27 (6), 426–432.

Silverstein, D.C., Hopper, K. (Eds.), 2009. Small Animal Critical Care Medicine. Elsevier, St Louis, pp. 81–86.

PLEURAL EFFUSION

Bonagura, J.D., Twedt, D.C. (Eds.), 2009. Kirk's Current Veterinary Therapy XIV. Elsevier, St Louis, pp. 646–649.

Silverstein, D.C., Hopper, K. (Eds.), 2009. Small Animal Critical Care Medicine. Elsevier, St Louis, pp. 125–130, 131–133, 134–137.

Traumatic emergencies

HBC (HIT BY CAR/AUTO ACCIDENT VICTIMS)

Diagnosis

History—Observed trauma, or sudden injury when unsupervised, or found injured.

Physical exam—Varies; often grease, dirt, plant material in the hair coat, abrasions, lacerations, road burns, bruising on skin, roughened nails, hyphema, variable fractures, variable mental conditions, dyspnea, variable degrees of shock.

As soon as the animal is or is thought to be stable, a thorough physical exam should be performed. The mnemonic (A CRASH PLAN) is useful for reminding the clinician not to exclude anything from the physical examination.

A = airway
Careful visualization, palpation and auscultation and examination of the oral cavity, pharynx and neck are performed;

C and R = cardiovascular and respiratory
Again, careful visualization, palpation and auscultation of the thorax *bilaterally* are performed. Percussion is added and the monitoring and recording of respiratory rate and depth is begun;

A = abdomen
Including examination of the inguinal, and caudal thoracic and paralumbar regions. This examination includes visualization, palpation, percussion and auscultation for bowel sounds, possible clipping of hair for the detection of bruises, punctures, red circles at the umbilicus, etc.;

S = spine
From C1 to the last coccygeal vertebra;

H = head
Including eyes, ears, nose, all cranial nerves and mouth, including the teeth and tongue;

P = pelvis
Including perineum, perianal and rectal examination. External genitalia of the male and female are also included;

L = limbs
Both pectoral and pelvic extremities, examining skin, muscles, tendons, bones and joints;

A = (peripheral) arteries
Including brachial and femoral pulses bilaterally, and also others such as cranial tibial, superficial palmar and caudal coccygeal;

N = (peripheral) nerves
Including the motor and sensory output to the limbs and tail.

Diagnostic procedures—

1. FAST (focused assessment with sonography for trauma) is an easy procedure to perform to look for and obtain samples of free abdominal fluid. Place the patient in left lateral recumbency for evaluation unless an injury (e.g. flail chest, fractures or injury to the vertebral column) precludes placement in this position, in which instance the patient should be placed in right lateral recumbency. A 2 × 2-inch (5 × 5 cm) area of hair should be clipped just caudal to the xiphoid process, just cranial to the pelvis, and over the right and left flanks caudal to the ribs at the most gravity-dependent location of the abdomen. Alcohol and acoustic coupling gel should be used at the ultrasound probe-to-skin interface. Use an ultrasound machine with either a 5 MHz or a 7.5 MHz curvilinear probe to obtain two ultrasonographic views (transverse and longitudinal) at the four prepared sites on the abdomen. If the patient has short hair, clipping is not necessary; just moisten the hair with isopropyl alcohol. Aspirates of fluid can be obtained and then analyzed.

2. TFAST (thoracic-focused assessment with sonography for trauma) is a procedure for the rapid diagnosis of pneumothorax and other thoracic injuries in traumatized patients. Place the patient in lateral recumbency to image one of the chest tube sites (7th–9th intercostal space on the dorsolateral thoracic wall) and the pericardial sites (5th–6th intercostal space on the ventrolateral thoracic wall). Then move the patient to sternal recumbency to image the other chest tube site. Evaluation for pleural and pericardial fluid at the pericardial sites includes imaging both transverse and longitudinal views. Imaging of only a single stationary longitudinal view at each chest tube site is required to evaluate for pneumothorax.

   Patients with significant respiratory distress may be imaged in sternal recumbency. The absence of the glide sign at the chest tube site indicates pneumothorax. The glide sign is the normal dynamic interface between lung margins gliding along the thoracic wall, forwards and backwards during respiration. If a glide sign is present that deviates from the normal linear continuity of the pulmonary–pleural interface, this is termed a 'step sign', and indicates concurrent thoracic injury. Subcutaneous emphysema over the thorax may also be evaluated.

3. Thoracic radiographs – the most common thoracic injuries that can be evaluated on thoracic radiographs of trauma patients include:
   A. Pneumothorax
   B. Pulmonary contusions
   C. Rib fractures
   D. Pleural fluid
   E. Pneumomediastinum
   F. Diaphragmatic hernia
   G. Sternal fracture.
4. Computed tomography is the gold standard imaging method to evaluate the stable trauma patient. Computed tomography allows for better distinction among specific tissue densities in the thorax and improved detection of subtle changes in organ position, size, shape and margin contour than conventional radiography.
5. ECG – various arrhythmias may occur; ventricular premature contractions are common.

Differential diagnosis

Dog bite wounds, other severe trauma.

Prognosis

The prognosis is good to grave.

Treatment (depending on severity of injuries)

1. Inform the client of the diagnosis, prognosis and the cost of treatment.
2. If the patient has mild abrasions or fractures, but no dyspnea, abdominal pain or signs of circulatory shock, hospitalize for observation for 12–24 hours.
   A. Clip and clean abrasions.
   B. Stabilize fractures if possible.
   C. Administer analgesics as indicated.
3. If the patient is in shock:
   A. Administer oxygen via a face mask, cover head with a plastic bag and run oxygen tubing into the bag, place a nasal oxygen catheter, use an Elizabethan collar oxygen hood ('Crowe collar'), or place the patient in an oxygen kennel.
   B. Place an intravenous catheter or an intraosseous catheter if necessary. Recommended IV catheter sizes are:
   <6.5 kg, 20 GA needle catheter
   6.5–10 kg, 18 GA needle catheter
   11–15 kg, 16 GA needle catheter
   16–21 kg, 14 GA needle catheter
   >21 kg, two or more 14 GA needle catheters.
   C. Start intravenous crystalloid therapy, with a balanced electrolyte replacement solution such as LRS, Plasma-Lyte or Normosol®-R:
      I. Canine – 90 mL/kg for the first hour
      II. Feline – 50 mL/kg for the first hour.

III. Re-evaluate the patient's cardiovascular and mental status every 15 minutes. Administer the fluids in ¼-shock boluses; repeat as needed to stabilize the patient. Generally decrease the rate to 20–40 mL/kg/h in dogs and 20–30 mL/kg/h in cats until the patient is stabilized. Continue at maintenance rates (1–2 mL/kg/h) when stable.

D. If the patient is in severe shock, administer Hetastarch or Dextran 70, 20 mL/kg IV. An additional 20 mL/kg of Hetastarch may be administered over the next 6–8h if needed for continued shock.

E. If the patient remains in severe shock, administer 7.5% NaCl, 4–5 mL/kg IV for dogs, and 2 mL/kg IV for cats, over 2–5 min (4 mL/kg for dogs with head trauma).

4. Administer analgesics, but avoid nonsteroidal anti-inflammatory agents initially in trauma patients.

A. Morphine sulfate
   I. Dog: 0.5 –1 mg/kg IM, SC q2–6h; 0.05–0.1 mg/kg IV q1–4h; 0.1–1 mg/kg/h IV CRI.
   II. Cat: 0.005–0.2 mg/kg IM, SC q2–6h
   III. Morphine, lidocaine and ketamine can be combined as an IV CRI for dogs
      a. Morphine: 0.1–1 mg/kg/h IV CRI.
      b. Lidocaine: 15–50 µg/kg/min IV CRI
      c. Ketamine: 2–5 µg/kg/min IV CRI
      d. Administer at maintenance fluid rates.

B. Hydromorphone
   I. Dog: 0.05–0.2 mg/kg IV, IM or SC q2–6h; 0.0125–0.05 mg/kg/h IV CRI
   II. Cat: 0.05–0.2 mg/kg IV, IM or SC q2–6h

C. Fentanyl
   I. Dog: 2–10 µg/kg IV to effect, followed by 1–10 µg/kg/h IV CRI
   II. Cat: 1–5 µg/kg/h to effect, followed by 1–5 µg/kg/h IV CRI

D. Buprenorphine
   I. Dog: 0.005–0.02 mg/kg IV, IM q4–8h; 2–4 µg/kg/h IV CRI; 0.12 mg/kg OTM
   II. Cat: 0.005–0.01 mg/kg IV, IM q4–8h; 1–3 µg/kg/h IV CRI; 0.02 mg/kg OTM

E. Lidocaine and ketamine can also be combined with hydromorphone or fentanyl in IV CRIs.

5. If severe or multiple wounds are present, or there is a high risk for the development of sepsis, administer broad-spectrum antibiotics, ampicillin or cefazolin, combined with enrofloxacin, cefoxitin, ampicillin sulbactam (Unasyn®) or ticarcillin-clavulanate (Timentin®).

6. Monitor urine output; normal = 1–2 mL/kg/h for dogs and cats.

7. Monitor body temperature; an external heat source may be necessary.

8. Thoracic trauma or dyspnea

A. Perform TFAST or bilateral thoracocentesis if a pneumothorax is suspected. Remove as much air as possible. Keep the needle or catheter against the chest wall to decrease iatrogenic pulmonary trauma. If pulmonary contusions are present, draw the air off as slowly as possible to allow for slow lung expansion.

B. Take thoracic radiographs.

Note: Radiographs are not therapeutic. The patient must be stabilized first, including thoracocentesis, or taking radiographs may become a terminal procedure.

Evaluate the external body wall, diaphragm, ribs, sternum and vertebrae. Look for subcutaneous emphysema and abnormal fluid accumulation. Evaluate the heart size, shape, and position, and mediastinal thickness, pulmonary tissue and vascular patterns. On radiographs, contusions appear as diffuse or patchy areas of alveolar and interstitial patterns that do not follow an anatomic pattern. Contusions may not be apparent radiographically for 4–6 hours following trauma.

C. Consider placing a thoracotomy tube. In patients with pneumothorax, use a Heimlich chest drain valve if the patient weighs more than 15 lb (6.8 kg). Thoracotomy tube placement is usually indicated if thoracocentesis is required more than twice in the treatment of pneumothorax.

9. Stabilization of flail chest

A. Immediately place the patient in lateral recumbent position with the flail side of the chest down.

B. Perform a peripheral nerve block with a local anesthetic.
   I. With a 22–25 gauge needle, inject 0.25–1 mL of the local anesthetic at the caudal border of the rib near the level of the intercostal foramen one to two intercostal spaces cranial and caudal to the flail segment.
   II. Also inject 0.25–1 mL of the local anesthetic at each fracture site.
   III. Bupivacaine (0.25–0.5%) can be administered every 6 hours or until other analgesics are administered. The total dose is 1–2 mg/kg for dogs and cats. The dose should not exceed 2.2 mg/kg.
   IV. Lidocaine (1–2%), 1–4 mg/kg, may be administered to dogs every 6–8 hours. Due to lidocaine sensitivity in cats, either avoid the use or cautiously administer 0.25–0.5 mg/kg.

C. An alternative to a peripheral nerve block is an intrapleural block. Following administration, place the patient with the affected side down for 20 minutes.

D. External stabilization of the flail segment may be performed.
   I. Secure the ribs to malleable plastic splinting material with 2-0 to 2 monofilament nonabsorbable suture passed percutaneously around the affected ribs. At least two sutures should be placed on each fractured rib, one dorsally and one ventrally, to avoid pivoting of the flail segment.
   II. Aluminum rods may be used as a splint.

E. Internal stabilization may be necessary in patients with an associated open pneumothorax, multiple unstable rib fractures or a large thoracic wall defect.

10. Pulmonary contusions
  A. Clinical signs include tachypnea, dyspnea, orthopnea, open-mouth breathing and hemoptysis. Moist rales and increased bronchial or bronchovesicular sounds are heard on thoracic auscultation.
  B. Thoracic radiographic changes typical of pulmonary contusion include an interstitial and / or alveolar lung infiltrate. The interstitial infiltrate may be localized to one lung lobe or may exist throughout the lung parenchyma. Alveolar infiltrate may be characterized as affecting one or multiple lung lobes.
  C. Mild – no treatment is necessary, other than confinement and rest. Arterial blood gas analysis is very useful. Pa_{O_2} is normally 80–100 mm Hg. Cyanosis normally occurs when Pa_{O_2} is less than 50 mm Hg.
  D. Moderate to severe – administer oxygen if the patient is in respiratory distress.
      I. Stabilize the patient and treat life-threatening injuries.
      II. Hospitalize for cage rest and observation.
      III. Administer intravenous fluids to restore tissue perfusion and optimum cardiac output. Monitor heart rate, respiratory rate, mucous membrane color and capillary refill time. Monitor urine output; minimum is 0.5–1 mL/kg/h in cats, 1–2 mL/kg/h in dogs.
      Monitor arterial blood pressure and CVP.
      IV. Monitor Sp_{O_2} and Pa_{O_2}. Administer oxygen to animals with overt respiratory distress and those with either a Pa_{O_2} of <65 mm Hg or a Sp_{O_2} of <91%. Oxygen may be administered via confinement in an oxygen kennel, with a 'Crowe collar' (Elizabethan collar with cellophane wrap over 80–90% of the opening), with oxygen brought in through a small line, or via nasopharyngeal catheter if there are no signs of head trauma. Nasal catheters may cause sneezing, which increases intracranial pressure and should be avoided in patients with head trauma.
      V. Mechanical ventilation with intermittent positive-pressure ventilation (IPPV) is indicated for patients with severe pulmonary contusions, as indicated by:
          a. Unconsciousness
          b. A large volume of blood in the airways
          c. Inability to maintain a patent airway
          d. Hypoventilation with a Pa_{CO_2} of >50 mm Hg, Pa_{O_2} of <60 mm Hg with greater than 50% oxygen content in the inhaled air
          e. Fatigue and respiratory weakness
          f. Increased intracranial pressure.
      VI. Monitor the heart for premature ventricular contractions by repeated auscultation and periodic ECGs.
      VII. Do not administer furosemide, glucocorticoids or antibiotics routinely to patients with pulmonary contusions.
      Bronchodilators are usually ineffective in these patients.

11. Abdominal trauma
    A. Monitor urine output; minimum is 1–2 mL/kg/h. If urine output is decreased or absent and the patient has abdominal pain, the patient possibly has a ruptured urinary bladder. Perform FAST ultrasound, abdominal radiography, and plain and contrast studies (pneumocystogram or water-soluble positive-contrast, intravenous pyelogram). Perform diagnostic peritoneal lavage or abdominocentesis. Obtain a fluid sample and save it for analysis.
    B. If a ruptured urinary bladder, or other urinary tract trauma, is causing intra-abdominal fluid accumulation, stabilization is required prior to exploratory surgery for dogs. Place a urinary catheter to keep peritoneal accumulation of urine low until surgery can be performed. Cats require surgical repair as soon as possible, or vigorous peritoneal lavage. Peritoneal dialysis will aid in stabilization and decrease uremia.
    C. Perform repeated PCV / TP (total protein), creatinine and potassium studies on both peripheral blood and abdominal fluid.
        I. PCV and TP. If the PCV is increasing, nearing that of peripheral blood, intraperitoneal hemorrhage is occurring. Nonclotting blood may be aspirated from the abdomen. Erythrophagocytosis may be observed.
        II. Creatinine or potassium if urinary tract leakage is suspected. An abdominal fluid creatinine concentration to peripheral blood creatinine concentration ratio of >2:1 was predictive of uroabdomen in dogs (specificity 100%, sensitivity 86%).
        III. An abdominal fluid potassium concentration to peripheral blood potassium concentration of >1.4:1 is also predictive of uroabdomen in dogs (specificity 100%, sensitivity 100%).
    D. If ecchymotic hemorrhaging is observed around the umbilicus (Cullen sign) or in the inguinal area, monitor the patient closely for intra-abdominal hemorrhaging.
    E. Take abdominal radiographs
        I. Look for the presence of free air in the abdomen.
        II. Look for a ground-glass appearance as seen with intra-abdominal fluid.
        III. Evaluate the normal placement and shape of abdominal organs.
        IV. Evaluate the integrity of the diaphragm and abdominal wall.
        V. Evaluate the appearance of the urinary bladder.
        VI. Evaluate the retroperitoneal region. Hemorrhage into the retroperitoneal space may reveal a depressed 'psoas line' or a depressed colon.
        VII. Look for fractures.
        VIII. Look for evidence of any other underlying health problems such as gastrointestinal foreign bodies or renal or cystic calculi.
    F. A diaphragmatic hernia is not a surgical emergency unless an abdominal organ is incarcerated and at risk of necrosis, or the patient's respiration is unable to be stabilized.

G. If abdominal trauma has occurred, perform abdominocentesis (either blindly or ultrasound guided) and / or a diagnostic peritoneal tap or diagnostic peritoneal lavage. Save any fluid sample in an EDTA tube for cytologic analysis, a serum tube for chemical analysis and another sterile tube for culture.

    I. To perform abdominocentesis, the patient should be placed in left lateral recumbency and the area surrounding the umbilicus subjected to clipping and full surgical preparation. Strict asepsis should be practiced at all times. A site should be chosen that is 2–3 cm caudal to the umbilicus and 2–3 cm left of the midline for sampling. The site should ideally be draped.

    II. If needle abdominocentesis reveals frank hemorrhage, look for clots in the sample. If the blood clots, it usually indicates that the needle entered a blood vessel or an organ. Abdominocentesis should be repeated in a different site.

    III. If needle abdominocentesis is negative, a four-quadrant abdominocentesis, diagnostic peritoneal tap or diagnostic peritoneal lavage can be performed.

    IV. Intra-abdominal hemorrhage into the retroperitoneal space usually goes undetected from abdominocentesis and should be considered in the patient with a negative tap and lavage but with continued signs of catastrophic hemorrhage.

    V. A negative tap does not rule out intra-abdominal hemorrhage.

H. If intra-abdominal hemorrhage is occurring, place a compressive wrap on the hindlimbs, pelvis and abdomen until ready to incise the abdomen on the surgical table.

I. If the patient's vital signs continue to decline despite resuscitative therapy, the patient's PCV drops while the PCV of the abdominal effusion rises, or the PCV of the abdominal effusion increases more than 5% from the original value, intra-abdominal hemorrhage is continuing.

J. If the patient cannot have exploratory surgery immediately, administer warmed, sterile 0.9% NaCl, 22 mL/kg (10 mL/lb) into the peritoneal space, to provide internal counter-pressure.

K. If the patient's PCV is rapidly dropping, if the patient exhibits signs of cardiovascular or respiratory distress, or the PCV is <20%, administer red blood cells (11 mL/kg, 5 mL/lb), a hemoglobin-based oxygen carrier, or whole blood (22 mL/kg, 10 mL/lb) intravenously and perform immediate exploratory surgery. (With chronic anemia, a lower PCV is tolerable.)

L. Ideally, administer blood and blood components after performing a cross match.

M. Example of the estimation of volume required in blood therapy: 30 kg dog with a PCV = 10%, desired PCV = 18%. Donor blood PCV = 50%. (Blood volume = 85–90 mL/kg for dogs and 65–75 mL/kg for cats.)

    I. Total blood volume = (90 mL/kg) × (30 kg) = 2700 mL

    II. Existing red cell mass = (2700 mL) × (10%) = 270 mL

    III. Desired red cell mass = (2700 mL) × (18%) = 490 mL

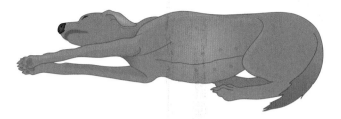

FIG. 5.1 **Schiff–Sherrington posture in a dog with spinal trauma between T2 and L3 vertebrae.** This is characterized by extensor rigidity of the forelimbs and flaccid paraplegia of the hindlimbs.

  IV. Required red cell mass = 490 mL − 270 mL = 220 mL
  V. Required blood volume = (220 mL) ÷ (50%) = 440 mL of fresh
     whole blood or 220 mL of packed red blood cells
  N. Usually administer whole blood at 10 mL/lb or 20 mL/kg of body
     weight. Administer packed red blood cells at 5 mL/lb or 10 mL/kg
     of body weight.
  O. The administration rate is usually 5–10 mL/kg/h, with the entire
     transfusion completed within 4 hours in stable patients. Blood
     components can be bolused in a crisis, after monitoring for
     transfusion reactions at a slow rate initially.
  P. Monitor the patient's response by assessing pulse rate and quality,
     respiratory rate and pattern, mucous membrane color and capillary
     refill time, blood pressure and with serial PCV / TPs.
12. Head trauma (see Ch. 13 Neurologic and ocular emergencies)
13. Spinal trauma
  A. Instruct the owners to keep the animal as quiet as possible and to
     tape or strap the animal to some kind of stretcher. The owners should
     also be advised to muzzle the animal to avoid personal injury.
  B. Evaluate patient status; institute emergency care for any life-
     threatening conditions such as shock, hemorrhage or pneumothorax.
  C. The presence of Schiff–Sherrington syndrome (extensor rigidity of
     the forelimbs, flaccid paraplegia of the hindlimbs and intact spinal
     reflexes caudal to the lesion, Fig. 5.1) indicates the potential presence
     of severe spinal trauma (compression or transection) somewhere
     from the third thoracic to the third lumbar vertebral segment. These
     signs, however, must be differentiated from pain and other
     neurologic problems.
  D. Administer intravenous fluids to treat shock and maintain systemic
     blood pressure which enables perfusion of the spinal cord.
  E. Administer an analgesic. Fentanyl CRI IV wears off quickly when the
     administration is stopped, facilitating repeat neurologic assessment.
  F. Administer methylprednisolone sodium succinate, 30 mg/kg IV,
     within 8 hours of the injury. Administer a subsequent dose of
     10 mg/kg IV 24 hours following the injury.
  G. Administer gastrointestinal protectants as the incidence of
     gastrointestinal ulcers increases with spinal trauma.
       I. Famotidine (Pepcid®), 0.5–1 mg/kg IV or PO q12–24h

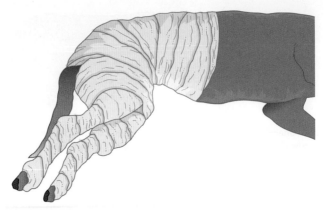

Fig. 5.2 Application of extremity wraps in the treatment of hypovolemic shock. If shock trousers are not available, any wide bandage material (such as ACE bandages) can be used to wrap the hindlimbs and the tail from the tips proximally over the pelvis and the entire abdomen. This causes an elevation of blood pressure in the cranial portion of the body to facilitate placement of an intravenous catheter. Once rapid intravenous fluid volume replacement is achieved, the extremity wraps should be released very slowly.

    II. Omeprazole (Prilosec®), 0.5–1.5 mg/kg PO q24h for dogs; 0.5–1 mg/kg PO q24h for cats

    III. Sucralfate, 0.5–1 g PO q8h for dogs; 0.25 g PO q8–12h for cats

  H. Stabilization and minimal handling and manipulation are essential and easily forgotten in the attempts to obtain diagnostic radiographs.

  I. Surgical reduction of spinal fractures should be performed as soon as the patient is stable enough to withstand surgery.

Four-quadrant peritoneal tap

1. Place the patient in lateral recumbency and provide sufficient restraint to prevent self-trauma.
2. Clip and surgically prepare the area surrounding the umbilicus.
3. Strict asepsis should be practiced at all times. The site should ideally be draped.
4. Four sites should be chosen that are 2–3 cm caudal to the umbilicus and 2–3 cm left of the midline for sampling.
5. Insert one 22 GA inch or 1½ inch needle in one site. Obtain any fluid that drips from the needle by gravity flow into red and purple topped blood tubes for analysis. If no fluid drips from the needle, insert a needle into the second site. Repeat until a needle is placed in each of the four sites. If no fluid is obtained, twirl one or more needles gently in place to stimulate fluid flow or gently aspirate with a small syringe.
6. Remove the needles from the abdominal wall.
7. A bandage is usually not necessary.

Diagnostic peritoneal tap

1. Sterile technique must be used, including sterile preparation of the infusion and collection sites.

2. Place the patient in right lateral recumbency.
3. Infuse warmed (body temperature) sterile 0.9% NaCl, 20–22 mL/kg (10 mL/lb) intraperitoneally through a 1.5-inch (3.8 cm) 22-gauge needle into the upper portion of the abdomen (away from the table). Place the needle into the mid- to caudal-third of the abdomen.
4. Allow a 5-minute dwell time, during which the abdomen may be gently manipulated to distribute the fluid throughout the abdomen.
5. Insert a standard IV catheter (not a jugular catheter) or 1.5-inch (3.8 cm) 22-gauge needle into the lower portion of the abdomen, nearest the table.
6. Obtain a 5–20 mL fluid sample for analysis either by gravity flow into collection tubes or by aspiration with a syringe. Place 2–4 mL of the peritoneal fluid in an EDTA tube and 3–10 mL in sterile red-top tubes.
7. If no fluid is obtained for analysis, administer another 22 mL/kg, 10 mL/lb, of warmed sterile 0.9% NaCl and repeat the collection attempt.
8. Remove the needles or catheters from the abdominal wall.
9. A bandage is usually not necessary.

Diagnostic peritoneal lavage

1. Sterile technique must be used, including sterile preparation of the infusion and collection sites.
2. Use a Cook peritoneal dialysis catheter, another multiholed peritoneal dialysis catheter, a pediatric Trocath®, or for cats use a 14 GA Teflon IV catheter with additional side holes, placed (with sterile technique) all on the same side to preserve the integrity of the catheter.
3. Make a stab incision (1 cm) through the linea alba 2–4 cm caudal to the umbilicus.
4. Aim the catheter towards the pelvic inlet.
5. Use **warm** (body temperature) saline (0.9% NaCl).
6. Add heparin, 250 u/L of dialysate.
7. Infuse 22 mL/kg, 10 mL/lb, warm dialysate solution intraperitoneally.
8. Roll the patient and remove 5–20 mL of fluid for analysis. Place 2–4 mL in an EDTA tube and 3–10 mL in sterile red-top tubes.
9. If no fluid is obtained for analysis, administer another 22 mL/kg, 10 mL/lb, of dialysate and repeat the collection attempt.
10. Remove the peritoneal catheter when finished, close the abdominal wall with one to two sutures, and apply a sterile abdominal wrap.

Peritoneal fluid analysis

1. PCV / TP. If the PCV is greater than 5%, intra-abdominal hemorrhage has occurred. Treat the patient supportively and repeat the tap in 30 minutes. Nonclotting blood may be aspirated from the abdomen. Erythrophagocytosis may be observed. If hemorrhaging continues, exploratory surgery is indicated.
2. Creatinine. If the abdominal fluid creatinine concentration is at least four times those of normal laboratory blood creatinine values, this indicates urinary tract leakage. An abdominal fluid creatinine concentration to

peripheral blood creatinine concentration ratio of >2:1 is predictive of uroabdomen in dogs.

3. Potassium. An abdominal fluid potassium concentration to peripheral blood potassium concentration of greater than 1.4:1 is predictive of uroabdomen in dogs.

4. Abdominal fluid lactate compared with serum lactate. In dogs, septic effusions have a peritoneal fluid lactate concentration of >2.5 mmol/L and a peritoneal fluid lactate concentration higher than blood lactate.

5. Abdominal fluid glucose level compared with blood glucose level. If the abdominal fluid glucose level is >20 mg/dL less than the peripheral blood glucose level from a sample obtained at the same time, in dogs and cats, this indicates septic peritonitis. These findings are 100% sensitive and 100% specific in diagnosing septic peritonitis in dogs and 86% sensitive and 100% specific in cats.

6. Bilirubin concentration higher in the abdominal fluid than in peripheral blood indicates hepatobiliary or proximal intestinal injury and exploratory surgery is indicated.

7. Microscopic examination

A. The presence of toxic or degenerative white blood cells, neutrophils with intracellular bacteria, observation of vegetable matter, or a WBC greater than 1000 cells/μL – indicates inflammation or suppuration and exploratory surgery is indicated.

B. Presence of bacteria – indicates bowel rupture has occurred and exploratory surgery is necessary.

C. Presence of vegetable matter – indicates visceral perforation requiring exploratory surgery.

D. Frank blood that does not clot – indicates intra-abdominal hemorrhage and requires exploratory surgery.

PNEUMOTHORAX

Diagnosis

History—May or may not have a history of trauma. The owner may observe sudden respiratory distress and restlessness, depression or cyanosis.

Physical exam—Dyspnea, open-mouthed breathing, dullness on thoracic auscultation, crepitation, cyanosis, diminished lung sounds, muffled heart sounds, and hyperresonance with chest percussion.

Thoracic radiographs—Lateral thoracic and ventrodorsal or dorsoventral view, *when stable.*

Note: Radiographs are not therapeutic. The patient must be stabilized first, including thoracocentesis, or taking radiographs may become a terminal procedure.

Radiographs may show elevation of the heart above the sternum, retraction of lung lobes from the periphery, and possibly signs of other thoracic injuries such as pulmonary contusions, hemothorax, fractures, diaphragmatic hernia, or pneumomediastinum.

TFAST (thoracic-focused assessment with sonography for trauma) is a procedure for the rapid diagnosis of pneumothorax and other thoracic injuries in traumatized patients. Place the patient in lateral recumbency to image one of the chest tube sites (7th–9th intercostal space on the dorsolateral thoracic wall) and the pericardial sites (5th–6th intercostal space on the ventrolateral thoracic wall). Then move the patient to sternal recumbency to image the other chest tube site. Evaluation for pleural and pericardial fluid at the pericardial sites includes imaging both transverse and longitudinal views. Imaging of only a single stationary longitudinal view at each chest tube site is required to evaluate for pneumothorax.

Patients with significant respiratory distress may be imaged in sternal recumbency. The absence of the glide sign at the chest tube site indicates pneumothorax. The glide sign is the normal dynamic interface between lung margins gliding along the thoracic wall, forwards and backwards during respiration. If a glide sign is present that deviates from the normal linear continuity of the pulmonary–pleural interface, this is termed a 'step sign', and indicates concurrent thoracic injury. Subcutaneous emphysema over the thorax may also be evaluated.

Prognosis

The prognosis is guarded.

Treatment

1. Emergency situation: if the patient has a tension pneumothorax (characterized by cyanosis, shock, shallow and rapid respiration, and a barrel-chested appearance), place an open 18-gauge needle *immediately* into the thorax to create an open pneumothorax. Proceed to treat the open pneumothorax.
2. Oxygen administration
   A. Oxygen cage or chamber oxygenation
   B. Nasal catheter oxygenation
   C. Elizabethan collar hood oxygenation
   D. Face mask oxygenation
   E. Endotracheal tube oxygenation
3. Inform the client of the diagnosis, prognosis and cost of the treatment.
4. Hospitalization of the patient for observation and enforced cage rest.
5. If only a small amount of air is present in the pleural cavity and the patient is not in respiratory distress, thoracocentesis is not necessary. However, closely monitor the patient for any adverse change.
6. Perform bilateral thoracocentesis in the dorsal third of the thorax between the ninth and eleventh ribs.
   A. Use a 20–22 GA 1 or 1.5 inch needle or a 19–21 GA butterfly needle attached to IV extension tubing, a three-way stop cock and a syringe.
   B. Use sterile technique (clip and scrub site, wear sterile gloves, use sterile equipment).
   C. Insert the needle near the cranial edge of the rib perpendicularly then once the pleural space is entered, gently direct the needle caudally.

D. Aspirate until negative pressure is obtained and the pleural cavity is empty or until the patient becomes uncooperative.

E. Repeat the procedure on the other side of the thorax.

7. A thoracostomy tube should be placed if negative pressure cannot be obtained via thoracocentesis, if thoracocentesis has to be performed for a total of 2 or 3 times, or to establish continuous drainage of the pleural space.

8. Apply an occlusive dressing. For cats, wrap the thorax with clear plastic food wrap as they tend to tolerate it better than heavy bandage materials.

9. Minimize stress.

10. Place an intravenous catheter, measure PCV and TP. Administer IV fluids if in shock.

11. Treat the cause of the pneumothorax.

12. Take thoracic radiographs, lateral and ventrodorsal or dorsoventral views, when stable.

    Note: Radiographs are not therapeutic. The patient *must* be stabilized first, including thoracocentesis, or taking radiographs may become a terminal procedure.

13. Perform an exploratory thoracotomy if unable to control leakage of air (very rare).

14. Placement of a thoracostomy tube

    A. General anesthesia is preferred.

    B. Provide supplemental oxygenation.

    C. Perform bilateral thoracocentesis.

    D. Clip, scrub and prepare the 9th or 10th intercostal space, midway to the ventral third of the height between the vertebrae and sternum.

    E. Perform a local anesthetic nerve block.

    F. Incise the skin with a scalpel blade (~½-inch long incision).

    G. Undermine the skin with the trocar thoracostomy tube, hold it perpendicular and point it slightly ventrally.

    H. Advance the thoracostomy tube ('walk if off') from the cranial border of the rib. Avoid the caudal border of the rib to prevent traumatizing the intercostal vessels and nerve.

    I. Vigorously thrust the trocar into the chest with a sudden, short blow.

    J. Remove the trocar, advance tube into the chest, and quickly attach a three-way stopcock and a cap or syringe or a Heimlich chest drain valve (if the patient weighs more than 15 lb or 6.8 kg). The stopcock can also be connected to a continuous thoracic drainage system such as a Pleura-Vac or Thora Seal Chest Drainage Unit.

    K. **Do not use a Foley catheter**.

    L. Check the tube placement with a thoracic radiograph.

    M. Suture the thoracostomy tube to the intercostal muscles and to skin.

    N. Place a purse-string suture in the skin around the placement site and a 'Chinese finger-lock' suture around the thoracostomy tube for additional security.

    O. Arrange the thoracostomy tube so that the valves and joints do *not* leak air. Beware of iatrogenic pneumothorax. Position the tube to protect it from trauma by the patient.

P. Instill bupivacaine 1.5 mg/kg flushed with 3–5 ml air or saline into the thoracic tube every 6–8 hours. A small amount of bicarbonate may be added to the bupivicaine at a 1:9 ratio just prior to administration to decrease the stinging sensation of the bupivicaine.

Q. Place occlusive antimicrobial ointment around the tube entry site and apply a bandage.

R. Verify proper tube placement with a thoracic radiograph.

Alternative method—

A. Clip, scrub and prepare the 9th or 10th intercostal space, midway to the ventral third of the height between the vertebrae and sternum.

B. Perform a local anesthetic nerve block.

C. Pull the skin forward; incise the skin with a scalpel blade (~ ½-inch long incision).

D. Make a small hole in the intercostal muscles with Metzenbaum scissors.

E. The thoracostomy tube may be a sterile red rubber urethral catheter or a long intravenous catheter. Utilizing a sterile technique, place multiple additional holes into the portion of the catheter that will be placed inside the pleural cavity. These holes should all be placed along the same side of the catheter. Use caution to avoid weakening the integrity of the catheter or creating jagged edges, which may cause tissue trauma.

F. Advance the thoracostomy tube through the hole, into the pleural cavity, with the aid of curved hemostats.

G. Advance the thoracostomy tube ('walk it off') from the cranial border of the rib. Avoid the caudal border of the rib to prevent traumatizing the intercostal vessels and nerve.

H. Suture the thoracostomy tube to the intercostal muscles and to skin.

I. Place a purse-string suture in the skin around the placement site and a 'Chinese finger-lock' suture around the thoracostomy tube for additional security.

J. Arrange the thoracostomy tube so that the valves and joints do *not* leak air. Beware of iatrogenic pneumothorax. Position the tube to protect it from trauma by the patient.

K. Place occlusive antimicrobial ointment around the tube entry site and apply a bandage.

15. The thoracostomy tube should be removed when the volume of air removed ceases or is less than 10 mL/kg/day. First clamp off the tube for several (12–24 hours) prior to removal to verify the tube is no longer needed.

16. Remove all sutures securing the tube then pull the tube while applying an occlusive antibiotic ointment and sterile dressing for 12–24 hours.

TRAUMATIC DIAPHRAGMATIC HERNIAS

Traumatic incidents can result in herniation of various areas of the body; the most common is a diaphragmatic hernia. Multisystemic trauma, hypovolemic shock, pulmonary contusions, pulmonary edema, traumatic myocarditis, fractured ribs and flail chest are common concurrent injuries in patients with traumatic diaphragmatic hernias.

Diaphragmatic hernias may be congenital but are more commonly secondary to blunt abdominal trauma, usually from an automobile. In dogs the most frequent area torn is the muscular portion of the diaphragm at its ventral and lateral aspects. Dorsal hernias are more common in cats.

Diagnosis

History—In acute cases, there may be a history of trauma. The most common presenting complaint is respiratory distress. Exercise intolerance, vomiting and difficulty lying down may also be observed. However, chronic traumatic cases may present with no history of recent trauma. A diaphragmatic hernia may be missed by a failure to radiograph the thorax following a traumatic incident, particularly vehicular trauma. The owner may observe weight loss, icterus, vomiting, diarrhea or respiratory distress.

Physical exam—The patient may exhibit expiratory dyspnea, tachypnea or abdominal breathing. The abdomen may appear 'tucked-up' and feel 'empty' upon palpation. The patient may sit or stand with elbows abducted and head extended. It may exhibit signs of hypovolemic shock, secondary to the acute trauma, or may exhibit weakness, icterus and poor body condition. Thoracic auscultation reveals muffled heart sounds, which may be abnormally positioned, and decreased lung sounds ventrally. Borborygmus may be auscultated in the thorax.

Thoracic radiographs—There is a loss of continuity of the diaphragm. Pleural effusion, fluid densities or bowel loops may be observed in the thoracic cavity. Fractured ribs and pulmonary contusions may also be present. The abdominal organs most commonly herniated into the thorax include the liver, small intestine, stomach, spleen, and omentum. Contrast radiography of the gastrointestinal tract or positive-contrast abdominal peritoneography may be useful. Dilute a sterile iodine based contrast agent 1:1 with sterile 0.9% NaCl and infuse 1.1–2.2 mL/kg into the peritoneal space near the umbilicus. Gently massage the abdomen then take radiographs.

Thoracic ultrasonography—The presence of pleural effusion enhances the ability to determine the presence of abdominal viscera in the thoracic cavity.

Differential diagnosis

Pulmonary contusions, pleural effusion (hemothorax, pyothorax, chylothorax, etc.), pulmonary thromboembolism, acute respiratory distress syndrome.

Prognosis

The prognosis varies from grave to good, depending upon the existence of concurrent complicating factors such as hypovolemic shock, cardiac dysrhythmias, adhesions, intestinal strangulation or obstruction, chronic liver disease, etc.

Treatment

1. Diaphragmatic herniorrhaphy is usually not an emergency procedure. Emergency surgery is performed only if the patient has life-threatening hypoventilation due to pulmonary compression, such as occurs following herniation of the stomach in left-sided diaphragmatic tears, or if a loop of bowel is strangulated or obstructed, vomiting, icterus, devitalized bowel is present, or fever of unknown origin develops.
   A. Gastric distention while entrapped in the thorax results in a tension pneumothorax.
   B. Emergency decompression is accomplished by inserting a needle through the left thoracic wall into the stomach or by passing an orogastric tube.
   C. Surgical repair should be performed as soon as possible.
2. Inform the client of the diagnosis, prognosis and cost of the treatment.
3. Administer oxygen.
4. Place an intravenous catheter and administer intravenous fluids to treat hypovolemic shock.
5. Administer intravenous antibiotics.
6. If the patient also has a fracture that requires surgical repair, herniorrhaphy should be performed first, to ensure adequate ventilation.
7. When the patient is stable, administer anesthesia and perform surgery.
   A. Anesthetic induction and intubation should be rapid and smooth.
   B. Pre-oxygenate the patient.
   C. If the patient is cardiovascularly stable, induce anesthesia with hydromorphone and midazolam, ketamine and diazepam, propofol, 2–6 mg/kg IV, or etomidate (Amidate®), 1–2 mg/kg IV. For dogs, combining lidocaine, 2 mg/kg IV, with the thiopental will decrease the dose needed and may protect against or treat ventricular arrhythmias.
   D. Maintain anesthesia with an inhalant anesthetic such as isoflurane (Forane®) or sevoflurane (Ultane®). Avoid nitrous oxide.
   E. Begin positive-pressure ventilation as soon as the endotracheal tube has been placed.
   F. Tilt the surgical table to lower the hindquarters and elevate the head.
8. Surgical procedure
   A. The repair must be performed quickly.
   B. For most diaphragmatic hernias, the ventral midline approach is indicated but the preparation for surgery should extend laterally to allow for sterile placement of a thoracostomy tube.
   C. If the diaphragmatic defect must be enlarged to return the viscera to the abdomen, make the incision in an accessible portion of the diaphragm to facilitate closure.
   D. Break down adhesions from chronic hernias carefully.
   E. Return herniated abdominal organs back to the abdominal cavity by applying gentle traction. Be particularly careful with the liver and spleen because incarceration leads to congestion, increased friability, and they are easily ruptured.

F. It is essential to replace the tissues to their normal anatomic location. If the wound is complicated, temporarily approximate the tissues with stay sutures.

G. Wrap the abdominal viscera in saline-moistened laparotomy sponges.

H. Examine the lungs for atelectasis; if observed, use low peak airway pressures, smaller tidal volume, or a faster respiratory rate.

I. Do not debride, freshen or resect the edges of the diaphragmatic tear.

J. Close the herniorrhaphy by suturing in a continuous pattern with 2-0 or 0 absorbable monofilament suture material such as polypropylene or polydioxanone suture (PDS) beginning in the most inaccessible area and progressing to the most accessible area of the defect.

K. Take large bites of tissue with each suture and do not pull the sutures too tight.

L. Avoid damaging the caudal vena cava.

M. If the defect was near the costal arch, incorporation of the ribs with the soft tissues may be necessary when suturing.

N. Reconstruction of the diaphragmatic defect with a mesh implant, may be necessary if there is not enough tissue to allow for primary closure. Omentum (double layers), muscle, liver or fascia may also be useful in some situations to aid in closure.

O. If there is evidence of pulmonary atelectasis, use low peak airway pressures, smaller tidal volume, or a faster respiratory rate. Otherwise, prior to tightening and tying the last one or two diaphragmatic sutures, inflate and re-expand the lungs to re-establish negative intrathoracic pressure.

P. Place a thoracostomy tube to re-establish negative intrathoracic pressure.

Q. Remove any remaining air from the pleural cavity either by needle aspiration or with a thoracostomy tube.

R. Inspect all abdominal organs for viability and return all abdominal organs to their normal anatomic positions.

S. Perform routine closure of the ventral midline incision, except just prior to tightening and tying the last two sutures in the linea alba; apply gentle pressure to both sides of the abdomen to expel residual air in the peritoneal cavity.

9. A thoracic radiograph may be taken prior to anesthetic recovery if there is concern regarding pleural effusion, collapsed lung lobes, position of the thoracostomy tube, or a persistent pneumothorax.

10. Continue to supplement oxygen until the patient has recovered from anesthesia.

11. Monitor for pulmonary edema and treat appropriately.

DEGLOVING INJURIES

Diagnosis

The diagnosis is usually obvious based on the physical exam.

Physical exam—

ALERT: When an animal with blood on it is presented for examination, all personnel having contact with the animal should wear

examination gloves and avoid direct contact with the blood until it is determined that the blood is actually the patient's and not from a human, who may have a contagious disease.

Apply a muzzle to most patients prior to beginning the physical exam, as they are in a heightened state of sensitivity and anxiety and are more prone to bite. Examine the patient as for all trauma situations; evaluate airway, breathing and circulation first. If a life-threatening abnormality is found involving the airway, breathing or circulation, temporarily stop performing the physical exam and address the life-threatening abnormality.

As soon as the animal is or is thought to be stable, a thorough physical exam should be performed. The mnemonic (A CRASH PLAN) is useful for reminding the clinician not to exclude anything from the physical examination. See the section at the start of this chapter on auto accident victims.

Radiographs—Radiographs should be taken of traumatized extremities to fully evaluate the extent of the injuries. Radiographs should also be taken of the thorax and any other area that may have been traumatized.

Laboratory procedures—
1. PCV, TS, lactate, BUN, creatinine and glucose should be evaluated in the patient with minor injuries.
2. Aged patients or patients with severe injuries warrant a complete CBC, biochemical profile, and possibly blood gas and coagulation panel.

Prognosis

The prognosis is guarded.

Treatment

1. Inform the client of the diagnosis, prognosis and cost of the treatment.
2. Evaluate as to possible need for amputation; if the injury is extensive, and if a guarded prognosis or a high risk of secondary infections, also consider the cost factor.
3. Control hemorrhage with pressure bandages if necessary.
4. If the patient is in shock, administer oxygen, place an intravenous catheter and administer intravenous fluids at 90 mL/kg/h to dogs, and 45–60 mL/kg/h to cats, for the first 30–60 minutes, then re-evaluate perfusion status.
5. Administer cefazolin IV, 40 mg/kg the first dose, then 20 mg/kg q6–8h.
6. Administer analgesics.
7. Apply a sterile water-soluble jelly to large wounds and bandage them until surgical repair can be performed.
8. Carefully assess the trauma patient before administering anesthesia. Treat shock and life-threatening problems first.
9. Anesthesia
   A. Local lidocaine block
   B. Injectable
      I. If the patient is cardiovascularly compromised, induce anesthesia with either oxymorphone or hydromorphone and diazepam

midazolam IV or diazepam and ketamine IV, then maintain on isoflurane or sevoflurane.

   II. If the patient is cardiovascularly stable, either induce with thiopental or propofol and maintain on isoflurane or sevoflurane, or induce with propofol and maintain with a propofol CRI IV.

10. Clip, scrub, flush and prep wounds.
11. Lavage contaminated wounds with copious amounts of water (tap, distilled or sterile).
12. After lavaging the gross contamination (grass, dirt, hair, plant debris) from the wounds, lavage with sterile LRS, Ringer's solution or physiologic saline. Use a 35 mL syringe and an 18-gauge needle, connected to a three-way stopcock and a bag of intravenous fluids for the lavage.
13. LRS causes less damage to fibroblasts and is the preferred lavage solution.
14. Debride wounds as thoroughly as possible. If possible, surgically close the wounds.
15. If additional debridement is needed, using sterile technique, apply a wet saline dressing consisting of wet saline-soaked gauze sponges, a Telfa Wet-Pruf® pad, gauze and Vetrap® for a wet-to-dry bandage.
16. An alternative therapy is to apply nonpasteurized honey or granulated sugar to the wound, then apply a bandage. Sugar is particularly effective and economical for large wounds. MediHoney is a commercially prepared wound paste and wound dressing. The bandages are less painful to change than wet-to-dry bandages.
17. Immobilize the limb to facilitate healing.
18. Bandages must be changed daily initially, then at decreasing frequency based upon the volume of exudate produced by the wounds. Sedation for bandage changes may be necessary. Changing wet-to-dry bandages can be painful.
19. After 4–5 days of daily bandage changes, when the volume of exudate decreases, bandage changes will decrease to every other day until a healthy granulation bed is achieved. At this time, third-intention healing is attempted; cover the wound with a nonadherent Telfa Wet-Pruf® pad, which needs to be changed two or three times per week.
20. Continue oral antibiotics for at least 7 days.

BITE WOUNDS AND LACERATIONS

Diagnosis

Usually obvious signs of external trauma; however, remember the external trauma is only 'the tip of the iceberg' and damage to underlying tissues may be much more severe than the external wounds would lead one to believe.

History—The patient may have been observed in a fight or attack, or may have been found with injuries after a period without supervision.
Physical exam—

   Alert: When an animal with blood on it is presented for examination, all personnel having contact with the animal should wear examination gloves and avoid direct contact with the blood until it is

determined that the blood is actually the patient's and not from a human, who may have a contagious disease.

Apply a muzzle to most patients prior to beginning the physical exam, as they are in a heightened state of sensitivity and anxiety and are more prone to bite. Examine the patient as for all trauma situations; evaluate airway, breathing and circulation first. If a life-threatening abnormality is found involving the airway, breathing or circulation, temporarily stop performing the physical exam and address the life-threatening abnormality.

As soon as the animal is or is thought to be stable, a thorough physical exam should be performed. The mnemonic (A CRASH PLAN) is useful for reminding the clinician not to exclude anything from the physical examination. See the section on auto accident victims at the beginning of this chapter.

Radiographs—Radiographs of the thorax and / or abdomen may be necessary even if no puncture wounds are observed over the chest or abdomen. Radiographs should be taken of traumatized extremities to fully evaluate the extent of the injuries.

Ultrasound—FAST and TFAST may be beneficial.

Laboratory procedures—
1. PCV, TS, BUN, creatinine, lactate and glucose should be evaluated on all bite wound victims.
2. A culture swab specimen for bacterial culture and antibiotic sensitivity of the wounds should be taken prior to the cleaning or administration of antibiotic medications.
3. Aged patients or patients with severe injuries warrant a complete CBC, biochemical profile, blood gas evaluation and coagulation panel.

Prognosis

The prognosis is excellent unless internal injuries, severe hemorrhage or other injuries are present.

Treatment

1. Advise a telephone caller to apply a clean cloth or dressing to the wounds, apply direct pressure to control serious hemorrhage, and to use extreme caution in handling the injured animal as they are prone to exhibit instinctive aggressive protective behavior. Recommend immediate evaluation by a veterinarian.
2. Inform the client of the diagnosis, prognosis and cost of the treatment.
3. Establish or maintain a patent airway.
4. Control hemorrhage with pressure bandages if necessary.
5. If the patient is in shock, administer oxygen, place an intravenous catheter and administer intravenous fluids at 90 mL/kg/h to dogs, and 45–60 mL/kg/h to cats, for the first 30–60 minutes, then re-evaluate perfusion status.
6. Administer a broad-spectrum parenteral antibiotic as soon as possible.
   A. Administer cefazolin IV, 40 mg/kg for the first dose, then 20 mg/kg q6–8h or ampicillin (10–50 mg IV, IM, SC q6–8h) or ampicillin sulbactam 20–50 mg/kg IV, IM q8h.

Traumatic emergencies

B. If there is penetration into the spinal canal, a sinus or the brain, also administer enrofloxacin (5–20 mg/kg IV, IM, SC, PO q24h for dogs, or 5 mg/kg IV, IM, SC, PO q24h for cats) or another quinolone in addition to cefazolin and ampicillin.

C. If there are wounds in the gastrointestinal tract, oral cavity or upper airway, administer metronidazole (10 mg/kg IV q8h), in addition to cefazolin; or administer a second-generation cephalosporin, such as cefoxitin (20 mg/kg IV q6–8h), as a single agent.

7. Administer analgesics.

8. Apply a sterile water-soluble jelly to large wounds and bandage them until surgical repair can be performed.

9. Carefully assess the trauma patient before administering anesthesia. Treat shock and life threatening problems first.

10. Anesthesia

A. Local lidocaine block

B. Injectable

I. If the patient is cardiovascularly compromised, induce anesthesia with either oxymorphone and diazepam IV, hydromorphone and midazolam, or diazepam and ketamine IV, then maintain on isoflurane or sevoflurane.

II. If the patient is cardiovascularly stable, either induce with thiopental or propofol and maintain on isoflurane or sevoflurane or induce with propofol and maintain with a propofol CRI IV.

11. Obtain a bacterial culture sample.

12. Clip, scrub, flush and prep wounds.

13. Lavage contaminated wounds with copious amounts of water (tap, distilled or sterile).

14. After lavaging the gross contamination (grass, dirt, hair, plant debris) from the wounds, lavage with sterile LRS, or physiologic saline. Use a 35 mL syringe and an 18- or 19-gauge needle, connected to a three-way stopcock and a bag of intravenous fluids for the lavage.

15. Surgically explore all wounds, especially those over the thorax or abdomen. If a wound perforates into the thorax, place a thoracostomy tube through the lesion and wrap the thorax (with cats, utilize clear plastic food wrap rather than bandage material), aspirate the air from the thorax and then perform exploratory surgery.

16. Take radiographs if questioning the presence of internal injuries. Contrast media (diatrizoate meglumine and diatrizoate sodium, Renografin-60®) might need to be injected into bite wounds to follow their track and determine their depth. TFAST may help assess for pneumothorax.

17. Debride wounds thoroughly. Flush with large amounts of sterile LRS. Place drains if indicated. Select wounds to be sutured closed carefully. Use monofilament absorbable suture in deep tissues and monofilament nonabsorbable sutures in the skin. Most small puncture wounds should be left open to drain.

18. If passive drains such as Penrose drains are used, they should be bandaged to avoid environmental contamination.

19. After the wounds have been thoroughly cleaned and debrided, the wounds may be bandaged with an antibacterial or antibiotic agent including:
    A. 0.1% gentamicin sulfate ointment
    B. Bacitracin, polymyxin, neomycin ointment
    C. Silver sulfadiazine ointment
20. Bite wounds to the neck may cause cervical spinal fractures, luxations, traumatic intervertebral disc prolapse, laryngeal or tracheal perforation, laryngeal paralysis, or severe hemorrhage.
21. Penetrating abdominal wounds are particularly serious and an exploratory laparotomy should be performed as soon as the patient is stabilized. Due to the compression and tearing forces, the underlying damage may be severe, including punctures to hollow organs, liver or splenic rupture, crushing of the pancreas, and damage to the urinary tract.
22. Postoperatively, monitor the patient for systemic complications such as renal failure, sepsis or peritonitis.
23. When the patient is stable and able to be discharged, dispense oral antibiotics for 5–10 days, and educate the client about wound care and complications to watch for:
    A. Cephalosporins and enrofloxacin
    B. Amoxicillin and clavulanate
    C. Cefpodoxime (Simplicef).
24. Re-examine the patient and remove drains in 2–3 days; re-examine the patient in 4–5 days if no drains. Remove sutures in 12–14 days.

GUNSHOT WOUNDS

Etiology

Most gunshot wounds are inflicted by handguns, in lower-income neighborhoods of urban areas, at night, on the weekend. Animals that have been left outside unsupervised or are allowed to freely roam are at an increased risk.

It can be assumed that a low-velocity weapon was used if the bullet remains in soft tissue without striking bone. If a high-velocity weapon was used, the bullet will usually be strong enough to shatter the dense bone of a large breed dog and exit the body.

Diagnosis

History—Observed or overheard gunfire immediately prior to the injury, or the animal was freely roaming or left outside unsupervised. Bleeding from the entry or exit wounds may or may not be observed. Respiratory distress, lameness or sudden death may occur.
Physical exam—The patient's mental attitude may range from alert to comatose, or dead. Dyspnea, lameness or severe hemorrhage may be observed. A puncture wound may be observed. There may be associated hemorrhage or bruising. Exit wounds are usually larger than entry wounds.
Radiographs—Radiographs should be taken of the affected area, to evaluate bone and soft tissue injuries, location of the projectile (if any portion remains in the patient) and type of projectile.

TFAST and/or FAST—These studies may help assess the patient for pneumothorax, pleural effusion or peritoneal effusion.

Differential diagnosis

Bite wounds or vehicular trauma.

Prognosis

The prognosis is good to grave, depending upon the location of the wounds, the velocity of the weapon and the extent of the damage.

Treatment

1. Inform the client of the diagnosis, prognosis and cost of the treatment.
2. Place an intravenous catheter and administer a balanced electrolyte replacement fluid, such as Normosol-R or LRS, at 80–90 mL/kg/h for the first hour in dogs, and 45–60 mL/kg/h for the first hour in cats. Administer the fluids in ¼-shock boluses and re-evaluate the patient every 15 minutes.
3. Administer oxygen.
4. Administer a synthetic colloid, such as Hetastarch, Pentastarch, or Dextran 70, in addition to crystalloid fluids if the patient is in severe hypovolemic shock.
5. Administer red blood cells, whole blood, or a hemoglobin-based oxygen carrier if there is extensive blood loss.
6. Administer broad-spectrum antibiotics.
7. Administer analgesics as indicated by the individual patient's needs.
8. Clip and clean the wounds.
9. Apply pressure wraps, if possible, to control hemorrhage during stabilization.
10. Hospitalize the patient for monitoring and continued treatment.
11. Re-evaluate the patient's cardiovascular status and fluid rate frequently. Make adjustments as indicated.
12. Head and neck injuries – if the patient is not dead on arrival, evaluate the patient's airway, breathing, mentation and cardiovascular status and treat accordingly.
    A. Jugular vein ligation may be required to control extensive hemorrhaging.
    B. Gunshot wounds to the brain are associated with a high mortality rate. Treat brain injuries as for head trauma.
    C. Ocular projectiles must be removed. Whenever the clinician is presented with an animal that has a ruptured orbit and a history of having been outside, a skull radiograph should be taken to ascertain the presence of a projectile foreign body.
    D. Perform a tracheostomy if necessary.
13. Thoracic wounds – hemothorax and pneumothorax are common sequelae to penetrating thoracic trauma. Laceration of the heart or a major vessel will usually result in sudden death. Pulmonary contusions may occur.

A. If the patient is not dead on arrival, evaluate the patient's airway, breathing, mentation and cardiovascular status and treat accordingly.

B. Perform thoracocentesis if indicated.

C. Thoracotomy may be necessary if the patient's status continues to decline.

14. Abdominal wounds – laceration of a major vessel may cause severe shock and rapid death. Wounds to the abdominal cavity should be surgically explored as soon as possible, due to the significant risk of peritonitis from perforation of the intestines or colon. Perforations tend to be multiple so thorough exploration is needed.

A. If the patient is not dead on arrival, evaluate the patient's airway, breathing, mentation and cardiovascular status and treat accordingly.

B. Administer broad-spectrum antibiotics and treat for peritonitis.

C. Apply a pressure wrap to control hemorrhage during stabilization.

D. Surgically explore abdominal wounds as soon as possible.

E. Administer RBC or a hemoglobin-based oxygen carrier if indicated.

15. Wounds to the spine or spinal cord – paralysis or tetraparesis may be observed, depending upon the location and severity of the injury.

A. If the patient is not dead on arrival, evaluate the patient's airway, breathing, mentation and cardiovascular status and treat accordingly.

B. Take radiographs prior to performing a thorough neurologic evaluation to avoid worsening any injuries.

C. Treat as for spinal trauma.

16. Limb wounds – evaluate the patient's airway, breathing, mentation and cardiovascular status and treat accordingly.

A. Apply compressive bandages to control hemorrhage.

B. Open fractures should be thoroughly lavaged and surgically explored as soon as possible.

C. Clip and clean the wounds.

D. Administer broad-spectrum antibiotics such as cefazolin, ampicillin-enrofloxacin, or amoxicillin-clavulanate.

E. Evaluate neurologic and soft-tissue damage to the affected limb.

F. Stabilize the limb with a splint if necessary.

G. If the damage is severe or hemorrhage cannot be controlled, amputate the affected limb.

17. Lead projectiles are toxic if they are lodged in the gastrointestinal tract, joints, central nervous system, or eye. Otherwise be cautious about removing lead projectiles. Do no harm.

Legal issues—

Police officers, attorneys, owners and other involved parties may request documentation of the injury. Photographs of the affected areas should be taken if possible. Medical records should be thorough and include documentation of all conversations. Radiographs should be taken.

If the projectiles are retrieved, they should be radiographed in place prior to removal. Projectiles should be handled carefully to avoid contamination or damage and saved for investigative personnel. Wrap forceps with tape prior to grasping a bullet, to avoid obliteration of the rifling marks used in identification. Wrap any projectile or fragment in facial tissues and place it in a vial or container and seal the container with tape. Label each container with the body region from which it was removed, the date, time, case number, owner's name and the initials of all present when the projectile was removed. Retain the projectile for law enforcement personnel; do not give it to the pet owner.

FRACTURES

There are three classifications of fractures, according to the need for repair:

1. *Critical fractures* – require immediate repair to maintain life or normal physiologic function of the structure involved. Includes skull fractures, spinal fractures, open fractures and certain types of luxation.
2. *Semicritical fractures* – may give rise to severe problems and abnormal function if not treated quickly. These fractures include those of joint surfaces or epiphyseal growth plates, luxation of the femoral head, shoulder and elbow; fractures of the mid and distal thirds of the humerus; pelvic fractures; and fractures of the os penis.
3. *Noncritical fractures* – do not require early reduction. Examples: scapular and pelvic fractures, greenstick fractures and closed fractures of the shafts of the long bones.

Diagnosis

History—Strenuous activity or trauma, aged patient, debilitated patient.
Physical exam—Variable degrees of lameness and swelling, abnormal angle, pain, may not palpate crepitation.
Radiographs—Take two views at 90°, i.e. lateral and anterior–posterior, as a minimum radiographic study. In young animals, differentiate fractures from growth plates.

The Salter–Harris evaluation system is beneficial for documentation of physeal fractures in young animals with open physes (Fig. 5.3).

Prognosis

The prognosis is usually good, except in multiple fractures and those complicated by infection.

Treatment

1. Inform the client of the diagnosis, prognosis, cost and the need for possible future surgical repair, which will add additional fees to the treatment costs.
2. Evaluate the patient closely for internal and other external injuries (ruptured bladder, fractured ribs, diaphragmatic hernia, etc.). **Always do a neurologic exam on all four limbs**.
3. Treat life-threatening injuries first.

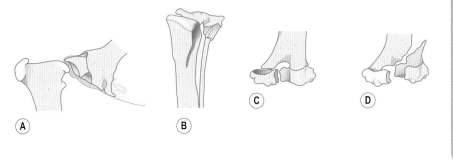

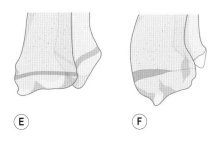

FIG. 5.3 **Salter–Harris classification of epiphyseal fractures involving the growth plate.** Adjacent metaphysis, and epiphysis. (A) Type I physeal fracture, with displacement of the epiphysis from the metaphysis at the growth plate. (B) Type II fracture of small corner of the metaphyseal bone, with displacement of the epiphysis from the metaphysis at the growth plate. (C) Type III fracture through the epiphysis and part of the growth plate; metaphysis is unaffected. (D) Type IV fracture through the epiphysis, growth plate and metaphysis. (E) Type V injury with soft-tissue swelling but no bony abnormalities seen immediately after injury. (F) Type V injury, 2 months after the trauma; closure and shortening of the ulna and partial closure with an angular deformity of the radius are evident. *From Piermattei DL, Flo GL, and DeCamp CE, Handbook of Small Animal Orthopedics and Fracture Repair, 4th edn, St. Louis, Saunders, 2006, Fig 22-5, p 742, with permission from Elsevier.*

4. Administer analgesics.
5. Clean any wounds. Open fractures require thorough cleaning and rapid surgical repair.
   A. Maintain strict asepsis when handling the open fracture.
   B. Use sterile gloves and instruments while cleaning and handling the open fracture wounds.
   C. Obtain a sample for bacterial culture and sensitivity testing.
   D. Debride all dead and damaged tissue with sharp dissection; avoid scrubbing of exposed soft tissues.
   E. Preserve bone fragments if possible.
   F. Lavage the wounds with a minimum of 1–2 liters of warm, sterile LRS using a lavage system of the liter of fluids connected to an intravenous fluid line with a three-way stopcock attaching the line to a 35 mL syringe with an 18- or 19-gauge needle used to deliver the solution.
   G. Apply a sterile dressing when the wound care is complete.
   H. Administer broad-spectrum antibiotics if wounds are present or severe soft tissue damage is suspected. Recommendations include

ticarcillin, amoxicillin sulbactam, or cephalosporins in combination with enrofloxacin. Include clindamycin or metronidazole if there is a concern regarding contamination by anaerobic bacteria.

   I. Open fractures should be repaired as soon as the patient is stable enough to survive anesthesia.

6. Immobilization
   A. Apply a soft padded wrap, with or without a splint, to immobilize the fracture and decrease swelling and pain. Splints are not recommended for humeral, femoral or pelvic fractures.
   B. Confinement, with or without sedation, for humeral, femoral and pelvic fractures.
7. Confinement and rest.
8. Repair the fracture(s) when the patient is stabilized.

AMPUTATIONS

Diagnosis

History—Emergency patients with a need for amputation usually have a history of severe trauma. Other indications for amputation include neoplasia, ischemic necrosis, severe orthopedic infection that is unresponsive to therapy, paralysis, congenital deformity, severe disability secondary to arthritis which is nonresponsive to therapy and, in some instances, due to financial limitations in cases of costly orthopedic repairs.
Physical exam—Evaluate the entire patient and treat life-threatening injuries as indicated.
Radiographs—Extensive orthopedic injury to a portion of the extremity, often with severe soft-tissue injury. In extremities that are considered candidates for amputation, the probability of the chances for successful repair should be small or the cost of repair not economically feasible.
Laboratory findings—Perform a complete biochemical, electrolyte and hematologic evaluation of the patient prior to surgery.

Prognosis

The prognosis is good to poor depending on the severity of systemic injuries.

Treatment

1. Inform the client of the diagnosis, prognosis and cost of the treatment.
2. Evaluate the entire patient and treat life-threatening injuries as indicated.
3. Shock, cardiovascular and respiratory problems must be resolved prior to administering anesthesia.
4. Place an intravenous catheter and administer intravenous fluids as indicated for shock.
5. Administer colloids if the patient is in a severe state of circulatory shock requiring large volume fluid replacement.
6. Administer analgesics.
7. If there is severe hemorrhaging from the affected extremity, apply a pressure wrap while stabilizing the patient for surgery.

8. In dogs that have suffered from severe blood loss, administer packed red blood cells or consider the administration of a hemoglobin-based oxygen carrier (HBOC).
9. In cats that have suffered from severe blood loss, administer fresh whole feline blood, packed RBCs, or consider the administration of a HBOC.
10. When determining the level of amputation, always amputate through normal tissue proximal to the diseased area to avoid leaving a dangling, useless stump.
    A. Tail – amputate proximal to the lesion. If the surgical site is near the base of the tail, exert caution to maintain perineal nerve function.
    B. Forelimb – removal of the scapula provides a more cosmetic appearance and is faster and easier than shoulder disarticulation.
    C. Hindlimb – amputation at the mid-thigh is easier and faster than disarticulation at the hip and leaves a stump that will help to protect the male genitalia.

COXOFEMORAL LUXATION

The usual displacement causes the femoral head to be displaced craniodorsally so that it rests against the lateral surface of the ilium. The limb appears rotated out and adducted. A caudodorsal luxation results in an inward rotation, whereas a ventral luxation results in an abducted position. With any luxation, movement is restricted. With a craniodorsal luxation, the luxated side will be comparatively shorter upon extension of the hindlimbs.

Radiographs are essential to confirm or deny the clinical diagnosis and to identify other injuries that may change or preclude treatment. Fractures of the acetabulum and fracture separation of the capital femoral physis, or fracture of the head and neck, all may appear as a luxated hip but necessitate very different prognoses and treatments. Additionally, hip luxation with concomitant fractures or avulsions, hip dysplasia, or Legg–Calvé–Perthes disease requires open reduction, or a salvage procedure and treatment will not be successful with closed reduction.

With no complicating factors, most luxations can be easily closed reduced within the first 3–4 days following the injury.

Closed reduction procedure (Fig. 5.4):

1. Administer general anesthesia.
2. Position the animal in lateral recumbency with the affected limb uppermost.
3. The hip is gently flexed and extended several times to relax muscles and break down any adhesions.
4. Have an assistant place a rope or towel in the inguinal region and provide counter-traction.
5. Grasp the leg at the stifle with one hand, and place the other hand on the greater trochanter.
6. While maintaining internal rotation and traction, the femur is abducted, and with strong downward pressure on the greater trochanter, the femoral head is popped into reduction.
7. Immediately after reduction, flex and extend the hip several times while maintaining pressure on the greater trochanter.

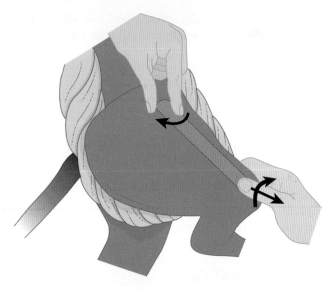

FIG. 5.4 Procedure for closed reduction of a coxofemoral luxation. This figure illustrates the right hand pulling and internally rotating the femur and the left hand directing the femoral head into the acetabulum. Continue abduction of the femur while pressure on the trochanter forces the femoral head into the acetabulum. The technique is described in detail in the text.

8. Apply an Ehmer sling (Fig. 5.5), which may be left in place for 2–14 days, depending on the stability of the reduction.
9. If closed reduction is not successful, or the hip continues to luxate, open surgical correction is needed.
10. For cats, open surgical correction is usually necessary.

ELBOW LUXATION

There is often severe soft-tissue and bone trauma associated with elbow luxation. Radiographic evaluation of the joint is essential prior to any attempts at closed reduction. Early reduction is mandatory. A delay of more than 2 days will make closed atraumatic reduction very difficult or impossible.

The radius and ulna generally luxate laterally, while the anconeal process may or may not be displaced to lie on the caudolateral aspect of the lateral epicondyle.

The animal is presented carrying the affected limb, with the antebrachium displaced slightly laterally and distal to the elbow. The radial head is easily palpated lateral to the humeral condyles, and there is a reduced range of flexion and extension in the joint.

Closed reduction procedure (Fig. 5.6):

1. Administer general anesthesia.
2. Place the patient in a lateral recumbent position with the affected limb uppermost.
3. The brachium is held in one hand and the lower limb in the other.
4. The joint is forced beyond 90° to relieve muscle spasms.

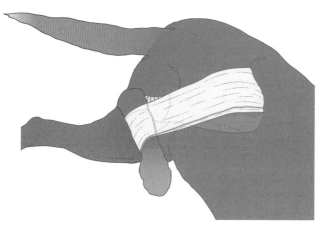

FIG. 5.5 **Application of an Ehmer sling.** With soft gauze, start on the medial surface of the metatarsus; wrap around the metatarsus, pass the gauze on the medial surface of the femur, come out over the lateral surface of the femur, back to the medial surface of the metatarsus. Pass the gauze around under the pes to the lateral surface of the metatarsus, continue once again to the medial surface of the femur and back laterally over the femur. Cover with adhesive tape. Additional support tape may be needed, passing over the lateral surface of the entire limb and encompassing the body. The finished bandage should result in inward rotation of the pes, and outward rotation of the femoral head into the acetabulum.

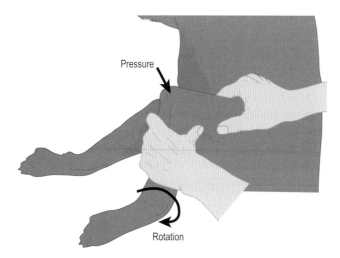

FIG. 5.6 **Procedure for closed reduction of an elbow luxation.** The elbow should be flexed at an approximately 100–110° angle. While twisting the antebrachium internally, slightly extend the joint and maintain continuous medial pressure on the head of the radius. The head of the radius is forced medially by applying gradual flexion and internal rotation of the antebrachium.

5. If the anconeal process is in the olecranon fossa, the only manipulation needed is full extension of the joint accompanied by internal rotation of the radius and ulna while abducting the limb.
6. When the anconeal process is lateral to the lateral epicondyle:
   A. The elbow joint is placed in full flexion and the carpal joint in 90° of flexion.

B. The metacarpal bones and the distal radius and ulna are grasped in one hand, while the elbow is held in the other hand.
C. The manus is rotated outwardly, which rotates the anconeal process caudal to the lateral humeral epicondyle.
D. Placement of digital pressure on the olecranon in a medial direction and abduction of the distal limb may help.
E. Once the anconeal process is entrapped caudal to the epicondyle, it is secured into position by fully extending the elbow joint.
F. If the elbow is relatively stable, then a support bandage is applied for 10–14 days, followed by leash exercise for 4 weeks.
7. If closed reduction is not successful or the joint is not stable, open surgical correction is needed.

DEHISCENCE

Etiology

Acute incisional hernias (dehiscence) result from poor holding strength of the sutured wound (suture type, size, knot security, suture pattern and strength of the tissues sutured); from excessive forces acting on the wound (tension, increased intra-abdominal pressure due to obesity, pregnancy, organ distention or abdominal effusions); or from exuberant activity, coughing, straining, or the patient chewing out or scratching out sutures.

Diagnosis

History and physical exam (usually obvious)—The owner may observe incisional swelling or a serosanguineous discharge from a surgical incision, usually within 4 days of surgery. These are impending signs of incisional herniation and warrant a physical examination immediately.

Note: When a telephone call is received sounding suspiciously like an abdominal wall dehiscence, instruct the client to wrap the abdomen in clean fabric and to carry the patient gently into the clinic. Advise them not to allow the patient to run or jump and transport the animal immediately to the clinic for treatment.

Laboratory—As quickly as possible, evaluate the PCV and TP, BUN, creatinine, lactate and blood glucose levels. As time allows, evaluate a CBC, full serum chemistry panel, blood gas analysis and coagulation panel. Conditions known to inhibit wound repair include anemia, uremia, hypoproteinemia, infection, diabetes mellitus, liver disease and hyperadrenocorticism.

Differential diagnosis

Excessive foreign body response to buried suture material, cellulitis, seroma and hematoma.

Prognosis

The prognosis is good to guarded. In one study of major abdominal eviscera-tion in dogs and cats, all 12 animals in the study survived with aggressive medical and surgical care.

Treatment

1. Apply a protective bandage until repair can be performed. If possible, depending on the site and the severity, attempt to stabilize for repair by the regular veterinarian.
2. Check if the referring veterinarian needs to be notified, and notify them if possible.
3. Inform the client of the diagnosis, prognosis and cost of the treatment.
4. Either sedate or anesthetize the patient.
5. Thoroughly lavage the exposed viscera thoroughly with sterile saline or LRS. Temporary closure of intestines can be made with skin staples. Perform a partial omentectomy if needed. Return the exposed viscera into the abdominal cavity, extending the abdominal wound if needed.
6. Place a sterile bandage over the abdominal wound.
7. Place an IV catheter, administer IV fluids and treat for shock if indicated.
8. Administer fresh-frozen plasma, packed RBCs, etc. if indicated.
9. Administer analgesics as indicated.
10. Perform surgery, including surgical exploration of the abdomen, repair or removal of traumatized organs, and replacement of abdominal viscera into the peritoneal cavity.
11. Obtain aerobic and anaerobic culture samples from the abdominal cavity at the time of surgery.
12. Administer broad-spectrum systemic antibiotics IV. Recommendations include cefoxitin or ampicillin and enrofloxacin, with or without metronidazole or clindamycin.
13. Prevent self trauma by placing an Elizabethan collar on the patient until the skin sutures or staples are removed.
14. Apply bandages as necessary.
15. Hospitalize the patient for recovery.
16. Discharge the patient with clear postoperative instructions, antibiotics, and an Elizabethan collar.

Note: Be extremely cautious in terminology and discussing the case with client. Do *not* under any circumstances imply incompetence or error on the part of the referring veterinarian.

REFERENCES/FURTHER READING

HBC (HIT BY CAR/AUTO ACCIDENT VICTIMS)

Crowe, D.T., 2006. Assessment and management of the severely polytraumatized small animal patient. Journal of Veterinary Emergency and Critical Care 16 (4), 264–275.

Culp, W.T.N., Silverstein, D.C., 2009. Abdominal trauma. In: Silverstein, D.C., Hopper, K. (Eds.), Small Animal Critical Care Medicine. Elsevier, St Louis, pp. 667–671.

Driessen, B., Brainard, B., 2006. Fluid therapy for the traumatized patient. Journal of Veterinary Emergency and Critical Care 16 (4), 276–299.

Hackner, S.G., 1995. Emergency management of thoracic pulmonary contusions. Compendium on Continuing Education 17 (5), 677–686.

Kyles, A.E., 1998. Transdermal fentanyl. Compendium on Continuing Education 20 (3), 721–726.

Lisciandro, G.R., Lagutchik, M.S., Mann, K.A., et al., 2009. DVM evaluation of an abdominal fluid scoring system determined using abdominal focused assessment with sonography for trauma in 101 dogs with motor vehicle trauma. Journal of Veterinary Emergency and Critical Care 19 (5), 426–437.

Muir, W., 2006. Trauma: physiology, pathophysiology, and clinical implications. Journal of Veterinary Emergency and Critical Care 16 (4), 253–263.

Powell, L.L., Rozanski, E.A., Tidwell, A.S., et al., 1999. A retrospective analysis of pulmonary contusion secondary to motor vehicular accidents in 143 dogs: 1994-1997 Department of Clinical Sciences. Journal of Veterinary Emergency and Critical Care 9 (3), 127–136.

Prittie, J., 2006. Optimal endpoints of resuscitation and early goal-directed therapy. Journal of Veterinary Emergency and Critical Care 16 (4), 329–339.

Schmiedt, C., Tobias, K.M., Otto, C.M., 2001. Evaluation of abdominal fluid: peripheral blood creatinine and potassium ratios for diagnosis of uroperitoneum in dogs. Journal of Veterinary Emergency and Critical Care 11 (4), 275–280.

Serrano, S., Boag, A.K., 2009. Pulmonary contusions and hemorrhage. In: Silverstein, D.C., Hopper, K. (Eds.), Small Animal Critical Care Medicine. Elsevier, St Louis, pp. 105–110.

Simpson, S.A., Syring, R., Otto, C.M., 2009. Severe blunt trauma in dogs: 235 cases (1997-2003). Journal of Veterinary Emergency and Critical Care 19 (6), 588–602.

Slensky, K., 2009. Thoracic trauma. In: Silverstein, D.C., Hopper, K. (Eds.), Small Animal Critical Care Medicine. Elsevier, St Louis, pp. 662–666.

Streeter, E.M., Rozanski, E.A., de Laforcade-Buress, A., et al., 2009. Evaluation of vehicular trauma in dogs: 239 cases (January-December 2001). Journal of the American Veterinary Medical Association 235, 405–408.

PNEUMOTHORAX

Lisciandro, G.R., Lagutchik, M.S., Mann, K.A., et al., 2008. Evaluation of a thoracic focused assessment with sonography for trauma (TFAST) protocol to detect pneumothorax and concurrent thoracic injury in 145 traumatized dogs. Journal of Veterinary Emergency and Critical Care 18 (3), 258–269.

McLaughlin, Jr., R.M., Roush, J.K. (guest eds), 1995. The Veterinary Clinics of North America, Small Animal Practice: Management of Orthopedic Emergencies 25 (5), 1032–1033.

Sauvé, V., 2009. Pleural space disease. In: Silverstein, D.C., Hopper, K. (Eds.), Small Animal Critical Care Medicine. Elsevier, St Louis, pp. 125 130.

Sigrist, N.E., 2009. Thoracentesis. In: Silverstein, D.C., Hopper, K. (Eds.), Small Animal Critical Care Medicine. Elsevier, St Louis, pp. 131–133.

Sigrist, N.E., 2009. Thoracostomy tube placement and drainage. In: Silverstein, D.C., Hopper, K. (Eds.), Small Animal Critical Care Medicine. Elsevier, St Louis, pp. 134–137.

Song, E.K., Mann, F.A., Wagner-Mann, C.G., 2008. Comparison of different tube materials and use of chinese finger trap or four friction suture technique for securing gastrostomy, jejunostomy, and thoracostomy tubes in dogs. Veterinary Surgery 37, 212–221.

TRAUMATIC DIAPHRAGMATIC HERNIAS

Fossum, T.W., 2002. Traumatic diaphragmatic hernias. In: Fossum, T.W. (Ed.), Small Animal Surgery, second ed. Mosby, St Louis, pp. 795–798.

Haskins, S.C., Klide, A.M. (guest eds), 1992. The Veterinary Clinics of North America, Small Animal Practice: Opinions in Small Animal Anesthesia 22 (2), 457.

Hunt, G.B., Johnson, K.A., 2003. Diaphragmatic, pericardial, and hiatal hernia. In: Slatter, D. (Ed.), Textbook of Small Animal Surgery, third ed. Saunders, Philadelphia, pp. 473–487.

McLaughlin, Jr., R.M., Roush, J.K. (guest eds), 1995. The Veterinary Clinics of North America, Small Animal Practice: Management of Orthopedic Emergencies 25 (5), 1034–1035.

Ricco, C.H., Graham, L., 2007. Undiagnosed diaphragmatic hernia – the importance of preanesthetic evaluation. Canadian Veterinary Journal 48, 615–618.

Sauvé, V., 2009. Pleural space disease. In: Silverstein, D.C., Hopper, K. (Eds.),

Small Animal Critical Care Medicine. Elsevier, St Louis, pp. 125–130.

Schmiedt, C.M., Tobias, K.M., Stevenson, M.A.M., 2003. Traumatic diaphragmatic hernia in cats: 34 cases (1991-2001). Journal of the American Veterinary Medical Association 222, 1237–1240.

BITE WOUNDS AND BITE WOUNDS

Garzotto, C.K., 2009. Wound management. In: Silverstein, D.C., Hopper, K. (Eds.), Small Animal Critical Care Medicine. Elsevier, St Louis, pp. 676–682.

Griffin, G.M., Holt, D.E., 2001. Dog-bite wounds: bacteriology and treatment outcome in 37 cases. Journal of the American Animal Hospital Association 37, 453–460.

Hedlund, C.S., 2002. Wound management. In: Fossum, T.W. (Ed.), Small Animal Surgery, second ed. Mosby, St Louis, pp. 134–148.

Meyers, B., Schoeman, J.P., Goddard, A., et al., 2008. The bacteriology and antimicrobial susceptibility of infected and non-infected dog bite wounds: Fifty cases. Veterinary Microbiology 127, 360–368.

Scheepens, E.T.F., Peeters, M.E., L'Eplattenier, H.F., et al., 2006. Thoracic bite trauma in dogs: a comparison of clinical and radiological parameters with surgical results. Journal of Small Animal Practice 47, 721–726.

Talan, D.A., Citron, D.M., Fredrick, B.S., et al., 1999. For the Emergency Medicine Animal Bite Infection Study Group. Bacteriologic Analysis of Infected Dog and Cat Bites. New England Journal of Medicine 340, 85–92.

Waldron, D.R., Zimmerman-Pope, N., 2003. Superficial skin wounds. In: Slatter, D. (Ed.), Textbook of Small Animal Surgery, third ed. Elsevier, St Louis, pp. 266–267.

DEGLOVING INJURIES

Basualdo, C., Sgroy, V., Finola, M.S., et al., 2007. Comparison of the antibacterial activity of honey from different provenance against bacteria usually isolated from skin wounds. Veterinary Microbiology 124, 375–381.

Garzotto, C.K., 2009. Wound management. In: Silverstein, D.C., Hopper, K. (Eds.), Small Animal Critical Care Medicine. Elsevier, St Louis, pp. 676–682.

Hedlund, C.S., 2002. Wound management. In: Fossum, T.W. (Ed.), Small Animal

Surgery, second ed. Mosby, St Louis, pp. 134–148.

Kirk, R.W., Bonagura, J.D. (Eds.), 1992. Current Veterinary Therapy XI. WB Saunders, Philadelphia, pp. 154–158.

Mathews, K.A., Binnington, A.G., 2002a. Wound management using sugar. Compendium for the Continuing Education of the Practicing Veterinarian 24 (1), 41–50.

Mathews, K.A., Binnington, A.G., 2002b. Wound management using honey. Compendium for the Continuing Education of the Practicing Veterinarian 24 (1), 53–60.

Waldron, D.R., Zimmerman-Pope, N., 2003. Superficial skin wounds. In: Slatter, D. (Ed.), Textbook of Small Animal Surgery, third ed. Elsevier, St Louis, p. 270.

GUNSHOT WOUNDS

Carr, B.G., Schwab, C.W., Branas, C.C., et al., 2008. Outcomes related to the number and anatomic placement of gunshot wounds. Journal of Trauma 64, 197–203.

Fullington, R.J., Otto, C.M., 1997. Characteristics, and management of gunshot wounds in dogs, and cats. Journal of the American Veterinary Medical Association 210 (5), 658–662.

McLaughlin, Jr., R.M., Roush, J.K. (guest eds), 1995. The Veterinary Clinics of North America, Small Animal Practice: Management of Orthopedic Emergencies 25 (5), 1111–1125.

Pavletic, M.M., 1996. Gunshot wound management. Compendium on Continuing Education 18 (12), 1285–1299.

Pavletic, M.M., 2004. Management of gunshot wounds in small animal practice standards of care. Emergency and Critical Care Medicine 6 (9), 1–10.

Waldron, D.R., Zimmerman-Pope, N., 2003. Superficial skin wounds. In: Slatter, D. (Ed.), Textbook of Small Animal Surgery, third ed. Elsevier, St Louis, p. 269.

FRACTURES

Boudrieau, R.J., 2003. Fractures of the radius and ulna. In: Slatter, D. (Ed.), Textbook of Small Animal Surgery, third ed. Elsevier, St Louis, pp. 1953–1973.

Boudrieau, R.J., 2003. Fractures of the tibia and fibula. In: Slatter, D. (Ed.), Textbook of Small Animal Surgery, third ed. Elsevier, St Louis, pp. 2144–2157.

Grant, G.R., Olds, R.B., 2003. Treatment of open fractures. In: Slatter, D. (Ed.), Textbook of Small Animal Surgery, third ed. Elsevier, St Louis, pp. 1793–1797.

Harasen, G., 2007. Pelvic fractures. Canadian Veterinary Journal April 48, 427–428.

Johnson, A.L., Hulse, D.A., 2002. Fundamentals of orthopedic surgery and fracture management. In: Fossum, T.W. (Ed.), Small Animal Surgery, second ed. Mosby, St Louis, pp. 821–1022.

McLaughlin, Jr., R.M., Roush, J.K. (guest eds), 1995. The Veterinary Clinics of North America, Small Animal Practice: Management of Orthopedic Emergencies 25 (5), 1093–1106.

Murtaugh, R.J., Kaplan, P.M., 1992. Veterinary Emergency, and Critical Care Medicine. Mosby, St Louis, pp. 138–143.

Piermattei, D.L., Flo, G.L., DeCamp, C.E., 2006. Handbook of Small Animal Orthopedics and Fracture Repair, fourth ed. Elsevier, St Louis, p. 742, Figure 22–745.

Piermattei, D.L., Flo, G.L., DeCamp, C.E., 2006. Handbook of Small Animal Orthopedics and Fracture Repair, fourth ed. Elsevier, St Louis, pp. 255–746.

Simpson, D.J., Lewis, D.D., 2003. Fractures of the femur. In: Slatter, D. (Ed.), Textbook of Small Animal Surgery, third ed. Elsevier, St Louis, pp. 2059–2089.

Tomlinson, J.L., 2003. Fractures of the humerus. In: Slatter, D. (Ed.), Textbook of Small Animal Surgery, third ed. Elsevier, St Louis, pp. 1905–1918.

Tomlinson, J.L., 2003. Fractures of the pelvis. In: Slatter, D. (Ed.), Textbook of Small Animal Surgery, third ed. Elsevier, St Louis, pp. 1989–2001.

AMPUTATIONS

Weigel, J.P., 2003. Amputations. In: Slatter, D. (Ed.), Textbook of Small Animal Surgery, third ed. Elsevier, St Louis, pp. 2180–2189.

COXOFEMORAL LUXATION

Holsworth, I.G., DeCamp, C.E., 2003. Coxofemoral luxation. In: Slatter, D.

(Ed.), Textbook of Small Animal Surgery, third ed. Elsevier, St Louis, pp. 2002–2008.

Johnson, A.L., Hulse, D.A., 2002. Coxofemoral luxation. In: Fossum, T.W. (Ed.), Small Animal Surgery, second ed. Mosby, St Louis, pp. 1102–1109.

Piermattei, D.L., Flo, G.L., DeCamp, C.E., 2006. Handbook of Small Animal Orthopedics and Fracture Repair, fourth ed. Elsevier, St Louis, pp. 461–467.

ELBOW LUXATION

Dassler, C.L., Vasseur, P.B., 2003. Elbow luxation. In: Slatter, D. (Ed.), Textbook of Small Animal Surgery, third ed. Elsevier, St Louis, pp. 1919–1926.

Johnson, A.L., Hulse, D.A., 2002. Traumatic elbow luxation. In: Fossum, T.W. (Ed.), Small Animal Surgery, second ed. Mosby, St Louis, pp. 1079–1022.

Piermattei, D.L., Flo, G.L., DeCamp, C.E., 2006. Handbook of Small Animal Orthopedics and Fracture Repair, fourth ed. Elsevier, St Louis, pp. 325–330.

DEHISCENCE

Fossum, T.W., 2002. Surgery of the abdominal cavity. In: Fossum, T.W. (Ed.), Small Animal Surgery, second ed. Mosby, St Louis, p. 258.

Fossum, T.W., 2002. Umbilical and abdominal hernias. In: Fossum, T.W. (Ed.), Small Animal Surgery, second ed. Mosby, St Louis, pp. 259–267.

Gower, S.B., Weisse, C.W., Brown, D.C., 2009. Major abdominal evisceration injuries in dogs and cats: 12 cases (1998-2008). Journal of the American Veterinary Medical Association 234, 1566–1572.

Hedlund, C.S., 2002. Wound management. In: Fossum, T.W. (Ed.), Small Animal Surgery, second ed. Mosby, St Louis, p. 144.

Netto, F.A., Hamilton, P., Rizoli, S.B., et al., 2006. Traumatic abdominal wall hernia: epidemiology and clinical implications. Journal of Trauma 61, 1058–1061.

Environmental emergencies

DROWNING (IMMERSION INJURY)

Diagnosis

History—The patient is found in or near water.

Physical exam—The patient is wet or damp, unless presentation for medical care has been delayed. The patient may have bradycardia, pale oral mucous membranes, weak femoral pulses, hypothermia, cyanosis, dyspnea, moist bronchovesicular sounds, epistaxis and a moist cough. Aspiration of fresh water may cause hyponatremia, hypervolemia and hypotonicity. By the time the patient reaches a veterinarian, the excess fluid has often redistributed, resulting in hypovolemia. Fresh water also alters surfactant ionic composition, altering surface tension within alveoli, which causes alveolar collapse, right-to-left intrapulmonary shunting and hypoxemia.

Aspiration of salt water may cause hypernatremia and hypovolemia. Salt water aspiration may wash out some of the surfactant but does not change the chemical properties. The hypertonic salt water draws fluid into the alveoli, again causing intrapulmonary shunting and hypoxemia. Obstruction of airways may be caused by particulate matter in aspirated water. Infection from contaminated water may cause pneumonia.

Thoracic radiographs—An alveolar pattern or a mixed interstitial–bronchial pulmonary pattern may be observed. Radiographic abnormalities may be delayed. Therapy should be initiated even if the pulmonary pattern is normal and should be based on the severity of clinical signs.

Laboratory evaluation—Measure blood gases, serum electrolytes, CBC and serum biochemical profile.

Supplemental oxygen therapy is indicated if the Pa_{O_2} is <90 mm Hg. Mechanical ventilation is indicated if the Pa_{O_2} is <60 mm Hg with an Fi_{O_2} of >50% or a Pa_{O_2} is <40 mm Hg at any FiO_2.

ECG—Bradycardia and various arrhythmias may occur.

Differential diagnosis

Acute respiratory distress syndrome, congestive heart failure, noncardiogenic pulmonary edema, pulmonary thromboembolism.

Prognosis

The prognosis is guarded, with a mortality rate of 37.5% for freshwater drowning victims. Only 11% of patients who required mechanical ventilation survived to be discharged from the hospital.

Treatment

1. Advise a telephone caller in the steps for cardiopulmonary resuscitation with mouth to nose resuscitation and external cardiac massage. Have them briefly hold the animal with its head down and compress the chest to clear the airway. Have them transport the pet immediately to the nearest open veterinary facility. The patient should be wrapped in a warm blanket if one is available.
2. Inform the client of the diagnosis, prognosis and cost of the treatment.
3. Hospitalization and observation for at least 24 hours.
4. Administer oxygen:
   A. Oxygen cage
   B. Elizabethan collar oxygen hood
   C. Nasal catheter
   D. Mask
   E. Place an endotracheal tube and provide mechanical ventilation, with positive end-expiratory pressure, if indicated; PEEP of 5 cm or higher is usually needed in cases of freshwater drowning because of surfactant damage and higher alveolar surface tension.
5. Place an intravenous catheter.
6. Administer intravenous fluid therapy with balanced electrolyte crystalloids, cautiously. Monitor carefully for pulmonary edema.
7. If the patient presents in severe shock and has pulmonary edema, administer Hetastarch or Dextran 70, 20 mL/kg IV. An additional 20 mL/kg of Hetastarch may be administered over the next 6–8 hours if needed for continued shock.
8. Monitor the patient's body temperature. Hypothermia is common.
   A. Submersion in ice water causes a 'diving reflex' in dogs, which results in apnea, bradycardia, selective vasoconstriction and shunting of blood to the brain and heart.
   B. If the patient's temperature is <89.5°F (<32°C), use warmed IV fluids, blankets, heating pads, warm water baths, warmed oxygen, etc. to carefully rewarm the patient.
   C. If resuscitative efforts are not successful, they should not be discontinued until the patient is normothermic. ('You're not dead until you are warm and dead.')
9. The administration of corticosteroids is not recommended.
10. Do not administer broad-spectrum systemic antibiotics unless bacterial pneumonia or sepsis occurs.

11. Consider the administration of pentoxifylline,15 mg/kg PO q8h, which has been shown to decrease neutrophil infiltration into lung tissue.

ELECTROCUTION

Diagnosis

History—Exposure to electrical cords or other electrical source, or observation by the owner.

Physical exam—Burns affecting the oral cavity may be tan, gray or pale yellow and may have blackened margins. They are usually found on the tongue and the buccal or lingual mucosa. There may be increased oral sensitivity, burns affecting the feet, and extensive tissue necrosis. Dyspnea, neurogenic pulmonary edema, respiratory arrest, seizures, cardiac arrhythmias, such as ventricular fibrillation, and gastrointestinal and musculoskeletal injuries may occur.

Thoracic radiographs—These may illustrate pulmonary edema in the perihilar region or in the caudal lung lobes. Radiographic changes may not appear for 18–24 hours. Consider repeating later.

Laboratory evaluation—

1. Immediately upon presentation, measure PCV, TS, blood gases, ACT or PT and PTT, BUN and blood glucose.
2. As time permits, evaluate the CBC, serum biochemical profile, including electrolytes, urinalysis and other individual tests as needed.
3. Repeatedly monitor ECG, blood pressure and blood gases for the first 48 hours.

Differential diagnosis

Acute respiratory distress syndrome, feline bronchial disease, pleural effusion, trauma.

Prognosis

The prognosis is guarded to poor.

Treatment

1. Quickly inform the client of the diagnosis, prognosis and cost of the treatment.
2. Assure a patent airway.
3. Administer oxygen if the patient is dyspneic or cyanotic.
4. Place an intravenous catheter.
5. Administer furosemide, 2–4 mg/kg IV in dogs, and 2 mg/kg IV in cats. Furosemide may not help patients with fulminating pulmonary edema.
6. If the patient has fulminating pulmonary edema, perform intubation and assisted ventilation.
7. Administer bronchodilators if pulmonary edema is present:
   A. Aminophylline, 6–10 mg/kg PO, IM or IV, q6–8h in dogs, or 4–8 mg/kg IM, SC, PO q12h in cats

B. Theophylline, 4–8 mg/kg PO, q6–8h

C. Long-acting theophylline (Theo-Dur®), 10–25mg/kg PO, q12h

D. Terbutaline (Brethine®):

   I. Dog: 1.25–5 mg PO q8–12h or 0.01 mg/kg SC q4h

   II. Cat: 0.625 mg PO q8h or 0.01 mg/kg SC q4h.

E. Albuterol (Proventil®), 0.02–0.05 mg/kg PO q8h.

8. If the patient presents in shock, administer balanced electrolyte crystalloids at 90 mL/kg for the first hour in dogs, and at 60 mL/kg for the first hour in cats. Monitor fluid therapy very closely, especially if the patient has pulmonary edema.

9. Avoid colloids and hypertonic saline administration unless the patient is in severe hypovolemic shock. During the first 6–8 hours following the electrical event, avoid the administration of plasma or synthetic colloids due to the increased susceptibility for pulmonary edema.

10. Monitor the heart with an ECG repeatedly. Treat cardiac arrhythmias as indicated.

11. Administer analgesics, such as morphine, oxymorphone, hydromorphone, or buprenorphine, as indicated by the patient's individual needs. Until the patient is stabilized and normal renal function is established, avoid the administration of nonsteroidal anti-inflammatory analgesics.

12. Monitor urine output. Minimal urine output should be 1–2 mL/kg/h in dogs, 0.5–1 mL/kg/h in cats.

13. To ease the patient's discomfort from oral burns, administer sucralfate suspension or a protective emollient such as triamcinolone acetonide paste (Orabase®) to the lesions.

14. Provide nutritional support, either orally or by the administration of partial parenteral nutrition. Place a feeding tube if the oral lesions are severe and long-term nutritional support is necessary.

HEAT STRESS AND HEAT STROKE

Diagnosis

Etiology—Heat stroke may be exertional or nonexertional in dogs and cats. There is often a history of excessive exposure to heat. The duration of exposure is variable, depending on environmental conditions and the animal's physical condition prior to the heat exposure. Heat stroke may occur owing to an increased metabolic rate, such as from exertion or malignant hyperthermia, as can occur secondary to other diseases and halothane anesthesia. Heat stroke may also occur in patients with a decreased cooling response from either respiratory depression or compromise (airway obstructions, cardiac or pulmonary disease), in patients with decreased convective heat loss such as in obesity or secondary to various medications (including diuretics, phenothiazines, and beta blockers) or due to a lack of acclimatization. Accidental entrapment inside an operating clothes dryer may cause heat stroke. Heat stroke also occurs in animals that are confined in areas with poor ventilation, especially in times of high humidity and high environmental temperature, combined with water deprivation. Brachycephalic dog breeds, such as bulldogs, are predisposed. Obesity, cardiorespiratory disease, including laryngeal paralysis, and advanced age are also predisposing factors.

History—Owners notice excessive panting, hypersalivation, listlessness, muscle tremors, vomiting diarrhea, ataxia, collapse, loss of consciousness and seizures.

Physical exam—Elevated body temperature (>104.9°F, 40.5°C) upon entry, congested mucous membranes, panting, tachycardia and hyperdynamic pulses are seen early in the disease process. If disseminated intravascular coagulopathy (DIC) occurs, petechia, hemoptysis, hematemesis and hematochezia may be observed. As the patient's condition worsens, gray mucous membranes, weak pulses, vomiting, bloody diarrhea, melena, depression, ataxia, cortical blindness, seizures, coma and death may occur. The patient's body temperature may be normal or low upon entry if the patient is in circulatory shock or the owner has taken steps to lower the temperature. Permanent brain damage may result at temperatures of 105.8°F (41°C).

Laboratory evaluation—Immediately upon entry, evaluate PCV, total solids, BUN, blood glucose, sodium, potassium, lactate and blood gases.

Evaluate a blood smear for the presence and number of NRBC (per 100 WBC). The morphology of the RBCs should be assessed, as schistocytes are common in DIC. PT, PTT, CBC, including platelet count, or thromboelastography may reveal DIC. During therapy, continue to re-evaluate ACT or PTT. A serum biochemical profile and urinalysis should also be evaluated.

Activated coagulation time—the normal ACT for a dog is 60–110 seconds and for a cat it is 50–75 seconds. In acute DIC, there is a slight to moderate prolongation in ACT (110–200 seconds in dogs, 75–120 seconds in cats). In end-stage DIC, there is marked prolongation of ACT (>200 seconds in dogs, >120 seconds in cats). The ACT tubes should be warmed to 37°C prior to and during the test procedure. Two tubes should be used; 2 mL of blood are taken by clean venipuncture with rapid aspiration from a large vein, directly into the first tube with a Vacutainer® system, or quickly transferred from a syringe into the first tube and discarded. Without removing the needle from the vein, additional blood is placed into the second tube and the test is performed. The time interval from injection of 2 mL of blood into the ACT tube until the first visible appearance of clot formation is determined to be the ACT.

The evaluation of the PTT can be substituted for the ACT and is available on in-house analyzers. Normal values depend upon methodology and are provided by the manufacturer.

An ECG should be evaluated every few hours initially. Ventricular arrhythmias are common.

Differential diagnosis

Malignant hyperthermia, strychnine toxicity, metaldehyde toxicity, amphetamine ingestion, macadamia nut ingestion, eclampsia, seizures of other etiologies, meningitis, encephalitis, other infectious or inflammatory disorders, and space-occupying lesions of the thermoregulatory center of the hypothalamus.

Prognosis

The prognosis varies with the severity and duration of hyperthermia. Negative prognostic indicators include persistent hypoglycemia, coma or progressively worsening neurologic status, presence of DIC, a higher relative NRBC count (over 18 NRBC/100 WBC versus an average of 2/100 WBC in survivors) and acute kidney injury. Death generally occurs within the first 24 hours. In one study, 64% of patients survived.

Treatment

1. Advise the telephone caller to spray cool water on their pet and bring the pet in for evaluation immediately. Do not have the caller apply ice water or induce rapid cooling as that is associated with an increased incidence of complications such as DIC.
2. Simultaneously provide supplemental oxygen administration (provide a patent airway if needed), administer IV fluids and initiate external cooling.
3. Inform the client of the diagnosis, prognosis and cost of the treatment.
4. Begin oxygen administration immediately upon entry, regardless of the patient's mental status. Place a nasal oxygen catheter or use Elizabethan collar hood oxygenation. Be cautious with oxygen cages as they tend to become hot and worsen the patient's condition.
5. Place an intravenous catheter, or two if the patient is a large breed dog.
6. Obtain pretreatment blood samples and obtain a minimum database.
7. Administer a balanced electrolyte crystalloid intravenous fluid rapidly IV, in shock doses (60–90 mL/kg/h in dogs, 45–60 mL/kg/h in cats).
8. Colloids may be administered in addition to crystalloids, but decrease the dose of crystalloids by 40–60%.
9. Slowly cool the patient by rinsing the body in cool water. The patient may be sprayed with water and placed in front of fans or immersed in a cool water bath. Avoid immersion in ice , which may induce DIC by causing vasoconstriction, capillary sludging and decreased cutaneous blood flow. Concentrate on the neck over the jugular veins and on the abdomen. An ice pack may be placed on the patient's head.
10. Internal cooling methods such as cold water gastric lavage and cold water enemas may enhance cooling but also interfere with monitoring of core temperature.
11. Monitor the patient's body temperature closely. Stop rinsing the body with cool water when the temperature reaches 103.0–103.5°F (39.5°C), to avoid hypothermia.
12. Provide supplemental dextrose in the IV fluids as needed to treat hypoglycemia.
13. Do not administer glucocorticoids or NSAIDs.

14. Administer sucralfate and famotidine or ranitidine to protect the gastrointestinal tract.
15. The administration of broad-spectrum systemic antibiotics is controversial, but may be considered to treat sepsis from bacterial translocation. A combination of ampicillin or cefazolin, enrofloxacin, and clindamycin or metronidazole is commonly recommended.
16. After the initial fluid resuscitation, treat electrolyte imbalances and acid–base disorders.
17. Perform repeated ECGs; monitor for cardiac arrhythmias. Treat cardiac arrhythmias as indicated, making sure electrolyte imbalances are corrected as a first step of therapy.
18. Monitor urine output; administer furosemide or mannitol if necessary after rehydration is achieved. Placement of a closed urinary collection system will facilitate monitoring.
19. Monitor and treat pulmonary edema. Administer furosemide if needed.
20. Administer diazepam as needed to control seizures.
21. Monitor the coagulation status with ACT, PTT or thromboelastography.
    A. If the patient has DIC, administer fresh frozen plasma. The dosage varies from 10 to 30 mL/kg IV.
    B. Heparin therapy is controversial, but should be considered.
       I. The dosage of unfractionated heparin is 100–200 IU/kg SC q8h or 10 IU/kg/h IV CRI for 2 hours. The goal of therapy is to prolong the PTT 1.5 times.
       II. Enoxaparin (Lovenox®), a low molecular weight heparin, is administered at the dosage of 0.8–1 mg/kg SC q6–8h in dogs and 1.0–1.25 mg/kg SC q8–12h in cats.
       III. Dalteparin (Fragmin®), another low molecular weight heparin, is administered at the dosage of 100–150 U/kg SC q8–12h in dogs and 180 IU/kg SC q4–6h in cats.

HYPOTHERMIA AND FROSTBITE

Lowering of the body temperature in nonhibernating animals causes the normal physiologic and metabolic processes to slow. Hypothermia (a body temperature less than 99.5°F (37.5°C) in dogs, and less than 100.0°F (37.8°C) in cats) may occur during a disease process; be caused by sedation, anesthesia or surgery; or may be caused by accidental exposure to a cold environment with inadequate shelter.

When the rectal temperature lowers to 82°F (27.8°C) or less, dogs and cats lose the ability to return their body temperature to normal, but with treatment they may survive. The extent of the injuries to body tissues varies with the actual temperature of the body and the duration of the hypothermic condition.

- Animals may survive conditions of mild hypothermia (30–32°C [86–90°F]) for 24–36 hours.
- Animals usually do not survive after 4–24 hours of moderate hypothermia (22–25°C [72–77°F]).
- The maximum survival time from severe hypothermia (less than 15°C [60°F]) is 6 hours.

Environmental emergencies

187

Frostbite (avascular necrosis) occurs following exposure to a cold environment, with body temperatures below 34°C (93°F); following freezing of any exposed body surface; or following contact with cold liquid, glass or metal. Exposure to cold causes destruction of superficial tissues secondary to the disturbances of blood flow through small surface blood vessels.

Frostbite occurs more commonly in the young or poorly nourished animal that is exposed to extreme cold and storms. The most commonly affected body areas in dogs and cats are the pinnae of the ears, the tail, the external genitalia and the footpads.

Diagnosis

Clinical signs of hypothermia
1. Clinical signs vary depending on body core temperature and the duration of the hypothermic condition.
2. Body temperature of less than 99.5°F (37.5°C) in dogs, and less than 100.0°F (37.8°C) in cats.
3. Altered mental state varying from depression to unconsciousness.
4. Bradycardia.
5. Hypotension.
6. Shivering may be observed but is absent in patients with body temperatures less than 87.8°F (31°C).
7. Respiration is slow and shallow.
8. Cardiac arrhythmias may be present, with ventricular arrhythmias being the most common.

Clinical signs of frostbite
1. Acute
   A. The patient has pale skin.
   B. The skin is cool to the touch.
   C. There may be hyperesthesia of affected body parts.
   D. Cyanosis may be apparent.
2. With thawing
   A. Tissue becomes erythematous.
   B. The patient may experience considerable pain.
   C. Localized swelling due to edema may be observed.
3. Chronic (several days later)
   A. Tissues may shrink.
   B. Discoloration may occur.
4. 20–30 days later
   A. Alopecia may occur.
   B. Sloughing of necrotic tissue may be observed.

Treatment

Treatment of hypothermia
1. Oxygen administration; intubate if necessary.
2. Place an intravenous catheter; begin rapid infusion of warmed (104–109°F, 43°C) balanced electrolyte crystalloid fluids.

3. Administer dextrose intravenously if the patient is very young or hypoglycemic.
4. Rapid return of the body core temperature is necessary.
   A. Move the patient from the cold environment into a warm room.
   B. Wrap the patient in warm blankets.
   C. Apply warm water bottles; be sure to have a towel or blanket between the bottle and the patient's skin to avoid thermal burns.
   D. Place the patient in an incubator or on a heating pad (use caution not to induce thermal burns).
   E. Turn a laterally recumbent patient from side to side every 2 hours.
   F. Immerse the patient in a warm water bath.
   G. Consider warm peritoneal dialysis if the hypothermic state has been prolonged or the body temperature is less than 32°C (89.6°F).
   H. Consider warm colonic lavage if the hypothermic state has been prolonged or the body temperature is less than 32°C (89.6°F).
   I. Consider warm gastric lavage if the hypothermic state has been prolonged or the body temperature is less than 32°C (89.6°F).
   J. Monitor and treat cardiac arrhythmias as necessary.

Treatment of frostbite
1. Remove the patient from the source of the cold.
2. Apply warm compresses to the affected areas.
3. Immerse the affected areas into warm (39–40°C (102–104°F)) water.
4. Do not rub the affected areas.
5. Gently dry the areas and apply cotton bandages, but do not apply pressure dressings.
6. Do not administer corticosteroids.
7. Administer prophylactic antibiotics.
8. Administer analgesics as needed for pain control.
9. Prevent self-trauma by applying an Elizabethan collar or bandages.
10. Do not allow affected areas to refreeze after the initial thawing.
11. Amputation is not appropriate in emergency clinic situations, as many tissues recover that do not appear viable initially.

SMOKE INHALATION

Diagnosis

History—Exposure to smoke and possibly fire.
Physical exam—Many physical changes will not be apparent for 24–48 hours after the incident. With all patients, evaluate the nose, mouth and upper airways, particularly the larynx for edema.
Stain both corneas with fluorescein, looking for corneal ulcers. Evaluate mucous membrane color: red mucous membranes indicate carbon monoxide toxicity; cyanotic mucous membranes indicate respiratory injury; pale mucous membranes indicate shock or destruction of red blood cells.
Examine the ears, neck, trunk, limbs, footpads, abdomen, urinary bladder, genitalia and anus. Look carefully under the hair coat. Pluck

some hair in several sites. If a partial or full-thickness burn is present, the hair may be easily epilated. Clip hair around visible wounds.

There are four classes of pulmonary injury:

I. *Minimal pulmonary injury* – the patient may smell of smoke, have singed whiskers, or have soot in its hair coat, saliva or nasal discharge. The patient is alert; respiratory rate is normal to slightly increased. The patient will rarely have facial burns or pale oral mucous membranes. Occasionally, there will be an oculonasal discharge. Thoracic radiographs are normal. The prognosis is good.

II. *Slight pulmonary injury* – the patient may smell of smoke, have singed whiskers, or have soot in its hair coat, saliva or nasal discharge. The patient is distressed. The respiratory rate is mildly to moderately increased. The patient will occasionally have burns, pale mucous membranes and oculonasal discharge. The oral mucous membranes will rarely be cherry red. Thoracic radiographs are usually normal. The prognosis is fair.

III. *Moderate pulmonary injury* – the patient may smell of smoke, have singed whiskers, or have soot in its hair coat, saliva or nasal discharge. The patient is highly distressed, has tachypnea, facial burns, oculonasal discharge, and often will have pale oral mucous membranes. Occasionally, the oral mucous membranes will be cherry red. Thoracic radiographs vary from normal to showing signs of pulmonary consolidation. The prognosis is guarded to poor.

IV. *Severe pulmonary injury* – the patient may smell of smoke, have singed whiskers, or have soot in its hair coat, saliva or nasal discharge. The patient is unconscious, with bradypnea or apnea. Facial burns are usually present. The patient usually has cherry red oral mucous membranes and an oculonasal discharge. Thoracic radiographs vary from normal to pulmonary consolidation. The prognosis is very poor.

Neurologic abnormalities—There are also reports of delayed-onset post-hypoxic neurologic symptoms associated with leukoencephalomalacia after exposure to smoke or carbon monoxide. In one case, a dog developed progressive neurologic signs 6 days after rescue from an apartment fire. At necropsy performed 3 days later, laminar necrosis of cerebrocortical neurons and leukoencephalomalacia of the central cerebral white matter was observed.

Thoracic radiographs—Abnormal findings may not appear until 16–24 hours after the injury; however, baseline radiographs will be useful for patient monitoring. Radiographic changes may be normal or abnormalities may range from a diffuse, patchy, interstitial infiltration or a mixed interstitial and alveolar pattern with air bronchograms to pulmonary consolidation.

ECG—May show signs of hypoxia or may be normal.

Laboratory evaluation—

1. Immediately upon presentation, measure PCV, TS, blood gases, lactate, PT and PTT or ACT, BUN and blood glucose.
2. As time permits, evaluate the CBC, serum biochemical profile including electrolytes, urinalysis and other individual tests as needed.

3. Repeatedly monitor ECG, blood pressure and blood gases for the first 48 hours.
4. The Pa_{O_2} of peripheral blood may be reported as falsely normal owing to interference by carbon monoxide. Carboxyhemoglobin levels can be measured by human laboratories or on a cooximeter.

Differential diagnosis

Aspiration pneumonia, pulmonary edema, acute respiratory distress syndrome, heart failure, bronchopneumonia, feline chronic bronchial disease.

Treatment

Class I—
1. Treat burns symptomatically.
2. Inform the client of the diagnosis, prognosis and cost of the treatment.
3. Stain both corneas with fluorescein; ulcerative keratitis is a common sequela. Treat with antibiotic ophthalmic preparations; avoid corticosteroid preparations.
4. Observation for 24–48 hours.

*Class II—*Treat as for Class I, and:
5. Provide a low-humidity oxygen-enriched environment (5–15%) for 1 6 hours, then re-evaluate.
6. Place an intravenous catheter in an unburned area on a limb.
7. Administer balanced electrolyte crystalloid intravenous fluids at 90 mL/kg for the first hour in dogs and at 50–60 mL/kg for the first hour in cats. Monitor fluid therapy very closely, especially if the patient has pulmonary edema.
8. After the shock dose of fluids has been administered, administer fluids at maintenance rates, plus replace losses by the following formula:
   2–4 mg/kg × % total body surface area (TBSA) of burn (dogs)
   1–2 mL/kg × % total body surface area (TBSA) of burn (cats).
   During the first 8 hours following shock fluid therapy, administer half of the fluids calculated by the above formula, the final half over the next 16 hours.
9. Avoid colloids and hypertonic saline administration unless the patient is in severe hypovolemic shock. During the first 6–8 hours following the injury, avoid the administration of plasma or synthetic colloids due to the increased susceptibility for pulmonary edema. If plasma is required to maintain albumin levels prior to 6 hours post-injury, administer at 2–3 mL/kg, doubled if necessary.
10. Avoid corticosteroid administration, unless needed for shock or pharyngeal or laryngeal edema.
11. Administer analgesics, intravenously if possible:
    A. Hydromorphone
       I. Dog: 0.05–0.2 mg/kg IV, IM, or SC q2–6h; 0.0125–0.05 mg/kg/h IV CRI
       II. Cat: 0.05–0.2 mg/kg IV, IM, or SC q2–6h

B. Fentanyl
   I. Dog: 2–10 μg/kg IV to effect, followed by 1–10 μg/kg/h IV CRI
   II. Cat: 1–5 μg/kg/h to effect, followed by 1–5 μg/kg/h IV CRI
C. Morphine
   I. Dog: 0.5–1 mg/kg IM, SC; 0.05–0.1 mg/kg IV
   II. Cat: 0.005–0.2 mg/kg IM, SC
D. Buprenorphine
   I. Dog: 0.005–0.02 mg/kg IV, IM q4–8h; 2–4 μg/kg/h IV CRI; 0.12 mg/kg OTM
   II. Cat: 0.005–0.01 mg/kg IV, IM q4–8h; 1–3 μg/kg/h IV CRI; 0.02 mg/kg OTM
E. Morphine, hydromorphone and fentanyl can each be combined with lidocaine (dogs only) and ketamine for a multimodal approach to analgesia.

Classes III and IV—Treat as for Classes I and II, and:
12. Administer 80–100% oxygen for at least 20–30 minutes, then provide an intermediately hydrated oxygen-enriched environment (15–30%).
    A. Intubate or place a tracheostomy tube if indicated.
    B. Administer oxygen for at least 4 hours. Intermittent positive-pressure ventilation (IPPV) or positive end-expiratory pressure (PEEP) may be beneficial in severely dyspneic patients.
13. Suction the upper airway if excessive secretions accumulate, but avoid damaging pharyngeal and laryngeal tissues.
14. If there are burns, cool the damaged areas with water or saline immersion, compresses or sprays for at least 30 minutes. Monitor the patient's body temperature and avoid hypothermia.
15. Apply silver sulfadiazine ointment and sterile occlusive dressings to wounds. Oxymorphone 0.04–0.06 mg/kg IV or hydromorphone 0.025–0.05 mg/kg/h IV CRI and ketamine 1–2 mg/kg IV may be useful for providing analgesia for wound care.
16. Lavage, debride and dress wounds at least once daily, using aseptic technique.
17. If the patient has severe pulmonary edema, administer furosemide, 2–4 mg/kg in dogs, 2 mg/kg in cats, IV.
18. If there is severe acute lung injury, with airway edema, exudation and possibly obstruction secondary to smoke inhalation, the nebulization of epinephrine may be beneficial. For an adult large dog (about 50 lbs / 23 kg), consider nebulization of 4 mg of epinephrine dissolved in saline over 30 minutes every 4 hours. This may help decrease airway erythema, edema and exudation, and improve air flow.
19. Administer bronchodilators:
    A. Aminophylline, 6–10 mg/kg PO, IM or IV, q6–8h in dogs or 4–8 mg/kg IM, SC, PO q12h in cats
    B. Theophylline, 4–8 mg/kg PO, q6–8h
    C. Long-acting theophylline (Theo-Dur®), 10–25 mg/kg PO, q12h
    D. Terbutaline (Brethine®)

I. Dogs: 1.25–5 mg PO q8–12h or 0.01 mg/kg SC q4h

II. Cats: 0.625 mg PO q8h or 0.01 mg/kg SC q4h

   E. Albuterol (Proventil®): 0.02–0.05 mg/kg PO q8h.

20. Promote airway secretion clearance.

   A. Maintain normal hydration status.

   B. Use a humidifier or vaporizer.

   C. Coupage or percussion of the chest.

   D. Consider the administration of an expectorant such as guaifenesin (Organidin®, 0.25–0.5 mL/10 lb (4.5 kg) PO q6h to dogs).

21. Administer antitussive medications cautiously, especially if the patient has excessive airway secretions:

   A. Hydrocodone, 0.25 mg/kg PO, q6–12h

   B. Butorphanol, 0.05–0.1 mg/kg SC, q6–12h, 0.5–1 mg/kg PO q6–12h

   C. Dextromethorphan, 1–2 mg/kg PO, q6–8h

     I. Robitussin® pediatric cough syrup contains 1.5 mg dextromethorphan/mL

     II. Vicks Formula 44® syrup contains 2 mg dextromethorphan/mL

     III. Mucinex Cough Mini-Melts for Children contains 5 mg dextromethorphan HBr and 100 mg guaifenesin per packet

   D. Codeine, 1–2 mg/kg PO, q6–12h.

22. Monitor ECG and arterial blood pressure continuously or frequently over the first 72 hours.

23. Monitor urine output. Normal urine output is 1–2 mL/kg/h. Acute renal failure is a common sequela.

24. Administer antibiotics as indicated by culture and sensitivity if infection occurs, or broad-spectrum antibiotics if the patient becomes septic.

25. Administer sucralfate, 0.5–1.0 g/dog or 0.25 g/cat PO q8h, or famotidine or ranitidine (0.5–1 mg/kg IV, dog; 2.5 mg/kg IV cat; q12h), to decrease gastric ulceration.

26. To ease the patient's discomfort from oral burns, administer sucralfate suspension or a protective emollient such as Orabase® (Squibb) to the lesions.

27. Provide nutritional support, either orally or by the administration of partial parenteral nutrition. Place a feeding tube if the oral lesions are severe and long-term nutritional support is necessary.

   A. The caloric needs are twice resting requirements.

   B. Avoid high-glucose administration, which increases CO_2 production and respiratory effort.

   C. Supplement with vitamins and minerals, especially A, C and zinc.

REFERENCES/FURTHER READING

DROWNING (IMMERSION INJURY)

Goldkamp, C.E., Schaer, M., 2008. Canine drowning. Compendium on Continuing Education for the Practicing Veterinarian 30 (6), 340–352.

Ibsen, L.M., Koch, T., 2002. Submersion and asphyxial injury. Critical Care Medicine 30 (suppl), S402–S408.

Powell, L.L., 2009. Drowning and submersion injury. In: Silverstein, D.C.,

Hopper, K. (Eds.), Small Animal Critical Care Medicine. Elsevier, St Louis, pp. 730–733.

ELECTROCUTION

Kirk, R.W., Bistner, S.I., Ford, R.B. (Eds.), 1990. Handbook of Veterinary Procedures and Emergency Treatment, fifth ed. WB Saunders, Philadelphia, p. 162.

Mathews, K.A., 1996. Veterinary Emergency and Critical Care Manual. Lifelearn Inc, Ontario, pp. 31–1 to 31–7.

Mann, F.A., 2009. Electrical and lightning injuries. In: Silverstein, D.C., Hopper, K. (Eds.), Small Animal Critical Care Medicine. Elsevier, St Louis, pp. 687–690.

Murtaugh, R.J., Kaplan, P.M., 1992. Veterinary Emergency and Critical Care Medicine. Mosby, St Louis, pp. 207–209.

Slatter, D.H. (Ed.), 1993. Textbook of Small Animal Surgery, vol. 1, second ed. WB Saunders, Philadelphia, pp. 365–367.

HEAT STRESS AND HEAT STROKE

Aroch, I., Segev, G., Loeb, E., et al., 2009. Peripheral nucleated red blood cells as a prognostic indicator in heatstroke in dogs. Journal of Veterinary Internal Medicine 23, 544–551.

Bouchama, A., Knochel, J.P., 2002. Heat stroke 1978–1988. New England Journal of Medicine 346 (25), 1978–1988.

Drobatz, K.J., 2009. Heat stroke. In: Silverstein, D.C., Hopper, K. (Eds.), Small Animal Critical Care Medicine. Elsevier, St Louis, pp. 723–726.

Drobatz, K.J., Macintire, D.K., 1996. Heat-induced illness in dogs: 42 cases (1976–1993). Journal of the American Veterinary Medical Association 209 (11), 1894–1899.

Johnson, S.L., McMichael, M., White, G., 2006. Heatstroke in small animal medicine: a clinical practice review. Journal of Veterinary Emergency and Critical Care 16 (2), 112–119.

HYPOTHERMIA AND FROSTBITE

Bonagura, J.D., Kirk, R.W. (Eds.), 1995. Current Veterinary Therapy XII. WB Saunders, Philadelphia, pp. 157–161.

Fenner, W.R., 1991. Quick Reference to Veterinary Medicine, second ed. JB Lippincott, Philadelphia, p. 629.

Hoskins, J.D., 1995. Veterinary Pediatrics, second ed. WB Saunders, Philadelphia, pp. 555–558.

Kirk, R.W. (Ed.), 1986. Current Veterinary Therapy IX. WB Saunders, Philadelphia, p. 551.

Kirk, R.W., Bistner, S.I., Ford, R.B. (Ed.), 1990. Handbook of Veterinary Procedures and Emergency Treatment, fifth ed. WB Saunders, Philadelphia, pp. 90–91.

Murtaugh, R.J., Kaplan, P.M., 1992. Veterinary Emergency, and Critical Care Medicine. Mosby Year Book, St Louis, pp.196–199, 210–211.

Todd, J., Powell, L.L., 2009. Hypothermia. In: Silverstein, D.C., Hopper, K. (Eds.), Small Animal Critical Care Medicine. Elsevier, St Louis, pp. 720–726.

SMOKE INHALATION

Jasani, S., Hughes, D., 2009. Smoke inhalation. In: Silverstein, D.C., Hopper, K. (Eds), Small Animal Critical Care Medicine. Elsevier, St Louis, pp. 118–121.

Kirk, R.W., Bonagura, J.D. (Eds), 1992. Current Veterinary Therapy XI. WB Saunders, Philadelphia, pp. 146–154.

Kirk, R.W., Bistner, S.I., Ford, R.B. (Ed.), 1990. Handbook of Veterinary Procedures and Emergency Treatment, fifth ed. WB Saunders, Philadelphia, pp. 210–211.

Lange, M., Hamahata, A., Traber, D.L., et al., 2011. Preclinical evaluation of epinephrine nebulization to reduce airway hyperemia and improve oxygenation after smoke inhalation injury. Critical Care Medicine 39 (5), 1–7.

Mariani, C.L., 2003. Full recovery following delayed neurologic signs after smoke inhalation in a dog. Journal of Veterinary Emergency and Critical Care 13 (4), 235–239.

Mathews, K.A., 1996. Veterinary Emergency, and Critical Care Manual. Lifelearn Inc, Ontario, pp. 31–1 to 31–7.

Murtaugh, R.J., Kaplan, P.M., 1992. Veterinary Emergency and Critical Care Medicine. Mosby, St Louis, pp. 410–411.

Dermatologic emergencies

ABSCESSATION

Diagnosis

History—The affected cat is usually an outside cat or living in a multiple cat household. Dogs can develop an abscess following inoculation of bacteria under the skin by trauma or foreign body perforation. The owner may observe lethargy, anorexia, lameness, swelling or a wound.
Physical exam—There may be a draining puncture wound or a fluctuant swelling, or the cat may exhibit nonspecific signs such as anorexia, lethargy and fever. Some cats will have severe cutaneous necrosis and extensive undermining of the subcutaneous tissues, resulting in a very large necrotic skin lesion. The cat may be lame if the injury is on a limb.
Laboratory evaluation—The cat should be tested for feline leukemia and feline immunodeficiency virus infections. Depending upon the physical status on entry, a CBC and a serum biochemical profile may also be indicated.

Prognosis

The prognosis is fair to good, depending on response to therapy, location and severity. If the cat has an immune system compromising disease such as feline leukemia or feline immunodeficiency virus infections, the incidence of complications, prolonged recovery, and recurrent infections increases and the prognosis worsens.

Treatment

1. Inform the client of the diagnosis, prognosis and cost of the treatment.
2. Administer parenteral antibiotics as soon as possible after admission. Recommendations include:
   A. Penicillin
   B. Amoxicillin

C. Amoxicillin-clavulanate
D. Third-generation cephalosporins such as cefpodoxime proxetil (Simplicef) or cefovecin sodium (Convenia)
E. Metronidazole
F. Clindamycin
G. Chloramphenicol.
3. Administer subcutaneous or intravenous fluids, if indicated. Be cautious when giving subcutaneous fluids; keep in mind the location of the abscess so that the cellulitis is not spread.
4. Provide anesthesia if necessary. Administer an analgesic.
5. Carefully assess the extent of the trauma before administering anesthesia.
6. Clip, scrub and flush wounds with sterile physiologic saline, LRS or Ringer's solution.
7. Surgically prepare a site over the ventral aspect of the mature abscess that has not drained, and surgically lance and drain the abscess if necessary. Lance the abscess in a ventrally dependent area if possible to promote drainage.
8. Flush, clean and debride the abscess of necrotic tissue. Remove a small piece of skin from the opening of the abscess to delay closure and promote drainage.
9. Suture abscesses closed and place Penrose drains only if there is a *large* defect in skin or if the anatomic location dictates closure.
10. Hospitalize the patient for recovery from anesthesia as needed.
11. Dispense 5–7 days of oral antibiotics.
12. Dispense wound care, feline leukemia virus and feline immunodeficiency virus handouts.
13. Instruct the client on wound care. Have the client clean the lesion and possibly flush open wounds daily.
14. Instruct the client not to give the patient aspirin, ibuprofen, acetaminophen or other over-the-counter medications.
15. Have the client take the patient in for re-evaluation in 3–4 days.

BURNS

Diagnosis

History—Exposure to hot water, grease or tar, or to fires, electrical cords, or wires.

Physical exam—Erythematous and edematous focal lesion with alopecia, varying degrees of inflammatory response, and possible eschar formation. Singed and burned hairs may be evident as well. The 'rule of nines' is applied to determine the total body surface area (TBSA) of the burns:
1. The head is counted as 9%.
2. The thorax is counted as 18%.
3. The abdomen is counted as 18%.
4. Each forelimb is counted as 9%.
5. Each hindlimb is counted as 18%.
6. $9 + 18 + 18 + 9 + 9 + 18 + 18 = 99\%$.

Classification of burns—
1. *First degree* – superficial: involves the entire epidermis; painful, erythematous, with or without vesicles. Hair may be singed but firmly attached. Healing is rapid once epithelial desquamation has occurred.
2. *Second degree* – partial thickness: involves the epidermis and the dermis. The lesion(s) is (are) painful but hair may be intact; severe subcutaneous edema develops. Heals slowly after sloughing.
3. *Third degree* – full thickness: involves the dermis and subcutaneous tissues. The lesion(s) is (are) painless, hair falls out, and skin may be black or pearly white. Healing is slow unless grafting is performed.
4. *Fourth degree* – involves muscle and bone.

Laboratory evaluation—
1. Immediately upon presentation, measure PCV, TS, blood gases, ACT or PT and PTT, BUN and blood glucose.
2. As time permits, evaluate the CBC, serum biochemical profile, including electrolytes, urinalysis and other individual tests as needed.
3. Repeatedly monitor ECG, blood pressure and blood gases for the first 48 hours.
4. Monitor albumin levels until granulation beds are formed.

Prognosis

Increased severity of burns on very young or very old patients, and burns that involve the head or joints worsen the prognosis. The prognosis is worse if >20% of the body is involved with second- to third-degree burns.

Burns require prompt evaluation of the extent and injury to other systems. They are usually very painful. Euthanasia should be a serious consideration if the injuries are severe.

Treatment

1. Inform the client of the diagnosis, prognosis and cost of the treatment.
2. If presented within 2 hours of the injury, cool the damaged areas with water or saline immersion, compresses or sprays for at least 30 minutes. Monitor the patient's body temperature and avoid hypothermia.
3. Treatment for first-degree burns
   A. Administer analgesics as needed:
      I. Ketamine CRI IV
      II. Morphine and lidocaine CRI IV
      III. Hydromorphone, morphine, or oxymorphone can be administered as needed or CRI IV
      IV. Fentanyl CRI IV
      V. Oxymorphone 0.04–0.06 mg/kg and ketamine 1–2 mg/kg IV may be useful for providing analgesia for wound care.
   B. Gently clip and clean the area.
   C. Lavage, debride and dress wounds at least once daily, using aseptic technique.
   D. Apply silver sulfadiazine (Silvadene®) ointment and sterile occlusive dressings to wounds.

Dermatologic emergencies

4. Treatment for second-degree burns
   A. Treat as for first-degree burns, and:
   B. Place an intravenous catheter, in an unburned area on a limb.
   C. Administer balanced electrolyte crystalloid intravenous fluids at 90 mL/kg for the first hour in dogs, and at 45–60 mL/kg for the first hour in cats. Monitor fluid therapy very closely, especially if the patient has pulmonary edema.
   D. After the shock dose of fluids has been administered, administer fluids at maintenance rates plus replace losses by the following formula known as the Parkland formula:
      I. % TBSA × 1–4 mL/kg = 24-hour maintenance fluid needs in dogs.
      II. % TBSA × 1–3 mL/kg = 24 hour maintenance fluid needs in cats.
      III. During the first 8 hours following shock fluid therapy, administer 50% of the fluids calculated by the above formula, with the remainder over the next 16 hours.
   E. The amount of fluid lost from evaporation is about 10 times the amount lost of normal skin and can be estimated by the following formula: evaporative loss (mL/h) = (%TBSA burned + 25) × total body surface area (m^2).
   F. During the first 8 hours following the injury, avoid colloids and hypertonic saline administration unless the patient is in severe hypovolemic shock. During this time, there is an increased risk of the development of pulmonary edema.
   G. Cleanse the wound(s) with cool saline compresses. Debride loose flesh.
   H. Apply antibiotic dressing (Silvadene®) and bandage the wound(s). Keep the patient warm, on a soft blanket.
   I. Skin grafts may be required.
   J. Temperature regulation is important.
5. Treatment of third-degree burns
   A. If extensive tissue damage has occurred, the prognosis is poor. Discuss euthanasia with the client.
   B. Treat as for second-degree burns.
   C. If there are small wounds, excise and suture, dress and cover them.
   D. If sepsis develops, administer a chloramphenicol injection below the eschar. Also administer broad-spectrum antibiotics intravenously.
   E. Hydrotherapy in a dilute povidone-iodine or chlorhexidine solution.
   F. Watch for septicemia, renal failure and hypoalbuminemia.
   G. Monitor serum total protein; protein loss occurs via devitalized skin.
   H. Temperature regulation is important.
   I. Provide nutritional support.
6. Hot tar can be removed by applying polyoxyethylene sorbitan or polysorbate, the emulsifying agents in Neosporin cream and other antibiotic ointments.
7. If the patient has suffered from smoke inhalation, refer to that section for treatment.
8. Monitor urine output. Normal urine output is 1–2 mL/kg/h. Acute renal failure is a common sequela.

9. Administer antibiotics as indicated by culture and sensitivity if infection occurs or broad-spectrum antibiotics if the patient becomes septic.
10. To ease the patient's discomfort from oral burns, administer sucralfate suspension or a protective emollient such as Orabase® to the lesions.
11. Provide nutritional support, either orally or by the administration of partial parenteral nutrition. Place a feeding tube if the oral lesions are severe and long-term nutritional support is necessary.
    A. The caloric needs are twice resting requirements.
    B. Avoid high glucose administration, which increases CO_2 production and respiratory effort.
    C. Supplement with vitamins and minerals, especially A, C and zinc.

CUTANEOUS FOREIGN BODIES

Etiology

Many items can become imbedded in an animal's skin, including plant material (cactus spines, thorns, foxtails, grass awns, the tips of palm or yucca leaves, etc.), metal objects (nails, tacks, pins, needles, slivers, bullets, fish hooks, clasps from leashes, etc.), wood materials (splinters) and miscellaneous items such as collars, rubber bands, bee stingers, porcupine quills and teeth.

Sometimes the items are intentionally driven into the animal, but most often they become imbedded accidentally.

Diagnosis

History—The owner may observe lameness, pain or swelling, or may be able to see a foreign body (or bodies) in the skin.

Physical exam—The animal may be covered with cactus spines, which makes the diagnosis obvious, but makes physical examination nearly impossible. In cases where actual contact with the animal is not possible, carefully assess the mental state and respiratory character, depth, rate and pattern. Look carefully for signs of external trauma such as bleeding or obvious fractures. In these cases, the patient will sometimes need to undergo anesthesia and have some of the cactus spines removed prior to performing a physical examination. Warn the owner of the potential complications from anesthesia, especially since physical evaluation of the patient is impossible.

Other patients may present with lameness. Upon close inspection of the interdigital spaces and plantar surface of the paw, a moist, erythematous, swollen area may be observed. There may be an open lesion, or a draining tract. In patients with a swelling, carefully palpate the area to determine whether there is an underlying foreign body. Look carefully at the skin surface for a protrusion or an opening. Perform a complete physical examination of the patient. If there are quills or cactus spines in the face, carefully examine the eyes for ocular foreign bodies.

Diagnostic imaging—Radiographs or MRI of the affected area may be helpful.

Differential diagnosis

Differentials depend upon the location of the lesion, but include infection (including osteomyelitis), neoplasia, seroma, hematoma and other causes of lameness.

Prognosis

The prognosis depends upon the location of the lesion and the removal of the foreign body. Grass awns have a tendency to migrate and can be particularly difficult to locate. Recurrent draining tracts will occur until the inciting cause is eliminated.

Treatment

1. Inform the client of the diagnosis, prognosis and cost of the treatment.
2. Administer analgesia.
3. Administer anesthesia if needed.
   A. Carefully examine the patient if possible prior to administering anesthesia.
   B. Perform a preoperative diagnostic work-up prior to inducing anesthesia.
   C. If anesthesia is necessary, consider administering a local anesthetic if possible.
   D. If the procedure is expected to be brief, an injectable anesthetic is acceptable.
   E. If the procedure is expected to be prolonged, such as for a cat entirely covered with cactus spines, an inhalant anesthetic is preferred.
3. Cactus spine and porcupine quill removal
   A. Do not clip the patient.
   B. Carefully grasp the cactus spine or quill just above the skin with a hemostat or needle holder and quickly jerk the spine or quill from the skin.
   C. Removal of the cactus spine from the hemostat or needle holder is facilitated by immersing the tip of the instrument with the spine on it into a bowl of water. It is quicker, easier and less of a hazard to the medical personnel, than wiping the instrument with a towel.
   D. Repeat the procedure until all visible spines or quills are removed.
   E. Carefully and gently run your hands over the entire skin surface of the patient. Remove any spines that are felt.
   F. If possible, have another staff member go over the patient to find any cactus spines that may have been missed.
   G. Advise the client to watch for any additional spines, quills or swellings as it is not possible to remove all of them from the patient.
   H. If excessive redness, drainage, or swelling occurs, indicating a possible infection, start the patient on antibiotics.
4. Removal of fish-hooks in skin
   A. Single hooks – due to the barb, the hook cannot be backed out.
      I. If the tip of the hook can be observed or felt, and the shank of the hook is protruding, grasp the shank with needle-nosed pliers.

     II. Cut off any excess hook or line with wire cutters. Be careful to cover the hook with your other hand when cutting it to avoid creating a hazardous projectile.

    III. Push the hook into the patient, directed in the manner in which it was heading, but push it up and out of the skin.

    IV. Grasp the tip as it comes through the skin.

    V. Occasionally, if the tip of the hook can be felt under the skin but not seen, it is useful to make a very small skin incision over the tip of the hook.

  B. Treble hooks – usually only one or two hooks will be imbedded in the patient.

    I. With wire cutters, cut off the shank that joins the three hooks together.

    II. Manage the individual hooks as advised above.

  C. Due to the low incidence of tetanus in dogs and cats, the administration of tetanus toxoid is not normally recommended.

  D. Advise the owner to clean the wound daily and monitor for redness, swelling or discharge.

  E. If excessive redness, drainage, or swelling occurs, indicating a possible infection, start the patient on antibiotics.

5. Other cutaneous foreign bodies

  A. If the foreign body is observed, gently grasp it and remove it from the patient.

  B. If the foreign body is not observed, such as in draining tracts from foxtails, gently clip and clean the surrounding area.

  C. Gently probe the lesion with mosquito hemostats or alligator forceps.

  D. Flush draining tracts with sterile saline.

  E. Radiographic contrast material may be injected and then the area can be radiographed to follow a tract.

  F. Bee stingers should be scraped off with a scalpel handle, tongue depressor or credit card, and not grasped as that may expel more venom into the patient.

6. Ocular foreign bodies are discussed in the section on Corneal foreign bodies.

(ACUTE MOIST) DERMATITIS (PYOTRAUMATIC DERMATITIS)

Diagnosis

History—Owner observed hair loss and reddened area or other skin lesion, scratching (excessive) or odor, usually with an acute onset and rapidly progressive. The lesion develops from the dog chewing and licking at a focal area of pain or pruritus.

The lesions may be secondary to allergies (flea, inhalant, food), ectoparasitisms, infections, foreign bodies, trauma, anal sacculitis or otitis externa.

Physical exam—The patient usually has a single localized, painful and pruritic, alopecic lesion. The lesion is usually an erythematous, erosive to ulcerative dermatosis with secondary superficial bacterial infection.

Prognosis

The prognosis is fair to good. The condition is generally not life threatening and is usually responsive to therapy.

Treatment

1. Inform the client of the diagnosis, prognosis and cost of the treatment.
2. Gently clip and clean the lesion with surgical scrub.
3. The patient may require sedation to clean the lesion.
4. Application of topical astringents, such as Gentamicin topical spray or DermaCool®, may be beneficial. Avoid sprays which contain alcohol because they burn.
5. Administer antibiotics, parenteral and oral for 2 weeks:
   A. Amoxicillin-clavulanate, 13.75–20 mg/kg PO q8–12h
   B. Cefadroxil, 22mg/kg PO q8–12h
   C. Cephalexin, 20mg/kg PO q8–12h
   D. Clindamycin, 5mg/kg PO q12h
   E. Cefpodoxime proxetil (Simplicef), 5–10 mg/kg PO once q24h for 5–7 days
   F. Cefovecin sodium (Convenia), 8 mg/kg SC once, may be repeated in 14 days.
6. If the patient is exhibiting intense pruritus:
   A. Prednisone, 0.25–0.5 mg/kg PO q12h for 2–3 days, then 0.25 mg/kg q24h for 2–3 days
   B. Topical spray containing a topical anesthetic such as lidocaine
   C. Topical spray containing an antihistamine such as diphenhydramine
   D. Some patients benefit from one injection of dexamethasone sodium phosphate 0.1–0.2 mg/kg IV, IM, SC.
7. Apply an Elizabethan collar or other method to reduce further self-trauma.

TOXIC EPIDERMAL NECROLYSIS AND ERYTHEMA MULTIFORME

Diagnosis

History—The dog or cat may have recently received levamisole, penicillins (ampicillin or hetacillin), cephalosporins, gentamicin, sulfonamides, griseofulvin, L-thyroxine, aurothioglucose, 5-fluorocytosine, diethylcarbamazine or antiserum. These diseases have also been associated with infections, toxins such as environmental insecticides, topical flea dips and D-limonene, neoplasia, systemic diseases such as endocarditis, hepatic necrosis and cholangiohepatitis, and may be idiopathic. The owner may observe lethargy, depression, anorexia and multiple skin lesions.

Physical exam—Toxic epidermal necrolysis (TEN) is more severe than erythema multiforme (EM). The lesions are painful and macular, papular, bullous, vesicular or target-like, with central areas of redness surrounded by an erythematous ring. Initially, the lesions are multifocal, but they eventually coalesce to cause full-thickness necrosis and dermal sloughing, and appear like burned skin. The lesions are nonpruritic and usually appear on the trunk of the patient, although stomatitis and footpad lesions can occur as well. The patient will usually have a fever. Nikolsky's sign, which is the ability to manually slip or push back areas of epidermis and create new ulcers, is often observed.

Laboratory findings—Perform a CBC, serum biochemical profile and urinalysis. Closely evaluate the serum liver enzymes. Test for systemic immune-mediated diseases by running a serum antinuclear antibody (ANA) analysis and Coombs' test. Perform liver function tests. Obtain skin biopsies.

Radiographs—If cutaneous lesions are suspected to be secondary to systemic disease or neoplasia, radiographs may be useful.

Ultrasonography—If cutaneous lesions are suspected to be secondary to systemic disease or neoplasia, ultrasonography may be beneficial.

Differential diagnosis

Neoplasia, burns, drug-induced necrosis, vasculitis, systemic lupus erythematosus, epitheliotropic lymphoma, TEN and EM.

Prognosis

TEN can be rapidly progressive, difficult to control or eliminate, and may be fatal. The prognosis is guarded to poor.

Treatment

1. Inform the client of the diagnosis, prognosis and cost of the treatment.
2. Discontinue the administration of any suspect medications.
3. Evaluate the patient closely for signs of neoplasia or systemic disease.
4. Administer intravenous fluids to replace estimated fluid losses.
5. Clean and debride the lesions.
6. Cover lesions with silver sulfadiazine cream.
7. Consider the administration of corticosteroids, which is controversial. The most common corticosteroid prescribed is prednisolone or prednisone, 2.2–4.4mg/kg q12h PO initially and then at reducing doses.
8. Administer analgesics as indicated by the patient.
9. Obtain blood cultures and administer the appropriate antibiotics to patients with sepsis.

JUVENILE CELLULITIS (JUVENILE PYODERMA, PUPPY STRANGLES)

Etiology

The etiology of this disease is unknown.

Diagnosis

History—The disease usually occurs in puppies less than 16 weeks of age. The owner may observe swelling around the face and neck, lethargy and anorexia. Several individuals in a litter may be affected. There may be an increased incidence in Golden Retrievers and Dachshunds. *Physical exam*—Swelling may be observed around the face, muzzle, pinnae and neck. At facial mucocutaneous junctions, there may be edema, papules, pustules and crusts. The puppy may have a mucopurulent ocular discharge and purulent otitis externa. The submandibular lymph nodes are usually enlarged. They may abscess and rupture. In some puppies, the submandibular lymph node swelling is so severe that respiratory compromise results from the tracheal compression. The puppy will usually have a fever, anorexia and lethargy. Dehydration may occur.

Differential diagnosis

Abscessation, acute allergic reaction with angioedema, sepsis, demodicosis, dermatophytosis.

Prognosis

The prognosis is fair to guarded, as some of these puppies will die. The cutaneous lesions may result in severe scarring.

Treatment

1. Inform the client of the diagnosis, prognosis and cost of the treatment.
2. Administer prednisone, 1 mg/kg PO q12h for 14 days, until the lesions resolve, and then taper the dose over an additional 2–4 weeks. If the condition is severe, administer dexamethasone sodium phosphate, 0.1–0.2 mg/kg IV, IM, SC then switch to oral prednisone.
3. Administer cephalexin, 20 mg/kg PO q8–12h, cefadroxil 22 mg/kg PO q8–12h, Cefpodoxime proxetil (Simplicef), 5–10 mg/kg PO once q24h for 5–7 days, or amoxicillin-clavulanate, 13.75–20 mg/kg PO q8–12h.
4. Administer fluid therapy if the patient appears dehydrated.
5. Evaluate and maintain a patent airway.
6. Lance and drain the submandibular lymph node if respiratory distress is present.
7. If the swelling is fluctuant, aspirate or lance and drain the purulent fluid.
8. Give symptomatic and supportive care as indicated.
9. Gently clean the face with warm water to decrease secondary infections and scarring.

AURAL (OR AURICULAR) HEMATOMA

Etiology

Pruritic or inflammatory conditions, such as otic foreign bodies, bacterial or fungal otitis externa, ear mites, atopy, food allergy, etc. may lead to the formation of aural hematomas secondary to self-trauma and rupture of branches of the auricular artery.

Diagnosis

History—The patient often has an ear infection or a history of head shaking and scratching at its ears. The problem is most common in dogs with pendulous ears.

Physical exam—There is visible and palpable swelling of the pinna. Examine the ear canal for the presence of *Otodectes cynotis*, yeast or bacterial otitis externa. Examine the feet and skin for other signs of allergic conditions.

Differential diagnosis

Acute allergic reaction with pinnal edema, abscess, neoplasia.

Prognosis

Although there may be detrimental cosmetic effects, the problem is not life threatening. Chronic and recurrent aural hematomas can lead to fibrosis and contraction of the pinnal cartilage and deformity of the ear.

Treatment

1. Inform the client of the diagnosis, prognosis and cost of the treatment.
2. Treat any underlying otitis.
3. Conservative therapy – for acute cases (less than 4 days' duration)
   A. Needle aspiration of the hematoma may be useful soon after hematoma formation.
   B. Sedation may be necessary.
   C. Clip and surgically prepare the concave (medial) surface of the pinna.
   D. Insert a 16- to 22-gauge needle into the fluctuant cavity and aspirate as much fluid as possible to drain the hematoma.
   E. After performing needle aspiration, apply a pressure wrap to secure the ear to the head.
   F. Recurrence is common.
   G. Aspiration is recommended as an emergency procedure, since delay in draining an aural hematoma causes the condition to worsen and leads to a permanently deformed, 'cauliflower' ear.
4. As an alternative, insert a teat canula into the hematoma to allow the hematoma to continue to drain.
   A. Sedation may be necessary.
   B. Clip and surgically prepare the concave (medial) surface of the pinna.
   C. Make a small 0.5 cm incision at the most distal and gravity-dependent portion of the hematoma.
   D. Make two small holes in the collar of the teat cannula with a 19- or 20-gauge needle.
   E. Insert the sterile teat cannula into the hematoma and aspirate as much fluid as possible to drain the hematoma.
   F. Suture the teat cannula in place with 1–2 sutures of 3-0 nylon or other nonabsorbable monofilament suture at the tip and another suture at the base through the opening in the teat cannula.

Dermatologic emergencies

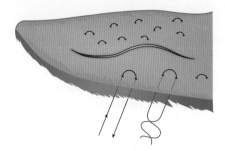

FIG 7.1 **'S' incision on the concave surface of the pinna.** *From Rosychuk, R.A., Merchant, S.R. (guest Eds.), 1994. The Veterinary Clinics of North America, Small Animal Practice. Ear, Nose and Throat 24 (5) ©Elsevier.*

    G. Have the owner clean the opening of the teat cannula and drain the hematoma daily.

    H. Apply an Elizabethan collar to decrease self-trauma.

    I. Remove the teat cannula in 3 weeks and allow the hole to heal by second intention.

5. Surgical therapy

    A. Administer anesthesia.

    B. Clip and surgically prepare the concave (medial) surface of the pinna.

    C. An 'S' incision is made with a number 10 scalpel blade on the inner surface of the pinna, over the hematoma (Fig. 7.1).

    D. The length of the 'S' should run the long axis of the pinna.

    E. Remove the fibrin clot.

    F. Flush the cavity with sterile saline.

    G. Close the cavity by placing *loosely* tied 1 cm wide vertical mattress sutures through the ear, avoiding major blood vessels. The sutures should run parallel to the long axis of the pinna. Use 3-0 or 4-0 monofilament nonabsorbable material. Leave the 'S' incision itself open to allow drainage.

    H. Pass the needle from the concave surface of the pinna and include both pinnal cartilages in the suture, but it is not necessary to penetrate the skin surface on the convex surface of the pinna.

    I. Stagger the mattress sutures to obliterate the dead space.

    J. Bandage the ear to the head, bringing the pendulous pinna up over the top of the dog's head.

    K. To allow cleaning and the application of medications, leave the ear canal exposed.

    L. Leave the bandage on for 10 days; remove the sutures after 14–21 days.

    M. Consider applying an Elizabethan collar to further prevent self-trauma or trauma to the bandage.

6. As an alternative, a Keyes biopsy punch can be used to create 5–6 mm holes in the proximal and distal ends of the hematoma.

ACUTE OTITIS EXTERNA

Etiology

Otitis externa is an inflammation of the epithelium of the external ear canal and may be caused by parasitic infestation or occurs secondary to many predisposing factors or disease states, including atopy, hypothyroidism, immune-mediated diseases, foreign bodies, parasites (*Otodectes cynotis, Otobius megnini, Sarcoptes, Notoedres* and *Demodex* spp.), trauma, adverse food reactions, neoplasia of the ear canals, inflammatory polyps in the ear canal, abnormally small ear canals, keratinization disorders such as primary idiopathic seborrhea and excessive moisture in the ears. Otitis externa can progress to otitis media, especially in the presence of a ruptured tympanum.

Diagnosis

History—The animal may have free access to fields or water. If the onset is gradual and otitis is confined to one ear, neoplasia is possible. If the condition is bilateral, it is often secondary to parasitic infestation or systemic disease. The animal has usually been scratching at its ears and shaking its head. The owner may notice pain when petting the animal near its ears or a foul odor from the ears. The animal may become listless or lethargic.

Physical exam—A thorough physical examination of the patient's entire body, as well as the ears, should be performed. Examine the pinna for redness, swelling, crusts, scabs or other lesions. Remove any hair that is growing in the ear canals. Normal ear wax may be present in small amounts and is pale yellow or yellow-brown. *Otodectes cynotis* may be observed grossly as white specks in a dark brown, waxy discharge, or may be visualized during cytology.

The tympanic membrane is normally slightly concave, glistening, pearl-gray and translucent. If the tympanic membrane is ruptured, the tear may be visible or it may be difficult to determine where the horizontal canal ends and the middle ear begins. Pathologic changes of the middle ear may be indicated by bulging or cloudiness, opacity and color change of the tympanic membrane.

Also evaluate the patient for the presence of vestibular signs, including head tilt, nystagmus, ataxia and a history of anorexia or occasional vomiting.

Laboratory evaluation—
1. Cytology – smears of otic exudate should be stained with modified Wright's stain or Gram's stain and examined for the number and type of yeast, bacteria, leukocytes, neoplastic cells, and parasites or their eggs or larva.
   A. Yeast is usually *Malassezia* pachydermatis or *Candida* spp.
   B. Gram-negative rods are usually *Pseudomonas, Proteus, Escherichia coli,* or *Corynebacterium* spp.
   C. Gram-positive cocci are usually *Staphylococcus* or *Streptococcus* spp.
2. Culture – is usually reserved for resistant infections.
3. Biopsy – a biopsy should be taken of a mass or area of proliferative tissue in the ear canal. Be sure to obtain a sample of normal and abnormal skin.

Diagnostic imaging—
Radiographs of the bullae may help diagnose otitis media.
CT may help evaluate for bone changes of the skull or bullae.

Dermatologic emergencies

MRI may be helpful to evaluate soft-tissue growths or fluid accumulation in the bullae.

Prognosis

Although otitis externa is not life threatening, it often becomes a chronic recurrent condition. Deafness, vestibular disease, cellulitis, facial nerve paralysis, otitis media, otitis interna and meningoencephalitis may occur if left untreated. Most cases of otitis externa resolve with appropriate therapy within 3–4 weeks. Cases of otitis media may require 6 weeks or more of therapy.

Treatment

1. Inform the client of the diagnosis, prognosis and the cost of treatment.
2. Sedate the animal if needed. General anesthesia is indicated in severe cases or uncooperative patients. Some patients benefit from the administration of an analgesic.
3. Thoroughly clean the horizontal and vertical external ear canals. Remove all hair, wax, foreign matter, debris and exudate.
4. If the tympanic membrane is ruptured, use sterile saline to clean the external ear canal.
5. If the tympanic membrane is intact, use a commercial ear cleanser with a ceruminolytic, antiseptic, and astringent.
   A. Ceruminolytics include carbamide peroxide and dioctyl sodium sulfosuccinate (DSS).
   B. Antiseptics include chlorhexidine gluconate and acetic acid.
   C. Astringents include salicylic acid, boric acid and isopropyl alcohol.
6. Install the cleaning solution, gently massage the ear and flush repeatedly with sterile saline until the ear is completely clean.
7. Topical antimicrobial medication is based on the evaluation of the otic exudate smear:
   A. Gram-positive cocci should be treated with chloramphenicol, neomycin or gentamicin. Gentamicin combined with tris-ethylenediaminetetraacetic acid (EDTA)-lysozyme has increased efficacy.
   B. Gram-negative rods should be treated with polymyxin B, gentamicin, amikacin or enrofloxacin.
   C. If the tympanic membrane is ruptured, do not use aminoglycosides.
   D. *Pseudomonas* infections benefit from the additional treatment of 2–5% acetic acid solutions.
   E. An additional antimicrobial treatment for *Pseudomonas* is a 1% silver sulfadiazine solution (mix 1.5 mL silver sulfadiazine cream with 13.5 mL distilled water, or 0.1 g of silver sulfadiazine powder with 100 mL of distilled water). Shake the solution well, and instill 4–12 drops into each ear canal twice a day. This therapy may be used in patients with a ruptured tympanic membrane.
   F. Yeast should be treated with topical clotrimazole or miconazole, thiabendazole or nystatin.

G. Posatex contains Orbifloxacin, Mometasone furoate monohydrate and posaconazole in an otic solution for dogs with otitis externa from a combined yeast and bacterial infection.

H. *Otodectes cynotis* infestation can be treated topically with Tresaderm or ivermectin otic suspension (Acarexx®).

   I. All animals in contact with the patient should be treated.

   II. Avoid the use of ivermectin in Collies, Shelties, Border Collies, Australian Shepherds, Old English Sheepdogs, German Shepherds, or mixes with these breeds or other breeds that commonly have an *MDR-1* gene mutation.

I. Topical glucocorticoid therapy, with fluocinolone acetonide in 60% dimethyl sulfoxide, may be helpful in reducing swelling, pruritus, exudation and tissue proliferation. Administer the solution and massage the ear canal for 30–60 seconds q8–12h. Additional corticosteroids, such as dexamethasone, betamethasone or triamcinolone, may also be beneficial in reducing inflammation. Corticosteroids may potentiate otitis and predispose the patient to a secondary yeast infection.

J. A bacterial culture and sensitivity should be performed if there is a lack of response to initial antimicrobial therapy.

8. Systemic therapy is indicated if the epithelium of the ear canal is ulcerated, if the tympanic membrane is ruptured, or if cytologic evaluation of the exudate reveals inflammatory cells that contain bacteria.

A. For bacterial infections, pending culture and sensitivity results, administer one of the following broad-spectrum antibiotics:

   I. Cephalexin, 20–30 mg/kg q8–12h PO

   II. Enrofloxacin, 2.5 mg/kg q12h PO

   III. Clindamycin, 7–10 mg/kg q12h PO

   IV. Cefpodoxime proxetil (Simplicef), 5–10 mg/kg PO q24h for 5–7 days.

B. For severe yeast or fungal infections, ketoconazole, 5–10 mg/kg PO q24h may be beneficial.

C. For *Otodectes* or other topical parasites, administer selamectin (Revolution®) as directed every 2 weeks for 3 applications.

D. If severe inflammation is present, prednisone 0.25–0.5 mg/kg PO q12h, may be useful for short-term therapy. If the patient has an autoimmune or hypersensitivity disease, long-term systemic glucocorticoid therapy may be essential.

9. Dispense cleansing solution for the owner to utilize every day initially, then every 3–7 days as the condition improves. Educate the client in the proper method for cleaning the animal's ears at home.

ANAL SAC DISEASE

ETIOLOGY

Although it is thought to occur secondary to conditions that cause inadequate emptying of the anal sacs during defecation, the cause of anal sac disease is unknown.

Diagnosis

History—The patient may be chewing or licking at the anal area, scooting or tail chasing. The patient may exhibit tenesmus, discomfort when standing or walking, or a change in temperament. The owner may observe a malodorous discharge from the perianal area.

Physical exam—The patient may exhibit discomfort when sitting or a reluctance to sit. There may be pain upon palpation of the perianal area or upon rectal palpation. The anal sacs may be swollen or a necrotic draining fistulous tract may be present. Palpation of the anal sacs is achieved by inserting a gloved index finger into the rectum and compressing the thumb against the skin ventrolateral to the anus.

Differential diagnosis

Anal sac neoplasia, perianal gland neoplasia, hematoma, perineal hernia, perianal fistula, other soft-tissue abscess, spider bite or other perianal trauma including bite wounds.

Prognosis

The individual incident carries a good prognosis for recovery; however, recurrences are common. Some patients benefit from surgical removal of the anal sacs.

Treatment

1. Inform the client of the diagnosis, prognosis and cost of the treatment.
2. For patients with anal sac impaction and mild sacculitis, the only required treatment is manual evacuation of the anal sac contents.
   A. Feeding a high-fiber diet may help prevent recurrence.
   B. The patient should be re-examined in 1–2 weeks.
   C. Instillation of an antibiotic ointment, such as otic or ophthalmic preparations, into the sac may be beneficial.
3. For patients with anal sac abscesses:
   A. Administer analgesics and/or anesthesia if necessary.
   B. Clip any excessive hair.
   C. Clean the perianal area.
   D. Lance the abscess, if necessary, with a number 15 or number 11 scalpel blade.
   E. Drain the anal sac contents.
   F. Flush the abscess with sterile saline or dilute povidone–iodine solution.
   G. Have the owner apply warm compresses to the perianal area for 10 minutes q12h for 3–5 days.
   H. Have the owner clean the area with antiseptics and administer antibiotics into the open lesion q12h for 5–7 days.
   I. Administer systemic antibiotics for 10–14 days.
   J. Dispense analgesics for administration at home for 3–5 days.
   K. If the patient persists in self-traumatizing the area, apply an Elizabethan collar.

ABSCESSES

Buriko, Y., Van Winkle, T.J., Drobatz, K.J., et al., 2008. Severe soft tissue infections in dogs: 47 cases (1996–2006). Journal of Veterinary Emergency and Critical Care 18 (6), 608–618.

Goldkamp, C.E., Levy, J.K., Edinboro, C.H., et al., 2008. Seroprevalences of feline leukemia virus and feline immunodeficiency virus in cats with abscesses or bite wounds and rate of veterinarian compliance with current guidelines for retrovirus testing. Journal of the American Veterinary Medical Association 232, 1152–1158.

Holzworth, J., 1987. Diseases of the Cat, Medicine, and Surgery, vol. 1. WB Saunders, Philadelphia, pp. 658–659.

Kunkle, G. (guest Ed.), 1995. Beale, K.M., Nodules and Draining Tracts. The Veterinary Clinics of North America, Small Animal Practice: Feline Dermatology 25 (4), 887–888.

Scott, D.W., Miller W.H. Jr., Griffin, C.E., 1995. Muller & Kirk's Small Animal Dermatology, fifth ed. WB Saunders, Philadelphia, p. 311.

Six, R., Cleaver, D.M., Lindeman, C.J., et al., 2009. Effectiveness and safety of cefovecin sodium, an extended-spectrum injectable cephalosporin, in the treatment of cats with abscesses and infected wounds. Journal of the American Veterinary Medical Association 234, 81–87.

Six, R., Cherni, J., Chesebrough, R., et al., 2008. Efficacy and safety of cefovecin in treating bacterial folliculitis, abscesses, or infected wounds in dogs. Journal of the American Veterinary Medical Association 233, 433–439.

BURNS

Garzotto, C.K., 2009. Thermal burn injury. In: Silverstein, D.C., Hopper, K. (Eds.), Small Animal Critical Care Medicine. Elsevier, St Louis, pp. 683–686.

Pope, E.R., 2003. Thermal, electrical, and chemical burns and cold injuries. In: Slatter, D. (Ed.), Textbook of Small Animal Surgery, third ed. Elsevier, St Louis, pp. 356–372.

(ACUTE MOIST) DERMATITIS (PYOTRAUMATIC DERMATITIS)

Birchard, S.J., Sherding, R.G., 1994. Saunders Manual of Small Animal Practice. WB Saunders, Philadelphia, p. 273.

Bonagura, J.D., Kirk, R.W. (Eds.), 1994. Current Veterinary Therapy XII. WB Saunders, Philadelphia, pp. 611–617.

Rosenkrantz, W.S., 2009. Pyotraumatic dermatitis ('hot spots'). In: Bonagura, J.D., Twedt, D.C. (Eds.), Kirk's Current Veterinary Therapy XIV. Elsevier, St Louis, pp. 446–449.

Scott, D.W., Miller W.H. Jr., Griffin, C.E., 1995. Muller & Kirk's Small Animal Dermatology, fifth ed. WB Saunders, Philadelphia, pp. 286–288.

TOXIC EPIDERMAL NECROLYSIS AND ERYTHEMA MULTIFORME

Birchard, S.J., Sherding, R.G., 1994. Saunders Manual of Small Animal Practice. WB Saunders, Philadelphia, pp. 330–334.

Kunkle, G., (guest Ed.), 1995. Angarano, D.W., Erosive and Ulcerative Skin Diseases. The Veterinary Clinics of North America, Small Animal Practice: Feline Dermatology 4 (25), 877.

Murtaugh, R.J., Kaplan, P.M., 1992. Veterinary Emergency and Critical Care Medicine. Mosby Year Book, St Louis, p. 392.

Scott, D.W., Miller W.H. Jr., Griffin, C.E., 1995. Muller & Kirk's Small Animal Dermatology, fifth ed. WB Saunders, Philadelphia, pp. 595–602.

JUVENILE CELLULITIS (JUVENILE PYODERMA, PUPPY STRANGLES)

Bonagura, J.D., Kirk, R.W., (Eds.), 1995. Current Veterinary Therapy XII. WB Saunders, Philadelphia, pp. 612–613.

Hoskins, J.D., 1995. Veterinary Pediatrics, second ed. WB Saunders, Philadelphia, pp. 266–267.

Scott, D.W., Miller W.H. Jr., Griffin, C.E., 1995. Muller & Kirk's Small Animal Dermatology, fifth ed. WB Saunders, Philadelphia, pp. 938–941.

AURAL (OR AURICULAR) HEMATOMA

Birchard, S.J., Sherding, R.G., 1994. Saunders Manual of Small Animal Practice. WB Saunders, Philadelphia, pp. 386–387.

Morgan, R.V., 1992. Handbook of Small Animal Practice, second ed. Churchill Livingstone, New York, pp. 1155–1156.

Rosychuk, R.A., Merchant, S.R., (guest Eds.), 1994. McCarthy, P.E. and McCarthy, R.J., Surgery of the Ear. The Veterinary Clinics of North America, Small Animal Practice: Ear, Nose and Throat 24 (5), 954–957.

Slatter, D.H., (Ed.), 1993. Textbook of Small Animal Surgery, vols I and II, second ed. WB Saunders, Philadelphia, pp. 1545–1546.

ACUTE OTITIS EXTERNA

Birchard, S.J., Sherding, R.G., 1994. Saunders Manual of Small Animal Practice. WB Saunders, Philadelphia, pp. 375–379, 391.

Bruyette, D.S., Lorenz, M.D., 1993. Otitis externa, and otitis media: diagnostic and medical aspects. In: Fingland, R.B. (guest Ed.), Seminars in Veterinary Medicine and Surgery (Small Animal): The Ear: Medical, Surgical, and Diagnostic Aspects, vol. 8, no 1. WB Saunders, Philadelphia, pp. 3–7.

Cole, L.K., 2009. Systemic therapy for otitis externa and media. In: Bonagura, J.D., Twedt, D.C. (Eds.), Kirk's Current Veterinary Therapy XIV. Elsevier, St Louis, pp. 434–436.

McKeever, P.J., 1996. Otitis externa. Compendium on Continuing Education 18 (7), 759–772.

Mendelsohn, C., 2009. Topical therapy of otitis externa. In: Bonagura, J.D., Twedt, D.C. (Eds.), Kirk's Current Veterinary Therapy XIV. Elsevier, St Louis, pp. 428–433.

Moriello, K.A., Diesel, A., 2010. Medical management of otitis. In: August, J.R. (Ed.), Consultations in Feline Internal Medicine, vol. 6. Elsevier, St Louis, pp. 347–357.

Rosychuk, R.A., Merchant, S.R. (guest Eds.), 1994. Rosychuk, R.A., Management of Otitis Externa. The Veterinary Clinics of North America, Small Animal Practice: Ear, Nose and Throat 24 (5), 921–949.

Scott, D.W., Miller W.H. Jr., Griffin, C.E., 1995. Muller & Kirk's Small Animal Dermatology, fifth ed. WB Saunders, Philadelphia, pp. 979–986.

ANAL SAC DISEASE

Birchard, S.J., Sherding, R.G., 1994. Saunders Manual of Small Animal Practice. WB Saunders, Philadelphia, no 72, p. 784.

Muse, R., 2009. Diseases of the anal sac. In: Bonagura, J.D., Twedt, D.C. (Eds.), Kirk's Current Veterinary Therapy XIV. Elsevier, St Louis, pp. 465–467.

Scott, D.W., Miller W.H. Jr., Griffin, C.E., 1995. Muller & Kirk's Small Animal Dermatology, fifth ed. WB Saunders, Philadelphia, no 122, pp. 969–970.

Tams, T.R., 1996. Handbook of Small Animal Gastroenterology. WB Saunders, Philadelphia, no 94, p. 366.

Hematologic emergencies

CANINE ANEMIA

Etiology

Regenerative anemia—Acute blood loss (trauma) after the first 48–96 hours, disseminated intravascular coagulopathy, chronic blood loss (hookworms, subinvolution of placental sites in the bitch, immune-mediated thrombocytopenia (ITP) with bleeding, tick infestation), hemolytic disease (immune-mediated hemolytic anemia [IMHA or IHA]), pyruvate kinase deficiency, phosphofructokinase deficiency, hypophosphatemia, hemobartonellosis, babesiosis, ehrlichiosis, heartworm disease, leptospirosis, onions, phenothiazines, vaccinations, vitamin K, sulfa antibiotics, anticonvulsants, penicillins, cephalosporins, zinc and lead poisoning.

Nonregenerative anemia—The first 48–96 hours following acute blood loss, nutritional deficiencies, iron deficiency, bone-marrow suppression secondary to malignancy, ionizing radiation, myelophthisis, myelodysplastic syndromes, myelofibrosis, osteosclerosis, osteopetrosis, chronic disease, renal disease, hypoadrenocorticism, hypothyroidism, ehrlichiosis, leishmaniasis, drug induced (vincristine, estrogens, chloramphenicol, phenylbutazone).

Diagnosis

History—The owner may observe anorexia, pica, lethargy, weakness, exercise intolerance, weight loss, syncope, or collapse. There may be a history of exposure to parasites, trauma, toxins, heat, or other ill animals. Inquire about medications currently or recently administered, including vaccinations and any recent illness or surgery. There may be an incidence of hematologic disorders in litter mates, parents or house mates. Inquire about the patient's current diet and nutritional status. Question the owner regarding any recent blood loss, including hematuria, melena, hematochezia, epistaxis or hemoptysis.

Physical exam—The patient may have pallor, icterus, ecchymoses or petechiae, and hypothermia. The patient may exhibit weakness, dyspnea, polypnea, tachycardia, pounding pulses, or a grade I / II systolic murmur. Upon palpation, lymphadenopathy, hepatomegaly and splenomegaly may be detected. The patient may also show signs of weight loss, cachexia, evidence of bleeding or trauma, or the presence of ticks or fleas. Rectal examination may show frank hemorrhage or melena.

Laboratory evaluation—

1. Look for autoagglutination in the blood tubes or on a microscope slide.
2. Evaluate the CBC.
   A. PCV <18% indicates severe anemia; 18–29% is moderate anemia; 30–36% is mild anemia.
   B. Regenerative anemias usually have macrocytic (increased MCV) and hypochromic (decreased MCHC) RBC indices.
   C. The normal reticulocyte count for a dog is 0–1%, or 0–60,000/μL. A reticulocyte count greater than 60,000, or >1% corrected reticulocyte count, is usually regenerative.
   D. A reticulocyte index greater than 2.5 indicates regenerative anemia.
   E. Hemolytic anemia patients will often have a strong to moderate regenerative response, leukocytosis characterized by neutrophilia with a left shift and monocytosis.
3. Blood smear evaluation:
   A. 8–12 platelets should be observed per high-power field (hpf). Less than 3–4 platelets per hpf indicates a clinically significant thrombocytopenia;1 platelet/hpf = 15,000 platelets.
   B. An increased number of nucleated RBCs may be seen.
   C. Evaluate RBC morphology, looking for spherocytosis, polychromasia or schistocytes.
   D. Look for intracellular parasites.
4. Direct Coombs' test—the result may be negative in 10–30% of dogs with IMHA.
5. Evaluate the serum or plasma protein concentration. Blood loss usually results in hypoproteinemia, but hemolysis does not.
6. Perform a serum biochemical profile.
7. Run the infectious disease titers for common regional illnesses.
8. Run a coagulation profile if there are signs of any bleeding abnormalities.
   A. ACT – evaluates the intrinsic and common pathway and can be performed in house; normal is 60–110s in the dog.
   B. PT – evaluates the extrinsic and common coagulation pathways.
   C. PTT – evaluates the intrinsic and common pathways.
   D. Fibrin (fibrinogen) degradation product (FDP) – elevation suggests diffuse coagulation or delayed hepatic clearance.
   E. D-dimers – elevation may indicate DIC and major vessel thrombosis.

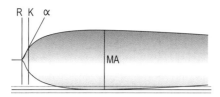

FIG 8.1 **Thromboelastography: a tool for measuring hypercoagulability, hypocoagulability and fibrinolysis.** Reaction time (R), clot formation time (K), angle (α), and maximal amplitude (MA). *Figure re-drawn from Donahue, S.M., Otto, C.M., 2005. Thromboelastography: a tool for measuring hypercoagulability, hypocoagulability, and fibrinolysis. Journal of Veterinary Emergency and Critical Care 15 (1), 9–16, with permission of John Wiley & Sons.*

9. Run thromboelastography (TEG) if available (Fig. 8.1).
   A. R = reaction time. It is measured from the start to detectable clot formation. Abnormalities are seen with defects of the intrinsic pathway, deficiencies of factors VIII, IX, XI and XII.
   B. K = kinetic time. It is the time to achieve a specific clot strength. It is influenced by hematocrit (HCT), platelet count / function, factor II, factor VIII, thrombin, fibrin and fibrinogen.
   C. α-angle is the rapidity of fibrin formation and cross linking. It is influenced by HCT, platelet count / function, factor II, factor VIII, thrombin, fibrin and fibrinogen.
   D. MA = maximum amplitude. It is a measure of maximum clot strength. It is influenced by HCT, platelet count / function, factor XII, thrombin, fibrin and fibrinogen.
   E. TMA = time to reach MA (minutes).
   F. CI = coagulation index – a formula for humans to determine whether the patient is hyper- or hypocoagulable.
10. Separate and freeze plasma for von Willebrand's disease testing, etc.
11. Perform a urinalysis and fecal examination.
12. Evaluate RBC fragility in house by adding 5 drops of patient blood to 5 mL 0.54% saline (made by mixing 3 volumes 0.9% NaCl with 2 volumes water), incubating for 30 minutes, then shaking the tube gently to agitate. Hemolysis indicates increased RBC osmotic fragility.

Radiographic evaluation—Thoracic and abdominal radiographs should be evaluated. A mass or organ enlargement may be observed. There may be evidence of internal hemorrhage, such as pericardial effusion, pleural effusion or abdominal effusion.

Ultrasonograph—Ultrasonographic evaluation of any abnormality noted on radiographs may be beneficial. Avoid obtaining ultrasound-guided biopsy samples until coagulation parameters have been evaluated.

Prognosis

The prognosis varies with the underlying etiology.

Treatment

1. Inform the client of the underlying etiologies, prognoses and cost of treatment.

2. Place an intravenous catheter.
3. Obtain blood samples (red-, purple- and blue-top tubes).
4. Pending the determination of a specific diagnosis, treat symptomatically and supportively.
   A. Attempt to find and stop any ongoing hemorrhage.
   B. Administer intravenous fluids to treat hypovolemic shock or renal disease (90 mL/kg/h for dogs initially, then readjusted for the patient's needs), or administer fluids at maintenance rates (2–4 mL/kg/h) if the patient is not in shock.
   C. Administer antiparasiticidal therapy as indicated:
      I. Fenbendazole (Panacur®), 50 mg/kg PO for 3 days.
      II. Pyrantel (Nemex®), 5 mg/kg PO, repeat in 7–10 days.
      III. Ivermectin, 200 µg/kg SC. (Ivermectin is not for use in Collies, Collie mixed-breed dogs, Shelties, Border Collies, Australian Shepherds, Old English Sheepdogs, other dogs with the mutant variant *MDR-1* gene, or in dogs with heartworm disease.)
   D. Treat topically for ticks or fleas. Nitenpyram (Capstar®) works rapidly and is very safe.
   E. Administer vitamin K_1 if there is a possibility of anticoagulant rodenticide toxicity or severe hepatic disease.
      I. For exposure to first-generation anticoagulant rodenticides, administer 0.25–1.25 mg/kg SC or PO q12h.
      II. For exposure to second-generation anticoagulant rodenticides, indanediones, and if the source is unknown, administer 5 mg/kg SC in several sites as an initial loading dose and then 2.5 mg/kg PO q12h.
   F. Administer H_2 blockers and gastric protectants if there is gastrointestinal hemorrhage.
      I. Ranitidine (Zantac®), 0.5–2 mg/kg IV, PO q8h
      II. Famotidine (Pepcid®), 0.5–1 mg/kg IV or PO q12–24h
      III. Omeprazole (Prilosec®), 0.5–1.5 mg/kg PO q24h
      IV. Pantoprazole (Protonix®), 0.7–1 mg/kg IV q24h
      V. Sucralfate, 0.5–1 g PO q8h; can start with a loading dose 4× higher.
   G. Administer doxycycline or tetracycline if the patient is suspected of having ehrlichiosis.
      I. Doxycycline, 5–10 mg/kg IV, PO q12h
      II. Tetracycline, 22 mg/kg PO q8–12h
   H. Administer imidocarb, 5 mg/kg IM once, if the dog is diagnosed with babesiosis.
5. Administer balanced electrolyte crystalloid fluids intravenously at maintenance rates, 2–4 mL/kg/h (1–2 mL/lb/h).
6. Administer oxygen if needed.
7. Administer corticosteroids if the patient may have immune-mediated hemolytic anemia (IHA or IMHA) or immune-mediated thrombocytopenia (ITP).
   A. Administer prednisolone at 2 mg/kg PO q12h for dogs <6 kg and 1.1 mg/kg or 30 mg/m² for dogs >30 kg, or
   B. Dexamethasone, 0.1–0.3 mg/kg (0.2–0.4 mg/lb) IV q12–24h, may be used initially, but should not be used for long-term therapy.

8. Administer packed RBCs or a hemoglobin-based oxygen carrier if the patient exhibits signs of cardiovascular or respiratory distress. Administer RBCs only after performing cross matching.
   A. Cross-match procedure
      I. Centrifuge samples collected into purple-topped tubes at $3400 \times G$ for 1 minute. Remove and retain the plasma.
      II. Wash the RBCs three times in isotonic saline, resuspend, centrifuge and discard supernatant, retaining the packed RBCs.
      III. Prepare 2% red cell saline suspension: 0.02 mL washed RBC, plus 0.98 mL of 0.9% NaCl.
      IV. Major cross match: 2 drops donor red cell suspension, 2 drops recipient plasma.
      V. Minor cross match: 2 drops recipient red cell suspension, 2 drops donor plasma.
      VI. Control: 2 drops recipient red cell suspension, 2 drops recipient plasma.
      VII. Incubate major, minor and control at 25°C for 30 minutes.
      VIII. Centrifuge all tubes at $3400 \times G$ for 1 minute.
      IX. A compatible sample will not show agglutination.
9. Use a blood filter and either an infusion pump manufactured to be safe for the administration of blood or gravity flow.
10. It is safe to piggy-back isotonic crystalloid fluids that do not contain calcium during blood or RBC administration. Do not piggy-back with LRS, 5% dextrose in water, 7.5% NaCl, or other hypotonic or hypertonic fluids.
11. Example of estimation of volume required in blood therapy: 30 kg dog with a PCV = 10%, desired PCV = 20%. Donor blood PCV = 50%. (Blood volume = 85–90 mL/kg for dogs.)
    A. Required whole blood volume to be administered:

$$\text{blood (mL)} = [BW\ (kg) \times 90] \times \left[\frac{\text{desired PCV} - \text{recipient PCV}}{\text{PCV of donor blood}} \right]$$
$$= [30 \times 90] \times [\{20\% - 10\%\} \div 50\%]$$
$$= 2700 \times [10\% \div 50\%]$$
$$= 2700 \times 0.2 = 540\ mL$$

$$\frac{\text{Desired RBC volume}}{\text{to be administered}} = 540 \div 2 = 270\,mL$$

12. Usually administer about 10 mL blood/lb (22 mL blood/kg) of body weight or 5 mL/lb (11 mL/kg) red blood cells.
13. Ideally, RBC or stored blood should be gently warmed to room temperature in a warm water bath or by sitting out of refrigeration for several minutes. However, warm saline may be added to the blood bag and the fluid line may be run through a fluid warmer if blood is needed in a crisis, without the time needed for warming.
14. Administer blood or RBC at the rate of 5–10 mL/kg/h (2.5–5 mL/lb/h) unless the patient's condition is critical, then rapid administration (20–80 mL/kg/h) is indicated. Blood or RBC transfusion should be completed within 4 hours to decrease bacterial growth in the unit of blood or RBC being administered.

Hematologic emergencies

A. Monitor for transfusion reactions.
    I. Urticaria
    II. Fever
    III. Vomiting
    IV. Dyspnea
    V. Hemoglobinemia, hemoglobinuria, hematuria
    VI. Restlessness
    VII. Pulmonary edema.

B. Treatment of transfusion reactions
    I. Stop the transfusion.
    II. Establish an airway; ensure adequate oxygenation.
    III. Antihistamines (diphenhydramine, 2 mg/kg IV or IM)
    IV. Shock therapy.

15. Monitor with serial PCV / TS at 1, 24 and 72 hours post-transfusion.

16. The recommended dosage for Oxyglobin®, a hemoglobin-based oxygen carrier which is not currently available, is 15–30 mL/kg IV, given at a rate of up to 10 mL/kg/h, but it can be rapidly administered if the dog is hypovolemic and in critical condition.

A. Do not administer other fluids or medications through the same IV line while administering Oxyglobin®.

B. No filter is needed.

C. A cross match is not needed.

D. The patient's hydration status should be normal prior to receiving Oxyglobin®.

E. Oxyglobin® is contraindicated in patients with congestive heart failure or anuric renal failure.

F. Post-administration monitoring of clinical pathology parameters will be affected. Check with the manufacturer for specific interference for the equipment utilized.

G. Post-administration, the dog will urinate orange for about 4 hours and the serum, skin, mucous membranes and sclera will become discolored a yellow to dark orange tone.

17. If the IMHA patient is critical, or the PCV continues to drop despite treatment, administer immunosuppressive drugs.

A. Azathioprine (Imuran®), 1–2 mg/kg PO q24h for 5–7 days, followed by 2 mg/kg every other day until prednisone therapy has been discontinued for 4 weeks. Taper the patient off azathioprine over 2–3 months by increasing the time period between doses by 1 day every 4 weeks.

B. Cyclophosphamide (Cytoxan®):
    I. 200–300 mg/m² IV bolus once, or
    II. 200 mg/m² PO divided over 4 days (50 mg/m²/day), stop for 3 days, repeat CBC and re-evaluate; or
    III. 50 mg/m² PO q24h for 4 days, stop for 3 days, repeat CBC and re-evaluate.

C. Discontinue immunosuppressive drugs for a few days if the segmented neutrophil count falls below 3,500/L or the platelet count is <30,000 L. Repeat the CBC, if the neutrophil count has increased, restart at a lower dose.

18. Therapy to prevent or diminish the incidence of thromboembolic disease is essential since about 80% of dogs that were necropsied following the diagnosis of IMHA had died from thromboembolism, not anemia.
    A. Aspirin 0.5 mg/kg PO q24h in dogs, q72h in cats
    B. Low doses of unfractionated heparin (UFH) 100–200 IU/kg SC q8h, or 5–10 U/kg/h IV CRI.
    C. Low molecular weight heparin (LMWH)
        I. Enoxaparin, 0.8 mg/kg SC q6–8h
        II. Dalteparin, 150 IU/kg SCq12h
    D. Clopidogrel 1.13 ± 0.17 mg/kg, PO, q24h or 1–5 mg/kg PO q24h in dogs and 18.75 mg/cat PO q24h.
19. Additional treatment for dogs with nonresponsive IMHA include:
    A. Danazol, 10–15 mg/kg PO q24h, may be hepatotoxic and is not recommended for chronic administration.
    B. Cyclosporine (ciclosporin) A, 5–10 mg/kg PO q24h. The plasma concentration should be monitored periodically. A safe trough level is 400–500 ng/mL. Cyclosporine A may be beneficial during the induction phase owing to its rapid onset of action.
    C. Leflunomide (Arava®) may be beneficial in refractory patients. The initial dose is 4 mg/kg PO q24h. A safe trough level of the active metabolite A77 1726 is 20 µg/mL plasma.
    D. Mycophenolate mofetil (MMF) may be administered at 10–20 mg/kg PO q12h.
    E. Mizoribine is a substitute for azathioprine in renal transplant patients in Japan and Europe. It has minimal hepatotoxicity and myelotoxicity.
    F. Human IV IgG (hIVIgG), 0.5–1 g/kg IV diluted in 0.9% NaCl, sterile water, or crystalloid IV fluid, delivered as an IV CRI over 6 hours. This dosage may be repeated daily for 3 consecutive days. These patients should receive aspirin and/or heparin therapy, as hIVIgG promotes hypercoagulability and inflammation.
    G. Splenectomy may be beneficial for patients that fail to respond to therapy or have severe adverse effects from therapy.

Long-term therapy
After 14 days with a stable or rising PCV and no clinical signs of anemia, the dose of prednisone may be decreased by 25% then decreased by 25% every 2 weeks until the patient is stable on 0.5 mg/kg q24h, then switch to alternate-day prednisone therapy. After no signs of relapse for 6 weeks, prednisone may be discontinued.

FELINE ANEMIA

Etiology

Regenerative anemia—Acute blood loss (trauma) after the first 48–96 hours, chronic blood loss (hookworms, flea infestation, immune-mediated thrombocytopenia (ITP) with bleeding, disseminated intravascular coagulopathy, hemolytic disease (immune-mediated hemolytic anemia [IMHA or IHA]), neonatal isoerythrolysis, hypophosphatemia, hemobartonellosis, babesiosis, ehrlichiosis, cytauxzoonosis, onions, acetaminophen, phenothiazines, benzocaine, methionine, methylene blue, propylene glycol, propylthiouracil, vitamin K, methimazole, sulfa antibiotics, penicillins and cephalosporins.

Nonregenerative anemia—Feline leukemia virus infection (FeLV), feline immunodeficiency virus (FIV) infection, feline infectious peritonitis (FIP) infection, feline panleukopenia virus infection, the first 48–96 hours following acute blood loss, renal disease, nutritional deficiencies, iron deficiency, flea infestation, bone-marrow suppression secondary to malignancy, ionizing radiation, myelophthisis, myelodysplastic syndromes, myelofibrosis, ostcosclerosis, osteopetrosis, chronic disease, hypoadrenocorticism, hypothyroidism, ehrlichiosis and chloramphenicol.

Diagnosis

History—The owner may observe anorexia, pica, lethargy, weakness, weight loss, syncope or collapse. There may be a history of exposure to parasites, trauma, toxins, heat or other ill animals. Inquire about medications currently or recently administered, and any recent illness or surgery. There may be an incidence of hematologic disorders in litter mates, parents or house mates. Inquire about the patient's current diet and nutritional status. Question the owner regarding any recent blood loss, including hematuria, melena, hematochezia, epistaxis or hemoptysis.

Physical exam—The patient may have pallor, icterus, ecchymoses or petechiae, and hypothermia. The patient may exhibit weakness, dyspnea, tachypnea, tachycardia, pounding pulses or a grade I / II systolic murmur. Upon palpation, lymphadenopathy, hepatomegaly and splenomegaly may be detected. The patient may also show signs of weight loss, cachexia, evidence of bleeding or trauma, or the presence of ticks or fleas.

Laboratory evaluation—

1. Look for autoagglutination in the blood tubes or on a microscope slide.
2. Evaluate the CBC.
   A. PCV <14% indicates severe anemia; 15–19% is moderate anemia; 20–24% is mild anemia.
   B. Regenerative anemias usually have macrocytic and hypochromic RBC indices.
   C. The normal reticulocyte count for a cat is 0–0.4% (0–40,000/μL) aggregated reticulocytes and less than 5% (<500,000/μL) punctate reticulocytes. Aggregate reticulocytes indicate the most active and recent form of regeneration. An aggregate reticulocyte count greater than 1% (100,000/μL) indicates regeneration.
   D. Hemolytic anemia patients will often have a strong to moderate regenerative response, leukocytosis characterized by neutrophilia with a left shift and monocytosis.

3. Blood smear evaluation
   A. 10–12 platelets should be observed per field under oil immersion. Less than 3–4 platelets per oil immersion field indicates a clinically significant thrombocytopenia.
   B. An increased number of nucleated RBCs may be seen.
   C. Evaluate RBC morphology; look for spherocytosis, polychromasia, schistocytes and Heinz bodies.
   D. Look for intracellular parasites, including hemobartonella organisms attached to RBCs, and *Cytauxzoon felis* organisms in macrophages and RBCs.
4. Direct Coombs' test—the result may be negative in 10–30% of cats with IMHA.
5. Evaluate the serum or plasma protein concentration. Blood loss usually results in hypoproteinemia, but hemolysis does not.
6. Perform a serum biochemical profile.
7. Run the infectious disease titers for common regional illnesses and feline viral disease, including FeLV, FIV and FIP.
8. Run a coagulation profile if there are signs of any bleeding abnormalities.
   A. ACT—evaluates the intrinsic and common pathway and can be performed in house; normal is 50–75 seconds in the cat.
   B. PT—evaluates the extrinsic and common coagulation pathways.
   C. PTT—evaluates the intrinsic and common pathways.
   D. FDP—elevation suggests diffuse coagulation or delayed hepatic clearance.
   E. D-dimers—elevation may indicate DIC and major vessel thrombosis.
9. Perform a urinalysis and fecal examination.
10. Evaluate RBC fragility in house by adding 5 drops of patient blood to 5 mL 0.54% saline (made by mixing 3 volumes 0.9% NaCl with 2 volumes water), incubating for 30 minutes, then shaking the tube gently to agitate. Hemolysis indicates increased RBC osmotic fragility.

Radiographic evaluation—Thoracic and abdominal radiographs should be evaluated. A mass or organ enlargement may be observed. There may be evidence of internal hemorrhage such as pericardial effusion, pleural effusion or abdominal effusion.

Ultrasonography—Ultrasonographic evaluation of any abnormality noted on radiographs may be useful. Avoid obtaining ultrasound-guided biopsy samples until coagulation parameters have been evaluated.

Prognosis

The prognosis varies with the underlying etiology.

Treatment

1. Inform the client of the underlying etiologies, prognoses and cost of the treatment.
2. Place an intravenous catheter.

3. Obtain blood samples (red-, purple- and blue-top tubes).
4. Pending the determination of a specific diagnosis, treat symptomatically and supportively.
   A. Attempt to find and stop any ongoing hemorrhage.
   B. Administer intravenous fluids to treat hypovolemic shock or renal disease (60 mL/kg/h initially then readjusted for the patient's needs), or administer fluids at maintenance rates (1–2 mL/kg/h) if the patient is not in shock.
   C. Administer antiparasiticidal therapy as indicated.
      I. Pyrantel (Nemex®), 20 mg/kg PO once
      II. Praziquantel (Droncit®), 6.3 mg/kg for cats <1.8 kg; 5 mg/kg for cats >1.8 kg PO
      III. Epsiprantel (Cestex®), 2.75 mg/kg PO
   D. Treat topically for fleas or ticks.
   E. Administer vitamin K_1 if there is a possibility of anticoagulant rodenticide toxicity or severe hepatic disease.
      I. For exposure to first-generation anticoagulant rodenticides, administer 0.25–1.25 mg/kg SC or PO q12h.
      II. For exposure to second-generation anticoagulant rodenticides, indanediones and if the source is unknown, administer 5 mg/kg SC in several sites as an initial loading dose and then 2.5 mg/kg PO q12h.
   F. Administer H_2 blockers and gastric protectants if there is gastrointestinal hemorrhage.
      I. Ranitidine (Zantac®), 1–2 mg/kg PO, IV, SC q12h
      II. Famotidine (Pepcid®), 0.5–1 mg/kg IV or PO q12–24h
      III. Omeprazole (Prilosec®), 0.5–1 mg/kg PO q24h
      IV. Pantoprazole (Protonix®), 0.7–1 mg/kg IV q24h
      V. Sucralfate, 0.25 g PO q8–12h
   G. Administer doxycycline or tetracycline if the patient is suspected of having an *Ehrlichiosis* sp. or *Hemobartonella* sp. infection until a negative result on a blood smear is confirmed by a reference laboratory.
      I. Doxycycline, 5–10 mg/kg IV, PO q12h
      II. Tetracycline, 22 mg/kg PO q8h
5. Administer balanced electrolyte crystalloid fluids intravenously at maintenance rates, 1–2 mL/kg/h.
6. Administer oxygen if needed.
7. Administer corticosteroids if the patient may have immune-mediated hemolytic anemia (IHA or IMHA) or immune-mediated thrombocytopenia (ITP).
   A. Administer prednisolone at 1–4 mg/kg IM or PO q12h; or
   B. Dexamethasone, 0.1–0.2 mg/kg (0.2–0.4 mg/lb) IV q12–24h may be used initially, but should not be used for long-term therapy.
8. Administer packed RBCs, whole blood, or a hemoglobin-based oxygen carrier if the patient exhibits signs of cardiovascular or respiratory distress. Administer blood only after performing a cross match. An in-house kit is also available to blood type the

patient prior to administration, to avoid potentially fatal transfusion reactions.

A. Cross matching

    I. Centrifuge samples at 3400 × G for 1 minute. Remove and retain plasma.

    II. Wash RBCs three times in isotonic saline, resuspend, centrifuge and discard supernatant, retaining packed RBCs.

    III. Prepare 2% red cell saline suspension: 0.02 mL washed packed RBC, plus 0.98 mL of 0.9% NaCl.

    IV. Major cross match: 2 drops donor red cell suspension, 2 drops recipient plasma.

    V. Minor cross match: 2 drops recipient red cell suspension, 2 drops donor plasma.

    VI. Control: 2 drops recipient red cell suspension, 2 drops recipient plasma.

    VII. Incubate major, minor, and control at 25°C for 30 minutes.

    VIII. Centrifuge all tubes at 3400 × G for 1 minute.

    IX. A compatible sample will lack agglutination.

B. Monitor for transfusion reactions including:

    I. Urticaria

    II. Fever

    III. Vomiting

    IV. Dyspnea

    V. Hemoglobinemia, hemoglobinuria, hematuria

    VI. Restlessness

    VII. Pulmonary edema.

C. Treatment of transfusion reactions

    I. Stop the transfusion.

    II. Establish an airway; ensure adequate oxygenation.

    III. Administer antihistamines (diphenhydramine, 2 mg/kg IV or IM).

    IV. Administer shock therapy.

9. Pretreat with diphenhydramine HCl at 1 mg/kg IV or IM, and dexamethasone sodium phosphate, 0.5–1 mg/kg IV, 20–40 minutes before starting the transfusion.

10. Example of estimation of volume required in blood therapy: 3 kg cat with a PCV = 10%, desired PCV = 20%. Donor blood PCV = 40%. (Blood volume = 65–75 mL/kg for cats). Blood volume to be administered (mL):

$$= [\text{BW (kg)} \times 70] \times [(\text{PCV desired} - \text{PCV recipient}) \div \text{PCV donor}]$$
$$= [3 \times 70] \times [(20\% - 10\%) \div 40$$
$$= 210 \times (10 \div 40) = 210 \times 0.25 = 52.5 \text{ mL}$$

11. Monitor with serial PCVs at 1, 24 and 72 hours post-transfusion.

12. Consider the administration of chlorambucil (Leukeran®, 20 mg/m² PO q2weeks) for cats with IMHA that is nonresponsive to corticosteroid therapy.

Diagnosis

History—The owner may notice spontaneous bleeding, including petechia, ecchymoses, mucosal bleeding and melena. The patient may suffer from an acute collapse episode, or may exhibit lethargy, anorexia and vomiting.

Obtain the history of any medications that may have been administered to the patient, including vaccinations. If possible, discontinue the medication and re-evaluate the platelet count in 2–6 days. If the platelet count returns to normal, the presumptive diagnosis is drug-induced thrombocytopenia.

Physical exam—The patient may be weak and lethargic. Pallor, gingival bleeding, petechiae and ecchymosis may be observed. Splenomegaly may be palpable. Perform a complete physical examination. Lymphadenopathy may be detected. Melena may be observed. The femoral pulse may be weak and thready.

Laboratory evaluation—

1. Evaluate the CBC.
   A. Platelet count of less than 100,000/µL indicates mild thrombocytopenia, less than 60,000/µL is moderate thrombocytopenia, and less than 30,000/µL is severe thrombocytopenia and is associated with an increased risk of hemorrhage.
   B. Expect to see 8–12 platelets/hpf; 1 platelet/hpf = 15,000 platelets.
   C. The patient may or may not be anemic.
   D. If IMHA (IHA) is associated with ITP (IMT), referred to as Evans's syndrome, a regenerative anemia with spherocytosis is usually present and the Coombs' test will usually be positive.
   E. Leukocytosis characterized by neutrophilia with a left shift may be observed.
2. Blood smear evaluation
   A. 11–25 platelets observed per oil immersion field are considered normal. A minimum of 10–12 platelets should be observed per oil immersion field. Less than 3–4 platelets per oil immersion field indicates a clinically significant thrombocytopenia.
   B. Evaluate RBC morphology, looking for spherocytosis, polychromasia or schistocytes.
   C. Look for intracellular parasites.
3. The buccal mucosal bleeding time (BMBT) should be measured if the platelet count is greater than 60,000/µL.
   A. Sedation may be required, particularly in cats.
   B. Evert the upper lip and apply a gauze muzzle to hold it in place and slightly engorge the buccal vessels.
   C. Make two incisions in the buccal mucosa of the everted lip with a template device such as the Simplate II® (Fig. 8.2).
   D. Soak up the hemorrhage by applying filter paper underneath the wound, but do not touch the wound.

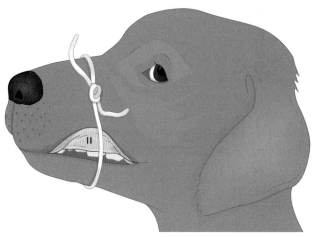

FIG 8.2 **Buccal mucosal bleed time site.** Evert the upper lip. Apply a gauze muzzle to hold the upper lip in place and to slightly engorge the buccal vessels. Make two incisions as shown in the buccal mucosa of the everted lip with a template device such as the Simplate II®.

   E Measure the time from making the incision until the bleeding stops.

   F. Normal BMBT is 2–3 minutes for dogs and cats.

   G. The BMBT is normal in patients with coagulation factor deficiencies and in some patients with DIC. The BMBT is prolonged in patients with thrombocytopenia, thrombocytopathia and von Willebrand's disease.

  4. Coagulation tests, including ACT, PTT and PT, may be slightly prolonged (<10%) if the platelet count is less than 10,000/µL. FDPs, D-dimers and fibrinogen concentration are normal.

  5. Evaluation of a bone-marrow aspirate or biopsy will usually show megakaryocytic hyperplasia, but sometimes megakaryocytic hypoplasia is observed.

  6. A direct megakaryocytic immunofluorescence assay (D-MIFA) may be performed on a bone-marrow smear.

  7. Platelet-bindable autoantibodies may be detected in patient serum or plasma by performing indirect assays, or direct assays may be performed to detect antibodies on the platelet surface (platelet surface–associated immunoglobulin G).

  8. Perform a serum biochemical profile.

  9. Run the infectious disease titers or PCR for common regional illnesses.

10. Perform a urinalysis and fecal examination.

Radiographic evaluation—Thoracic and abdominal radiographs should be evaluated. A mass or organ enlargement may be observed. There may be evidence of internal hemorrhage, such as pericardial effusion, pleural effusion or abdominal effusion.

Ultrasonography—Ultrasonographic evaluation of any abnormality noted on radiographs may be useful. Avoid obtaining ultrasound-guided biopsy samples until coagulation parameters have been evaluated.

Differential diagnosis

1. Decreased platelet production—immune-mediated megakaryocytic hypoplasia, retroviral infection (FeLV and FIV), ehrlichiosis, Rocky Mountain spotted fever, babesiosis, cyclic thrombocytopenia, myelophthisis, idiopathic bone-marrow aplasia, and drug-induced megakaryocytic hypoplasia (beta-lactam antibiotics, estrogens, melphalan, phenylbutazone).
2. Increased platelet destruction, sequestration, or utilization—immune-mediated thrombocytopenia (ITP), live-viral vaccines, disseminated intravascular coagulation, vasculitis, splenomegaly, splenic torsion, endotoxemia, acute hepatic necrosis, neoplasia, hemolytic uremic syndrome, microangiopathy, and drug-induced thrombocytopenia (including acetaminophen, amrinone, antihistamines, aspirin, benzodiazepines, chloramphenicol, cimetidine, phenytoin (Dilantin®), ethanol, erythromycin, furosemide, heparin, lidocaine, nitroglycerin, phenothiazines, prednisone, propranolol, quinidine, tetracyclines and thiazides).
3. Thrombocytopathia—aspirin, Chediak–Higashi syndrome in cats, Glanzmann's thrombasthenia in Otterhounds and Great Pyrenees dogs.

Prognosis

The prognosis is fair, with a reported survival rate of 70–75%. A decreased probability of survival was noted in patients with melena or a high BUN at the time of hospital admission.

Treatment

1. Inform the client of the underlying etiologies, prognoses and cost of the treatment.
2. Place an intravenous catheter.
3. Obtain blood samples (red- purple- and blue-top tubes).
4. Pending the determination of a specific diagnosis, treat symptomatically and supportively.
   A. Attempt to find and stop any ongoing hemorrhage.
   B. Administer intravenous fluids to treat hypovolemic shock or renal disease (90 mL/kg/h initially for dogs, 60 mL/kg/h initially for cats, delivered in $\frac{1}{4}$-shock dose boluses then readjusted for the patient's needs), or administer fluids at maintenance rates (2–4 mL/kg/h for dogs, 1–2 mL/kg/h for cats) if the patient is not in shock.

C. Treat topically for ticks or fleas.
D. Administer H_2 blockers and gastric protectants if there is gastrointestinal hemorrhage or during long-term glucocorticoid therapy.
   I. Ranitidine (Zantac®), 0.5–2 mg/kg IV, PO q8h (dogs), 1–2 mg/kg PO, IV, SC q12h (cats)
   II. Famotidine (Pepcid®), 0.5–1 mg/kg IV or PO q12–24h
   III. Omeprazole (Prilosec®)
      a. Dogs: 0.5–1.5 mg/kg PO q24h
      b. Cats: 0.5–1 mg/kg PO q24h
   IV. Pantoprazole (Protonix®), 0.7–1 mg/kg IV q24h
   V. Sucralfate
      a. Dogs: 0.5–1 g PO q8h; can start with a loading dose 4× higher
      b. Cats: 0.25 g PO q8–12h
E. Administer doxycycline or tetracycline if the patient is suspected of having ehrlichiosis.
   I. Doxycycline, 5–10 mg/kg IV, PO q12h
   II. Tetracycline, 22 mg/kg PO q8–12h
F. Administer imidocarb, 5 mg/kg IM, once if the dog is diagnosed with babesiosis.
5. Administer balanced electrolyte crystalloid fluids intravenously at maintenance rates, 2–4 mL/kg/h.
6. Administer oxygen if needed.
7. Administer corticosteroids if the patient may have immune-mediated thrombocytopenia (ITP).
   A. Administer prednisolone at 1–2 mg/kg PO q12h; or
   B. Dexamethasone, 0.1–0.2 mg/kg (0.2–0.4 mg/lb) IV q12–24h, may be used initially but should not be used for long-term therapy.
8. Administer vincristine, 0.02 mg/kg IV once.
9. Administer azathioprine (Imuran®), 50 mg/m² or 2 mg/kg PO q24h for 14 days then 2 mg/kg PO every other day.
10. Platelet transfusion may be beneficial for the patient with a life-threatening hemorrhagic crisis. The circulating half life of transfused platelets is short and the platelet count of the recipient is usually not increased.
11. Administer packed RBCs or a hemoglobin-based oxygen carrier if the patient exhibits signs of cardiovascular or respiratory distress. If the patient is severely and acutely hemorrhaging, administer fresh whole blood.
12. The use of a blood filter is not recommended for the administration of platelet concentrates.
13. Additional treatment for dogs with nonresponsive ITP
    A. Cyclosporine, 5–10 mg/kg PO q12h
    B. Human gamma globulin (hIVIgG), 0.5–1 g/kg IV once over 6–12 hours
    C. Mycophenolate mofetil, 10–20 mg/kg PO q12h
14. Consider performing a splenectomy.

Hematologic emergencies

COAGULOPATHIES

Etiology

1. Factor I deficiency (hypofibrinogenemia or dysfibrinogenemia in Saint Bernards, Vizslas, Collies and Borzois)
2. Factor II deficiency (hypoprothrombinemia in Boxers, Cocker Spaniels, and Devon Rex cats)
3. Factor VII deficiency (in Beagles, Alaskan Malamutes, miniature Schnauzers, Boxers and English Bulldogs)
4. Factor VIII deficiency (hemophilia A in many dog breeds, mixed-breed dogs, and Devon Short Hair cats)
5. Factor IX deficiency (hemophilia B in many breeds of dogs and cats)
6. Factor X deficiency (Stuart–Prower trait in Cocker Spaniels, Jack Russell Terriers and Devon Rex cats)
7. Factor XI deficiency (hemophilia C) (plasma thromboplastin antecedent deficiency in Springer Spaniels, Kerry Blue Terriers, Weimaraner and Great Pyrenees)
8. Factor XII deficiency (Hageman factor deficiency in cats and many dog breeds, including German short-haired Pointers and Poodles)
9. Von Willebrand's disease in many dog and cat breeds
10. Vitamin K deficiency or antagonism, such as with anticoagulant rodenticide toxicity
11. Hepatic disease
12. Disseminated intravascular coagulation
13. Circulating anticoagulants such as heparin.

Diagnosis

History—The patient may have a history of present and past bleeding episodes, bleeding amounts inappropriate to the injury, inciting cause of hemorrhaging, familial history, toxin exposure, environmental factors, drug administration including vaccinations and nonsteroidal anti-inflammatory drugs and the age at onset. A diagnosis must be pursued as treatment varies considerably according to etiology.

Physical exam—Deep hemorrhages into body cavities, subcutaneous tissues, muscles, hematoma formation, petechia, or ecchymotic hemorrhages (check oral, penile, vulvar, conjunctival mucous membranes, sclera, retinas and skin), epistaxis, melena, joint pain or swelling, hematuria, icterus, evidence of trauma, intrapulmonary hemorrhage (Table 8.1).

Laboratory tests—

1. CBC with platelet count
2. Coagulation profile
   A. Intrinsic and common pathways
      I. PTT – normal is less than 25% elevation above control values.
      II. ACT – normal in the dog is 60–110 seconds; normal in the cat is 50–75 seconds.
   B. Extrinsic and common pathways: PT – normal is less than 25% elevation above control values (Fig. 8.3).

Table 8.1 *Useful clinical features in differentiating between coagulation factor abnormalities and platelet or vascular abnormalities*

Coagulation factor abnormalities	Vascular or platelet abnormalities
Petechiae are rare	Petechiae are common
Hematomas are common	Hematomas are rare
Bleeding is often localized	Bleeding usually occurs at multiple locations
Bleeding commonly occurs into muscles and joints	Bleeding frequently involves mucous membranes
Bleeding may be delayed at onset, or stop, then start again (rebleed)	Prolonged bleeding from cuts

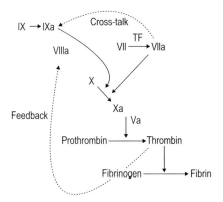

FIG 8.3 **The coagulation system pathway.** TF = tissue factor. The diagram illustrates how coagulation factors interact with one another. Activated factors are designated with an "a", as in "IXa". *Reprinted from Aird, WC, critical Care Medicine, 2005, Vol 33, No 12 (suppl.) S485-487, with permission of Wolters Kluwer Health.*

C. Fibrinogen – levels increase during acute inflammation.

D. Fibrin degradation products – an increase is compatible with ongoing systemic fibrinolysis as usually seen with DIC. Normal is <10 g/mL in cats and dogs. FDPs occur in patients with hepatic failure, major focal vascular thrombosis, dysfibrinogenemia, excessive fibrinolysis and DIC.

E. The D-dimer test measures the amount of a fragment of fully polymerized, cross-linked fibrin that occurs due to active fibrinolysis. Increased levels of this fragment may be pathognomonic for major vessel thrombosis and DIC.

F. Thromboelastography (TEG) (see Fig. 8.1)

   I. R = reaction time. It is measured from the start to detectable clot formation. Abnormalities are seen with defects of the intrinsic pathway, deficiencies of factors VIII, IX, XI, and XII.

   II. K = kinetic time. It is the time to achieve a specific clot strength. It is influenced by HCT, platelet count / function, factor II, factor VIII, thrombin, fibrin and fibrinogen.

   III. α-angle is the rapidity of fibrin formation and cross linking. It is influenced by HCT, platelet count / function, factor II, factor VIII, thrombin, fibrin and fibrinogen.

IV. MA = maximum amplitude. It is a measure of maximum clot
strength. It is influenced by HCT, platelet count / function,
factor XII, thrombin, fibrin and fibrinogen.

V. TMA = time to reach MA (minutes).

VI. CI = coagulation index, a formula for humans to determine
whether the patient is hyper- or hypocoagulable.

3. Serum chemistry profile–especially renal and hepatic function (BUN,
creatinine, serum alanine aminotransferase (ALT) alkaline phosphatase,
bilirubin)

4. Urinalysis

5. Fecal examination

6. Coombs' test, von Willebrand disease (VWD) (collect blood for VWD
in a blue-top tube, separate the plasma and immediately freeze the
plasma for testing. Dogs at risk from excessive surgical hemorrhage
are usually those with 30% or less of the normal level of von
Willebrand factor.)

7. Infectious disease serology testing as indicated by common regional
illnesses, history and clinical signs

Differential diagnosis

Immune-mediated thrombocytopenia, immune-mediated hemolytic anemia,
VWD, inherited coagulopathies, anticoagulant rodenticides, disseminated
intravascular coagulation

Prognosis

The prognosis is fair to poor.

Treatment

1. Inform the client of the differential diagnoses, prognosis and cost of the
treatment.

2. Hospitalize the patient for observation and treatment.

3. Pursue the diagnosis, treat the specific disease entity, trauma, toxin
exposure, etc.

4. Place an intravenous catheter in the cephalic or saphenous veins, as
jugular bleeding is hard to control following catheter placement.

5. Obtain blood samples for laboratory evaluation using the smallest
gauge needle possible and apply pressure to the venipuncture site for a
minimum of 5 minutes.

6. Monitor PCV/TP and ACT or coagulation profile.

7. Administer fresh whole blood or blood component therapy as indicated
if the patient is presented in circulatory shock or the patient is
exhibiting severe uncontrollable hemorrhage. (See Appendix III.)

   A. Cryoprecipitate is the preferred component to treat VWD, factor VIII
   deficiency (hemophilia A), hypofibrinogenemia and
   dysfibrinogenemia. If cryoprecipitate is not available, fresh frozen
   plasma is a useful alternative.

B. Stored plasma is recommended for the treatment of prothrombin deficiency, factor VII deficiency, factor IX deficiency (hemophilia B), factor X deficiency, and factor XI deficiency (hemophilia C).

8. Avoid intramuscular or subcutaneous injections.
9. Avoid drugs known to interfere with hemostasis (e.g. aspirin).
10. Administer vitamin K_1 if anticoagulant rodenticide toxicity or vitamin K deficiency is suspected.
    A. For exposure to first-generation anticoagulant rodenticides, administer 0.25–1.25 mg/kg SC or PO q12h.
    B. For exposure to second-generation anticoagulant rodenticides, indanediones, and if the source is unknown, administer 5 mg/kg SC in several sites as an initial loading dose and then 2.5 mg/kg PO q12h.
11. Consider administration of corticosteroids if suspect IMHA, ITP, etc.
    A. Administer prednisolone at 1–4 mg/kg SC or PO q12h; or
    B. Dexamethasone, 0.1–0.2 mg/kg IV q12–24h, may be used initially, but should not be used for long-term therapy.
12. Administer vincristine, 0.5–0.75 mg/m² IV, if the patient may have ITP and the platelet count remains low.
13. Additional treatment recommendations for patients with VWD include:
    A. Administration of deamino 8-D-arginine vasopressin (DDAVP®):
        I. Use the nasal preparation, which contains 0.1 mg/mL of DDAVP®.
        II. Administer DDAVP® SC at 1.0 mcg/kg for von Willebrand factor.
        III. Administer DDAVP® SC at 0.4 mcg/kg for maximal effect on factor VIII.
        IV. The coagulation response begins almost immediately, reaches maximal levels within 30 minutes and remains elevated for 4 hours.
        V. Not all dogs will respond to DDAVP®.
    B. DDAVP® can also be administered to the donor dog, at the dose of 0.6–1.0 mcg/kg SC 20–120 minutes prior to the collection of whole blood.

EPISTAXIS

Etiology

Ehrlichiosis, *Rickettsia rickettsii*, Rocky Mountain spotted fever, heartworm disease, leptospirosis, chronic feline viral upper respiratory disease, trauma, nasal foreign body, rhinitis, sinusitis, periapical abscess, thrombocytopenia, hypertension, neoplasia (including adenocarcinoma, squamous cell carcinoma, chondrosarcoma, hemangiosarcoma, melanoma, lymphosarcoma, neuroblastoma, and multiple myeloma), anticoagulant rodenticide toxicity, aspirin-induced thrombocytopathia, coagulopathy and idiopathic causes have been noted.

Diagnosis

History—The owner has usually observed active epistaxis or has found evidence of bleeding. Determine the frequency of hemorrhagic episodes and whether the hemorrhage is bilateral or unilateral. Obtain information regarding previous trauma, tick infestation, anorexia, lethargy, weight loss, nasal discharge, playing in grass or bushes or hunting, and possible toxin (anticoagulant rodenticide) exposure.

Large breed dogs with dolichocephalic faces, such as Collies, Irish Setters and German Shepherds, have a higher incidence of sinonasal neoplasia. In younger patients, trauma, foreign bodies and congenital coagulopathy are more common, whereas in older patients neoplasia is more common. VWD is more common in some breeds such as Doberman Pinschers and German Shepherds.

Physical exam—Note the patient's age, whether the hemorrhage is bilateral or unilateral, mucus membrane color, and capillary refill time. Pay particular attention to the anatomy of the muzzle, face and mouth (especially hard palate). Look for ticks. The patient may have a fever, lymphadenopathy, muscle wasting, icterus, petechiation and / or ecchymosis, hematomas and hemarthroses. Check for the presence of blood in feces and urine. Examine the sclera and retina. Measure arterial blood pressure.

Laboratory procedures—
1. CBC including platelet count
2. Reticulocyte count if anemic
3. Coagulation profile including PT, PTT or ACT, fibrinogen, and fibrin degradation products and possibly D-dimers. Thromboelastography would also be helpful if available (see Fig. 8.1).
4. Evaluate a complete serum chemistry profile. Carefully evaluate serum protein levels. Protein plasmapheresis may be indicated.
5. Infectious disease serology testing, including fungal titers, as indicated by common regional illnesses, history and clinical signs.
6. Run a PT test if anticoagulant rodenticide toxicity is suspected.

Nasal and thoracic radiographs—
1. Nasal radiographs may reveal increased fluid density, asymmetry, bone destruction or loss of turbinate structure.
2. Thoracic radiographs may reveal abnormal densities, masses, foreign bodies or fluid accumulation.

Other diagnostic procedures—
1. Oral and nasal examination under sedation
2. Endoscopic exam of the caudal nasal cavity
3. Nasal biopsy, flushing and cytology.

Prognosis

The prognosis is variable depending on the underlying etiology.

Treatment

1. Inform the client of the diagnosis, prognosis and the cost of treatment.
2. If moderate and decreasing or mild epistaxis, hospitalization and observation is indicated.
3. If moderate and increasing or severe epistaxis, hospitalize the patient for observation.
   A. Administer a *low* dose of acepromazine, 0.1–1 mg SC, or butorphanol, 0.2–0.4 mg/kg SC.
   B. Administer Yunan Paiyao or Baiyao. On the first day of therapy, give the small round red pill provided in the package and 1 or more capsules, based on body weight. Give the capsules for 5 days, then stop for 5 days, and repeat if needed. Do not administer daily for prolonged time periods.
      I. For dogs under 10 lbs, give 1 capsule by mouth one time a day.
      II. For dogs from 10 to 30 lbs, give 1 capsule by mouth two times a day.
      III. For dogs above 30 but less than 60 lbs, give 2 capsules two times a day.
      IV. For dogs above 60 lbs, give 2 capsules three times a day.
   C. Gently pack the nasal cavity with epinephrine-soaked gauze or umbilical tape.
   D. Flush the nasal sinuses with 1:1000 epinephrine.
   E. Apply cold compresses to muzzle.
   F. Administer blood component therapy as indicated, red blood cells for anemia, fresh frozen plasma for albumin and clotting factors, platelet-rich plasma if severe thrombocytopenia, or fresh whole blood transfusion if necessary for anemia thrombocytopenia and clotting factor deficiency (Appendix III).
4. If ehrlichiosis is the suspected etiology, administer tetracycline, 22–44 mg/kg PO q8h, or doxycycline, 5–10 mg/kg IV or PO q12h.
5. If immune-mediated thrombocytopenia is the suspected etiology, administer prednisone, 1–2 mg/kg PO q12h. Dexamethasone 0.1–0.2 mg/kg IV q12–24h, may be used initially but should not be used for long-term therapy.

DISSEMINATED INTRAVASCULAR COAGULATION (DIC)

Diagnosis

History—Predisposing disease, trauma, acidosis, anoxia, hypoxia, stasis of blood flow, and hypotension (bacterial sepsis, viremia, allergic vasculitis, snake bites, immune-mediated hemolytic anemia, acute hemolytic transfusion reaction, feline infectious peritonitis, gastric dilatation-volvulus, malignancy (including hemangiosarcoma), hepatic disease, amyloidosis, nephrotic syndrome, uremia, congestive heart failure, shock, surgery, pancreatitis, hemorrhagic gastroenteritis, babesiosis, dirofilariasis, heat stroke, etc.).
Clinical signs—In addition to the clinical signs of the underlying disease, the patient exhibits a combination of hemolytic and thrombolytic signs, including petechiae, ecchymoses, excessive bleeding from venipuncture

Table 8.2 *Diagnostic indicators of disseminated intravascular coagulation*

Stage	Platelets	ACT	ATIII	FSPs	Fibrinogen
Peracute	Decreased	Normal	Decreased	Normal	Normal
Acute	Decreased	Decreased	Decreased	Increased	Decreased
Chronic	Normal or decreased	Normal or increased	Normal or decreased	Increased or normal	Normal

Data from Kristensen AT, Feldman BF (1995), with permission of WB Saunders.

sites, bleeding from the genitourinary tract and / or the gastrointestinal tract.

Laboratory evaluation (Table 8.2)—

1. CBC
   A. The platelet count is usually decreased. The normal platelet count is 200,000–500,000/μL.
   B. The patient may be anemic if the underlying etiology is a hemolytic disorder or excessive blood loss has occurred.
   C. The white blood cell count may be increased if the underlying condition is infectious or inflammatory, or decreased if the etiology is sepsis.
2. Blood smear – schistocytes (fragmented cells) may be observed.
3. A complete serum chemistry profile may reveal the underlying etiology or complications of DIC.
4. Coagulation profile
   A. The PT and PTT are usually prolonged.
   B. Fibrin split products (FSPs or FDPs) will be observed only when the mononuclear phagocytic system is saturated. FSPs may never be observed in some cases of fulminant DIC, and may be observed in thrombotic disease without complicating DIC.
   C. Fibrinogen level is usually decreased.
   D. Activated coagulation time.
      I. Normal ACT for dogs is 60–110 seconds, and for cats it is 50–75 seconds. In DIC, the ACT will usually become prolonged, fibrinogen concentrations will diminish and platelet numbers will be reduced.
      II. Procedure – the ACT tubes should be warmed to 37°C prior to and during the test procedure. Two tubes should be used; 2 mL of blood are taken by clean venipuncture with rapid aspiration from a large vein, directly into the first tube with a Vacutainer® system, or quickly transferred from a syringe into the first tube and discarded. Without removing the needle from the vein, additional blood is placed into the second tube and the test is performed. The time interval from injection of 2 mL of blood into the ACT tube until the first visible appearance of clot formation is determined to be the ACT.

5. Decreased concentrations of ATIII (<80%), when accompanied by clinical signs and other laboratory test abnormalities, can help to confirm a diagnosis of DIC.
6. The D-dimer test measures the amount of a fragment of fully polymerized, cross-linked fibrin that occurs due to active fibrinolysis. Elevation of this fragment may indicate major vessel thrombosis and DIC.
7. Thromboelastography (TEG)
   A. R = reaction time. It is measured from the start to detectable clot formation. Abnormalities are seen with defects of the intrinsic pathway, deficiencies of factors VIII, IX, XI and XII.
   B. K = kinetic time. It is the time to achieve a specific clot strength. It is influenced by HCT, platelet count / function, factor II, factor VIII, thrombin, fibrin and fibrinogen.
   C. α-angle is the rapidity of fibrin formation and cross linking. It is influenced by HCT, platelet count / function, factor II, factor VIII, thrombin, fibrin and fibrinogen.
   D. MA = maximum amplitude. It is a measure of maximum clot strength. It is influenced by HCT, platelet count / function, factor XII, thrombin, fibrin and fibrinogen.
   E. TMA = time to reach MA (minutes).
   F. CI = coagulation index. A formula for humans to determine if the patient is hyper- or hypocoagulable.

Prognosis

The prognosis is guarded to poor.

Treatment

1. Inform the owner of the underlying etiologies, diagnosis, prognosis and cost of the treatment.
2. Treat the underlying condition causing DIC.
3. Administer high-volume intravenous fluid therapy with a balanced electrolyte solution, such as LRS, Plasma-Lyte®, or Normosol®-R, to prevent stasis and organ ischemia
   A. Dogs: 90 mL/kg the first hour IV, then re-evaluate. Administer in ¼-shock boluses (22–23 mL/kg) and re-evaluate after each aliquot.
   B. Cats: 45–60 mL/kg first hour IV, then re-evaluate. Administer in ¼-shock boluses (11–15 mL/kg) and re-evaluate after each aliquot.
   C. Every 15 minutes, re-evaluate the patient's cardiovascular status. Generally decrease the rate to 20–40 mL/kg/h in dogs and 20–30 mL/kg/h in cats until the patient is stabilized. Continue at maintenance rates (1–2 mL/kg/h) when stable.
4. Administer oxygen therapy as indicated.
5. Administer systemic broad-spectrum antibiotics if an underlying infection is suspected.
6. Repeated monitoring of ACT or PTT measurements.
7. Administer fresh frozen plasma, 20–30 mL/kg IV, or red blood cells, or fresh whole blood as indicated by the individual patient's needs.

HEMOPERITONEUM

Etiology

The most common cause of intra-abdominal hemorrhage is blunt trauma inflicted by an automobile. Other traumatic incidences that cause intra-abdominal hemorrhage include a kick to the abdomen by a person or a large animal, gunshot wounds, dog bite wounds, and penetrating foreign objects such as arrows or knives. Intra-abdominal hemorrhage can also occur following rupture of vessels due to gastric dilatation and volvulus, splenic or intestinal torsion, and from neoplasia. Anticoagulant rodenticide toxicity and other coagulopathies can cause intra-abdominal hemorrhage. Post-surgical complications, such as slipped ovarian ligatures, can also result in intra-abdominal hemorrhage.

Diagnosis

History—Obtain information regarding the possibility of trauma. Question the owner about confinement of the patient to the owner's property, the environment, the presence of large animals, previous illness, recent surgery, and toxin exposure.

Physical exam—The patient may present in various stages of hypovolemic shock. The mental status will vary from alert to comatose. Heart rate, respiratory rate, mucous membrane color, capillary refill time, pulse pressure and blood pressure will reflect the severity of the stage of shock. Jugular distention or external wounds may be observed. Bleeding from other sites or petechiation or ecchymosis may be seen. Look for bruising around the umbilicus and the presence of blood around the vulva or prepuce. The abdomen may be distended, fluctuant and tender; however, distention of the abdomen is not observed until 40mL/kg of blood has accumulated in the peritoneal cavity.

Four-quadrant abdominocentesis or a diagnostic peritoneal tap may reveal the presence of blood in the abdominal cavity. If blood is obtained by performing abdominocentesis, it indicates that a large volume of blood (>5 mL/kg) is present in the peritoneal cavity.

Abdominal radiographs—Initially, there may not be enough blood present in the peritoneal cavity to be visible on a radiograph. Evaluate the retroperitoneal space, diaphragm, chest, scapulae, sternebrae, spine, pelvis and femurs for signs of trauma or fluid accumulation.

In patients that may have a bleeding abdominal mass, thoracic radiographs should be evaluated for the presence of metastatic neoplasia prior to abdominal surgery.

Abdominal and thoracic ultrasonography—FAST ultrasonography may allow for detection of smaller amounts of intra-abdominal blood accumulation than radiographs. Masses may be observed on the spleen, liver, auricular appendages, etc.

Laboratory evaluation—

1. PCV and TS should be monitored frequently (every 15–30 minutes). It is important to take into account the effects of hemodilution from fluid therapy for shock.

2. Blood gas evaluation may be beneficial, especially in patients that are exhibiting respiratory distress.
3. A CBC (including a platelet count), biochemical profile and urinalysis, should be performed in all patients to provide a minimum database.
4. A coagulation panel and TEG should be considered in patients with a history of anticoagulant rodenticide toxicity or signs of a coagulopathy. ACT, PT and PTT can be monitored in house.
5. The PCV and TS of fluid obtained by abdominocentesis or diagnostic peritoneal tap should be compared with that of peripheral blood.

Differential diagnosis

Acute abdominal pain, peritonitis, hypovolemic shock.

Prognosis

The prognosis is fair to guarded, depending on the source of the hemorrhage.

Treatment

1. Inform the client of the diagnosis, prognosis and cost of the treatment.
2. Administer oxygen.
3. Obtain pretreatment blood samples.
4. Place an intravenous catheter and administer a balanced electrolyte crystalloid solution at moderate rates IV unless the patient presents in critical condition.
    A. Administer fluids at 30–40 mL/kg/h in dogs, and 25 mL/kg/h in cats.
    B. Re-evaluate blood pressure and perfusion every 5 minutes.
    C. Avoid hypertension, which may dislodge a clot, until the hemorrhage is controlled.
5. If the patient presents with life-threatening hemorrhage, administer intravenous fluids at the rate of 90 mL/kg/h in dogs, and 50–60 mL/kg/h in cats.
    A. Also administer a colloid such as Hetastarch or Pentastarch at the dose of 20 mL/kg in dogs, and 15 mL/kg in cats.
    B. Re-evaluate blood pressure and perfusion every 5 minutes.
    C. When the patient's cardiovascular status improves, decrease the rate by 50% and continue to monitor the patient.
6. Clip the abdomen, looking for wounds, bruising and signs of trauma.
7. If penetrating abdominal wounds are observed, administer systemic antibiotics.
8. Apply external counterpressure to the hindlimbs, tail, pelvis and abdomen by placing folded towels in the inguinal areas, over the ventral abdomen and between the hindlimbs, and wrapping with a bandage from the hind paws toward the diaphragm.

A. Apply some pressure, but not a tourniquet-like effect.
B. Do not compromise diaphragmatic expansion.
C. Avoid making a lumpy bandage.

9. Administer RBCs or a hemoglobin-based oxygen carrier if the PCV decreases below 25%. Administer plasma if the TS decreases below 4.0 mg/dL.
   A. The dose of RBC is 11 mL/kg (5 mL/lb).
   B. The dose of whole blood is 22 mL/kg (10 mL/lb).
   C. The dosage of Oxyglobin®, a hemoglobin-based oxygen carrier, which is not currently available is:
      I. Dogs: 15–30 mL/kg (6.8–13.6 mL/lb) IV
      II. Cats: 5–20 mL/kg (2.3–9 mL/lb) IV, administered in increments of 5 mL/kg (2.3 mL/lb).
   D. The dose of plasma varies from 5 to 30 mL/kg (2.3–13.6 mL/lb) IV.

10. Clean and bandage wounds if indicated.

11. Administer general anesthesia and perform an exploratory laparotomy if hemorrhage continues, the patient continues to deteriorate despite therapy, or in the presence of penetrating abdominal wounds.

12. Administer analgesics if indicated.

REFERENCES/FURTHER READING

CANINE ANEMIA

Al-Ghazlat, S., 2009. Immunosuppressive therapy for canine immune-mediated hemolytic anemia. Compendium for the Continuing Education of the Practicing Veterinarian. 33–44.

Bianco, D., Hardy, R.M., 2009. Treatment of Evans' syndrome with human intravenous immunoglobulin and leflunomide in a diabetic dog. Journal of the American Animal Hospital Association 45:147–150.

Cohn, L.A., 2009. Acute hemolytic disorders. In: Silverstein, D.C., Hopper, K. (Eds.), Small Animal Critical Care Medicine. Elsevier, St Louis, pp. 523–528.

Cotter, S.M. (Ed.), 1991. Advances in Veterinary Science, Comparative Medicine, Comparative Transfusion Medicine, vol 36. Academic Press, London, pp. 188–218.

Donahue, S.M., Otto, C.M., 2005. Thromboelastography: a tool for measuring hypercoagulability, hypo-coagulability, and fibrinolysis. Journal of Veterinary Emergency and Critical Care 15 (1), 9–16.

Duncan, J.R., Prasse, K.W., 1986. Veterinary Laboratory Medicine, Clinical Pathology, second ed. Iowa State University Press, Ames, pp. 19–24.

Fenty, R.K., deLaforcade, A.M., Shaw, S.P., et al., 2011. Identification of hypercoagulability in dogs with primary immune-mediated hemolytic anemia by means of thromboelastography. Journal of the American Veterinary Medical Association 238, 463–467.

Giger, U., 2009. Anemia. In: Silverstein, D.C., Hopper, K., (Eds.), Small Animal Critical Care Medicine. Elsevier, St Louis, pp. 518–523.

Helmond, S.E., Polzin, D.J., Armstrong, P.J., et al., 2010. Treatment of immune-mediated hemolytic anemia with individually adjusted heparin dosing in dogs. Journal of Veterinary Internal Medicine 24, 597–605.

Hohenhaus, A.E. (guest ed.), 1992. Problems in Veterinary Medicine: Transfusion Medicine, vol 4, no 4. J B Lippincott, Philadelphia, pp. 612–622.

Horgan, J.E., Roberts, B.K., Schermerhorn, T., 2009. Splenectomy as an adjunctive treatment for dogs with immune-mediated hemolytic anemia: ten cases (2003–2006). Journal of Veterinary Emergency and Critical Care 19 (3), 254–261.

McManus, P.M., Craig, L.E., 2001. Correlation between leukocytosis and necropsy findings in dogs with immune-mediated hemolytic anemia:

34 cases (1994–1999). Journal of the American Veterinary Medical Association 218, 1308–1313.

Orcutt, E.S., Lee, J., Bianco, D., 2010. Immune-mediated hemolytic anemia and severe thrombocytopenia in dogs: 12 cases (2001–2008). Journal of Veterinary Emergency and Critical Care 20 (3), 338–345.

Piek, C.J., Junius, G., Dekker, A., et al., 2008. Idiopathic immune-mediated hemolytic anemia: treatment outcome and prognostic factors in 149 dogs. Journal of Veterinary Internal Medicine 22, 366–373.

Prittie, J.E., 2010. Controversies related to red blood cell transfusion in critically ill patients. Journal of Veterinary Emergency and Critical Care 20 (2), 167–176.

Sinnott, V.B., Otto, C.M., 2009. Use of thromboelastography in dogs with immune mediated hemolytic anemia: 39 cases (2000–2008). Journal of Veterinary Emergency and Critical Care 19 (5), 484–488.

Weinkle, T.K., Center, S.A., Randolph, J.F., et al., 2005. Evaluation of prognostic factors, survival rates, and treatment protocols for immune-mediated hemolytic anemia in dogs: 151 cases (1993–2002). Journal of the American Veterinary Medical Association 226, 1869–1880.

Whelan, M.F., O'Toole, T.E., Chan, D.L., et al., 2009. Use of human immunoglobulin in addition to glucocorticoids for the initial treatment of dogs with immune-mediated hemolytic anemia. Journal of Veterinary Emergency and Critical Care 19 (2), 158–164.

FELINE ANEMIA

Bacek, L.M., Macintire, D.K., 2011. Treatment of primary immune-mediated hemolytic anemia with mycophenolate mofetil in two cats. Journal of Veterinary Emergency and Critical Care 21 (1), 45–49.

Bighignoli, B., Owens, S.D., Froenicke, L., et al., 2010. Blood types of the domestic cat. In: August, J.R. (Ed.), Consultations in Feline Internal Medicine, vol 6. Saunders Elsevier, St Louis, pp. 628–638.

Cohn, L.A., 2009. Acute hemolytic disorders. In: Silverstein, D.C., Hopper, K. (Eds.), Small Animal Critical Care Medicine. Elsevier, St Louis, pp. 523–528.

Cotter, S.M. (Ed.), 1991. Advances in Veterinary Science, Comparative Medicine, Comparative Transfusion Medicine, vol 36. Academic Press, London, pp. 189–218.

Duncan, J.R., Prasse, K.W., 1986. Veterinary Laboratory Medicine, Clinical Pathology, second ed. Iowa University Press, Ames, pp. 19–24.

Giger, U., 2009. Anemia. In: Silverstein, D.C., Hopper, K. (Eds.), Small Animal Critical Care Medicine. Elsevier, St Louis, pp. 518–523.

Giger, U., 2009. Transfusion medicine. In: Silverstein, D.C., Hopper, K. (Eds.), Small Animal Critical Care Medicine. Elsevier, St Louis, pp. 281–286.

Hohenhaus, A.E. (guest ed.), 1992. Problems in Veterinary Medicine: Transfusion Medicine, vol 4, no 4. J B Lippincott, Philadelphia, pp. 600–610.

Kohn, B., 2010. Immune mediated hemolytic anemia. In: August, J.R. (Ed.), Consultations in Feline Internal Medicine, vol 6. Saunders Elsevier, St Louis, pp. 617–627.

Sherding, R.G. (Ed.), 1994. The Cat: Diseases and Clinical Management, second ed. WB Saunders, Philadelphia, pp. 702–716.

Wong, C., Haskins, S.C., 2007. The effect of storage on the P50 of feline blood. Journal of Veterinary Emergency and Critical Care 17 (1), 32–36.

IMMUNE-MEDIATED THROMBOCYTOPENIA

Appleman, E.H., Sachais, B.S., Patel, R., et al., 2009. Cryopreservation of canine platelets. Journal of Veterinary Internal Medicine 23, 138–145.

Bianco, D., Armstrong, P.J., Washabau, R.J., 2009. A prospective, randomized, double-blinded, placebo-controlled study of human intravenous immunoglobulin for the acute management of presumptive primary immune-mediated thrombocytopenia in dogs. Journal of Veterinary Internal Medicine 23, 1071–1078.

Callan, M.B., Appleman, E.H., Sachais, B.S., 2009. Canine platelet transfusions. Journal of Veterinary Emergency and Critical Care 19 (5), 401–415.

Cotter, S.M. (Ed.), 1991. Advances in Veterinary Science, Comparative Medicine, Comparative Transfusion Medicine, vol 36. Academic Press, London, pp. 101–109, 116–119, 209–211.

EMERGENCY PROCEDURES FOR THE SMALL ANIMAL VETERINARIAN

deGopegui, R.R., Feldman, B.F., 1995. Use of blood and blood components in canine and feline patients with hemostatic disorders. In Kristensen, A.T., Feldman, B.F., (guest eds.). The Veterinary Clinics of North America, Small Animal Practice: Canine, and Feline Transfusion Medicine 25 (6), 1387–1402.

Dircks, B.H., Schuberth, H.J., Mischke, R., 2009. Underlying diseases and clinicopathologic variables of thrombocytopenic dogs with and without platelet-bound antibodies detected by use of a flow cytometric assay: 83 cases (2004–2006). Journal of the American Veterinary Medical Association 235, 960–966.

Drellich, S., Tocci, L.J., 2009. Thrombocytopenia. In: Silverstein, D.C., Hopper, K. (Eds.), Small Animal Critical Care Medicine. Elsevier, St Louis, pp. 515–518.

Duncan, J.R., Prasse, K.W., 1986. Veterinary Laboratory Medicine, Clinical Pathology, second ed. Iowa State University Press, Ames, pp. 19–24.

Hohenhaus, A.E., (guest ed.), 1992. Problems in Veterinary Medicine: Transfusion Medicine, vol 4, no 4. J B Lippincott, Philadelphia, pp. 598, 618–619.

O'Marra, S.K., Delaforcade, A.M., Shaw, S.P., 2011. Treatment and predictors of outcome in dogs with immune-mediated thrombocytopenia. Journal of the American Veterinary Medical Association 238, 346–352.

Putsche, J.C., Kohn, B., 2008. Primary immune-mediated thrombocytopenia in 30 dogs (1997–2003). Journal of the American Animal Hospital Association 44, 250–257.

Sullivan, P.S., Evans, H.L., McDonald, T.P., 1994. Platelet concentration, and hemoglobin function in Greyhounds. Journal of the American Veterinary Medical Association 205 (6), 838–841.

Wondratschek, C., Weingart, C., Kohn, B., 2010. Primary immune-mediated thrombocytopenia in cats. Journal of the American Animal Hospital Association 46, 12–19.

COAGULOPATHIES

Brooks, M.B., Erb, H.N., Foureman, P.A., et al., 2001. von Willebrand disease phenotype and von Willebrand factor marker genotype in Doberman

Pinschers. American Journal of Veterinary Research 62, 364–369.

Cotter, S.M. (Ed.), 1991. Advances in Veterinary Science, Comparative Medicine, Comparative Transfusion Medicine, vol 36. Academic Press, London, pp. 97–136.

deGopegui, R.R., Feldman, B.F., 1995. Use of blood and blood components in canine and feline patients with hemostatic disorders. In Kristensen, A.T., Feldman, B.F., (guest eds.). The Veterinary Clinics of North America, Small Animal Practice: Canine, and Feline Transfusion Medicine 25 (6), 1387–1402.

Hackner, S.G., 1995. Approach to the Diagnosis of Bleeding Disorders. Compendium on Continuing Education 17 (3), 331–347.

Hackner, S.G., 2009. Bleeding disorders. In: Silverstein, D.C., Hopper, K. (Eds.), Small Animal Critical Care Medicine. Elsevier, St Louis, pp. 507–514.

Hohenhaus, A.E., (guest ed.), 1992. Problems in Veterinary Medicine: Transfusion Medicine, vol 4, no 4. J B Lippincott, Philadelphia, pp. 618–622, 636–645.

Hopper, K., Bateman, S., 2005. An updated view of hemostasis: mechanisms of hemostatic dysfunction associated with sepsis. Journal of Veterinary Emergency and Critical Care 15 (2), 83–91.

Meyers, K.M., Wardrop, J., Meinkoth, J., 1992. Canine von Willebrand's disease: pathobiology, diagnosis, and short-term treatment. Compendium on Continuing Education 14 (1), 13–21.

Yaxley, P.E., Beal, M.W., Jutkowitz, L.A., 2010. Comparative stability of canine and feline hemostatic proteins in freeze-thaw-cycled fresh frozen plasma. Journal of Veterinary Emergency and Critical Care 20 (5), 472–478.

EPISTAXIS

Bissett, S.A., Drobatz, K.J., McKnight, A., et al., 2007. Prevalence, clinical features, and causes of epistaxis in dogs: 176 cases (1996–2001). Journal of the American Veterinary Medical Association 231, 1843–1850.

Dhupa, N., Littman, M.P., 1992. Epistaxis. Compendium on Continuing Education 14 (8), 1033–1041.

Mylonakis, M.E., Saridomichelakis, M.N., Lazaridis, V., et al., 2008. A retrospective study of 61 cases of spontaneous canine epistaxis (1998– to 2001). Journal of Small Animal Practice 49, 191–196.

DISSEMINATED INTRAVASCULAR COAGULATION

Bateman, S.W., 2009. Hypercoagulable states. In: Silverstein, D.C., Hopper, K. (Eds.), Small Animal Critical Care Medicine. Elsevier, St Louis, pp. 502–506.

Bateman, S., Mathews, K.A., Abrams-Ogg, C.G., 1998. Disseminated intravascular coagulation in dogs: review of the literature. Journal of Veterinary Emergency and Critical Care 8, 29–45.

Bruchim, Y., Aroch, I., Saragusty, J., 2008. Disseminated intravascular coagulation. Compendium on Continuing Education for the Practicing Veterinarian 30 (10), E1–E16.

deGopegui, R.R., Feldman, B.F., 1995. Use of blood and blood components in canine and feline patients with hemostatic disorders. In Kristensen, A.T., Feldman, B.F., (guest eds.). The Veterinary Clinics of North America, Small Animal Practice: Canine, and Feline Transfusion Medicine 25 (6), 1387–1402.

Estrin, M.A., Spangler, E.A., 2010. Disseminated intravascular coagulation. In: August, J.R. (Ed.), Consultations in Feline Internal Medicine, vol 6. Saunders Elsevier, St Louis, pp. 639–651.

Estrin, M.A., Wehausen, C.E., Jessen, C.R., et al., 2006. Disseminated intravascular coagulation in cats. Journal of Veterinary Internal Medicine 20, 1334–1339.

Levi, M., 2007. Disseminated intravascular coagulation. Critical Care Medicine 35, 2191–2195.

Otto, C.M., Rieser, T.M., Brooks, M.B., et al., 2000. Evidence of hypercoagulability in dogs with parvoviral enteritis. Journal of the American Veterinary Medical Association 217, 1500–1504.

Wiinberg, B., Jensen, A.L., Johansson, P.I., et al., 2008. Thromboelastographic evaluation of hemostatic function in dogs with disseminated intravascular coagulation. Journal of Veterinary Internal Medicine 22, 357–365.

HEMOPERITONEUM

Aronsohn, M.G., Dubiel, B., Roberts, B., et al., 2009. Prognosis for acute nontraumatic hemoperitoneum in the dog: a retrospective analysis of 60 cases (2003–2006). Journal of the American Animal Hospital Association 45, 72–77.

Hammond, T.N., Pesillo-Crosby, S.A., 2008. Prevalence of hemangiosarcoma in anemic dogs with a splenic mass and hemoperitoneum requiring a transfusion: 71 cases (2003–2005). Journal of the American Veterinary Medical Association 232, 553–558.

Herold, L.V., Devey, J.J., Kirby, R., et al., 2008. Clinical evaluation and management of hemoperitoneum in dogs. Journal of Veterinary Emergency and Critical Care 18 (1), 40–53.

Johannes, C.M., Henry, C.J., Turnquist, S.E., et al., 2007. Hemangiosarcoma in cats: 53 cases (1992–2002). Journal of the American Veterinary Medical Association 231, 1851–1856.

Jutkowitz, L.A., 2009. Massive transfusion. In: Silverstein, D.C., Hopper, K. (Eds.), Small Animal Critical Care Medicine. Elsevier, St Louis, pp. 691–693.

Jutkowitz, L.A., Rozanski, E.A., Moreau, J.A., et al., 2002. Massive transfusion in dogs: 15 cases (1997–2001). Journal of the American Veterinary Medical Association 220, 1664–1669.

O'Kelley, B.M., Whelan, M.F., Brooks, M.B., 2009. Factor VIII inhibitors complicating treatment of postoperative bleeding in a dog with hemophilia A. Journal of Veterinary Emergency and Critical Care 19 (4), 381–385.

Pintar, J., Breitschwerdt, E.B., Hardie, E.M., et al., 2003. Acute nontraumatic hemoabdomen in the dog: a retrospective analysis of 39 cases (1987–2001). Journal of the American Animal Hospital Association 39, 518–522.

Gastrointestinal emergencies

SALIVARY MUCOCELES AND RANULAS

Etiology

Damage to a salivary duct or gland that results in leakage of saliva into the surrounding tissues results in the formation of a salivary mucocele or sialocele. The trauma may be blunt trauma or penetration by a foreign body. A ranula is a sublingual mucocele. The sublingual and mandibular salivary glands are the most commonly involved.

Diagnosis

History—The owner may observe swelling in the cervical area, loss of appetite, difficulty in swallowing, blood-tinged saliva, or difficulty in breathing.

Physical exam—A nonpainful, soft, fluctuant mass may be observed in the cervical area, orbital area or sublingual area. The animal may exhibit abnormal movements of the tongue, dyspnea or dysphagia. Aseptic aspiration of the swelling with an 18- to 20-gauge needle and syringe yields a clear, gray, honey-colored or blood-tinged, thick, sticky and stringy fluid-like saliva.

Ultrasound—Ultrasound may be useful to assess the salivary glands, lymph nodes, and muscles in the area for masses, cystic lesions, sialoliths, inflammation and in obtaining guided biopsies or aspirates.

Differential diagnosis

Abscess, neoplasia, rattlesnake bite, spider bite, insect bite, scorpion sting, localized inflammatory reaction, seroma, hematoma, cyst.

Prognosis

Although usually not life threatening, recurrence may happen.

Emergency treatment

1. Inform the client of the diagnosis, prognosis and cost of the treatment.
2. Aseptic aspiration may be indicated if the patient is exhibiting dyspnea or discomfort.
3. Administer oxygen if indicated.
4. Administer anesthesia and perform endotracheal intubation if necessary to establish a patent airway.
5. Administer broad-spectrum antibiotics if an infectious component is present.
6. Administer an NSAID if needed to decrease inflammation.
7. Recommend the patient be fed a soft diet for 1 week.
8. Refer the patient to the daytime veterinarian for surgical removal of the mucocele.

ESOPHAGEAL FOREIGN BODIES

Diagnosis

History—The owner may have observed the animal chewing on a bone or playing with a ball, coin, wooden stick, needle or pin, or chewing on a foreign object. The animal may have swallowed a fish hook. A piece of a toy may be missing. The owner may observe acute respiratory distress, excessive salivation, difficulty swallowing, agitation including pawing at the mouth, regurgitation, restlessness, lethargy and anorexia.

Esophageal foreign bodies occur more frequently in dogs than in cats, owing to the indiscriminate eating habits of dogs. The condition occurs more commonly in toy and non-sporting breeds of dogs, with Terriers (including West Highland White Terriers, Yorkshire Terriers and Shih Tzus) having the highest incidence.

Physical exam—

Caution: Wear examination gloves during the physical examination and avoid contact with the patient's saliva until the diagnosis of rabies is ruled out.

The patient may present with an upper airway obstruction if the esophageal foreign body is compressing the trachea. The patient may be cyanotic, have a weak and rapid pulse, and may have increased lung sounds due to aspiration pneumonia. The patient may exhibit agitation by shaking its head or pawing at the mouth. There may be stridor, ptyalism and persistent gulping. A fishing line may be observed in the mouth. Carefully examine under the base of the tongue, particularly in cats that may have swallowed a linear foreign body.

Most esophageal foreign bodies become trapped in the caudal esophagus just cranial to the cardiac sphincter, at the thoracic inlet or in the heart base area.

Radiographs—Radiographs of the cervical and thoracic esophagus may reveal the presence of a foreign body or a mass effect in the esophagus. Evaluate for signs of aspiration pneumonia or esophageal tears, pneumomediastinum and pleural effusion. Look for additional gastrointestinal foreign bodies. If contrast radiography is performed, use an iodinated compound rather than barium.

Laboratory evaluation—A CBC should be evaluated. If the patient is to undergo sedation or anesthesia, the appropriate pre-anesthetic blood screening should be performed.

Differential diagnosis

Rabies, dysfunction of cranial nerves IX and X, trigeminal neuropathy, myasthenia gravis, periodontal disease, stomatitis, tracheal or oropharyngeal foreign body, esophageal mass, esophageal stricture, mediastinal mass, or insect bite to the oropharyngeal region.

Prognosis

The prognosis varies from good to poor, depending upon the foreign body, duration of obstruction, severity of obstruction, location, surrounding tissue damage including esophageal perforation, and associated problems such as aspiration pneumonia and mediastinitis.

Treatment

1. Inform the client of the diagnosis, prognosis and cost of the treatment. If the situation is critical due to airway obstruction, quickly obtain the owner's permission for sedation, an attempt at foreign body removal or tracheostomy tube placement.
2. Sedation may be necessary.
   A. Acepromazine, 0.05 mg/kg IV, ketamine and diazepam, or propofol should be administered.
   B. Place the patient in left lateral recumbency.
3. The Heimlich maneuver may be beneficial. It may be possible to manipulate the mass towards the mouth by applying pressure rostrally with one hand around the ventral aspect of the neck caudal to the foreign body, while inserting the other hand into the mouth and grasping the foreign body with the other hand. Racquetballs sometimes need to be cut while in place and then grasped with sponge forceps.
4. If removal is not successful and the patient is in a state of severe respiratory distress due to tracheal compression, perform a tracheostomy.
5. If the object has sharp edges, is pointed or is causing the patient distress, sedation and endoscopic removal of the foreign body within 4–6 hours of presentation should be attempted, unless signs of esophageal perforation are present.
   A. General anesthesia should be administered.
   B. Place the patient in left lateral recumbency.
   C. Place an endotracheal tube.
   D. **Caution: Insufflation of air into a perforated esophagus during endoscopy can result in acute respiratory distress and death.**

E. Gentle manipulation of the foreign body is important to avoid further esophageal trauma.

F. If possible, remove pointed or sharp objects with the sharp end exiting the oral cavity last.

G. After the foreign body has been removed, evaluate the esophageal mucosa for erosion, ulceration and perforation.

6. If the esophageal foreign body is not pointed, does not have sharp edges and is not causing patient distress, removal is not a true emergency procedure and can be delayed until the availability of adequate equipment and personnel can be arranged.

7. Removal of fish hooks

A. If the hook is free within the lumen of the esophagus, grasp the point or curve, with the point facing caudally, and gently retract the hook through the mouth.

B. If the hook is superficially embedded in the submucosa or mucosa of the esophageal wall but the point of the hook is observed penetrating into the lumen of the esophagus, grasp the point and pull the entire hook through the esophageal wall. Once it is freed from the wall, retract the hook through the mouth.

C. If fishing line is attached to the hook, a deep esophageal laceration or perforation may result from pulling the hook through the esophageal wall. This procedure should be avoided.

D. If the point appears to be embedded in the mucosa or submucosa but is not visible, it can be pulled gently out. A superficial tear will result, but will usually heal without complications.

8. In some cases, it is best to attempt to push the esophageal foreign body gently into the stomach and then perform a gastrotomy rather than an esophagotomy.

9. Following esophageal endoscopy, survey thoracic radiographs should be evaluated for signs of esophageal perforation including pneumomediastinum.

10. Surgery of the esophagus should be performed if there are signs of esophageal perforation or the foreign body cannot be removed or dislodged into the stomach.

11. If the esophageal damage is mild, feed blended soft food from an elevated position for 3–5 days.

12. If the esophageal damage is moderate:

A. Feed blended soft food.

B. Administer a mucosal protectant, sucralfate 0.5–1 g PO q8h in dogs and 0.25–0.5 g PO q8h in cats.

C. Administer an H_2-blocker.
 I. Famotidine 0.5–1 mg/kg PO q12h in dogs, 0.5 mg/kg PO q12h in cats
 II. Ranitidine 1–2 mg/kg PO q12h in dogs, 3.5 mg/kg PO q12h in cats

D. Administer a proton-pump inhibitor.
 I. Omeprazole (Prilosec®), 0.7–1 mg/kg PO q24h in dogs, 0.7–1.5 mg/kg PO q12–24h in cats
 II. Pantoprazole (Protonix®), 0.7–1 mg/kg IV q24h

Gastrointestinal emergencies

E. Administer a prokinetic medication.
   I. Cisapride (Propulsid®) 0.25–0.5 mg/kg PO q8–12h in dogs, 1.25–2.5 mg/cat PO q8–12h in cats
   II. Metoclopramide 0.2–0.4 mg/kg PO q8h in dogs, 0.2–0.4 mg/kg PO q8h in cats

13. If the esophageal damage is severe:
   A. Withhold food and water for 5–7 days.
   B. Place a gastrotomy tube. Feed blended food and water through the tube.
   C. Administer antibiotics (cephalosporins, amoxicillin, ampicillin) in a liquid form via the gastrotomy tube.
   D. Administer a mucosal protectant, sucralfate 0.5–1 g PO q8h in dogs and 0.25–0.5 g PO q8h in cats.
   E. Administer an H_2-blocker.
      I. Famotidine 0.5–1 mg/kg PO q12h in dogs, 0.5 mg/kg PO q12h in cats
      II. Ranitidine 1–2 mg/kg PO q12h in dogs, 3.5 mg/kg PO q12h in cats
   F. Administer a proton-pump inhibitor.
      I. Omeprazole 0.7–1 mg/kg PO q24h in dogs, 0.7–1.5 mg/kg PO q12–24h in cats
      II. Pantoprazole (Protonix®), 0.7–1 mg/kg IV q24h
   G. Administer a prokinetic medication.
      I. Cisapride 0.25–0.5 mg/kg PO q8–12h in dogs, 1.25–2.5 mg/cat PO q8–12h in cats
      II. Metoclopramide 0.2–0.4 mg/kg PO q8h in dogs, 0.2–0.4 mg/kg PO q8h in cats

14. Esophageal foreign bodies may cause early complications such as esophagitis, esophageal perforation, mediastinitis, pneumothorax and aortic perforation. Delayed complications that may develop include esophageal stricture, diverticulum formation and development of bronchoesophageal fistulas.

15. Repeat thoracic radiographs immediately, 12 hours and 24 hours after foreign body removal to evaluate for signs of perforation (including pneumothorax and pneumomediastinum).

16. If pleural effusion is observed on the thoracic radiographs, perform thoracocentesis to obtain a fluid sample. Fluid analysis, including culture, should be performed. A thoracotomy should be performed as soon as the animal is stabilized.

17. Endoscopically re-evaluate the esophagus in 3–5 days. Esophagitis may lead to stricture formation and gastroesophageal reflux.

18. If an esophageal stricture develops that interferes with swallowing, dilation is necessary.
   A. Inject triamcinolone acetonide or dexamethasone at three or four sites around the inflamed area or stricture, especially before or immediately after attempting dilation.
   B. Bougienage involves the use of a long, narrow, rigid instrument (a bougie) that is gently pushed through the stricture to progressively break down and stretch the scar tissue.

C. The procedure of esophageal balloon dilation involves passing an inflatable balloon into the stricture under endoscopic or fluoroscopic guidance.

D. The outcome of either bougienage or balloon dilation will need to be re-evaluated endoscopically months later, and repeat sessions may be needed.

ACUTE ABDOMINAL PAIN

Etiology

There are numerous causes of acute abdominal pain; the following is a partial list.

1. Hepatobiliary—acute hepatitis (toxic or infectious), hepatic abscess, hepatic rupture, hepatic neoplasia, cholecystitis, common bile duct obstruction, biliary calculi, bile duct or gallbladder rupture, cholangiohepatitis
2. Splenic—abscess, perforation, ruptured neoplasm, torsion
3. Gastrointestinal—gastric dilatation and volvulus, gastroenteritis, hemorrhagic gastroenteritis, parvovirus gastroenteritis, panleukopenia, other viral or bacterial gastroenteritis, garbage intoxication, intestinal obstruction by a foreign body or neoplasia, intussusception, gastric or duodenal ulceration, perforated viscus, herniation with incarcerated bowel, obstipation, trauma, neoplasia, mesenteric volvulus, mesenteric avulsion, mesenteric thrombosis, mesenteric lymphadenitis
4. Pancreatic—pancreatic abscess, acute pancreatitis, neoplasia
5. Urogenital—pyelonephritis, acute nephritis, acute tubular necrosis, calculi (renal, ureteral, cystic, or urethral), obstruction of the urethra or ureter, trauma or avulsion (renal, ureteral, bladder, or urethral), bladder rupture, thrombosis of a renal artery, acute metritis, pyometra, uterine torsion, acute prostatitis, prostatic abscess, testicular torsion, orchitis
6. Peritonitis—chemical (bile, pancreatic enzymes, gastric juices, blood, urine), or septic (penetrating wound, ruptured abscess, ruptured viscous)
7. Extra-abdominal—myositis, steatitis, rectus abdominus hematoma, intervertebral disc disease, ethylene glycol toxicity, heavy metal toxicity, arsenic toxicity

Diagnosis

History—Attention should be given to the age, species, breed and sex of the patient. Young animals swallow foreign bodies more commonly than older animals. Young dogs are also more likely to become infected with contagious diseases such as parvovirus. An intact male dog with only one scrotal testicle may have testicular torsion. Pyometra is usually not painful, unless rupture and septic peritonitis have occurred. Acute pancreatitis is most common in middle-aged obese female dogs. Linear foreign bodies are more common in cats. Intestinal volvulus occurs most commonly in young adult German Shepherd dogs. The animal will usually present with a history of vomiting and abdominal pain. It is important to differentiate between regurgitation and vomiting.

Question the owner regarding the possible ingestion of a foreign body, toxin or other dietary indiscretion. What is the normal diet? Is the animal fed bones: if so, what kind and when? Is the animal fed people food: if so, what kind and when? Are other animals ill? Any history of medical problems? Is the patient receiving any medication, including over-the-counter drugs such as aspirin, ibuprofen, etc.? Is there a possibility of trauma? Has there been exposure to any other animals? Is the patient current on vaccinations?

When was the patient last normal? Have the owner describe the first sign of abnormality and the progression of abnormal signs. Have the owner describe the appearance and volume of the contents of the vomitus and the frequency of vomiting. Are there other signs besides vomiting? Is the patient defecating, urinating, acting normally? When did the patient last eat?

Physical exam—Perform a complete physical examination, starting with evaluation of a patent airway, respiratory rate and pattern, lung sounds, perfusion status, heart rate and rhythm, mucous membrane color, capillary refill time, pulse rate and character, mental attitude and rectal temperature.

Perform a thorough oral examination, including looking under the tongue for the presence of a linear foreign body. Carefully palpate the abdomen, evaluating organomegaly, gaseous distention, fluid wave, uterine distention, any palpable masses, urinary bladder size, and localization of pain. Look for signs of external trauma. Auscultate the abdomen for the presence and amount of borborygmus, which is usually increased in patients with acute enteritis, toxicity and acute intestinal obstruction, and decreased in patients with peritonitis, ileus and chronic intestinal obstruction. Perform a rectal examination to assess the prostate and feces.

Laboratory evaluation—Initially upon presentation, a critical patient should have a minimum database evaluated, including PCV, TS, dipstick BUN, PT and PTT or ACT and blood glucose. As time allows, the following further diagnostic parameters should be evaluated.
1. Electrolytes
2. Blood gases
3. Lactate
4. CBC
5. Complete serum biochemical profile, including ALT, ALP, BUN, creatinine
6. Spec cPL (canine pancreatic-specific lipase) for pancreatitis in dogs and fPLI (feline pancreatic lipase immunoreactivity) for cats
7. Coagulation profile – PT, PTT, FSPs, D-dimers and possibly TEG if available
8. Urinalysis
9. Fluid obtained from abdominocentesis (blind or ultrasound guided) or diagnostic peritoneal lavage should be evaluated for:

A. Cytology—toxic or degenerative white blood cells, WBC count. The presence of vegetable fibers indicates perforation and the need for immediate exploratory laparotomy.
B. Creatinine or potassium if urinary tract leakage is suspected. An abdominal fluid creatinine concentration to peripheral blood creatinine concentration ratio of >2:1 was predictive of uroabdomen in dogs (specificity 100%, sensitivity 86%). An abdominal fluid potassium concentration to peripheral blood potassium concentration of >1.4:1 is also predictive of uroabdomen in dogs (specificity 100%, sensitivity 100%). If the abdominal fluid creatinine concentration is at least four times those of normal laboratory blood creatinine values, this also indicates urinary tract leakage.
C. Abdominal fluid lactate compared with serum lactate. In dogs, septic effusions had a peritoneal fluid lactate concentration >2.5 mmol/L and a peritoneal fluid lactate concentration higher than blood lactate.
D. Abdominal fluid glucose level compared with blood glucose level. If the abdominal fluid glucose level was >20 mg/dL less than the peripheral blood glucose level from a sample obtained at the same time, in dogs and cats, this indicates septic peritonitis. These findings are 100% sensitive and 100% specific in diagnosing septic peritonitis in dogs and 86% sensitive and 100% specific in cats.
E. PCV and TS. If the PCV is increasing, nearing that of peripheral blood, intraperitoneal hemorrhage is occurring. Nonclotting blood may be aspirated from the abdomen. Erythrophagocytosis may be observed.

Abdominal radiographs—Should be carefully reviewed for the presence of free abdominal gas, organomegaly, foreign bodies, fluid accumulation, intestinal obstruction, renal calculi, ureteral calculi, cystic calculi, diaphragmatic hernia, body-wall herniation, abnormalities of the prostate or uterus, gastric dilatation and volvulus or loss of detail.
Abdominal ultrasonography—Accumulation of free peritoneal fluid may be observed. Assess the hepatobiliary system, spleen, urogenital system, prostate gland, pancreas, adrenal glands, and mesenteric lymph nodes. Look for masses and septic foci. Ultrasound-guided aspirates or biopsies may be obtained if indicated. Focused assessment with sonography for trauma (FAST) is an easy procedure to perform to look for and obtain samples of free abdominal fluid. Place the patient in left lateral recumbency for evaluation unless an injury (e.g. flail chest, fractures or injury to the vertebral column) precludes placement in this position, in which instance the patient should be placed in right lateral recumbency. A 2 × 2-inch (5 × 5 cm) area of hair should be clipped just caudal to the xiphoid process, just cranial to the pelvis, and over the right and left flanks caudal to the ribs at the most gravity-dependent location of the abdomen. Alcohol and acoustic coupling gel should be used at the ultrasound probe-to-skin interface. Use an ultrasound machine with either a 5- or 7.5-MHz curvilinear probe to obtain two ultrasonographic views (transverse and longitudinal) at the four prepared sites on the

abdomen. If the patient has short hair, clipping is not necessary; just moisten the hair with isopropyl alcohol.

Prognosis

The prognosis varies with the etiology, duration, severity of clinical signs on presentation, and response to therapy.

Treatment

1. Inform the client of the underlying etiologies, diagnosis, prognosis and cost of the treatment.
2. Attempt to find and treat the underlying condition causing pain.
3. Anticipation of complications, not reaction to clinical signs, is necessary for patient survival.
4. Administer oxygen supplementation.
5. Place an intravenous catheter and obtain blood and urine samples.
6. Administer high-volume intravenous fluid therapy with a balanced electrolyte solution such as LRS, Plasma-Lyte® or Normosol®-R to prevent stasis and organ ischemia.
   A. Dogs: 90–100 mL/kg for the first 1–2 hours IV, then re-evaluate.
   B. Cats: 45–60 mL/kg for the first 1–2 hours.
   C. Every 15–30 minutes, re-evaluate the patient's cardiovascular status. Generally decrease the rate to 20–40 mL/kg/h in dogs and 20–30 mL/kg/h in cats until the patient is stabilized. Continue at 10–20 mL/kg/h to maintain perfusion. Fluid rate requirements may range from 2 to 7 times normal maintenance rates.
   D. Monitor for fluid overload or continued hypotension.
      I. Monitor blood pressure. Maintain systolic pressure above 90 mm Hg and mean arterial pressure above 60 mm Hg.
      II. Monitor central venous pressure (maintain between 8 and 10 cm of water).
      III. Monitor urine output (minimum should be 1–2 mL/kg/h).
7. Administration of 7.5% hypertonic saline, 4 mL/kg IV, will help to achieve peracute volume resuscitation, but should be followed by, or accompanied by, either crystalloid fluid therapy or crystalloid and colloid fluid therapy.
8. Administer colloid therapy to improve perfusion and expansion of the vascular space while avoiding peripheral edema.
   A. Hetastarch
      I. Dogs: administer a 20 mL/kg IV bolus, possibly followed by an additional 20 mL/kg IV over 4–6 hours daily for at least 3 days.
      II. Cats: administer a 10–15 mL/kg IV bolus, possibly followed by an additional 10–15 mL/kg IV over 4–6 hours daily as needed.
      III. Reduce the crystalloid fluid volume administered by 40–60%.
   B. Dextran 70 (avoid in patients with thrombocytopenia or coagulopathy)
      I. Dogs: administer 14–20 mL/kg IV.
      II. Cats: administer 10–15 mL/kg IV.

C. Plasma—administer if the patient is exhibiting clinical signs of coagulopathy.

9. Administer analgesics as indicated by the individual patient's needs.
    A. Hydromorphone
        I. Dogs: 0.05–0.2 mg/kg IV, IM, or SC q2–6h; 0.0125–0.05 mg/kg/h IV CRI
        II. Cats: 0.05–0.2 mg/kg IV, IM, or SC q2–6h
    B. Fentanyl
        I. Dogs: 2–10 µg/kg IV to effect, followed by 1–10 µg/kg/h IV CRI
        II. Cats: 1–5 µg/kg/h to effect, followed by 1–5 µg/kg/h IV CRI
    C. Morphine
        I. Dogs: 0.5–1 mg/kg IM, SC; 0.05–0.1 mg/kg IV
        II. Cats: 0.005–0.2 mg/kg IM, SC
    D. Buprenorphine
        I. Dogs: 0.005–0.02 mg/kg IV, IM q4–8h; 2–4 µg/kg/h IV CRI; 0.12 mg/kg OTM
        II. Cats: 0.005–0.01 mg/kg IV, IM q4–8h; 1–3 µg/kg/h IV CRI; 0.02 mg/kg OTM

10. Administer antibiotic therapy if the suspected cause of the pain is infectious and also prophylactically for gastrointestinal and hepatic translocation.
    A. When the source of infection is unknown or a mixed population of bacteria is suspected:
        I. Administer clindamycin, 10 mg/kg q12h or 11 mg/kg q8h IV, and enrofloxacin, 5–10 mg/kg q12h IV or 5–20 mg/kg q24h IV
            a. Administer enrofloxacin only at the dose of 10–20 mg/kg twice then decrease the dose, as seizures may occur with high doses.
            b. Avoid the use of enrofloxacin in all puppies less than 8 months of age and in giant breed puppies less than 18 months of age.
        II. Administer a combination of ampicillin (20–40 mg/kg q8h IV), or a first-generation cephalosporin (cefazolin (20 mg/kg q8h IV)), with a fluoroquinolone (enrofloxacin (dosage for dogs = 5–10 mg/kg q12h, IV or 5–20 mg/kg q24h IV; dosage for cats = 5 mg/kg q24h IV), ciprofloxacin (5–15 mg/kg q12h PO or 5–20 mg/kg q24h PO)), and an aminoglycoside (amikacin (10–15 mg/kg q24h IV), gentamicin (6–8 mg/kg q24h IV), or tobramycin (2–4 mg/kg q8h IV)), or a third-generation cephalosporin (ceftizoxime (25–50 mg/kg IV, IM, SC q6–8h), cefotaxime (20–80 mg/kg IV, IM q6–8h)).
            a. The penicillins have been combined with a β-lactamase inhibitor (ticarcillin-clavulanate (Timentin®) 30–50 mg/kg q6–8h IV, ampicillin-sulbactam (Unasyn®) 50 mg/kg q6–8h IV, and piperacillin-tazobactam (Zosyn®, dose = 50 mg/kg IV, IM q4–6h) for increased efficacy.
            b. Aminoglycosides should be avoided in the presence of dehydration or azotemia as they may cause renal failure.

Gastrointestinal emergencies

    c. Aminoglycosides administered once every 24 hours are more effective and cause less renal toxicity.

    d. If furosemide is utilized, aminoglycosides should be discontinued, as the combination increases the risk of inducing iatrogenic renal failure.

    e. When the patient is on aminoglycosides, urine sediment should be evaluated at least daily for casts and cellular debris.

    f. If an anaerobic infection is suspected, add either metronidazole (10 mg/kg IV CRI over 1h, q8–12h), clindamycin, cefoxitin or penicillin G to the above combinations.

  III. Administer imipenem, 2–5 mg/kg IV CRI over 1 hour, q8h.

    a. Imipenem may cause seizures in young animals.

    b. Nausea, diarrhea and allergic reactions may occur.

  B. For translocation and hepatic or gastrointestinal infections, administer cefoxitin, 40 mg/kg IV initially and continued at 20 mg/kg IV q6–8h in the dog and q8h in the cat.

12. If there is no improvement in the patient's status, fever, white blood cell count or band count after 36–48 hours, consider changing the antibiotic therapy. Reassess the patient and review the history and diagnostic data.

13. Administer vasopressor and positive inotropic agents if the cardiovascular status is still compromised following volume replacement.

  A. Dobutamine, 2–20 µg/kg/min IV CRI in dogs, 1–5 µg/kg/min IV CRI in cats

  B. Dopamine, 5–10 µg/kg/min IV CRI in dogs

  C. Norepinephrine, 0.05–2 µg/kg/min IV CRI

14. Monitor PCV, maintain at a minimum of 20%. Administer red blood cells or whole blood if necessary.

15. Monitor serum glucose levels and maintain between 100 and 140 mg/dL.

16. Monitor blood gases and optimize the patient's pH.

17. Monitor serum electrolytes q2–4h initially as rapid changes occur.

18. Monitor serum magnesium levels and serum potassium levels, as magnesium reduces the loss of potassium.

  A. If serum magnesium is <0.7 mmol/L, supplementation is indicated.

  B. Administer magnesium intravenously at the rate of 30 mg/kg over 4 hours as a CRI IV.

  C. Supplementation can be repeated as needed up to three times in a 24-hour period.

  D. The maximum amount of magnesium that should be administered is 125 mg/kg/24h.

19. Monitor coagulation parameters for disseminated intravascular coagulation (DIC), which should be expected to occur.

  A. Recheck the platelet count and ACT or PTT daily.

  B. Trends should be followed, rather than one test at a point in time.

C. Treat DIC, as discussed in that chapter, with fluid therapy, oxygenation, treatment of the underlying disorder, plasma administration and possibly, heparin therapy.
20. Antiemetic therapy may be indicated.
   A. Ondansetron (Zofran®), 0.1–0.18 mg/kg IV q6–8h.
   B. Dolasetron (Anzemet®), 0.6–1 mg/kg IV q24h.
   C. Maropitant (Cerenia®),1 mg/kg SC q24h.
   D. Chlorpromazine, 0.05–0.1 mg/kg slowly IV q4h in dogs, and 0.01–0.025mg/kg slowly IV q4h in cats, if the patient has been adequately fluid volume replaced.
   E. Prochlorperazine, 0.13 mg/kg IM or SC q6h.
   F. Metoclopramide, 0.01–0.02 mg/kg/h CRI IV or 0.2–0.4 mg/kg q8h SC or IV.
   G. Butorphanol, 0.2–0.4 mg/kg q2–4h IV, provides some antiemetic benefit.
   H. Auscultate and palpate the abdomen two to three times a day.
21. Gastric protection should be provided by treating prophylactically.
   A. Ranitidine (Zantac®), 0.5–2 mg/kg IV, PO q8h (dogs), 2.5 mg/kg IV q12h (cats) or 3.5 mg/kg PO q12h (cats)
   B. Famotidine (Pepcid®), 0.5–1 mg/kg IV or PO q12–24h
   C. Omeprazole (Prilosec®)
      I. Dogs: 0.5–1.5 mg/kg PO q24h
      II. Cats: 0.5–1 mg/kg PO q24h
   D. Pantoprazole (Protonix®), 0.7–1 mg/kg IV q24h
   E. Sucralfate
      I. Dogs: 0.5–1 g PO q8h; can start with a loading dose 4× higher
      II. Cats: 0.25 g PO q8–12h
22. If the patient develops oliguria:
   A. Review fluid therapy and provide adequate fluid volume replacement.
   B. Measure central venous pressure and mean arterial pressure. Maintain central venous pressure between 8 and 10 cm of water and mean arterial pressure above 60 mm Hg.
   C. Administer mannitol, 0.1–1 g/kg IV, or furosemide, 1 mg/kg/h CRI IV for 4 h, if the patient is not volume overloaded. Use mannitol carefully in SIRS because, in the presence of vasculitis, mannitol can leak into interstitial tissues and worsen interstitial edema.
23. Perform exploratory surgery or definitive surgery if the etiology is isolated and surgery is indicated.
   A. Perform a thorough and symptomatic exploration of the abdominal cavity.
   B. Surgically correct any gross abnormality observed.
   C. If no gross abnormalities are observed, obtain biopsies of the liver, kidney, pancreas, stomach, small intestine, mesenteric lymph node and abdominal muscle.
   D. Remove all irrigation fluid by suctioning and sponging the abdominal cavity.
   E. During surgery, place a gastrotomy tube or jejunostomy tube if indicated.

F. If there is severe contamination of the peritoneal cavity or septic peritonitis, consider open peritoneal drainage.

24. Nutritional support should be initiated within 12 hours of presentation.
   A. Provide a minimum of 25% of the patient's protein and energy requirements within the first 12 hours.
   B. Provide a minimum of 75% of the patient's protein and energy requirements within 72–96 hours.
   C. After the patient has been rehydrated, administer a 3.5% amino acid solution with glycerine (Procalamine® 45–50 mL/kg/day IV). The amino acid solution should make up 25–50% of the patient's maintenance fluid needs and can be administered through a peripheral vein, 'piggy-backed' on the maintenance fluid line.
   D. The patient can then be eased onto an enteral nutrition program, orally, through a nasogastric tube, gastrotomy tube, or jejunostomy tube. Oral supplementation with electrolytes, glucose, and glutamine supplementation is available in commercial products, including Resorb® and Vivonex TEN®.
      I. For dogs and cats, the package of Vivonex TEN® should be diluted with double the amount of fluid recommended on the package for human consumption.
      II. The dose is 40–45 mL/kg/day.
      III. The first day, administer 33% of the recommended dose, in divided feedings given every 1–2 hours.
      IV. The second day, administer 66% of the recommended dose, in divided feedings given every 1–2 hours.
      V. The third day, administer the recommended dose, in divided feedings given every 1–2 hours.
   E. If no vomiting occurs, a bland diet can be given.
      I. It may be beneficial to administer a liquid diet, such as CliniCare®, first, to see if the patient can tolerate oral feeding.
      II. CliniCare® should initially be diluted to a 50% solution to decrease the incidence of osmotic diarrhea.
      III. Hills i/d®, or a/d®, Eukanuba recovery formula®, and Purina EN® are examples of diets that may be considered.
   F. Patients that have anorexia, pancreatitis, or gastroduodenal pathology can receive nutritional supplementation via various feeding tubes.
      I. Nasogastric tube
      II. Esophagostomy tube
      III. Gastrotomy tube
      IV. Jejunostomy tube – the preferred method for patients with pancreatitis
   G. Total parenteral nutrition can be utilized as an adjunct, but the benefits are greater and the risks are reduced by utilizing enteral nutrition if at all possible.

25. Monitor the patient's mentation status. If the patient becomes depressed, check the serum osmolality and glucose levels. Provide appropriate nursing care, including elevation of the head, prevention of aspiration, lubrication of the eyes, turn the patient every 4h, etc.

26. Provide comfort and general nursing care.
    A. Turn the recumbent animal over from one side to the other every 4 hours.
    B. Keep the patient clean and dry.
    C. Provide padding, towels, pillows, etc. to provide comfort.
    D. Check the intravenous catheter site frequently.
    E. Provide kind words and affection.
    F. Allow the patient to rest, when possible, by decreasing the light and noise levels.

PERITONITIS

Peritonitis may occur as the primary disease process, as with feline infectious peritonitis or bacterial peritonitis (from periodontal disease, from the ovarian bursa in a patient with pyometra, and through the lumbocostal arch from the pleural cavity). More commonly, peritonitis is a secondary disease process, such as peritonitis caused by the transmural migration of endogenous intestinal bacteria, which occurs during localized bowel ischemia or a state of systemic shock. Peritonitis causes sepsis and SIRS and is often fatal.

Forms of secondary peritonitis

1. Aseptic peritonitis
   A. Mechanical trauma that results in mild peritonitis occurs during every surgery in the peritoneal cavity, from sponges, lint, suture material, glove powder, contamination by room air, etc. The long-term effects are usually minimal in a patient with a normal immune system.
   B. Foreign-body peritonitis results when sponges or surgical instruments are left in the peritoneal cavity following surgery. Other causes include penetration of the peritoneum by bullets, animal bites, arrows, or other sharp objects, which bring hair and dirt into the peritoneal cavity, in addition to causing trauma to abdominal organs. Foreign bodies such as toothpicks, needles, bones, wood splinters, vegetable material, and linear foreign bodies may perforate the gastrointestinal tract and result in contamination of the peritoneal cavity.
   C. Chemical peritonitis is caused by barium sulfate, enema solutions, antibacterial powders, antiseptics, urine, bile, gastric fluid, and pancreatic secretions. Gastric and pancreatic secretions are particularly irritating and cause immediate cellular damage, the release of vasoactive substances, superoxides and other cellular toxins. As the damage progresses, SIRS develops.
2. Septic peritonitis
   A. Bacterial peritonitis often involves a mixture of anaerobes (*Clostridium* spp., *Peptostreptococcus* spp., and *Bacteroides* spp.) and aerobes (*Escherichia coli*, *Klebsiella* spp., and *Proteus* spp.).
   B. The source of the bacterial contamination is often ischemic intestine, from strangulation, secondary to mechanical obstruction and

distention, transmural migration of endogenous intestinal bacteria during bowel ischemia caused by systemic shock, or leakage from the gastrointestinal tract (due to neoplasia, previous surgery, necrosis, foreign body perforation, or penetrating abdominal trauma).

Diagnosis

History—The history is usually vague, consisting of inappetence, depression, vomiting, or other nonspecific signs. There may be a history of recent trauma or abdominal surgery. The patient may exhibit a 'praying position' or kyphosis.

Physical exam—The patient may appear depressed, 'tucked up' in the abdomen, and may exhibit abdominal tenderness upon palpation. Subnormal temperature is observed more commonly than fever. The patient may present in a state of hypodynamic shock, with dehydration, hypovolemia, tachycardia and weak peripheral pulses. Wounds or erythema may be observed on the caudal thorax or abdomen. An intra-abdominal mass or discomfort may be found upon abdominal palpation. The patient may have injected mucous membranes and slow capillary refill time. There may be abdominal distention, secondary to ileus, and diminished bowel sounds.

Laboratory evaluation—

1. Evaluate the CBC. Initially, neutropenia and thrombocytopenia are observed. As the septic process continues, neutrophilia with a left shift is expected.
2. The blood glucose level may be decreased.
3. Total solids and albumin may be decreased due to protein loss into the peritoneal cavity.
4. Evaluate the following.
   A. Electrolytes
   B. Blood gases
   C. Complete serum biochemical profile, including ALT, ALP, BUN, and creatinine
   D. Coagulation profile
      I. Platelet count
      II. ACT or PT, PTT, TEG if available
   E. Urinalysis
5. Evaluation of peritoneal fluid obtained by abdominocentesis or diagnostic peritoneal lavage.
   A. Measure the glucose level of the peritoneal fluid and compare it to the patient's blood glucose level. If the peritoneal fluid glucose level is >20 mg/dL lower than the blood glucose level, septic peritonitis is strongly suspected.
   B. In dogs, comparison of the lactate level of the peritoneal fluid with the serum lactate level may be helpful.
      If the peritoneal lactate level is >2.5 mmol/L higher than serum lactate level, septic peritonitis is strongly suspected.
   C. Measure the creatinine level of the peritoneal fluid and compare it to the patient's serum creatinine level. If the peritoneal creatinine

level is two times higher than that of serum, it indicates urine is leaking into the abdominal cavity and exploratory surgery is necessary.
D. A bilirubin concentration higher in the peritoneal fluid than in serum indicates the presence of hepatobiliary or proximal intestinal disease or injury and exploratory surgery is indicated.
E. Measure the PCV and TS of the peritoneal fluid and compare it to peripheral blood. If the PCV is greater than 5%, intra-abdominal hemorrhage has occurred. Treat the patient supportively and repeat the peritoneal tap in 30 min. If the PCV has increased, exploratory surgery is indicated.
F. Microscopic examination
   I. Cytology – intracellular bacteria in neutrophils or a high leukocyte count indicates infection and exploratory surgery is indicated.
      a. WBC, greater than 1,000 cells/µL, indicates inflammation or suppuration and exploratory surgery is indicated.
      b. An increase in neutrophils (less than 100,000/µL) commonly occurs in the peritoneal fluid of animals without peritonitis that have had recent abdominal surgery. However, these neutrophils should not contain bacteria and should not be toxic or degenerate.
   II. The presence of bacteria indicates septic peritonitis and exploratory surgery is necessary.
   III. The presence of vegetable matter indicates bowel perforation has occurred and exploratory surgery is required.
G. Bacterial culture of septic peritoneal effusion most commonly identifies the presence of the following bacteria: *Escherichia coli*, *Enterococcus* spp., *Clostridium* spp., *Pseudomonas* spp., *Acinetobacter* spp., and coagulase-negative *Staphylococcus* spp., *Enterobacter* spp., α-hemolytic *Streptococcus* spp., *Pasteurella multocida*, and *Proteus* spp. Polymicrobial infections are common.

Abdominal radiographs—
1. Survey films may show a loss of serosal detail from peritoneal effusion or pneumoperitoneum. Pneumoperitoneum may be observed in normal patients for 1–5 weeks following abdominal surgery, so this should be taken into account in postoperative patients with signs of peritonitis. Intraluminal accumulation of gas and generalized intestinal ileus may be observed. The presence of free peritoneal gas in a patient that has not had previous abdominal surgery and has clinical signs of peritonitis is an absolute indication for immediate exploratory surgery, as it indicates rupture of an abdominal viscus, penetrating abdominal trauma or a ruptured urinary bladder. Additional diagnostic imaging studies of the abdomen are not necessary.
2. Contrast studies
   A. Evaluation of the urinary tract utilizing contrast studies may be useful.

B. Evaluation of the gastrointestinal tract utilizing contrast studies, with either barium sulfate or hyperosmolar iodinated contrast materials is not recommended.
   I. There is an increased risk for contamination of the peritoneal cavity.
   II. Both types of contrast agents increase the severity of peritonitis.
   III. Ileus causes contrast agents in the stomach to remain there for many hours.
   IV. An early exploratory laparotomy is more revealing and more beneficial to the welfare of the patient.

Abdominal ultrasonography—This may reveal previously undetected pockets of fluid accumulation, abscess, neoplastic masses, organomegaly, bile duct obstruction, the presence of calculi, and aid in obtaining samples for culture.

Differential diagnosis

Acute abdominal pain without peritonitis, ascites, SIRS, gastroenteritis.

PROGNOSIS

The prognosis is generally guarded to poor, but varies depending upon the underlying etiology, the patient's previous health status, early surgical correction, establishment of effective drainage, antibiotic administration, and nutritional and hemodynamic support. The presence of severe shock, coagulation abnormalities, or hypoglycemia indicate a poorer prognosis.

Treatment

1. Inform the client of the underlying etiologies, diagnosis, prognosis, and cost of the treatment.
2. Attempt to find and treat the underlying etiology.
3. Anticipation of complications, not reaction to clinical signs, is necessary for patient survival.
4. Administer oxygen supplementation.
5. Place an intravenous catheter and obtain blood and urine samples.
6. Administer high-volume intravenous fluid therapy with a balanced electrolyte solution such as LRS, Plasma-Lyte® or Normosol®-R to prevent stasis and organ ischemia.
   A. Dogs: 90–100 mL/kg for the first 1–2 hours IV, then re-evaluate.
   B. Cats: 45–60 mL/kg for the first 1–2 hours.
   C. After the first 1–2 hours, re-evaluate the patient's cardiovascular status. Generally decrease the rate to 20–40 mL/kg/h in dogs and 20–30 mL/kg/h in cats until the patient is stabilized. Continue at 10–20 mL/kg/h to maintain perfusion. Fluid rate requirements may range from 2 to 7 times normal maintenance rates.
   D. Monitor for fluid overload or continued hypotension.

     I. Monitor blood pressure. Maintain systolic pressure above 100 mm Hg and mean arterial pressure above 75 mm Hg.

    II. Monitor central venous pressure (maintain between 3 and 5 cm H_2O).

   III. Monitor urine output (minimum should be 1–2 mL/kg/h).

7. Administration of 7.5% hypertonic saline, 4–5 mL/kg IV in the dog, 2 mL/kg IV in the cat, will help to achieve peracute volume resuscitation, but should be followed by, or accompanied by, either crystalloid fluid therapy or crystalloid and colloid fluid therapy.

8. Administer colloid therapy, along with crystalloid fluid therapy, to improve perfusion and expansion of the vascular space while avoiding peripheral edema

  A. Hetastarch

     I. Dogs: administer a 20 mL/kg IV bolus, followed by an additional 20 mL/kg IV over 4–6 hours daily for at least 3 days.

    II. Cats: administer a 5–10 mL/kg IV bolus, followed by an additional 5–10 mL/kg IV over 4–6 hours daily as needed.

   III. Reduce the crystalloid fluid volume administered by 40–60%.

  B. Plasma: 10–40 mL/kg IV, administer when the patient exhibits clinical signs of peripheral edema or consider when the serum albumin level is less than 2.0 mg/dL.

    Other recommended therapies for hypoalbuminemia in dogs include canine albumin and 25% human serum albumin (HSA) (2 mL/kg IV). The administration of HSA has been associated with life-threatening anaphylactic shock and type III hypersensitivity reactions in dogs. HSA should not be administered to dogs with normal albumin levels.

9. Perform abdominocentesis or diagnostic peritoneal lavage and obtain peritoneal fluid samples for cytologic evaluation and culture. Ultrasound may also be used to localize fluid pockets for aspiration.

  A. Sterile technique must be utilized.

  B. Administer systemic broad-spectrum antibiotics.

  C. Use a Cook peritoneal dialysis catheter, another multiholed peritoneal dialysis catheter, or a pediatric trocath, or for cats, use a 14GA Teflon IV catheter with additional side holes, placed (with sterile technique) all on the same side to preserve the integrity of the catheter.

  D. Make a stab incision (1 cm) through the linea alba 2–4 cm caudal to the umbilicus.

  E. Aim the catheter towards the pelvic inlet.

  F. Infuse *warm* (body temperature) sterile saline (0.9% NaCl) 22 mL/kg (10 mL/lb), intraperitoneally.

  G. Roll the patient to disperse the fluid, then remove 5–20 mL of fluid for analysis. Place 2–4 mL of peritoneal fluid in an EDTA tube and 3–10 mL in sterile red top tubes.

  H. Remove the peritoneal catheter when finished, close the abdominal wall with one to two sutures, and apply a sterile abdominal wrap.

10. Administer analgesics as indicated by the individual patient's needs.
   A. Hydromorphone
      I. Dogs: 0.05–0.2 mg/kg IV, IM, or SC q2–6h; 0.0125–0.05 mg/kg/h IV CRI
      II. Cats: 0.05–0.2 mg/kg IV, IM, or SC q2–6h
   B. Fentanyl
      I. Dogs: 2–10 µg/kg IV to effect, followed by 1–10 µg/kg/h IV CRI
      II. Cats: 1–5 µg/kg/h to effect, followed by 1–5 µg/kg/h IV CRI
   C. Morphine
      I. Dogs: 0.5–1 mg/kg IM, SC; 0.05–0.1 mg/kg IV
      II. Cats: 0.005–0.2 mg/kg IM, SC
   D. Buprenorphine
      I. Dogs: 0.005–0.02 mg/kg IV, IM q4–8h; 2–4 µg/kg/h IV CRI; 0.12 mg/kg OTM
      II. Cats: 0.005–0.01 mg/kg IV, IM q4–8h; 1–3 µg/kg/h IV CRI; 0.02 mg/kg OTM

11. Administer broad-spectrum antibiotic therapy pending culture and sensitivity. Include coverage for anaerobic infections.
   A. Administer a combination of a first-generation cephalosporin (cefazolin (20 mg/kg q8h IV)), with an aminoglycoside (amikacin (for dogs 15–30 mg/kg q24h IV, IM, SC, for cats 10–14 mg/kg q24h IV, IM, SC), gentamicin (for dogs 9–14 mg/kg q24h IV, IM, SC, for cats 5–8 mg/kg q24h IV, IM, SC), or tobramycin (for dogs 9–14 mg/kg q24h IV, IM, SC, for cats 5–8 mg/kg q24h IV, IM, SC)), or a third-generation cephalosporin (ceftizoxime (25–50 mg/kg IV, IM, SC q6–8h) or cefotaxime (20–80 mg/kg IV, IM q6–8h)) and metronidazole, 10 mg/kg IV CRI over 1 hour, q8–12h.
      I. Aminoglycosides should be avoided in the presence of dehydration or azotemia as they may cause renal failure.
      II. Aminoglycosides administered once every 24 hours are more effective and cause less renal toxicity.
      III. If furosemide is utilized, aminoglycosides should be discontinued, as the combination increases the risk of inducing iatrogenic renal failure.
      IV. When the patient is on aminoglycosides, urine sediment should be evaluated at least daily for casts and cellular debris.
      V. The penicillins have been combined with a β-lactamase inhibitor (ticarcillin-clavulanate (Timentin®, 30–50 mg/kg q6–8h IV), ampicillin-sublactam (Unasyn®, 22–50 mg/kg q6–8h IV), and piperacillin-tazobactam (Zosyn®, 50 mg/kg IV, IM q4–6h) for increased efficacy.
   B. Administer a combination of cefoxitin, (40 mg/kg IV initially and continued at 20 mg/kg IV q6–8h in the dog and q8h in the cat), and metronidazole, 10 mg/kg IV CRI over 1h, q8–12h.

12. The administration of corticosteroids in septic shock is no longer recommended. Some patients with persistent hypotension that is not responsive to IV fluid and vasopressor therapy may have relative adrenal insufficiency. These patients may benefit from the

administration of hydrocortisone 2.9–4.3 mg/kg q24h, dexamethasone 0.1–0. 4 mg/kg q24h IV, or prednisone 0.7–1 mg/kg PO q24h.

13. Perform an exploratory laparotomy or definitive abdominal surgery if the etiology is isolated.
    A. Perform a thorough and symptomatic exploration of the peritoneal cavity.
    B. Surgically correct any gross abnormality observed.
    C. Control leakage from a hollow viscus by debridement and closure, resection or serosal patch application.
    D. Remove all foreign material, necrotic tissue, and blood clots from the peritoneal cavity.
    E. Perform peritoneal irrigation with large volumes of warm lavage fluid and remove all lavage fluid from the peritoneal cavity prior to closure.
    F. Place a gastrotomy tube or jejunostomy tube if indicated.
    G. If there is severe contamination of the peritoneal cavity or septic peritonitis, placement of a suction drain such as a Jackson–Pratt drain is recommended.
    H. If possible, in 1–2 days, perform exploratory surgery again to re-examine the peritoneal cavity. Repair damaged viscera, debride necrotic tissue, and irrigate the peritoneal cavity.
    I. Monitor albumin levels at least once daily. Extensive protein and fluid loss occurs from peritoneal effusion and repeated plasma administration may be necessary.

14. Nutritional support should be initiated within 6 hours of presentation
    A. Provide a minimum of 25% of the patient's protein and energy requirements within the first 12 hours.
    B. Provide a minimum of 75% of the patient's protein and energy requirements within 72–96 hours.
    C. After the patient has been rehydrated, administer a 3.5% amino acid solution with glycerine (Procal Amine®). The normally recommended dose is 40–45 mL/kg/day. The amino acid solution should make up ¼ to ½ of the patient's maintenance fluid needs and can be administered through a peripheral vein, 'piggy-backed' on the maintenance fluid line.
    D. The patient can then be eased onto an enteral nutrition program, either orally, through a nasogastric tube, gastrotomy tube, or jejunostomy tube. Oral supplementation with electrolytes, glucose, and glutamine supplementation is available in commercial products including Resorb® and Vivonex, TEN®.

       For dogs and cats, the package of Vivonex, TEN®, 40–45 mL/kg/day, should be diluted with double the amount of fluid recommended on the package for human consumption.
       I. The first day, administer 33% of the recommended dose, in divided feedings given every 1–2 hours.
       II. The second day, administer 66% of the recommended dose, in divided feedings given every 1–2 hours.
       III. The third day, administer the recommended dose, in divided feedings given every 1–2 hours.

Gastrointestinal emergencies

E. If vomiting does not occur, a bland diet can be given.
   I. It may be beneficial to administer a liquid diet, such as CliniCare®, first, to see if the patient can tolerate oral feeding.
   II. CliniCare® should initially be diluted to a 50% solution to decrease the incidence of osmotic diarrhea.
   III. Hills i/d®, or a/d®, Purina EN, or Eukanuba recovery formula® are examples of diets that may be considered.
F. Patients that have anorexia, pancreatitis, or gastroduodenal pathology can receive nutritional supplementation via various feeding tubes.
   I. Nasogastric tube
   II. Esophagostomy tube
   III. Gastrotomy tube
   IV. Jejunostomy tube—the preferred method for patients with pancreatitis
G. Total parenteral nutrition can be utilized as an adjunct, but the benefits are greater and the risks are reduced by utilizing enteral nutrition if at all possible.

15. If there is no improvement in the patient's status, fever, white blood cell count or band count after 36–48 hours, consider changing the antibiotic therapy. Reassess the patient and review the history and diagnostic data.
16. Administer vasopressor and positive inotropic agents if the cardiovascular status is still compromised following volume replacement.
   A. Dopamine, 5–10 µg/kg/min IV CRI
   B. Dobutamine, 2–20 µg/kg/min IV CRI in dogs, 1–5 µg/kg/min IV CRI in cats
   C. Norepinephrine 0.05–2 µg/kg/min IV CRI
   D. Vasopressin 0.5–2 mU/kg/min IV CRI
   E. Epinephrine, 0.005–1 µg/kg/min IV CRI
17. Monitor PCV, maintain at a minimum of 20%. Administer red blood cells or whole blood if necessary.
18. Monitor serum glucose levels and maintain between 80–150 mg/dL.
19. Monitor blood gases and optimize the patient's pH.
20. Monitor serum electrolytes q2–4h initially as rapid changes occur.
21. Monitor serum magnesium levels and serum potassium levels, as magnesium reduces the loss of potassium.
22. Monitor coagulation parameters for disseminated intravascular coagulation (DIC), which should be expected to occur.
   A. Recheck the platelet count and ACT or PTT (or TEG if available) daily.
   B. Trends should be followed, rather than one test at a point in time.
   C. Treat DIC, as discussed in that chapter, with fluid therapy, oxygenation, treatment of the underlying disorder, plasma administration, and possibly, heparin therapy.
23. Antiemetic therapy may be indicated.
   A. Ondansetron (Zofran®), 0.1–1 mg/kg IV or PO q24h.
   B. Dolasetron (Anzemet®), 0.6–1 mg/kg IV, SC or PO q24h.

C. Maropitant (Cerenia®), 1 mg/kg SC or 2 mg/kg PO q24h for up to 5 days (dogs only, not labeled for use in cats).
D. Metoclopramide (Reglan®), 0.2–0.5 mg/kg SC, IM, or PO q6h, 1–2 mg/kg/day as a CRI IV, or 0.01–0.02 mg/kg/h CRI IV.
E. Chlorpromazine (Thorazine®), 0.05–0.1 mg/kg IV, or 0.2–0.5 mg/kg IM, or SC q6–8h.
F. Prochlorperazine (Compazine®), 0.1–0.5 mg/kg IM or SC q6–8h.
G. Butorphanol, 0.2–0.4mg/kg q2–4h IV, provides some antiemetic benefit.
24. Gastric protection should be provided by treating prophylactically.
A. Ranitidine (Zantac®), 0.5–2 mg/kg IV, PO q8h (dogs), 2.5 mg/kg IV q12h (cats) or 3.5 mg/kg PO q12h (cats)
B. Famotidine (Pepcid®), 0.5–1 mg/kg IV or PO q12–24h
C. Omeprazole (Prilosec®)
   I. Dogs: 0.5–1.5 mg/kg PO q24h
   II. Cats: 0.5–1 mg/kg PO q24h
D. Pantoprazole (Protonix®), 0.7–1 mg/kg IV q24h
E. Sucralfate
   I. Dogs: 0.5–1 g PO q8h; can start with a loading dose 4× higher
   II. Cats: 0.25 g PO q8–12h
25. Regurgitation is a common complication. Therapy includes the administration of prokinetic agents, placement of a nasogastric tube and intermittent suction, or intermittent passage of an orogastric tube to drain excessive gastric fluid.
26. Auscultate and palpate the abdomen two to three times a day.
27. If the patient develops oliguria:
A. Review fluid therapy and provide adequate fluid volume replacement.
B. Consider the administration of a fluid bolus of 5–10 mL/kg IV over 10 minutes, which may help assess the patient's response and the potential for fluid overload.
C. Measure central venous pressure and mean arterial pressure. Maintain central venous pressure between 8 and 10 cm H_2O and mean arterial pressure above 80 mmHg.
D. Mannitol (10% or 20%), 0.1–0.5g/kg administered IV over 10–15 minutes, if there are no contraindications (vasculitis, bleeding disorders, hyperosmolar syndrome, congestive heart failure, volume overload). If no increase in urine production within 30 minutes, the same dose may be repeated. Do not exceed a mannitol dose of 2 g/kg/day.
E. Furosemide is usually given as a bolus of 1–6 mg/kg IV followed by a constant rate infusion of 0.25–1 mg/kg/h IV. If the bolus (repeated 1-2 times total) does not lead to urine production then the CRI may not help either. **Avoid furosemide administration in patients with ARF due to aminoglycoside administration, as furosemide has been shown to exacerbate aminoglycoside toxicity.**
28. Monitor the patient's mentation status. If the patient becomes depressed, check the serum osmolality and glucose levels. Provide

appropriate nursing care, including elevation of the head, prevention of aspiration, lubrication of the eyes, turn the patient every 4h, etc.

29. Provide comfort and general nursing care.
    A. Turn the recumbent animal over from one side to the other every 4 hours.
    B. Keep the patient clean and dry.
    C. Provide padding, towels, pillows, etc. to provide comfort.
    D. Check the intravenous catheter site frequently.
    E. Provide kind words and affection.
    F. Allow the patient to rest, when possible, by decreasing the light and noise levels.

GASTRIC DILATATION AND VOLVULUS (GDV)

Etiology

Although several factors, including breed, have been investigated, the etiology is unknown. Although most common in large or giant breed, deep-chested dogs, GDV can occur in any breed of dog, in cats and in other species.

Diagnosis

History—The patient may have recently been fed. The owner may observe repeated unproductive retching, restlessness, abdominal distention and hypersalivation. The patient may have been found in a state of collapse. Question the owner about any treatment they may have attempted, including orogastric decompression or gastric trocarization.

Physical exam—The patient will often present with obvious distention of the abdomen that is tympanic. Abdominal palpation reveals varying degrees of gastric distention and splenomegaly. The patient may retch with an inability to vomit. Often the patient is presented in a state of hypovolemic shock. Occasionally, the only finding is spreading of the forelimbs and hind limbs so as to stretch the abdomen, an enlarged and displaced spleen, or tachycardia.

Abdominal radiographs—Take right lateral recumbency and dorsoventral abdominal radiographs. If the patient resists the position for the dorsoventral view, a left lateral view can be utilized in its place. If the stomach is normal, the right lateral view will illustrate fluid in the pylorus, and with the left lateral view, the pylorus will contain gas. If a gastric torsion is present, the pylorus will be displaced cranially and to the left. The right lateral abdominal radiograph will typically display the 'double bubble', 'reverse C' or 'Popeye sign' in cases with classic GDV. See Figure 9.1.

Thoracic radiographs may be considered part of a thorough evaluation of an elderly patient, to check for concurrent metastatic pulmonary neoplasia.

Laboratory evaluation—Initially upon presentation, a critical patient should have a minimum database evaluated, including PCV, TS, lactate, BUN, creatinine, glucose, PT and PTT or ACT. As time allows, further diagnostic parameters should be evaluated, including:

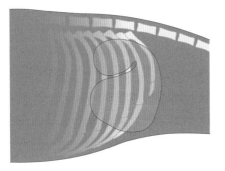

FIG 9.1   Radiographic demonstration of gastric dilatation and volvulus. This figure depicts the classic compartmentalization that occurs with displacement of the pylorus to the left of midline and craniodorsally within the abdomen. Small intestinal distention often occurs simultaneously.

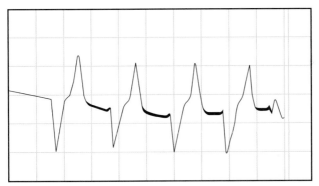

FIG 9.2   Premature ventricular contractions on an ECG strip. These are the most common arrhythmias that occur in gastric dilatation and volvulus patients.

1. Electrolytes
2. Blood gases
3. CBC
4. Complete serum biochemical profile, including ALT, alkaline phosphate (Alk Phos), BUN, creatinine
5. Coagulation profile (if indicated)—PT, PTT, FSPs, D-dimers, platelet count, TEG (if available)
6. Measure preoperative plasma lactate levels in a heparinized blood sample obtained prior to the administration of intravenous fluids. The normal range of plasma lactate levels in dogs is about 0.3–2.5 mmol/L.

Electrocardiography—Various arrhythmias may be observed, but the most common are premature ventricular contractions (PVCs). See Figure 9.2.

Prognosis

The prognosis is guarded to grave, depending on the physical status of the patient upon presentation. The mortality rate is reported to be from 33% to 43%. A plasma lactate level >6.0 mmol/L has been proposed to be associated with gastric necrosis, severe systemic hypoperfusion, and a worse prognosis in dogs with gastric dilatation and volvulus, but further study has not supported this finding.

Treatment

1. Inform the client of the diagnosis, prognosis and cost of the treatment.
2. Obtain pretreatment blood samples.
3. Place the largest-diameter possible intravenous catheter, or two intravenous catheters in the front limbs, and administer high-volume intravenous fluid therapy with a balanced electrolyte solution such as LRS, Plasma-Lyte® or Normosol®-R to correct stasis and organ ischemia.
   A. Dogs: 90–100 mL/kg, administered in ¼-shock boluses over 5–10 minutes, followed by re-evaluation after each bolus. Continue with the shock boluses as needed until the patient begins to stabilize then decrease the IV fluid rate.
   B. Cats: 45–60 mL/kg, also administered in ¼-shock boluses as described above.
   C. When the patient stabilizes, decrease the IV fluid rate to 10–20 mL/kg/h to maintain perfusion during anesthesia. Fluid rate requirements may range from 2 to 7 times normal maintenance rates.
   D. Monitor for fluid overload or continued hypotension.
      I. Monitor blood pressure. Maintain systolic pressure above 100 mm Hg and mean arterial pressure above 75 mm Hg.
      II. Monitor central venous pressure (maintain between 3 and 5 cm of water).
      III. Monitor urine output (minimum should be 1–2 mL/kg/h).
4. For rapid resuscitation or patients with hypotension despite crystalloid fluid therapy, administer Hetastarch, 5–10 mL/kg IV boluses up to 20 mL/kg then CRI of 20 mL/kg/day IV.
5. Consider the administration of 7.5% NaCl IV, 4–5 mL/kg in dogs, 2 mL/kg in cats, over 2–5 minutes if the patient is in severe hypovolemic shock and there is no indication of intra-abdominal hemorrhage. Hypertonic saline in Hetastarch may also be administered to contribute to rapid volume restoration in the treatment of hypovolemic shock.
6. Administer supplemental oxygen while treating for shock.
7. If the patient presents with severe gastric distension, immediate transcutaneous gastrocentesis may be performed to decompress the stomach.
   A. Clip and surgically prepare an area caudal to the right or left 13th rib (wherever the most tympany is detected) and trocarize the stomach with one or two 18- or 20-GA needles or over-the-needle catheters.
   B. If the area is on the left side, be cautious to avoid needle puncture of the spleen.
8. If surgery is going to be delayed, orogastric decompression may be performed.

A. Administer narcotic analgesics, which also act as premedication agents for anesthesia. Commonly administered combinations include butorphanol, 0.2–0.4 mg/kg IV, oxymorphone or hydromorphone, 0.02–0.05 mg/kg IV, fentanyl, 2–5 μg/kg IV, with diazepam, 0.2–0.5 mg/kg IV.

B. Pass the largest-diameter smooth-surfaced orogastric tube possible.

C. Perform gastric lavage with warm tap water to empty the stomach.

9. Do not spend a long time attempting to pass an orogastric tubing. Immediate surgical intervention is desired.

10. Take abdominal radiographs after initiating intravenous fluid therapy, unless euthanasia is an option being more heavily considered by the owner than surgery.

11. Recommend and perform surgery as soon as possible if the stomach is distended. Do not waste time trying to differentiate volvulus from simple bloat as volvulus is an extension of the clinical progression of bloat. A bloated stomach causes significant vascular compromise to the gastric mucosa and adversely affects systemic circulation. A distended stomach causes up to a 75% reduction in arterial flow to the gastric mucosa and is a surgical emergency.

12. Administer preoperative antibiotics, ampicillin, 20–40 mg/kg IV q6–8h, cefoxitin, 40 mg/kg IV initially and continued at 20 mg/kg IV q6–8h in the dog and q8h in the cat, or cefazolin, 20 mg/kg IV q6–8h combined with enrofloxacin 5–20 mg/kg IV q24h.

13. Monitor the ECG. If any arrhythmias are observed, treat accordingly.

14. Pre-anesthetic medications are usually not necessary, due to tachycardia and depression of the patient. Avoid phenothiazine derivatives. Do not administer atropine unless bradycardia occurs during induction or under anesthesia.

15. Induce anesthesia with:
    A. Propofol, 2–6 mg/kg IV, titrated to effect
    B. Diazepam, 0.2–0.5 mg/kg IV, and ketamine, 10 mg/kg IV, titrated to effect
    C. Oxymorphone, 0.2 mg/kg IV, and diazepam, 0.2 mg/kg IV, titrated to effect
    D. Fentanyl, 0.02 mg/kg IV, and diazepam, 0.2 mg/kg IV, titrated to effect
    E. Place an endotracheal tube.
    F. Place an orogastric tube as soon as possible after induction to decrease the risk of gastric reflux and aspiration.

16. Maintain anesthesia with isoflurane or sevoflurane and oxygen—**no nitrous**!
    A. Supplement with either oxymorphone, 0.05–0.2 mg/kg IV, or fentanyl, 2–5 μg/kg IV as needed.
    B. Positive-pressure ventilation is often needed.
    C. Fluid administration needs often exceed 10–20 mL/kg/h.
    D. Boluses of Hetastarch, 5 mL/kg IV, are often helpful in stabilization of the hypotensive patient during surgery.
    E. Administer dopamine 5–10 μg/kg/min IV CRI or dobutamine 2–20 μg/kg/min IV CRI in dogs (1–5 μg/kg/min IV CRI in cats) if a

positive inotropic agent is needed. If dopamine and dobutamine are ineffective, administer norepinephrine, 0.05–0.3 µg/kg/min IV.

17. Surgery

A. Make a *long* midline incision beginning at the xyphoid process.

B. If the stomach is grossly distended, pass an orogastric tube, or perform needle decompression.

C. Reposition the stomach. As the patient lies in dorsal recumbency on the surgery table most GDVs are rotated with the pylorus positioned ventrally and to the left, so one hand is used to press the right side of the dilated stomach down while grasping the pyloric region with the other hand and gently pulling the pyloric region up (ventrally) and to the right.

D. Partial gastrectomy may be necessary to remove areas of the stomach that are pale greenish to grayish in color, which result from ischemia or necrosis, or black to blue-black areas which result from venous occlusion and hemorrhage. Areas that are questionable in appearance should be re-evaluated 10–15 minutes after returning the stomach to normal position. Tissue with questionable viability should be resected. Recent literature states that the survival of dogs following gastric resection is 70–74%.

E. Perform a gastrotomy only if absolutely necessary, to remove large gastric foreign bodies or large quantities of ingesta.

F. Perform a serosal gastropexy, permanent incisional gastropexy, belt-loop gastropexy, or circumcostal gastropexy to the right ventrolateral abdominal wall, caudal to the 12th rib, near the level of the costochondral junction. (See Figure 9.3.) Use 2-0 monofilament nonabsorbable or absorbable suture for the gastropexy.

G. Suture the deeper (dorsal-cranial) margins of the gastropexy incision first.

H. Avoid incorporation of the pexy with closure of the abdominal wall due to the potential for damage during future abdominal surgery.

I. Evaluate the spleen. Return it to its normal anatomic position and remove it only if necessary due to infarction and thrombosis. Removal of the spleen is associated with an increased mortality rate.

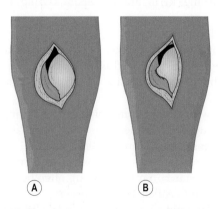

FIG 9.3 Technique for performing serosal gastropexy. (A) Illustrates the surgical approach; (B) illustrates the purse-string sutures opposing the circular incisions in the parietal peritoneum and the gastric serosa.

J. Evaluate the other abdominal organs quickly, but thoroughly. An enterotomy is occasionally necessary to remove an intestinal foreign body.

K. If gastric resection is performed or pancreatic trauma is evident, place a jejunostomy tube.

L. Lavage and suction the peritoneal cavity.

M. Rapid closure of the linea alba is facilitated by using a simple continuous pattern with a monofilament nonabsorbable or slowly absorbable suture such as Prolene or PDS.

    I. 0 for animals <14 kg (30 lb)

    II. 1 for animals 14–36 kg (31–80 lb)

    III. 2 for animals >36 kg (81 lb)

N. Close the subcutaneous tissue and skin with continuous patterns, consider using staples in the skin to further decrease the surgical time.

18. Monitor the ECG throughout surgery and for the next 3–4 days postoperatively (every 2–6 hours as indicated). Arrhythmias occur in 40–50% of the patients. In patients that do not have arrhythmias upon initial presentation or during surgery, it is not uncommon for arrhythmias to occur about 12–24 hours after surgery.

19. Continue IV fluids at maintenance levels, 40–60 mL/kg/day, until the patient can be weaned off fluids.

20. Provide post-operative analgesia with fentanyl, hydromorphone, or morphine with or without lidocaine CRI IV or with intermittent injections of a narcotic analgesic. The patient can be changed to oral tramadol when possible, but nonsteroidal anti-inflammatory medications should be avoided.

21. Monitor serum potassium levels and supplement fluids with potassium chloride as needed.

22. Monitor serum electrolytes, acid-base status, PCV, TS, blood glucose level, and renal function.

23. Treat cardiac arrhythmias if necessary. Administer oxygen if an arrhythmia is observed.

A. The most common arrhythmia is the premature ventricular contraction (PVC).

B. Treat PVCs if:

    I. They are multifocal in origin.

    II. They are increasing in the frequency of occurrence.

    III. The heart rate is >180 bpm.

    IV. R on T phenomenon is observed.

    V. There is evidence of impaired cardiac output (mean arterial blood pressure ≤60 mm Hg) or a lack of a palpable femoral pulse during tachycardia.

C. Administer a lidocaine bolus, 2–4 mg/kg, slowly IV, repeat once or twice over 10–15 minutes, while monitoring the ECG. Follow the bolus administration by administering a lidocaine CRI.

    I. Place 1 mg of lidocaine per milliliter of fluid in the fluid bag. To make a 1 mg/mL concentration, add 50 mL of 2% lidocaine to 1 liter of fluids.

II. Administer lidocaine IV as a CRI at 30–80 μg/kg/min.

D. If there is no response to lidocaine, administer procainamide, 6–10 mg/kg IV in 2 mg increments every 5 minutes to a maximum of 20 mg/kg, to avoid hypotension, while monitoring the ECG. If procainamide is effective at controlling the ventricular arrhythmia, continue procainamide at 25–40 μg/kg/min as an IV CRI or administer 6–10 mg/kg IM every 6 hours.

E. If there is no response or limited response to lidocaine or procainamide, check the serum potassium level.

    I. If the serum potassium level is low, increase the potassium supplementation in the intravenous fluids and continue to monitor the ECG.

    II. If the serum potassium level is normal, administer magnesium sulfate IV at 0.15–0.3 mEq/kg (12.5–35 mg/kg) over 2–4 hours as an IV CRI, which can be repeated for a total of three doses within 24 hours. In life-threatening situations, magnesium sulfate, 0.15–0.3 mEq/kg may be administered IV over 15–20 minutes.

    III. If there is no response to procainamide therapy, include propranolol, diluted to 0.1 mg/mL, administer at 0.1 mg/min until effect is observed or maximum dose of 0.06 mg/kg is reached.

24. Esophagitis is a common postoperative malady. Administer an H_2 blocker.

A. Ranitidine (Zantac®), 0.5–2 mg/kg IV, PO q8h (dogs), 2.5 mg/kg IV q12h (cats) or 3.5 mg/kg PO q12h (cats)

B. Famotidine (Pepcid®), 0.5–1 mg/kg IV or PO q12–24h

C. Omeprazole (Prilosec®):

    I. Dogs: 0.5–1.5 mg/kg PO q24h

    II. Cats: 0.5–1 mg/kg PO q24h

D. Pantoprazole (Protonix®), 0.7–1 mg/kg IV q24h

25. Consider the administration of metoclopramide to stimulate normal gastric motility postoperatively, 0.2–0.5 mg/kg SC, IM, or PO q6h, 1–2 mg/kg/day as a CRI IV, or 0.01–0.02 mg/kg/h CRI IV.

26. Gradually reintroduce the patient back to food and water.

A. Start the patient on small amounts of oral liquids 8–12 hours after surgery, unless a gastrotomy or enterotomy was performed.

B. Initially, offer small amounts of a low-fat canned dog food made into a slurry.

C. Gradually switch the patient to a good quality canned dog food with divided meals offered 4–5 times each day.

D. With time the patient can switch to dry dog food but should always be feed at least 3 divided meals each day to prevent gorging.

E. Recommend that exercise be avoided after the dog is fed.

ACUTE CANINE (VIRAL) GASTROENTERITIS

Diagnosis

History—The patient may have a history of vomiting and/or diarrhea, anorexia, lethargy, foreign-body ingestion, dietary indiscretion, poor vaccination history, exposure to ill or multiple dogs, abdominal pain, or a previous illness.

Canine parvovirus (CPV) gastroenteritis is probably the most common and severe viral enteritis causing severe illness in puppies. Many different diseases cause acute gastroenteritis, which can all be clinically managed in a similar manner to CPV, since the treatment is symptomatic and supportive.

The incubation period of CPV is 2–14 days, with most clinical cases occurring 4–7 days after exposure. CPV is most commonly observed in puppies from 6 weeks to 6 months of age. Dog breeds that are reported to be at an increased risk include Rottweilers, Doberman Pinschers, Labrador Retrievers, American Pit Bull Terriers, German Shepherds, Springer Spaniels and Yorkshire Terriers.

Active shedding of the virus in feces generally occurs for about 2 weeks post-inoculation, but in rare cases has persisted for 1 year. Normally, recovered dogs do not transmit disease to their susceptible kennel mates, even when they have lived together for several months. Subclinical infections probably play a significant role in the spread of infection. If conditions are favorable, CPV can remain infectious for 5 months or more in ground that has been contaminated with fecal material.

Physical exam—The patient may present with signs of vomiting and/or diarrhea and may vomit or have diarrhea in the waiting room or examination room. The patient may have an elevated body temperature and may appear dehydrated. Abdominal palpation may reveal abdominal pain. Always do rectal exam. If the patient is too small, use a rectal thermometer to gently evaluate the rectum, rectal contents, and stool appearance and consistency. The rectal exam may reveal diarrhea, which may be mucoid, watery or bloody.

The patient may present with variable degrees of depression and hypovolemic shock. Septic shock and systemic inflammatory response syndrome (SIRS) may occur secondary to bacterial translocation across the diseased gastrointestinal lining.

Laboratory evaluation—Initially upon presentation, a critical patient should have a minimum database evaluated, including PCV, TS, BUN and glucose. As time allows, further diagnostic parameters should be evaluated:

1. Electrolytes—hypokalemia, hyponatremia, hypernatremia and hypochloremia are common abnormalities.
2. Blood gases—the patient may exhibit a variety of acid–base disturbances. Metabolic acidosis is often the most prominent abnormality but metabolic alkalosis may occur from excessive loss of gastric fluid with recurrent vomiting.
3. CBC with differential usually reveals a transient lymphopenia.
   A. Neutropenia and panleukopenia may be seen in patients with severe disease.
   B. Anemia may be seen secondary to intestinal parasitism or a concurrent rickettsial infection such as ehrlichiosis.
4. Complete serum biochemical profile, including ALT, albumin, phosphorus, BUN, creatinine and glucose.

5. Perform an in-house CPV fecal antigen test such as an ELISA test. There may be false negatives due to serum neutralizing antibodies in bloody diarrhea. False positives may occur shortly after parvovirus vaccination due to fecal shedding of the vaccine virus. PCR testing can differentiate the vaccine virus from clinical parvovirus infection. If desired, the ELISA result can be verified by submitting a CPV serum antibody hemagglutination inhibition (HI) test to a reference lab. A high IgM titer with a low-to-negative IgG titer helps to determine acute CPV infection in dogs with hemorrhagic diarrhea. There are specialized ELISAs and double-antibody sandwich ELISA tests currently being developed which will reportedly be more sensitive than HI for detecting CPV specific antibodies in serum.
6. Fecal examination.
7. Urinalysis.
8. Coagulation profile (if indicated) – measure ACT, or PT and PTT, FSPs, D-dimers and thromboelastography. Puppies infected with Parvovirus gastroenteritis are often in a hypercoagulable state.

Abdominal radiographs—These should be evaluated if there is a palpable mass, such as an intussusception, severe abdominal pain, a localized gas distended bowel loop, or a history of foreign-body ingestion. Gas- and fluid-filled bowel loops are usually observed in puppies with canine parvovirus infections.
Abdominal ultrasonography—Generally, it is not needed; however, it may be useful if free abdominal fluid, possible intussusception, or an abdominal mass is detected.

Differential diagnosis

Intestinal parasitism, gastrointestinal foreign-body, dietary indiscretion, salmonellosis, *Clostridium* spp. infection, pancreatitis, protozoan infestation, rickettsial disease (salmon poisoning disease, ehrlichiosis), viral infections (coronavirus, distemper, parvovirus, etc.), and toxicity.

Prognosis

The prognosis is variable, depending on the etiology and duration of illness at the time of presentation.

Treatment

1. Inform the client of the differential diagnoses, prognosis and cost of the treatment.
2. Give the client the appropriate client education handouts.
3. Isolate the patient from other canine patients, and follow strict sanitary guidelines to avoid spreading the viral infection in the hospital. Clean all contaminated surfaces with a 1:30 dilution of household bleach or other appropriate virucidal cleanser.
4. Obtain pretreatment blood samples.
5. Assess the degree of dehydration.

A. Severe dehydration, 10–12%—the patient is usually moribund and in a state of hypovolemic shock.
B. Moderate dehydration, 7–10%—the patient usually has sunken eyeballs, skin tenting and slow capillary refill time (>1.5 seconds).
C. Mild dehydration, 5–7%—the patient has dry, tacky mucous membranes.

6. Place the largest-diameter possible intravenous catheter and administer high-volume intravenous fluid therapy with a balanced electrolyte solution such as LRS, Plasma-Lyte® or Normosol®-R to prevent stasis and organ ischemia
   A. The initial fluid rate if the patient presents in hypovolemic shock is 90–100 mL/kg the first 1–2 hours IV, then re-evaluate.
   B. After the first 1–2 hours, re-evaluate the patient's cardiovascular status. Generally decrease the rate to 20–40 mL/kg/h until the patient is stabilized. Continue at rates as high as 5–10 mL/kg/h to maintain perfusion. Fluid rate requirements may range from 2–7 times normal maintenance rates (44–66 mL/kg/day). Fluids such as Multilyte-M® or Plasma-Lyte-M® may be utilized for maintenance.
   C. The maintenance fluid rate for pediatric patients (6–12 weeks of age) = 120–200 mL/kg/day. The preferred IV fluid for pediatric patients may be LRS due to the ability of lactate to act as a metabolic fuel in the hypoglycemic pediatric patient.
   D. If the patient has a mild degree of dehydration, replace the deficit over 2–6 hours. The volume of the deficit can be calculated as follows: deficit (in mL) = dehydration (%) × body weight (kg).
   E. Monitor for fluid overload or continued hypotension.
      I. Monitor blood pressure. Maintain systolic pressure above 90 mm Hg and mean arterial pressure above 60 mm Hg.
      II. Monitor central venous pressure (maintain between 8 and 10 cm H_2O).
      III. Monitor urine output (minimum should be 1–2 mL/kg/h) and urine specific gravity (which should be 1.015–1.020).

7. Consider the administration of Dextran 70 or Hetastarch, 14–20 mL/kg IV bolus.

8. Consider the administration of 7.5% NaCl IV, 4–5 mL/kg over 2–5 minutes if the patient is in severe hypovolemic shock.
   A. Hypertonic saline in Dextran 70 (HSD) may also be administered to contribute to rapid volume restoration in the treatment of hypovolemic shock.
   B. 7.5% NaCl should not be administered to dehydrated patients or those with increased serum sodium levels.
   C. All patients that receive 7.5% NaCl should also receive crystalloid fluids either prior to or simultaneously with the administration of 7.5% NaCl.

9. Administer antibiotics.
   A. Sodium ampicillin, 20–40 mg/kg IV q6–8h
   B. Cefoxitin, 40 mg/kg IV initially and continued at 20–25 mg/kg q6–8h IV
   C. Ticarcillin-clavulanate (Timentin®), 30–50 mg/kg q6–8h IV

D. In patients that are well-hydrated, amoxicillin, 15–30 mg/kg q12h SC or IM, and amikacin, 3.5–5 mg/kg q8h IV or 10–15 mg/kg q24h IV

   I. Aminoglycosides should be avoided in the presence of dehydration or azotemia as they may cause renal failure.

   II. If furosemide is utilized, aminoglycosides should be discontinued, as the combination increases the risk of inducing iatrogenic renal failure.

   III. When the patient is on aminoglycosides, urine sediment should be evaluated at least daily for casts and cellular debris.

E. Sodium ampicillin, 20–40 mg/kg q6–8h IV, and amikacin, 3.5–5 mg/kg q8h IV or 10–15 mg/kg q24h IV

F. Sodium ampicillin, 20–40 mg/kg q6 8h IV, and ceftizoxime (25–50 mg/kg q6–8h, IV, IM, SC), or cefotaxime, 20–80 mg/kg q6–8h IV or IM

G. If an anaerobic infection is suspected, administer metronidazole, 10 mg/kg IV CRI over 1 hour, q8h, or clindamycin, 10 mg/kg q12h IV, in addition to one of the above antibiotic regimens.

H. Trimethoprim and sulfadiazine (15–30 mg/kg SC q12h) (avoid in Dobermans and Rottweilers)

I. Enrofloxacin, 5–10 mg/kg q12h IV, and sodium ampicillin, 20–40 mg/kg q6–8h IV

   I. Avoid enrofloxacin in young large breed dogs with incomplete closure of epiphyseal growth plates. One study has shown no detrimental effects to the use of enrofloxacin for 3–5 days in young large breed dogs.

   II. Dilute enrofloxacin 1:1 with sterile water and administer it slowly intravenously over 15–20 minutes.

10. If the patient exhibits excessive, repeated vomiting, or nausea, repeat the physical examination including palpation of the abdomen for an intussusception. Consider the administration of antiemetics, after volume replacement is achieved.

A. Chlorpromazine, 0.05–0.1 mg/kg IV q4–6h as needed, 0.2–0.5 mg/kg SC, IM q6–8h, or 1 mg/kg diluted in 1 mL of 0.9% NaCl and administered rectally q8h via a plastic catheter

B. Prochlorperazine, 0.25–0.5 mg/kg SC, IM q6–8h

C. Ondansetron (Zofran®), 0.1–0.2 mg/kg IV q6–12h

D. Dolasetron (Anzemet®), 0.6–1 mg/kg IV, SC or PO q24h

E. Maropitant (Cerenia®), 1 mg/kg SC or 2 mg/kg PO q24h for up to 5 days

F. Metoclopramide (Reglan®), 0.2–0.5 mg/kg SC, IM, or PO q6h, 1–2 mg/kg/day as a CRI IV, or 0.01–0.02 mg/kg/h CRI IV. If the patient is on metoclopramide, it is very important to palpate the abdomen every 2–4 hours and closely monitor for intussusception. Avoid metoclopramide if a mechanical obstruction is suspected, or if the patient has a history of seizures.

G. Butorphanol, 0.2–0.4 mg/kg IV, IM q2—6h, has been shown to exhibit an antiemetic effect as well as an analgesic effect.

H. Place a nasogastric tube, suction gastric fluid every few hours and reduce the stimulus to vomit.

I. Monitor for signs of a gastrointestinal foreign body, intussusception, acute pancreatitis, or reflux esophagitis. Palpate the abdomen every 4 hours.

11. If hematemesis or signs of nausea (drooling, exaggerated swallowing motions) occur, administer:

A. Famotidine (Pepcid®), 0.5–1 mg/kg IV q12h.

B. Ranitidine, 2–5 mg/kg IV or SC q12h.

C. Omeprazole (Prilosec®), 0.5–1.5 mg/kg PO q24h.

D. Pantoprazole (Protonix®), 0.7–1 mg/kg IV q24h.

E. Sucralfate, 0.5–1 g PO q8h.

F. Consider the administration of an oral therapeutic dose of barium sulfate, 0.55–1.1 mL/kg (0.25–0.5 mL/lb) PO q12h.

12. Administer medications for the control of abdominal pain as indicated. Butorphanol also has an antiemetic effect. For analgesia, buprenorphine or fentanyl CRI IV are alternatives.

13. Monitor blood glucose levels, maintain at 100–130 mg/dL with IV boluses of 25% dextrose (1 mL/kg) as necessary. Dilute the dextrose solution to 12.5% if the patient is less than 16 weeks of age.

A. If the hydration status is normal, consider adding dextrose to the crystalloid intravenous fluid to make a 2.5–5% dextrose solution for CRI. Continue to monitor hydration status.

B. Avoid rebound hypoglycemia by tapering the patient off of the dextrose drip.

14. If the patient is severely anemic, rule out concurrent rickettsial or parasitic infections and consider the administration of canine red blood cells, 5–10 mL/kg IV over 3–4 hours, through a filter. Cross match prior to the administration of RBCs.

15. Evaluate a fecal sample for hookworms, roundworms, whipworms, coccidia and giardia. Treat accordingly. Consider the administration of an antiparasiticidal agent to all affected puppies, regardless of fecal examination findings.

A. Ivermectin, 250 µg/kg SC, can be given to all breeds of dogs except those with MDR-1 gene mutation, including Collies, Collie mixed-breed dogs, Shelties, Border Collies, Australian Shepherds, Old English Sheepdogs, German Shepherds, Silken Windhounds, Long-Haired Whippets, their mixes, or in dogs with heartworm disease.

B. Fenbendazole (Panacur®), 50 mg/kg PO for 3 days.

C. Pyrantel (Nemex®), 5 mg/kg PO, repeat in 7–10 days.

16. Monitor protein losses. Recheck TS and / or albumin levels at least once a day.

A. If the TS is <3.5 mg/dL, administer Hetastarch or Dextran 70, 14–20 mL/kg IV. The beneficial colloidal effects of Hetastarch increase with repeated, serial, daily administration.

B. Administer plasma, 5–30 mL/kg IV if the patient has a coagulopathy, is in DIC or has severe hypoalbuminemia and has peripheral edema and other clinical signs of volume overload. Administer plasma through a filter.

Table 9.1 Suggested potassium¹ maximum infusion rate

Estimated potassium losses	(mEq/L)	(mL/kg per hour)
Maintenance (serum level = 3.6–5.0)	20	25
Mild (serum level = 3.1–3.5)	30	17
Moderate (serum level = 2.6–3.0)	40	12
Severe (serum level = 2.1–2.5)	60	8
Life threatening (serum level <2.0)	80	6

¹Potassium supplementation should not exceed 0.5 mEq/kg per hour.

17. Supplement intravenous fluids with additional potassium depending on the laboratory potassium level or the severity and duration of vomiting (Table 9.1).
18. Provide nutritional support.
    A. A partial parenteral nutritional solution, such as Procalamine®, which contains 3% amino acids, glycerol and electrolytes, can be administered IV through a peripheral vein and should be administered to puppies that have been anorectic for more than 3 days.
    B. The dose of Procalamine® is 40–45 mL/kg/day, administered at maintenance fluid rates.
    C. The Procalamine® infusion line can be 'piggy-backed' into the balanced electrolyte fluid infusion line to ease administration.
    D. As an alternative to a commercially prepared product, a partial parenteral solution may be prepared by adding 300 mL of an 8.5% amino acid solution to 700 mL of LRS with 5% dextrose. Lipid emulsion administration is controversial and has been associated with immunosuppression.
    E. When administering partial parenteral solutions, it is important to aseptically place and maintain the intravenous catheter. Monitor the catheter daily for pain, redness or swelling.
19. Administer oral glutamine, in the form of either glutamine powder (250 mg/kg q12h) or Vivonex TEN®.
    A. Glutamine is essential for normal enterocyte function and must be absorbed across the intestinal lining to be effective. A lack of glutamine for as few as 3 days will result in microscopic damage to enterocyte function and intestinal integrity.
    B. Administer Vivonex TEN® PO q1–2h or via CRI through a nasogastric tube.
    C. The dose of Vivonex TEN® is 40–45 Kcal/kg/day (1 Kcal = 1 mL).
    D. Mix Vivonex TEN® as a 50% solution by adding 500 mL of water to a single packet rather than 250 mL as stated in the packet instructions.
    E. Give $\frac{1}{3}$ or 33% of the recommended dose on the first day, $\frac{2}{3}$ or 66% the second day, and the full dose the third and following days, until the puppy resumes eating.

    F. The administration of Vivonex TEN® orally every 1–2 hours is recommended, unless emesis is uncontrollable and unrelenting, hematemesis is present, a gastrointestinal obstruction is present, or the patient is so depressed that aspiration pneumonia may occur following emesis.

20. Consider adding vitamin B complex, 4 mL/L, to intravenous fluids.

21. Consider the administration of antiserum against LPS endotoxin (SEPTI-Serum®).

    A. The dose is 4.4 mL/kg (2 mL/lb) diluted in a crystalloid intravenous fluid, administered in a CRI over 1 hour IV.

    B. The dose of antiserum to be administered must be diluted in an equal amount of a crystalloid intravenous fluid.

    C. The patient must be closely monitored for signs of anaphylactic reactions during and shortly following administration.

    D. Antiserum administration is generally recommended only once per patient, but it may be repeated within 5–7 days, with an increased incidence of anaphylactic reactions.

    E. This therapy is controversial, but has been beneficial in some septic patients that were unresponsive to other therapeutic manipulations.

22. Oseltamivir phosphate (Tamiflu®) is an antiviral developed for the treatment of influenza A and B in people. Oseltamivir may be effective in the treatment of canine parvovirus infections. The recommended dose is 2.2 mg/kg PO q12h. It should be started as soon as the puppy is recognized to be ill. It may be diluted in the attempt to improve the taste. One study found that puppies given Oseltamivir did not experience the same severity of weight loss or decrease in white blood cell count as the control group of puppies.

23. Monitor the PCV, TS and blood glucose levels every 12 hours or more frequently.

24. Monitor the CBC and serum chemistries (albumin, ALT, creatinine, potassium and additional chemistries as indicated by the patient) every 24–48 hours. Adjust therapy accordingly.

25. Monitor blood gases as indicated by the patient's clinical status, initial evaluation and progression of signs.

26. Monitor urine output, color and USG at least once daily. The minimum volume of urine output should be 1–2 mL/kg/h. USG should be between 1.015 and 1.020. If administering aminoglycoside antibiotics, check for the presence of casts daily.

27. Monitor body weight and repeat a physical examination every 12–24 hours.

28. If the puppy's rectal temperature is above 106°F (41.3°C):

    A. Increase intravenous fluid rate (use room temperature fluids or cool fluids slightly) and recheck the temperature.

    B. If no reduction in temperature, administer acetaminophen elixir, 10 mg/kg PO once.

    C. Or administer ketoprofen, 0.5–1 mg/kg IV, once.

    D. Or administer dipyrone, 10–15 mg/kg IV, once.

29. As time allows, give the puppy some tender loving nursing care. Nourish its emotional needs as well as its physical needs. Take time just

to pet the puppy and play, if it feels up to it, so that future visits to the veterinarian will not be perceived as threatening and frightening.

30. NPO while vomiting, except for administering an oral glutamine-containing electrolyte solution every 1–2 hours.
31. If the puppy maintains for 12 hours without vomiting, offer Pedialyte® or CliniCare®.
    A. Dilute CliniCare® to 50% when first offered, to avoid an osmotic diarrhea.
    B. Increase CliniCare® to full strength after 24 hours.
    C. If the puppy tolerates CliniCare® or Pedialyte® for 12–24 hours then offer a gruel of Hill's i/d® and water, Hill's a/d®, or Eukanuba Nutritional Recovery Formula®. If the patient is able to eat the gruel without vomiting, over the next 24 hours, decrease the amount of water in the mixture. Continue to feed a bland diet for 3 days, then gradually switch the puppy to its normal puppy food.

GASTROINTESTINAL OBSTRUCTION AND INTUSSUSCEPTION

Etiology

Intraluminal foreign bodies (bones, rocks, items of clothing, balls, toys, string, tinsel, thread, dental floss, fishing line, etc.) can cause obstruction. Mural lesions of the gastrointestinal tract (neoplasia, hematoma, hyperplasia) can cause obstruction. Extraluminal conditions involving the gastrointestinal tract (gastric dilatation and volvulus, intestinal volvulus or torsion, strictures, hernias, and intussusception) can cause obstruction.

Diagnosis

History—The owner may have observed the dog or cat swallowing or chewing on a foreign object. The patient usually presents with a history of vomiting. The patient may have anorexia and depression. There may be a decrease in the frequency of defecation and the owner may observe blood in the feces. Intussusception occurs secondary to numerous conditions that cause enteritis, including canine parvovirus gastroenteritis, intestinal parasitism and organophosphate toxicity.

Linear foreign bodies are more commonly seen in cats. They cannot be ruled out in cats lacking a history of playing with thread, string or tinsel.

Physical exam—The physical examination is usually normal in patients with gastric foreign bodies. Abdominal palpation cannot detect most gastric foreign bodies. Some intestinal foreign bodies may be detected by abdominal palpation, as can some intussusceptions. An intussusception is usually described as being 'sausage-shaped'. Other abnormal findings in patients with intestinal foreign bodies or intussusception include dehydration, weakness, abdominal tenderness, distended bowel loops, and decreased or absent borborygmus.

It is important to thoroughly examine the oral cavity, including underneath the tongue, in cats that may have ingested a linear foreign body (i.e. in any vomiting or dysphagic cat).

Laboratory evaluation—Initially upon presentation, a critical patient should have a minimum database evaluated, including PCV, TS, lactate, BUN, creatinine and glucose. As time allows, further diagnostic parameters should be evaluated:

1. Electrolytes – hyponatremia, hypochloremia and hypokalemia are common.
2. Blood gases – the patient may exhibit a variety of acid–base disturbances, from metabolic acidosis to metabolic alkalosis.
3. CBC – leukocytosis may be present.
4. Complete serum biochemical profile, including ALT, alkaline phosphatase, albumin, phosphorus, glucose, BUN, and creatinine. Pre-renal azotemia and alterations of hepatic enzymes secondary to sepsis may be observed.
5. Perform an in-house canine Parvovirus (CPV) fecal antigen test, such as an ELISA test, if the patient is a young dog.
6. Run a SNAP cPL or fPL, or submit cPLI or fPLI tests to check for pancreatitis.
7. Fecal examination.
8. Urinalysis.
9. Abdominocentesis and cytologic evaluation of peritoneal fluid may be helpful in evaluating if bowel leakage and peritonitis have occurred.

Abdominal radiographs—May be normal unless there is a radiopaque foreign body or a gas-distended bowel loop. Bowel distention occurs proximal to the foreign body. The common areas for gastrointestinal foreign bodies to cause obstruction are the pylorus, distal duodenum and proximal jejunum. Bowel perforation is indicated by the presence of free abdominal gas, fluid opacity in the abdominal cavity and loss of abdominal visceral detail.

Linear foreign bodies may cause a plication, pleating, or gathering of small intestinal loops, which may appear as numerous end-on loops on survey radiographs. This should not be confused with the normal 'string of beads' appearance of cat intestines, which is a symmetric narrowing and widening of the intestinal lumen.

Contrast studies with air, carbon dioxide or positive-contrast agents, or double-contrast studies, may be helpful. Barium should be avoided in patients suspected of gastrointestinal perforation. Gastric retention is diagnosed by the observation of contrast media retained in the stomach longer than 12 hours. Normal gastric emptying begins less than 30 minutes after ingestion.

An ileocolic intussusception may appear as a tubular soft-tissue mass, with an oval or rounded leading edge on survey films. The intussusceptum (the invaginated segment) may be surrounded by intestinal gas. On contrast films, the intussusception appears as a radiolucent filling defect, there is delayed intestinal transit time, abrupt narrowing of the intestinal lumen at the entrance to the intussusceptum, and dilation of the intestine proximal to the intussusception. A barium enema is most helpful in diagnosing an ileocolic intussusception.

Gastroscopy—It may be beneficial in the diagnosis and removal of gastric foreign bodies.

Abdominal ultrasonography—This may help determine the presence of an intussusception, which appears as a double-concentric, hypoechoic ring with a hyperechoic center on cross section. The appearance of foreign bodies will be variable with ultrasonography, depending on the degree of obstruction and the composition of the foreign body. Areas of small bowel distention should be investigated for the presence of an obstruction.

Exploratory celiotomy—This is a useful diagnostic tool in patients with persistent vomiting, abdominal pain, intestinal distention, or peritonitis. Obstructions or foreign bodies cannot always be observed with other diagnostic methods.

Differential diagnosis

Gastric mucosal hypertrophy, gastric ulceration, gastric neoplasia, pyloric stenosis, pancreatitis, acute gastritis, acute gastroenteritis, paralytic ileus, inflammatory bowel disease, mesenteric volvulus.

Prognosis

The prognosis varies depending on the duration of the obstruction, the location of the obstruction, and the amount of tissue compromised. Some patients with a simple, early obstruction with normal gastrointestinal integrity will have a good prognosis; others with a prolonged duration of intussusception will have extensive bowel necrosis and peritonitis and will not survive. The prognosis for intestinal volvulus or torsion is grave.

Treatment

1. Inform the client of the diagnosis, prognosis and cost of the treatment.
2. Emesis can be induced with apomorphine, 0.03–0.04 mg/kg IV, 1–5 mg SC or in the conjunctival fornix, in dogs or with xylazine, 1 mg/kg IM, in cats to attempt removal of rounded gastric foreign bodies with a smooth surface.
3. Endoscopy can be attempted for removal of small gastric foreign bodies such as hooks, needles, etc.
4. Large gastric foreign bodies or those with a rough surface that may result in esophageal trauma should be removed by gastrotomy.
5. Place an intravenous catheter.
6. Administer intravenous fluids based on the patient's acid–base balance and electrolyte status. Correct dehydration and treat for hypovolemic shock if indicated.
7. Administer antibiotics to decrease the occurrence of sepsis in anticipation of bacterial translocation across the compromised gastrointestinal barrier.

A. Cefazolin, 20 mg/kg q8h IV, or sodium ampicillin, 20–40 mg/kg q6–8h IV and amikacin, 3.5–5 mg/kg q8h IV or 10–15 mg/kg q24h IV, or gentamicin, 6–9 mg/kg q24h IV or 2–3 mg/kg q8h IV

   I. Aminoglycosides should be avoided in the presence of dehydration or azotemia as they may cause renal failure.

   II. If furosemide is utilized, aminoglycosides should be discontinued, as the combination increases the risk of inducing iatrogenic renal failure.

   III. When the patient is on aminoglycosides, urine sediment should be evaluated at least daily for casts and cellular debris.

B. Sodium ampicillin, 20–40 mg/kg q6–8h IV, and ceftizoxime, 25–50 mg/kg q6–8h, IV, IM, SC, or cefotaxime, 20–80 mg/kg q6–8h IV or IM

C. Cefoxitin, 40 mg/kg IV initially and continued at 20–25 mg/kg q6–8h IV

D. Ticarcillin-clavulanate (Timentin®), 30–50 mg/kg q6–8h IV

E. Ampicillin sulbactam (Unasyn), 20–50 mg/kg IV, IM q6–8h

F. Enrofloxacin, 5–10 mg/kg q12h IV or 5–15 mg/kg q24h IV in dogs, maximum of 5 mg/kg/day in cats, and sodium ampicillin, 20–40 mg/kg q6–8h IV

   I. Avoid enrofloxacin in young large breed dogs with incomplete closure of epiphyseal growth plates. One study has shown no detrimental effects to the use of enrofloxacin for 3–5 days In young large breed dogs.

   II. Dilute enrofloxacin 1:1 with saline and administer it slowly intravenously.

   III. Do not exceed the dosage of 5 mg/kg/day of enrofloxacin in cats due to the possible development of blindness.

G. If an anaerobic infection is suspected, administer metronidazole, 10 mg/kg IV CRI over 1 hour, q8h, or clindamycin, 10 mg/kg q12h IV, in addition to one of the above antibiotic regimens.

8. Avoid the administration of metoclopramide if an obstruction is suspected. Other antiemetics, such as dolasetron, ondansetron, or maropitant, may be administered but emesis will generally continue until the obstruction is relieved.

9. Immediate surgery is indicated, as delay may increase the severity of intestinal necrosis and possible perforation.

10. Surgical correction of any lesion should be performed, foreign bodies should be removed and thorough exploration of all abdominal organs should be performed. If no lesion is grossly observed, intestinal biopsies of the jejunum and ileum at least should be taken.

11. Linear foreign-body removal

A. With the patient under general anesthesia, examine thoroughly under the tongue and cut the string if present.

B. Gently examine the entire intestinal tract.

C. Perform a gastrotomy if indicated to remove a gastric foreign body.

D. Make an enterotomy incision midway along the length of the obstruction.

E. Gently pull the string from the mesenteric side of the intestinal lumen.

F. Remove as much string as possible through each enterotomy site, cut the ends when necessary and make another enterotomy incision further down the length of the obstruction.

G. Where there are signs of perforation and peritonitis along the mesenteric border of the intestine, intestinal resection and anastomosis are indicated.

   I. Use a simple interrupted suture pattern with either apposing or crushing sutures or a simple continuous pattern with appositional sutures.

   II. Use synthetic monofilament absorbable or nonabsorbable suture or synthetic multifilament absorbable suture of size 3-0 or 4-0 in dogs and 4-0 or 5-0 in cats.

H. Wrap the anastomosis site with omentum.

I. Perform peritoneal lavage with warmed sterile saline and carefully aspirate all lavage fluid from the abdomen prior to closure of the abdominal cavity.

J. If malabsorption is expected owing to the length of intestine that must be removed (generally when more than 75% of the small intestine is resected), the prognosis is guarded.

12. Reduction of an intussusception

   A. Gently squeeze the intussuscipiens (the enveloping segment) while applying gentle traction to the proximal segment (the intussusceptum or invaginated section).

   B. If the intussusception is reduced, examine the serosal surface for signs of trauma. Simple lacerations may be repaired with synthetic absorbable 3-0 sutures, placed in a simple interrupted pattern.

   C. If the intussusception cannot be reduced, or the involved intestinal segments are not viable, resection and anastomosis are indicated.

   D. Wrap the anastomosis site with omentum.

   E. Enteropexy, suturing of the site of the intussusception to the abdominal wall, or enteroplication, suturing the intestine in accordion-like folds, is recommended to decrease the incidence of recurrence.

   F. Perform peritoneal lavage with warmed sterile saline and carefully aspirate all lavage fluid from the abdomen prior to closure of the abdominal cavity.

13. If peritonitis has occurred secondary to bowel perforation, delayed abdominal closure should be utilized to facilitate abdominal drainage.

14. If the viability of a section of bowel is in doubt, a second exploratory laparotomy 24 hours later is indicated to reassess the viability.

15. Offer the patient a small amount of water to drink 24 hours after surgery. If no vomiting occurs for 8–12 hours on liquids, offer a small amount of bland food. Continue the patient on a bland diet for 3–5 days, then gradually switch back to the regular diet.

16. Complications following intestinal surgery include breakdown of the enterotomy or anastomosis site with subsequent peritonitis, peritonitis, abscessation, adhesion formation, stricture formation, and malabsorption syndromes from the resection of large portions (75% or more) of the small intestine.

17. Signs of peritonitis following gastrointestinal surgery
    A. Increased abdominal pain
    B. Depression
    C. Persistent vomiting
    D. Fever and leukocytosis
    E. Absence of normal borborygmus
    F. Ileus
    G. Abdominal radiographs may show an accumulation of fluid and gas throughout the intestinal tract, a lack of intestinal detail, and a ground-glass appearance of the abdominal cavity. Free air will be present in the abdominal cavity normally following abdominal surgery, so the presence of free abdominal air cannot be used to evaluate for signs of intestinal perforation postoperatively.
    H. Abdominocentesis or diagnostic peritoneal lavage and fluid analysis is usually the most valuable diagnostic tool. Ultrasound may assist in location of fluid pockets.
        I. Cytology – toxic or degenerative white blood cells, WBC count. The presence of vegetable fibers indicates perforation and the need for immediate exploratory laparotomy. An increase in neutrophils ($\geq 10\,000/mm^3$) commonly occurs in the lavage fluid of animals without peritonitis that have had recent abdominal surgery. However, these neutrophils should not contain bacteria and should not be degenerate.
        II. Creatinine or potassium if urinary tract leakage is suspected. An abdominal fluid creatinine concentration to peripheral blood creatinine concentration ratio of >2:1 was predictive of uroabdomen in dogs (specificity 100%, sensitivity 86%). An abdominal fluid potassium concentration to peripheral blood potassium concentration of >1.4:1 is also predictive of uroabdomen in dogs (specificity 100%, sensitivity 100%). If the abdominal fluid creatinine concentration is at least four times those of normal laboratory blood creatinine values, this also indicates urinary tract leakage.
        III. Abdominal fluid lactate compared with serum lactate. In dogs, septic effusions had a peritoneal fluid lactate concentration >2.5 mmol/L and a peritoneal fluid lactate concentration higher than blood lactate.
        IV. Abdominal fluid glucose level compared with blood glucose level. If the abdominal fluid glucose level was >20 mg/dL less than the peripheral blood glucose level from a sample obtained at the same time, in dogs and cats, this indicates septic peritonitis. These findings are 100% sensitive and 100% specific in diagnosing septic peritonitis in dogs and 86% sensitive and 100% specific in cats.
        V. PCV and TS—if the PCV is increasing, nearing that of peripheral blood, intraperitoneal hemorrhage is occurring. Nonclotting blood may be aspirated from the abdomen. Erythrophagocytosis may be observed.
18. If peritonitis is suspected, a second exploratory celiotomy should be performed immediately.

FELINE DIARRHEA

Etiology

1. Anatomic abnormalities – congenital abnormally short colon; surgical resection of a large portion of either the small or large intestine; a thick, persistent pancreaticomesojejunal ligament; portosystemic shunts; obstructive lesions; traumatic or congenital diaphragmatic or pericardial hernias
2. Infectious agents
   A. Viral enteritis—feline panleukopenia, enteric coronavirus, FIP, rotavirus, astrovirus, feline calicivirus, FeLV and FIV
   B. Bacterial enteritis—*Campylobacter jejuni, Salmonella* spp., *Escherichia coli, Bacillus piliformis, Clostridium perfringens* (enterotoxic diarrhea / garbage gastroenteritis)
   C. Fungal enteritis—*Histoplasma capsulatum* and *Aspergillus fumigatus*
   D. Parasitic enteritis—*Isospora* spp., *Giardia, Toxoplasma gondii, Cryptosporidium* spp., *Toxocara cati, Ancylostoma tubaeforme* and *caninum, Uncinaria stenocephala, Strongyloides tumefaciens* and *planiceps, Dyplidium caninum, Spirometra mansonoides, Taenia taeniaeformis,* and *Dirofilaria immitis*
3. Immune-mediated disease—food intolerance and / or sensitivity
4. Inflammatory—plasmacytic lymphocytic, eosinophilic, granulomatous, histiocytic or ulcerative gastroenteritis, suppurative enterocolitis, inflammatory bowel disease
5. Metabolic and endocrine disorders—hyperthyroidism, diabetes, pancreatic exocrine insufficiency, pancreatitis and hepatic disease
6. Neoplastic diseases—lymphosarcoma, intestinal mast cell tumors, systemic feline mastocytosis, intestinal adenocarcinoma (especially in male Siamese cats) and other intestinal tumors
7. Medications and toxins—a variety of medications, chemicals, and plant materials having direct irritative effects on the bowel or altering gut motility and causing diarrhea
8. Miscellaneous – idiopathic feline colitis especially in 'nervous breeds' (Siamese, Abyssinian, Burmese), dietary indiscretion or overload, abrupt dietary change or stress

Diagnosis

History—The owner may observe vomiting and diarrhea, intermittent diarrhea, anorexia and lethargy. There may have been a sudden diet change within 1–3 days prior to the onset of diarrhea.

Physical exam—Perform a complete and thorough physical examination; however, performing a rectal exam on an unsedated feline patient is not recommended. The patient may appear dehydrated. Abdominal tenderness may be elicited upon abdominal palpation. An abdominal mass may be palpable.

Laboratory evaluation—

1. Fecal examinations (gross and microscopic)
2. CBC

3. Complete serum biochemistry profile
4. Urinalysis
5. FeLV and FIV tests
6. Thyroid tests
7. Empirical treatment for *Giardia*
8. A controlled elimination diet
9. Further testing may be necessary (oxygen-specific function tests, SNAP fPL, fPLI, fecal cultures, absorption tests).

Abdominal radiographs—These may reveal a gastrointestinal foreign body, an area of thickened intestine, an obstructive pattern or an intra-abdominal mass.

Abdominal ultrasonography—This may help determine the presence of thickened bowel walls or abdominal masses.

Anesthesia, endoscopy and intestinal biopsies may contribute to the diagnosis. Exploratory celiotomy is a useful diagnostic tool in patients with persistent vomiting and diarrhea, abdominal pain, intestinal distention, or peritonitis. Intramural lesions, obstructions or foreign bodies cannot always be observed with other diagnostic methods.

Prognosis

The prognosis is variable, depending on the etiology and the patient's condition at presentation.

Treatment

1. Inform the client of the diagnosis, prognosis and cost of the treatment.
2. Acute diarrhea (mild)
   A. Maintain NPO for 24–36 hours unless the patient is less than 8 weeks of age.
   B. Maintain hydration with oral fluids unless the patient is vomiting.
   C. Begin bland food (such as boiled chicken or turkey, cottage cheese, potato and rice). Avoid baby foods that contain onion powder, as onion powder has been linked to Heinz body anemia in cats. If the diarrhea resolves, gradually return the patient to its regular diet over 2–3 days.
   D. Empirically treat the patient for coccidia and/or *Giardia*.
      I. The recommended treatment for coccidiosis in cats is sulfadimethoxine (Albon®), 55 mg/kg initial dose, followed by 25 mg/kg q24h for 14 days.
      II. The recommended treatment for giardiasis in cats is metronidazole, 10 mg/kg PO q8h for 7–10 days.
   E. The recommended treatment of *Toxocara* and *Ancylostoma* infection in cats is pyrantel (Nemex®), 20 mg/kg PO given once and repeated in 3 weeks.
   F. Treat the specific cause as needed.
3. Acute diarrhea (severe) – treat as for canine parvovirus gastroenteritis.
   A. Administer either intravenous or subcutaneous balanced electrolyte crystalloid fluids such as Normosol®-R or LRS. Intravenous fluid therapy is preferred.

Gastrointestinal emergencies

B. Potassium supplementation is usually necessary. Check serum potassium levels and treat accordingly. Empirically, add 30 mEq of potassium chloride to each liter of intravenous fluids.

C. Administer antibiotics if the patient has a fever, leukocytosis or severe hemorrhagic enteritis. Recommendations include amoxicillin, enrofloxacin, metronidazole and trimethoprim-sulfa.

D. Monitor blood glucose levels; maintain blood glucose between 100 and 150 mg/dL with a 5% dextrose drip if necessary.

E. Administer antiemetics if necessary.

F. Administer colloids or plasma if the patient develops hypoproteinemia or hypoalbuminemia.

G. Provide nutritional support, consider the administration of Procalamine®, 40–45 mL/kg/day IV, for partial parenteral nutrition.

H. Treat the specific cause as needed. If the patient only has mild diarrhea, avoid the administration of antibiotics, which may promote the development of a carrier state.

   I. If campylobacteriosis is suspected, administer erythromycin, 10–15 mg/kg PO q8h, or tetracycline or chloramphenicol.

   II. If salmonellosis is suspected, administer enrofloxacin, trimethoprim-sulfa, or chloramphenicol if the patient is septic.

   III. If clostridial overgrowth is suspected, administer amoxicillin, clindamycin, chloramphenicol or tylosin.

I. The use of antidiarrheal agents is contraindicated.

J. If the patient is not vomiting, feed a bland diet such as cottage cheese, boiled chicken and potato.

4. Chronic diarrhea (3–4 weeks' duration)

A. Provide the patient with nutritional support. Often a diet change to Iams Veterinary Formula Intestinal Low-Residue Feline, Purina EN Feline®, Hill's Feline i/d® or Hill's Feline Science Diet® may be beneficial.

B. Administer metronidazole (10–20 mg/kg PO q8h), tylosin powder ⅟₁₆ teaspoon q12h mixed with food) or sulfasalazine (3–4.5 mg/kg q8–12h for 7–10 days). Use sulfasalazine cautiously in cats due to the salicylate (aspirin) content.

C. Treat the specific cause as needed.

D. Treatment of inflammatory bowel disease in cats

   I. Prednisone, 0.5–1 mg/kg PO q12h for 2–4 weeks, then gradually decreased at 50% increments at 2-week intervals

   II. Metronidazole, 10–15 mg/kg PO q12h, for several months

   III. Budesonide, 1 mg PO q24h

   IV. If there is a lack of response to the above medications, the addition of azathioprine (Imuran®), 0.3–0.5 mg/kg PO once q48h for 3–9 months, may be beneficial in some cats.

HEMORRHAGIC GASTROENTERITIS (HGE)

Diagnosis

History—HGE is usually seen in young adult small breed dogs (Poodles, Dachshunds, Miniature Schnauzers). There is usually an acute onset of vomiting, hematemesis, fetid diarrhea, hematochezia, a 'jam-like' consistency to the feces, and tenesmus.

Physical exam—The patient is usually presented with depression and dehydration and no marked abdominal pain. The patient has profuse hematemesis and / or hematochezia. The condition can progress into a state of severe hypovolemic shock.

Laboratory evaluation—Often, there are no significant abnormalities other than an elevated PCV (often 55–70%), with little or no change in TS; however, a stress leukogram is possible. The normal PCV for a Dachshund may be up to 55%.

Differential diagnosis

1. Acute parvovirus or coronavirus gastroenteritis
2. Parasitic infestations of the intestinal tract
3. Nonsteroidal anti-inflammatory or corticosteroid administration-related gastrointestinal ulceration
4. Toxicities such as arsenic or lead
5. *Salmonella* gastroenteritis.

Prognosis

The prognosis is favorable to poor, depending upon the patient's physical status at the time of presentation.

Treatment

1. Inform the client of the diagnosis, prognosis and cost of the treatment.
2. Administer a balanced electrolyte crystalloid intravenous fluid such as Normosol®-R or LRS, at the rate of 40–60 mg/kg/h, until the PCV is <50%. If the patient is in hypovolemic shock, administer the fluids at the rate of 60–90 mL/kg/h for 1 hour and then re-evaluate the hydration and perfusion status. Fluid therapy is usually needed for 24–48 hours.
3. Antimicrobial therapy with penicillins (ampicillin, amoxicillin) is usually recommended.
4. Consider the administration of hetastarch, 10–20 mL/kg/day IV, to improve profusion status.
5. Observe the patient closely for disseminated intravascular coagulation (DIC). Treat the patient appropriately with fresh frozen plasma, etc. if DIC occurs.
6. If the patient exhibits excessive, repeated vomiting, or nausea, consider the administration of antiemetics after volume replacement is achieved:
   A. Maropitant (Cerenia), 1 mg/kg IV, SC q24h for up to 5 days.
   B. Dolasetron (Anzemet) 0.6–1 mg/kg IV, SC q24h.
   C. Odansetron (Zofran®), 0.1–0.18 mg/kg IV q8–12h.
7. If hematemesis or signs of nausea (drooling, exaggerated swallowing motions) occur, administer:
   A. Famotidine (Pepcid®), 0.5–1 mg/kg IV q12h
   B. Ranitidine, 2–5 mg/kg IV or SC q12h
   C. Cimetidine, 5–10 mg/kg IV or IM q8–12h

D. If severe hematemesis is present, administer omeprazole (Prilosec®), 0.2–0.7 mg/kg PO q24h

E. Sucralfate, 1 g dissolved in 10 mL of water; administer 250–500 mg for a dog <20 kg PO q6–8h and 1g PO q6–8h for a dog >20 kg

F. Consider the administration of an oral therapeutic dose of barium sulfate, 0.55–1.1 mL/kg (0.25–0.5 mL/lb) PO q12h.

8. Continue the patient on maintenance intravenous fluids; NPO for 12–24 hours. Start on oral liquids after 12–24 hours with no vomiting. Feed a bland diet after 24–48 hours and continue for 3 days, then gradually switch back to the regular dog food.

COLITIS

Diagnosis

History—The owner may notice an increased frequency of defecation of a low volume of stool with tenesmus, dyschezia and urgency. Mucus or blood, or both, are commonly seen in the stool. Frequent vomiting and weight loss are rare, but can occur in chronic or recurrent cases.

Physical exam—The patient is usually normal, except for the presence of mucus and possibly blood in the feces. A rectal examination is critical. Rectal discomfort, hematochezia or a thickened, irregular rectal mucosal surface may be detected. Some patients may have gravel or bone chips impacted in the rectum.

Laboratory evaluation—A CBC and serum biochemical profile should be performed to rule out other abdominal conditions.

1. The CBC is usually normal; however, some patients will have an iron deficiency anemia, neutrophilia, eosinophilia and / or hypoproteinemia.
2. The serum biochemical profile is usually normal.
3. Fecal flotation and direct smears may show parasites.
4. Rectal cytology should be performed.
   A. Use a gloved finger, a conjunctival spatula, or a moistened cotton swab to gently scrape the rectal mucosa to collect rectal epithelial cells.
   B. Transfer the sample to a glass slide.
   C. Normal findings include colonic epithelial cells, various types of debris and a mixed population of yeast and bacteria.
   D. Abnormal findings include neoplastic cells, inflammatory cells and infectious organisms such as *Clostridium perfringens* endospores or *Histoplasma capsulatum*.
5. Cats should be tested for feline leukemia virus and feline immunodeficiency virus.
6. T_4 testing is also recommended in middle-aged to older cats.

Abdominal radiographs—These should be evaluated to rule out other abdominal conditions. Look for masses, intestinal foreign bodies and luminal obstruction of the colon.

Dietary trial—Involving feeding a highly digestible diet exclusively for 4–6 weeks.

1. Sample diets include Hill's Prescription Diet i/d®, Eukanuba Low Residue®, Royal Canin Intestinal HE® and Purina EN®.
2. After 4–6 weeks, if the diet change is not effective at eliminating clinical signs, supplement the diet with 1.33 g/kg/day of soluble fiber, such as psyllium (Metamucil®).
3. Novel protein diets or hydrolyzed diets may be effective for some patients.
4. Supplementation with omega-3 fatty acids has been beneficial for some patients.

Colonoscopy and biopsy of the colon are helpful for establishing the diagnosis.

Differential diagnosis

1. Inflammatory (lymphocytic—plasmacytic, histiocytic ulcerative, eosinophilic, granulomatous or suppurative colitis)
2. Parasitic (*Trichuris vulpis, Giardia, Tritrichomonas foetus, Ancylostoma* spp., *Uncinaria stenocephala, Entamoeba histolytica* and *Balantidium coli* infestations)
3. Neoplasia (benign polyp, leiomyoma, adenocarcinoma, lymphosarcoma, mast cell tumor, leiomyosarcoma, plasmacytoma)
4. Noninflammatory conditions (irritable bowel syndrome, cecal inversion, ileocolic intussusception, small bowel malassimilatory disorder)
5. Infections (*Histoplasma capsulatum, Salmonella* spp., *Yersinia enterocolitica, Prototheca* spp., *Heterobilharzia americana, Clostridium perfringens* or *Cl. difficile, Histoplasma capsulatum, Pythium insidiosum*)
6. Metabolic disorders (uremia, pancreatitis, hypoadrenocorticism, hypothyroidism, hyperthyroidism)
7. Dietary indiscretion
8. Food allergy or intolerance
9. Stress.

Prognosis

The prognosis is variable depending on the underlying etiology and is good for idiopathic colitis.

Treatment

1. Inform the client of the diagnosis, prognosis and cost of the treatment.
2. Treat the underlying cause if determined.
3. Administer sulfasalazine (Azulfidine®, Salazopyrin®), 20–30 mg/kg PO every 8 hours for dogs and 10–20 mg/kg PO every 24 hours for cats short term (avoid due to the salicylate component in sulfasalazine). Also avoid the use of sulfasalazine for Doberman Pinschers.
4. Administer prednisone or prednisolone. The starting dose for dogs is 2 mg/kg/day PO or 20 mg/m² PO q12h for dogs ≥25 kg. Administer

this dose for 2 weeks after resolution of clinical signs, then start a slow tapering schedule.

5. An alternative to prednisone or prednisolone is budesonide, at 1 mg PO q24h in cats and small dogs and 2 mg PO q24h in large dogs.

6. Administer an antimicrobial agent.
   A. Metronidazole (Flagyl®), 10–15 mg/kg PO q12h
   B. Tylosin, 10–40 mg/kg PO q12h

7. Motility modifiers – these medications are contraindicated in cases of invasive and toxigenic bacterial infections of the bowel and gastric outlet obstruction associated with atony.
   A. Anticholinergics (propantheline bromide (Pro-Banthine®), Darbazine®) – are not recommended.
      I. They may decrease bowel spasms and tenesmus.
      II. Side effects include ileus, xerostomia, tachycardia, urinary retention and glaucoma.
   B. Narcotic analgesics
      I. Paregoric, attapulgite (Donnagel-PC®, Parapectolin®) – increase segmentation by a direct action on the circular smooth muscle of the intestine, decrease transit time, and analgesia. These medications are not safe in small dogs and are not recommended in cats.
      II. Diphenoxylate (Lomotil®), 0.05–0.2 mg/kg PO q8–12h in dogs, increases segmentation of smooth muscle and decreases peristalsis. Diphenoxylate should not be used in cats.
      III. Loperamide (Imodium®), 0.1–0.2 mg/kg PO q8–12h in dogs and 0.08–0.16 mg/kg PO q12h in cats, increases segmentation of smooth muscle and decreases peristalsis. Loperamide should be used cautiously in cats. It should also not be administered to dogs with MDR1 mutation, including Border Collies, Australian Shepherds, Collies, Shetland Sheepdogs, Old English Sheepdogs, German Shepherds, etc. and their mixes. It may increase water absorption by the bowel. Loperamide may also increase the risk for bacterial proliferation in the intestinal lumen.

8. Immunosuppressive agents – azathioprine, chlorambucil and cyclosporine have been used in some patients but have multiple serious side effects.

RECTAL PROLAPSE

Etiology
Rectal prolapse commonly occurs in dogs or cats that are experiencing habitual or continual straining; therefore, obvious causes of straining to void feces or urine should be evaluated.

Diagnosis

Differentiation between a rectal prolapse and an intussusception, which is rare, is made by attempting to insert a finger or a blunt probe between the mucocutaneous junction of the anus and the protruding bowel. If the finger

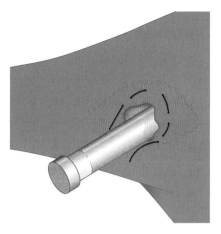

FIG 9.4 Reduction of a rectal prolapse. A blood sample tube or a thermometer can be used to maintain the proper diameter anal opening, depending upon the size of the patient. A purse-string suture of nonabsorbable, monofilament suture material is tied around the anus, applying enough pressure to inhibit rectal prolapse.

or blunt probe passes easily, an intussusception is present; if resistance is met, a rectal prolapse has occurred.

Prognosis

The prognosis is fair to guarded, depending upon the underlying etiology, severity and duration.

Treatment

1. Inform the client of the diagnosis, prognosis and cost of the treatment.
2. Successful treatment requires identification and treatment of the cause.
3. Administer fluid replacement therapy for dehydration and electrolyte disturbances.
4. Symptomatic control of diarrhea.
5. Treatment of the causative illness (antibiotics, parasiticides, etc.).
6. Application of hypertonic glucose solutions or granulated sugar to the rectal mucosa to reduce edema.
7. Under general anesthesia, manually reduce a minor rectal prolapse, and maintain with a purse-string suture in the anus for 2–3 days. Draw the suture closed around a 4-inch (10 cm) rectal thermometer or object of similar diameter in puppies and kittens; use a blood sample tube in mature animals. Once the suture has been tied, remove the item which helped to assess the size. (See Figure 9.4) Application of an Elizabethan collar may be needed in some patients.
8. Topical anesthetic ointment with 1% dibucaine (Nupercainal Ointment®) can be instilled in the rectum or a hydrocortisone retention enema, Cortenema®, 20–60 mL can be administered rectally q24h postoperatively for 2–3 days.

9. A nonreducible rectal prolapse with necrosis of the mucosa is best managed by full-thickness amputation and anastomosis.
10. If a rectal prolapse becomes recurrent, nonreducible or intractable to treatment, celiotomy and colopexy should be performed.

PERINEAL HERNIA

Diagnosis

History—Perineal hernias occur most commonly in male dogs from 7 to 9 years of age. There appears to be an increased incidence in Boston Terriers, Boxers, Corgis, Dachshunds, Old English Sheepdogs and Pckingese. Between 10 and 14 years of age there appears to be an increased incidence in Collies and mixed-breed dogs.

The owner may observe a perineal swelling, constipation, obstipation, tenesmus and dyschezia. Stranguria may occur. Other signs that may be observed include fecal incontinence, urinary incontinence, diarrhea, ulceration of the skin overlying the swelling, a change in the way the tail is held, and depression and vomiting secondary to post-renal uremia.
Physical exam—Most cases of perineal hernia are unilateral, on the right side, but it can occur on the left side and also bilaterally. Usually the swelling is ventral and lateral to the anus, but it may not be obvious.

Contents of the hernia usually include retroperitoneal fat, connective tissue, fluid, the prostate gland, and sacculation or flexure of the rectum. The urinary bladder, colon, jejunum or a prostatic cyst may occasionally be found in the hernial sac.

Rectal examination may reveal a rectal diverticulum, rectal deviation or lack of muscular support in the perineal region.

Radiographs may provide beneficial information regarding the anatomic structures present within the hernia. Positive- or negative-contrast studies may be useful to demonstrate the position of the urinary bladder. Oral barium administration followed by radiographs taken about 5 hours after ingestion of barium, or 24 hours if the patient is constipated, may reveal the presence of rectal sacculation or a rectal flexure in the perineal hernia.
Laboratory evaluation—Patients should be evaluated for dehydration, sepsis and post-renal uremia.

Differential diagnosis

Neoplasia, seroma, hematoma, abscess, perianal fistula, anal sac abscess.

Prognosis

The prognosis is fair to guarded with recurrence in about 30–45% of surgical patients. Fecal incontinence occurs in less than 10% of surgical patients. Persistent tenesmus occurs in 10–25% of surgical patients. Anuria or urinary incontinence that typically resolves about 1 week after surgery occurs in 15% of patients.

Treatment

1. Inform the client of the diagnosis, prognosis and the cost of treatment.
2. Surgical treatment is recommended, unless straining to defecate occurs infrequently. However, surgery is rarely an emergency.
3. Attempt urethral catheterization. If catheterization is unsuccessful, perform transcutaneous perineal cystocentesis to empty the urinary bladder. Once the bladder is evacuated, attempt manual reduction of the hernia by applying gentle pressure to the perineal swelling.
4. If the patient is dehydrated, administer intravenous fluid therapy.
5. If surgery is to be performed, administer warm water enemas with stool softeners 12–18 hours prior to surgery and withhold food for 24 hours prior to surgery.
6. If medical management is elected:
   A. Feed the patient a high-fiber diet with an increased moisture content.
   B. Give the patient bulk-forming laxatives, such as methylcellulose and psyllium.
   C. Administer dioctyl sodium sulfosuccinate either orally or as an enema.
7. If the patient has concurrent prostatic hyperplasia, castration is recommended.

ACUTE HEPATIC FAILURE

Etiology

In most cases, the etiology is idiopathic. The following is a list of some of the known causes of acute hepatic failure, but it is not complete.

1. Chemical induced (arsenic, heavy metals, carbon tetrachloride, tannic acid, selenium)
2. Medications
   A. Analgesics (acetaminophen, salicylates, phenylbutazone, carprofen)
   B. Anticonvulsants (phenobarbital, phenytoin, primidone)
   C. Miscellaneous (antineoplastics, azathioprine, diazepam, glucocorticoids, griseofulvin, itraconazole, ketoconazole, mebendazole, megestrol acetate, methimazole, mibolerone, trimethoprim-sulfa, tetracycline)
3. Anesthetics (halothane, methoxyflurane)
4. Biologic toxins (aflatoxin, blue-green algae endotoxin, amanita mushroom toxin, pennyroyal oil)
5. Infectious agents
   A. Fungal – Histoplasmosis, Coccidioidomycosis, Blastomycosis
   B. Viral – canine herpesvirus, infectious canine hepatitis (Adenovirus 1), feline infectious peritonitis (Coronavirus)
   C. Bacterial – *Leptospira* spp., *Clostridium piliforme*, *Ehrlichia* spp., *Rickettsia* spp., *Yersinia pseudotubercularis*, *Francisella tularensis*, *E. coli*, *Listeria*, *Salmonella*, hepatic abscess, cholangiohepatitis
   D. Protozoa – *Babesia*, *Toxoplasma*, *Heterobilharzia americana* (canine Schistosomiasis)
   E. Parasitic – *Dirofilaria immitis*

6. Systemic conditions that may lead to hepatic failure – shock, heat stroke, acute pancreatitis, hemolytic anemia, sepsis, extrahepatic infections, inflammatory bowel disease, colitis, neoplasia, copper storage diseases, and secondary to surgical hypotension or hypoxia
7. Other toxins (xylitol, sago palm, iron, lead, zinc)

Diagnosis

History—The owner may be able to provide a history of drug administration, toxin exposure, infection, seizures, etc. The owner may observe vomiting, anorexia, weight loss, lethargy, diarrhea, polyuria (PU) and polydipsia (PD), jaundice, excessive bleeding, abdominal distention, or signs of hepatic encephalopathy (depression, behavioral changes, seizures, coma).

Physical exam—The patient may appear depressed. There may be signs of vomiting and diarrhea. The rectal temperature may vary. Abdominal palpation may reveal cranial abdominal pain, ascites and hepatomegaly. Jaundice and edema may be observed. There may be petechia or other signs of a bleeding disorder. The patient may have seizures.

Laboratory evaluation—

1. CBC – mild to moderate anemia may occur. Target cells, acanthocytes and erythrocytic microcytosis may be observed. Thrombocytopenia may occur, as may thrombocytopathia.
2. Urinalysis – the urine specific gravity may be hyposthenuric or isosthenuric. Bilirubinuria may be present.
3. A complete serum biochemical profile should be evaluated. Abnormalities associated with hepatic disease include:
   A. Increased alanine aminotransferase (ALT) – ALT is considered to be liver specific in dogs and cats. Increases are seen with hepatocellular necrosis and inflammation, increased hepatocyte membrane permeability, cholestasis and production by regenerating hepatocytes during resolution on an initial injury
      I. Medications, such as anticonvulsant drugs and corticosteroids, or hyperadrenocorticism, can result in mild to moderate (2–10 times normal) increases in ALT levels.
      II. Severe skeletal muscle injury may cause increases in ALT levels of 5–25 times normal.
   B. Increased aspartate aminotransferase (AST) – AST is not liver specific in dogs and cats. It is also present in significant quantities in skeletal muscle.
   C. Increased alkaline phosphatase (ALP) – increases in ALP are a result of cholestasis or drug induction. Liver, bone and corticosteroid-induced isoenzymes are reflected in measurement of serum ALP levels:
      I. Mild increases occur in young animals or animals with severe bone disease.
      II. Small increases in serum ALP levels in cats suggest significant cholestasis.

III. The corticosteroid-induced isoenzyme does not occur in cats.
IV. Anticonvulsant drug therapy in dogs, but not in cats, can also increase serum levels of ALP.
D. Increased gamma glutamyltransferase (GGT) – increases in GGT indicate cholestasis and increased production by hepatocytes. GGT levels usually resemble ALP levels, except in cats, in which GGT activity usually exceeds ALP activity. Mild increases (2–3 times normal) in GGT may be related to anticonvulsant drug therapy.
E. Increased serum bilirubin concentration – can be due to either hemolysis or cholestasis. Check the CBC.
F. Hypoalbuminemia indicates chronic hepatic disease and a reduction of 70–80% of the functional hepatic mass.
G. Decreased BUN concentration may occur because of impaired hepatic ability to convert ammonia to urea. A decreased BUN can also occur in patients on a low-protein diet, those receiving fluid diuresis and patients with PU / PD.
H. Hypoglycemia may occur secondary to decreased hepatic glycogen stores, impaired hepatic gluconeogenesis and decreased hepatic insulin degradation. However, severe liver dysfunction must be present. Except in dogs and cats with congenital portosystemic shunts, hypoglycemia indicates a poor prognosis. Other causes of hypoglycemia, including sepsis, insulinoma and hypoadrenocorticism, should be ruled out.

4. A coagulation panel should be evaluated. PT and PTT may be prolonged in patients with liver disease.
5. Blood gas analysis should be performed as the acid–base imbalances associated with hepatic disease vary from respiratory alkalosis, metabolic alkalosis, metabolic acidosis, and mixed acid–base disturbances.
6. Liver function tests may be beneficial.
   A. Fasting and postprandial serum bile acid concentration evaluation is particularly helpful in detection of portosystemic shunt patients.
   B. Increased levels of blood ammonia may indicate hepatic encephalopathy due to portosystemic shunt, but normal levels do not exclude this diagnosis.
   C. If the blood ammonia levels are normal, an ammonia tolerance test may be performed. In dogs with portosystemic shunts, the blood ammonia level will increase to up to 10 times baseline values.
7. Analysis of ascitic abdominal fluid usually reveals a transudate or modified transudate with a protein concentration >2.5 g/dL. If the biliary tract has ruptured, the abdominal fluid may appear yellow or green and the concentration of bilirubin in the abdominal fluid will usually exceed that of serum.
8. Serologic antibody titers for infectious diseases may be beneficial.

Abdominal radiographs—These may allow for evaluation of liver size, the presence of abscesses or choleliths, and the presence of abdominal effusion.

Abdominal ultrasonography—This may reveal focal parenchymal abnormalities, including cysts, abscesses and masses or diffuse parenchymal abnormalities including hepatic lipidosis and cirrhosis. Ultrasonography can allow evaluation of the biliary tract and gallbladder and investigation of vascular lesions such as portosystemic shunts, hepatic venous congestion and hepatic arteriovenous fistulae. Ultrasound-guided biopsies may also be obtained, allowing the clinician to obtain tissue from focal lesions and avoid structures as desired.

Prognosis

The prognosis is guarded to poor.

Treatment
1. Inform the client of the diagnosis, prognosis and cost of the treatment.
2. Whenever possible, implement treatment for the specific underlying etiology.
3. Obtain pre-treatment blood and urine samples.
4. Place an intravenous catheter if the patient is dehydrated, vomiting, is uremic, has hepatic encephalopathy, DIC, or is in shock.
5. Administer intravenous fluids as needed, using 0.9% NaCl, 2.5% dextrose in 0.45% NaCl or Ringer's solution (avoid LRS in patients with severe hepatic failure). Avoid dehydration and pre-renal azotemia. Monitor for signs of primary renal failure, which may occur associated with hepatic failure.
6. Supplement potassium in the intravenous fluids as indicated by the serum potassium level.
7. Administer 25% dextrose IV boluses as needed to correct hypoglycemia. Add dextrose to the intravenous fluids to make a 2.5–5% dextrose concentration.
8. Administer hepatoprotective agents.
   A. *N*-acetylcysteine, 50 mg/kg IV or PO every 6 hours for 24 hours; dilute *N*-acetylcysteine to a 5% solution in 0.9% NaCl, administer IV slowly over 30 minutes
   B. *S*-adenosylmethionine (SAM-e), 18–20 mg/kg PO q24h
   C. Silymarin (milk thistle), 20–50 mg/kg PO q24h
   D. Vitamin E, 10 U/kg PO q24h
9. Colchicine is an antifibrotic agent that may improve the biochemical markers of canine hepatic disease. It should not be used in cats. Overdosage can be fatal. The recommended dosage of colchicine in dogs is 0.014–0.03 mg/kg PO q24h.
10. Ursodeoxycholic acid (UDCA, Ursodiol®, Actigall®) has been recommended to assist with the breakdown of bile acids, provide antioxidant effects and provide immunomodulating effects in the treatment of cholestatic disorders, sclerosing cholangitis and chronic hepatopathies. The recommended dosage is 10–15 mg/kg/day for dogs and cats.
11. Administer antibiotics to control extrahepatic infections and sepsis.
    A. **Avoid** chloramphenicol, tetracyclines, lincomycin, erythromycin, streptomycin, sulfonamides and hetacillin.

B. Commonly recommended antibiotics
   I. Ampicillin, 22 mg/kg PO, SC, IV, q8h
   II. Amoxicillin, 11 mg/kg PO, SC, q12h
   III. Cefazolin, 20 mg/kg IV q8h
   IV. Cefoxitin, 20–25 mg/kg IV q6–8h
   V. Metronidazole, 7.5–10 mg/kg IV CRI over 1h, q8h or 10–15 mg/kg PO q12h.
12. Administer a gastrointestinal protectant.
   A. Ranitidine (Zantac®), 0.5–2 mg/kg IV, PO q8h (dogs), 2.5 mg/kg IV q12h (cats) or 3.5 mg/kg PO q12h (cats)
   B. Famotidine (Pepcid®), 0.5–1 mg/kg IV or PO q12–24h
   C. Omeprazole (Prilosec®)
      I. Dogs: 0.5–1.5 mg/kg PO q24h
      II. Cats: 0.5–1 mg/kg PO q24h
   D. Pantoprazole (Protonix®), 0.7–1 mg/kg IV q24h
13. Provide nutritional support.
   A. If the patient is not vomiting, offer a low-protein, low-fat, highly digestible carbohydrate diet such as Hill's Prescription l/d® or h/d®, or offer cottage cheese and rice or potato. Avoid feeding meat.
   B. If the patient is reluctant to eat, place a feeding tube, such as a gastrostomy tube or jejunostomy tube, and tube feed.
14. If the patient presents in an hepatic coma:
   A. Administer retention enemas every 6 hours containing neomycin (15 mg/kg) and lactulose (diluted 1:2 with water, 50–200 mL total dose).
   B. An alternative retention enema is povidone-iodine solution, diluted 1:10 with water, administered at 50–200 mL total dose.
   C. Possibly the most effective enema solution is lactulose (diluted 3:7 with water, 20 mL/kg). Instill the lactulose solution into the colon with a Foley catheter and leave the solution in place for 15–20 minutes. Repeat every 4–6 hours.
   D. When the patient is awake enough to swallow, continue on maintenance therapy of neomycin, 10–20 mg/kg PO q6–8h or metronidazole, 7.5 mg/kg PO q8h, and lactulose, 0.5 mL/kg PO q6–8h or 3–10 mL PO q8h in dogs and 1–3 mL PO q8h in cats.
15. **Avoid corticosteroid** administration in most cases.
16. Add vitamins B and C to the intravenous fluids.
17. If the patient has biliary obstruction or prolonged PT, administer vitamin K_1, 0.5–2 mg/kg SC q12h for 2 or 3 dosages then PO daily.
18. Administer lactulose if blood ammonia levels are increased or the patient exhibit signs of hepatic encephalopathy.
   A. 0.5 mL/kg PO q8–12h
   B. Dogs: 1–10 mL PO q8h
   C. Cats: 0.25–1 mL PO q8–12h
19. Consider performing a bile acids test.
   A. Take a serum sample after a 12-hour fast.
   B. Feed p/d (dogs) or c/d (cats).
   C. Take a second serum sample 2 hours after feeding.
20. Thiamine supplementation is recommended for any anorectic cat, 100 mg PO or IM then 50 mg PO q12h.

Gastrointestinal emergencies

21. Avoid the use of diazepam, especially as an appetite stimulant, as it may cause profound sedation. Also avoid acepromazine, as it may also cause excessive sedation.

HEPATIC ENCEPHALOPATHY

Etiology

Either a reduction in functional hepatic mass or a reduction in portal blood flow, which results in a reduction of detoxification of gastrointestinal toxins, can lead to hepatic encephalopathy. The substances associated with the development of abnormal mentation and neurologic dysfunction in dogs and cats include ammonia, indoles, methionine, octopamine, serotonin, short-chained fatty acids, aromatic amino acids, skatoles and tryptophan. Portosystemic shunts may be microscopic and congenital or arise secondary to sustained portal hypertension or severe primary hepatobiliary disease.

Diagnosis

History—The owner may observe nausea, hypersalivation, vomiting, anorexia, lethargy, depression, weight loss, diarrhea and fever. Neurologic signs of hepatic encephalopathy may be precipitated by eating, especially of a high-protein meal, and by azotemia, dehydration, constipation and infection. The signs include trembling, circling, head pressing, ataxia, dementia, personality change, cortical blindness, seizures and coma.

Physical exam—The patient may appear depressed. There may be signs of vomiting and diarrhea. The rectal temperature may vary. Abdominal palpation may reveal cranial abdominal pain, ascites and hepatomegaly. Jaundice and edema may be observed. There may be petechia or other signs of a bleeding disorder. The patient may seizure.

Laboratory evaluation—

1. CBC – mild to moderate anemia may occur. Target cells, acanthocytes and erythrocytic microcytosis may be observed. Thrombocytopenia may occur, as may thrombocytopathia.
2. Urinalysis – the urine specific gravity may be hyposthenuric or isosthenuric. Bilirubinuria may be present.
3. A complete serum biochemical profile should be evaluated. Abnormalities associated with hepatic disease include:
   A. Increased alanine aminotransferase (ALT) – ALT is considered to be liver specific in dogs and cats. Increases are seen with hepatocellular necrosis and inflammation, increased hepatocyte membrane permeability, cholestasis and production by regenerating hepatocytes during resolution of an initial injury.
      I. Medications such as anticonvulsant drugs and corticosteroids, or hyperadrenocorticism, can result in mild to moderate (2–10 times normal) increases in ALT levels.
      II. Severe skeletal muscle injury may cause increases in ALT levels of 5–25 times normal.

B. Increased aspartate aminotransferase (AST) – AST is not liver specific in dogs and cats. It is also present in significant quantities in skeletal muscle.

C. Increased alkaline phosphatase (ALP) – increases in ALP are a result of cholestasis or drug induction. Liver, bone and corticosteroid-induced isoenzymes are reflected in measurement of serum ALP levels.
   I. Mild increases occur in young animals or animals with severe bone disease.
   II. Small increases in serum ALP levels in cats suggest significant cholestasis.
   III. The corticosteroid-induced isoenzyme does not occur in cats.
   IV. Anticonvulsant drug therapy in dogs, but not in cats, can also increase serum levels of ALP.

D. Increased gamma glutamyltransferase (GGT) – increases in GGT indicate cholestasis and increased production by hepatocytes. GGT levels usually resembles ALP levels, except in cats, in which GGT activity usually exceeds ALP activity. Mild increases (2–3 times normal) in GGT may be related to anticonvulsant drug therapy.

E. Increased serum bilirubin concentration – can be due to either hemolysis or cholestasis. Check the CBC.

F. Hypoalbuminemia indicates chronic hepatic disease and a reduction of 70–80% of the functional hepatic mass.

G. Decreased BUN concentration may occur because of impaired hepatic ability to convert ammonia to urea. A decreased BUN can also occur in patients on a low-protein diet, those receiving fluid diuresis, and patients with PU / PD.

H. Hypoglycemia may occur secondary to decreased hepatic glycogen stores, impaired hepatic gluconeogenesis and decreased hepatic insulin degradation. However, severe liver dysfunction must be present. Except in dogs and cats with congenital portosystemic shunts, hypoglycemia indicates a poor prognosis. Other causes of hypoglycemia, including sepsis, insulinoma and hypoadrenocorticism, should be ruled out.

4. A coagulation panel should be evaluated. PT and PTT may be prolonged in patients with liver disease.

5. Blood gas analysis should be performed as the acid–base imbalances associated with hepatic disease vary from respiratory alkalosis, metabolic alkalosis, metabolic acidosis and mixed acid–base disturbances.

6. Liver function tests may be beneficial.
   A. Fasting and postprandial serum bile acid concentration evaluation is particularly helpful in detection of portosystemic shunt patients.
   B. Increased levels of blood ammonia may indicate hepatic encephalopathy due to portosystemic shunt, but normal levels do not exclude this diagnosis.
   C. If the blood ammonia levels are normal, an ammonia tolerance test may be performed. In dogs with portosystemic shunts, the blood ammonia level will increase up to 10 times baseline values.

7. Analysis of ascitic abdominal fluid usually reveals a transudate or modified transudate with a protein concentration >2.5 fg/dL. If the biliary tract has ruptured, the abdominal fluid may appear yellow or green and the concentration of bilirubin in the abdominal fluid will usually exceed that of serum.
8. Serologic antibody titers for infectious diseases may be beneficial.

Abdominal radiographs—These may allow for evaluation of liver size, the presence of abscesses or choleliths, and the presence of abdominal effusion.

Abdominal ultrasonography—This may reveal focal parenchymal abnormalities, including cysts, abscesses and masses or diffuse parenchymal abnormalities including hepatic lipidosis and cirrhosis. Ultrasonography can allow evaluation of the biliary tract and gallbladder and investigation of vascular lesions such as portosystemic shunts, hepatic venous congestion and hepatic arteriovenous fistulae. Ultrasound-guided biopsies may also be obtained, allowing the clinician to obtain tissue from focal lesions and avoid structures as desired.

Prognosis

The prognosis is guarded to poor.

Treatment

1. Inform the client of the diagnosis, prognosis and cost of the treatment.
2. Whenever possible, implement treatment for the specific underlying etiology.
3. Obtain pre-treatment blood and urine samples.
4. Give the patient nothing by mouth.
5. Place an intravenous catheter.
6. Administer intravenous fluids as needed, using 2.5% dextrose in 0.45% NaCl, 0.9% NaCl or Ringer's solution (avoid LRS in patients with severe hepatic failure). Avoid dehydration and prerenal azotemia. Monitor for signs of primary renal failure, which may occur associated with hepatic failure.
7. Supplement potassium in the intravenous fluids as indicated by the serum potassium level.
8. Administer 25% dextrose IV boluses as needed to correct hypoglycemia. Add dextrose to the intravenous fluids to make a 2.5–5% dextrose concentration.
9. Administer retention enemas every 4–6 hours containing lactulose (diluted 3:7 with water, 20 mL/kg). Instill the lactulose solution into the colon with a Foley catheter and leave the solution in place for 15–20 minutes.
10. When the patient is awake enough to swallow, continue on maintenance therapy of neomycin, 10–20 mg/kg PO q6–8h or metronidazole, 7.5 mg/kg PO q8h, and lactulose, 0.5 mL/kg PO q6–8h.
11. Administer antibiotics to control extrahepatic infections and sepsis.

A. **Avoid** Chloramphenicol, tetracyclines, lincomycin, erythromycin, streptomycin, sulfonamides and hetacillin.
B. Commonly recommended antibiotics
   I. Ampicillin, 22 mg/kg PO, SC, IV, q8h
   II. Amoxicillin, 11 mg/kg PO, SC, q12h
   III. Neomycin sulfate, 20 mg/kg PO q8h
   IV. Metronidazole, 7.5–10 mg/kg PO or IV CRI over 1 hour, q8h
12. Administer a gastrointestinal protectant.
   A. Ranitidine (Zantac®), 0.5–2 mg/kg IV, PO q8h (dogs), 2.5 mg/kg IV q12h (cats) or 3.5 mg/kg PO q12h (cats)
   B. Famotidine (Pepcid®), 0.5–1 mg/kg IV or PO q12–24h
   C. Omeprazole (Prilosec®)
      I. Dogs: 0.5–1.5 mg/kg PO q24h
      II. Cats: 0.5–1 mg/kg PO q24h
   D. Pantoprazole (Protonix®), 0.7–1 mg/kg IV q24h
13. Flumazenil (Romazicon®), 0.02 mg/kg IV, may improve the neurologic status in some dogs.
14. Mannitol 20%, 100–1000 mg/kg IV over 15–20 minutes, repeated q4h as needed and furosemide, 1–2 mg/kg IV q8–12h, may be indicated if there is a failure to respond to therapy or rapid central nervous system deterioration suggestive of cerebral edema.
15 For long-term management, the ideal diet should be high in digestible carbohydrates and contain highly digestible protein of high biologic value.
   A. Hill's Prescription Diets l/d®
   B. Pro-Plan CNM NF-Formula®
   C. Homemade diet using low-fat cottage cheese, possibly small amounts of egg, with rice, pasta or potato, supplemented with vegetables and fruits
   D. If the patient is reluctant to eat, an esophagostomy or gastrotomy tube may be placed.
16. Thiamine supplementation is recommended for any anorectic cat, 100 mg PO or IM then 50 mg PO q12h.
17. Arginine should also be supplemented for any anorectic cat, 1 g per day.
18. Avoid the use of diazepam, especially as an appetite stimulant, as it may cause profound sedation. Also avoid acepromazine, as it may also cause excessive sedation.

FELINE HEPATIC LIPIDOSIS

Etiology

The underlying pathophysiology is poorly understood, but the condition has been associated with nutritional, metabolic, hormonal, toxic and hypoxic liver injury. Diabetes mellitus and pancreatitis may cause hepatic lipidosis. Arginine and / or taurine deficiency may be involved. It usually develops in obese cats after a period of prolonged anorexia.

Diagnosis

History—The owner may observe anorexia, lethargy, depression, weight loss with a previous history of obesity, vomiting, diarrhea or constipation. There may be a history of a stressful event, such as boarding, surgery, introduction of a new pet into the household, abrupt dietary change or a move.

Physical exam—Abnormalities that may be detected by physical examination include jaundice, dehydration, weakness, poor hair coat, variable body condition (normal to cachectic), hepatomegaly and pallor.

Laboratory evaluation—

1. The CBC may reveal a nonregenerative, normocytic, normochromic anemia with poikilocytosis. The WBC count is usually normal. Heinz bodies may be observed.
2. A complete serum biochemical profile with electrolytes. Abnormalities include:
   A. Pre-renal azotemia from dehydration
   B. Increased total bilirubin
   C. Increased ALP (5–15 times normal levels)
   D. Mildly increased or normal GGT
   E. Increased ALT (2–5 times normal levels)
   F. Increased AST
   G. Increased fasting and postprandial serum bile acid concentrations
   H. Hypokalemia, hypomagnesemia, hypophosphatemia, hypochloremia
   I. Hypoalbuminemia
   J. Hypoglycemia.
   K. Hyperammoniemia.
3. Blood gas evaluation.
4. A coagulation panel should be evaluated and may reveal a marked prolongation of PT and PTT and hypofibrinogenemia.
5. The cat should also be tested for FeLV and FIV.

Abdominal radiographs—These may reveal mild hepatomegaly and a diffuse loss of abdominal detail.

Abdominal ultrasonography—This may reveal a diffuse increased hepatic parenchymal echogenicity and hepatomegaly. In conjunction, there is decreased visualization of the walls of the portal vein. Peritoneal effusion and a hypoechoic irregular pancreas suggest the presence of concurrent pancreatitis.

An ultrasound-guided hepatic biopsy may confirm vacuolation of hepatocytes. Hepatic biopsy specimens from a patient with hepatic lipidosis when placed in a buffered 10% formalin solution will usually float.

Differential diagnosis

Diabetes mellitus, cholangiohepatitis, other hepatic diseases.

Prognosis

The prognosis is good to guarded, depending on the length and severity of the illness at the time of presentation and the underlying etiology.

Treatment

1. Inform the client of the diagnosis, prognosis and cost of the treatment.
2. Avoid stress.
3. Administer intravenous fluids with a balanced electrolyte solution, such as Normosol®-R or Ringer's solution to correct dehydration, then administer fluids at maintenance rates (20–30 mL/kg/day). Do not administer dextrose solutions unless the patient has hypoglycemia that has been documented. Dextrose administration can stimulate hepatic fat synthesis and block fat oxidation for energy.
4. Supplement intravenous fluids with potassium chloride as indicated by serum potassium levels.
5. Place a feeding tube to administer nutritional therapy.
    A. A 5–6 Fr. nasogastric tube is useful only for short-term therapy, but is preferable to force-feeding.
    B. An esophagostomy tube is very easy to place and does not require expensive equipment or involvement of the abdominal cavity with a risk of peritonitis. Esophagostomy tubes may be managed long term by the owner at home.
        I. Administer general anesthesia.
        II. Place an endotracheal tube.
        III. Clip and surgically prepare the lateral cervical area on the left side.
        IV. Through the mouth, place the tip of a curved forceps into the proximal esophagus and position the tip so that the skin overlying the esophagus is tented outward. The site of the tube placement should be about ⅓ to ½ of the distance down the neck.
        V. Incise the skin, subcutaneous tissue and esophagus just enough to fit a red rubber feeding tube of at least 10 Fr. in size.
        VI. Push the tip of the forceps through the incision and grasp the tip of the feeding tube.
        VII. Retract the tip of the feeding tube out through the mouth, with the syringe end of the feeding tube remaining percutaneously outside the esophageal incision.
        VIII. Direct the tip of the feeding tube into the esophagus and feed the tube down the esophagus until the tip lies in the distal third of the esophagus. Do not have the tip pass the cardia.
        IX. The position of the tube can be confirmed radiographically.
        X. Suture the feeding tube to the skin, with a Chinese finger-lock pattern.
        XI. Place a support wrap around the neck.
    C. A gastrostomy tube can also be managed long term by the owner at home.
        I. Blind method
            a. Administer general anesthesia.
            b. Place the patient in right lateral recumbency.

c. Place an endotracheal tube.

d. Clip and surgically prepare the skin caudal to the last rib.

e. Lubricate a flexible, curved polyvinyl placement tube and pass it through the mouth into the stomach.

f. Grasp the tube through the body wall and push a 14 g over-the-needle catheter into the placement tube lumen in the stomach. Remove the stylet from the catheter.

g. Pass a guide wire with a no. 1 or 2 polyester suture attached through the catheter that is long enough to pass through the length of the placement tube.

h. Remove the placement tube, guide wire and suture from the stomach through the mouth.

i. Pass the suture retrograde through another catheter and secure it to the modified end of a 14–24 Fr. Pezzar-type (mushroom-tipped) catheter or a low-profile gastrostomy device.

j. Carefully enlarge the entry wound in the body wall with a scalpel.

k. Lubricate the catheter and feeding tube then gently pull them into the stomach and through the body wall.

l. Pull the mushroom tip until it rests against the gastric mucosa.

m. Secure the tube by suturing tape tabs and using a Chinese finger-lock suture.

n. Place a light abdominal bandage over the tube exit site.

II. Endoscopic method

a. Administer general anesthesia.

b. Place the patient in right lateral recumbency.

c. Place an endotracheal tube.

d. Clip and surgically prepare the skin caudal to the last rib.

e. Insufflate the stomach with air, with the endoscope placed in the stomach.

f. Push an 18 g over-the-needle catheter through the body wall into the stomach where the illuminated tip of the endoscope is observed.

g. With the endoscope, position the catheter in the stomach and remove the stylet.

h. Insert no. 1 or 2 polyester suture through the catheter and grasp it with the endoscope.

i. Withdraw the endoscope and suture from the stomach.

j. Pass the suture retrograde through another catheter and secure it to the modified end of a 14–24 Fr. Pezzar-type (mushroom-tipped) catheter or a low-profile gastrostomy device.

k. Carefully enlarge the entry wound in the body wall with a scalpel.

l. Lubricate the catheter and feeding tube, then gently pull them into the stomach and through the body wall.

m. Pull the mushroom tip until it rests against the gastric mucosa.

   n. Secure the tube by suturing tape tabs and using a Chinese finger-lock suture.
   o. Place a light abdominal bandage over the tube exit site.
6. Provide nutritional support (60–80 kcal/kg/day).
   A. CliniCare® diluted to 200–300 mOsm/L initially and gradually increased over 1 week.
   B. Human liquid diets (Pulmocare®) with protein (Pro-Magic® or dehydrated cottage cheese) and taurine added. Mix with warm water and blend prior to each meal.
   C. Blenderized Hill's Prescription Diet l/d®.
   D. Hill's Prescription Diet a/d® or Eukanuba Nutritional Recovery Diet®.
   E. Continuous infusion is recommended. Start at 3 mL/kg/h and progressively increase to 10–15 mL/kg/h.
   F. If continuous feeding is not feasible, feed 4–6 times daily.
7. Cats with hepatic encephalopathy require a lower-protein diet such as Hill's Prescription Diet l/d or RenalCare®.
8. Administer a B vitamin complex at double the daily maintenance dose, 4 mL/L.
9. Supplement thiamine by administering 100 mg IM q12h initially for several days, then 50–100 mg q12–24h PO.
10. Supplement taurine, 500 mg/day initially.
11. Administer vitamin K_1 (0.5–2 mg/kg SC q12h for usually 2–3 doses then PO daily).
12. Administer metoclopramide if the patient exhibits persistent vomiting, 0.2–0.5 mg/kg PO q6–8h through the feeding tube or SC 30 minutes prior to feeding.
13. Do not attempt to feed the cat for 1 week. Then offer food other than the desired maintenance diet, as the initial response of nausea may be remembered and the cat may become conditioned to avoid the first diets offered during bouts of nausea.
14. When feeding is to be attempted, administer an appetite stimulant.
   A. Cyproheptadine, 1–2 mg per cat PO q12h
   B. Mirtazapine 3 mg per cat PO q72h
15. Avoid the administration of glucocorticoids.

FELINE CHOLANGIOHEPATITIS

Etiology

The etiology is unknown. An immune-mediated disorder may be involved. Other causes associated with feline cholangiohepatitis include toxins, bacterial infection ascending from the gastrointestinal tract to the biliary tract, systemic infections, cholelithiasis, pancreatitis, nephrotic syndrome, hepatobiliary parasites (including *Platynosomum concinnum* or *P. fastosum*), anatomic abnormalities of the biliary tract, and periductal biliary fibrosis.

There are two major types of cholangiohepatitis in cats. They are classified by the histopathologic findings as either lymphocytic (nonsuppurative) or neutrophilic (suppurative).

Feline triaditis syndrome is a condition in cats involving concurrent pancreatitis, inflammatory bowel disease and cholangitis.

Diagnosis

History—The condition is more common in young to middle-aged cats, but can occur at any age. There is no apparent breed or sex predisposition. The owner may observe anorexia, vomiting, diarrhea, lethargy, weight loss and jaundice. The signs may be intermittent or persistent and acute or chronic.

Physical exam—The patient may be febrile, dehydrated and jaundiced. Ascites or hepatomegaly, and abdominal pain or discomfort may be present.

Laboratory evaluation—

1. The CBC may reveal a mild nonregenerative anemia, neutrophilia with a left shift and lymphopenia.
2. A complete serum biochemical profile with electrolytes. Abnormalities include:
   A. Pre-renal azotemia from dehydration
   B. Increased conjugated bilirubin
   C. Increased ALP
   D. Increased GGT
   E. Increased ALT
   F. Increased AST
   G. Fasting serum bile acid concentrations are normal in 50% of the patients
   H. Postprandial serum bile acid concentrations are usually increased
   I. Hypokalemia
   J. Signs of advanced hepatic disease include hypoalbuminemia, hypoglycemia, hyperammonemia and a decreased BUN.
3. Blood gas evaluation.
4. Urinalysis may reveal bilirubinuria.
5. A coagulation panel should be evaluated and may reveal a marked prolongation of PT and PTT and hypofibrinogenemia.
6. The cat should also be tested for FeLV and FIV.

Abdominal radiographs—These may reveal mild hepatomegaly and a diffuse loss of abdominal detail. Occasionally, a radiopaque cholelith may be visible.

Abdominal ultrasonography—This may reveal hepatomegaly. The hepatic surface may be irregular and nodular. Peritoneal effusion and a hypoechoic irregular pancreas suggest the presence of concurrent pancreatitis.

Biopsy—A hepatic biopsy may reveal diffuse hepatic disease consisting of infiltrates of lymphocytes, lymphocytes and plasma cells, or neutrophils in the portal triads. Other histologic changes commonly observed include portal triad fibrosis, bile duct proliferation, and centrilobular accumulation of bile with bile casts in canalicular areas. A culture of bile or hepatic tissue is often positive for *E. coli*, but that may be either a primary or secondary infection.

Differential diagnosis

Diabetes mellitus, feline hepatic lipidosis, other hepatic diseases.

Prognosis

The prognosis is guarded to poor. Relapses occur in 25–50% of cats, requiring intermittent or continual therapy for months or years.

Treatment

1. Inform the client of the diagnosis, prognosis and cost of the treatment.
2. The lymphocytic form should be treated with prednisone.
   A. The initial prednisone dose is 2–4 mg/kg q24–48h.
   B. Taper the prednisone dose over 2–3 months, if there are signs of remission.
   C. Also consider the administration of ursodeoxycholic acid (UDCA, Ursodiol®, Actigall®), 10–15 mg/kg q24h PO.
   D. Also administer antibiotics if the hepatic biopsy culture result is positive.
3. The neutrophilic form should be treated with antibiotics, ideally based on the results of the hepatic biopsy culture.
   A. For empiric antibiotic therapy or if the culture is negative, administer ampicillin, 20 mg/kg q8h, amoxicillin, 11–22 mg/kg q8–12h, cefazolin 10–20 mg/kg q8h, or cephalexin, 11–22 mg/kg q8h, or amoxicillin-clavulanic acid, 62.5 mg/cat PO q12h.
   B. Also administer metronidazole, 10–15 mg/kg q12h, in combination with one of the above antibiotics.
   C. The antibiotics should be administered for 4–8 weeks.
   D. If there is a transient response or failure of a response to antibiotic therapy, administer prednisone, 1–2 mg/kg q24h PO, in addition to antibiotics.
      I. If the patient improves, increase the dosage to 1 mg/kg q12h for 2 weeks then start tapering the dosage.
      II. A dosage as low as 0.5 mg/kg PO q48h may be maintained for 4 weeks or longer.
4. UDCA, (Ursodiol®, Actigall®), 10–15 mg/kg PO q24h, may be beneficial for patients with cholangiohepatitis with biliary stasis and inspissated bile.
5. Furosemide may be beneficial to reduce ascites.
6. Administer a hepatic protective agent.
   A. N-acetylcystine, 50 mg/kg IV or PO every 6 hours for 24 hours; dilute N-acetylcysteine to a 5% solution in 0.9% NaCl, administer IV slowly over 30 minutes
   B. S-adenosylmethionine (SAM-e), 18–20 mg/kg PO q24h
   C. Silymarin (milk thistle), 20–50 mg/kg PO q24h
7. Intravenous fluids and other symptomatic therapy should be administered based on the needs of the individual patient.
8. Vitamin K, 0.5–2 mg/cat SC or PO q12h, may be beneficial if the patient exhibits signs of a coagulopathy.

9. Nutritional support
    A. Cats without signs of hepatic encephalopathy should be fed a diet of 30–40% protein. A balanced, high-protein maintenance diet is sufficient.
    B. Cats with signs of hepatic encephalopathy require a reduced-protein diet such as boiled rice and cottage cheese or Hill's Prescription Feline l/d®.
    C. If the cat is anorectic or vomiting, the appropriate feeding tube may be placed.

PANCREATITIS

Etiology

The etiology is often idiopathic. Predisposing factors include:

1. Obesity
2. A high-fat diet
3. Ingestion of a high-fat meal
4. Hyperlipidemia – hyperadrenocorticism, diabetes mellitus, hypothyroidism, or idiopathic in Miniature Schnauzers
5. Hypercalcemia (>15 mg/dL) – malignancy, hyperparathyroidism, vitamin D intoxication
6. Corticosteroid therapy and hyperadrenocorticism
7. Infection
8. Abdominal surgery or trauma
9. Duodenal reflux into the pancreatic duct
10. Biliary tract disease
11. Pancreatic duct obstruction
12. Hyperstimulation – scorpion venom, cholinesterase inhibitors, cholinergic agonists, caerulein
13. Pancreatic ischemia – thrombosis, hypovolemia, localized stasis of pancreatic microvasculature
14. Pancreatic neoplasia.

Diagnosis

History—The patient may have a history of dietary indiscretion, getting into the trash the week before admission, a diet consisting of table food or treats from the table, or a report of the dog having been present at a large gathering with food during the week. The owner may have observed vomiting, diarrhea, anorexia, restlessness, panting, trembling, weakness and abdominal pain. Pancreatitis occurs most commonly in the middle-aged to older neutered male dog, with Miniature Schnauzers, Yorkshire Terriers and Terriers as a group being more commonly affected.

In cats with pancreatitis, the signs are usually subtle and include anorexia and weight loss, with or without vomiting. Cholangitis / cholangiohepatitis often occurs concurrently with feline pancreatitis.
Physical exam—The patient may have a fever and a depressed mental attitude. There may be signs of dehydration. The patient may assume an

unnatural, 'praying', posture or a hunched-up abdomen. There may be
pain detected upon palpation of the cranioventral abdomen, which may
vary from mild to intense. Diarrhea may be present and may be
hemorrhagic. A mass may be palpable in the right cranial abdomen.
Jaundice, arrhythmias or external signs of hemorrhage, including
petechiae or ecchymoses, may be evident.

Laboratory evaluation—

1. CBC
   A. The CBC may reveal a neutrophilic leukocytosis, with or without a
      left shift.
   B. Neutropenia with a degenerative left shift may be seen in patients
      with severe pancreatic necrosis, sepsis or endotoxemia.
   C. An elevated PCV, due to dehydration, is common. Anemia may
      occur, especially in cats.
   D. Patients with DIC may have thrombocytopenia, macroplatelets and
      RBC fragments.
   E. The plasma may be icteric or lipemic.
2. Complete serum chemical evaluation, including electrolytes.
   Abnormalities may include:
   A. Elevated ALP – rule out hepatic disease
   B. Elevated ALT – rule out hepatic disease
   C. Elevated bilirubin – rule out hepatic or hemolytic disease
   D. Elevated amylase – may also occur in patients with
      gastrointestinal, hepatic and neoplastic disease, or from delayed
      renal clearance
   E. Elevated lipase – may also occur in patients with gastrointestinal,
      hepatic and neoplastic disease, or from delayed renal clearance
   F. Elevated BUN – may be pre-renal or renal
   G. Elevated creatinine – may be pre-renal or renal
   H. Hyperglycemia – may have concurrent diabetes mellitus or
      diabetic ketoacidosis
   I. Hypokalemia
   J. Hypocalcemia
   K. Fasting hyperlipidemia
   L. Hypoalbuminemia.
3. To distinguish between renal disease and pancreatitis, perform a
   urinalysis. A USG >1.025 indicates adequate renal tubular function
   and helps to rule out advanced renal disease. Ketones and glucose in
   the urine may indicate concurrent diabetic ketoacidosis.
4. Blood–gas analysis – metabolic acidosis is the most common
   acid–base disturbance, although acid–base status is unpredictable
   and should be evaluated in each individual patient.
5. Coagulation profile – a prolonged ACT, prolonged PTT, prolonged PT,
   increased FSPs, decreased fibrinogen, elevated D-dimer level, and
   thrombocytopenia indicate DIC.
6. Serum canine pancreatic lipase immunoassay (Spec cPL, Idexx
   Laboratories) concentration can now be measured by in-house ELISA.
   The cut-off value suggested for pancreatitis is above 400 µg/L,
   with values above 200 µg/L being equivocable. It is currently

Gastrointestinal emergencies

recommended to use the Spec cPL result in conjunction with abdominal ultrasound and blood test results to make an assumed diagnosis of canine pancreatitis. A feline Spec fPL test has just been introduced for in-house use which has 80% specificity and 79% sensitivity per Idexx.

7. Serum trypsin-like immunoreactivity (TLI) assay is specific for pancreatic disease. Elevations in trypsin and trypsinogen (>35 mg/L) are associated with acute pancreatitis. Measurement of TLI in dogs must be done very early in the course of the disease process, because the half life is short and it tends to rise early in the course of the disease and then rapidly decline.

Serum fTLI (feline trypsin-like immunoreactivity) in cats with pancreatitis was determined to be clinically useful and suitable for the diagnosis of acute and chronic pancreatitis in cats, with a sensitivity of 86, 62, 48 or 33% by means of cut-off values of 49, 82, 88 or 100 mg/L, respectively. It is recommended to utilize measurement of serum fTLI in concert with other diagnostic tests until better tests can be developed.

A new enzyme-linked immunosorbent assay (ELISA) for serum fTLI in serum has been developed and validated. The reported reference range for serum fTLI ELISA is 12–82 mg/L, which is slightly higher than the control range of the fTLI radioimmune assay.

8. Analysis of peritoneal fluid may indicate an intra-abdominal infection or inflammation.

Diagnostic imaging

Thoracic radiographs—These may reveal pleural effusion or pulmonary edema.

Abdominal radiographs—May reveal increased density, loss of abdominal detail, and contrast in the right cranial quadrant of the abdomen. A ground-glass appearance indicates the presence of peritonitis. The descending segment of the duodenum may be displaced to the right and the pyloric antrum may be displaced to the left on ventrodorsal views. The duodenum may be displaced ventrally on lateral views. Ileus in the duodenum or transverse colon and gastric distension may be observed. Barium passage from the stomach and through the duodenum may be delayed.

Abdominal ultrasonography—This may reveal irregular pancreatic enlargement and a decreased or mottled pancreatic echogenicity. Pancreatic cavitary lesions, or a mass effect such as pseudocysts and abscesses, may be observed. Fluid accumulation around the pancreas and generalized abdominal effusion may be observed. A dilated major duodenal papilla may be observed. In patients with concurrent hepatic disease, obstruction of the common bile duct may be seen. The highest reported sensitivity of abdominal ultrasonography for canine pancreatitis is 68%.

Abdominal computed tomography— Contrast-enhanced computed tomographic examination of the abdomen may reveal pancreatic necrosis or other evidence of pancreatitis.

Complications and sequelae

1. Acute complications
   A. Hypovolemic and endotoxic shock – may be indicated by hypothermia, collapse and circulatory shock
   B. Peritonitis and necrosis of intra-abdominal fat
   C. Sepsis
   D. DIC – associated with thrombosis, bleeding and infarction
   E. Jaundice – indicating biliary obstruction, intrahepatic cholestasis, and / or hepatocellular necrosis
   F. Acute oliguric renal failure
   G. Respiratory distress – possibly due to pleural effusion or noncardiogenic pulmonary edema
   H. Cardiac arrhythmias – due to myocardial ischemia or necrosis from the release of myocardial depressant factor
   I. Hyperglycemia
   J. Hypocalcemia – signs of tetany are rare
   K. Intestinal hypomotility
   L. Hypernatremia
2. Chronic complications and sequelae
   A. Pancreatic abscesses and pseudocysts
   B. Chronic recurring pancreatitis
   C. Diabetes mellitus and / or exocrine pancreatic insufficiency from end-stage pancreatic fibrosis and atrophy
   D. Hepatic disease secondary to common bile duct obstruction following chronic fibrosing pancreatitis

Differential diagnosis

Early in the onset of mild pancreatitis, one of the main differentials is thoraco-lumbar intervertebral disc disease. Additional differentials include gastrointestinal disease (enteritis, gastrointestinal obstruction, inflammatory bowel disease), hypoadrenocorticism, hepatic disease, cholangitis / cholangiohepatitis, renal disease, intra-abdominal neoplasia, pyometra, peritonitis and sepsis.

Prognosis

The prognosis is guarded to poor. The disease often has a prolonged and unpredictable clinical course. Patients with concurrent disease, such as diabetic ketoacidosis, acute renal failure, sepsis, hepatic or cholestatic disease, or bowel infarction, have a poor prognosis. Advise the owner about the possibility of the development of complications such as secondary diabetes mellitus, peritonitis, severe circulatory shock, DIC and sudden death. Mortality rates range from 27% to 42%.

Treatment

1. Inform the client of the diagnosis, prognosis and cost of the treatment. Advise the owner that the clinical course is often prolonged and unpredictable.

2. Hospitalize the patient for treatment and monitoring.
3. Place an intravenous catheter.
4. Administer balanced electrolyte crystalloid fluids, such as Normosol®-R or LRS, IV.
   A. If the patient is in shock, administer the fluids at the following rates:
      I. Dogs: 90 mL/kg for the first hour, administered in ¼-shock boluses, with patient re-evaluation performed every 15 minutes.
      II. Cats: 60 mL/kg for the first hour, administered in ¼-shock boluses, with patient re-evaluation performed every 15 minutes.
      III. After the first 1–2 hours, re-evaluate the patient's cardiovascular status.
      Generally decrease the rate to 20–40 mL/kg/h in dogs and 20–30 mL/kg/h in cats until the patient is stabilized.
   B. For rehydration and maintenance, administer intravenous crystalloid fluids at the rate of 60 mL/kg/24h for dogs and 40 mL/kg/24h for cats, plus the deficit plus losses.
   C. If the patient is in shock, administer Hetastarch or Dextran 70, 20 mL/kg IV. An additional 20 mL/kg of Hetastarch may be administered over the next 6–8 hours if needed for continued shock.
   D. If the patient is in severe circulatory shock and the serum sodium level is normal to low, administer 7.5% NaCl, 4–5 mL/kg IV for dogs, and 2 mL/kg IV for cats, over 2–5 minutes.
5. Currently, clear evidence is lacking regarding the benefit of replacing antiproteases including α_2-macroglobulins with fresh frozen plasma (FFP). FFP, 10–20 mL/kg IV, should be administered to patients with documented coagulopathy.
6. Consider the administration of red blood cells (11 mL/kg, 5 mL/lb) or whole blood (22 mL/kg, 10 mL/lb) if the patient is in severe shock or in hemorrhagic shock. For blood components, perform a cross match and administer blood components through a filter.
7. Supplement potassium as indicated by the serum potassium level.
8. Although the routine administration of antibiotics is not recommended in dogs, for dogs with documented pancreatic infection and in protracted cases of acute pancreatitis that fail to respond to supportive measures, antibiotic use is justified. The recommended antibiotics include clindamycin (5–11 mg/kg IV q12h), metronidazole (10 mg/kg IV CRI over 1h, q8h), chloramphenicol (40–50 mg/kg IV, SC, IM or PO q8h), and ciprofloxacin (5–15 mg/kg PO q12h, 10–20 mg/kg PO q24h), all of which achieve therapeutic tissue levels in canine models of acute pancreatitis.
9. Administer analgesics as indicated by the individual patient's needs.
   A. Hydromorphone
      I. Dogs: 0.05–0.2 mg/kg IV, IM, or SC q2–6h; 0.0125–0.05 mg/kg/h IV CRI
      II. Cats: 0.05–0.2 mg/kg IV, IM, or SC q2–6h
   B. Fentanyl
      I. Dogs: 2–10 µg/kg IV to effect, followed by 1–10 µg/kg/h IV CRI
      II. Cats: 1–5 µg/kg/h to effect, followed by 1–5 µg/kg/h IV CRI

C. Morphine
   I. Dogs: 0.5–1 mg/kg IM, SC; 0.05–0.1 mg/kg IV
   II. Cats: 0.005–0.2 mg/kg IM, SC
D. Buprenorphine
   I. Dogs: 0.005–0.02 mg/kg IV, IM q4–8h; 2–4 µg/kg/h IV CRI;
      0.12 mg/kg OTM
   II. Cats: 0.005–0.01 mg/kg IV, IM q4–8h; 1–3 µg/kg/h IV CRI;
       0.02 mg/kg OTM
10. If the patient exhibits excessive, repeated vomiting, or nausea,
    administer an antiemetic.
    A. Ondansetron (Zofran®), 0.1–1 mg/kg IV or PO q24h
    B. Dolasetron (Anzemet®), 0.6–1 mg/kg IV, SC or PO q24h
    C. Maropitant (Cerenia®), 1 mg/kg SC, IV or 2 mg/kg PO q24h for up
       to 5 days
    D. Metoclopramide (Reglan®), 0.2 – 0.5 mg/kg SC, IM, or PO q6h,
       1–2 mg/kg/day as a CRI IV, or 0.01–0.02 mg/kg/h CRI IV
    E. Chlorpromazine (Thorazine®, Largactil®), 0.05–0.1 mg/kg IV, or
       0.2–0.5 mg/kg IM, or SC q6–8h
    F. Prochlorperazine (Compazine®), 0.1–0.5 mg/kg IM or SC q6–8h
11. If hematemesis or signs of nausea (drooling, exaggerated swallowing
    motions) occur, administer a gastroprotectant agent.
    A. Ranitidine (Zantac®), 0.5–2 mg/kg IV, PO q8h (dogs), 2.5 mg/kg IV
       q12h (cats) or 3.5 mg/kg PO q12h (cats)
    B. Famotidine (Pepcid®), 0.5–1 mg/kg IV or PO q12–24h
    C. Omeprazole (Prilosec®)
       I. Dogs: 0.5–1.5 mg/kg PO q24h
       II. Cats: 0.5–1 mg/kg PO q24h
    D. Pantoprazole (Protonix®), 0.7–1 mg/kg IV q24h
12. Administer enteral nutrition as soon as possible. In patients with
    moderate to severe acute pancreatitis, enteral nutrition delivered via a
    nasojejunal tube may be successful. If vomiting is frequent, severe, or
    hematemesis occurs, restrict oral intake for 1–2 days. If longer dietary
    restriction is required, provide nutritional support with partial
    parenteral nutrition, total parenteral nutrition (TPN) or via a surgically
    placed jejunostomy tube. Because of the frequent complications that
    may occur, TPN should be initiated only in patients who do not tolerate
    enteral nutrition.
13. When it is advisable to offer food, begin by offering the patient small
    amounts of water. If water is well tolerated, gradually reintroduce the
    patient to food. The initial diet should be Hill's Prescription i/d low
    fat GI restore®, rice, pasta, potato or other low-fat and low-protein diet.
    Then maintain the patient on a low-fat diet such as Hill's Prescription
    i/d low fat GI restore® or w/d® for several weeks.
14. Repeat analysis of acid–base status, blood glucose level and electrolytes
    every 24–48 hours. Adjust fluid therapy as needed based on the
    acid–base status and electrolyte levels.
15. If the patient has concurrent diabetic ketoacidosis, the pancreatitis must
    be brought under control before regulation of the diabetic condition
    may be initiated. These patients will require prolonged hospital stays.

Table 9.2 *Insulin therapy adjustments: use an insulin dose of 2 U/kg for dogs and 1.1 U/kg for cats*

If glucose is: (mg/dL)	Fluids	Insulin in 250 mL (mL/h)
>250	0.9% NaCl	10
200–250	0.45% NaCl + 2.5% dextrose	7
150–200	0.45% NaCl + 2.5% dextrose	5
100–150	0.45% NaCl + 5% dextrose	5
<100	0.45% NaCl + 5% dextrose	Stop insulin infusion

From Macintire DK: Emergency therapy of diabetic crises: insulin overdose, diabetic ketoacidosis and hyperosmolar coma. The Veterinary Clinics of North America, Small Animal Practice: Diabetes Mellitus, Vol. 25. No. 3, 1995 ©Elsevier.

A. Control hyperglycemia (blood glucose >250 mg/dL) with short-acting regular crystalline insulin. Either the IM or SC method or an insulin CRI IV infusion may be utilized. (See Table 9.2.)

B. After rehydration, recheck the blood glucose level.

C. There are three methods for insulin administration: the IM hourly method, the CRI method and the subcutaneous insulin method. With all methods, it is important to lower blood glucose levels slowly, at a rate of 50–75 mg/dL/h, over 24–48 hours, to decrease the development of cerebral edema.

D. After the pancreatitis has resolved, **when the patient can and will eat, without vomiting, and the urine ketones are negative,** the patient may be switched from a short-acting regular crystalline insulin to a longer-lasting insulin.

16. Monitor for oliguric renal failure. The minimum volume of urine output should be 1–2 mL/kg/h. If oliguria occurs, administer furosemide.

17. Consider the administration of unfractionated heparin, 250 units/kg SC q8h, to prevent microthrombi formation and the initiation of DIC.

18. Monitor for cardiac arrhythmias. Provide treatment if necessary.

19. If the patient shows signs of peritonitis, perform abdominocentesis, diagnostic peritoneal lavage or ultrasound-guided abdominocentesis and obtain peritoneal fluid samples for cytologic evaluation and culture.

20. Surgery is necessary for the treatment of pancreatic abscesses, biliary obstruction or for the management of septic peritonitis.

REFERENCES/FURTHER READING

SALIVARY MUCOCOELES AND RANULAS

Birchard, S.J., Sherding, R.G., 1994. Saunders Manual of Small Animal Practice. WB Saunders, Philadelphia, pp. 627–629.

Morgan, R.V., 1992. Handbook of Small Animal Practice, second ed. Churchill Livingstone, New York, pp. 353–356.

Slatter, D.H. (Ed.), 1993. Textbook of Small Animal Surgery, second ed. WB Saunders, Philadelphia, pp. 516–517.

Willard, M.D., 2009. Sialocele, digestive system disorders. In: Nelson, R.W., Couto, C.G. (Eds.), Small Animal Internal Medicine, fourth ed. Mosby Elsevier, St Louis, p. 414.

ESOPHAGEAL FOREIGN BODIES

Bissett, S.A., Davis, J., Subler, K., et al., 2009. Risk factors and outcome of bougienage for treatment of benign esophageal strictures in dogs and cats: 28 cases (1995–2004). Journal of the American Veterinary Medical Association 235, 844–850.

Glazer, A., Walters, P., 2008. Esophagitis and esophageal strictures. Compendium for the Continuing Education of the Practicing. Veterinarian 30 (5), 281–292.

Han, E., 2003. Diagnosis and management of reflux esophagitis. Clinical Techniques in Small Animal Practice 18 (4), 231–238.

Leib, M.S., Sartor, L.L., 2008. Esophageal foreign body obstruction caused by a dental chew treat in 31 dogs (2000–2006). Journal of the American Veterinary Medical Association 232, 1021–1025.

Rousseau, A., Prittie, J., Broussard, J.D., et al., 2007. Incidence and characterization of esophagitis following esophageal foreign body removal in dogs: 60 cases (1999–2003). Journal of Veterinary Emergency and Critical Care 17 (2), 159–163.

Sale, C.S.H., Williams, J.W., 2006. Results of transthoracic esophagotomy retrieval of esophageal foreign body obstructions in dogs: 14 cases (2000–2004). Journal of the American Animal Hospital Association 42, 450–456.

Willard, M.D., 2009. Esophageal foreign objects, digestive system disorders. In: Nelson, R.W., Couto, C.G. (Eds.), Small Animal Internal Medicine, fourth ed. Mosby Elsevier, St Louis, pp. 423–424.

ACUTE ABDOMINAL PAIN

Amsellem, P.M., Seim, H.B., MacPhail, C.M., et al., 2006. Long-term survival and risk factors associated with biliary surgery in dogs: 34 cases (1994–2004). Journal of the American Veterinary Medical Association 229, 1451–1457.

Beal, M.W., 2005. Approach to the acute abdomen. Veterinary Clinics in Small Animals 35, 375–396.

Drobatz, K.J., 2009. Acute abdominal pain. In: Silverstein, D.C., Hopper, K. (Eds.), Small Animal Critical Care Medicine. Elsevier, St Louis, pp. 534–537.

Gorman, S.C., Freeman, L.M., Mitchell, S.L., et al., 2006. Extensive small bowel resection in dogs and cats: 20 cases (1998–2004). Journal of the American Veterinary Medical Association 228, 403–407.

Mann, F.A., 2009. Acute abdomen: evaluation and emergency treatment. In: Bonagura, J.D., Twedt, D.C. (Eds.), Kirk's Current Veterinary Therapy XIV. Saunders Elsevier, St Louis, pp. 67–72.

Schwartz, S.G.H., Mitchell, S.L., Keating, J.H., et al., 2006. Liver lobe torsion in dogs: 13 cases (1995–2004). Journal of the American Veterinary Medical Association 228, 242–247.

Worley, D.R., Hottinger, H.A., Lawrence, H.J., 2004. Surgical management of gallbladder. Mucoceles in dogs: 22 cases (1999–2003). Journal of the American Veterinary Medical Association 225, 1418–1422.

PERITONITIS

Baker, S.G., Mayhew, P.D., Mehler, S.J., 2011. Choledochotomy and primary repair of extrahepatic biliary duct rupture in seven dogs and two cats. Journal of Small Animal Practice 52, 32–37.

Bentley, A.M., Otto, C.M., Shofer, F.S., 2007. Comparison of dogs with septic peritonitis: 1988–1993 versus 1999–2003. Journal of Veterinary Emergency and Critical Care 17 (4), 391–398.

Burkitt, J.M., Haskins, S.C., Nelson, R.W., et al., 2007. Relative adrenal insufficiency in dogs with sepsis. Journal of Veterinary Internal Medicine 21, 226–231.

Costello, M.F., Drobatz, K.J., Aronson, L.R., et al., 2004. Underlying cause, pathophysiologic abnormalities, and response to treatment in cats with septic peritonitis: 51 cases (1990–2001). Journal of the American Veterinary Medical Association 225, 897–902.

Grimes, J.A., Schmiedt, C.W., Cornell, K.K., et al., 2011. Identification of risk factors for septic peritonitis and failure to survive following gastrointestinal surgery in dogs. Journal of the American Veterinary Medical Association 238, 486–494.

Lawson, A.K., Seshadri, R., 2007. Two cases of planned relaparotomy for severe peritonitis secondary to gastrointestinal pathology. Journal of the American Animal Hospital Association 43, 117–121.

Levin, G.M., Bonczynski, J.J., Ludwig, L.L., 2004. Lactate as a diagnostic test for septic peritoneal effusions in dogs and cats. Journal of the American Animal Hospital Association 40, 364–371.

Ruthrauff, C.M., Smith, J., Glerum, L., 2009. Primary bacterial septic peritonitis in cats: 13 cases. Journal of the American Animal Hospital Association 45, 268–276.

Saxon, W.D., "The Acute Abdomen". In: Kirby, R.D., Crowe, D.T., Jr (guest eds.), 1994. The Veterinary Clinics of North America, Small Animal Practice: Emergency Medicine 24 (6), 1207–1224.

Volk, S.W., 2009. Peritonitis. In: Silverstein, D.C., Hopper, K. (Eds.), Small Animal Critical Care Medicine. Elsevier, St Louis, pp. 579–583.

GASTRIC DILATATION AND VOLVULUS

Beck, J.J., Staatz, A.J., Pelsue, D.H., et al., 2006. Risk factors associated with short-term outcome and development of perioperative complications in dogs undergoing surgery because of gastric dilatation-volvulus: 166 cases (1992–2003). Journal of the American Veterinary Medical Association 229, 1934–1939.

Brourman, J.D., Schertel, E.R., Allen, D.A., et al., 1996. Factors associated with perioperative mortality in dogs with surgically managed gastric dilatation-volvulus: 137 cases (1988–1993). Journal of the American Veterinary Medical Association 208 (11), 1855–1858.

Buber, T., Saragusty, J., Ranen, E., et al., 2007. Evaluation of lidocaine treatment and risk factors for death associated with gastric dilatation and volvulus in dogs: 112 cases (1997–2005). Journal of the American Veterinary Medical Association 230, 1334–1339.

de Papp, E., Drobatz, K.J., Hughes, D., 1999. Plasma lactate concentration as a predictor of gastric necrosis and survival among dogs with gastric dilatation-volvulus: 102 cases (1995–1998). Journal of the American Veterinary Medical Association 215 (1), 49–52.

Green, T.I., Tonozzi, C.C., Kirby, R., et al., 2011. Evaluation of initial plasma lactate values as a predictor of gastric necrosis and initial and subsequent plasma lactate values as a predictor of survival in dogs with gastric dilatation-volvulus: 84 dogs (2003–2007). Journal of

Veterinary Emergency and Critical Care 21 (1), 36–44.

Hammel, S.P., Novo, R.E., 2006. Recurrence of gastric dilatation-volvulus after incisional gastropexy in a Rottweiler. Journal of the American Animal Hospital Association 42, 147–150.

Leib, M.S., Konda, L.J., Wingfield, W.E., et al., 1985. Circumcostal gastropexy for prevention of recurrence of GDV in the dog: an evaluation of 30 cases. Journal of the American Veterinary Medical Association 187 (3), 245–248.

Mackenzie, G., Barnhart, M., Kennedy, S.A., 2010. Retrospective study of factors influencing survival following surgery for gastric dilatation-volvulus syndrome in 306 dogs. Journal of the American Animal Hospital Association 46, 97–102.

Mathews, K.A., 2009. Gastric dilation-volvulus. In: Bonagura, J.D., Twedt, D.C. (Eds.), Kirk's Current Veterinary Therapy XIV. Saunders Elsevier, St Louis, pp. 77–82.

Parton, A.T., Volk, S.W., Weisse, C., 2006. Gastric ulceration subsequent to partial invagination of the stomach in a dog with gastric dilatation-volvulus. Journal of the American Veterinary Medical Association 228, 1895–1900.

Schertel, E.R., Allan, D.A., Muir, W.W., et al., 1997. Evaluation of a hypertonic saline-dextran solution for treatment of dogs with shock induced by gastric dilatation-volvulus. Journal of the American Veterinary Medical Association 210 (2), 226–230.

Streeter, E.M., Rozanski, E.A., Berg, J., et al., 2004. Esophageal perforation in a dog following an acute episode of gastric dilatation with 360 degree volvulus. Journal of Veterinary Emergency and Critical Care 14 (2), 125–127.

Volk, S.W., 2009. Gastric dilatation-volvulus and bloat. In: Silverstein, D.C., Hopper, K. (Eds.), Small Animal Critical Care Medicine. Elsevier, St Louis, pp. 584–588.

Whitney, W.O., Scavelli, T.D., Matthiesen, D.T., et al., 1989. Belt-loop gastropexy: technique and surgical results in 20 dogs. Journal of the American Animal Hospital Association 25 (1), 75–83.

Zacher, L.A., Berg, J., Shaw, S.P., et al., 2010. Association between outcome and changes in plasma lactate concentration during presurgical treatment in dogs with gastric dilatation-volvulus: 64 cases (2002–2008). Journal of the American Veterinary Medical Association 236, 892–897.

ACUTE CANINE (VIRAL) GASTROENTERITIS

Humm, K.R., Hughes, D., 2009. Canine parvovirus infection. In: Silverstein, D.C., Hopper, K. (Eds.), Small Animal Critical Care Medicine. Elsevier, St Louis, pp. 482–485.

Lobetti, R.G., Joubert, K.E., Picard, J., et al., 2002. Bacterial colonization of intravenous catheters in young dogs suspected to have parvoviral enteritis. Journal of the American Veterinary Medical Association 220, 1321–1324.

Macintire, D.K., 2008. Pediatric fluid therapy. The Veterinary Clinics of North America, Small Animal Practice 38, 621–627.

Macintire, D.K., Smith-Carr, S., 1997. Canine parvovirus. Part II. Clinical signs, diagnosis and treatment. Compendium for the Continuing Education of the Practicing Veterinarian 19 (3), 291–301.

Mantione, N.L., Otto, C.M., 2005. Characterization of the use of antiemetic agents in dogs with parvoviral enteritis treated at a veterinary teaching hospital: 77 cases (1997–2000). Journal of the American Veterinary Medical Association 227, 1787–1793.

McMichael, M.A., Lees, G.E., Hennessey, J., et al., 2005. Serial plasma lactate concentrations in 68 puppies aged 4 to 80 days. Journal of Veterinary Emergency and Critical Care 15 (1), 17–21.

Otto, C.M., Drobatz, K.J., Soter, C., 1997. Endotoxemia and tumor necrosis factor activity in dogs with naturally occurring parvoviral enteritis. Journal of Veterinary Internal Medicine 11 (2), 65–70.

Prittie, J., 2004. Canine parvoviral enteritis: a review of diagnosis, management, and prevention. Journal of Veterinary Emergency and Critical Care 14 (3), 167–176.

Savigny, M.R., Macintire, D.K., 2010. Use of oseltamivir in the treatment of canine parvoviral enteritis. Journal of Veterinary Emergency and Critical Care 20 (1), 132–142.

Smith-Carr, S., Macintire, D.K., Swango, L.J., 1997. Canine parvovirus. Part I. Pathogenesis and vaccination. Compendium for the Continuing Education of the Practicing Veterinarian 19 (2), 125–133.

Trotman, T.K., 2009. Gastroenteritis. In: Silverstein, D.C., Hopper, K. (Eds.), Small Animal Critical Care Medicine. Elsevier, St Louis, pp. 558–561.

Willard, M.D., 2009. Antiemetics. In: Silverstein, D.C., Hopper, K. (Eds.), Small Animal Critical Care Medicine. Elsevier, St Louis, pp 778–780.

Willard, M.D., 2009. Canine parvoviral enteritis, digestive system disorders. In: Nelson, R.W., Couto, C.G. (Eds.), Small Animal Internal Medicine, fourth ed. Mosby Elsevier, St Louis, pp. 443–445.

GASTROINTESTINAL OBSTRUCTION AND INTUSSUSCEPTION

Adams, W.M., Sisterman, L.A., Klauer, J.M., et al., 2010. Association of intestinal disorders in cats with findings of abdominal radiography. Journal of the American Veterinary Medical Association 236, 880–886.

Burkitt, J.M., Drobatz, K.J., Saunders, H.M., et al., 2009. Signalment, history, and outcome of cats with gastrointestinal tract intussusception: 20 cases (1986–2000). Journal of the American Veterinary Medical Association 234, 771–776.

Oliveira-Barros, L.M., Costa-Casagrande, T.A., Cogliati, B., et al., 2010. Histologic and immunohistochemical evaluation of intestinal innervation in dogs with and without intussusception. American Journal of Veterinary Research 71, 636–642.

Pastore, G.E., Lamb, C.R., Lipscomb, V., 2007. Comparison of the results of abdominal ultrasonography and exploratory laparotomy in the dog and Cat. Journal of the American Animal Hospital Association 43, 264–269.

Penninck, D., Mitchell, S.L., 2003. Ultrasonographic detection of ingested and perforating wooden foreign bodies in four dogs. Journal of the American Veterinary Medical Association 223 (2), 206–209.

Ralphs, S.C., Jessen, C.R., Lipowitz, A.J., 2003. Risk factors for leakage following intestinal anastomosis in dogs and cats: 115 cases (1991–2000). Journal of the American Veterinary Medical Association 223, 73–77.

Tams, T.R., 1996. Handbook of Small Animal Gastroenterology. WB Saunders, Philadelphia, pp. 232–234, 265.

Willard, M.D., 2009. Intestinal obstruction, digestive system disorders. In: Nelson, R.W., Couto, C.G. (Eds.), Small Animal Internal Medicine, fourth ed. Mosby Elsevier, St Louis, pp. 462–466.

FELINE DIARRHEA

Adams, W.M., Sisterman, L.A., Klauer, J.M., et al., 2010. Association of intestinal disorders in cats with findings of abdominal radiography. Journal of the American Veterinary Medical Association 236, 880–886.

German, A.J., 2009. Inflammatory bowel disease. In: Bonagura, J.D., Twedt, D.C. (Eds.), Kirk's Current Veterinary Therapy XIV. Saunders Elsevier, St Louis, pp. 501–506.

Reed, N., Gunn-Moore, D., Simpson, K., 2007. Cobalamin, folate and inorganic phosphate abnormalities in ill cats. Journal of Feline Medicine and Surgery 9, 278–288.

Tams, T.R., 1996. Handbook of Small Animal Gastroenterology. WB Saunders, Philadelphia, pp. 286–290.

Washabau, R.J., Day, M.J., Willard, M.D., et al., 2010. The WSAVA International Gastrointestinal Standardization Group. Endoscopic, Biopsy, and Histopathologic Guidelines for the Evaluation of Gastrointestinal Inflammation in Companion Animals, ACVIM Consensus Statement. Journal of Veterinary Internal Medicine 24, 10–26.

Willard, M.D., Moore, G.E., Denton, B.D., et al., 2010. Effect of tissue processing on assessment of endoscopic intestinal biopsies in dogs and cats. Journal of Veterinary Internal Medicine 24, 84–89.

Willard, M.D., 2009. Small intestinal inflammatory bowel disease, digestive system disorders. In: Nelson, R.W., Couto, C.G. (Eds.), Small Animal Internal Medicine, fourth ed. Mosby Elsevier, St Louis, pp. 458–459.

Wolf, A.M., 1989. Diarrhea in the cat. In: Willard, M.D. (Ed.), Seminars in Veterinary Medicine and Surgery Small Animal, vol 4, no 3. WB Saunders, Philadelphia, pp. 212–218.

HEMORRHAGIC GASTROENTERITIS

Boysen, S.R., 2009. Gastrointestinal hemorrhage. In: Silverstein, D.C., Hopper, K. (Eds.), Small Animal Critical Care Medicine. Elsevier, St Louis, pp. 566–570.

Tams, T.R., 1996. Handbook of Small Animal Gastroenterology. WB Saunders, Philadelphia, pp. 263–264.

Willard, M.D., 2009. Gastrointestinal protectants. In: Silverstein, D.C., Hopper, K. (Eds.), Small Animal Critical Care Medicine. Elsevier, St Louis, pp. 775–777.

Willard, M.D., 2009. Hemorrhagic gastroenteritis, digestive system disorders. In: Nelson, R.W., Couto, C.G. (Eds.), Small Animal Internal Medicine, fourth ed. Mosby Elsevier, St Louis, p. 428.

COLITIS

Jergens, A.E., 2004. Clinical assessment of disease activity for canine inflammatory bowel disease. Journal of the American Animal Hospital Association 40, 437–445.

Leib, M.S., 2000. Treatment of chronic idiopathic large-bowel diarrhea in dogs with a highly digestible diet and soluble fiber: a retrospective review of 37 cases. Journal of Veterinary Internal Medicine 14, 27–32.

Parnell, N.K., 2009. Chronic colitis. In: Bonagura, J.D., Twedt, D.C. (Eds.), Kirk's Current Veterinary Therapy XIV. Saunders Elsevier, St Louis, pp. 515–520.

Willard, M.D., 2009. Acute colitis, digestive system disorders. In: Nelson, R.W., Couto, C.G. (Eds.), Small Animal Internal Medicine, fourth ed. Mosby Elsevier, St Louis, p. 468.

RECTAL PROLAPSE

Hoskins, J.D., 1995. Veterinary Pediatrics, second ed. WB Saunders, Philadelphia, pp. 181–182.

Kirk, R.W., Bistner, S.I., Ford, R.B. (Eds.), 1990. Handbook of Veterinary Procedures and Emergency Treatment, fifth ed. WB Saunders, Philadelphia, p. 108.

Tams, T.R., 1996. Handbook of Small Animal Gastroenterology. WB Saunders, Philadelphia, pp. 362–363.

Webb, C.B., 2009. Anal-rectal disease. In: Bonagura, J.D., Twedt, D.C. (Eds.), Kirk's Current Veterinary Therapy XIV. Saunders Elsevier, St Louis, pp. 527–531.

Willard, M.D., 2009. Rectal prolapse, digestive system disorders. In: Nelson,

R.W., Couto, C.G. (Eds.), Small Animal Internal Medicine, fourth ed. Mosby Elsevier, St Louis, pp. 468–469.

PERINEAL HERNIA

Gilley, R.S., Caywood, D.S., Lulich, J.P., et al., 2003. Treatment with a combined cystopexy-colopexy for dysuria and rectal prolapse after bilateral perineal herniorrhaphy in a dog. Journal of the American Veterinary Medical Association 222 (12), 1717–1722.

Head, L.L., Francis, D.A., 2002. Mineralized paraprostatic cyst as a potential contributing factor in the development of perineal hernias in a dog. Journal of the American Veterinary Medical Association 221 (4), 533–535.

Tams, T.R., 1996. Handbook of Small Animal Gastroenterology. WB Saunders, Philadelphia, pp. 363–364.

Webb, C.B., 2009. Anal-rectal disease. In: Bonagura, J.D., Twedt, D.C. (Eds.), Kirk's Current Veterinary Therapy XIV. Saunders Elsevier, St Louis, pp. 527–531.

Willard, M.D., 2009. Perineal hernia, digestive system disorders. In: Nelson, R.W., Couto, C.G. (Eds.), Small Animal Internal Medicine, fourth ed. Mosby Elsevier, St Louis, pp. 470–471.

ACUTE HEPATIC FAILURE

Aguirre, A.L., Center, S.A., Randolph, J.F., et al., 2007. Gallbladder disease in Shetland Sheepdogs: 38 cases (1995–2005). Journal of the American Veterinary Medical Association 231, 79–88.

Al-Khafaji, A., Huang, D.T., 2011. Critical care management of patients with end-stage liver disease. Critical Care Medicine 39 (5), 1157–1166.

Berent, A.C., Rondeau, M.P., 2009. Hepatic failure. In: Silverstein, D.C., Hopper, K. (Eds.), Small Animal Critical Care Medicine. Elsevier, St Louis, pp. 552–558.

Center, S.A., 2007. Interpretation of liver enzymes. The Veterinary Clinics of North America, Small Animal Practice 37, 297–333.

Fernandez, N.J., Kidney, B.A., 2007. Alkaline phosphatase: beyond the liver. Veterinary Clinical Pathology 36, 223–233.

Flatland, B., 2009. Hepatic support therapy. In: Bonagura, J.D., Twedt, D.C. (Eds.), Kirk's Current Veterinary Therapy XIV. Saunders Elsevier, St Louis, pp. 554–557.

Pike F.S., Berg, J., King, N.W., et al., 2004. Gallbladder mucocele in dogs: 30 cases (2000–2002). Journal of the American Veterinary Medical Association 224, 1615–1622.

Poldervaart, J.H., Favier, R.P., Penning, L.C., et al., 2008. Primary hepatitis in dogs: a retrospective review (2002–2006). Journal of Veterinary Internal Medicine 23 (1), 72–80.

Sepesy, L.M., Center, S.A., Randolph, J.F., et al., 2006. Vacuolar hepatopathy in dogs: 336 cases (1993–2005). Journal of the American Veterinary Medical Association 229, 246–252.

Wagner, K.A., Hartmann, F.A., Trepanier, L.A., 2007. Bacterial culture results from liver, gallbladder, or bile in 248 dogs and cats evaluated for hepatobiliary disease: 1998–2003. Journal of Veterinary Internal Medicine 21, 417–424.

Watson, P.J., Bunch, S.E., 2009. Treatment of complications of hepatic disease and failure, hepatobiliary and exocrine pancreatic disorders. In: Nelson, R.W., Couto, C.G. (Eds.), Small Animal Internal Medicine, fourth ed. Mosby Elsevier, St Louis, pp. 520–527.

Webster, C.R.L., Cooper, J.C., 2009. Diagnostic approach to hepatobiliary disease. In: Bonagura, J.D., Twedt, D.C. (Eds.), Kirk's Current Veterinary Therapy XIV. Saunders Elsevier, St Louis, pp. 543–549.

Willard, M.D., 2009. Acute hepatitis, digestive system. In: Nelson, R.W., Couto, C.G. (Eds.), Small Animal Internal Medicine, fourth ed. Mosby Elsevier, St Louis, pp. 552–553.

HEPATIC ENCEPHALOPATHY

Buob, S., Johnston, A.N., Webster, C.R.L., 2011. Portal hypertension: pathophysiology, diagnosis, and treatment. Journal of Veterinary Internal Medicine 25, 169–186.

d'Anjou, M., 2007. The sonographic search for portosystemic shunts. Clinical Techniques of Small Animal Practice 22, 104–114.

Mertens, M., Fossum, T.W., Willard, M.D., 2010. Diagnosis of congenital portosystemic shunt in Miniature Schnauzers 7 years of age or older (1997–2006). Journal of the American Animal Hospital Association 46, 235–240.

Tobias, K.M., 2009. Portosystemic shunts. In: Bonagura, J.D., Twedt, D.C. (Eds.), Kirk's Current Veterinary Therapy

XIV. Saunders Elsevier, St Louis, pp. 581–586.

Watson, P.J., Bunch, S.E., 2009. Hepatic encephalopathy, hepatobiliary and exocrine pancreatic disorders. In: Nelson, R.W., Couto, C.G. (Eds.), Small Animal Internal Medicine, fourth ed. Mosby Elsevier, St Louis, pp. 491–494.

FELINE HEPATIC LIPIDOSIS

Biourge, V., MacDonald, M.J., King, L., 1990. Feline hepatic lipidosis. Compendium for the Continuing Education of the Practicing Veterinarian 12 (2), 1244–1258.

Center, S.A., 2005. Feline hepatic lipidosis. The Veterinary Clinics of North America, Small Animal Practice 35, 225–269.

Holan, K.M., 2009. Feline hepatic lipidosis. In: Bonagura, J.D., Twedt, D.C. (Eds.), Kirk's Current Veterinary Therapy XIV. Saunders Elsevier, St Louis, pp. 570–575.

Watson, P.J., Bunch, S.E., 2009. Hepatic lipidosis, hepatobiliary and exocrine pancreatic disorders. In: Nelson, R.W., Couto, C.G. (Eds.), Small Animal Internal Medicine, fourth ed. Mosby Elsevier, St Louis, pp. 520–527.

FELINE CHOLANGIOHEPATITIS

Berent, A.C., 2009. Acute biliary diseases of the dog and cat. In: Silverstein, D.C., Hopper, K. (Eds.), Small Animal Critical Care Medicine. Elsevier, St Louis, pp. 542–546.

Eich, C.S., Ludwig, L.L., 2002. The surgical treatment of cholelithiasis in cats: a study of nine cases. Journal of the American Animal Hospital Association 38, 290–296.

Rondeau, M.P., 2009. Hepatitis and cholangiohepatitis. In: Silverstein, D.C., Hopper, K. (Eds.), Small Animal Critical Care Medicine. Elsevier, St Louis, pp. 547–551.

Twedt, D.C., 2009. Armstrong PJ, Feline inflammatory liver disease In: Bonagura, J.D., Twedt, D.C. (Eds.), Kirk's Current Veterinary Therapy XIV. Saunders Elsevier, St Louis, pp. 576–581.

Watson, P.J., Bunch, S.E., 2009. Cholangitis, hepatobiliary and exocrine pancreatic disorders. In: Nelson, R.W., Couto, C.G. (Eds.), Small Animal Internal Medicine, fourth ed. Mosby Elsevier, St Louis, pp. 527–531.

PANCREATITIS

Anderson, J.R., Cornell, K.K., Parnell, N.K., et al., 2008. Pancreatic abscess in 36 dogs: a retrospective analysis of prognostic indicators. Journal of the American Animal Hospital Association 44, 171–179.

DeCock, H.E.V., Forman, M.A., Farver, T.B., et al., 2007. Prevalence and histopathologic characteristics of pancreatitis in cats. Veterinary Pathology 44, 39–49.

Gerhardt, A., Steiner, J.M., Williams, D.A., et al., 2001. Comparison of the sensitivity of different diagnostic tests for pancreatitis in cats. Journal of Veterinary Internal Medicine 15, 329–333.

Gaynor, A.R., 2009. Acute pancreatitis. In: Silverstein, D.C., Hopper, K. (Eds.), Small Animal Critical Care Medicine. Elsevier, St Louis, pp. 537–542.

Holm, J.L., Chan, D.L., Rozanski, E.A., 2003. Acute pancreatitis in dogs. Journal of Veterinary Emergency and Critical Care 13 (4), 201–213.

Johnson, M.D., Mann, F.A., 2006. Treatment for pancreatic abscesses via omentalization with abdominal closure versus open peritoneal drainage in dogs: 15 cases (1994–2004). Journal of the American Veterinary Medical Association 228, 397–402.

Lem, K.Y., Fosgate, G.T., Norby, B., et al., 2008. Associations between dietary factors and pancreatitis in dogs. Journal of the American Veterinary Medical Association 233, 1425–1431.

Mansfield, C.S., James, F.E., Robertson, I.D., 2008. Development of a clinical severity index for dogs with acute pancreatitis. Journal of the American Veterinary Medical Association 233, 936–944.

Neilson-Carley, S.C., Robertson, J.E., Newman, S.J., et al., 2011. Specificity of a canine pancreas-specific lipase assay for diagnosing pancreatitis in dogs without clinical or histologic evidence of the disease. American Journal of Veterinary Research 72, 302–307.

Ruaux, C.G., 2003. Diagnostic approaches to acute pancreatitis. Clinical Techniques in Small Animal Practice 18 (4), 245–249.

Son, T.T., Thompson, L., Serrano, S., et al., 2010. Surgical intervention in the management of severe acute pancreatitis in cats: 8 cases (2003–2007). Journal of Veterinary Emergency and Critical Care 20 (4), 426–435.

Steiner, J.M., 2009. Canine pancreatic disease. In: Bonagura, J.D., Twedt, D.C. (Eds.), Kirk's Current Veterinary Therapy XIV. Saunders Elsevier, St Louis, pp. 534–538.

Steiner, J.M., Newman, S.J., Xenoulis, P.G., 2008. Sensitivity of serum markers for pancreatitis in dogs with macroscopic evidence of pancreatitis. Veterinary Therapeutics 9 (4), 263–273.

Thompson, L.J., Seshadri, R., Raffe, M.R., 2009. Characteristics and outcomes in surgical management of severe acute pancreatitis: 37 dogs (2001–2007). Journal of Veterinary Emergency Critical Care 19 (2), 165–173.

Watson, P.J., Bunch, S.E., 2009. Pancreatitis, the exocrine pancreas. In: Nelson, R.W., Couto, C.G. (Eds.), Small Animal Internal Medicine, fourth ed. Mosby Elsevier, St Louis, pp. 579–606.

Weatherton, L.K., Streeter, E.M., 2009. Evaluation of fresh frozen plasma administration in dogs with pancreatitis: 77 cases (1995–2005). Journal of Veterinary Emergency and Critical Care 19 (6), 617–622.

Williams, D.A., 2009. Feline exocrine pancreatic disease. In: Bonagura, J.D., Twedt, D.C. (Eds.), Kirk's Current Veterinary Therapy XIV. Saunders Elsevier, St Louis, pp. 538–543.

9

Gastrointestinal emergencies

Metabolic and endocrine emergencies

DIABETES MELLITUS

Diagnosis

History—Most dogs with diabetes mellitus are 4–14 years of age, with a majority of the patients presenting between 7 and 9 years of age. Females are twice as likely to be affected than males. Commonly affected breeds include Keeshonds, Puliks, Cairn Terriers, Miniature Pinschers, Miniature Poodles, Miniature Schnauzers, Dachshunds and Beagles. Most diabetic cats are diagnosed at greater than 6 years of age. Diabetes mellitus appears most frequently in neutered male cats.

The owner may notice polyuria, polydipsia, weight loss and polyphagia. The owner may complain about the dog urinating in the house, or having to frequently change the litter. The owner may observe sudden blindness or rear limb weakness.

Physical exam—Many diabetic patients are obese. Abdominal palpation may reveal hepatomegaly due to hepatic lipidosis. The patient may have cataracts and a poor hair coat. A plantigrade posture and hindlimb weakness may be observed. Patients with diabetic ketoacidosis (DKA) may exhibit dehydration, an acetone odor to the breath, lethargy and weakness.

Laboratory evaluation—
1. Measure the fasting blood glucose level. The patient with diabetes mellitus will have a persistent fasting hyperglycemia (>200 mg/dL). Cats can exhibit a stress hyperglycemia of 300–400 mg/dL.
2. Perform a urinalysis. Abnormal findings may include the following.
   A. Glycosuria is present.
      (Caution: Persistent glycosuria accompanied by euglycemia does not indicate diabetes mellitus. It does, however, indicate primary renal glycosuria, a tubular defect involving the reabsorption of glucose. The syndrome is most common in Basenjis and Norwegian Elkhounds.)
   B. Proteinuria, bacteriuria, hematuria and pyuria may be seen in patients with cystitis.

C. Large amounts of ketones in the urine indicate ketoacidosis.
D. Submit cystocentesis samples for urine culture and sensitivity testing.
3. CBC may reveal a mild polycythemia if the patient is dehydrated. Concurrent infection or inflammation may result in a leukocytosis.
4. Evaluate a complete serum biochemical profile, including electrolytes. Abnormal findings may include:
A. An increased ALT and ALP secondary to hepatic lipidosis
B. Increased amylase and lipase secondary to pancreatitis
C. Increased BUN and creatinine secondary to dehydration or primary renal failure as a result of glomerulosclerosis.
5. Perform a blood gas analysis.
6. The serum thyroxine (T_4) concentration should be evaluated in all geriatric diabetic cats and dogs. Due to the occurrence of the euthyroid sick syndrome, low T_4 levels are not diagnostic of hypothyroidism, whereas high levels are diagnostic of hyperthyroidism.
7. Glycosylated hemoglobin levels are not valid in dogs and cats.
8. Serum fructosamine levels may be elevated and may be beneficial in differentiating between transient stress hyperglycemia and diabetic hyperglycemia in cats.

Differential diagnosis

1. Hypoadrenocorticism
2. Pituitary diabetes insipidus
3. Hyperadrenocorticism
4. Chronic renal failure
5. Hyperthyroidism
6. Pyometra / endometritis
7. Chronic hepatic disease
8. Fanconi syndrome
9. Excessive sodium intake
10. Psychogenic water drinking.

Prognosis

The prognosis is fair. Long-term therapy is usually necessary.

Treatment

1. Inform the client of the diagnosis, prognosis and cost of the treatment.
2. Feeding two to three times daily, close to the time of insulin administration and at the expected time of peak insulin activity (8–10 hours after administration), or in the morning, afternoon and evening, is recommended
A. Avoid semi-moist foods owing to the high sugar content.
B. Diets containing an increased fiber concentration, a maintenance protein concentration and a fat content of 17% or less of dry matter are recommended.

C. Hill's Prescription Diet r/d® or w/d®, Science Diet Maintenance Light®, Iams Less Active®, Protocol Canine Five®, Purina Fit and Trim® and Waltham Canine High Fiber® diets are among those recommended.

D. Feeding several small meals within the time frame of insulin action is beneficial.

E. Dogs and cats that are 'nibblers' and eat small amounts throughout the day may be continued to be allowed free access to food, but gluttonous patients should have their feedings restricted.

F. Weight reduction should be gradual for obese patients.

G. Provide the patient with consistent rations and feeding times.

3. Provide the patient with consistent daily exercise.

4. If the patient is an intact female, ovariohysterectomy is recommended.

5. Insulin therapy for dogs

A. Administration of an intermediate-acting insulin twice a day or a long-acting insulin once a day is the recommended insulin therapy for dogs. Beef insulins are more antigenic in dogs than is human recombinant or porcine insulin.

B. Vetsulin®, a porcine lente insulin, is the only insulin approved by the US FDA for dogs. The recommended starting dose is 0.25 U/kg SC every 12 hours. The average dose is 0.75–0.78 U/kg per injection every 12 hours, with most dogs requiring between a range of 0.28–1.4 U/kg. If Vetsulin® is to be administered once a day, the average dose is 1.09 U/kg per injection every 24 hours, with most dogs requiring 0.43–2.18 U/kg.

C. The other preferred insulin for dogs is recombinant human neutral protamine Hagedorn (NPH) insulin. The starting dose is 0.25 U/kg SC every 12 hours.

D. Based upon the patient's response to therapy and blood glucose curves, the insulin dose should be adjusted by 1–5 U per injection and allowed to equilibrate over 5–7 days.

E. The goal is to obtain a blood glucose nadir of 80–150 mg/dL and to maintain the blood glucose concentration at less than 250–300 mg/dL.

6. Insulin therapy for cats

A. Glargine, a long-acting insulin, is the recommended insulin for cats. Protamine zinc insulin (PZI) is the second choice.

B. The recommended starting dose of glargine insulin is 0.5 U/kg SC every 12 hours with monitoring of urine glucose concentration, blood glucose level and the amount of water being drunk. The maximum starting dose should be less than or equal to 3 U/cat. If monitoring is not feasible, the starting dose should be 1 U/cat every 12 hours. In one study (Roomp & Rand), the median maximum glargine insulin dose for cats was 2.5 U/cat every 12 hours.

C. The cat should be re-examined and blood glucose re-checked once a week for the first 4–8 weeks. If the pre-insulin blood glucose concentration is ≥216 mg/dL, the insulin dose should be increased by 0.25–1 U/injection. If the blood glucose nadir is ≥180 mg/dL, the dose should be increased by 0.5–1 U/injection. If the pre-insulin blood glucose concentration is ≤180 mg/dL, decrease the dose by 0.5–1 U/injection. If the blood glucose nadir is <54 mg/dL, decrease the dose by 1 U/injection.

D. Some cats require a dose of 6–10 U/cat SC every 12 hours. These cats usually need the dose decreased after glycemic control is achieved. If the dose is very high, such as >25 U/cat every 12 hours, the source of treatment failure should be investigated. Causes of treatment failure include acromegaly and hyperadrenocorticism.

E. If PZI insulin is used, the initial dose is 1–3 U SC in the morning. Increase to q12h administration if problems occur with glycemic regulation.

7. Prior to administration, insulin should be slowly warmed to room temperature by gentle rolling or agitation. Do not shake the insulin bottle. Glargine is good for 6 months if it is kept refrigerated.

8. The recommended diets for diabetic dogs include Hill's prescription diet w/d®, Hill's Science Diet® adult, Purina veterinary diet DCO®, Purina Pro Plan® small breed adult or weight management, Royal Canin diabetic HF® and Royal Canin Hifactor® formula.

9. The recommended diets for diabetic cats include Hill's prescription diet m/d®, Purina veterinary diet DM® and Royal Canin diabetic DS®.

10. Monitor for the development of hypoglycemia and diabetic remission.

DIABETIC KETOACIDOSIS

Diagnosis

History—The patient may have previously been diagnosed to be diabetic. The owner may observe polyuria / polydipsia, weight loss, vomiting, diarrhea, lethargy, weakness, anorexia or a ravenous appetite.

Physical exam—The clinical appearance of patients with diabetic ketoacidosis varies from emaciated and dehydrated to obese to nonremarkable. The patient may have an acetone ('fruity') odor to the breath and may present comatose. The patient may present with dehydration, cataracts and / or hepatomegaly. Evaluate for signs of infection, hepatic lipidosis, pancreatitis and chronic renal failure.

Laboratory evaluation—

1. Urinalysis may reveal glycosuria (4+), ketonuria, pyuria and a urine specific gravity ≥1.030. Beta hydroxybutyrate is not detected by urine test strips, but may be converted to acetoacetate, which is detectable, by adding several drops of hydrogen peroxide to the urine sample. Ketones may also be detected in serum samples.

2. A urine culture and sensitivity should be performed on a sample obtained by sterile cystocentesis.

3. A complete serum chemistry profile may reveal:
   A. Hyperglycemia (>300 mg/dL)
      I. For serial monitoring, use a 25-GA needle or obtain samples from a central venous catheter
      II. For serial monitoring, the Accu-Check II® using the Chemstrip bG® reagent strips, the Glucometer III®, Accu-check III®, Tracer

II® and the One Touch® were the glucometers rated to have an accuracy above average
B. Elevated BUN and creatinine (prerenal azotemia)
C. Elevated liver enzymes and total bilirubin
D. Hyponatremia
E. Hypophosphatemia
F. Hypomagnesemia
G. Hypokalemia, normokalemia or hyperkalemia
H. Increased serum osmolality, normal = 285–310 mOsm (serum osmolality = 2[Na + K] + glucose/18 + BUN/2.8)
I. Increased anion gap, normal is 15–25 mEq/L (anion gap = [Na + K] – [Cl + TCO_2])
J. Increased total protein (TP)
K. Lipemia.
4. CBC may reveal dehydration, leukocytosis, anemia and Heinz body anemia.
5. Blood gas analysis may reveal metabolic acidosis.

Abdominal and thoracic radiographs—These may reveal concurrent disease states such as pyometra, neoplasia or cardiac disease.
Abdominal ultrasound—This may be beneficial as part of a thorough work-up in an ill patient.
ECG monitoring—This may be helpful to monitor the cardiac effects of hypokalemia and hyperkalemia.
1. Hypokalemia may cause ventricular and supraventricular arrhythmias, depression of the T-wave amplitude, prolongation of the Q–T interval, and depression of the S–T segment.
2. Hyperkalemia may cause cardiac arrest, complete heart block, bradycardia, ventricular arrhythmias, spiked T-waves, flattened P-waves, prolongation of the P–R interval, prolongation of the QRS interval and a decreased amplitude of the R-wave.

Prognosis

The prognosis is fair to guarded. The mortality rate of patients with DKA is 30–40%. If the patient has a concurrent serious illness, such as pancreatitis, sepsis or hyperadrenocorticism, the prognosis is guarded.

Treatment

1. Inform the client of the diagnosis, prognosis and cost of the treatment.
2. Hospitalize the patient and repeatedly monitor blood and urine glucose levels.
3. If the patient is severely dehydrated, the administration of insulin is usually delayed for 2–4 hours while initiating fluid therapy. Administer intravenous fluids, 0.9% NaCl, Plasma-Lyte® 148 or Normosol®-R, at the rate of 40–60 mL/kg/h until rehydration is achieved, then continue at a rate of 1.5–2 times maintenance rates to replace losses and maintain hydration.

4. If the patient is vomiting, administer antiemetics. If the patient has pancreatitis, provide supportive therapy.
   A. Ondansetron (Zofran®), 0.1–1 mg/kg IV or PO q24h
   B. Dolasetron (Anzemet®), 0.6–1 mg/kg IV, SC or PO q24h
   C. Maropitant (Cerenia®), 1 mg/kg SC or 2 mg/kg PO q24h for up to 5 days (dogs only, not labeled for use in cats)
   D. Metoclopramide (Reglan®), 0.2–0.5 mg/kg SC, IM, or PO q6h, 1–2 mg/kg/day as a CRI IV, or 0.01–0.02 mg/kg/h CRI IV
   E. Chlorpromazine (Thorazine®), 0.05–0.1 mg/kg IV, or 0.2–0.5 mg/kg IM, or SC q6–8h
   F. Prochlorperazine (Compazine®), 0.1–0.5 mg/kg IM or SC q6–8h
5. Supplement potassium as needed, based on the serum potassium level (see Table 10.1).
6. If hypokalemia persists despite therapy, check the ionized magnesium level. If the magnesium is <1.2 mg/dL, administer magnesium chloride or magnesium sulfate, 0.75–1 mEq/kg/day as an IV CRI in 5% dextrose in saline or water. Magnesium is incompatible with sodium bicarbonate and calcium.
7. Monitor serum phosphorus levels. Hemolytic anemia and neuromuscular weakness can result from low levels of serum phosphorus, which cause inadequate ATP and 2,3-DPG production, crenation, and lysis of RBCs. If the phosphorus level is ≤2 mg/dL, supplementation is necessary.
   A. If the serum phosphorus level is 1–2 mg/dL, administer 0.03 mmol/kg/h of sodium phosphate, or use potassium phosphate if the patient is also hypokalemic.
   B. If the serum phosphorus level is <1 mg/dL, administer 0.1 mmol/kg/h of sodium phosphate.
8. Administer $NaHCO_3$ if the pH is <7.0.
9. Search for and treat any infection. The urogenital tract is a common location. Administer a broad-spectrum antibiotic such as a cephalosporin.
10. After rehydration, recheck the blood glucose level.
11. If the patient is receiving supplemental oxygen therapy, the blood glucose level may be falsely low owing to the increased oxygen partial pressure.

Table 10.1   *Suggested potassium[1] maximum infusion rate*

Estimated potassium losses	(mEq/L)	(mL/kg per hour)
Maintenance (serum level = 3.6–5.0)	20	25
Mild (serum level = 3.1–3.5)	30	17
Moderate (serum level = 2.6–3.0)	40	12
Severe (serum level = 2.1–.5)	60	8
Life threatening (serum level <2.0)	80	6

[1]Potassium supplementation should not exceed 0.5 mEq/kg per hour.

12. There are three methods for regular insulin administration: the IM hourly method, the CRI method and the subcutaneous insulin method. With all methods, it is important to lower blood glucose levels slowly, at a rate of 50–75 mg/dL/h, over 24–48 hours, to decrease the development of cerebral edema.

13. IM hourly method for regular insulin administration – administer regular insulin into the muscles of the hindlegs.
   A. Administer regular insulin, 0.2 U/kg IM.
   B. Then administer hourly injections of regular insulin, 0.1 U/kg IM until the blood glucose level is ≤250 mg/dL.
   C. Recheck the blood glucose level every 1–2 hours.
   D. When the blood glucose level = 150–250 mg/dL, change the IV fluids to 5% dextrose with 4–8 mEq/L KCl added and then decrease the frequency of administration of regular insulin, 0.1–0.4 U/kg IM q4–6h, or 0.5 U/kg SC q6–8h.
   E. Maintain the blood glucose level at 100–200 mg/dL at 4 hours after the last insulin injection.
   F. Continue the patient on regular insulin until the ketonuria, acidemia, electrolyte imbalances and fluid imbalances have resolved and the patient is eating on its own.

14. CRI method for insulin administration
   A. Add regular crystalline insulin to a 250 mL bag of 0.9% NaCl.
   B. The dose of regular crystalline insulin to add is 2.2 U/kg for dogs and 1.1 U/kg for cats.
   C. Insulin binds to plastic, so 50 mL of the solution should be run through the IV line and discarded.
   D. Either 'piggy-back' the insulin infusion line onto regular IV fluids or place a separate intravenous catheter.
   E. Adjust the insulin infusion as shown in Table 10.2.
   F. Monitor the urine or serum for ketones.
   G. **When the patient can and will eat without vomiting**, when concurrent pancreatitis has resolved, if present, **and when the urine or serum ketones are negative**, the patient may be switched from a short-acting regular crystalline insulin to a longer-lasting insulin.

Table 10.2 *Insulin therapy adjustments: use an insulin dose of 2 U/kg for dogs and 1.1 U/kg for cats*

If glucose is: (mg/dL)	Fluids	Insulin in 250 mL (mL/h)
>250	0.9% NaCl	10
200–250	0.45% NaCl + 2.5% dextrose	7
150–200	0.45% NaCl + 2.5% dextrose	5
100–150	0.45% NaCl + 5% dextrose	5
<100	0.45% NaCl + 5% dextrose	Stop insulin infusion

From MacIntyre DK: Emergency therapy of diabetic crises: insulin overdose, diabetic ketoacidosis and hyperosmolar coma. The Veterinary Clinics of North America, Small Animal Practice: Diabetes Mellitus, Vol. 25. No. 3, 1995 ©Elsevier.

15. Subcutaneous insulin method may be used once a normal hydration status has been established. The blood glucose level should drop at a rate of 50–75 mg/dL/h to a level of 200–250 mg/dL.
    A. Administer regular insulin, 0.25 U/kg, SC q4–6h.
    B. Measure the serum glucose level in 4–6 hours.
    C. If the blood glucose level is >500 mg/dL, increase the insulin dose by 50–100% of the initial dose.
    D. If the blood glucose level is 400–500 mg/dL, repeat the initial dose.
    E. If the blood glucose level is 250–400 mg/dL, reduce the insulin dose to 50% of the initial dose.
    F. If the blood glucose level is ≤250 mg/dL, decrease the insulin dose to 25% of the initial dose and change the intravenous fluids to a 2.5–5% dextrose solution.
16. Glargine can be combined with regular insulin to treat diabetic ketoacidosis.
    A. Administer the recommended initial dose of glargine insulin SC every 12 hours and also administer regular insulin IM, 1 U every 2–4 hours.
    B. The goal is to maintain the blood glucose level between 145 and 250 mg/dL.
    C. Regular insulin administration should continue until dehydration is resolved and the appetite returns, which usually takes 24–48 hours.
17. When the blood glucose level is stabilized at 150–250 mg/dL and the patient is stabilized (ketonuria is resolved and the patient is eating on its own), begin Vetsulin®, NPH, glargine or PZI insulin therapy.
    A. Vetsulin®, a porcine lente insulin, is the only insulin approved by the US FDA for dogs. The recommended starting dose is 0.25 U/kg SC every 12 hours. The average dose is 0.75–0.78 U/kg per injection every 12 hours, with most dogs requiring between a range of 0.28–1.4 U/kg. If Vetsulin® is to be administered once a day, the average dose is 1.09 U/kg per injection every 24 hours, with most dogs requiring 0.43–2.18 U/kg.
    B. The other preferred insulin for dogs is recombinant human NPH insulin. The starting dose is 0.25 U/kg SC every 12 hours.
    C. Based upon the patient's response to therapy and blood glucose curves, the insulin dose should be adjusted by 1–5 U per injection and allowed to equilibrate over 5–7 days.
    D. The goal is to obtain a blood glucose nadir of 80–150 mg/dL and to maintain the blood glucose concentration at less than 250–300 mg/dL.
18. Insulin therapy for cats
    A. Glargine, a long-acting insulin, is the recommended insulin for cats. PZI is the second choice.
    B. The recommended starting dose of glargine insulin is 0.5 U/kg SC every 12 hours with monitoring of urine glucose concentration, blood glucose level, and the amount of water being drank. The maximum starting dose should be less than or equal to 3 U/cat. If the monitoring is not feasible, the starting dose should be 1 U/cat every 12 hours. In one study (Roomp & Rand), the median

maximum glargine insulin dose for cats was 2.5 U/cat every 12 hours.

C. The cat should be re-examined and blood glucose re-checked once a week for the first 4–8 weeks. If the pre-insulin blood glucose concentration is ≥216 mg/dL, the insulin dose should be increased by 0.25–1 U/injection. If the blood glucose nadir is ≥180 mg/dL, the dose should be increased by 0.5–1 U/injection. If the pre-insulin blood glucose concentration is ≤180 mg/dL, decrease the dose by 0.5–1 U/injection. If the blood glucose nadir is <54 mg/dL, decrease the dose by 1 U/injection.

D. Some cats require a dose of 6–10 U/cat SC every 12 hours. These cats usually need the dose decreased after glycemic control is achieved. If the dose is very high, such as >25 U/cat every 12 hours, the source of treatment failure should be investigated. Causes of treatment failure include acromegaly and hyperadrenocorticism.

E. If PZI insulin is used in the treatment of a diabetic cat, the initial dose is 1–3 U SC in the morning. Increase to q12h administration if problems occur with glycemic regulation.

19. Repeatedly offer the patient a high-fiber diet such as Hill's Prescription Diet w/d® and encourage the patient to eat as soon as possible, unless the patient also has pancreatitis.

20. If the patient presents in a hyperosmolar diabetic coma:

A. Place an intravenous catheter and administer Normosol®-R or LRS with potassium supplemented as necessary based on the serum potassium level.

B. Do not administer insulin for approximately the first 12 hours of therapy, unless the patient is ketoacidotic, then begin *slowly* after about 4 hours of fluid therapy.

C. Decrease blood glucose very slowly or risk the onset of cerebral edema.

HYPERGLYCEMIA HYPEROSMOLAR NONKETOTIC SYNDROME OF DIABETES MELLITUS (HHS)

This condition is rare. It occurs in both cats and dogs. The syndrome is due to hyperglycemia and osmotic diuresis, which result in prerenal azotemia. This results in severe hyperosmolality of the extracellular fluid. Associated diseases include congestive heart failure, asthma, renal failure, sepsis, pancreatitis, inflammatory bowel disease, urinary tract infection, neoplasia, hyperadrenocorticism, hyperthyroidism and glucocorticoid administration.

History—The patient may exhibit polyphagia, polydipsia, polyuria and weight loss for days or weeks. The owner may notice anorexia, lethargy, progressive weakness and a decrease in water consumption.

Physical exam—The patient may present with severe dehydration, depression, hypothermia and decreased capillary refill. Neurologic signs include restlessness, ataxia, disorientation, abnormal papillary light reflexes or other cranial nerve abnormalities, twitching, mental dullness, seizures and coma.

Laboratory findings—
1. Blood glucose >600 mg/dL (may be as high as 1600 mg/dL)
2. Hyperosmolality, >350 mOsm/kg; normal serum osmolality = 285–310 mOsm (serum osmolality = 2[Na + K] + glucose/18 + BUN/2.8
3. Prerenal or renal azotemia
4. Severe *clinical* dehydration (may not be reflected in blood work due to intracellular fluid shift)
5. Lack of serum or urine ketones
   A. 'Real' hyperosmolar nonketotic syndrome—acidosis due to lactic acidosis
   B. 'False' hyperosmolar nonketotic syndrome—presence of β-hydroxybutyrate ketones (traditional dipsticks or tablets will not measure beta hydroxybutyrate)
6. Mild or absent metabolic acidosis

Prognosis

The prognosis is guarded to poor.

Treatment

1. Inform the client of the diagnosis, prognosis and cost of the treatment.
2. Hospitalize the patient for observation and therapy.
3. Place an IV catheter. Placement of a long catheter, central line or triple lumen catheter may be beneficial as multiple blood samples will be needed during monitoring.
4. Fluid chosen for the patient should have less sodium than the serum sodium.
   A. In acute cases, fluids containing large amounts of water are the best options to quickly reduce serum sodium. Examples would include 5% dextrose in water or hypotonic saline (0.45% saline).
   B. In chronic cases, fluids with higher sodium contents are used to more slowly reduce the serum sodium. Examples would include 0.9% saline, Normosol®-R, Plasma-Lyte®, or LRS.
   C. Animals should be given intravenous fluids with the intent of replacing water lost from the body and / or diluting the sodium.
      I. Calculate the corrected serum sodium level. For every 100 mg/dL increase in glucose above normal, the measured serum sodium level decreases by 1.6 mEq/dL.
      $$Na^+_{(corr)} = Na^+_{(measured)} + 1.6([measured\ glucose - normal\ glucose] \div 100)$$
      II. Calculate the water deficit = weight (kg) × [(patient current corrected Na/normal Na) − 1]
         Usually shortened to water deficit = weight (kg) × [(patient current Na/140) −1]
         Water deficit is in *liters*.
      III. Determine the time frame over which to replace the water deficit. This is usually dependent upon the chronicity of the hypernatremia.

a. If there is acute development of hypernatremia (i.e. <6–12 hours), replace the water deficit over 6–12 hours. Add the water deficit replacement per hour to the patient's maintenance fluids for that hour.

b. If there is a more chronic or unknown time frame for development of hypernatremia, replace the water deficit more slowly, often over 24–48 hours.

D. Recheck the sodium concentration every 4–6 hours and try to lower the sodium at a rate of no more than 0.5 mEq/L/h.

I. Try to avoid causing cerebral edema by replacing fluid too fast. With chronic hypernatremia, the brain forms idiogenic osmoles within brain cells that will draw water into the cells and cause edema. Slow replacement of fluid will allow the body to break down the idiogenic osmoles to protect brain cells.

II. Recheck the serum sodium concentrations regularly during treatment (every 4–12 hours depending on the case). Chronic hypernatremia requires more frequency of rechecks. With acute hypernatremia, sodium levels do not need to be checked until after administration of full water deficit.

5. Administer potassium supplementation based on measured serum potassium levels. The patient may have hypokalemia, normokalemia or hyperkalemia. Frequent serum potassium monitoring is important.

6. Administer phosphorus supplementation based on measured serum phosphorus levels. The patient may have hypophosphatemia, normophosphatemia or hyperphosphatemia.

7. Gradual glucose reduction is essential. Rapid reduction may precipitate cerebral edema. If the blood glucose is rapidly decreased, coma may be induced.

A. It is important *not* to assume that, in the absence of ketones, the diabetes is not severe.

B. Use one of the insulin regimens as designated for severe DKA.

C. Use a slightly lower insulin dose. With the insulin CRI IV method, use regular insulin at the dose of 1.1 U/kg/24h for dogs rather than 2.2 U/kg/24h as recommended for the treatment of DKA.

D. Do not initiate insulin therapy until adequate fluid therapy has been administered. Generally, insulin therapy is not initiated until the patient has been receiving intravenous fluids for 12–24 hours.

8. Treat any underlying or associated medical disorders (sepsis, pancreatitis, renal failure, congestive heart failure, etc.).

9. Monitor urine output, urine glucose, BUN, serum electrolytes, acid–base balance and CVP frequently.

10. When the patient has stabilized, the patient can be managed as a DKA patient, with regular insulin administered SC q6–8h.

HYPOGLYCEMIA

Diagnosis

History—The owner may notice a decreased appetite or illness in a young animal or weakness, incoordination, lethargy, abnormal behavior or seizures. There may have been a period of excessive activity or stress.

Physical exam—The clinical signs may vary from ataxia, depression, weakness, trembling or seizures to coma.

Laboratory evaluation—

1. The blood glucose level is less than 60 mg/dL.
2. Evaluate a CBC and complete serum chemistry profile, including electrolytes.
3. Perform a urinalysis.
4. Assess the patient's acid–base status.
5. Perform a fecal examination.
6. If insulinoma is the suspected cause, assess the patient's insulin level from a blood sample drawn while the patient is hypoglycemic. Evaluate an amended insulin-to-glucose ratio (AIGR):

   $$AIGR = (insulin \times 100) \div (plasma\ glucose - 30)$$

   If the plasma glucose level is <30 mg/dL, the denominator of 1 is used.

   An AIGR over 30 suggests insulinoma.

Abdominal ultrasound may be part of a thorough evaluation of an adult patient with hypoglycemia.

Differential diagnosis

1. Increased glucose utilization
   A. Insulin overdose
   B. Insulinoma (functional β-cell pancreatic tumor)
   C. Ingestion of hypoglycemic drugs
   D. Renal glycosuria
   E. Sepsis
   F. Severe polycythemia
   G. Idiopathic
      I. Neonatal
      II. Juvenile, as commonly occurs in toy breeds
      III. Hunting dogs
   H. Exocrine pancreatic neoplasia
2. Decreased glucose production
   A. Glycogen storage diseases
   B. Functional hypoglycemia
   C. Starvation
   D. Malabsorption
   E. Hepatic disease
      I. Hepatic neoplasia
      II. Portocaval shunts
      III. Cirrhosis or fibrosis
      IV. Hepatic enzyme deficiency
   F. Hypoadrenocorticism
   G. Hypopituitarism
3. Xylitol intoxication
4. Error or artifact

A. Prolonged sample storage (the serum or plasma glucose concentration decreases at the rate of about 7 mg/dL/h if the serum or plasma is not separated from the red and white blood cells)

B. Glucometer error

C. Laboratory error.

Prognosis

The prognosis is variable, depending upon the underlying etiology. The prognosis for dogs with β-cell tumors is very guarded to poor.

Treatment

1. Advise a telephone caller whose puppy, kitten or diabetic patient is having hypoglycemic seizures at home to rub or pour ½–2 teaspoons of honey or light corn (Karo) syrup on the pet's buccal mucosa and bring the pet to the veterinarian. If the pet revives enough to eat, a small meal may be fed prior to heading to the veterinary office.
2. Inform the client of the differential diagnoses, prognosis and cost of the treatment.
3. Obtain blood samples; measure the blood glucose level.
4. Place an intravenous catheter.
5. Administer 2–20 mL 25% dextrose IV (1 mL/kg).
   A. If the patient is less than 16 weeks of age, further dilute the dextrose bolus to 10%.
   B. If the patient is alert with no history of vomiting, administer 50% dextrose PO.
   C. Caution should be utilized when administering dextrose to patients suspected of having an insulinoma. Rebound hypoglycemia may make their condition worse.
6. Hospitalize the patient for observation and treatment.
7. Administer a 5% dextrose drip IV, 10–20 mL/kg every 6–8 hours.
8. Maintain the blood glucose level at a minimum of 90 mg/dL.
9. When the patient has recovered, encourage eating, unless the patient is vomiting. If the patient is vomiting, maintain NPO and administer a continuous IV glucose infusion.
10. Pursue the underlying etiology.
11. Treatment for a patient with insulinoma is as follows.
    A. The treatment of choice for Insulinoma is surgical excision.
    B. Administer lower doses of 25% dextrose slowly intravenously over 10–15 minutes when needed.
    C. Place the patient on a CRI of 2.5–5% dextrose in water IV at 1.5–2 times the patient's maintenance fluid rate.
    D. Administer dexamethasone, 0.1–0.2 mg/kg IV, or prednisone, 0.25–0.5 mg/kg PO q12h.
    E. Administer diazoxide (Proglycem®), 5–30 mg/kg PO q12h.
    F. The doses of prednisone and diazoxide may need to be increased over time.

G. If the seizures are still uncontrollable, anesthetize the patient with a pentobarbital CRI for 4–8 hours and continue the above therapy.

I. Administer an initial bolus of pentobarbital at 2 mg/kg or higher slowly IV to effect.

II. Following the bolus, begin a constant rate infusion of pentobarbital in a balanced electrolyte solution at 5 mg/kg/h.

III. Adjust to fit the needs of the individual patient, within the normal dose range of 3–10 mg/kg/h.

IV. Continue at a constant level of anesthesia for 3 hours, then decrease the dose by 1 mg/kg/h every hour.

V. The pentobarbital CRI should be administered for approximately 4–8 hours, unless seizures resume.

12. Patients with xylitol intoxication may develop coagulopathy and hepatic failure.

A. Administer fresh frozen plasma if the patient has coagulopathy or DIC.

B. Administer medications to support hepatic function.

I. *N*-acetylcystine, 50 mg/kg IV or PO every 6 hours for 24 hours; dilute *N*-acetylcysteine to a 5% solution in 0.9% NaCl, administer IV slowly over 30 minutes

II. *S*-adenosylmethionine (SAM-e), 18–20 mg/kg PO q24h

III. Silymarin (milk thistle), 20–50 mg/kg PO q24h

HYPOADRENOCORTICISM (ADDISONIAN CRISIS)

Diagnosis

History—The owner may observe anorexia, weight loss, lethargy, intermittent vomiting and diarrhea which may become severe, hematemesis, melena, hematochezia , shivering, polyuria, polydipsia, waxing and waning weakness, muscle cramps, pain, shaking and acute collapse. The patient may have a history of treatment for hyperadrenocorticism. The condition occurs more frequently in female dogs and is rare in cats. It occurs most commonly in the young to middle-aged female dog. The most commonly affected dogs are mixed breeds and the Portuguese Water Dog, Great Dane, West Highland White Terrier, Standard Poodle, Wheaton Terrier and Rottweiler.

Physical exam—The patient may exhibit signs of dehydration, weakness, hypothermia and depression. The patient may have bradycardia and weak femoral pulses. Abdominal pain may be detected upon abdominal palpation. Melena or hematochezia may be found on rectal exam. The patient may present in a state of hypovolemic shock.

Laboratory evaluation—

1. Normochromic normocytic nonregenerative anemia

2. Neutrophilic leukocytosis, mild neutropenia, eosinophilia or lymphocytosis may be revealed by a CBC

3. Prerenal azotemia

4. Marginally depressed blood glucose is occasionally seen
5. Mild metabolic acidosis
6. Hyponatremia (often <140 mEq/L)
7. Hypochloremia (<105 mEq/L)
8. Hyperkalemia (often >6.0 mEq/L)
9. Sodium : potassium ratio = ≤27 : 1 (normal varies from 27 : 1 to 40 : 1)
10. Hyperphosphatemia may be present.
11. Hypercalcemia may be present.
12. Urinalysis may show isosthenuria and hypersthenuria.
13. Resting serum cortisol level will be very low in these patients.
14. ACTH stimulation test with the synthetic adrenocorticotropin cosyntropin (Cortrosyn®)
    A. Obtain a plasma sample.
    B. Administer 0.25 mg (250 µg) of cosyntropin (Cortrosyn®) to a dog IM or 5 µg/kg to a dog IV or 0.125 mg (125 µg) to a cat IM or IV.
    C. Obtain plasma samples 1 hour post-ACTH administration in dogs and 30 and 60 minutes post-ACTH administration in cats.
    D. An abnormally decreased post-ACTH plasma cortisol concentration (<2.0 mg/dL) aids in the diagnosis of hypoadrenocorticism.
15. If cosyntropin (Cortrosyn®) is unavailable, ACTH gel may be used.
    A. Obtain a plasma sample.
    B. Administer 2.2 IU/kg ACTH gel IM in dogs and cats.
    C. Obtain another blood sample 2 hours post-ACTH gel administration in dogs and 1 and 2 hours' post-ACTH gel administration in cats.
16. The measurement of the blood aldosterone concentration after ACTH administration may also aid in the diagnosis of hypoadrenocorticism.

Thoracic radiographs—These may reveal microcardia and megaesophagus.
Electrocardiography—This may reveal changes reflecting hyperkalemia.
1. Peaked T-wave, which usually responds to fluid therapy and corticosteroid administration
2. Absent P-wave
3. Widening ORS complex
4. Irregular R–R intervals
5. Heart block
6. Sine wave

Abdominal ultrasound—This may reveal small adrenal glands bilaterally.

Differential diagnosis

The differential diagnoses include severe gastrointestinal disease, pancreatitis, diabetic ketoacidosis, renal failure, urethral obstruction, ruptured urinary tract and severe hepatic failure.

Prognosis

The prognosis is good to excellent with medical management.

1. Inform the client of the diagnosis, prognosis and cost of the treatment.
2. Place an intravenous catheter.
3. Administer intravenous fluid therapy, 0.9% NaCl at the rate of 4–12 mL/kg/h IV initially in dogs, 45–60 mL/kg/h IV initially in cats.
4. If the patient is hypoglycemic, add dextrose to the intravenous fluids to make a 5% dextrose solution. Add 100 mL of 50% dextrose to 1 liter of IV fluids.
5. Treatment of severe hyperkalemia (>8.5 mEq/L) includes:
   A. Sodium bicarbonate, 1–2 mEq/kg IV over 15–20 minutes
   B. Dextrose, 0.5–1.0 g/kg IV over 30–60 minutes
   C. Regular crystalline insulin, 0.5 U/kg IV with 2–3 g of dextrose per unit of insulin IV. Monitor the patient for severe hypoglycemia with this method.
   D. The administration of calcium gluconate, 0.5–1.5 mL/kg slow IV may help stabilize the heart temporarily, while IV fluids are diluting the serum potassium level and the other medications are taking effect.
6. Sodium bicarbonate administration should be considered if the serum bicarbonate level is <12 mEq/L.
   A. The bicarbonate deficit in mEq/L= body weight (kg) × 0.5 × base deficit (mEq/L)
   B. Administer 25% of the calculated dose in IV fluids during the first 6 hours.
7. An ACTH stimulation test must be done to confirm the diagnosis and prior to glucocorticoid administration. The priority treatment is IV fluid therapy, most patients can wait until an ACTH stimulation test in completed for glucocorticoids to be administered.
8. Administer glucocorticoids.
   A. Hydrocortisone 1.25 mg/kg IV once then 0.5–1 mg/kg q6h tapering off
   B. Prednisolone sodium succinate, 4 mg/kg IV bolus, then prednisone 0.2–0.3 mg/kg IV or PO q12h tapering off
   C. Dexamethasone sodium phosphate, 0.5 mg/kg IV followed by 0.05–0.1 mg/kg q12h tapering off
9. Administer mineralocorticoids.
   A. Desoxycorticosterone pivalate (DOCP®), 2.2 mg/kg IM or SC. Repeat every 25 days or as indicated by monitoring the individual patient's sodium and potassium levels.
   B. Administer fludrocortisone acetate (Florinef®), 0.01–0.02 mg/kg PO q12–24h q12h PO.
10. Monitor urine output.
11. If the patient is vomiting, do not offer food, water or administer oral medications. Administer antiemetics as needed.
    A. Ondansetron (Zofran®), 0.1–1 mg/kg IV or PO q24h
    B. Dolasetron (Anzemet®), 0.6–1 mg/kg IV, SC or PO q24h
    C. Maropitant (Cerenia®), 1 mg/kg SC or 2 mg/kg PO q24h for up to 5 days

D. Metoclopramide (Reglan®), 0.2–0.5 mg/kg SC, IM, or PO q6h, 1–2 mg/kg/day as a CRI IV, or 0.01–0.02 mg/kg/h CRI IV
12. Administration of prednisone or prednisolone, 0.1–0.22 mg/kg q12–24h PO, may be necessary as long-term therapy. Patients receiving DOCP usually need daily glucocorticoid supplementation. About 50% of patients receiving fludrocortisone do not require daily glucocorticoids.

SHAR PEI FEVER SYNDROME

Shar Pei fever syndrome or Shar Pei hock syndrome is a familial, progressive condition involving renal amyloidosis and polyarthritis. It is thought to be an immune-based polyarthritis.

Diagnosis

History—The condition occurs in puppies or adults. The owner may observe anorexia, lethargy and swelling of the tarsal or carpal joints. Mild vomiting and diarrhea may be noted. Weight loss, polyuria, polydipsia and vomiting may be seen when renal dysfunction occurs. Renal or hepatic failure usually occurs between 3 and 5 years of age.
Physical exam—The patient may present with a fever that often exceeds 105°F (40.5°C). There may be visible swelling in the tarsal or carpal joints. Palpable cellulitis may be present around the joints. The patient may also have a swollen and painful muzzle. The patient may have poor body condition, a poor hair coat, ascites or edema.
Laboratory evaluation—
1. CBC may reveal dehydration. The WBC may be elevated to 26 000–30 000, with a left shift.
2. A complete serum biochemical profile should be evaluated, with special emphasis placed on evaluation of renal and hepatic enzyme levels.
3. Hypoalbuminemia may be present.
4. A urinalysis should be performed to assess the degree of proteinuria.
5. The urine protein / creatinine ratio should be monitored.

Differential diagnosis

Fever of other origins, such as viral infections or fungal infections, Lyme disease, panosteitis and infectious polyarthritis.

Prognosis

These patients often progress into renal or hepatic failure due to amyloidosis; therefore, the prognosis is poor.

Treatment

1. Inform the client of the diagnosis, prognosis and cost of the treatment.
2. Place an intravenous catheter.

3. Administer a room-temperature balanced electrolyte solution such as Normosol®-R or LRS IV.
4. Avoid the administration of corticosteroids. They may hasten the development of amyloidosis.
5. Nonsteroidal anti-inflammatory medications, such as dipyrone or ketoprofen, may be administered if hydration and renal function are adequate.
   A. Dipyrone, 11 mg/kg of 50% dipyrone, SC, IM, or IV
   B. Ketoprofen, 0.25–0.5 mg/kg/day SC, IM, IV, or PO
6. The administration of DMSO, 10–20% solution, may be beneficial. The recommended dose varies up to 250 mg/kg PO, IV, SC, topically or intra-articularly.
7. The administration of colchicine, 0.03 mg/kg q24h PO, may be beneficial. Human ingestion must be avoided. Gloves should be worn when handling colchicine.
8. Antibiotic administration should be considered in the patient with severe systemic illness, owing to the immune system involvement, but antibiotics are not useful in the relatively healthy patient with hyperthermia.
9. Most patients will recover spontaneously within 36–48 hours without treatment.

REFERENCES/FURTHER READING

DIABETES MELLITUS

Alt, N., Kley, S., Haessig, M., et al., 2007. Day-to-day variability of blood glucose concentration curves generated at home in cats with diabetes mellitus. Journal of the American Veterinary Medical Association 230, 1011–1017.

Durocher, L.L., Hinchcliff, K.W., DiBartola, S.P., et al., 2008. Acid-base and hormonal abnormalities in dogs with naturally occurring diabetes mellitus. Journal of the American Veterinary Medical Association 232, 1310–1320.

Feldman, E.C., Nelson, R.W., 2004. Canine diabetes mellitus. In: Feldman, E.C., Nelson, R.W. (Eds.), Canine and Feline Endocrinology and Reproduction, third ed. Saunders Elsevier, St Louis, pp. 486–538.

Feldman, E.C., Nelson, R.W., 2004. Feline diabetes mellitus. In: Feldman, E.C., Nelson, R.W. (Eds.), Canine and Feline Endocrinology and Reproduction, third ed. Saunders Elsevier, St Louis, pp. 539–579.

Gilor, C., Graves, T.K., 2010. Synthetic insulin analogs and their use in dogs and cats. In: Graves, T.K. (guest ed.), The Veterinary Clinics of North America, Small Animal Practice. Saunders Elsevier, Philadelphia, vol 40, no 2, pp. 309–317.

Greco, D.S., 2009. Complicated diabetes mellitus. In: Bonagura, J.D., Twedt, D.C. (Eds.), Kirk's Current Veterinary Therapy XIV. Saunders Elsevier, St Louis, pp. 214–218.

Kley, S., Casella, M., Reusch, C.E., 2004. Evaluation of long-term home monitoring of blood glucose concentrations in cats with diabetes mellitus: 26 cases (1999–2002). Journal of the American Veterinary Medical Association 225, 261–266.

Monroe, W.E., 2009. Canine diabetes mellitus. In: Bonagura, J.D., Twedt, D.C. (Eds.), Kirk's Current Veterinary Therapy XIV. Saunders Elsevier, St Louis, pp. 196–199.

Nelson, R.W., Henley, K., Cole, C., the PZIR Clinical Study Group, 2009. Field Safety and Efficacy of Protamine Zinc Recombinant Human Insulin for Treatment of Diabetes Mellitus in Cats. Journal of Veterinary Internal Medicine 23, 787–793.

Nelson, R.W., Lynn, R.C., Wagner-Mann, C.C., et al., 2001. Efficacy of protamine zinc insulin for treatment of diabetes mellitus in cats. Journal of the American

Veterinary Medical Association 218, 38–42.

Plotnick, A.N., Greco, D.S., Diagnosis of diabetes mellitus in dogs and cats, contrasts and comparisons. In Greco, D.S., Peterson, M.E. (guest eds.), 1995. The Veterinary Clinics of North America, Small Animal Practice: Diabetes Mellitus 25 (3), 563–570.

Rand, J.S., 2009. Feline diabetes mellitus. In: Bonagura, J.D., Twedt, D.C. (Eds.), Kirk's Current Veterinary Therapy XIV. Saunders Elsevier, St Louis, pp. 199–204.

Reusch, C.E., 2009. Diabetic monitoring. In: Bonagura, J.D., Twedt, D.C. (Eds.), Kirk's Current Veterinary Therapy XIV. Saunders Elsevier, St Louis, pp. 209–213.

Roomp, K., Rand, J.S., 2009. Evaluation of detemir in diabetic cats managed with a protocol for intensive blood glucose control [abstract]. Journal of Veterinary Internal Medicine 23 (3), 697.

Rucinsky, R., Cook, A., Haley, S., et al., 2010. AAHA diabetes management guidelines for dogs and cats. Journal of the American Animal Hospital Association 46, 215–224.

Scott-Moncrieff, J.C., 2010. Insulin resistance in cats. In: Graves, T.K. (guest ed.), The Veterinary Clinics of North America, Small Animal Practice. Saunders Elsevier, Philadelphia, vol 40, no 2, pp. 241–257.

Van de Maele, I., Rogier, N., Daminet, S., 2005. Retrospective study of owners' perception on home monitoring of blood glucose in diabetic dogs and cats. Canadian Veterinary Journal 46, 718–723.

DIABETIC KETOACIDOSIS

Chastain, C.B., 1981. Intensive care of dogs and cats with diabetic ketoacidosis. Journal of The American Veterinary Medical Association 179 (10), 972–978.

Feldman, E.C., Nelson, R.W., 2004. Diabetic ketoacidosis. In: Feldman E.C., Nelson R.W. (Eds.), Canine and Feline Endocrinology and Reproduction, third ed. Saunders Elsevier, St Louis, pp. 580–615.

Greco, D.S., 2009. Complicated diabetes mellitus. In: Bonagura, J.D., Twedt, D.C. (Eds.), Kirk's Current Veterinary Therapy XIV. Saunders Elsevier, St Louis, pp. 214–218.

Hess, R.S., 2009. Diabetic ketoacidosis. In: Silverstein, D.C., Hopper, K. (Eds.),

Small Animal Critical Care Medicine. Elsevier, St Louis, pp. 288–291.

Hoenig, M., Dorfman, M., Koenig, A., 2008. Use of a hand-held meter for the measurement of blood beta-hydroxybutyrate in dogs and cats. Journal of Veterinary Emergency and Critical Care 18 (1), 86–87.

Hume, D.Z., Drobatz, K.J., Hess, R.S., 2006. Outcome of dogs with diabetic ketoacidosis: 127 dogs (1993–2003). Journal of Veterinary Internal Medicine 20, 547–555.

O'Brien, M.A., 2010. Diabetic emergencies in small animals. In: Graves, T.K. (guest ed.), The Veterinary Clinics of North America, Small Animal Practice. Saunders Elsevier, Philadelphia, vol 40, no 2, pp. 317–333.

HYPEROSMOLAR NONKETOTIC SYNDROME OF DIABETES MELLITUS

Feldman, E.C., Nelson, R.W., 2004. Hyperosmolar nonketotic diabetes mellitus. In: Feldman, E.C., Nelson, R.W. (Eds.), Canine and Feline Endocrinology and Reproduction, third ed. Saunders Elsevier, St Louis, pp. 612–614.

Koenig, A., 2009. Hyperglycemic hyperosmolar syndrome. In: Silverstein, D.C., Hopper, K. (Eds.), Small Animal Critical Care Medicine. Elsevier, St Louis, pp. 291–294.

Koenig, A., Drobatz, K.J., Beale, A.B., et al., 2004. Hyperglycemic, hyperosmolar syndrome in feline diabetics: 17 cases (1995–2001). Journal of Veterinary Emergency and Critical Care 14 (1), 30–40.

Nichols, R., Crenshaw, K.L., Complications and concurrent disease associated with diabetic ketoacidosis and other severe forms of diabetes mellitus. In Greco, D.S., Peterson, M.E. (guest eds.), 1995. The Veterinary Clinics of North America, Small Animal Practice: Diabetes Mellitus 25 (3), 617–624.

O'Brien, M.A., 2010. Diabetic emergencies in small animals. In Graves, T.K. (guest ed.), The Veterinary Clinics of North America, Small Animal Practice. Saunders Elsevier, Philadelphia, vol 40, no 2, pp. 317–333.

HYPOGLYCEMIA

Feldman, E.C., Nelson, R.W., 2004. Beta-cell neoplasia: insulinoma. In: Feldman, E.C., Nelson, R.W., Canine and Feline Endocrinology and Reproduction, third ed. Saunders Elsevier, St Louis, pp. 616–644.

Koenig, A., 2009. Hypoglycemia. In: Silverstein, D.C., Hopper, K. (Eds.), Small Animal Critical Care Medicine. Elsevier, St Louis, pp. 295–299.

Watson, P.J., Bunch, S.E., 2009. Hypoglycemia, disorders of the endocrine pancreas. In: Nelson, R.W., Couto, C.G. (Eds.), Small Animal Internal Medicine, fourth ed. Mosby Elsevier, St Louis, pp. 765–767.

HYPOADRENOCORTICISM (ADDISONIAN CRISIS)

Adler, J.A., Drobatz, K.J., Hess, R.S., 2007. Abnormalities of serum electrolyte concentrations in dogs with hypoadrenocorticism. Journal of Veterinary Internal Medicine 21, 1168–1173.

Burkitt, J.M., 2009. Hypoadrenocorticism. In: Silverstein, D.C., Hopper, K. (Eds.), Small Animal Critical Care Medicine. St Louis, Elsevier, pp. 321–324.

Feldman, E.C., Nelson, R.W., 2004. Hypoadrenocorticism In: Feldman, E.C., Nelson, R.W. (Eds.), Canine and Feline Endocrinology and Reproduction, third ed. Saunders Elsevier, St Louis, pp. 394–439.

Greco, D.S., 2007. Hypoadrenocorticism in small animals. Clinical Techniques in Small Animal Practice 22, 32–35.

Kintzer, P.P., Peterson, M.E., 2009. Hypoadrenocorticism. In: Bonagura, J.D., Twedt, D.C. (Eds.), Kirk's Current Veterinary Therapy XIV. Saunders Elsevier, St Louis, pp. 231–235.

Lennon, E.M., Boyle, T.E., Hutchins, R.G., et al., 2007. Use of basal serum or plasma cortisol concentrations to rule out a diagnosis of hypoadrenocorticism in dogs: 123 cases (2000–2005). Journal of the American Veterinary Medical Association 231, 413–416.

Meeking, S., 2007. Treatment of acute adrenal insufficiency. Clinical Techniques in Small Animal Practice 22, 36–39.

Schaer, M., 2001. The treatment of acute adrenocortical insufficiency in the dog. Journal of Veterinary Emergency Critical Care 11 (1), 7–14.

Thompson, A.L., Scott-Moncrieff, J.C., Anderson, J.D., 2007. Comparison of classic hypoadrenocorticism with glucocorticoid-deficient hypoadrenocorticism in dogs: 46 cases (1985–2005). Journal of the American Veterinary Medical Association 230, 1190–1194.

SHAR PEI FEVER SYNDROME

Bonagura, J.D., Twedt, D.C. (Eds.), 2009. Kirk's Current Veterinary Therapy XIV. Saunders Elsevier, St Louis, pp. 1188–1195

Kirk, R.W., Bonagura, J.D. (Eds.), 1992. Current Veterinary Therapy XI. WB Saunders, Philadelphia, pp. 823–826.

Osborne, C.A., Finco, D.R., 1995. Canine and Feline Nephrology and Urology. Williams & Wilkins, Philadelphia, pp. 400–415.

Taylor, S.M., 2009. Familial Chinese Shar Pei fever, disorders of the joints. In: Nelson, R.W., Couto, C.G. (Eds.), Small Animal Internal Medicine, fourth ed. Mosby Elsevier, St Louis, p. 1137.

Urinary emergencies and electrolyte disorders

Elizabeth J Thomovsky DVM, MS, DACVECC
and Signe J Plunkett DVM

ACUTE RENAL FAILURE (ARF)

Etiology

The four main causes of ARF are:

1. Renal ischemia (induced by hypotension, severe dehydration, hypovolemia, hypoperfusion to kidneys, thrombosis or microthrombosis to renal vessels from DIC or other causes, avulsion of renal vessels, hypertension).
2. Nephrotoxicity.
3. Primary renal diseases (pyelonephritis, leptospirosis, infectious canine hepatitis, immune-mediated disease, lymphoma).
4. Other systemic disease (feline infectious peritonitis, sepsis, borreliosis, babesiosis, leishmaniasis, bacterial endocarditis, pancreatitis, DIC, heart failure, systemic lupus erythematosus, hepatorenal syndrome, hyperviscosity syndrome, hypothermia, hyperthermia, burns, transfusion reactions).

Known nephrotoxins include:

1. Therapeutic agents
   A. Analgesics—ibuprofen, naproxen, phenylbutazone, piroxicam, and other nonsteroidal anti-inflammatory agents (NSAIDs)
   B. Antiprotozoals—thiacetarsamide, pentamidine, sulfadiazine, trimethoprim-sulfamethoxazole, dapsone
   C. Antifungals—amphotericin B
   D. Antimicrobials—aminoglycosides, cephalosporins, nafcillins, sulfonamides, tetracyclines, penicillins, fluoroquinolones, carbapenems, rifampin, tetracyclines, vancomycin, aztreonam
   E. Antiviral drugs—acyclovir, foscarnet
   F. ACE inhibitors—enalapril
   G. Diuretics—mannitol

H. Miscellaneous—Dextran 40, allopurinol, cimetidine, apomorphine, deferoxamine, streptokinase, penicillamine, tricyclic antidepressants
2. Anesthetics—methoxyflurane
3. Chemotherapeutic agents—cisplatin, doxorubicin, methotrexate, carboplatin, adriamycin, azathioprine
4. Immunosuppressive drugs—cyclosporine
5. Heavy metals—cadmium, chromium, lead, mercury, uranium, bismuth salts, arsenic, gold, thallium, copper, silver, nickel, antimony
6. Miscellaneous agents—snake venom, lilies (cats), grapes and raisins (dogs), gallium nitrate, diphosphonates, mushrooms, calcium antagonists (hypercalcemia), bee venom, illicit drugs
7. Organic compounds—carbon tetrachloride, chloroform, ethylene glycol, herbicides, pesticides, solvents
8. Pigments—hemoglobin, myoglobin
9. Radiographic contrast agents. (If radiographic contrast agents must be used in patients susceptible to developing ARF, do not exceed the dose of 1.5 mL/kg/24 h.)

Diagnosis

History—The owner may observe increased drinking, changes in urine volume (increased or decreased), vomiting, diarrhea, anorexia, lethargy and weight loss.

Physical exam—The patient may present with signs of lethargy, vomiting, diarrhea, and dehydration. The patient may have halitosis due to uremic breath, and uremic oral ulcers may be present. Patients with acute renal failure are generally in good body condition and have enlarged or swollen and often painful kidneys. Patients with chronic renal failure are often thin and muscle wasted.

Perform a rectal exam to detect any pelvic, prostatic, or urethral disorders, and to assess the color and character of feces. Melena or coffee-ground vomitus may occur due to upper gastrointestinal hemorrhage secondary to uremic gastropathy.

Look for petechiation and ecchymoses, which would indicate platelet dysfunction secondary to uremia.

If indicated (history of straining to urinate, large inexpressible bladder on exam), pass a urethral catheter to assess the patency of the lower urinary tract. The patient may be polyuric, oliguric (<0.5 mL/kg/h of urine output) or anuric.

Some patients are presented in a stupor or may be comatose.

It is important to always establish blood pressure and treat any diagnosed hypertension (systolic blood pressure >180 mm Hg in dogs and >200 mm Hg in cats).

A fundic exam should be performed to detect retinal hemorrhage or retinal detachment secondary to hypertension.

Laboratory evaluation—
1. The CBC may be normal or there may be a leukocytosis +/− stress leukogram. The patient can be hemoconcentrated which can hide

Table 11.1 *Indices that may help differentiate pre-renal azotemia from acute renal failure (ARF)*

Indices	Pre-renal azotemia	ARF
Urine specific gravity	Hypersthenuric	Isosthenuric or minimally concentrated
Urine sodium (mEq/L)	<10–20	>25
Fractional excretion of sodium (%)	<1	>1
Urine creatinine to plasma creatinine ratio	>20 : 1	<10 : 1
Renal failure index (urine Na/urine to plasma creatinine ratio)	>1	>2

From Grauer GF, Fluid therapy in acute and chronic renal failure. The veterinary clinics of North America: small animal practice, Advances in Fluid and Electrlyte Disorders, Vol. 28, No. 3, 1998 ©Elsevier, with permission.

underlying true anemia secondary to decreased erythropoietin production.
2. The serum biochemical profile may reveal numerous abnormalities:
   A. Serum BUN is increased. (Rule out BUN elevation due to dehydration, gastrointestinal hemorrhage, increased protein intake.)
   B. Serum creatinine is increased.
   C. Serum phosphorus level is usually increased.
   D. Serum sodium level may be normal, increased, or decreased.
   E. Serum potassium level may be normal, increased or decreased.
3. Urinalysis (Table 11.1)
   A. Pre-treatment urine specific gravity isosthenuric = 1.007–1.015.
   B. Renal tubular casts or granular casts may be observed.
4. Evaluate blood gases. Metabolic acidosis is the most common acid–base disorder with ARF.

Abdominal radiography—May assist in the evaluation of renal size, and may also assist in the identification of radiopaque uroliths associated with urinary tract infection or urinary tract obstruction. If ureteral calculi are noted, the radiographs may be consistent with obstruction and secondary hydronephrosis leading to renal failure (usually requires bilateral ureteral calculi).

Contrast radiography may assist in the identification of urinary tract obstruction or rupture. For evaluation of the upper urinary tract, perform excretory urography (an intravenous pyelogram – IVP). The dose of iodinated contrast medium in the form of sodium iothalamate or sodium diatrizoate, is 180 mg/kg body weight. For evaluation of the urinary bladder and urethra, perform a voiding cystourethrogram or IVP.

The patient should be well-hydrated prior to the intravenous administration of contrast agents. Excretory urography is often of limited value in patients with ARF, because the kidneys cannot excrete the contrast media well enough to produce diagnostic-quality films.

Abdominal ultrasonography—May be useful in the detection of renal parenchymal disease and the presence and location of uroliths and ureteroliths. Ultrasonography is also useful as a guide when obtaining renal aspirates or biopsies.

Ethylene glycol toxicity results in a mild to dramatic diffuse increase in renal echogenicity due to the deposition of intratubular and interstitial refractile oxalate crystals. The crystalline deposits are usually in the cortex but may be present in the medulla in severe cases. The crystals may accumulate in a band-like zone of the medulla just inside the corticomedullary junction and create a medullary rim sign, known as the 'halo sign'. If the 'halo sign' is observed, the prognosis is grave. Nephrocalcinosis and hypercalcemic nephropathy may also increase renal echogenicity, but to a lesser extent than ethylene glycol toxicity.

Renal biopsy is unnecessary in the initial stabilization of patients with ARF that have clinical and laboratory evidence of the condition and a history compatible with ARF. Renal biopsy may be beneficial in patients with ARF in order to determine the etiology of renal failure in patients that do not respond to therapy, when peritoneal dialysis or hemodialysis is contemplated and when the distinction between ARF and CRF (chronic renal failure) cannot be made. There is some research currently being conducted to determine future therapeutics based on the results of renal biopsies.

Differential diagnosis

1. Pre-renal azotemia
2. Post-renal azotemia
3. Diabetes mellitus
4. Hypoadrenocorticism
5. Hyperadrenocorticism
6. Pyometra
7. Chronic renal failure
8. Psychogenic polydipsia
9. Hepatic insufficiency
10. Portosystemic shunt
11. Pituitary diabetes insipidus
12. Hyperthyroidism
13. Iatrogenic or drug-induced polyuria.

Prognosis

The prognosis is dependent upon whether the renal failure is polyuric (>2 mL/kg/h urine production) or oliguric/anuric.

1. Polyuric renal failure can typically be managed successfully in the hospital although many patients require continued therapies at home (fluid therapy, special diets).
2. Oliguric/anuric renal failure has a guarded to poor prognosis but improves to fair to good if the patient becomes polyuric.
3. In all cases of ARF, patients may continue to improve over a 6–8 week period wherein the kidneys undergo renal regeneration and compensation. In some cases, patients need to be supported in the hospital for several weeks, which can become cost prohibitive.
4. Anuric patients are unlikely to survive.

5. If dialysis is necessary, the prognosis worsens and the cost significantly increases.

Treatment

1. Inform the client of the diagnosis, prognosis and cost of the treatment.
2. Obtain pre-treatment blood and urine samples.
3. Thoroughly question the owner about possible exposure to ethylene glycol. If ethylene glycol cannot be ruled out, discuss treatment of ethylene glycol toxicity with the owner, the prognosis, and the risks of therapy.
4. Discontinue the administration of all potentially nephrotoxic drugs.
5. Initiate specific antidotal therapy, if applicable, such as for ethylene glycol toxicosis.
6. Place an intravenous catheter. Jugular catheterization is particularly useful as it will allow monitoring of central venous pressure.
7. Administer intravenous fluids, usually at 2–3 times maintenance fluid rates. Usually a balanced electrolyte crystalloid fluid, such as LRS or Normosol®-R, is indicated initially.
   A. Administer the dehydration deficit over the first 4–6 hours.
      % dehydration × body weight in kg × 1000 = volume of fluid to be replaced in milliliters
   B. A fluid bolus of 20 mL/kg IV over 10 minutes may help assess the patient's response and the potential for fluid overload.
8. If the patient presents in severe hypovolemic shock, administer fluids rapidly. In dogs, administer fluids at up to 70–90 mL/kg IV over the first hour. In cats, administer fluids at 50–60 mL/kg IV over the first hour. Typically when resuscitating for shock, administer a bolus of ¼–⅓ of the entire shock dose over 5–10 minutes, reassess the patient's vital statistics and administer another bolus if indicated only. Many patients respond after one to two boluses and do not require the full shock dose of fluids.
9. If the patient presents in severe hypovolemic shock, consider the administration of Hetastarch (15–20 mL/kg IV), in addition to the crystalloid fluids. As with crystalloids, administer the Hetastarch divided into boluses of 5–10 mL/kg and reassess after each bolus to determine if more is required. If a patient is oliguric or anuric, administration of Hetastarch is more likely to lead to fluid overload than administration of crystalloids.
10. During the rehydration phase, monitor the central venous pressure (CVP), urine production and body weight frequently.
    A. The CVP should not increase more than 5–7 cm H_2O. Greater increases might indicate possible fluid overload / overhydration.
    B. Other signs of overhydration include serous nasal discharge, tachypnea, tachycardia, restlessness, shivering, chemosis, dyspnea, increased bronchovesicular sounds, pulmonary crackles and edema, decreased mentation, nausea, vomiting, diarrhea, ascites, polyuria, and subcutaneous edema (appearing first in the tarsal joints and intermandibular space). Body weight increases greater than the estimated dehydration percent might indicate overhydration as well.

C. If overhydration occurs, slow or discontinue fluid administration. Administer diuretics and oxygen if indicated.

11. In cases of oliguric or anuric renal failure, it is best to have an indwelling urinary catheter from which urine production can be measured. It is helpful to have an indwelling catheter in polyuric renal failure but these cases can much more easily be managed without knowing exact urine production amounts. Minimum urine output should be 1–2 mL/kg/h after a patient is rehydrated. Strict aseptic technique and a closed collection system must be utilized when placing a urinary catheter.

12. Monitor the patient's body weight every 6–12 hours. Monitor the patient closely for signs of overhydration.

13. After rehydration, if urine output is insufficient, administer an IV fluid bolus of at least 5–10 mL/kg. If monitoring CVPs, attempt to increase the CVP by 5–7 cm H_2O with fluid boluses. If this does not improve urine production consider other agents:

A. Mannitol (10% or 20%), 0.1–0.5g/kg administered IV over 10–15 minutes, if there are no contraindications (vasculitis, bleeding disorders, hyperosmolar syndrome, congestive heart failure, volume overload). If no increase in urine production within 30 minutes, the same dose may be repeated. Do not exceed a mannitol dose of 2 g/kg/day.

B. Hypertonic dextrose (10–20% solutions) may be used as an alternative to mannitol. Check the patient's blood glucose level first. Do not administer hypertonic dextrose if the patient is hyperglycemic. The dose of 10–20% dextrose is 25–50 mL/kg as an intermittent slow IV bolus over 1–2 hours, repeated q8–12h.

Mannitol and hypertonic dextrose may be more helpful in patients with renal tubular damage leading to filling of the renal tubules with debris that will be forced out by the osmotic effects of these drugs.

C. Furosemide is usually given as a bolus followed by a constant rate infusion. If the bolus (repeated 1–2 times total) does not lead to urine production then the CRI will not help either. Bolus dose= 1–6 mg/kg IV. **Avoid furosemide administration in patients with ARF due to aminoglycoside administration, as furosemide has been shown to exacerbate aminoglycoside toxicity.**

Constant rate infusion at the dose of 0.25–1 mg/kg/h CRI IV.

D. Dopamine administration may be beneficial in dogs:

I. To increase renal blood flow and urine volume, administer dopamine, 0.5–5 µg/kg/min in 0.9% NaCl CRI IV. Do *not* add dopamine to alkaline fluids.

II. It does *not* help in cats due to reduced or absent dopaminergic receptors in cat kidneys.

E. Diltiazem has been shown to have a positive effect in the treatment of leptospirosis. Diltiazem was administered 0.1–0.5 mg/kg IV over 30 minutes followed by 1–5 µg/kg/min as a CRI to induce urine production in patients with leptospirosis. Diltiazem was added to patients' treatment regimes in addition to IV crystalloid fluid therapy, ampicillin, +/– furosemide, and +/– dopamine.

14. If diuresis cannot be induced, perform peritoneal dialysis or hemodialysis. Indications for dialysis include:

A. Exposure to dialyzable toxins
B. Treatment of overhydration
C. Severe persistent uremia, acidosis or hyperkalemia
D. Oliguria / anuria.

15. Placement of a peritoneal dialysis catheter (see Fig. 14.2)
    A. Administer a general anesthetic, being cautious to avoid hypotension.
    B. Consider performing an omentectomy or partial omentectomy, to decrease omental plugging of the peritoneal dialysis catheter, particularly in the cat.
    C. The surgeon *must* use sterile technique. Every junction of the peritoneal catheter set must be covered with a povidone-iodine wrap, which is changed daily.
    D. Use a peritoneal dialysis catheter, a pediatric trocar, or for cats, use a 14-GA Teflon IV catheter with additional side holes placed all on the same side to preserve the integrity of the catheter.
    E. Consider obtaining a renal biopsy at the time the peritoneal dialysis catheter is placed.
    F. Make a stab incision (1 cm) through the linea alba 2–4 cm caudal to the umbilicus.
    G. Aim the catheter towards the pelvic inlet.
    H. Secure the catheter by suturing to the abdominal wall, not just to skin. Use a purse-string suture at the entry site and a 'Chinese finger-lock' suture on the catheter to secure it in position.
    I. Cover the entry site into the abdomen with a povidone-iodine patch and a sterile bandage.
    J. Use *warm* 1.5%, 4.0%, or 7% dextrose dialysate solution, LRS, or 0.9% NaCl. (The preferable solution, if commercial dialysate solution is not available, is 1.5% dextrose in LRS; made by adding 30 mL 50% dextrose to 1000 mL LRS.)
    K. Add 250 units heparin/liter of dialysate.
    L. Infuse 20–30 mL/kg intraperitoneal (IP).
    M. Dwell time = 45 minutes.
    N. Drainage time = 15 minutes.
    O. Repeat *continuously*, or every 2 hours until the BUN, creatinine and hydration status approach normal values, then decrease the frequency of dialysis.
    P. Flush the peritoneal catheter with 5–10 mL heparinized saline after each infusion or drainage to diminish clogging of peritoneal catheter.
    Q. Monitor the patient's CBC, TP, serum electrolytes, PT, PTT, body temperature, urine (sediment and dipstick) and the dialysate for signs of infection.
    R. When peritoneal lavage is no longer necessary, sedate or anesthetize the patient, remove the peritoneal catheter and close the abdominal incision with one to two sutures in the linea alba, then close the skin. Apply a sterile abdominal wrap.

16. Maintenance of the peritoneal dialysis catheter
    A. Sterility is very important.

Table 11.2 *Suggested potassium¹ maximum infusion rate*

Estimated potassium losses	Suggested potassium (mEq/L)	Maximum infusion rate (mL/kg per hour)
Maintenance (serum level = 3.6–5.0)	20	25
Mild (serum level = 3.1–3.5)	30	17
Moderate (serum level = 2.6–3.0)	40	12
Severe (serum level = 2.1–2.5)	60	8
Life threatening (serum level <2.0)	80	6

¹Potassium supplementation should not exceed 0.5 mEq/kg per hour.

B. Wash hands thoroughly prior to wearing sterile gloves when handling the peritoneal dialysis catheter.

C. Flush the catheter with heparinized saline after every installation and drainage.

D. Wipe every connection and injection port with chlorhexidine or povidone-iodine solution every time prior to manipulation.

E. Cover the entry site into the abdomen with a sterile bandage.

F. Keep a clean, dry and sterile bandage on the abdomen, over the catheter entry site. Check the bandage, the entry site and bandage every 12–24 hours. Change the bandage every 2 days.

G. If at all possible, perform the installation and drainage of the peritoneal lavage fluid in the surgical suite to keep contamination to a minimum.

17. Supplement intravenous fluids with additional potassium as indicated by frequent monitoring of the serum potassium level (Table 11.2).

18. Hypocalcemia often occurs with renal failure. It is important to monitor ionized serum calcium, and supplement if needed. The recommended dosage of calcium gluconate 10% IV is 1–1.5 mL /kg IV over 15–20 minutes.

19. Treat specific diseases that have led to the ARF.

A. Hypercalcemia may cause acute renal failure. The treatment is:

   I. Administer intravenous fluid therapy with 0.9% NaCl.

   II. Administer furosemide, 2–5 mg/kg IV or PO q12h, in dogs and cats. Alternatively, administer 5 mg/kg bolus IV and follow with 5 mg/kg/h CRI.

   III. Administer prednisone, 1–1.5 mg/kg IM or PO q12h.

   IV. Bisphosphonates (ex. pamidronate): 1.3–2 mg/kg in 150 mL of 0.9% NaCl give over 2 hours (IV infusion). Dose patients once.

B. Leptospirosis

   I. Ampicillin 22 mg/kg IV q8h for at least the first 3 days (or until the patient is eating). This eliminates the circulating bacteria.

   II. Tetracycline (usually doxycycline) 5 mg/kg PO q12h for 2 weeks to eliminate carrier state.

C. Lymphoma: chemotherapy (various options)

D. Pyelonephritis: antibiotics based on culture (see pyelonephritis section)

    E. Ethylene glycol: 4-methylpyrazole or ethanol (see ethylene glycol section for complete discussion)

    F. Lyme disease (borreliosis): doxycycline 5 mg/kg PO or IV q12h, ampicillin 22 mg/kg IV q12h, or amoxicillin 22 mg/kg PO q12h. All treatment for 21–28 days total.

20. Hyperphosphatemia is common and may adversely affect appetite. Administer oral phosphate-binding agents if vomiting is controlled and *patients are eating*. Administer aluminum hydroxide 30–90 mg/kg/day PO.

21. Hypokalemia

    A. Supplement the intravenous fluids with potassium (see Table 11.2).

    B. Administer oral potassium, 2–5 mg potassium chloride per day.

22. Monitor blood gases and correct acid-base abnormalities as needed. Administer sodium bicarbonate **only** if *measured* serum bicarbonate [HCO_3] is 12 mEq/L or less and pH <7.1

23. Treat hypertension:

    A. Amlodipine 0.625–1.25 mg/cat PO q24h or 0.05–0.2 mg/kg PO q12–24h in dogs

    B. Diltiazem: 0.5 mg/kg PO q6h

    C. Hydralazine: 0.5–2 mg/kg PO q8–12h

    D. Nitroprusside: 0.5–2 µg/kg/min IV (titrate dose as needed to control blood pressure). Use only in severe hypertension (>230 mm Hg). Ideally monitor blood pressure continuously with an arterial catheter and invasive blood pressure measurements during this treatment.

24. For maintenance fluid therapy after rehydration, use balanced electrolyte solutions such as Normosol®-M. If not available, LRS, Normosol®-R, or 0.9% NaCl may be utilized, while carefully monitoring serum electrolyte levels. Administer fluids at a volume to match urine volume and other losses, including insensible losses (20 mL/kg/day) and continuing losses (from vomiting or diarrhea)

    A. Hourly fluid rate should match hourly urine production (typically at least 1–2 mL/kg/h).

    B. Replace continuing losses from vomiting and diarrhea over 24 hours.

    C. Replace insensible losses over 24 hours.

25. Treat nausea and gastric hyperacidity with H_2 blockers and gastric protectants.

    A. Ranitidine (Zantac®), 0.5–2 mg/kg IV, PO q8h (dogs), 1–2 mg/kg q12h PO, IV (cats)

    B. Famotidine (Pepcid®), 0.5–1 mg/kg IV or PO q12–24h

    C. Omeprazole (Prilosec OTC®), 0.5–2 mg/kg PO q24h

    D. Pantoprazole (Protonix®, Pantoloc®), 1 mg/kg IV q24h

26. Xylocaine (lidocaine) Viscous Solution®, 2–10 mL, may be applied orally prior to feeding to decrease the discomfort of oral ulcerations. Consider flushing the mouth 2–3 times daily with a lidocaine, diphenhydramine and aluminum hydroxide mixed together in equal parts to reduce discomfort and aid in healing of ulcerations.

27. Control vomiting with antiemetics.
    A. Metoclopramide (Reglan®), 0.2–0.3 mg/kg SC or IM q8h or 1–2 mg/kg/24h (0.04–0.08 mg/kg/h) CRI IV. If the patient is on metoclopramide, it is very important to palpate the abdomen every 2–4 hours and closely monitor for intussusception. Avoid metoclopramide if a mechanical obstruction is suspected, or if the patient has a history of seizures.
    B. Chlorpromazine (Thorazine®), 0.05–0.1 mg/kg IV q4–6h as needed, 0.2–0.5 mg/kg SC, IM q6–8h, or 1 mg/kg diluted in 1mL of 0.9% aCl and administered rectally q8h via a plastic catheter.
    C. Prochlorperazine, 0.25–0.5 mg/kg SC, IM q6–8h.
    D. Ondansetron (Zofran®), 0.1–0.2 mg/kg IV q6–12h.
    E. Maropitant (Cerenia®), 1 mg/kg SQ q24h or 2 mg/kg PO q24h. Do not administer for more than 4–5 days in succession.
    F. Dolasetron (Anzemet®), 0.6 mg/kg IV q24h.
28. Eventually, the fluid needs decrease, usually after 5–6 days of profound diuresis and intravenous fluid therapy. Signs that the fluid volume should be decreased include:
    A. The patient is feeling better and showing interest in eating and drinking
    B. The vomiting and diarrhea have been controlled
    C. There have been significant decreases in the blood urea nitrogen (BUN), creatinine and phosphorus concentrations.
29. To taper the intravenous fluid administration volume, decrease the maintenance fluids administered by 25% per day. Return to prior volume administration for at least 48 hours if the PCV, TP, BUN and / or creatinine levels increase or if the patient loses weight. In some cases patients can be weaned off fluids despite increases in blood values and supplemented with SQ fluids in preparation for discharge from the hospital.
30. All patients should be discharged with oral H_2 blockers, phosphate binders, and instructions for a protein-restricted diet (see following section on Chronic Renal Failure). In some cases, patients should also go home with subcutaneous fluids (preferably LRS if available). This would include patients with creatinine levels persistently >5 mg/dL, those with minimal decreases in their creatinine after fluid diuresis, or those whose creatine levels increase as IV fluids are weaned.
31. It is important that patients have recheck bloodwork 3–7 days after discharge from the hospital in order to determine if the patients require more aggressive at-home treatment to maintain their well-being.

CHRONIC RENAL FAILURE (CRF)

Etiology

CRF is defined as kidney damage that has existed for more than 3 months or a reduction of glomerular filtration rate of more than 50% for at least 3 months. Chronic renal failure may be congenital or may be acquired. A specific etiology often cannot be identified and management is not dependent upon the etiologic agent. Any disease that causes renal failure can lead to CRF.

Some documented causes of acquired CRF include:

1. Infectious diseases—ehrlichiosis, brucellosis, dirofilariasis, leptospirosis, borreliosis (Lyme disease), systemic mycoses, pyelonephritis, bacterial endocarditis, pyometra, feline infectious peritonitis, feline leukemia virus infection, infectious canine hepatitis
2. Immunologic disorders—chronic glomerulonephritis, immune complex deposition, systemic lupus erythematosus, polyarthritis, vasculitis
3. Inflammatory diseases—chronic pyoderma, chronic pancreatitis, pyelonephritis
4. Amyloidosis
5. Nephrotic syndrome
6. Neoplastic diseases—multiple myeloma, renal carcinoma, renal lymphosarcoma, mast cell tumors, etc.
7. Nephrotoxins—including NSAIDs, aminoglycoside antibiotics, and hypercalcemia
8. Hypertension
9. Hereditary and congenital disorders—renal dysplasia, renal hypoplasia, polycystic renal disease, familial nephropathies
10. Urinary outflow obstruction
11. Idiopathic

Diagnosis

History—The owner may observe anorexia, lethargy, weight loss, polyuria, polydypsia, nocturia, a coarse, dull hair coat, depression, vomiting, diarrhea, halitosis, weakness and exercise intolerance. The history may reveal a possible etiologic factor.

Physical exam—The physical exam findings vary with the progression of the disease. The patient may present with weakness, dehydration, lethargy, pallor, a dull hair coat, oral ulcers, glossitis, stomatitis, and loose teeth. The patient may exhibit signs of depression, neuromuscular twitches, coma or seizures. If the patient has extreme hypoproteinemia, edema, ascites or pleural effusion may be present. The kidneys may be small and firm, and may have an irregular surface. Some patients with CRF will have abnormally large kidneys due to FIP, polycystic renal disease, or renal lymphosarcoma. A rectal examination should be performed to evaluate the trigonal area of the urinary bladder, pelvic urethra, and the prostate gland, and also to evaluate the color and consistency of feces. Systemic blood pressure measurements may reveal hypertension. Ophthalmic examination may reveal retinal hemorrhages, retinal detachment, and vessel tortuosity.

Laboratory evaluation—

1. Urinalysis
   A. Urine specific gravity <1.025, often 1.008–1.013.
   B. Possibly proteinuria (>2+ in dilute urine is significant).
   C. May show concurrent urinary tract infection (pyuria, hematuria, bacturia).

    D. Urine obtained by cystocentesis should be submitted for bacterial culture.
2. CBC
    A. Lymphopenia may be present.
    B. Normocytic, normochromic, nonregenerative anemia is a common finding.
    C. May have leukocytosis with concurrent pyelonephritis, pyometritis, or other infectious disease.
    D. Thrombocytopenia may be present in patients with concurrent rickettsial disease or immune-mediated disease.
3. Serum biochemical profile
    A. Azotemia
       I. The serum creatinine is elevated. Gradual increases from 1.0 to 2.0 are significant.
       II. The serum BUN is elevated.
    B. Hyperphosphatemia is a common finding.
    C. The serum calcium level may be increased or decreased.
    D. Hypoalbuminemia may be observed.
    E. Hyperlipemia and hyperamylasemia may occur secondary to reduced renal clearance or due to concurrent pancreatitis.
    F. Hypercholesterolemia is seen in many patients with nephrotic syndrome.
    G. Potassium levels can be increased, decreased or normal
4. Blood gas evaluation commonly reveals a metabolic acidosis.
5. Serologic testing for the commonly occurring infectious diseases in the area should be performed (most commonly leptospirosis).

Systemic blood pressure should be measured.

1. Hypertension in dogs is defined as: systolic pressure >180 mm Hg.
2. Hypertension in cats is defined as: systolic pressure >200 mm Hg.
    Abdominal radiographs—May demonstrate renal osteodystrophy, the presence of radiopaque uroliths or ureteroliths, and allow evaluation of renal size. Decreased renal excretory function may reduce the effectiveness of excretory urography (intravenous pyelogram – IVP) procedures.
    Abdominal ultrasonography—Is useful to evaluate renal size and to determine the presence of polycystic renal disease, hydronephrosis and urolithiasis. Facilitates renal aspiration or biopsy. Consider platelet counts and coagulation parameters prior to obtaining renal biopsies.

Differential diagnosis

1. Hypoadrenocorticism
2. Hyperadrenocorticism
3. Pituitary diabetes insipidus
4. Diabetes mellitus
5. Hyperthyroidism

Table 11.3 *Parameters that may help differentiate acute from chronic renal failure*

ARF	CRF
History	
Ischemic episode or toxicant exposure	Previous renal disease or renal insufficiency
	Longstanding polydipsia/polyuria
	Chronic weight loss, vomiting, diarrhea
Physical examination	
Good body condition	Poor body condition
Smooth, swollen, painful kidneys	Small, irregular kidneys
Relatively severe clinical signs for level of dysfunction	Relatively mild clinical signs for level of dysfunction
Clinicopathologic findings	
Normal or increased hematocrit	Osteodystrophy
Active urine sediment	Nonregenerative anemia
Normal to increased serum potassium	Inactive urine sediment
More severe metabolic acidosis	Normal to low serum potassium
	Less severe metabolic acidosis

From Grauer GF, Fluid therapy in acute and chronic renal failure. The veterinary clinics of North America: small animal practice, Advances in Fluid and Electrlyte Disorders, Vol. 28, No. 3, 1998 ©Elsevier, with permission.

6. Acute renal failure (Table 11.3)
7. Pyometra (pyometritis)
8. Chronic hepatic disease
9. Fanconi syndrome
10. Excessive sodium intake
11. Psychogenic water drinking.

Prognosis

The prognosis is guarded to poor for the long term. Cats tend to have a better and longer prognosis with CRF than dogs.

Treatment

1. Inform the client of the diagnosis, prognosis and cost of the treatment.
2. Obtain pretreatment blood and urine samples (cystocentesis preferred).
3. Provide unlimited access to water, unless it promotes acute vomiting.
4. Place an intravenous catheter.
5. Administer intravenous fluids:
   A. Correct dehydration within 6–8 hours and provide for losses.
   B. Institute diuresis at up to three times daily fluid requirements if indicated. Use LRS, Normosol®-R, Plasma-Lyte® or 0.9% NaCl to institute diuresis.
   C. If the patient is oliguric or anuric, see the previous section on acute renal failure.
6. Treat the underlying cause, if known; e.g. administer antibiotics for pyelonephritis (ampicillin is very safe for kidneys), antidote for toxins if known.
   A. Dosage adjustment of many antibiotics is recommended for patients with severe renal failure – see Appendices XII and XIII.

B. A simple method to calculate a beneficial dosage adjustment is to divide the normal dose by the patient's serum creatinine level.

7. Correct metabolic imbalances as necessary.
   A. Hyperphosphatemia
      I. Rehydrate the patient.
      II. Decrease the dietary protein and phosphorus intake.
         a. Dogs with renal disease should be fed a diet of 0.13–0.28% phosphorus, on a dry-matter basis.
         b. Cats with renal disease should be fed a diet of <1.0 mg/kcal of phosphorus, on a dry-matter basis.
      III. Consider the administration of oral phosphate binders, such as aluminum carbonate or aluminum hydroxide, before meals. Do not administer if patient is anorexic.
         Administer aluminum hydroxide 30–90 mg/kg/day PO.
   B. Hypercalcemia (especially >14 mg/dL total calcium or iCa >1.5 mg/dL)
      I. This usually resolves with fluid therapy.
      II. The preferred intravenous fluid is 0.9% NaCl.
      III. Administer furosemide, 5 mg/kg IV +/– CRI 5 mg/kg/h IV.
      IV. Bisphosphonates (ex. pamidronate): 1.3–2 mg/kg in 150 mL of 0.9% NaCl give over 2 hours (IV infusion). Dose patients once every 2 weeks.
      V. The administration of glucocorticoids is not as effective as in other causes of hypercalcemia.
   C. Hypocalcemia
      I. Restrict dietary phosphorus intake.
      II. Use Vitamin D and calcium supplements *only if* total calcium <10 mg/dL and phosphorus >5 mg/dL *and* calcium:phosphorus ratio <55.
         a. Calcium carbonate, 100 mg/kg/day
         b. Vitamin D 0.06 µg/kg/day
   D. Hypokalemia
      I. Supplement the intravenous fluids with potassium (see Table 11.2).
      II. Administer oral potassium, 2–5 mg potassium chloride per day.
   E. Hyperglycemia – treat the uremia.
   F. Hypercholesterolemia – treat the uremia.
   G. Hypermagnesemia – avoid magnesium-containing antacids. Typically not clinically significant
   H. Metabolic acidosis – treat if the plasma bicarbonate is <12 mmol/L or the pH of blood is <7.1 or these parameters do not improve within 8–12 hours of IV fluid therapy.
      I. If the patient can tolerate oral supplementation, give sodium bicarbonate, 8–12 mg/kg PO q8–12h. (One teaspoon of baking soda contains 2000 mg of bicarbonate. Usually administer 0.2–1 tsp sodium bicarbonate PO q8–12h.)
      II. If the patient is vomiting or NPO:
         Calculate bicarbonate deficit = 0.5 × body weight (kg) × (desired HCO_3 – current HCO_3).

Give $\frac{1}{3}$–$\frac{1}{2}$ of calculated dosage over 3–4 hours IV. Recheck HCO_3 and consider repeating dosage.

III. Monitor blood gas values. Stop bicarbonate administration when the plasma bicarbonate level is >14 mmol/L, blood pH >7.2, and total CO_2 >15 mmol/L.

IV. Monitor urine pH, maintain at pH of 6–7.5.

V. **Do not use sodium bicarbonate if the patient has concurrent hypertension, congestive heart failure, hypoproteinemia or oliguria.**

VI. Consider the administration of calcium lactate, calcium carbonate, or potassium bicarbonate if the patient does not have hyperkalemia.

VII. Use caution if hypocalcemia is present; the administration of sodium bicarbonate to patients with hypocalcemia may induce hypocalcemic tetany.

9. Treat nausea and gastric hyperacidity with H_2 blockers and gastric protectants.

A. Ranitidine (Zantac®), 0.5–2 mg/kg IV, PO q8h in dogs, 1–2 mg/kg IV, SC, PO q12h in cats

B. Famotidine (Pepcid®), 0.5–1 mg/kg IV or PO q12–24h

C. Cimetidine (Tagamet®), 2.5–5 mg/kg IV, IM, PO q8–12h

10. If the patient has oral ulcers, administer an H_2 blocker and also administer Xylocaine Viscous®, 2–10 mL, prior to feeding. Consider flushing mouth 2–3 times daily with mixture of lidocaine, diphenhydramine and aluminum hydroxide in equal parts to decrease pain and help in healing.

11. Control vomiting with antiemetics.

A. Metoclopramide (Reglan®), 0.2–0.3 mg/kg SC or IM q8h or 1 mg/kg/24h (0.04–0.08 mg/kg/h) CRI IV. If the patient is on metoclopramide, it is very important to palpate the abdomen every 2–4 h and closely monitor for intussusception. Avoid metoclopramide if a mechanical obstruction is suspected, or if the patient has a history of seizures.

B. Chlorpromazine (Thorazine®), 0.05–0.1mg/kg IV q4–6h as needed, 0.2–0.5 mg/kg SC, IM q6–8h, or 1mg/kg diluted in 1 mL of 0.9% NaCl and administered rectally q8h via a plastic catheter.

C. Prochlorperazine, 0.25–0.5 mg/kg SC, IM q6–8h.

D. Ondansetron (Zofran®), 0.1–0.2 mg/kg IV q6–12h.

E. Maropitant (Cerenia®), 1 mg/kg SQ q 24h or 2 mg/kg PO q24h. Do not administer for more than 4-5 days in succession.

F. Dolasetron (Anzemet®), 0.6 mg/kg IV q24h.

12. Ensure adequate nutrient intake for caloric needs. Use high-quality, low-quantity protein, restricted phosphorus diets as necessary to maintain BUN < 60 mg/dL.

A. The diet should also be low in phosphorus and sodium.

B. The minimum protein requirements for the dog with chronic renal disease are 2–2.2 g/kg/day, and for cats, 3.3–3.5 g/kg/day.

C. Dogs

    I. Feed a diet containing a minimum of 9–16% protein, depending upon the severity of clinical signs.

    II. Dogs with renal disease should be fed a diet of 0.13–0.28% phosphorus, on a dry-matter basis.

    III. Recommended diets include Hill's prescription diet k/d®, Purina NF©-formula diets and Royal Canin Renal LP©.

D. Cats

    I. Feed a diet containing a minimum of 21% protein.

    II. Cats with renal disease should be fed a diet of < 1.0 mg/kcal of phosphorus, on a dry-matter basis.

    III. Recommended diets include Hill's prescription diet feline k/d®, Purina NF®, or Royal Canin Renal LP modified®.

13. The administration of calcitriol (1,25-dihydroxyvitamin D), 1.5–3.5 ng/kg/day PO, combined with phosphorus restriction and oral phosphate binders may help to lower serum parathyroid hormone (PTH), with the following reported effects. Will help to control hypocalcemia associated with renal failure. Benefits include:

A. Decreased central nervous system depression, allowing the patient to appear brighter, more alert, and more interactive with the owner

B. Improved appetite

C. Increased physical activity

D. Lengthening of life span:

    I. Decreased susceptibility to infection

    II. Slowed progression of renal failure.

14. Human recombinant erythropoietin can be used in the treatment of non-regenerative anemia in dogs and cats secondary to chronic renal disease

A. The dose is 50–100 µg/kg SC two to three times per week until the patient's PCV is ≥30% in cats and ≥35% in dogs, then decrease administration to once every 4–5 days.

B. The hematocrit must be monitored as polycythemia may be induced.

C. Potentially fatal immune-mediated reactions may be induced with human erythropoietin.

D. Often given with iron concurrently.

15. Maintain systolic blood pressure at 120–160 mm Hg.

A. Restrict dietary sodium intake (commercial renal diets).

B. Pharmacologic management of hypertension. Suggested medications include:

    I. Hydralazine, 1–2 mg/kg PO q12h

    II. Diltiazem 0.5 mg/kg q6–8h in dogs and cats

    III. Amlodipine 0.625–1.25 mg PO q24h in cats, 0.1–0.25 mg/kg PO q12–24h in dogs

    IV. Emergency therapy – administer sodium nitroprusside, 1–5 mg/kg/min CRI IV in dogs and cats. Must monitor blood pressure continuously, ideally with invasive arterial blood pressure monitoring.

C. If the blood pressure remains elevated with single agent therapy, anti-hypertensive medications can be used in combination.

16. Appetite stimulation in patients with renal disease
    A. Offer different types of food.
    B. Warm, moist foods, or add warm water to dry foods.
    C. Add liquid enteral diets, clam juice, bouillon, dehydrated cottage cheese, garlic, carnitine, or brewer's yeast to the food.
    D. Allow the patient to eat anything it wants.
    E. Place a feeding tube.
    F. Chemical appetite stimulation in cats includes:
        I. Cyproheptadine, 2–4 mg/kg PO q12h
        II. Mirtazapine 3–4 mg/cat PO q72h
        III. Prednisone 0.25 mg/kg PO q24h.

PYELONEPHRITIS

Diagnosis

History—Since pyelonephritis is a common cause of acute uremia, owners will observe signs consistent with that condition including polyuria and polydipsia, vomiting, lethargy and inappetence. Owners may also feel that their pet in pain, specifically arching its back and reluctant to move around or 'walking on eggshells.' However, in some cases, the clinical signs associated with this condition are extremely vague and therefore it is difficult to diagnose. Always question the owner as to whether a fever was documented at any point in the past.

Physical exam—Assess the hydration status and perform a full physical examination. Commonly, patients have a fever when examined. One finding consistent with pyelonephritis is an elevated body temperature either at the time of the exam or historically. During abdominal palpation, be sure to palpate the kidneys for signs of pain, asymmetry, enlargement, or irregular contours. Be aware that pain in the kidney region can mimic spinal pain in the T3–L3 region. Palpate the urinary bladder to assess distention, bladder wall thickness, the presence of cystic calculi, or pain upon palpation. In dogs, perform a rectal examination to detect prostatic disease, urethral masses, or urethral calculi. Observe ambulation and micturition. Palpate the urinary bladder after micturition to assess residual bladder volume. Consider passing a urethral catheter to quantify and evaluate the urine.

Laboratory evaluation—
1. Perform a CBC, serum chemistry and urinalysis prior to any treatment. Consistent findings would be an inflammatory leukogram +/– a left shift, azotemia and indications of pyuria. An animal does not have to have ANY of these findings with pyelonephritis.
2. Collect urine aseptically or in a sterile fashion to facilitate culturing the urine. Typically, bacteria cultured from the bladder will be the same as that in the kidney. The best sample to reflect kidney infection would be obtained by pyelocentesis (typically ultrasound-guided and under anesthesia or deep sedation). In most cases, treatment is initiated for any bacteria in the bladder and pyelocentesis is only pursued when cultures from the bladder are negative and kidney

infection is still strongly suspected or there is a strong suspicion that different organisms are present in each location.

3. Abdominal imaging – radiographs can be performed and may show indications of renomegaly that could be consistent with pyelonephritis. Abdominal ultrasound is the diagnostic of choice. Dilation of the renal pelvices +/– the proximal portion of the ureter (prior to any fluid therapy) is consistent with and suggestive of pyelonephritis. A lack of renal pelvic / ureteral dilation does *not* rule out pyelonephritis.

4. Excretory urography can be considered but has largely been superceded by ultrasound. Dilation of the renal pelvices and / or proximal ureter is consistent with pyelonephritis. There may also be decreased opacity during the nephrogram and pyelogram phases or prolongation of dye retention in the renal pelvis. Excretory urography can be normal in patients with pyelonephritis.

5. Predisposing causes of pyelonephritis include anatomic abnormalities (ectopic ureters, vaginal strictures), kidney or bladder urolithiasis or neoplasia, an indwelling urinary catheter, vesicoureteral reflex, abnormal micturition due to lower or upper motor neuron disorders, glucosuria, or systemic immunosuppression (iatrogenic or secondary to hyperadrenocorticism). Most of these causes can be determined from patient history, bloodwork / urinalysis, and imaging of the kidneys / bladder. However, contrast studies or a neurologic examination may be required to ensure normal urine flow.

Differential diagnosis

1. Other causes of thoracolumbar pain including intervertebral disc disease, discospondylitis, a spinal tumor, or meningitis
2. Acute renal failure
3. Chronic renal failure
4. Other causes of fever including infection of another organ system, sterile inflammatory disease (typically immune-mediated disease) or pyometra
5. Pre-renal azotemia
6. Post-renal azotemia
7. Glomerulonephropathies
8. Nephrolithiasis
9. Neoplasia
10. Trauma

Prognosis

In most cases, if pyelonephritis is diagnosed early and appropriate antibiotic therapy is initiated, animals respond well to treatment. In cases with resistant bacteria or other predisposing causes that cannot be remedied, it can be difficult to completely clear up infections and avoid re-infection during treatment or immediately thereafter.

Treatment

1. Inform the client of the differential diagnoses, prognosis and cost of the treatment.
2. Hospitalize the patient to provide intravenous fluids and other supportive care. Provide fluid therapy with a balanced electrolyte crystalloid replacement fluid for diuresis and rehydration.
3. Administer prophylactic intravenous antibiotic therapy with an antibiotic with good renal penetration and clearance through the kidneys. Antibiotics include amoxicillin with clavulanic acid, fluoroquinolones, trimethoprim-sulfa or aminoglycosides. Antibiotics are usually continued for a minimum of 4 weeks. Change antibiotics based on results of culture. It is important to re-culture the urine and / or perform pyelocentesis in order to ensure that the infection has been completely cleared.
4. Identify and treat any underlying predisposing factors.
5. Animals can be sent home on oral antibiotics once their fever has broken and they are eating and drinking.

HEMATURIA AND HEMOGLOBINURIA

Diagnosis

History—The owner may observe bloody urine, lethargy, anorexia, vomiting, stranguria, dysuria, pollakiuria, or urinary incontinence. If the hematuria is accompanied by stranguria, dysuria, or pollakiuria, lower urinary tract infection should be suspected. If the patient exhibits lethargy, depression, anorexia, diarrhea, vomiting, weight loss, fever or abdominal pain, upper urinary tract disease should be suspected. Spontaneous hemorrhage that is not associated with voiding may indicate genital tract disease or trauma.

Physical exam—Assess the hydration status. Palpate the kidneys for signs of pain, asymmetry, enlargement, or irregular contours. Be aware that pain in the kidney region can mimic spinal pain in the T3–L3 region. Palpate the urinary bladder to assess distention, bladder wall thickness, the presence of cystic calculi, or pain upon palpation. In dogs, perform a rectal examination to detect prostatic disease, urethral masses, or urethral calculi. In larger female dogs, perform a digital vaginal examination and a visual vaginal examination with the aid of a vaginal speculum. Observe ambulation and micturition. Palpate the urinary bladder after micturition to assess residual bladder volume. Pass a urethral catheter to quantify residual urine volumes and to assess patency of the urethra. Cystocentesis may help to differentiate lower urinary tract or genital tract disease from upper urinary tract disease.

Perform a thorough physical examination. Evaluate mucous membrane color, splenic size, and lymph nodes. Look for other signs of hemorrhage, pallor, icterus, petechiation or ecchymosis.

Laboratory evaluation—

1. Obtain pretreatment blood and urine samples.
2. Perform a CBC and serum biochemical profile with electrolytes.

3. Perform an ACT or PT / PTT on patients with a suspected bleeding disorder.
  A. Activated coagulation time – the normal ACT for a dog is 60–110 seconds, and for a cat is 50–75 seconds. Prolongation of the ACT indicates abnormalities of the secondary coagulation cascade (deficiency or malfunction of the clotting factors). The ACT tubes should be warmed to 37°C prior to and during the test procedure. Two tubes should be used. A total of 2 mL of blood is taken by clean venipuncture with rapid aspiration from a large vein, directly into the first tube with a vacutainer system, or quickly transferred from a syringe into the first tube and discarded. Without removing the needle from the vein when using a vacutainer system, additional blood is placed into the second tube and the test is performed. The time interval from injection of 2 mL of blood into the ACT tube until the first visible appearance of clot formation is the ACT.
  B. In many clinics, benchside PT / PTT analyzers are available. Similar to the ACT, blood should be aspirated via a clean venipuncture from a large vein. Blood is used to fill a sodium citrate tube (blue top tube) either via a vacutainer system or from a syringe. It is important that the tubes are filled completely in order to allow for appropriate dilution and accurate results.
4. Perform a urinalysis – differentiate hemoglobinuria from hematuria by centrifugation of a urine sample. In hemoglobinuria, the urine will retain its deep red color.
5. Submit a urine sample, preferably obtained by cystocentesis, for urine culture and sensitivity testing.

Abdominal radiographs—Evaluate abdominal radiographs. Survey films may not be diagnostic. In male dogs, always take a lateral caudal abdominal radiograph with the rear legs pulled cranially in order to allow for complete evaluation of the urethra as it exits the pelvis and extends into the penis. Consider performing a retrograde urethrogram or contrast cystography. Look for signs of trauma, abdominal distention, free fluid in the peritoneal cavity, masses or calculi on the radiographs.
Abdominal ultrasonography—Beneficial to better elucidate intravesicular masses and evaluate the kidneys for morphologic changes. The majority of the time, ultrasound is the diagnostic of choice for bladder neoplasia.
Cystotomy—It is helpful to obtain bladder wall biopsies for histopathology and bladder wall cultures.

Differential diagnosis

1. Upper urinary tract (renal) hematuria
   A. Glomerulonephropathies
   B. Infections (pyelonephritis)
   C. Nephrolithiasis
   D. Neoplasia
   E. Renal cystic disease
   F. Trauma
   G. Idiopathic

2. Lower urinary tract hematuria
   A. Infections
   B. Inflammation
   C. Cystic calculi
   D. Neoplasia
   E. Trauma
   F. Cyclophosphamide-induced sterile cystitis
3. Prostatic hematuria
   A. Infection
   B. Neoplasia
   C. Hyperplasia
4. Hematuria secondary to a systemic condition
   A. Coagulopathies including anticoagulant rodenticide toxicity
   B. Thrombocytopenia
   C. Thrombocytopathia
   D. Ehrlichiosis
5. Hemoglobinuria
   A. Autoimmune hemolytic anemia
   B. Transfusion reaction
   C. Heat stroke
   D. Splenic torsion
   E. Post-caval syndrome (dirofilariasis)
   F. DIC
   G. Rattlesnake envenomation
   H. Babesiosis
6. Myoglobinuria – due to muscle damage

Prognosis

The prognosis is good to guarded, depending upon the underlying etiology.

Treatment

1. Inform the client of the differential diagnoses, prognosis and cost of the treatment.
2. Perform cystocentesis or urethral catheterization to obtain urine samples. Cystocentesis must be performed with extreme care since the integrity of the urinary bladder wall at this time is often questionable. Do not perform cystocentesis if there is concern of a neoplastic mass in the bladder; it is possible to seed the abdomen with tumor cells via a cystocentesis.
3. Perform retrograde urohydropropulsion of urethral calculi if necessary.
4. Hospitalize the patient to monitor urine output.
5. Attempt to diagnose the underlying etiology and treat appropriately. Administer vitamin K_1 for treatment of anticoagulant rodenticide toxicities, corticosteroids for immune-mediated disorders, perform surgery to remove calculi, etc.

6. Administer intravenous fluid therapy with a balanced electrolyte crystalloid replacement fluid for diuresis and promotion of potassium excretion. In cases associated with obstruction, fluid therapy may need to be delayed until after the obstruction has been relieved.
7. Administer antibiotics if the patient has an infectious disease or peri-operatively.
8. Patients with myoglobinuria from excessive exertion, such as occurs in hunting dogs or other causes of excessive muscle damage like dog fights, may have dark urine that is brownish rather than red tinged. Treatment includes the administration of intravenous fluids until the urine clears. Myoglobin is nephrotoxic so fluid therapy should induce diuresis and renal function should be monitored via bloodwork.

FELINE LOWER URINARY TRACT DISEASE (FLUTD) (NOT OBSTRUCTED)

Etiology

The disease is usually idiopathic and involves inflammation of the bladder wall. This inflammation in turn changes the pH of the urine and can lead to crystalluria, which perpetuates bladder wall inflammation. Alternatively, crystalluria in some cats will secondarily lead to inflammation of the bladder wall and therefore continued crystal formation. In many cases, FLUTD is linked to environmental stress in cats (new pets, intercat aggression, new people in household, etc.) Cats will become obstructed secondarily to FLUTD when plugs of mucous and inflammatory cells +/− crystals become lodged in the urethra. An increased incidence of FLUTD has been shown in indoor only multi-cat household cats, those that are obese, and in cats eating a high-magnesium diet. Bouts of FLUTD typically last 7–14 days unless complicated by urinary calculi or obstruction (mainly male cats).

Diagnosis

History—The owner may observe hematuria, dysuria, stranguria, lethargy, decreased appetite and excessive licking of the perineal region. The patient may urinate in inappropriate places, often on cool smooth surfaces such as tile, sinks, or bathtubs.
Physical exam—Pain may be detected upon caudal abdominal palpation. Usually at least a small stream of urine can easily (cautiously) be expressed but the bladder is typically very small. The cat is alert and responsive. The heart rate is normal. Femoral pulses are strong and regular.
Laboratory evaluation—
1. Evaluate the serum BUN, creatinine, potassium, glucose, PCV and TS as a minimum database. If the client allows, evaluate a CBC and complete biochemical profile with electrolytes.
2. Perform a urinalysis to check for bactiuria, crystalluria, casts, etc.

Table 11.4 Criteria for interpreting quantitative urine culture results obtained from cats

	Level of bacteriuria (organisms/mL) indicating	
Urine collection method	Contamination	Infection
Cystocentesis	<1000	>1000
Catheterization	<1000	≥1000
Voiding	<10 000	≥10 000

From Lees GE, Bacterial urinary tract infections. The veterinary clinics of North America, Small Animal Practice, Disorders of the Feline Lower Urinary Tract I, Biology and Pathophysiology, Vol. 26, No. 2, 1996. ©Elsevier, with permission.

3. Submit urine obtained by cystocentesis for bacterial culture and sensitivity (Table 11.4).
4. Perform serology tests for FeLV and FIV.

Abdominal radiography—May be beneficial for patients with chronic or recurrent FLUTD in order to look for uroliths.
Abdominal ultrasonography—May be beneficial for patients with chronic or recurrent LUTD to look for radiodense uroliths and bladder masses.

Prognosis

The prognosis is typically good for resolution of individual bouts unless cats become obstructed. Patients often have recurrent signs.

Treatment

1. Inform the client of the diagnosis, prognosis and cost of treatment. Give the client an education handout.
2. If the patient has an elevated BUN, creatinine or PCV, administer a balanced electrolyte crystalloid replacement fluid, such as LRS or Normosol®-R, either SC or IV.
3. Administer antibiotics based on urinalysis and urine culture and sensitivity results.
   Antibiotics that are commonly used to treat urinary tract infections in cats include:
   A. Amoxicillin and clavulanate, 12.5 mg/kg q12h
   B. Cephalexin, 20 mg/kg q8h
   C. Enrofloxacin, 2.5 mg/kg q12h or 5 mg/kg q24h
   D. Trimethoprim and sulfonamide, 15 mg/kg q12h
4. The administration of amitriptyline, 5–10 mg/cat/q24h PO, may be beneficial in some cases and is believed to reduce bladder wall inflammation. This medication is bitter to the taste and often leads to hypersalivation in cats.
5. For longer term maintenance, glucosamine supplementation can be pursued to improve the health of the mucous layer lining the bladder.
6. Meloxicam 0.1 mg/kg PO as a single dose is often used in an attempt to reduce bladder wall inflammation. Do not use this medication in cats

that have concurrent metabolic abnormalities (specifically liver or renal) or in animals that are not eating well. Corticosteroid administration is currently not recommended as an anti-inflammatory.

7. If crystalluria is observed, feeding a special diet formulated to reduce crystal formation is indicated. Examples of diets include Hill's Science Diet c/d®, Purina UR® and Royal Canin Urinary SO®. However, some veterinarians believe that such diets will help in all cases of FLUTD.

8. Hospitalize the patient for observation or advise the owner that it is critical to observe the patient closely in the next few days' time to ensure that the cat is continuing to urinate. Be sure to explain to the owner that the (male) cat may develop a urethral obstruction and require catheterization at any time. It might be prudent to inform them of the estimate of charges to relieve the obstruction for the cat at this time to avoid surprises for the client later.

9. Monitor closely for urinary bladder distention, stranguria and lack of urination, which could indicate urethral obstruction.

10. Upon discharge, dispense the appropriate antibiotics if indicated and a therapeutic diet +/– a bladder wall anti-inflammatory drug.

FELINE LOWER URINARY TRACT DISEASE (FLUTD) (URETHRAL OBSTRUCTION)

Etiology

The etiology of a urethral obstruction is typically a plug made of mucous and inflammatory cells formed during FLUTD. In some cases, the obstruction is a calculus and in still other cases, it is believed that urethral spasm is the true cause of the cat's inability to urinate.

Diagnosis

History—The owner may observe stranguria +/– vocalization during attempts at voiding, dysuria, lack of urination, hematuria, inappropriate voiding, vocalization, vomiting, lethargy, aggressiveness and / or pain when the abdomen is handled. The owner often presents the cat because of perceived 'constipation'.

Physical exam—Perform a thorough physical examination. Assess the mental state. Evaluate the hydration status and cardiovascular status. Auscultate the heart for arrhythmias. Palpate femoral pulses for strength and character. Palpate the abdomen for a distended urinary bladder that cannot be expressed (unless the bladder has ruptured), thickened urinary bladder wall, or the presence of cystic calculi. Examine the penis and preputial area. The penis may be edematous, hyperemic, cyanotic or necrotic. In some cases, visible crystalline material can be seen obstructing the tip of the penis.

The patient may be severely depressed or comatose if the obstruction is chronic. Bradycardia, hypothermia, hyperpnea, halitosis and pale mucous membranes with a prolonged capillary refill time indicate chronic obstruction, which is more severe.

Laboratory evaluation—

1. The emergency minimum database that should be evaluated includes:
   A. PCV / TS
   B. Azostick BUN, or serum BUN and serum creatinine
   C. Electrolytes (especially potassium)
   D. Serum glucose
   E. Venous blood gases – metabolic acidosis is the most common acid–base disturbance
2. When time allows, evaluate a routine minimum database:
   A. CBC
   B. Serum biochemical profile
   C. Urinalysis with culture and cytology
3. Perform urolith analysis if the patient has urolithiasis to determine the type of calculus.

ECG evaluation—Lead II is sufficient. Abnormalities due to poor perfusion and hyperkalemia include a lack of P-waves, a wide QRS, a prolonged QT interval, and tall spiked T-waves. These changes can progress to atrial standstill and eventually ventricular arrest.
Abdominal radiographs—May be helpful to evaluate urolithiasis, cystic neoplasia and other abnormalities. Most may be detected on standard radiographs or possibly with the aid of contrast studies.
Abdominal ultrasound—May be useful to evaluate the bladder lumen as well as the proximal urethra and kidneys.

Prognosis

The prognosis is good to grave, depending on the presence or absence of vomiting, hypothermia, obtundation, azotemia / uremia or cardiac arrhythmias.

Treatment

1. Inform the client of the diagnosis, prognosis, cost of treatment and the possibility of recurrence.
2. Place an intravenous catheter.
3. Evaluate an ECG. If the patient has bradycardia and hyperkalemia, the heart will usually return to normal once the obstruction is relieved and fluid administration is underway.
4. Treatment of hyperkalemia. The only treatment that will reverse hyperkalemia is to unblock the cat so expedite that process.
   A. If hyperkalemia is mild, up to 7 mEq/L, treat with LRS, Normosol®-R or PlasmaLyte and work on relieving the obstruction.
   B. If hyperkalemia is moderate, 7–8 mEq/L, consider using 0.9% NaCl as the intravenous fluid choice and work on relieving the obstruction.
   C. If the serum potassium level exceeds 7.5–8 mEq/L and / or the patient shows evidence of bradycardia or ECG abnormalities, additional therapy is indicated:
      I. Administer 10% calcium gluconate, 0.2–0.5 mL/kg IV over 15 minutes while monitoring the ECG. The effect lasts about 10–15

minutes. While this protects the heart from the cardiotoxic effects of potassium, the serum potassium level is not decreased, so an additional therapy is also indicated and / or the patient needs to be unblocked.

II. Administer sodium bicarbonate, 0.5–1 mEq/kg, slow IV over 2–5 minutes then infuse an additional 1–2 mEq/kg slowly IV over 30–60 minutes. The serum potassium level is decreased within minutes, and the effect may last up to several hours.

III. An alternative method is to administer 20% glucose, 1–2 mL/kg IV over 30–60 minutes. Glucose administration will stimulate endogenous insulin production and force potassium into cells to reduce serum potassium levels.

IV. If desired, insulin administration may follow glucose administration. Administer regular insulin, 0.2–0.4 U/kg IV and 50% dextrose, 2 g (4 mL per unit of dextrose per unit of administered insulin). Administer IV fluids with 2.5% dextrose to the patient.

V. Terbutaline can also be used to temporarily reduce serum potassium levels. The recommended dose for dogs is 0.2 mg/kg PO q8–12h and for cats 0.625 mg PO q8–12h.

   D. Monitor serum electrolytes q2–4h as needed.

5. Initiate intravenous fluid therapy. Start LRS, Normosol®-R or Plasma-Lyte® at the rate of 10 mL/kg/h or more, depending upon urine output.

A. To calculate the hydration deficit (mild dehydration is 5%, moderate is 8%, severe or shock is 12%): % dehydration × BW (kg) = liters of fluid needed.

B. If the patient is mildly dehydrated, administer the hydration deficit over 12 hours.

C. If the patient is moderately dehydrated, administer the hydration deficit within 4 hours.

D. If the patient is severely dehydrated or in hypovolemic shock, administer the hydration deficit over 1–2 hours or faster.

E. In addition to correcting dehydration, administer fluids at 1.5–3 times maintenance rates of 1–2 mL/kg/h. Keep up with post-obstructive diuresis losses and match 'ins' with 'outs'.

F. The fluid rate for each individual patient will vary but depends on the patient's vital signs, degree of azotemia, urine production, hydration and mentation.

G. Monitor closely to avoid fluid overload and medullary washout.

6. Do not attempt to relieve the urethral obstruction by passing a urethral catheter without anesthesia unless the patient is severely obtunded to stuporous / comatose! Do not attempt to express the urinary bladder until the obstruction is relieved. Some veterinarians believe in a therapeutic cystocentesis prior to placing a urinary catheter to relieve the pressure in the bladder and thus facilitate urethra catheterization.

7. The general anesthetic utilized depends on the condition of the cat:

A. If the patient is extremely depressed, attempt urethral catheterization without anesthesia

B. Isoflurane via box induction or mask induction

C. Diazepam, 0.5 mg/kg, and ketamine, 5–10 mg IV or IM

D. Propofol, 2–6 mg/kg IV given to effect.

8. Relieve the urethral obstruction by gently massaging the penis between the thumb and forefinger. Extend the penis caudally to make the urethra as straight as possible. Avoid inflicting iatrogenic trauma to the penis or prepuce. Gently insert an open-ended 3.5 Fr. polypropylene Tomcat catheter and flush the urethra with sterile saline or LRS. If the Tomcat catheter cannot be passed up the urethra, gently insert an ophthalmic lacrimal duct flush cannula.

9. If unable to relieve the obstruction, clip, prep, and perform cystocentesis, then reattempt urethral catheterization.

A. Use a 22-gauge needle attached to a flexible intravenous extension set which is attached to a large capacity syringe (20–60 mL).

B. Insert the needle through the ventral or ventrolateral wall of the bladder.

C. Direct the needle through the bladder wall at a 45° angle with the tip of the needle tilted away from the trigone region.

10. If the obstruction is very easy to relieve and a good stream of apparently normal urine is obtained, express the bladder, flush with sterile saline and remove the urethral catheter. Replace the Tomcat catheter with a red rubber catheter for longer term catheterization (usually 12–24 hours).

11. If the obstruction was difficult to relieve, the urine stream is of a poor size, the cat is uremic, the urine is very bloody, the urine contains large amounts of crystalline debris, or detrusor dysfunction secondary to bladder overdistention is present, suture a 3.5 Fr. red rubber urethral catheter in place for at least 24 hours (Fig. 11.1). Measure the distance to the bladder prior to passing the red rubber urethral catheter to avoid iatrogenic bladder trauma.

12. Flush the urinary bladder with LRS or sterile 0.9% NaCl until the urine is clear. Empty the bladder. Mark 'Time 0' on the medical record to facilitate monitoring of urine output.

13. If the urinary bladder does not distend when the bladder is flushed with sterile saline, consider that either a urinary bladder rupture or a urethral tear has occurred. Perform contrast cystography to diagnose this condition. Surgical repair may be indicated but an indwelling urinary catheter left in place for several days' time can be used to keep the bladder from becoming distended and allow for bladder wall or urethral healing without surgery and / or allow for stabilization of the patient's metabolic condition prior to surgery.

14. Connect the urinary catheter to a sterile urine collection apparatus and maintain a closed urinary collection system. Monitor urine output and adjust fluid therapy as needed. Post-obstruction diuresis may occur wherein cats produce profound amounts of urine. Make sure to match intravenous fluid amounts with urine fluid production until the post-obstructive diuresis resolves (usually at least 12 hours but can be several days). Urine output must be at least 1–2 mL/kg/h. Monitor for acute renal failure.

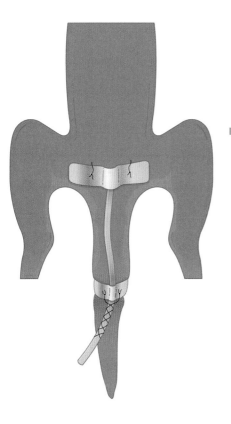

FIG 11.1 **Securing an indwelling urethral catheter in a male cat with urethral obstruction.** Note two structures are placed through the skin of the perineal region laterally to the prepuce and through a piece of tape securely fastened around the catheter as it leaves the prepuce. Another piece of tape is used to secure the catheter to the tail, and a Chinese 'fingerlock' suture is used to secure the catheter to this piece of tape.

A. If the patient is not producing enough urine through the catheter (<1–2 mL/kg/hr), check the patency and positioning of the urethral catheter. Catheters may become dislodged, punctured or kinked.

B. Administer a fluid bolus of 10–15 mL/kg IV if the patient is still dehydrated or normovolemic.

C. Administer furosemide, 1–2 mg/kg IV, or mannitol, 0.25–0.5 g/kg IV if the patient is fully hydrated and is oliguric or anuric.

D. If the patient has fluid overload, stop the intravenous fluids, administer furosemide (1–2 mg/kg/ IV) and consider initiating a furosemide CRI at the rate of 0.5–2 µg/kg/h. Alternatively, consider administering mannitol 0.5 g/kg IV as a bolus to facilitate urine production.

15. Provide supportive nursing care. Many cats require an Elizabethan collar to prevent dislodgement of the urethral catheter.

16. The administration of antibiotics is controversial. Amoxicillin 10–20 mg/kg SC, then PO q12h is often administered if an infection is strongly suspected or proved via culture. There is concern that administering antibiotics while an indwelling urinary catheter is in place will create resistant organisms. It is best to wait to give antibiotics until the urinary catheter has been removed unless it is believed that

the patient will not do well without them (i.e. in cases of pyelonephritis or other systemic infectious disease).

17. If considerable inflammation exists, administer meloxicam 0.1 mg/kg PO q24h. Do not use this medication if there are concerns about renal function or the patient is dehydrated.

18. Provide nutritional support. After recovering from sedation, offer Hill's prescription diet feline c/d® Purina UR®, Royal Canin Urinary SO® or other similar diets and distilled water.

19. Recheck the PCV, TP, serum BUN, serum creatinine, serum potassium and serum glucose levels in 24 hours. Re-check potassium levels sooner (i.e. 1–2 hours after unblocking an animal) if they were greater than 7.5–8 mEq/L to ensure that they have normalized.

20. Post-obstructive diuresis may lead to hypokalemia and may require potassium supplementation. If that condition occurs, monitor potassium levels daily and supplement potassium as needed.

21. Remove the urethral catheter when the urine appears visually clear of hemorrhage and post-obstructive diuresis is not present. In cases where neither of these conditions occurred, catheterization is usually recommended for 12–24 hours prior to removal of the catheter. Keep the cat hospitalized for an additional 12–24 hours for observation to ensure that he does not immediately re-obstruct.

22. Culture the urine at the time of urethral catheter removal by aspirating 3–5 mL of urine through the urethral catheter, discarding it, and then aspirating 7–10 mL of urine through the urethral catheter for testing. Alternatively, collecting a cystocentesis sample after the urinary catheter has been removed is probably a more representative sample for culture. It is rare to have true infection in the bladder after urethral obstruction.

23. To decrease urethral spasm, if no obstruction is present, administer:
    A. Prazosin 0.25–0.5 mg/cat PO q8–12h
    B. Phenoxybenzamine (Dibenzylene®) 2.5–5 mg PO q12–24h.

24. When the patient is discharged, dispense the appropriate antibiotic as indicated by the urine culture for 7–14 days of treatment and also dispense a therapeutic prescription diet.

25. Repeat the urine culture 7–14 days after the antibiotic therapy is complete to confirm a negative urine culture.

CANINE UROLITHIASIS

Etiology

Magnesium ammonium phosphate uroliths in dogs are usually the result of a bacterial urinary tract infection. Dalmatians and English Bulldogs are predisposed to urate urolithiasis due to metabolic abnormalities. Animals with portal vascular anomalies are predisposed to the development of urate urolithiasis. Hyperparathyroidism may lead to calcium phosphate uroliths. Silica uroliths occur in animals fed diets with large amounts of soybean hulls or corn gluten. Calcium phosphate uroliths occur more often in animals with excessive dietary calcium or phosphorus intake. Calcium oxalate, sterile struvite and silica urolithiasis formation are often idiopathic.

Diagnosis

History—Uroliths are found most often in the urinary bladder or urethra. Less than 10% of uroliths are found in the renal pelvis. In dogs with nephrolithiasis or ureterolithiasis, the owner may observe hematuria, sublumbar or abdominal discomfort, depression, anorexia, and vomiting. The owner may observe dysuria, hematuria, stranguria, pollakiuria, cloudy urine, or notice a foul odor to the urine in dogs with cystourolithiasis or urethral urolithiasis.

Physical exam—Perform a thorough physical exam. Assess the mental state. Evaluate the hydration status and cardiovascular status. Auscultate the heart for arrhythmias. Palpate femoral pulses for strength and character. Carefully palpate the abdomen. Evaluate the renal size and shape. Monitor for a pain response during renal palpation. Evaluate the size of the urinary bladder (unless the bladder has ruptured), bladder wall thickness and feel for obvious cystouroliths. Examine the penis and preputial area. Perform a rectal examination in all dogs and palpate the extrapelvic urethra in male dogs. During an attempt to pass a urethral catheter, the feeling of passing through grit or sand may be felt and inability to pass a urethral catheter indicates urethral obstruction.

Characteristics of canine uroliths (Fig. 11.2)—

1. Struvite (magnesium ammonium phosphate) uroliths
   A. There is an increased incidence in Miniature Schnauzers, Miniature Poodles, Bichon Frises and Cocker Spaniels.
   B. 80–97% of the uroliths that occur in female dogs are struvite.
   C. They are radiopaque.
   D. The urine is usually alkaline.
   E. There is a high incidence of concurrent urinary tract infection, especially with *Staphylococcus* and *Proteus* spp.
   F. Dogs less than 1 year of age that develop uroliths usually have struvite uroliths.
2. Calcium oxalate uroliths
   A. There is an increased incidence in Miniature Schnauzers, Miniature Poodles, Bichon Frises, Yorkshire Terriers, Lhasa Apsos and Shih Tzus.
   B. There is an increased incidence in male dogs.
   C. They are radiopaque.
   D. The urine is usually acidic to neutral.
   E. A contributing factor may be the presence of hypercalcemia.
3. Cystine uroliths
   A. There is an increased incidence in Chihuahuas, Yorkshire Terriers, Dachshunds, English Bulldogs, Basset Hounds, Mastiffs and Rottweilers.
   B. There is an increased incidence in male dogs.
   C. Radiodensity of the uroliths is variable, but they are most often radiolucent.
   D. The urine is usually acidic.
4. Ammonium acid urate uroliths
   A. There is an increased incidence in Dalmatians and English Bulldogs.

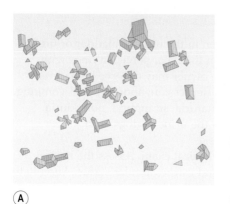

A

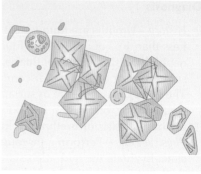

B

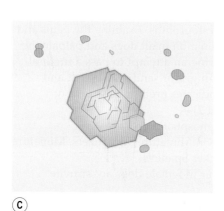

C

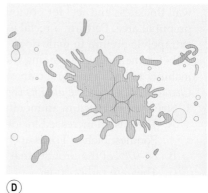

D

FIG 11.2 **Urinary crystals:** (A) struvite, (B) calcium oxalate, (C) cystine and (D) ammonium acid urate.

B. There is an increased incidence in male dogs.
C. The uroliths are radiolucent in relation to the surrounding tissue densities.
D. The urine is usually acidic to neutral.
E. Dogs with severe hepatic insufficiency, such as patients with portosystemic shunts, have an increased incidence.

5. Silicate uroliths
   A. There is an increased incidence in Golden Retrievers, Labrador Retrievers and German Shepherds.
   B. There is an increased incidence in male dogs.
   C. Radiodensity of the uroliths is variable, but they are most often radiolucent.
   D. The urine is usually acidic to neutral.
   E. A possible predisposing factor is a high dietary intake of silicates, as found in corn gluten and soybean hulls.

Laboratory evaluation—
1. Urinalysis may indicate inflammation of the urinary tract (proteinuria, hematuria, pyuria, and increased numbers of epithelial cells).
2. Measure urine pH.

3. Evaluate a urine sediment sample microscopically. Urolithiasis may occur without crystalluria, and crystalluria may be observed in the absence of urolithiasis. However, if both conditions are present, the composition of the uroliths is usually the same as that of the crystals observed in the urine. Be aware that exceptions do occur.
4. Submit a urine sample, preferably obtained by cystocentesis, for bacterial culture.
5. A small section of the urolith and the bladder mucosa should be submitted for bacterial culture if a cystotomy is performed to remove cystouroliths. Submit an entire stone(s) for analysis and identification if removed surgically.
6. Evaluate a CBC for signs of dehydration or infection.
7. Evaluate a serum biochemical profile for signs of post-renal or renal azotemia, hyperkalemia and other abnormalities.
8. Evaluate the acid–base balance of the patient. Metabolic acidosis is the most common abnormality.
9. Perform abdominocentesis if a urinary tract rupture is suspected. Measure the creatinine level of the peritoneal fluid and compare it to the patient's serum creatinine level. If the peritoneal creatinine level is higher than that of serum, it indicates that urine is leaking into the abdominal cavity and exploratory surgery may be necessary. Also measure the peritoneal fluid potassium level versus that of the serum. If the peritoneal potassium level is higher than that of serum, it is consistent with urine leakage.

ECG evaluation—May reveal bradycardia and signs compatible with hyperkalemia if there is uroabdomen (flattened P-waves, a prolonged PR interval, widened QRS complexes, and tall or spiked T-waves).
Abdominal radiography—May reveal nephrolithiasis or urolithiasis. Double-contrast-enhanced cystography or retrograde positive contrast-enhanced urethrography should be performed in patients which exhibit the clinical signs of urolithiasis but lack visibly radiopaque uroliths on plain radiographs. If the abdominal contents possess a ground glass appearance and the urinary bladder is not visible on the plain films, a urinary tract rupture with free abdominal fluid should be suspected.
Abdominal ultrasonography—May be helpful to confirm the presence of cystouroliths, nephrolithiasis, hydronephrosis, ureterolithiasis, urethral obstruction and dilation, urolithiasis, or the presence of free fluid (urine) in the abdominal cavity.

Differential diagnosis

1. Nephrolithiasis – Renal cell carcinoma, transitional cell carcinoma, embryonal nephroblastoma, renal metastatic neoplasia (hemangiosarcoma, melanoma, mast cell tumors, carcinomas), pyelonephritis
2. Ureterolithiasis – ureteral leiomyosarcoma, leiomyoma, extension of bladder neoplasia, compression by intra-abdominal neoplasia, ureteral blood clots, ureteral strictures

3. Cystolithiasis – cystitis (sterile or bacterial) cystic neoplasia (including transitional cell carcinoma, rhabdomyosarcoma, fibrosarcoma, adenocarcinoma, and hemangiosarcoma)
4. Urethrolithiasis – mucous plug, blood clot, urethritis, fractured os penis, urethral foreign body

Prognosis

Recurrence is common. The prognosis depends on the degree and duration of the obstruction and the severity of concurrent renal disease. A permanent pelvic urethrostomy may be beneficial to decrease the severity of life-threatening urethral obstruction.

Treatment

1. Inform the client of the diagnosis, prognosis and cost of the treatment.
2. Attempt urethral catheterization under deep sedation or general anesthesia to relieve abdominal distention.
3. If urethral catheterization is unsuccessful and the urinary bladder distention must be immediately relieved, perform cystocentesis.
   A. Use a 22–20-gauge over-the-needle catheter.
   B. After placing the catheter into the bladder, remove the needle and attach extension tubing with a three-way stopcock. Carefully aspirate urine, avoiding cystic iatrogenic trauma.
   C. Re-attempt urethral catheterization.
4. If urethral catheterization is unsuccessful and the uroliths are located proximal to the os penis, perform urethrohydropropulsion.
   A. Evaluate the shape and size of the uroliths in relation to the patient size. Smooth uroliths pass easier than those with irregular surfaces. The urolith must be smaller than the smallest diameter of the patient's urethra.
   B. Assess the size of the urinary bladder.
   C. Administer sedatives with analgesic and muscle-relaxing effects or administer general anesthesia.
   D. Pass a soft flexible catheter aseptically into the urethra until contact is made with the urolith.
   E. Occlude the urethral orifice while injecting sterile saline into the urethra as an assistant compresses the urethra proximal to the obstruction with digital pressure, usually by rectal palpation.
   F. The assistant should quickly release the urethral compression as the urethra is dilated by the hydrostatic force of the injected saline. This causes a gradual retropulsion of the urolith into the urinary bladder.
   G. Take follow-up radiographs or double-contrast-enhanced cystograms to assess complete urolith removal.
5. Treatment of urolithiasis may be either medical or surgical. The medical dissolution of cystine, struvite and urate uroliths has been successful. The treatment of urolith-induced obstructive uropathy is either surgical, by voiding urohydropropulsion or by catheter urolith removal.

6. Urohydropropulsion technique is used in patients when stones are present in the bladder (not the urethra) and one wishes to avoid surgical removal of stones.
   A. Evaluate the urolith shape and size in relation to the patient size. Smooth uroliths pass easier than those with irregular surfaces. The urolith must be smaller than the smallest diameter of the patient's urethra.
   B. Administer sedatives with analgesic and muscle-relaxing effects leading to deep sedation or administer general anesthesia:
      I. An opioid (oxymorphone, morphine, hydromorphone, fentanyl, etc) followed by propofol IV to effect +/− gas anesthesia
      II. Alternatively, administer an opioid with dexmedetomidine or another tranquilizer to sedate the patient. In most cases, better relaxation of sphincters is obtained with general anesthesia (CRI of propofol or gas anesthesia).
   C. Pass a urethral catheter into the urinary bladder.
   D. Moderately distend the urinary bladder with sterile saline, by administering 4–6 mL/kg of body weight. Monitor bladder distention by abdominal palpation.
   E. Remove the urethral catheter.
   F. Hold the front end of the patient up so that the vertebral column is vertical.
   G. With abdominal palpation, gently agitate the urinary bladder to move uroliths into the trigone region.
   H. Express urine and uroliths by applying steady digital pressure to the urinary bladder.
   I. Repeat steps (C) through (H) as needed.
   J. Take follow-up radiographs or double-contrast-enhanced cystograms to assess complete urolith removal. If unsuccessful, surgical removal of the uroliths is indicated.
7. Place an intravenous catheter and begin intravenous fluid therapy. If a urinary tract obstruction is present, intravenous fluid therapy should be conservative until the obstruction is relieved. Administer intravenous fluids at the rate of 10 mL/kg/h or more, depending upon urine output.
   A. Replace any dehydration. To calculate the hydration deficit (mild dehydration is 5%, moderate is 8%, severe or shock is 12%):
      % dehydration × BW (kg) = liters of fluid needed.
   B. If the patient is mildly dehydrated, administer the hydration deficit over 12 hours.
   C. If the patient is moderately dehydrated, administer the hydration deficit within 4 hours.
   D. If the patient is severely dehydrated or in hypovolemic shock, administer the hydration deficit over 1–2 hours.
   E. In addition to correcting dehydration, administer fluids at 1.5–3 times maintenance rates of 1–2 mL/kg/h. Keep up with post-obstructive diuresis losses.
   F. The fluid rate of each individual patient will vary, but depends on the patient's vital signs, degree of azotemia, urine production, hydration, and mentation.
   G. Monitor closely to avoid fluid overload and medullary washout.

8. Treat metabolic acidosis if the serum HCO_3 <12 mmol/L, pH <7.1, or if the patient has a bradyarrhythmia.
   A. Use the following formula to determine the bicarbonate deficit: [HCO_3 normal (20) – HCO_3 actual] × 0.3 × body weight in kg.
   B. Give 50% of the bicarbonate deficit as sodium bicarbonate, over 3–6 hours.
   C. Re-evaluate the blood gas status. If the pH is still critical (pH ≤7.1 or HCO_3 <12), repeat another aliquot of the bicarbonate deficit over 3–6 hours.
   D. Monitor blood gases q2–6h as needed.
9. Treatment of hyperkalemia
   A. If hyperkalemia is moderate, 7–8 mEq/L, relieve the obstruction and administer 0.9% NaCl to re-establish hydration and then re-evaluate the serum potassium level.
   B. If the serum potassium level exceeds 7.5–8 mEq/L, additional therapy is indicated.
      I. Administer 10% calcium gluconate, 0.2–0.5 mL/kg IV over 15 minutes while monitoring the ECG. The effect lasts about 10–15 minutes. Although this protects the heart from the cardiotoxic effects of potassium, the serum potassium level is not decreased, so an additional therapy is also indicated.
      II. Administer sodium bicarbonate, 0.5–1 mEq/kg, slow IV over 2–5 minutes, then infuse an additional 1–2 mEq/kg slow IV over 30–60 minutes. The serum potassium level is decreased within minutes, and the effect may last up to several hours.
      III. An alternative method is to administer 20% glucose, 1–2 mL/kg IV over 30–60 minutes to stimulate endogenous insulin production, which drives potassium into the cells.
      IV. If desired, insulin administration may follow glucose administration. Administer regular insulin, 0.2–0.4 U/kg IV, and 50% dextrose, 2 g (4 mL per unit of dextrose per unit of administered insulin). Administer IV fluids with 2.5% dextrose to the patient. Be very cautious to avoid severe, prolonged, potentially fatal hypoglycemia.
   C. Monitor serum electrolytes q2–4h as needed.
10. Recommendations for prevention
   A. Struvite uroliths
      I. Hill's prescription s/d® or c/d® diets, Royal Canin Urinary SO® diet
      II. Control urinary tract infections.
   B. Calcium oxalate uroliths
      I. Hill's prescription u/d®, w/d® or k/d® diets
      II. NF-Formula® (Purina CNM)
      III. Royal Canin Urinary SO® diet
      IV. Potassium citrate, 40–75 mg/kg PO q12h
      V. Vitamin B_6 (pyridoxine hydrochloride), 2 mg/kg/day, has been recommended but is not proven to be beneficial.
      VI. Hydrochlorothiazide (Hydro Diuril®), 2–4 mg/kg PO q12h, may be administered but is contraindicated in patients with hypercalcemia.

VII. The administration of neutral phosphate, 250 mg/day PO, has been recommended but the dosage should be adjusted to maintain a normal serum phosphorus level.

C. Cystine uroliths
   I. Hill's prescription u/d® diet
   II. Royal Canin Urinary UC® diet
   III. Thiol-containing drugs
   IV. D-penicillamine (10–15 mg/kg q12h PO), or N-(2-mercaptoproprionyl)-glycine (10–15 mg/kg q12h PO)

D. Ammonium acid urate uroliths
   I. Hill's prescription u/d® or k/d® diets
   II. Royal Canin Urinary UC® diet
   III. Allopurinol (7–10 mg/kg q8–24h PO)
   IV. Control infection
   V. Add potassium chloride (light salt) to the diet to increase water consumption.
   VI. Potassium citrate, 50 mg/kg q12h.

E. Silicate uroliths
   I. Hill's prescription u/d® diet
   II. Prevent consumption of dirt and grass.

11. Monitor urine output. The minimum urine output should be 2 mL/kg/h.

A. Post-obstructive diuresis may necessitate an increased intravenous fluid rate to keep up with urine output.

B. Acute renal failure may occur. Monitor for oliguria or anuria and treat early and aggressively.

C. Consider re-obstruction, bladder atony, urethral damage, urinary tract rupture, urethral spasms, or reflex dyssynergia if the patient is unable to urinate after calculus removal.
   I. Urethritis has been treated with dexamethasone sodium phosphate, 0.25 mg/kg, one or two doses, 12 hours apart. This is controversial and may lead to urinary tract infection. Newer recommendations involve administration of NSAIDs rather than steroids but effect has not been proved to be beneficial.
   II. Reflex dyssynergia may respond to phenoxybenzamine, 5–15 mg/dog once daily, or prazosin 1 mg/15 kg of weight q8h for 5–7 days.
   III. Bladder atony may respond to bethanechol, 1.25–5 mg PO q8h in combination with phenoxybenzamine or prazosin. These medications should be avoided if there is a possibility of urethral obstruction.

UROABDOMEN

Etiology

Urine leakage from the bladder is most commonly associated with trauma to the bladder. Trauma can take the form of exogenous trauma such as that suffered by animals hit by a car, or iatrogenic trauma. Iatrogenic trauma can occur during urethral catheterization, cystocentesis, vigorous palpation of the bladder, or attempts to express the bladder. In rare cases, chronic severe urolithiasis can cause severe enough inflammation and irritation to the bladder wall as to cause leakage of urine. In most cases, iatrogenic trauma does not lead to bladder leakage unless there is severe disease of the bladder that is pre-existent such as urolithiasis, infection of the bladder, or neoplasia.

Diagnosis

History—Owners may report trauma such as the patient having been hit by a car. Alternatively, the patient may have been receiving treatment involving the bladder that would have led to uroabdomen. Examples include cystocentesis, urethral catheterization, palpation of the bladder, etc. In most cases, any trauma that might have caused uroabdomen typically occurred several days prior to the onset of clinical signs. Patients are anorexic and often have a fever, abdominal pain, and may vomit.

Physical exam—A full physical examination should be performed. Patients often have abdominal pain, especially in the caudal abdomen. A fluid wave or distention of the abdomen may be noted. Many animals have fevers secondary to chemical burning of the peritoneal cavity. During abdominal palpation of especially cats and small dogs, it may be difficult to palpate a bladder. In some cases, during palpation of the bladder and expression of the bladder, the bladder size will shrink but no urine will escape the urethra.

Laboratory evaluation—

1. Uroabdomen is suspected when there is free fluid in the abdomen, specifically in the caudal abdominal region. Free fluid is diagnosed via radiographs or abdominal ultrasound.
   A. Radiographs – it is usually difficult to distinguish the outline of all parts of the bladder on a radiograph and a generalized lack of detail is found in especially the caudal abdomen. Radiographs allow diagnosis of uroliths either in the bladder or free in the abdomen.
   B. Abdominal ultrasound – free fluid can be visualized directly with ultrasound, typically in the region of the bladder but it also can be found generalized in the abdomen if there is a large enough volume.
2. Obtain a sample of the free fluid via a four-quadrant tap or ultrasound or radiograph-guided abdominocentesis. The fluid will cytologically be acellular if acute and contain inflammatory cells if more chronic and there is associated chemical peritonitis.
   A. A creatinine level and potassium level should be performed on the fluid along with a creatinine level and potassium level on a peripheral blood sample.
   B. Uroabdomen is diagnosed when the levels of creatinine in the free fluid is at least *twice* that of the peripheral blood. Similarly, potassium levels are at least 1.9 times that of the peripheral blood.
3. Excretory urography or a retrograde cystourethrogram can be used to identify the bladder rent definitively by looking for contrast leakage into the abdominal cavity. Contrast agents within the peritoneal cavity

may cause worsening irritation of the peritoneal lining. The fundus of the bladder is the most common site for a rupture.

4. A full CBC and serum chemistry can be performed to evaluate the patient for any other systemic disease. A urine sample can be collected via catheterization and submitted for culture to look for concurrent disease of the urinary system (aside from the rupture in the bladder).

Differential diagnoses

1. Urine leakage from ureters, kidneys or urethra rather than bladder.
2. Free fluid due to blood, ascites, bile, etc.
3. Peritonitis due to leakage from the gastrointestinal tract, gallbladder, etc.

Prognosis

In most cases uroabdomen can be successfully managed as long as the patient's other concurrent injuries can be managed.

Treatment

1. Treat any shock or other life-threatening conditions in the patient.
2. Definitive treatment of large bladder wall rents causing uroabdomen involves an abdominal exploratory and repair of the bladder wall. This *should not* be pursued until the patient's condition has been deemed otherwise stable and other life threatening injuries have been managed. Small rents in the bladder wall are managed by diversion of urine for 7–10 days (see below).
3. While awaiting definitive treatment of large rents or when managing small rents medically, urine should be re-directed out of the abdomen.
   A. Urethral catheterization with a Foley indwelling catheter will allow drainage of urine.
   B. Peritoneal catheterization with a mushroom-tipped catheter (tube cystostomy) can be pursued to divert urine from the abdomen. This catheter can be introduced along the ventral midline although newer techniques also describe placement of the catheter in the patient's flank.
   C. Urinary diversion should occur until either:
      I. 7–10 days have elapsed allowing for small bladder wall rents to heal, or
      II. A patient is deemed stable enough for an abdominal exploratory procedure.
4. If uroliths, neoplasia or bacterial infection of the bladder are believed to have contributed to the bladder wall rupture, patients should have stones removed surgically and / or treated medically with diets (see urolithiasis section), neoplasia should be biopsied in order to determine appropriate treatment, or antibiotics should be started pending culture results.

Urinary emergencies and electrolyte disorders

Etiology

1. Neoplasia (including lymphoma, anal sac apocrine gland adenocarcinoma, and other neoplasms)
2. Hypoadrenocorticism
3. Chronic renal failure
4. Primary hyperparathyroidism
5. Hypervitaminosis D
6. Cholecalciferol-containing rodenticide intoxication
7. Septic osteomyelitis, and other disorders.

Diagnosis

History—The history will vary depending upon the underlying etiology. The patient may be asymptomatic or present with severe systemic illness, often due to secondary renal failure. The owner may observe anorexia, weight loss, vomiting, constipation, polyuria, polydypsia, weakness, depression or seizures.

Physical exam—The patient may appear depressed and weak. Bradycardia may be present. There may be signs of vomiting. The patient may be stuporous, comatose or may have seizures. Rectal examination may reveal constipation or a perianal mass. Be sure to express the anal glands prior to palpation to avoid missing a mass in the anal glands. Perform a thorough rectal and perianal examination.

Laboratory evaluation—
1. Evaluate a CBC.
2. Evaluate a complete serum biochemical profile, and pay particular attention to the BUN, creatinine, and serum phosphorus concentrations. While total calcium levels can be used to screen for hypercalcemia, verify hypercalcemia by measuring ionized calcium levels (iCa greater than 1.4 in dogs and cats)
3. Perform a urinalysis.

Radiographic evaluation—Evaluation of the thorax, abdomen, and skeleton should be performed.

ECG—This may reveal arrhythmias, prolongation of the PR interval and shortening of the QT interval.

Prognosis

The prognosis is variable depending on underlying disease and whether renal failure is present.

Treatment

1. Inform the client of the diagnosis, prognosis and cost of the treatment.
2. Pursue identification of the underlying etiology.
3. Correct any associated metabolic, endocrine, inflammatory, toxicologic or iatrogenic disorders.
4. Place an intravenous catheter.
5. Administer intravenous fluid therapy. The fluid of choice is 0.9% NaCl.

6. Once fluid volume has been restored, administer furosemide, 2–4 mg/kg IV, IM or PO q12h.
7. Administer calcitonin, 4 U/kg IV, then 4–8 U/kg SC q12–24h.
8. Administer bisphosphonates such as pamidronate 1.3–2 mg/kg in 150 mL of 0.9% NaCl (give over 2 hours) once. Dose can be repeated in 1–3 weeks' time. Pamidronate has been shown to cause or exacerbate renal failure.
9. Once samples for potential lymphoma have been collected (ex. lymph node aspirates, aspirates of liver or spleen) initiate glucocorticoid therapy. Administer prednisolone or prednisone, 2–4 mg/kg PO q12h.
10. Feed the patient a low-calcium diet, such as Hill's prescription diet k/d®, u/d®, or s/d®.
11. If the patient has hyperphosphatemia and is eating, administer a calcium-free intestinal phosphorus binder such as aluminum hydroxide to bind dietary calcium. Phosphate binders should only be given to animals who are eating.

HYPOCALCEMIA

Etiology

1. Eclampsia (puerperal tetany or milk fever)
2. Hypoparathyroidism
3. Ethylene glycol toxicity
4. Nutritional secondary hyperparathyroidism
5. Malabsorption
6. Renal failure
7. Hypoproteinemia
8. Pancreatitis
9. Acute hyperphosphatemia
10. Administration of phosphate enemas.

Diagnosis

History—The owner may observe lethargy, anorexia, increased excitability, nervousness, focal muscle twitching (especially of the ear and facial muscles), intense facial rubbing, panting, a stiff gait, tetany or seizures. Eclampsia usually occurs 2–3 weeks after delivery of a large litter. It may occur prior to delivery or at any time during lactation and has been seen in any breed of dog as well as cats, although small breed dogs are over-represented.

Physical exam—The patient may exhibit behavioral aberrations, restlessness, ataxia, paresis, hypersensitivity to light and sound, muscle tremors or fasciculations, tetany or generalized motor seizures. Hyperthermia, a painful abdomen, tachyarrhythmias, muffled heart sounds and a weak femoral pulse may be present.

Laboratory findings—

1. The total serum calcium level is less than 9 mg/dL in adult dogs and cats, and less than 7 mg/dL in dogs and cats that are less than 6 months of age. Clinical signs usually occur in adult animals with serum total calcium levels <7.5 mg/dL. Typically clinical signs occur

when ionized calcium is less than 1.00 mg/dL (normal ranges of ionized calcium are often 1.2–1.4 nmol/L). In general, ionized calcium is far more accurate than total calcium and should be used to verify low total calcium levels measured on blood panels.
2. Hypomagnesemia may be present in some patients.
3. Evaluate a CBC.
4. Evaluate a complete serum biochemical profile.
5. Perform a urinalysis.

Prognosis

The prognosis is usually excellent for eclampsia and varies for the other underlying etiologies.

Treatment

1. Inform the client of the diagnosis, prognosis and cost of the treatment.
2. Guidelines for initiating therapy
   A. Hypocalcemia does not always require treatment and is contraindicated in some cases. Specific therapeutic intervention is *not* indicated for those conditions characterized by a decrease in total serum calcium, but a normal quantity of ionized calcium. This is most likely to occur in conditions accompanied by hypoalbuminemia, as in malabsorption syndromes, protein-losing enteropathies, nephrotic syndrome and liver disease.
   B. Mild decreases in serum calcium that are due to some other transient condition, such as acute pancreatitis, which are not associated with hypocalcemic signs should not be treated.
   C. Asymptomatic hypocalcemia associated with renal failure should not be treated as long as hyperphosphatemia prevails.
3. Place an intravenous catheter.
4. Administer 2–15 mL 10% calcium gluconate slowly IV (0.5–1.5 mL/kg at 1 mL/min) or place the calcium gluconate into a 5% dextrose solution and administer slowly IV. Calcium chloride may be administered IV at the dose of 5–15 mg/kg/h IV. Beware of perivascular extravasation because calcium chloride is very irritating.
5. Monitor the heart during calcium administration via auscultation and ECG. Stop the calcium administration if the patient's heart rate decreases. Nausea, vomiting and cardiac arrhythmias are potential side effects of calcium administration.
6. If the patient with tetany fails to respond to the high dose of calcium, either check the serum ionized magnesium level or administer magnesium chloride, 0.15–0.3 mEq/kg slowly IV over 5–15 minutes. Magnesium chloride contains 9.25 mEq of magnesium per gram.
7. Once the signs of tetany are controlled, administer calcium either orally or subcutaneously
   A. Calcium gluconate can be given SC diluted 1:1 but irritation can lead to skin necrosis. Better to administer oral calcium.

B. Calcium carbonate tablets are administered 25–50 mg/kg/day (most common formulation).
C. Calcium lactate tablets may be administered PO at the dose of 25–50 mg/kg/day in 3–4 divided doses.
8. It is a good idea to administer oral vitamin D in many cases to improve absorption of intestinal calcium, especially in cases of chronic hypocalcemia (renal failure, intestinal malabsorptive disorders).
A. Vitamin D_2 4000–6000 U/kg/day initially and later 1000–2000 U/kg/day once daily to once weekly.
B. Calcitriol 20–30 ng/kg/day for 3–4 days and later 5–15 ng/kg/day.
9. If tetany persists, check blood glucose levels, and treat as indicated.
10. If tetany persists, administer methocarbamol to try to slow or stop muscle fasciculations. Diazepam or pentobarbital IV can also be administered.
11. Pursue the diagnosis, and treat for the specific condition as soon as possible.
12. Hospitalize and observe the patient after calcium administration (preferably for 12–24 hours) to ensure that the patient is able to maintain her calcium levels and is eating and drinking normally.
13. For patients with eclampsia, advise the owner to wean the puppies or kittens. Dispense milk replacer and nurser bottles. Instruct the owner about the care of the puppies or kittens.
14. In cases of eclampsia, advise the owner to have the patient and her litter re-examined by her regular veterinarian and to obtain nutritional counseling.

HYPERKALEMIA

Hyperkalemia: the serum potassium concentration exceeds 5.5 mEq/L. Serum potassium concentrations of 7.5 mEq/L or greater are considered life threatening and require rapid treatment.

Etiology

1. Urinary tract disorders
   A. Anuric or oliguric renal failure
   B. Urethral obstruction
   C. Ruptured urinary bladder or ureter
2. Gastrointestinal disorders
   A. Various gastrointestinal diseases such as trichuriasis and salmonellosis
   B. Perforated duodenal ulcer
3. Endocrine disorders
   A. Hypoadrenocorticism
   B. Hyporeninemic hypoaldosteronism (with renal failure or diabetes mellitus)
   C. Diabetic ketoacidosis

4. Drug induced
   A. Potassium-sparing diuretics (spironolactone, etc.)
   B. Heparin
   C. Prostaglandin inhibitors
   D. ACE inhibitors (enalapril, etc.)
   E. Non-specific beta blockers (propanolol, etc.)
   F. Excessive administration of potassium supplements
   G. Trimethoprim-sulfa
5. Miscellaneous causes
   A. Chylothorax
   B. Acute inorganic acidosis (ammonium chloride, hydrogen chloride)
   C. Hyperkalemia periodic paralysis
   D. Acute tumor lysis syndrome
   E. Crush injuries (massive tissue trauma)
   F. Feline aortic thromboembolism (during reperfusion of affected extremities)
6. Pseudohyperkalemia
   A. Hemolysis in certain breeds (Akitas, Shiba Inu, Kindo, English Springer Spaniels), neonates, or certain individuals with high intracellular potassium concentrations
   B. Leukocytosis >100 000 cells/μL
   C. Thrombocytosis.

Diagnosis

History—There may be a history compatible with renal failure, abdominal trauma, urethral obstruction, gastroenteritis, polyuria, polydipsia, polyphagia, medication, neoplasia, breed association or other etiology. If urine output and renal function are normal, hyperkalemia is uncommon.

Physical exam—The most common clinical sign of hyperkalemia is muscular weakness. Paresthesia and paralysis may also occur. Cardiac conduction abnormalities are common when the serum potassium level is higher than 7.5 mEq/L.

Electrocardiographic changes are related to the increase in serum potassium level, including:
1. High, peaked or deep T-waves
2. Prolonged PR interval
3. Decreased amplitude and widening of the P-wave to complete disappearance of the P-wave
4. Prolonged QRS complex
5. Complete heart block
6. Bradycardia
7. Atrial standstill
8. Ectopic beats
9. Sine wave complexes (fusion of the QRS complex with the T-wave)
10. Ventricular fibrillation or standstill

Laboratory findings—
1. Evaluate a serum biochemical profile.
2. Evaluate a CBC.
3. Evaluate acid–base status.
4. Perform a urinalysis.
5. Evaluate baseline cortisol level and / or run an ACTH stimulation test.
   A. Dogs with basal cortisol concentrations >2 μg/dL that are not receiving corticosteroids, mitotane or ketoconazole are highly unlikely to have hypoadrenocorticism.
   B. ACTH stimulation test with the synthetic adrenocorticotropin cosyntropin (Cortrosyn®)
      I. Obtain a plasma sample.
      II. Administer 0.25 mg (250 μg) of cosyntropin (Cortrosyn®) to a dog IM or 5 μg/kg to a dog IV or 0.125 mg (125 μg) of cosyntropin (Cortrosyn®) to a cat IM or IV.
      III. Obtain plasma samples 1 hour post-ACTH administration in dogs and 30 and 60 minutes post-ACTH administration in cats.
      IV. An abnormally decreased post-ACTH plasma cortisol concentration (<2.0 mg/dL) aids in the diagnosis of hypoadrenocorticism.
   C. If cosyntropin (Cortrosyn®) is unavailable, ACTH gel may be used.
      I. Obtain a plasma sample.
      II. Administer 2.2 IU/kg ACTH gel IM in dogs and cats.
      III. Obtain another blood sample 2 hours post-ACTH gel administration in dogs and 30 minutes and 1 hour post-ACTH gel administration in cats.
6. Perform other tests based on history and potential etiology.

Prognosis

ECG abnormalities of the QRS complex have the potential to cause fatal arrhythmias and require immediate treatment.

Treatment

1. Inform the client of the diagnosis, prognosis and cost of treatment.
2. Place an intravenous catheter.
3. If mild hyperkalemia (5.5– 7.0 mEq/L) is present, administer a crystalloid fluid such as LRS, Normosol®-R or 0.9% NaCl IV. If the patient is not in renal failure and is not dehydrated, furosemide administration may enhance potassium excretion.
4. Treat the underlying etiology.
   A. If a urinary tract obstruction is present, relieve the obstruction.
   B. Administer fluid therapy for the dehydrated oliguric or anuric patient.
   C. Administer 0.9% NaCl and mineralocorticoids for patients with hypoadrenocorticism.
5. For severe hyperkalemia (7.5 mEq/L or higher) and/or the patient shows evidence of bradycardia or ECG abnormalities, additional therapy is indicated.
   A. Administer 10% calcium gluconate, 0.5–1.5 mL/kg IV, over 5–15 minutes.

I. Calcium immediately counteracts the direct cardiotoxic effects of hyperkalemia by decreasing the membrane potential and decreasing excitability of the cardiac membrane.

II. Monitor the heart during calcium administration via auscultation and ECG. Stop the calcium administration if the patient's heart rate decreases. Nausea, vomiting, and cardiac arrhythmias are potential side effects of calcium administration.

III. If 10% calcium gluconate is not available and 10% calcium chloride must be used, administer one-third of the calcium gluconate dose and do not allow perivascular extrusion.

IV. The effects occur within minutes and response lasts possibly 30 minutes.

B. Administer sodium bicarbonate ($NaHCO_3$ 40 mEq, 90 mOsm), 0.5–2 mEq/kg slowly IV over 15–30 minutes.

I. Sodium bicarbonate administration causes extracellular alkalosis, which attracts hydrogen ions from the intracellular space and causes an exchange of potassium ions from the extracellular space into the intracellular space.

II. Large volumes of sodium bicarbonate may cause a paradoxical cerebrospinal fluid acidosis.

III. Sodium bicarbonate administration may also decrease the availability of calcium ions and neutralize the stabilizing effect of calcium administration.

IV. The effects occur within 15 minutes and last about 30 minutes.

C. Administer glucose 20%, 1–2 mL/kg IV over 30–60 minutes.

I. Glucose administration will stimulate endogenous insulin production and force potassium into cells to reduce serum potassium levels.

II. Hypertonic dextrose can worsen cellular dehydration in severely dehydrated patients.

III. The effects occur within 1 hour and last for a few hours.

D. If desired, insulin administration may follow glucose administration. Administer regular insulin, 0.2–0.4 U/kg IV and 50% dextrose, 2 g (4 mL per unit of dextrose per unit of administered insulin). Administer IV fluids containing 2.5% dextrose to the patient.

I. Insulin facilitates the transport of glucose into cells, and potassium shifts in the same direction.

II. Insulin also stimulates the Na^+–H^+ antiporter and the Na^+,K^+-ATPase pump, which cause insulin to enter cells.

III. The effects occur within 30 minutes and last 30–60 minutes.

E. Terbutaline can also be used to temporarily reduce serum potassium levels.

I. Administer 0.2 mg/kg PO q8–12h in dogs and 0.625 mg PO every 8–12 in cats.

II. The beta agonist stimulates Na^+,K^+-ATPase activity, which increases cellular uptake of potassium.

F. Peritoneal dialysis and hemodialysis are effective at decreasing serum potassium concentrations.

Hypokalemia: the serum potassium concentration is less than 3.5 mEq/L.

Etiology

1. Urinary tract disorders
   A. Chronic renal failure
   B. Post-obstructive diuresis
   C. Excessive urinary losses
   D. Distal (type 1) renal tubular acidosis
   E. Proximal (type 2) renal tubular acidosis following sodium bicarbonate therapy
2. Gastrointestinal disorders
   A. Various gastrointestinal diseases that cause diarrhea
   B. Vomiting of gastric contents
3. Endocrine disorders
   A. Diabetes-mellitus-induced diuresis without adequate potassium supplementation
   B. Diabetic-ketoacidosis-induced diuresis without adequate potassium supplementation
   C. Mineralocorticoid excess
   D. Hyperadrenocorticism
   E. Primary hyperaldosteronism
4. Drug induced
   A. Loop diuretics (furosemide, etc.)
   B. Thiazide diuretics (hydrochlorothiazide, chlorothiazide)
   C. Penicillin
   D. Total parenteral nutrition
   E. Administration of potassium-free or potassium-deficient IV fluids
   F. Administration of glucose-containing IV fluids, with or without insulin
   G. Insulin
   H. Sodium bicarbonate
   I. Mineralocorticoid supplementation
5. Miscellaneous causes
   A. Diet-induced hypokalemic nephropathy in cats
   B. Dialysis
   C. Hypokalemia periodic paralysis in Burmese cats
6. Pseudohyperkalemia.

Diagnosis

History—There may be a history compatible with renal failure, abdominal trauma, urethral obstruction, gastroenteritis, polyuria, polydipsia and polyphagia, medication, neoplasia, breed association or other etiology.

Physical exam—Clinical signs usually are not observed until the serum potassium level is less than 2.5 mEq/L. Muscle weakness is the most common sign. Other clinical signs, depending upon the severity of hypokalemia include anorexia, cardiac conduction abnormalities, vomiting, decreased intestinal motility, lethargy, confusion, paresthesia, muscle cramps, paralysis and respiratory muscle impairment.

Electrocardiographic changes may occur when the serum potassium level is less than 2.5 mEq/L, including:

1. Depressed ST segment
2. Lowering, flattening, or inversion of the T-wave
3. Presence of an elevated U-wave (in human beings)
4. Increased P-wave amplitude
5. Prolonged PR interval
6. Prolonged QRS interval
7. Sinus bradycardia, primary heart block, paroxysmal atrial tachycardia and atrioventricular dissociation may also occur.

Laboratory findings—
1. Evaluate a serum biochemical profile.
2. Evaluate a CBC.
3. Evaluate acid–base status.
4. Perform a urinalysis.
5. Perform other tests based on history and potential etiology.

Prognosis

Hypokalemia is rarely fatal. The focus should be on supportive treatment and correction of the underlying disorder.

Treatment

1. Inform the client of the diagnosis, prognosis and cost of the treatment.
2. If hypokalemia is chronic and mild (3.0–3.5 mEq/L), the ingestion of potassium may be increased:
   A. By adding potassium rich foods such as oranges, bananas, or nuts, to the diet
   B. By administration of an oral potassium supplement, 0.5–1 mEq/kg mixed in food every 12– 24 hours.
3. If hypokalemia is acute or severe, potassium chloride should be administered in intravenous fluids.
   A. Generally, the rate should not exceed 0.5 mEq/kg/h IV.
   B. In a crisis situation, under direct ECG monitoring, the rate may be increased to 1.5 mEq/kg/h.
   C. The rate should not exceed 10 mEq/h, as the effects of higher concentrations on the right ventricular wall may have fatal results.
   D. See Table 11.2 for the recommended doses and rates of potassium chloride administration.
4. Potassium therapy requires close monitoring, titration and gradual return to normal levels.

5. If hypokalemia persists despite therapy, check the ionized magnesium level.
   A. If the magnesium is <1.2 mg/dL, administer magnesium chloride or magnesium sulfate, 0.75–1 mEq/kg/day as an IV CRI in 5% dextrose in saline or water.
   B. Magnesium is incompatible with sodium bicarbonate and calcium.

HYPERNATREMIA

Etiology

Causes of hypernatremia are divided into two categories: loss of water or hypotonic fluid from the body or gain of sodium. Water loss occurs from diabetes insipidus, lack of water intake, fever, vomiting, diarrhea, cutaneous loss through the skin, or third space loss (examples: peritonitis or pancreatitis). Water can also be lost through the kidneys during renal failure, a post-obstructive diuresis, or while undergoing an osmotic diuresis during diabetes mellitus or after receiving mannitol. Sodium gain occurs during hypertonic fluid administration (examples: hypertonic saline, sodium bicarbonate, sodium phosphate enemas, parenteral nutrition), hyperaldosteronism, or hyperadrenocorticism.

Diagnosis

History—Clinical signs typically only occur when the hypernatremia is severe (usually greater than 180 mEq/L) or at lower sodium levels if the hypernatremia is acute (within a few hours). Owners may notice either decreased drinking (leading to the high serum sodium) or they may notice increased drinking in response to pre-existent hypernatremia. Patients may similarly be polyuric (leading to hypernatremia) or oliguric due to retention of water in response to the hypernatremia. In some cases, patients have neurologic signs ranging from abnormal behavior to ataxia to seizures. Animals are often anorexic, vomiting, lethargic, and weak, largely due to hypertonicity from the hypernatremia. However, some animals do not show any clinical signs.

Physical exam—Always complete a full physical examination looking for indications of dehydration, which would occur in water losses. Some animals show signs consistent with the underlying cause for hypernatremia including hypersalivation due to nausea, diarrhea staining in the perianal region, dropped hocks due to diabetic neuropathy, fever, or signs of hyperadrenocorticism such as a pot-bellied appearance or bilateral flank alopecia. Often there are no significant physical examination findings.

Laboratory findings—
1. CBC, serum chemistry (including electrolytes), urinalysis. Obtain all samples prior to fluid therapy. Hypernatremia will be documented on the chemistry panel.
2. Consider confirmatory testing for other underlying causes such as a urine culture if diabetes mellitus is diagnosed, an ACTH stimulation test or low-dose dexamethasone suppression test for hyperadrenocorticism, etc.

3. Consider abdominal radiographs or ultrasound if GI disease is suspected.

Prognosis

Typically the hypernatremia itself can be managed successfully. Longer term outcomes are dependent upon the underlying disease process.

Treatment

1. Inform the owner of the cost of treatment and prognosis.
2. Animals should be given intravenous fluids with the intent of replacing water lost from the body and / or diluting the sodium.
   A. Calculate the water deficit = weight (kg) × [(patient current Na ÷ normal Na) − 1]
   B. Usually shortened to water deficit = weight (kg) × [(patient current Na ÷ 140) −1]
   C. Water deficit is in *liters*.
   D. Determine the time frame over which to replace the water deficit. This is usually dependent upon the chronicity of the hypernatremia.
      I. If acute development of hypernatremia (i.e. <6–12 hours), replace the water deficit over 6–12 hours. Add the water deficit replacement per hour to the patient's maintenance fluids for that hour.
      II. If more chronic or unknown time frame for development of hypernatremia, replace the water deficit more slowly, often over 24–48 hours.
         a. Recheck the sodium concentration every 4–6 hours and try to lower the sodium at a rate of no more than 0.5 mEq/L/h.
         b. Try to avoid causing edema of the brain by replacing fluid too fast. With chronic hypernatremia, the brain forms idiogenic osmoles within brain cells that will draw water into the cells and cause edema. Slow replacement of fluid will allow the body to break down the idiogenic osmoles to protect brain cells.
   E. Recheck the serum sodium concentrations regularly during treatment (every 4–12 hours depending on the case). Chronic hypernatremia requires more frequency of rechecks. With acute hypernatremia, sodium levels do not need to be checked until after administration of full water deficit.
   F. Fluid chosen for the patient should have less sodium than the serum sodium.
      I. In acute cases, fluids containing large amounts of water are the best options to quickly reduce serum sodium. Examples would include 5% dextrose in water or hypotonic saline (0.45% saline).
      II. In chronic cases, fluids with higher sodium contents are used to more slowly reduce the serum sodium. Examples would include 0.9% saline, Normasol® / Plasma-Lyte®, or LRS.
3. Attempt to identify and treat any underlying diseases (diabetes mellitus, GI disease, etc.). Treatments for those disorders are tailored to the conditions.

Etiology

Causes of hyponatremia are divided into three categories depending on the plasma osmolality (i.e. normal, high or low osmolality):

1. Normal plasma osmolality: hyperlipidemia, hyperproteinemia
2. High plasma osmolality: hyperglycemia, mannitol infusion
3. Low plasma osmolality: liver disease, congestive heart failure, nephrotic syndrome, renal failure, psychogenic polydipsia, syndrome of inappropriate antidiuretic hormone (SIADH), myxedema coma, hypotonic fluid administration, GI disease (vomiting, diarrhea), third space loss (pancreatitis, peritonitis, uroabdomen, pleural effusion, peritoneal effusion, cutaneous loss (burns), hypoadrenocorticism and administration of diuretics.

Diagnosis

History—Clinical signs typically only occur in acute cases rather than in chronic disorders. Neurologic signs can occur due to hypotonic fluid flux into brain cells in acute disorders leading to ataxia, weakness, abnormal behaviors, or possibly seizure activity. In more chronic disorders, the brain cells can adjust to changes in serum osmolality. Systemically, in acute hyponatremia (i.e. water intoxication), animals might be lethargic, vomit, or increase significantly in body weight. The owners might notice signs consistent with the patient's underlying disease such as polyuria / polydipsia from renal failure, vomiting / diarrhea from GI disease, etc. Most animals do not have clinical signs specifically due to their hyponatremia. Be sure to obtain a good drug history from the owners including diuretic administration.

Physical exam—Always complete a full physical examination looking for indications of overhydration from excess water retention. Some animals show signs consistent with the underlying cause for hyponatremia including hypersalivation due to nausea, diarrhea staining in the perianal region, signs of hypothyroidism such as a poor haircoat or flank alopecia, signs of pleural effusion or peritoneal effusion (fluid wave in abdomen, muffled lung sounds in chest). There may not be any significant physical examination findings.

Laboratory findings—

1. CBC, serum chemistry (including electrolytes), urinalysis. Obtain all samples prior to fluid therapy. Hyponatremia will be documented on the chemistry panel as will things such as hyperlipidemia or hyperproteinemia.
2. Consider confirmatory testing for other underlying causes such as an ACTH stimulation test for hypoadrenocorticism, thyroid testing, etc.
3. If free fluid is present in a body cavity, perform thoracocentesis or abdominocentesis to obtain a sample. Perform cytology and a cell count on the fluid to diagnose its source.
4. Consider abdominal radiographs or ultrasound if GI disease is suspected.

Prognosis

Typically the hyponatremia itself can be managed successfully. Longer term outcomes are dependent upon the underlying disease process.

Treatment

1. Inform the owner of the cost of treatment and prognosis.
2. If severe acute hyponatremia (<24–48 hours' duration), consider correcting sodium levels. Animals should be given intravenous fluids with the intent of replacing body sodium. Use only 0.9% saline or other crystalloids (do not use hypertonic solutions).
   A. If acute development of hyponatremia (i.e. <24–48 hours), these patients need to have their sodium corrected. Recheck the sodium concentration every 4–6 hours and try to increase the sodium at a rate of no more than 0.5 mEq/L/h.
   B. If more chronic or unknown time frame for development of hyponatremia, do not be concerned about correcting sodium by itself. Focus on treating the underlying condition.
3. Try to avoid causing myelinolysis of the brain cells by correcting the sodium too fast. With chronic hyponatremia, the brain cells lose osmoles to avoid edema. As the serum sodium is corrected, brain cells can lose fluid rapidly to the serum causing myelinolysis. Slow replacement of sodium will allow the brain to replace its lost osmoles to avoid losing too much fluid.
4. Attempt to identify and treat any underlying diseases (hypoadrenocorticism, GI disease, etc). Treatments for those disorders are tailored to the conditions.

HYPOPHOSPHATEMIA

Etiology

Causes of hypophosphatemia are due to translocation of phosphorus within the body, loss, decreased intake, or laboratory error. Translocation occurs during treatment for conditions such as diabetic ketoacidosis, insulin release (exogenously or endogenously), respiratory alkalosis, administration of parenteral nutrition, refeeding syndrome, or hypothermia. Loss of phosphorus occurs with hyperparathyroidism, renal tubular disease, eclampsia, possibly hyperadrenocorticism and after diuretic administration. Decreased intake of phosphorus is largely due to phosphate binder administration or dietary vitamin D deficiency.

Concerns with hypophosphatemia are that cells (specifically red blood cells) become deficient in ATP causing red blood cells to become more fragile, leading to hemolysis. This occurs when serum phosphorus concentrations are <1.0 mg/dL. Erythrocyte 2,3 DPG levels also become too low with severe hypophosphatemia, impeding oxygen delivery to cells. Platelets may be less functional with hypophosphatemia and muscles are weaker due to hypophosphatemia.

Diagnosis

History—Owners may not notice any clinical signs or patients may show weakness, lethargy, anorexia, and vomiting. Alternatively, owners may notice signs attributable to the patient's underlying disease such as polyuria / polydipsia from renal disease or diabetes mellitus. Question owners about whelping in intact female dogs, and obtain a complete drug history.

Physical exam—Always complete a full physical examination. Most animals do not show any specific physical findings consistent with hypophosphatemia. Some animals show signs consistent with the underlying cause such as dropped hocks due to diabetic neuropathy, indications of recent whelping, or bilateral flank alopecia attributable to hyperadrenocorticism.

Laboratory findings—

1. CBC, serum chemistry (including electrolytes), urinalysis. Obtain all samples prior to fluid therapy. Hypophosphatemia will be documented on the chemistry panel.
2. Be sure to note any hemolysis in the blood samples as hypophosphatemia (usually <1.0 mg/dL) can lead to red blood cell fragility and hemolysis.
3. Consider confirmatory testing for other underlying causes such as an ACTH stimulation test or low dose dexamethasone stimulation test for hyperadrenocorticism, parathyroid levels, etc.
4. Consider abdominal radiographs or ultrasound to evaluate the kidney parenchyma.

Prognosis

Typically the hypophosphatemia itself can be managed successfully. Longer term outcomes are dependent upon the underlying disease process.

Treatment

1. Inform the owner of the cost of treatment and prognosis.
2. Prevention of hypophosphatemia is the most important to avoid side effects. Be aware of situations when hypophosphatemia can occur in order to anticipate and treat it. Supplement fluid therapy with KPO_4 during parenteral nutrition supplementation, when treating diabetic ketoacidosis, or when administering insulin for other reasons.
   A. Supplement phosphorus when serum concentrations <1.5 mg/dL.
   B. Oral phosphorus can be given in the form of potassium-phosphorus (K-Phos) or in various other formats. It is slow to correct phosphorus but is typically safe. Oral phosphorus may cause vomiting.
   C. Intravenous phosphorus can be given in two ways:
      I. Determine the amount of potassium that the patient requires (see Table 11.2 for potassium supplementation recommendations). Give ½ of the total amount of potassium as KCl and ½ as KPO_4 to supplement phosphorus.

II. Administer 0.01–0.06 mmol/kg/h of KPO$_4$ as a constant rate infusion IV. Recheck the serum phosphorus level every 6–8 hours to determine whether the rate of administration is appropriate.

   a. Dilute the phosphorus in 0.9% sodium chloride.

   b. Note that calculation is in mmol/L rather than mEq/L. Typically, potassium phosphate has 3 mmol/L of phosphorus and 4.4 mEq/L of potassium.

3. Attempt to identify and treat any underlying diseases. Treatments for those disorders are tailored to the conditions.

HYPOMAGNESEMIA

Etiology

Causes of hypomagnesemia are typically related to loss through the GI tract or kidneys. With GI disease, there is typically pathology such as malabsorption or chronic diarrhea although reduced intake can also cause hypomagnesemia. With renal disease, any cause of diuresis (renal failure, diabetes mellitus, hyperaldosteronism, post-obstructive diuresis, osmotic agent or diuretic administration) can lead to hypomagnesemia. Also, administration of drugs such as gentamicin, cisplatin, carbenicillin, ticarcillin, or cyclosporin have been linked to hypomagnesemia via renal loss of magnesium. In some cases, lactation, pancreatitis, or insulin administration can lead to hypomagnesemia due to loss of magnesium or redistribution of the electrolyte in the body.

In most cases, magnesium deficits do **not** exist by themselves but are present with concurrent hypercalcemia (from hyperparathyroidism), hypocalcemia, hypokalemia, or hypophosphatemia. Magnesium levels tend to mimic potassium levels very closely.

Diagnosis

History—Typically in small animals there are no historical findings consistent with hypomagnesemia itself. Owners may report whelping and lactation or administration of drugs that could contribute to hypomagnesemia. Polyuria / polydipsia could indicate renal disease or diabetes mellitus. Owners may also report vomiting or diarrhea consistent with pre-existent GI disease or pancreatitis.

Physical exam—Always complete a full physical examination. Most animals do not show any specific physical findings consistent with hypomagnesemia. Some animals show signs consistent with the underlying cause such as dropped hocks due to diabetic neuropathy, indications of recent whelping, or weakness due to other electrolyte disorders. Abdominal pain and nausea might indicate GI disease or pancreatitis. Since many of the underlying diseases can lead to dehydration, make note of the patient's hydration status.

Laboratory findings—

1. CBC, serum chemistry (including electrolytes), urinalysis. Obtain all samples prior to fluid therapy. In-house lab machines rarely report

magnesium and therefore samples may need to be sent out to a reference laboratory. In many cases, if hypokalemia exists, magnesium is likely to be low as well (but true magnitude of magnesium decrease is not known without having a serum magnesium level).

2. There is no level below which hypomagnesemia is known to become clinically significant.
3. Consider abdominal radiographs or ultrasound to evaluate the kidney parenchyma, GI system, or pancreas.
4. Consider urine culture in diabetic patients.

Prognosis

Typically the hypomagnesemia itself can be managed successfully, usually without direct treatment. Longer term outcomes are dependent upon the underlying disease process.

Treatment

1. Inform owner of the cost of treatment and prognosis.
2. Since 99% of magnesium is stored within tissues, it is difficult to determine when to supplement magnesium based on blood levels. Usually treating the underlying cause and other electrolyte abnormalities will lead to normalization of magnesium.
3. If magnesium supplementation is deemed important (questionable if this is ever the case):
   A. Oral magnesium can be given at 1–2 mEq/L
   B. Parenteral magnesium is available in $MgSO_4$ or $MgCl_2$ formats:
      I. Give at 0.75–1.0 mEq/kg/day for faster replacement or 0.3–0.5 mEq/kg/day for slower replacement.
      II. Emergent/loading doses of magnesium are 20–30 mEq/kg/day.
4. Attempt to identify and treat any underlying diseases. Treatments for those disorders are tailored to the conditions.

REFERENCES/FURTHER READING

ACUTE RENAL FAILURE

Abuelo, J.G., 2007. Normotensive ischemic acute renal failure. New England Journal of Medicine 357, 797–805.

Chew, D.J., Gieg, J.A., 2006. Fluid therapy during intrinsic renal failure. In: diBartola, S.P. (Ed.), Fluid, Electrolyte, and Acid-Base Disorders in Small Animal Practice, third ed. Elsevier, St Louis, pp. 518–540.

Grauer, G., 2009. Acute renal failure. In: Nelson, R.W., Couto, C.G. (Eds.), Small Animal Internal Medicine, fourth ed. Mosby Elsevier, St Louis, pp. 645–653.

Langston, C., 2010. Acute intrinsic renal failure. In: Drobatz, K.J., Costello, M.F. (Eds.), Feline Emergency and Critical Care Medicine. Wiley-Blackwell, Ames, pp. 303–312.

Langston, C., 2010. Acute uremia. In: Ettinger, S.J., Feldman, E.C. (Eds.), Textbook of Veterinary Internal Medicine Diseases of the Dog and Cat, seventh ed. Elsevier Saunders, St Louis, pp. 1969–1981.

Urinary emergencies and electrolyte disorders

Langston, C.E., 2009. Acute renal failure. In: Silverstein, D.C., Hopper, K. (Eds.), Small Animal Critical Care Medicine. Elsevier, St Louis, pp. 590–594.

Langston, C., May 2008. Managing fluid and electrolyte disorders in renal failure. Advances in fluid, electrolyte, and acid-base disorders. In: deMorais, H.A., DiBartola, S.P. (Eds.), Veterinary Clinics: Small Animal Practice, vol. 38. Elsevier, St Louis, no 3, pp. 677–697.

Mathews, K., 2006. Management of acute renal failure. In: Mathews, K.A. (Ed.), Veterinary Emergency and Critical Care Manual, second ed. Lifelearn Inc., Guelph, Canada, pp. 709–726.

Mathews, K.A., Monteith, G., 2007. Evaluation of adding diltiazem to therapy to standard treatment of acute renal failure caused by leptospirosis: 18 dogs (1998-2001). Journal of Veterinary Emergency Critical Care 17 (2), 149–158.

Mehta, R.L., Pascual, M.T., Soroko, S., et al, 2002. Diuretics, mortality, and non-recovery of renal function in acute renal failure. Journal of the American Medical Association 288 (20), 2547–2553.

Ross, L., 2009. Acute renal failure. In: Bonagura, J.D., Twedt, D.C. (Eds.), Kirk's Current Veterinary Therapy XIV. Elsevier Saunders, St Louis, pp. 879–882.

Seshadri, R., Crump, K., 2010. Acute renal failure. In: Mazzaferro, E.M. (Ed.), Blackwell's Five Minute Veterinary Consult Clinical Companion Small Animal Emergency and Critical Care. Wiley-Blackwell, Ames, pp. 13–20.

Sigrist, N.E., 2007. Use of dopamine in acute renal failure. Journal of Veterinary Emergency and Critical Care 17 (2), 117–126.

Simmons, J.P., Wohl, J.S., Schwartz, D.D., et al, 2006. Diuretic effects of fenoldopam in healthy cats. Journal of Veterinary Emergency and Critical Care 16 (2), 96–103.

Stokes, J.E., 2009. Diagnostic approach to acute azotemia. In: Bonagura, J.D., Twedt, D.C. (Eds.), Kirk's Current Veterinary Therapy XIV. Elsevier Saunders, St Louis, pp. 855–860.

CHRONIC RENAL FAILURE

Acierna, M.J., 2009. Systemic Hypertension in Renal Disease. In: Bonagura, J.D., Twedt, D.C. (Eds.), Kirk's Current Veterinary Therapy XIV. Elsevier Saunders, St Louis, pp. 910–912.

Cortadellas, O., del Palacio, M.J.F., Talavera, J., et al, 2010. Calcium and phosphorus homeostasis. In: Dogs with spontaneous chronic kidney disease at different stages of severity. Journal of Veterinary Internal Medicine 24, 73–79.

Elliott, J., Watson, A.D.J., 2009. Chronic kidney disease: staging and management. In: Bonagura, J.D., Twedt, D.C. (Eds.), Kirk's Current Veterinary Therapy XIV. Elsevier Saunders, St Louis, pp. 883–892.

Grauer, G., 2009. Chronic renal failure. In: Nelson, R.W., Couto, C.G. (Eds.), Small Animal Internal Medicine, fourth ed. Mosby Elsevier, St Louis, pp. 653–659.

Jepson, R.E., Brodbelt, E., Vallance, C., et al, 2009. Evaluation of predictors of the development of azotemia in cats. Journal of Veterinary Internal Medicine 23, 806–813.

Kerl, M.E., Langston, C.E., 2009. Treatment of anemia in renal failure. In: Bonagura, J.D., Twedt, D.C. (Eds.), Kirk's Current Veterinary Therapy XIV. Elsevier Saunders, St Louis, pp. 914–918.

King, J.N., Tasker, S., Gunn-Moore, D.A., et al, 2007. Prognostic factors in cats with chronic kidney disease. Journal of Veterinary Internal Medicine 21, 906–916.

Langston, C.E., 2009. Chronic renal failure. In: Silverstein, D.C., Hopper, K. (Eds.), Small Animal Critical Care Medicine. Elsevier, St Louis, pp. 594–598.

Polzin, D.J., 2010. Chronic kidney disease. In: Ettinger, S.J., Feldman, E.C. (Eds.), Textbook of Veterinary Internal Medicine Diseases of the Dog and Cat, seventh ed. Elsevier Saunders, St Louis, pp. 1990–2021.

Schaer, M. (Ed.), 1989. The Veterinary Clinics of North America, Small Animal Practice: Fluid and Electrolyte Disorders 19 (2), 343–359.

PYELONEPHRITIS

Barsanti, J.A., 2009. Management of drug resistant urinary tract infections. In: Bonagura, J.D., Twedt, D.C. (Eds.), Kirk's Current Veterinary Therapy XIV. Elsevier Saunders, St Louis, pp. 921–925.

Brown, S.A., Grauer, G.F., 1997. Pyelonephritis. In: Morgan, R.V. (Ed.), Handbook of Small Animal Practice, third ed. Saunders, Philadelphia, pp. 500–502.

Grauer, G., 2009. Pyelonephritis. In: Nelson, R.W., Couto, C.G. (Eds.), Small

Animal Internal Medicine, fourth ed. Mosby Elsevier, St Louis, pp. 660–666.

Labato, M.A., 2009. Uncomplicated urinary tract infections. In: Bonagura, J.D., Twedt, D.C. (Eds.), Kirk's Current Veterinary Therapy XIV. Elsevier Saunders, St Louis, pp. 918–921.

Langston, C., 2010. Acute uremia. In: Ettinger, S.J., Feldman, E.C. (Eds.), Textbook of Veterinary Internal Medicine Diseases of the Dog and Cat, seventh ed. Elsevier Saunders, St Louis, pp. 1969–1981.

Malouin, A., 2010. Pyelonephritis. In: Drobatz, K.J., Costello, M.F. (Eds.), Feline Emergency and Critical Care Medicine. Wiley-Blackwell, Ames, pp. 299–300.

Pressler, B., Bartges, J.W., 2010. Urinary tract infections. In: Ettinger, S.J., Feldman, E.C. (Eds.), Textbook of Veterinary Internal Medicine Diseases of the Dog and Cat, seventh ed. Elsevier Saunders, St Louis, pp. 2036–2047.

HEMATURIA AND HEMOGLOBINURIA

Ettinger, S.J. (Ed.), 1989. The Textbook of Veterinary Internal Medicine, Diseases of the Dog and Cat, third ed. WB Saunders, Philadelphia, pp. 160–163.

Grauer, G., 2009. Urinary Tract Disorders. In: Nelson, R.W., Couto, C.G. (Eds.), Small Animal Internal Medicine, fourth ed. Mosby Elsevier, St Louis, pp. 611–614.

Stone, E., 2006. Hematuria. In: Mathews, K.A. (Ed.), Veterinary Emergency and Critical Care Manual, second ed. Lifelearn Inc., Guelph, Canada, pp. 731–735.

FELINE LOWER URINARY TRACT DISEASE: NOT OBSTRUCTED

Grauer, G., 2009. Feline Lower urinary tract disease. In: Nelson, R.W., Couto, C.G. (Eds.), Small Animal Internal Medicine, fourth ed. Mosby Elsevier, St Louis, pp. 677–681.

Kruger, J.M., Osborne, C.A., 2009. Management of feline nonobstructed idiopathic cystitis. In: Bonagura, J.D., Twedt, D.C. (Eds.), Kirk's Current Veterinary Therapy XIV. Elsevier Saunders, St Louis, pp. 944–950.

Kruger, J.M., Osborne, C.A., Lulich, J.P., 2010. Feline lower urinary tract disease (FLUTD). In: Mazzaferro, E.M. (Ed.), Blackwell's Five Minute Veterinary Consult Clinical Companion Small Animal Emergency and Critical Care. Wiley-Blackwell, Ames, pp. 273–280.

Lees, G.E., 1996. Bacterial urinary tract infections. The Veterinary Clinics of North America, Small Animal Practice: Disorders of the Feline Lower Urinary Tract I, Biology and Pathophysiology 26 (2), 300.

Malouin, A., 2010. Urologic emergencies. In: Drobatz, K.J., Costello, M.F. (Eds.), Feline Emergency and Critical Care Medicine. Wiley-Blackwell, Ames, pp. 282–283.

Osborne, C.A., Kruger, J.M., Lulich, J.P. (guest eds), 1996. The Veterinary Clinics of North America, Small Animal Practice: Disorders of the Feline Lower Urinary Tract I.: Etiology and Pathophysiology 26 (2), 300–301.

FELINE LOWER URINARY TRACT DISEASE: OBSTRUCTED

Drobatz, K.J., 2009. Urethral obstruction in cats. In: Bonagura, J.D., Twedt, D.C. (Eds.), Kirk's Current Veterinary Therapy XIV. Elsevier Saunders, St Louis, pp. 951–954.

Gerber, B., Eichenberger, S., Reusch, C.F., 2008. Guarded long-term prognosis in male cats with urethral obstruction. Journal of Feline Medicine and Surgery 10, 16–23.

Grauer, G., 2009. Feline lower urinary tract disease. In: Nelson, R.W., Couto, C.G. (Eds.), Small Animal Internal Medicine, fourth ed. Mosby Elsevier, St Louis, pp. 681–683.

Malouin, A., 2010. Urologic emergencies. In: Drobatz, K.J., Costello, M.F. (Eds.), Feline Emergency and Critical Care Medicine. Wiley-Blackwell, Ames, pp. 283–289.

Mathews, K.A., 2006. Feline lower urinary tract obstruction. In: Mathews, K.A. (Ed.), Veterinary Emergency and Critical Care Manual, second ed. Lifelearn Inc., Guelph, Canada, pp. 745–750.

Osborne, C.A., Kruger, J.M., Lulich, J.P. (guest eds), 1996. The Veterinary Clinics of North America, Small Animal Practice: Disorders of the Feline Lower Urinary Tract I: Etiology and Pathophysiology 26 (3), 500–511.

Westropp, J.L., Buffington, C.A.T., 2010. Lower urinary tract disorders in cats. In: Ettinger, S.J., Feldman, E.C. (Eds.), Textbook of Veterinary Internal Medicine Diseases of the Dog and Cat, seventh ed. Elsevier Saunders, St Louis, pp. 2069–2086.

CANINE UROLITHIASIS

Adams, L.G., Lulich, J.P., 2009. Laser lithotripsy for uroliths. In: Bonagura, J.D., Twedt, D.C. (Eds.), Kirk's Current Veterinary Therapy XIV. Elsevier Saunders, St Louis, pp. 940–943.

Adams, L.G., Syme, H.M., 2010. Canine ureteral and lower urinary tract diseases. In: Ettinger, S.J., Feldman, E.C. (Eds.), Textbook of Veterinary Internal Medicine Diseases of the Dog and Cat, seventh ed. Elsevier Saunders, St Louis, pp. 2086–2109.

Bartges, J.W., Kirk, C.A., 2009. Interpreting and managing crystalluria. In: Bonagura, J.D., Twedt, D.C. (Eds.), Kirk's Current Veterinary Therapy XIV. Elsevier Saunders, St Louis, pp. 850–854.

Dolinsek, D., 2004. Calcium oxalate urolithiasis in the canine: Surgical management and preventative strategies. Canadian Veterinary Journal 45, 607–609.

Grauer, G., 2009. Canine urolithiasis. In: Nelson, R.W., Couto, C.G. (Eds.), Small Animal Internal Medicine, fourth ed. Mosby Elsevier, St Louis, pp. 667–676.

Houston, D.M., Moore, A.E.P., Favrin, M.G., et al, 2004. Canine urolithiasis: A look at over 16 000 urolith submissions to the Canadian Veterinary Urolith Centre from February 1998 to April 2003. Canadian Veterinary Journal 45, 225–230.

UROABDOMEN

Anderson, R.B., Aronson, L.R., Drobatz, K.J., et al, 2006. Prognostic factors for successful outcome following urethral rupture in dogs and cats. Journal of the American Animal Hospital Association 42, 136–146.

Bray, J.P., Doyle, R.S., Burton, C.A., 2009. Minimally invasive inguinal approach for tube cystotomy. Veterinary Surgery 38 (3), 411–416.

Culp, W.T.N., Silverstein, D.C., 2009. Abdominal trauma. In: Silverstein, D.C., Hopper, K. (Eds.), Small Animal Critical Care Medicine. Elsevier, St Louis, pp. 669–670.

Halling, J., 2006. Urine leakage – abdomen / perineum / dorsum. In: Mathews, K.A. (Ed.), Veterinary Emergency and Critical Care Manual, second ed. Lifelearn Inc., Guelph, Canada, pp. 727–730.

Lulich, J.P., Osborne, C.A. (Eds.), 1997. Bladder Trauma in Handbook of Small Animal Practice, third ed. Rhea V. Morgan. WB Saunders, Philadelphia, pp. 542–543.

Malouin, A., 2010. Uroabdomen. In: Drobatz, K.J., Costello, M.F. (Eds.), Feline Emergency and Critical Care Medicine. Wiley-Blackwell, Ames, pp. 294–295.

Meige, F., Sarrau, S., Autefage, A., 2008. Management of traumatic urethral rupture in 11 cats using primary alignment with a urethral catheter. Veterinary Comparative Orthopedics and Traumatology 21, 76–84.

Osborne, C.A., Sanderson, S.L., Lulich, J.P., et al, 1996. Medical management of iatrogenic rents in the wall of the feline urinary bladder. Veterinary Clinics of North America Small Animal Practice 26 (3), 551–562.

Zhang, J.T., Wang, H.B., Shi, J., et al, 2010. Laparoscopy for percutaneous tube cystostomy in dogs. Journal of the American Veterinary Medical Association 236 (9), 975–977.

HYPERCALCEMIA

Feldman, E.C., 2010. Disorders of parathyroid glands. In: Ettinger, S.J., Feldman, E.C. (Eds.), Textbook of Veterinary Internal Medicine Diseases of the Dog and Cat, seventh ed. Elsevier Saunders, St Louis, pp. 1744–1751.

Green, T., Chew, D.J., 2009. Calcium disorders. In: Silverstein, D.C., Hopper, K. (Eds.), Small Animal Critical Care Medicine. Elsevier, St Louis, pp. 233–238.

Messinger, J.S., Windham, W.R., Ward, C.R., 2009. Ionized hypercalcemia in dogs: a retrospective study of 109 cases (1998-2003). Journal of Veterinary Internal Medicine 23, 514–519.

Rinkhardt, N., 2006. Hypercalcemia. In: Mathews, K.A. (Ed.), Veterinary Emergency and Critical Care Manual, second ed. Lifelearn Inc., Guelph, Canada, pp. 373–376.

Schaer, M., May 2008. Hypercalcemia. Advances in fluid, electrolyte, and acid-base disorders. In: deMorais, H.A., DiBartola, S.P. (Eds.), Veterinary Clinics: Small Animal Practice, vol. 38. Elsevier, St Louis, no 3, pp. 525–528.

Schenck, P.A., Chew, D.J., Nagode, et al, 2006. Disorders of calcium: hypercalcemia and hypocalcemia. In: diBartola, S.P. (Ed.), Fluid, Electrolyte, and Acid-Base Disorders in Small Animal Practice, third ed. Elsevier, St Louis, pp. 122–194.

HYPOCALCEMIA

Feldman, E.C., 2010. Disorders of parathyroid glands. In: Ettinger, S.J., Feldman, E.C. (Eds.), Textbook of Veterinary Internal Medicine Diseases of the Dog and Cat, seventh ed. Elsevier Saunders, St Louis, pp. 1744–1751.

Green, T., Chew, D.J., 2009. Calcium disorders. In: Silverstein, D.C., Hopper, K. (Eds.), Small Animal Critical Care Medicine. Elsevier, St Louis, pp. 238–239.

Holowaychuk, M.K., Hansen, B.D., DeFrancesco, T.C., et al, 2009. Ionized hypocalcemia in critically ill dogs. Journal of Veterinary Internal Medicine 23, 509–513.

Rinkhardt, N., 2006. Hypocalcemia. In: Mathews, K.A. (Ed.), Veterinary Emergency and Critical Care Manual, second ed. Lifelearn Inc., Guelph, Canada, pp. 377–380.

Schaer, M., May 2008. Hypocalcemia, advances in fluid, electrolyte, and acid-base disorders. In: deMorais, H.A., DiBartola, S.P. (Eds.), Veterinary Clinics: Small Animal Practice, vol. 38. Elsevier, St Louis, no 3, 521 525.

Schenck, P.A., Chew, D.J., Nagode, et al, 2006. Disorders of calcium: hypercalcemia and hypocalcemia. In: diBartola, S.P. (Ed.), Fluid, Electrolyte, and Acid-Base Disorders in Small Animal Practice, third ed. Elsevier, St Louis, pp. 122–194.

Wills, T.B., Bohn, A.A., Martin, L.G., 1995. Hypocalcemia in a critically ill patient. Journal of Veterinary Emergency and Critical Care 15 (2), 136–142.

HYPERKALEMIA

diBartola, S.P., deMorais, H.A., 2006. Disorders of potassium: hypokalemia and hyperkalemia. In: diBartola, S.P. (Ed.), Fluid, Electrolyte, and Acid-Base Disorders in Small Animal Practice, third ed. Elsevier, St Louis, pp. 91–121.

Kogika, M.M., deMorais, H.A., May 2008. Hyperkalemia. Advances in fluid, electrolyte, and acid-base disorders. In: deMorais, H.A., DiBartola, S.P. (Eds.), Veterinary Clinics: Small Animal Practice, vol. 38. Elsevier, St Louis, no 3, 477–480.

Mathews, K.A., 2006. Hypokalemia / hyperkalemia. In: Mathews, K.A. (Ed.), Veterinary Emergency and Critical Care Manual, second ed. Lifelearn Inc., Guelph, Canada, pp. 394–399.

Riordan, L.L., Schaer, M., 2009. Potassium disorders. In: Silverstein, D.C., Hopper, K. (Eds.), Small Animal Critical Care Medicine. Elsevier, St Louis, pp. 231–233.

Schaer, M., May 2008. Therapeutic approach to electrolyte emergencies. Advances in fluid, electrolyte, and acid-base disorders. In: deMorais, H.A., DiBartola, S.P. (Eds.), Veterinary Clinics: Small Animal Practice, vol. 38. Elsevier, St Louis, no 3, 515–518.

Willard, M., May 2008. Therapeutic approach to chronic electrolyte disorders. Advances in fluid, electrolyte, and acid-base disorders. In: deMorais, H.A., DiBartola, S.P. (Eds.), Veterinary Clinics: Small Animal Practice, vol. 38. Elsevier, St Louis, no 3, 537–539.

HYPOKALEMIA

diBartola, S.P., deMorais, H.A., 2006. Disorders of potassium: hypokalemia and hyperkalemia. In: diBartola, S.P. (Ed.), Fluid, Electrolyte, and Acid-Base Disorders in Small Animal Practice, third ed. Elsevier, St Louis, pp. 9–121.

Kogika, M.M., deMorais, H.A., May 2008. Hypokalemia. Advances in fluid, electrolyte, and acid-base disorders. In: deMorais, H.A., DiBartola, S.P. (Eds.), Veterinary Clinics: Small Animal Practice, vol. 38. Elsevier, St Louis, no 3, pp. 481–484.

Mathews, K.A., 2006. Hypokalemia / hyperkalemia. In: Mathews, K.A. (Ed.), Veterinary Emergency and Critical Care Manual, second ed. Lifelearn Inc., Guelph, Canada, pp. 394–399.

Riordan, L.L., Schaer, M., 2009. Potassium disorders. In: Silverstein, D.C., Hopper, K. (Eds.), Small Animal Critical Care Medicine. Elsevier, St Louis, pp. 229–231.

Schaer, M., May 2008. Therapeutic approach to electrolyte emergencies. Advances in fluid, electrolyte, and acid-base disorders. In: deMorais, H.A., DiBartola, S.P. (Eds.), Veterinary Clinics: Small Animal Practice, vol. 38. Elsevier, St Louis, no 3, 512–515.

Willard, M., May 2008. Therapeutic approach to chronic electrolyte disorders. Advances in fluid, electrolyte, and acid-base disorders. In: deMorais, H.A., DiBartola, S.P. (Eds.), Veterinary

Urinary emergencies and electrolyte disorders

Clinics: Small Animal Practice, vol. 38.
Elsevier, St Louis, no 3, 535–541.

HYPERNATREMIA

Burkitt, J.M., 2009. Sodium disorders. In:
Silverstein, D.C., Hopper, K. (Eds.),
Small Animal Critical Care Medicine.
Elsevier, St Louis, pp. 224–229.

DiBartola, S.P., 2006. Disorders of sodium
and water: hypernatremia and
hyponatremia. In: diBartola, S.P. (Ed.),
Fluid, Electrolyte, and Acid-Base
Disorders in Small Animal Practice, third
ed. Elsevier, St Louis, pp. 47–79.

Goldkamp, C., Schaer, M., 2007.
Hypernatremia in dogs. Compendium
on Continuing Education for the
Practicing Veterinarian 29 (3), 152–162.

Mathews, K.A., 2006.
Hypernatremia / hyponatremia. In:
Mathews, K.A. (Ed.), Veterinary
Emergency and Critical Care Manual,
second ed. Lifelearn Inc., Guelph,
Canada, pp. 381–385.

Schaer, M., 1999. Disorders of serum
potassium, sodium, magnesium and
chloride. Journal of Veterinary
Emergency and Critical Care 9 (4),
209–217.

Schaer, M., May 2008. Hypernatremia.
Advances in fluid, electrolyte, and
acid-base disorders. In: deMorais, H.A.,
DiBartola, S.P. (Eds.), Veterinary Clinics:
Small Animal Practice, vol. 38. Elsevier,
St Louis, no 3, pp. 522–524.

HYPONATREMIA

Burkitt, J.M., 2009. Sodium disorders. In:
Silverstein, D.C., Hopper, K. (Eds.),
Small Animal Critical Care Medicine.
Elsevier, St Louis, pp. 226–229.

DiBartola, S.P., 2006. Disorders of sodium
and water: hypernatremia and
hyponatremia. In: diBartola, S.P. (Ed.),
Fluid, Electrolyte, and Acid-Base
Disorders in Small Animal Practice, third
ed. Elsevier, St Louis, pp. 47–79.

Mathews, K.A., 2006.
Hypernatremia / hyponatremia. In:
Mathews, K.A. (Ed.), Veterinary
Emergency and Critical Care Manual,
second ed. Lifelearn Inc., Guelph,
Canada, pp. 386–389.

Schaer, M., 1999. Disorders of serum
potassium, sodium, magnesium and
chloride. Journal of Veterinary
Emergency and Critical Care 9 (4),
209–217.

Schaer, M., May 2008. Hyponatremia.
Advances in fluid, electrolyte, and
acid-base disorders. In: deMorais, H.A.,
DiBartola, S.P. (Eds.), Veterinary Clinics:
Small Animal Practice, vol. 38. Elsevier,
St Louis, no 3, 518–522.

HYPOPHOSPHATEMIA

Aldrich, J., 2009. Phosphate disorders. In:
Silverstein, D.C., Hopper, K. (Eds.),
Small Animal Critical Care Medicine.
Elsevier, St Louis, pp. 244–247.

Bates, J.A., May 2008. Phosphorus: a quick
reference. Advances in fluid, electrolyte,
and acid-base disorders. In: deMorais,
H.A., DiBartola, S.P. (Eds.), Veterinary
Clinics: Small Animal Practice, vol. 38.
Elsevier, St Louis, no 3, 471–475.

DiBartola, S.P., Willard, M.D., 2006.
Disorders of phosphorus:
hypophosphatemia and
hyperphosphatemia. In: diBartola, S.P.
(Ed.), Fluid, Electrolyte, and Acid-Base
Disorders in Small Animal Practice, third
ed. Elsevier, St Louis, pp. 195–209.

Schropp, D.M., Kovacic, J., 2007.
Phosphorus and phosphate metabolism
in veterinary patients. Journal of
Veterinary Emergency and Critical Care
17 (2), 127–134.

HYPOMAGNESEMIA

Bateman, S., 2006. Disorders of
magnesium: magnesium deficit and
excess. In: diBartola, S.P. (Ed.), Fluid,
Electrolyte, and Acid-Base Disorders in
Small Animal Practice, third ed. Elsevier,
St Louis, pp. 210–228.

Dhupa, N., Proulx, J., May 2008.
Hypocalcemia and hypomagnesemia.
Advances in fluid, electrolyte, and
acid-base disorders. In: deMorais, H.A.,
DiBartola, S.P. (Eds.), Veterinary Clinics:
Small Animal Practice, vol. 38. Elsevier,
St Louis, no 3, 587–608.

Schaer, M., 1999. Disorders of serum
potassium, sodium, magnesium and
chloride. Journal of Veterinary
Emergency and Critical Care 9 (4),
209–217.

Willard, M., May 2008. Therapeutic
approach to chronic electrolyte
disorders. Advances in fluid, electrolyte,
and acid-base disorders. In: deMorais,
H.A., DiBartola, S.P. (Eds.), Veterinary
Clinics: Small Animal Practice, vol. 38.
Elsevier, St Louis, no 3, 535–541.

Reproductive emergencies

DYSTOCIA

Etiology

The causes of dystocia include uterine inertia, fetopelvic disproportion, fetal maldisposition, birth canal abnormalities, fetal death and other causes.

Diagnosis

History—No delivery of a fetus for more than 24 hours after the onset of stage 1 labor, including a rectal temperature drop below 37.8°C (100°F); greater than 30–60 minutes of active labor with no fetus delivered; fetal membrane visibility for 15 minutes or longer; greater than 3–4 hours between deliveries; more than 24 hours of labor to deliver the entire litter of puppies or more than 36 hours of labor to deliver the entire litter of kittens; weak and infrequent labor contractions; crying or biting at the vulvar area or flanks; depression, weakness, signs of toxemia, excessive or abnormal vaginal hemorrhaging or discharge. Dystocia is also present if the bitch or queen has gone >70–72 days since the first breeding, >68–70 days since the last breeding, or >58 days of diestrus.

Dystocia occurs commonly in brachycephalic breeds of dogs and miniature and small breeds of dogs, although it can occur in any breed of dog and in cats.

Physical exam—Perform a thorough patient examination. Palpation of the abdomen should include assessment of abdominal distention, abdominal shape, presence of palpable fetuses, and fetal movement. Evaluate the mammary glands for health and the presence of milk. Evaluation of the vulva may reveal abnormal discharge, odor, damage or constriction. Lochia, or uteroverdin, is a green vulvar discharge that indicates placental separation has occurred. Delivery of a fetus should normally occur within 2 hours of the appearance of lochia. A hygienic, gentle vaginal exam should be performed to assess vaginal tone, possible presence of a fetus in the birth canal, presence of an amniotic vesicle, fetal position, possibly a complicating factor such as a previous pelvic fracture, or inadequate or absent contractions. The cervix cannot be palpated in most small animal patients.

Laboratory evaluation—

1. Assessment of the patient's serum calcium level may reveal hypocalcemia. If possible, assess ionized calcium levels.
2. Assessment of the patient's blood glucose level may reveal hypoglycemia.
3. If the patient is systemically ill, a CBC and complete serum biochemical profile and urinalysis should be evaluated.

*Abdominal radiographs—*Abdominal radiographs may confirm pregnancy after 35 days of pregnancy following completion of organogenesis. The fetal skeletons will be visible after 40 days of pregnancy. Radiographs are valuable in determining the number of fetuses present, their positioning, their size in relation to the pelvic canal, the presence of an obstruction in the birth canal and, possibly, the presence of fetal death. Signs of fetal death that may be apparent radiographically include intrafetal gas patterns (especially in the fetal heart and stomach), collapse of the fetal spinal column, overlapping or misalignment of fetal cranial bones (Spalding's sign), or fetal positioning that is abnormal.

*Abdominal ultrasonography—*This may be valuable in assessing fetal age, size, number, position and viability. At about 21 days of pregnancy, a fetal heart beat may be detected with Doppler ultrasound. At about 35 days of pregnancy, the presence of fetuses may be detected, fetal hearts may be observed and the heart rates counted. The normal fetal heart rate should be twice the maternal rate or higher, normally 200 beats per minute or higher in dogs, 200 to 250 beats per minute or higher in cats. A decrease in heart rate to less than 170–180 beats per minute indicates fetal distress and less than 150 beats per minute indicates emergency intervention is needed.

Prognosis

The prognosis is excellent to guarded.

Treatment

1. Inform the client of the diagnosis, prognosis and cost of the treatment.
2. Perform a vaginal exam; attempt manipulation of the fetus.
   A. Apply lubricants liberally.
   B. Use gauze sponges to aid in manipulation of the fetus. Do not pull on the distal fetal extremities or jaw.
   C. Position the bitch or queen in a standing position.
   D. Apply traction on the fetus gently in a posterior and ventral direction.
   E. Sometimes it is beneficial to turn the fetus to one side or the other.
   F. An episiotomy may be necessary if the vaginal vault is too small to allow vaginal delivery.
   G. If instruments are needed to assist deliver, use a spay hook, nonratcheted sponge forceps or placental forceps.

3. Administer an intravenous balanced electrolyte solution IV if the patient is dehydrated.
4. If the serum ionized calcium level is decreased, administer calcium gluconate 10% 0.5–1.5 mL/kg slowly IV, while monitoring the heart for bradycardia or arrhythmias.
5. Administer dextrose 25% IV if the patient is hypoglycemic.
6. Administer oxytocin 0.25–2.0 IU IM or SC (maximum 4 IU). If the bitch or queen is systemically ill or obvious reasons are apparent that will prohibit vaginal delivery, do not administer oxytocin. Start medical treatment (fluid therapy, etc.) and perform a cesarean section as soon as the bitch or queen is stable.
7. Oxytocin can be repeated in 30–60 minutes for a total of two doses, with intermittent vaginal exams and feathering. If no results, recommend a cesarean section. If the patient delivers a fetus, wait another hour between fetuses.
8. Anesthesia and surgery
   A. Place an IV catheter; begin administration of LRS or Normosol®-R IV, 10–20 mL/kg/h until recovered from anesthesia.
   B. Administer a broad-spectrum systemic antibiotic such as cefazolin, 22–30 mg/kg IV, if an infection is suspected.
   C. Use minimal anesthesia, avoid ketamine.
      I. Canine anesthesia
         a. Premedicate the bitch with butorphanol, 0.45 mg/kg IM; diazepam, 0.45 mg/kg IM; and atropine, 0.045mg/kg IM, or glycopyrrolate, 0.005–0.011 mg/kg IM, SC, if desired.
         b. Epidural analgesia may be administered following sedation.
            i. Lidocaine, not to exceed 5 mg/kg
            ii. Bupivacaine, 1 mL/3.5 kg, and/or morphine, 0.1 mg/kg
         c. Mask induction is performed with isoflurane or sevoflurane and then the bitch is intubated and maintained on isoflurane or sevoflurane.
         d. Small doses of diazepam or midazolam with oxymorphone or hydromorphone, or propofol may be administered IV for induction and followed by isoflurane or sevoflurane maintenance.
      II. Feline anesthesia
         a. Premedicate the queen with glycopyrrolate, 0.005–0.011 mg/kg IM or SC 15 minutes prior to administering anesthetics.
         b. Induce anesthesia with diazepam, 0.027 mg/kg IV or 0.4 mg/kg IM and ketamine, 5.5–6 mg/kg IM or IV. Then place an endotracheal tube and maintain with isoflurane or sevoflurane inhalation.
         c. Intubation may also be facilitated by spraying the vocal folds with 0.5% lidocaine.
         d. An alternative method is to inject 0.5–1% lidocaine at a maximum dose of 10 mg/kg subcutaneously along the ventral midline incision site after the diazepam and ketamine combination has taken effect. Once the kittens are removed from the uterus, isoflurane may be administered if more anesthetic time is required for completion of the surgery.

   e. If the patient is depressed or ill prior to surgery, pre-oxygenate the queen, then administer diazepam, 0.027 mg/kg IV or 0.4 mg/kg IM, or midazolam, 0.2 mg/kg IM, combined with either butorphanol, 0.4 mg/kg IM, or oxymorphone, 0.2 mg/kg IM. If additional anesthesia is needed, administer ketamine, 1 mg/kg IV, or thiopental, 1 mg/kg IV.

   D. Remove fetuses as quickly and gently as possible. Clean debris from the nose and mouth of the neonate(s) with a bulb syringe or use the One Puff breathing device.

   E. Administer oxygen to newborns, give 1–2 drops doxapram (Dopram®) under the tongue if needed to stimulate respiration. Respiration may also be stimulated by stimulating the acupuncture governing point GV26. Reverse narcotics with 1–2 drops naloxone (Narcan®) under the tongue. Stimulate and warm newborns, but do not shake them forcefully. (Forceful shaking may displace surfactant and decrease the ability of the pulmonary alveoli to expand.) Ligate the umbilical cords.

   F. Perform an ovariohysterectomy, if the client so desires, or if complications dictate.

   G. The administration of a post-whelping oxytocin injection ('a clean-out shot') is controversial. Oxytocin at 0.25–2 U IM may be administered upon client request.

   H. Complete surgery; hospitalize the bitch or queen for recovery *separated* from the newborns until she is alert, then gradually introduce the offspring to the bitch or queen.

   I. If an episiotomy was performed, remember to close it up as soon as delivery is complete.

   J. Dispense 3–5 days' oral antibiotic therapy if a uterine infection or dead fetus is present.

   K. Give the client post-operative instructions (suture removal, monitor temperature and vaginal discharge, etc.).

9. Instruct the client to have the bitch and puppies or queen and kittens re-examined by their regular veterinarian in 3–5 days and to call the regular veterinarian's office the next business day regarding care of the dewclaws and tails.

FADING NEONATAL SYNDROMES (NEONATAL MORTALITY)

Etiology

There are two categories of the causes of neonatal death: noninfectious and infectious. The noninfectious causes include maternal malnutrition, hypothermia, hypoglycemia, neonatal isoerythrolysis in kittens, trauma, stillbirth and anatomic abnormalities. The infectious diseases that result in neonatal mortality include the following:

1. Viral infections – herpesvirus, canine and feline parvoviruses, calicivirus, feline leukemia virus, morbillivirus, coronavirus, canine adenovirus 1, and canine distemper virus

2. Bacterial infections – *Bacteroides* spp., *Bordetella* spp., *Brucella* spp., *Campylobacter* spp., *Clostridium* spp., *Enterobacter* spp., *Escherichia coli*, *Fusobacterium* spp., *Klebsiella* spp., *Pasteurella* spp., *Pseudomonas* spp., *Salmonella* spp., St*aphylococcus* spp. and hemolytic and nonhemolytic *Streptococcus* spp.
3. Parasitic infestations – *Ancylostoma* spp., *Coccidium* spp., *Cryptosporidium* spp., *Giardia* spp., and *Toxocara* spp.

Diagnosis

History—The highest death rate occurs during the first 3 days, but the first 2 weeks of life are very hazardous for puppies and kittens. Typically 15–40% of all full-term neonates die within this time period. Neonatal mortality increases in litters born to older, heavier dams and queens that are older than 3 years of age at the time the first litter is delivered. Postpartum illnesses, such as metritis and mastitis, also increase the rate of neonatal deaths.

The environment should be kept at about 29.4°C (85°F) and 55–65% humidity. Heavy-coated breeds and many house pets are better at 21.1–23.0°C (70–75°F) with an ambient humidity. Heat lamps can be utilized to warm one portion of the whelping box. A clean, private, quiet and familiar environment is essential. Exposure to infectious diseases should be restricted.

The normal rectal temperature at birth is 35.6–36.1°C (96–97°F). By 7 days of age, the normal rectal temperature has increased to 37.8°C (100°F). The normal birth weight of kittens is 90–110 g. The kitten should gain a minimum of 7–10 g/day and weigh at least 500 g at 6 weeks of age. Puppies should gain 5–10% of their birth weight per day. They should have doubled their birth weight by 10–12 weeks of age.

Persistent crying (for longer than 20 minutes) is the most common sign of neonatal illness. Other signs include decreased nursing, decreased activity, failure to gain weight, decreased muscle tone and a dry, rough hair coat.

Physical exam—The neonates may pile on top of one another if they are hypothermic, or lay widely spaced and avoid contact if they are hyperthermic. Dehydration, abdominal bloating, cyanosis and pallor may be observed. Weakness, bradycardia, respiratory distress, convulsions and coma may be observed in neonates suffering from hypoglycemia. Trauma may result in puncture wounds or crushing injuries.

Laboratory evaluation—
1. Always measure the blood glucose level when presented with an ill neonate.
2. If an adequate blood sample can be obtained, perform a CBC and serum biochemical profile.
3. Consider performing a blood culture.
4. Urinalysis and urine culture.
5. Lactate levels are normally higher in the neonate.
An ECG may be beneficial.

Radiographs and ultrasound—These may be helpful.

The most useful diagnostic test in litter situations is to perform a necropsy.

Prognosis

Due to the rapid onset and progression of clinical signs, and the generally poor response to treatment, the prognosis is guarded to poor, regardless of the underlying etiology.

Treatment

1. Inform the client of the diagnosis, prognosis and cost of the treatment.
2. Warm the hypothermic neonate slowly, over 1–3 hours, to a rectal temperature of 36.1–36.7°C (97–98°F).
   A. Provide external heat support with a Bair Hugger, or very carefully positioned and monitored circulating hot water blanker, hot water bottle, or heated rice bag. Avoid excessive heat and burns.
   B. Turn the patient over hourly.
   C. Record the patient's rectal temperature hourly.
3. Treat hypoglycemia with oral or intravenous glucose solutions.
   A. Dilute IV glucose solutions to a concentration of 12.5% or less, to avoid phlebitis.
   B. If the patient is receiving intravenous fluid therapy, the fluids should contain a concentration of 5% dextrose.
   C. Maintain the blood glucose concentration between 100 and 140 mg/dL.
4. Parenteral fluid therapy – LRS is the recommended IV fluid because the neonate with hypoglycemia prefers lactate as a metabolic fuel source.
   A. Administer fluid therapy either SC, IV, or through an intraosseous catheter.
   B. Supplement IV and IO fluids with dextrose to a concentration of 5% dextrose. Do not give Dextrose 5% or higher concentrations SC.
   C. Supplement the fluids with potassium chloride if the patient is hypokalemic.
   D. Administer warmed intravenous fluids.
   E. The fluid needs for a neonate are much higher than an adult. The recommended maintenance fluid rate for a neonatal puppy is 80–100 mL/kg/day.
   F. Weigh the neonate every 6–12 hours to help monitor hydration.
   G. If severe dehydration is present, bolus warm LRS IV, 40–45 mL/kg to a puppy and 25–30 mL/kg to a kitten, then try to keep up with ongoing losses.
5. Identify and treat the underlying etiology if possible.
6. Antibiotic therapy
   A. Antibiotics that are safe to administer to neonates, or to nursing bitches or queens, include amoxicillin, amoxicillin-clavulanate, cephalosporins, erythromycin, penicillins and tylosin.
   B. Antibiotics to avoid include aminoglycosides, chloramphenicol, ciprofloxacin, enrofloxacin, polymyxin, sulfonamides, tetracyclines and trimethoprim.

7. Provide nutritional support.
    A. When the neonate has been warmed and rehydrated, it may be tube-fed with a commercial milk replacer, unless it is vomiting.
    B. If the patient is vomiting, provide nutritional support with PPN, TPN, or placement of a feeding tube.
8. Treat traumatic injuries and abscesses as with an adult patient.

MASTITIS

Diagnosis

History—The owner may observe swelling of the mammary gland(s). The bitch or queen may be febrile, listless, reluctant to nurse and have a decreased appetite. The puppies or kittens may be weak, crying and ill. Death of the bitch, queen, puppies or kittens may occur.

Physical exam—The involved mammary gland(s) is / are warm, painful and feel firm or hard. The milk from the affected gland(s) is / are abnormal in color and texture. The bitch or queen may have a fever, may be dehydrated and may exhibit signs of sepsis.

Laboratory evaluation—

1. A milk sample may be submitted for cytologic evaluation and bacterial culture and sensitivity. Fluid aspirated from the affected gland may be submitted for cytologic evaluation and bacterial culture and sensitivity.
2. The CBC may reveal leukocytosis with a neutrophilia, and degenerative left shift or leukopenia may occur with sepsis.
3. The serum biochemical profile may reveal hypoglycemia and additional changes associated with sepsis or dehydration.
4. Culture and susceptibility is recommended.

Differential diagnosis

Hematoma, seroma, abscess, galactostasis, neoplasia.

Prognosis

If presented early in the disease course, the prognosis is good.

Treatment

1. Inform the client of the diagnosis, prognosis and cost of the treatment.
2. Ampicillin, amoxicillin, amoxicillin-clavulanate or cephalosporins are recommended unless the bacterial sensitivity results indicate another antibiotic would be more appropriate. Administer antibiotics for 10–14 days beyond the resolution of inflammation.
3. Administer intravenous fluids to the bitch or queen if dehydration is evident.
4. Treat the bitch or queen for sepsis if indicated.
5. If the infection is mild, encourage nursing from the affected glands to promote drainage.

Reproductive emergencies

6. If the mammary gland is severely infected and necrotic, do not allow the puppies or kittens to nurse. In these patients, manual milking should be performed to keep the affected gland(s) empty.
7. Supplement the neonates with commercial milk replacement to assure adequate nutritional support.
8. Apply warm compresses or run warm water over the infected mammary glands several times a day to promote drainage.
9. If the infected mammary gland is abscessed, lancing, draining, and flushing with dilute (1%) povidone-iodine is indicated. Surgical debridement and closure may be necessary in severe infections.

PYOMETRA (PYOMETRITIS)

Diagnosis

History—Suspect pyometra as the underlying etiology in any ill intact female dog or cat. The owner may observe lethargy, vomiting, polyuria, polydipsia, abdominal distention, abdominal pain or a foul odor. The owner may possibly observe a vaginal discharge and think the dog is 'in heat'.

Physical exam—The physical examination varies from alert and no significant findings to depressed, with abdominal distention, abdominal pain, and dehydration. A purulent vaginal discharge may be observed in some patients with an 'open' pyometra.

Laboratory tests—
1. CBC – may reveal leukocytosis with neutrophilia and a degenerative left shift. The PCV may be elevated owing to dehydration. The PCV may be decreased owing to a nonregenerative anemia of chronic illness.
2. Complete serum biochemical profile – may reveal elevations of the BUN and creatinine due to prerenal or secondary renal azotemia, elevated ALT and ALP, and electrolyte abnormalities.
3. Urinalysis – the urine specific gravity is variable; pyuria and bacturia may be present. Cystocentesis is not recommended.
4. Vaginal smear and cytology – degenerative neutrophils, macrophages and bacteria may be observed.

Abdominal radiographs—These may reveal a fluid-dense tubular structure in the ventrocaudal abdomen. Patients with an open-cervix pyometra may not have an enlarged uterus visible radiographically.

Abdominal ultrasonography—This will assist in evaluation of the uterine size and thickness of the uterine wall. It also helps to confirm that the intrauterine material is of fluid density rather than fetal tissues.

Differential diagnosis

Pregnancy, vaginitis, mucometra, hydrometra, uterine neoplasia, neoplasia of other caudal abdominal organs, gastrointestinal disease, pancreatitis, sepsis, renal failure.

Prognosis

The prognosis is variable, depending on the severity of the systemic illness. The reported mortality rate varies from 4% to 20%.

Treatment

1. Inform the client of the diagnosis, prognosis and cost of the treatment.
2. Place an intravenous catheter.
3. Administer balanced electrolyte replacement intravenous fluids, such as LRS or Normosol®-R. The rate needed will vary with the patient's status, from shock rates to twice maintenance rates.
4. Administer broad-spectrum antibiotics. Avoid aminoglycosides if possible. Utilize second-generation cephalosporins, trimethoprim-sulfa, or enrofloxacin.
   A. Administer cefoxitin, 40 mg/kg IV, initially, and continued at 20 mg/kg IV q6–8h in the dog and q8h in the cat.
   B. Administer trimethoprim-sulfa, 15 mg/kg IM q12h.
   C. Administer enrofloxacin, 5–10 mg/kg IV q12h or 5–20 mg/kg IV q24h.
   D. For severely ill patients, administer a combination of ampicillin (20–40 mg/kg q8h IV), or a first-generation cephalosporin (cefazolin (20 mg/kg q8h IV) or cephalothin (20–30 mg/kg q6h IV), with a fluoroquinolone (enrofloxacin, ciprofloxacin), and a third-generation cephalosporin (ceftizoxime ([25–50 mg/kg IV, IM, SC q6–8h]), cefotaxime ([20–80 mg/kg IV, IM q6–8h]).
5. Ovariohysterectomy
   A. If the patient is *stable* with an open pyometra, it is not essential to perform surgery immediately, but recommend surgery as soon as possible owing to the potential for uterine rupture and peritonitis.
   B. If the patient has a closed pyometra, immediate ovariohysterectomy is recommended.
6. If the patient has an open pyometra and the owner wishes to breed the patient during the next heat cycle, medical therapy with prostaglandin $PGF_{2\alpha}$ may be attempted.
   A. $PGF_{2\alpha}$ is not approved for use in dogs and cats.
   B. $PGF_{2\alpha}$ should not be used in animals older than 8 years of age.
   C. $PGF_{2\alpha}$ should not be used in animals that are critically ill.
   D. $PGF_{2\alpha}$ should not be used in patients with concurrent diseases or pre-existing uterine pathology.
   E. The patient should be hospitalized during therapy, as uterine rupture or retrograde expulsion of uterine contents into the abdominal cavity may occur.
   F. The product preferred is dinoprost (Lutalyse®).
   G. Broad-spectrum bactericidal antibiotics should be administered simultaneously.
   H. The Lutalyse® dose for dogs is 0.1–0.25 mg/kg SC q24h for 5–7 days.
   I. The Lutalyse® dose for cats is 0.10 mg/kg SC q24h for 5–7 days.
   J. Side effects that commonly occur include restlessness, panting, hypersalivation, vomiting, defecation, abdominal cramping, fever and

tachycardia. Hemorrhagic shock may be caused by administering an overdose.

K. After treatment with PGF$_{2\alpha}$ pyometra may recur.

VAGINAL EDEMA (HYPERPLASIA) OR PROLAPSE AND UTERINE PROLAPSE

Diagnosis

History—Vaginal prolapse occurs most frequently in large breed bitches 3 years of age or less. It appears to be most common in Boxers and Mastiffs. It usually occurs when the bitch is in, or has just been through, proestrus or estrus. The patient is usually presented when the owner notices tissue protruding from the vulva. The bitch may be observed licking at the tissue or refuse to allow intromission. Vaginal prolapse may occur following forced separation during mating.

Uterine prolapse is a rare complication of delivery. The cervix or one or both uterine horns may be involved. The owner may observe straining, licking, vaginal discharge or a mass protruding from the vulva.

Physical exam—Vaginal prolapse appears clinically as either swelling in the perineum or a mass projecting from the vulva. The tissue is usually soft, large, smooth, glistening, pale pink to opalescent in color, rounded and reducible. Usually the prolapse originates from the ventral floor of the vaginal vault cranial to the urethral orifice. If the vaginal prolapse is severe it may resemble a doughnut and may include the entire circumference of the vaginal wall. The prolapse may be partial or complete. In complete vaginal prolapse, the cervix projects through the vulvar labia.

The appearance of a mass protruding from the vulva in a bitch or queen that has delivered within the last 48 hours is diagnostic for uterine prolapse.

Differential diagnosis

Benign polyp, neoplasia (leiomyoma or transmissible venereal tumor) and clitoral enlargement.

Prognosis

The prognosis for resolution is good, if the ability to urinate is maintained and necrotic tissue is debrided. Spontaneous regression of vaginal prolapse occurs during diestrus.

Treatment

1. Inform the client of the diagnosis, prognosis and cost of the treatment.
2. Vaginal prolapse treatment
   A. Administer a hyperosmotic agent such as 50% dextrose topically to the extruded and engorged mass to decrease swelling and ease manual tissue reduction.

B. If urination is not possible, an indwelling urethral catheter should be placed.

C. Administer general anesthesia.

D. Attempt manual reduction of the vaginal tissue. An episiotomy may allow for increased exposure and easier reduction.

E. Keep the tissue clean with saline washes or with hexachlorophene (pHisoHex®).

F. Lubricate the mass with water-soluble jelly.

G. Prevent trauma to the mass.

    I. Apply topical antibiotic ointments or antibiotic-steroid creams.

    II. Apply a 'diaper'.

    III. Apply an Elizabethan collar.

    IV. Keep the patient inside on padded and smooth surfaces.

H. Debridement of necrotic tissue is necessary.

I. Ovariohysterectomy does not hasten mass shrinkage, but will prevent recurrence.

J. Surgical excision of the prolapsed tissue may be attempted if the bitch is unable to urinate, if vascular compromise of the bladder, uterus or vaginal tissue is suspected, or if the vaginal tissue is extremely necrotic.

K. If the patient is septic or hypotensive, intravenous fluids, antibiotics and additional therapy should be administered as needed.

3. Uterine prolapse treatment

A. Administer a hyperosmotic agent such as 50% dextrose topically to the extruded and engorged mass to decrease swelling and ease manual tissue reduction.

B. Administer general anesthesia or epidural anesthesia.

C. Rinse the prolapsed tissue with warm saline, then with an antibiotic rinse.

D. Lubricate the prolapsed tissue with water-soluble jelly.

E. Attempt manual reduction of the uterine tissue if the tissue has not been traumatized and appears viable. Use gloved fingers, a long glass tube, or a sterile smooth syringe plunger to assist in reduction.

F. If the prolapsed uterine tissue is replaced, administer systemic antibiotics to treat metritis.

G. Surgical removal of the uterine tissue should be performed if the tissue has been traumatized or does not appear viable.

    I. Ovariohysterectomy should be performed after manual reduction of the uterine prolapse.

    II. If manual reduction is impossible, amputate the uterus and reduce the uterine stump.

PARAPHIMOSIS

Diagnosis

History—The owner observes that the penis of the male dog is protruding for a long period of time. The penis may appear swollen or abnormal in color. The owner may observe straining to urinate or difficulty in urinating. The dog may be observed licking at its penis. Paraphimosis occurs more commonly in the intact male dog, following sexual excitement. It may also occur in long-haired cats, but is uncommon.

Physical exam—The male dog presents with an engorged protruding penis. The penis may be dry or necrotic. The patient may have hematuria, stranguria or anuria. Strangulation of the penis due to string, hair or a foreign object may be observed.

Ultrasonography—Doppler evaluation of the penis may be helpful to determine the presence of active blood flow.

Differential diagnosis

The presence of a hematoma or foreign debris within the prepuce may prevent retraction of the penis into the prepuce, paralysis of the retractor penis muscles, malformation or fracture of the os penis, chronic priapism, an abnormally large preputial orifice, or congenital shortening of the prepuce.

Prognosis

Although not generally life threatening, paraphimosis is an emergency condition. The prognosis for penile tissues depends upon the severity of the vascular compromise and secondary trauma. If the condition has been prolonged, necrosis and gangrene of the penile tissues with secondary systemic complications may become life threatening.

Treatment

1. Inform the client of the diagnosis, prognosis and cost of the treatment.
2. Evaluate the patient's cardiovascular status and treat for shock if necessary.
3. Gently rinse the penis with saline or tap water.
4. Apply a hyperosmotic agent, such as 50% dextrose, topically to the extruded and engorged portion of the penis to decrease swelling and edema.
5. Application of a cold pack to the extruded and engorged portion of the penis may also aid in decreasing swelling and edema.
6. Administer sedation or general anesthesia.
7. Clean the exposed portion of the penis. Remove all hair and foreign debris.
8. Debride necrotic tissue if necessary.
9. Heavily lubricate the exposed portion of the penis and attempt manual replacement.
10. In some cases, a preputial incision may be required.
11. If the penis is severely traumatized and urethral involvement is suspected, place an indwelling soft rubber urethral catheter for 7–14 days.
12. Place a purse-string suture in the tip of the prepuce to hold the penis within it for 1–24 hours.

13. Place an Elizabethan collar on the patient.
14. Infuse antibiotic and steroid ointments into the prepuce daily for 7–14 days.
15. After 1–24 hours, remove the purse-string suture and re-evaluate the penis. If the penis appears normal, manually extrude the penis from the prepuce daily for 7–14 days to decrease adhesion formation.
16. If penile necrosis occurs, penile resection and urethrotomy are necessary. Castration will also be necessary.

ACUTE PROSTATITIS

Diagnosis

History—The dog usually has an acute onset of abdominal pain or back pain, fever, vomiting, lethargy, malaise, polyuria, polydipsia and anorexia. The owner may observe a hemorrhagic preputial discharge or hematuria.

Physical exam—The patient may have a fever, varying degrees of dehydration, palpable caudal abdominal pain, discomfort upon rectal examination, and a hemorrhagic preputial discharge or hematuria. The patient may walk with stiff rear limbs. During the rectal examination, it may not be possible to appreciate a change in prostatic size. If the patient has a prostatic abscess then prostatomegaly, asymmetry and fluctuant areas may be detected. The patient may exhibit tachycardia, injected mucous membranes and weak or thready femoral pulses if in septic shock.

Laboratory evaluation—
1. The CBC may reveal a neutrophilic leukocytosis with or without a left shift, toxic neutrophils and monocytosis.
2. Culture of prostatic fluid may be beneficial, but obtaining a prostatic fluid sample is hazardous in patients with acute prostatitis or a prostatic abscess. Instead, obtain urine by cystocentesis. The most commonly isolated bacteria from a patient with prostatitis are *Enterobacter*, *Escherichia coli*, *Klebsiella*, *Mycoplasma*, *Proteus*, *Pseudomonas*, *Staphylococcus* and *Streptococcus* spp.

3. Urinalysis may show pyuria, bacteriuria and hematuria.

Abdominal radiographs—May reveal prostatomegaly.

Abdominal ultrasonography—May reveal prostatomegaly. If a prostatic abscess is present, ultrasound may reveal intraparenchymal fluid-filled spaces.

Differential diagnosis

Benign prostatic hypertrophy, prostatic neoplasia, periprostatic cysts.

Prognosis

The prognosis is guarded to poor depending on the severity of clinical signs at presentation.

Treatment

1. Inform the owner of the diagnosis, prognosis, and cost of the treatment.
2. Obtain samples for bacterial culture and sensitivity testing.
3. Pending culture and sensitivity results, administer broad-spectrum antibiotics. Recommendations include enrofloxacin, ciprofloxacin, erythromycin, clindamycin, trimethoprim-sulfonamide and chloramphenicol.
4. If the patient is dehydrated or in shock, administer intravenous fluids.
5. If the patient is severely ill, the antibiotics should be administered intravenously.
6. Prostatic abscesses should be surgically drained.
7. Antibiotics should be administered for 3–4 weeks. A few days after discontinuing antibiotic therapy, another urine or prostatic fluid sample should be submitted for culture.
8. Castration should be performed when the patient is stable.

REFERENCES/FURTHER READING

DYSTOCIA

Davidson, A.P., 2009. Dystocia management. In: Bonagura, J.D., Twedt, D.C. (Eds.), Kirk's Current Veterinary Therapy XIV. Saunders Elsevier, St Louis, pp. 992–998.

Feldman, E.C., Nelson, R.W., 2004. Dystocia. In: Feldman, E.C., Nelson, R.W. (Eds.), Canine and Feline Endocrinology and Reproduction, third ed. Saunders Elsevier, St Louis, pp. 816–826.

Funquist, P.M.E., Nyman, G.C., Lofgren, J., et al, 1997. Use of propofol-isoflurane as an anesthetic regimen for cesarean section in dogs. Journal of the American Veterinary Medical Association 211 (3), 313–317.

Gendler, A., Brourman, J.D., Graf, K.E., 2007. Canine dystocia: medical and surgical management. Compendium for the Continuing Education of the Practicing Veterinarian 551–563.

Johnson, C.A., 2009. Dystocia, False pregnancy, disorders of pregnancy and parturition, and mismating. In: Nelson, R.W., Couto, C.G. (Eds.), Small Animal Internal Medicine, fourth ed. Mosby Elsevier, St Louis, pp. 931–935.

Kutzler, M.A., 2009. Dystocia and obstetric crises. In: Silverstein, D.C., Hopper, K. (Eds.), Small Animal Critical Care Medicine. Elsevier, St Louis, pp. 611–615.

Moon, P.F., Erb, H.N., Ludders, J.W., et al, 2000. Perioperative risk factors for puppies delivered by cesarean section in the United States and Canada. Journal of the American Animal Hospital Association 36, 359–368.

FADING NEONATAL SYNDROMES (NEONATAL MORTALITY)

Bonagura, J.D., Kirk, R.W. (Eds.), 1995. Current Veterinary Therapy XII. WB Saunders, Philadelphia, pp. 30–33.

Hoskins, J.D., 1995. Veterinary Pediatrics, second edn. WB Saunders, Philadelphia, pp. 51–55.

McMichael, M., 2009. Critically ill pediatric patients. In: Silverstein, D.C., Hopper, K. (Eds.), Small Animal Critical Care Medicine. Elsevier, St Louis, pp. 747–751.

Murtaugh, R.J., Kaplan, P.M., 1992. Veterinary Emergency and Critical Care Medicine. Mosby, St Louis, pp. 466–468.

MASTITIS

Dosher, K.L., 2009. Mastitis. In: Silverstein, D.C., Hopper, K. (Eds.), Small Animal Critical Care Medicine. Elsevier, St Louis, pp. 619–621.

Feldman, E.C., Nelson, R.W., 2004. Mastitis. In: Feldman, E.C., Nelson, R.W. (Eds.), Canine and Feline Endocrinology and Reproduction, third ed. Saunders Elsevier, St Louis, pp. 831–832.

Johnson, C.A., 2009. Mastitis, postpartum and mammary disorders. In: Nelson, R.W., Couto, C.G. (Eds.), Small Animal Internal Medicine, fourth ed. Mosby Elsevier, St Louis, pp. 946.

Kutzler, M.A., 2009. Canine postpartum disorders. In: Bonagura, J.D., Twedt, D.C. (Eds.), Kirk's Current Veterinary Therapy XIV. Saunders Elsevier, St Louis, pp. 1001.

PYOMETRA (PYOMETRITIS)

Crane, M.B., 2009. Pyometra. In: Silverstein, D.C., Hopper, K. (Eds.), Small Animal Critical Care Medicine. Elsevier, St Louis, pp. 607–611.

Johnson, C.A., 2009. Pyometra, Disorders of the Vagina and Uterus. In: Nelson, R.W., Couto, C.G. (Eds.), Small Animal Internal Medicine, fourth ed. Mosby Elsevier, St Louis, pp. 852–867.

Smith, F.O., 2009. Pyometra. In: Bonagura, J.D., Twedt, D.C. (Eds.), Kirk's Current Veterinary Therapy XIV. Saunders Elsevier, St Louis, pp. 1008–1009.

VAGINAL EDEMA (HYPERPLASIA) OR PROLAPSE AND UTERINE PROLAPSE

Feldman, E.C., Nelson, R.W., 2004. Vaginal hyperplasia / vaginal prolapse. In: Feldman, E.C., Nelson, R.W. (Eds.), Canine and Feline Endocrinology and Reproduction, third ed. Saunders Elsevier, St Louis, pp. 906–909.

Feldman, E.C., Nelson, R.W., 2004. Uterine prolapse. In: Feldman, E.C., Nelson, R.W. (Eds.), Canine and Feline Endocrinology and Reproduction, third ed. Saunders Elsevier, St Louis, pp. 915.

Johnson, C.A., 2009. Vaginal hyperplasia / prolapse, disorders of the vagina and uterus. In: Nelson, R.W., Couto, C.G. (Eds.), Small Animal Internal Medicine, fourth ed. Mosby Elsevier, St Louis, pp. 918–919.

Kutzler, M.A., 2009. Canine postpartum disorders. In: Bonagura, J.D., Twedt, D.C. (Eds.), Kirk's Current Veterinary Therapy XIV. Saunders Elsevier, St Louis, pp. 999–1000.

Novo, R.E., 2009. Surgical repair of vaginal anomalies in the bitch. In: Bonagura, J.D., Twedt, D.C. (Eds.), Kirk's Current Veterinary Therapy XIV. Saunders Elsevier, St Louis, pp. 1012–1018.

PARAPHIMOSIS

Feldman, E.C., Nelson, R.W., 2004. Phimosis and paraphimosis. In: Feldman, E.C., Nelson, R.W. (Eds.), Canine and Feline Endocrinology and Reproduction, third ed. Saunders Elsevier, St Louis, pp. 954–955.

Johnson, C.A., 2009. Paraphimosis, disorders of the penis, prepuce, and testes. In: Nelson, R.W., Couto, C.G. (Eds.), Small Animal Internal Medicine, fourth ed. Mosby Elsevier, St Louis, pp. 969–970.

Rochat, M.C., 2009. Paraphimosis and priapism. In: Silverstein, D.C., Hopper, K. (Eds.), Small Animal Critical Care Medicine. Elsevier, St Louis, pp. 615–618.

ACUTE PROSTATITIS

Feldman, E.C., Nelson, R.W., 2004. Prostatitis. In: Feldman, E.C., Nelson, R.W. (Eds.), Canine and Feline Endocrinology and Reproduction, third ed. Saunders Elsevier, St Louis, pp. 977–986.

Johnson, C.A., 2009. Acute bacterial prostatitis and prostatic abscess, disorders of the prostate gland. In: Nelson, R.W., Couto, C.G. (Eds.), Small Animal Internal Medicine, fourth ed. Mosby Elsevier, St Louis, pp. 978–979.

Sirinarumitr, K., 2009. Medical treatment of benign prostatic hypertrophy and prostatitis in dogs. In: Bonagura, J.D., Twedt, D.C. (Eds.), Kirk's Current Veterinary Therapy XIV. Saunders Elsevier, St Louis, pp. 1046–1048.

Neurologic and ocular emergencies

HEAD TRAUMA

Diagnosis

History—The owner may have observed head trauma, or be suspicious of head trauma. Determine whether the patient lost consciousness, whether it was observed walking after the incident and whether the patient was aware of its surroundings.

Physical exam—

1. Keep cranial and cervical manipulation to a minimum until the extent of the injuries has been determined.
2. Evaluate the patient for level of consciousness (LOC), airway integrity, respiratory pattern, otic and / or nasal hemorrhage, ocular injuries, lacerations, abrasions, dental and oral trauma, posture, and limb movements.
3. Very carefully palpate the skull to locate any fractures.
4. Proceed with a thorough, full-body examination.
5. The clinical signs of head trauma may include:
   A. Altered mentation—obtundation, dementia, stupor, coma, seizures or death
   B. Traumatic injuries—(abrasions, lacerations, epistaxis, oral or dental trauma, skull fractures)
   C. Neurologic signs—opisthotonos, fixed pupils, anisocoria, pathologic nystagmus, cranial nerve deficits, proprioceptive deficits, circling, head tilt.
6. Neurologic exam (repeat frequently)
   A. LOC—trauma to the cerebrum or brainstem may result in stupor or coma. The level of consciousness changes from alert and awake, to dull, obtunded, stuporous and then comatose with deterioration of the patient. Patients with forebrain dysfunction may have delirium or dementia. Patients with lesions of the brain stem or severe forebrain lesions may exhibit obtundation, stupor or coma.

B. Posture
  I. Decerebrate rigidity is a sign of a brainstem lesion. The appearance is a stuporous or comatose animal with four rigid limbs and cervical dorsiflexion.
  II. Patients with unilateral cerebral or thalamic injuries may exhibit the aversive syndrome. With arousal, the animal circles or adopts the posture of circling the head and neck toward the body side of the affected cerebral hemisphere.
  III. A patient that has a cerebellar lesion may exhibit decerebellate rigidity, characterized by opisthotonus, extension of the forelimbs and flexion of the hindlimbs. These patients have normal consciousness.
  IV. A patient with a lesion from C1 to C5 will have normal consciousness (unless respiratory failure occurs) and additional signs depending upon the severity of the lesion, ranging from cervical pain to tetraplegia, ataxia, and upper motor neuron weakness of all four limbs. Usually the degree of proprioceptive ataxia and weakness is comparable in all four limbs, or ipsilateral limbs are comparable. A patient with a lesion of the spinal cord from T2 to L3 vertebrae in dogs or from T3 to L4 vertebrae in cats, which contain the T3 to L3 spinal segments, may exhibit Schiff–Sherrington posture (extension of the thoracic limbs with increased extensor tone of the thoracic limbs and paralysis or paresis of the pelvic limbs).
C. Pupil size and pupillary light reflexes—rule out primary ocular injury. Damage to cerebral or midbrain white matter results in miotic pupils, or pupils that respond readily to light. Damage to CN III results in dilated, unresponsive pupils. A rapid change from normal pupils to miosis or mydriasis is a sign of a rapid increase in intracranial pressure (ICP), necessitating emergency treatment. The pupillary light reflex evaluates CN II (optic nerve) and CN III (oculomotor nerve).
D. Palpebral reflexes—presence of a normal blink reflex when the medial canthus of the eyes is touched is an evaluation of the ophthalmic branch of CN V (trigeminal nerve). The maxillary branch of CN V is evaluated by touching the lateral canthus of the eyes.
E. Corneal reflex—gentle touching of the cornea with a cotton-tipped applicator moistened with saline causes a blink, which evaluates the ophthalmic branch of the trigeminal nerve (CN V) and retraction of the globe, which evaluates the abducens nerve (CN VI) and motor function of the facial nerve (CN VII).
F. Respiratory pattern
  I. Midbrain injury may result in neurogenic hyperventilation, with an increased depth and rate of respiration.
  II. Tentorial herniation following a deep bilateral cerebral injury may result in periodic hyperpnea alternating with periods of apnea, referred to as Cheyne–Stokes breathing.
  III. Brainstem injury may lead to apnea.

Prognosis

The prognosis is variable and may be correlated to the appearance of the pupils:

1. Fixed pupils / nonresponsive pupils—midbrain lesion, guarded prognosis
2. Fixed, dilated pupils, pupillary light response—cerebral edema or hemorrhage, fair prognosis
3. Anisocoria—cerebral edema, better prognosis
4. Fixed constricted pupils—cerebral, diencephalic / pontine lesions, better prognosis. Be sure to differentiate from pupillary constriction due to ocular injury.

Treatment

1. Inform the client of the diagnosis, prognosis and cost of the treatment.
2. Hospitalize the patient for close observation and treatment. Place the patient on a board or firm surface and elevate the cranial end by 30%. Avoid applying pressure to the neck or kinking of the neck. Position the head normally, with nose in a neutral position, rather than head flexed and nose tucked, which may compromise the airway. Monitor temperature, pulse, and respiration. Avoid hyperthermia. Also monitor for arrhythmias, which may occur due to brainstem lesions.
3. Ventilate the patient with oxygen.
   A. Use an oxygen cage, a mask, or a hood made from an Elizabethan collar. Avoid applying pressure to the neck. Also avoid the use of a nasal catheter or nasal prongs as they may cause sneezing, which increases ICP.
   B. If facial damage is severe, consider transtracheal catheterization or tracheostomy.
   C. Administer humidified oxygen at 100 mL/kg/min. Avoid the administration of 100% for longer than 24 hours. Ideally decrease the oxygen concentration as quickly as possible to avoid oxygen toxicity. Monitor oxygen saturation (SPO$_2$) with a pulse oximeter; maintain SPO$_2$ at 90% or higher. If therapy is not able to maintain SPO$_2$, Pa_{CO_2} is >50 mm Hg, total CO$_2$ is above normal, or the patient is apneic, mechanical ventilation is indicated.
      I. If the patient requires mechanical ventilation and is stuporous or semi-comatose, administer 2% lidocaine, 0.75 mg/kg IV, to the dog to prevent coughing during intubation. If the patient is a cat, spray the larynx with lidocaine (lidocaine is toxic to cats, so only a minimal amount should be administered).
      II. If the patient requires sedation for intubation, administer IV sedation. Avoid ketamine in patients with head trauma.
      III. Administer 2% lidocaine, 0.75 mg/kg IV, in dogs, prior to extubation.
      IV. Naloxone, 0.01–0.04 mg/kg IV, IM, SC, may be administered if narcotic-induced hypoventilation occurs.

4. Place an intravenous catheter; avoid the jugular veins.
5. Administer Hetastarch, 14–20 mL/kg, and 7.5% NaCl, 4 mL/kg IV for dogs, and 2 mL/kg IV for cats, then start on a balanced electrolyte solution such as PlasmaLyte®, Normosol®-R or LRS, at 40 mL/kg/h in dogs and 20 mL/kg/h in cats, or 60–70 mL/kg/h in dehydrated dogs and 20–40 mL/kg/h in dehydrated cats. Do not administer 7.5% NaCl to a dehydrated patient.
6. Monitor mean arterial blood pressure or systolic pressure.
   A. Mean arterial pressure $= \dfrac{(\text{Systolic pressure} - \text{diastolic pressure})}{3}$
   $+ \text{diastolic pressure.}$
   B. Maintain mean arterial blood pressure at 80–100 mm Hg, to maintain normal cerebral perfusion pressure. Maintain systolic pressure at 120–140 mm Hg.
   C. Avoid hypertension if hemorrhage is occurring in a noncompressible body region (abdomen, thorax, or cranium).
      I. Hypertension in dogs is defined as: systolic pressure >180 mm Hg.
      II. Hypertension in cats is defined as: systolic pressure >160 mm Hg.
      III. Reassess the neurological status for signs of increased ICP.
      IV. Administer an opioid analgesic to decrease pain induced hypertension.
         a. Morphine (dogs only), 0.3–0.5 mg/kg IM, SC
         b. Oxymorphone, 0.05–0.2 mg/kg IM, SC, IV
         c. Hydromorphone 0.05–0.2 mg/kg IM, SC, IV
   D. If hypotension persists in the face of volume replacement, without ongoing blood loss, administer dobutamine, 2–20 µg/kg/min IV CRI in dogs (1–5 µg/kg/min IV CRI in cats) or dopamine, 5–10 µg/kg/min IV CRI (µg) in dogs. Start at the lower dose and increase gradually to the higher dose as needed for effect. If tachycardia develops, stop. Gradually wean the patient off pressor agents.
   E. If the patient is normotensive and normovolemic, continue IV fluids at a maintenance rate of 2–3 mL/kg/h.
7. Administer furosemide, 1–2 mg/kg IV or IM q6–12 h in dogs, and 0.5–1.0 mg/kg IV or IM q6–12 h in cats.
8. If an osmotic agent is required, administer either mannitol or hypertonic saline (7.5% NaCl) if it has not already been administered. Recent studies have shown hypertonic saline to be superior to mannitol in decreasing cerebral edema.
   A. Hypertonic saline, NaCl 7.5%, 4 mL/kg in dogs, and 2 mL/kg in cats, slow IV over 10–15 min
   B. Mannitol, 250–1000 mg/kg IV, over 20 minutes
      I. Repeat mannitol every 4 hours as needed.
      II. **Mannitol is contraindicated in a dehydrated patient or one with anuric renal failure, congestive heart failure, volume overload, hyperosmolar conditions, and in patients with intracranial hemorrhage**. In these patients, utilize furosemide, 1–2 mg/kg IV.

Neurologic and ocular emergencies

9. Sedation—if seizures occur then administer diazepam, 0.5–1.0 mg/kg IV, or phenobarbital, 2–4 mg/kg IV.
10. Skull radiographs and computerized tomography (CT) or magnetic resonance imaging (MRI) should be performed when the patient is stable.
11. Craniotomy may be indicated if rapid deterioration occurs.
12. Avoid ketamine, corticosteroids and glucose-containing solutions in head trauma patients.
   A. Ketamine increases intracranial pressure.
   B. Corticosteroids are contraindicated in head trauma.
   C. Glucose-containing solutions are contraindicated unless the patient has a documented low blood glucose level.

(ACUTE) MYELOPATHIES (PARAPARESIS/PARAPLEGIA)

Diagnosis

History—The patient may have a history of trauma or be found injured. There may be a history of acute pain or distress and an inability to walk after jumping, running or lying about at home.
Physical exam—
1. Spinal cord lesions or disorders do not cause signs of cranial disorders. They do not cause altered mentation, cranial nerve deficits or cerebellar or vestibular ataxia.
2. Lesions of the cervical spinal cord (C1–C5) usually present with upper motor neuron (UMN) hemiplegia if the lesion is asymmetric or UMN tetraplegia.
3. Cervicothoracic lesions (C6–T2) usually cause UMN signs (exaggerated myotatic reflexes) in the hindlimbs and lower motor neuron (LMN) signs (decreased or absent myotatic reflexes) in the forelimbs. Signs may be asymmetrical. If the lesion is not severe, the signs may be UMN to the forelimbs only.
4. Thoracolumbar lesions (T3–L3) usually cause UMN signs to the hindlimbs, with paraplegia or hemiplegia. Pelvic limb spinal reflexes are preserved and usually hyperactive. Schiff–Sherrington syndrome may be present, as characterized by extensor rigidity of the forelimbs and flaccid paraplegia of the hindlimbs.
5. Lesions of the spinal cord segments L4–L6 cause paresis or paralysis of the hindlimbs or one hindlimb, normal forelimbs, postural reaction deficits in one or both hindlimbs, upper motor neuron signs of one or both hindlimbs (decreased to absent patellar reflexes, intact withdrawal reflex, urinary retention, decreased to absent extensor muscle tone of the hindlimbs).
6. Lesions of the L6–S3 spinal cord segments cause paraparesis or monoparesis of the hindlimbs with normal forelimbs. Paralysis or paresis of the tail may be present. Postural reaction deficits will be present in one or both hindlimbs. Lower motor neuron signs to the hindlimbs and/or perineal region will be present (decreased withdrawal reflexes, hyper-reflexic patellar reflexes, decreased to

absent perianal or perineal reflex, decreased pelvic limb and tail muscle tone, and urinary and fecal incontinence).

Radiographs—Severe spinal cord lesions may not always appear on radiographs. Myelography, CT or MRI may be useful and should be performed preoperatively on all surgical candidates. Radiographs may be helpful in the diagnosis of patients with congenital spinal malformations, including atlantoaxial subluxation, hemivertebrae, discospondylitis, spinal trauma (with fractures or luxations) and spinal neoplasia.

Radiographic changes that are compatible with intervertebral disc disease include:
1. Narrowing or dorsal wedging of the intervertebral disc space and interarticular facet space
2. Opacification and reduction in size of the intervertebral foramen
3. Narrowing of the interarticular facet space
4. Appearance of mineralized disc material within the vertebral canal or displaced dorsally within the disc space.

Differential diagnosis

1. Neuromuscular junction diseases
2. Thromboembolism
3. Fibrocartilaginous embolism (FCE)
4. Intervertebral disc herniation (IVDD)
5. Vertebral trauma
6. Meningitis (bacterial or steroid-responsive)
7. Meningomyelitis—infectious or noninfectious
8. Hemorrhage within the spinal cord
9. Cervical spondylomyelopathy (Wobbler syndrome)
10. Spinal neoplasia
11. Degenerative myelopathy
12. Atlantoaxial subluxation
13. Discospondylitis (bacterial or fungal)
14. Chiari-like malformation and syringomyelia

Prognosis

The prognosis is guarded to poor.

Treatment

1. Localize the lesion; if possible note especially the presence of motor function and of deep pain
2. Inform the client of the diagnosis, prognosis and the cost of treatment.
3. If motor function and deep pain are present, confinement, monitoring and medical therapy may be an option. If there is an absence of motor function and of deep pain, surgery within 24 hours is highly recommended.

4. Depending on the degree of vertebral displacement, spinal fractures may be treated by confinement or by surgery.

5. *Always* provide the owner with three options for suspected intervertebral disc herniations.

    A. Immediate referral to a surgeon or neurologist for contrast myelography, CT or MRI, and / or decompressive laminectomy; if disc herniation has resulted in paralysis, immediate surgery should be performed. The absence of pain perception provides a poorer prognosis than patients who still perceive pain.

    B. Conservative management includes hospitalization, IV fluid therapy and anti-inflammatory therapy.

        I. Non-steroidal anti-inflammatory medications appear to improve the outcome and decrease complications when compared with glucocorticoids.

            a. Meloxicam, 0.1–0.2 mg/kg IV, SC, PO once then 0.1 mg/kg PO q24h (dogs), 0.1 mg/kg IV, SC, PO once in cats

            b. Carprofen, 4 mg/kg IV, IM, SC once, then 0.5–2.2 mg/kg IV, IM, SC, PO q12h for dogs, 4 mg/kg IV or SC once in cats

            c. Ketoprofen, 1–2 mg/kg IV, then 1 mg/kg IV, IM, SC, PO q24h up to 5 days in dogs, 1–2 mg/kg IV or SC then 1 mg/kg IV, IM, SC, PO q24h up to 3 days in cats

            d. Deracoxib (Deramaxx®) 3–4 mg/kg PO q24h in dogs for up to 7 days

        II. If glucocorticoids are selected, it is preferred to administer methylprednisolone sodium succinate within 8 hours of the primary injury at the dosage of 30 mg/kg IV, once, followed by an IV CRI of 5.4 mg/kg/h for 24–48 hours.

        III. If NSAIDs are contraindicated and glucocorticoid administration is selected, but methylprednisolone sodium succinate is not available, dexamethasone sodium phosphate (0.2–0.3 mg/kg IV initially), followed by prednisone (0.5 mg/kg q12h) may be administered. The only glucocorticoid proven to be beneficial to patients with spinal cord trauma is methylprednisolone sodium succinate. Dexamethasone sodium phosphate has been shown to be less effective in some experimental trials.

        IV. Analgesia should be provided. Options include hydromorphone, morphine / lidocaine CRI, fentanyl CRI, oral tramadol, or for cats, buprenorphine.

        V. Methocarbamol (15–20 mg/kg IV or PO q8h) may decrease the pain from muscle spasms.

        VI. Sucralfate (0.5–1 g per dog PO q8–12 h or 33 mg/kg PO q8h in dogs, 0.25–0.5 g per cat PO q8–12 h), to decrease gastrointestinal ulceration.

        VII. Prazosin, 1 mg/15 kg body weight (0.067 mg/kg) PO q8h in dogs or 0.25–0.5 mg/cat PO q12–24 h, may decrease urethral internal sphincter spasms.

    C. Humane euthanasia—if the owner is unwilling or unable to care for the pet, 'see him suffer', etc.

6. Suspected meningitis or meningoencephalitis cases should be started on trimethoprim-sulfa (15 mg/kg PO q12h), clindamycin (10–12.5 mg/kg PO q12h), and doxycycline (5–10 mg/kg IV or PO q12h) and infectious disease titers should be submitted to the laboratory.
7. Nursing care
   A. Monitor for frank hemorrhage in the feces or for melena. If gastrointestinal hemorrhage develops, decrease the dosage and frequency of the corticosteroids and treat with amoxicillin, misoprostol, and omeprazole or famotidine orally.
   B. Express the urinary bladder q4–6 h or pass a urethral catheter.
   C. Administer enemas if necessary.
   D. Perform physical therapy to maintain muscle tone and strength.
   E. Reassess the patient's neurologic status frequently. Postural reactions, hopping, and gait assessment are not recommended as they may increase the severity of the lesion. Pain perception and flexor and extensor reflexes should, however, be reassessed frequently.

LOWER MOTOR NEURON DISEASES

I. POLYRADICULONEURITIS ('COONHOUND PARALYSIS')

Polyradiculoneuritis is an immune-mediated disorder of axons or myelin or both. It occurs following exposure to a specific antigen combined with an altered immune system response. Immunosuppressive drugs do not improve recovery.

History—The client may report acute or peracute onset of diffuse LMN paresis. There may be a history of a possible raccoon bite. A vocal change may be noted. The paresis is rapidly progressive to tetraplegia.
Physical exam—The cranial nerves are usually normal. Megaesophagus is not associated with this disease. Flaccid progressive weakness from the hindlimbs to involve all four limbs is observed. The patellar reflexes will be diminished or absent. Muscle tone will be decreased. Muscle atrophy may occur.
Laboratory evaluation—There are no tests to confirm the diagnosis of polyradiculoneuritis. CSF analysis may reveal an elevated protein level, and pleocytosis may or may not be present.

Prognosis

Many patients recover. Repeat episodes in the same patient are common.

Treatment

1. Inform the client of the diagnosis, prognosis and cost of treatment.
2. Long-term treatment (weeks to months) will be necessary for recovery.
3. The patient should rest on a water bed or similar bedding to prevent pressure sores.
4. The patient should be turned from side to side hourly.

Neurologic and ocular emergencies

5. The patient may need abdominal compression to assist defecation and urination.
6. The patient may need support to eat and drink.
7. Physical therapy should be provided to prevent muscle atrophy.
8. If respiratory compromise is severe, long-term ventilator therapy may be needed.

II. MYASTHENIA GRAVIS

Myasthenia gravis is a neuromuscular junction disorder with two forms: congenital and acquired. The congenital form is an acetylcholine receptor developmental disorder observed in puppies less than 8 weeks of age. Breeds affected include the smooth Fox Terrier and the Jack Russell terrier. The acquired form is an autoimmune disease that may occur in any breed of dog and in cats, particularly the Siamese and Abyssinian. The more commonly affected dog breeds include Golden Retrievers, German Shepherds, Labrador Retrievers and Dachshunds. Antibodies bind to the acetylcholine receptor and prevent attachment of acetylcholine.

History—There are three clinical syndromes in dogs: generalized, focal and fulminating. The generalized form begins with hind limb paresis, followed by thoracic limb paresis. The patient may have a short stride and crouched posture, then the neck may become flexed, and collapse may occur. The signs are described as exercise-induced fatigue. Brief periods of exercise induce the clinical signs that then resolve following 30–60 minutes of rest.

The focal form usually causes regurgitation due to megaesophagus; however, weakness of the facial muscles may also be present and seen as weak and drooping lips and eyelids.

The fulminating form is an acute onset of severe clinical signs including profound weakness.

Physical exam—The cranial nerves are usually normal. Eyelid and lip paresis with drooling and dyspnea may be observed. Megaesophagus may occur. Flaccid progressive weakness from the hindlimbs to involve all four limbs is observed. The spinal reflexes will be normal. Muscle tone will be decreased. Muscle atrophy does not usually occur.

The Tensilon test is a procedure helpful in establishing the diagnosis of generalized myasthenia gravis. The patient is exercised to the point of lower motor neuron paresis being observed, then edrophonium (Tensilon®) is injected, 0.1–0.2 mg/kg in dogs, 0.25–0.5 mg/cat, IV. If the patient rises and is able to walk normally for 2–3 minutes, this is considered a positive response. Focal and fulminant myasthenia gravis patients cannot be diagnosed with this procedure.

Laboratory evaluation—Acetylcholine receptor antibodies may be detected by immunoprecipitation radioimmunoassay. Immune complexes bound to acetylcholine receptors may be evaluated in muscle biopsies with immunocytochemical methods. This test is often more rewarding and more effective in the congenital and focal forms of myasthenia gravis. Thyroid tests are recommended in these patients as many have underlying hypothyroidism and, with supplementation, the clinical signs resolve.

EMG and CSF analysis are usually normal.

Diagnostic imaging—Thoracic radiographs should be evaluated in all patients suspected to have myasthenia gravis, to evaluate for the presence of megaesophagus and to look for aspiration pneumonia.

Prognosis

This is usually a lifelong condition, with recurrent episodes of aspiration pneumonia. Some puppies appear to outgrow the congenital form. Some patients undergo spontaneous remission about 6.4 months following the diagnosis.

Treatment

1. Inform the client of the diagnosis, prognosis and cost of treatment.
2. Lifelong therapy is usually required for maintenance.
3. Pyridostigmine bromide (Mestinon®), 0.5–3.0 mg/kg PO q8–12h in dogs, 0.25 mg/kg PO q8–12h in cats; for cats, it is recommended to dilute the pyridostigmine syrup 1:1 to decrease gastric irritation.
4. Prednisone 0.5 mg/kg PO q12h in dogs initially, then gradually increased to immunosuppressive levels over the next 1–2 weeks. Cats are usually given prednisone at the dosage of 1–4 mg/kg PO q12h.
5. Dogs may be given azathioprine 1 mg/kg q12h PO, but azathioprine should not be administered to a cat.
6. Mycophenolate mofetil (CellCept®) 10–20 mg/kg PO q12h may also be administered to dogs, in combination with prednisone and azathioprine, but should not be administered to cats.
7. The patient should be fed with the head and forequarters elevated. It is often helpful to feed the patient 2 hours following administration of pyridostigmine, when the drug is at its peak effect. The patient should be kept in an upright position for 10–15 minutes after eating to facilitate gravity flow into the stomach.

III. BOTULISM

History—The dog may have ingested carrion or spoiled food containing a preformed type C neurotoxin produced by the bacterium *Clostridium botulinum*. The dog may walk with a short-strided, shuffling gate. Weakness rapidly progresses to recumbency and to paralysis within 24 hours. More than one dog may be involved.

Physical exam—Cranial nerve dysfunction, including loss of the pupillary light reflex, dilated pupils, facial weakness, dysphagia, decreased jaw tone and an altered voice may be observed. Megaesophagus may occur, resulting in regurgitation and potentially aspiration pneumonia. Flaccid progressive weakness from the hindlimbs to involve all four limbs is observed. Spinal reflexes will be diminished or absent. Muscle tone will be decreased. The dog is usually still able to wag its tail. Respiratory muscle paralysis may occur, leading to death.

Laboratory evaluation—Botulinum toxin type C may be identified in the stomach contents, blood, vomitus or feces of affected animals. CSF analysis is usually normal. Electromyography (EMG) reveals diminished amplitude of spontaneous activity, loss of denervation potentials and diminished amplitude of muscle action potential in response to a stimulus of supramaximal strength.

Prognosis

Most dogs recover within 3 weeks, with supportive therapy.

Differential diagnosis

Patients infected with Rabies virus appear similar but usually have altered mentation. If in doubt, place the patient into isolation.

Treatment

1. Inform the client of the diagnosis, prognosis and cost of treatment.
2. If type C antitoxin is available, administer 10000 units IM twice, 4 hours apart.
3. The patient should rest on a water bed or similar bedding to prevent pressure sores.
4. The patient should be turned from side to side hourly.
5. The patient may need abdominal compression to assist defecation and urination.
6. The patient may need support to eat and drink.
7. Physical therapy should be provided to prevent muscle atrophy.
8. Aspiration is a common complication.
9. If respiratory compromise is severe, long-term ventilator therapy may be needed.
10. Most dogs recover within 3 weeks.

IV.   TICK PARALYSIS

History—Within 4–9 days following exposure to a female of certain strains of *Dermacentor andersoni, Dermacentor variablis, or Amblyomma americanum* ticks, the client may report an acute onset of a rapidly ascending motor paresis or paralysis. These ticks are usually encountered in the central Mid-Atlantic coastal states including North Carolina. The patient may have developed a hoarse bark.

Physical exam—The cranial nerves are usually normal; however, facial weakness, dysphagia, decreased jaw tone and an altered voice may be observed. Megaesophagus is not associated with this disease. Flaccid progressive weakness from the hindlimbs to involve all four limbs is observed. Spinal reflexes will be diminished or absent. Muscle tone will be decreased. Respiratory muscle paralysis may occur, leading to death. A tick may be found on the patient. The diagnosis is confirmed if the patient rapidly improves (within 72 hours) following removal of the tick.

Laboratory evaluation—There are no tests to confirm the diagnosis of tick paralysis. CSF analysis is usually normal. EMG is usually normal.

Prognosis

Many patients recover. The prognosis is good if the tick is removed.

Treatment

1. Inform the client of the diagnosis, prognosis and cost of treatment.
2. Thoroughly examine the patient for ticks.
3. If no tick is found, consider tick dipping the patient in an insecticidal solution.
4. Long-term treatment for weeks to months, including ventilator therapy, may be necessary for recovery if no tick is found.
5. The patient should rest on a water bed or similar bedding to prevent pressure sores.
6. The patient should be turned from side to side hourly.
7. The patient may need abdominal compression to assist defecation and urination.
8. The patient may need support to eat and drink.
9. Physical therapy should be provided to prevent muscle atrophy.

V.   OTHER ILLNESSES

Those that should be considered include rattlesnake envenomation, organophosphate toxicity and *Neospora caninum* (in puppies <12 weeks of age, localized to the lumbosacral roots).

TETANUS

Tetanus is a disease that results from contamination of a wound with spores of *Clostridium tetani*, a gram-positive, anaerobic spore-forming bacillus. The spores produce tetanospasmin and tetanolysin (or tetanolepsin), which are toxins. Tetanospasmin causes the neurologic signs, and tetanus antitoxin is aimed at neutralizing this toxin. Tetanolysin causes tissue damage and lysis of erythrocytes, producing an environment prime for bacterial growth. Tetanospasmin inhibits the release of glycine and gamma aminobutyric acid (GABA) (inhibitory neurotransmitters) from the neuromuscular endplate, which causes irreversible blockade of skeletal muscle neuronal inhibition, alterations of autonomic control and generalized muscle spasms. Sprouting of new axon terminals is required for recovery and takes at least 3 weeks.

Dogs and cats are much more resistant, 200 and 2400 times, respectively, than humans.

Diagnosis

History—There may be a history of a wound such as a penetrating injury, gunshot or bite wound, or the wound may not be found. Clinical signs develop 3–18 days after the wound is infected. There are two forms observed in animals: the localized form and the generalized form.

1. The localized form results from a lower toxin load and at the site of infection causes muscle rigidity; it may spread and progress into the generalized form.
2. The generalized form causes extreme muscle rigidity with sustained tonic contraction of the extended limbs and all muscles, resulting in a stiff gait, elevated outstretched tail, erect ears, and contraction of the facial muscles (risus sardonicus). The client may observe anorexia, as a result of trismus (lockjaw), laryngeal spasm and dysphagia.

Physical exam—The patient may exhibit hypertonic myotactic reflexes, normal conscious proprioception, a stiff gait, elevated outstretched tail and erect ears. As the disease progresses, cranial nerve signs become apparent, including trismus, risus sardonicus, protrusion of the third eyelid, enophthalmos, erect ears, dysphagia and laryngeal spasm. Recumbency with extensor rigidity of all four limbs and opisthotonus develop as the condition worsens. Seizures may occur. Death is usually due to respiratory or cardiac failure. The patient will be hypersensitive to all external stimuli including light, sound and touch. Autonomic dysfunction is noted in humans and causes severe complications. Excess sympathetic activity and catecholamine levels occur due to the loss of inhibition of autonomic discharge, from the loss of glycine and GABA release. The clinical signs include tachypnea and tachycardia, hypertension, ptyalism and increased protein catabolism. Other complications include arrhythmias, hypotension, and thrombosis. The veterinary patient should be monitored for these complications.

Laboratory evaluation—It is difficult to isolate *C. tetani* from wounds and to identify tetanospasmin, so diagnosis is based upon the clinical signs, with or without the presence of a wound, as the wounds may be hidden or unable to be found. It is important to start aggressive treatment as quickly as possible whenever a case of tetanus is suspected. Common changes observed in the CBC and serum chemistry profile include neutrophilic leukocytosis and elevated creatine kinase and aspartate aminotransferase.

Differential diagnosis

Other causes of extensor rigidity and opisthotonus include decerebrate rigidity from severe brainstem disease due to neoplasia, infection or trauma, but these patients usually have altered mentation. Decerebellate rigidity, as occurs following trauma to the rostral cerebellum, may result in extensor rigidity and opisthotonos, with normal mentation. Myoclonus may be mistaken for tetanus and is usually caused by canine distemper meningoencephalomyelitis.

Prognosis

The prognosis for generalized tetanus varies with the severity of clinical signs. About 50% of dogs survive with intensive care for 3–4 weeks.

Treatment

1. Inform the client of the diagnosis, prognosis and cost of the treatment.
2. Hospitalization in an ICU that provides 24-hour care is essential to improving survival.
3. Place an intravenous catheter.
4. Provide maintenance IV fluid therapy.
5. Administer one dose of tetanus immunoglobulin to neutralize the circulating toxin.
   A. Equine anti-tetanus serum (ATS), 500–1000 IU IM once (may also be administered IV* or SC) (*should not contain thimerosal [thiomersal]; a test dose is recommended prior to IV administration.)
   B. Administer human tetanus immune globulin (TIG), 500–1000 IU IM once.
   C. Intrathecal administration may improve recovery.
   D. Monitor for adverse reactions.
      I. Anaphylactic reactions have the signs of vomiting, hypotension, tachycardia, urticaria, angioedema, pulmonary edema and neurologic dysfunction. Treatment includes stopping the administration of the antitoxin and the administration of epinephrine, antihistamines and glucocorticoids.
      II. Anaphylactoid reactions have the signs of mild fever, restlessness, and urticaria. Treatment includes stopping the administration of the antitoxin, administration of diphenhydramine, and then restarting the administration of the antitoxin at a more dilute concentration and / or a slower rate.
      III. Serum sickness may occur within weeks of administration of the antitoxin. The clinical signs include urticaria, vasculitis, erythema, lymphadenopathy, swollen joints and, on lab evaluation, neutropenia, proteinuria, and glomerulonephritis may be present. Treatment is symptomatic.
6. Until recovery is nearly complete, most medications should be administered IV if possible, through the IV fluid line, to decrease patient stimulation. The exception is the anti-tetanus serum, which has decreased complications when administered IM, and the human tetanus immune globulin, which is approved only for IM administration.
7. Administer antibiotics to stop the development of clostridial spores and further toxic generation and release. The antibiotic preferred in human medicine is metronidazole. The following are the options.
   A. Metronidazole, 10 mg/kg IV q8h or 15 mg/kg IV q12h
   B. Penicillin G, 20 000–100 000 U/kg IV q6–12 h (increases the risk of convulsions)
   C. Clindamycin, 5–11 mg/kg IV q8–12 h
   D. Tetracycline, 22 mg/kg PO q8h
8. Wound management—debride and thoroughly clean all visible wounds to eliminate an anaerobic environment.

9. Administer parasympatholytics (atropine or glycopyrrolate) to control bradycardia and decrease airway secretions.
   A. Atropine sulfate, 0.02 mg/kg IV, IM, SC
   B. Glycopyrrolate, 0.01 mg/kg IV, IM, SC
10. Administer benzodiazepines or phenobarbital as needed for seizures.
    A. Diazepam, 0.5–1 mg/kg IV as needed
    B. Midazolam, 0.2–0.4 mg/kg IV
    C. Phenobarbital, 2–4 mg/kg q8h
    D. Pentobarbital, 3–15 mg/kg IV to effect
11. Administer phenothiazines and methocarbamol to reduce muscle spasms.
    A. Acepromazine, 0.1–0.2 mg/kg IM or IV q6h
    B. Chlorpromazine, 0.5–1 mg/kg IV q8h
    C. Methocarbamol, 55–220 mg/kg IV, not to exceed 330 mg/kg/day. Administer one-half of the calculated dose, observe the patient, then administer the remaining half slowly as needed.
12. Provide nutritional support.
    A. Gastrotomy tube (percutaneous endoscopic gastrotomy tube)—may be the best choice. General anesthesia is required. There is a risk of peritonitis.
    B. Esophagostomy tube—second choice. General anesthesia is required. Reflux esophagitis and aspiration pneumonia may occur.
    C. Nasoesophageal or nasogastric tube—may cause constant laryngeal and nasal irritation. Reflux esophagitis and aspiration pneumonia may occur. Only small volumes of limited types of nutritional support may be administered.
    D. Elevate the head of the bed by 30° during feeding to decrease the risk of reflux and aspiration.
13. Place the patient in a well-padded, quiet, dark environment to diminish stimulation.
14. Consider the administration of dantrolene, 0.2–1 mg/kg IV, to diminish muscle spasms.
15. In patients with adequate renal function, consider the administration of magnesium to allow the patient to regain autonomic control and reduce muscle spasms. Maintain the patient at between 2 and 4 mmol/L (normal = 0.7–1.05 mmol/L), which is a supranormal level. Monitor for severe hypocalcemia and for magnesium toxicity. An early sign of magnesium toxicity is loss of the patellar tendon reflex.
16. A tracheostomy may be needed in patients with severe laryngospasm.
17. Positive pressure ventilation may be needed for patients with respiratory failure.
18. The patient should be turned from side to side every 2–4 hours.
19. Intermittent passage of a sterile urethral catheter may be needed to drain the urinary bladder in patients with urinary retention.
20. Occasional enemas and manual assistance with evacuation of feces may be needed.
21. Use oral 0.1% chlorhexidine acetate rinses periodically to moisten and clean the mouth.

22. Improvement may be observed within 1 week. Recovery usually requires 3–4 weeks of therapy.

VESTIBULAR DISORDERS

Diagnosis

History—The owner may describe an acute onset of head tilt, circling, nystagmus and falling or rolling. The patient may appear dizzy, or have a history of vomiting, anorexia and possibly depression. There may be a history of previous ear infections or throat infections, head trauma or aminoglycoside administration.

Physical exam—(see Table 13.1)
1. Peripheral vestibular system—head tilt, circling and rolling are toward the lesion; horizontal and rotary nystagmus are possible, with the fast phase away from the side of the head tilt. An increase in extensor tone of the contralateral limbs in relation to the head tilt and a decrease in extensor tone of the ipsilateral limbs may also be observed. Postural reactions are usually normal.
2. Central vestibular system—Head tilt may be either toward or away from the lesion; horizontal, rotary or vertical nystagmus may be present; hemiparesis or tetraparesis, conscious proprioceptive deficits, hypermetria, head bobbing and tremors may be observed. Mentation may range from normal to comatose.

Laboratory evaluation—
1. Evaluate a CBC and complete serum biochemical profile.
2. Consider measuring serum antibody titers for local rickettsial and fungal infections.

Skull radiographs (under anesthesia)—The open-mouthed view to evaluate the tympanic bullae may be particularly useful.

Additional diagnostic procedures that may be helpful in certain cases include CSF tap, CSF analysis, and a CT or MRI of the brain and tympanic bullae.

Table 13.1 *Differentiation of peripheral versus central vestibular disease*

	Central	Peripheral
Nystagmus		
Spontaneous	Horizontal	Horizontal
	Rotary	Rotary
	Vertical	
Positional	Changing	Constant
Head tilt	Present	Present
Cranial nerve deficits	Any other than VII	VII
Horner's syndrome	+/−	+/−
Postural reaction (abnormalities or conscious proprioception deficits)	Present	Absent

From Bagley, RS, The veterinary clinics of North America: small animal practice, intracranial disease, Vol. 26, No. 4, 1996: 697 ©Elsevier, with permission.

Differential diagnosis

1. Peripheral—otitis interna / media, head trauma, inner ear trauma, idiopathic feline vestibular syndrome, idiopathic canine vestibular syndrome, congenital vestibular disease, hypothyroidism, aminoglycoside or other otoxicity, naso- or otopharyngeal polyps, aural neoplasia or neoplasia of cranial nerves VII or VIII.
2. Central—granulomatous meningoencephalitis, necrotizing meningoencephalitis, viral (FIP, canine distemper), protozoal (toxoplasmosis, neosporosis), bacterial (bartonellosis, ehrlichiosis, other rickettsial disease, abscess), or mycotic (blastomycosis, cryptococcosis, coccidioidomycosis, other), hydrocephalus, cerebrovascular disease, intracranial neoplasia (meningioma, glioma, lymphoma, metastatic neoplasia, other), infarction, brainstem trauma, metronidazole toxicity.

Prognosis

The prognosis varies, being better for disease of the peripheral vestibular system than for central vestibular system. Dogs with geriatric vestibular syndrome generally recover within 2–3 weeks and recurrences are uncommon.

Treatment

1. Inform the client of the diagnosis, prognosis and cost of the treatment.
2. Place an intravenous catheter.
3. Perform an otoscopic exam and treat ear problem(s) as needed.
   A. Clean ears with sterile saline or sterile water, until an intact tympanic membrane can be confirmed. Avoid the administration of oily ear medications.
   B. Administer chloramphenicol, enrofloxacin, or trimethoprim-sulfa and cephalexin PO or IV for inner-ear infections
   C. Perform a myringotomy and obtain a culture and sensitivity sample if an inner-ear infection is present. If the emergency clinician plans to refer the patient for a myringotomy to a specialist the following day; do not initiate antibiotics. Waiting 24 hours will not generally be detrimental, but initiating antibiotics prior to obtaining the culture sample may affect the results.
4. Corticosteroids are contraindicated and antibiotics are not helpful in the treatment of geriatric (benign idiopathic) vestibular disease.
5. Antihistamines may antagonize vestibular stimulation of the vomiting center of the brain and decrease the patient's nausea.
   A. Meclizine (Bonine®): 12.5–25 mg PO q24h
   B. Dimenhydrinate (Dramamine®): 4–8 mg/kg PO q8h ($\frac{1}{4}$ of a 50 mg tablet q8–24 h in cats, $\frac{1}{4}$–1 tablet q8–24 h in dogs, $\frac{1}{8}$ tablet in puppies weighing 1–4 kg)
   C. Diphenhydramine (Benadryl®): 2–4 mg/kg PO, IM q8h
   D. Maropitant (Cerenia®) 8 mg/kg PO q24h for 2 days in dogs

6. Administer fluid therapy as needed.
7. Provide sedation as needed to prevent self-trauma.
   A. Cats and small dogs <5 kg: diazepam, 1–2 mg IV
   B. Dogs >5–12 kg: diazepam, 5 mg IV
   C. Dogs >12 kg: diazepam, 10–15 mg IV
8. A dark, quiet environment is beneficial.

SHAKING AND TREMORS

Definitions

A tremor is an involuntary, rhythmic, regular movement of either a localized body part or generalized and affecting the entire body. It is caused by alternating contraction and relaxation of agonist and antagonist muscles.

An intention tremor develops during voluntary movement and is worsened by voluntary movement. It is especially prominent in highly controlled movements such as eating. Intention tremors may be seen with cerebellar disease.

A fine tremor involving the head, neck, trunk and forelimbs that disappears when the patient is not supporting itself is referred to as a postural tremor. Postural tremor is seen with metabolic diseases.

Muscle fasciculations do not produce the rhythmic limb or body movements as seen with tremor. Associated with motor unit disease, they are contractions of muscle fibers.

Myoclonus is characterized by a localized area of muscle contraction that results in a jerking motion, as associated with canine distemper virus infections.

Diagnosis

History—The onset, progression, and severity of tremors vary according to the etiology. Tremor may vary from mild and localized to severe and generalized. The patient may appear anxious. The ability to stand or walk may be inhibited.

Physical exam—Hyperthermia may occur. Ataxia, hypermetria, head tilt and decreased menace response may be observed. Tremors of variable severity and ranging from localized to generalized may be observed, and may be exaggerated with excitement. An abnormal eye movement caused by tremor of the extraocular muscles, referred to as opsoclonus, may occur.

Laboratory evaluation—Evaluate the CBC and complete serum biochemical profile, including electrolytes. Perform additional blood tests as indicated (toxicity and infectious disease screens).

Differential diagnoses

1. Congenital abnormal myelin formation as seen in Chow Chows, Dalmatians, Springer Spaniels, Scottish Terriers, Weimaraners, Samoyeds, Bernese Mountain Dogs and Lurchers
   A. Hypomyelination
   B. Dysmyelination

2. Toxicity (mycotoxins following dietary indiscretion, hexachlorophene, lead, organophosphates, carbamates, pyrethrins and pyrethroids, ivermectin, bromethalin, theobromine [chocolate], metaldehyde, and strychnine)

3. Inflammation
   A. Steroid-responsive tremor syndrome (SRTS) ('white dog shaker syndrome')—a corticosteroid-responsive meningoencephalitis that causes mild to incapacitating tremors in all coat colors of dogs, usually occurring in young, adult, small to medium breeds; consists of generalized tremor, which is acute in onset and rapidly progressive
   B. Granulomatous meningoencephalitis
   C. Meningoencephalitis of unknown etiology

4. Metabolic disease
   A. Hepatic encephalopathy
   B. Uremic encephalopathy

5. Infectious diseases

6. Drug therapy (fentanyl, droperidol, epinephrine, isoproterenol, 5-fluorouracil).

Prognosis

The prognosis varies with the underlying etiology; it is generally excellent for the steroid-responsive tremor syndrome.

Treatment

1. Inform the client of the diagnosis, prognosis and cost of the treatment.
2. Obtain pretreatment blood samples.
3. Place an intravenous catheter.
4. Treat the patient for nonspecific toxicity if suspected or possible.
   A. Administer sedation, intubate the patient and perform gastric lavage.
   B. Administer activated charcoal PO.
   C. Initiate intravenous fluid therapy.
5. Administer diazepam (0.5–3.0 mg/kg slowly) or pentobarbital sodium (4–8 mg/kg) intravenously as needed to relieve tremors.
6. A constant rate intravenous infusion of diazepam may be needed (0.1–0.5 mg/kg/h).
7. If SRTS is suspected, administer prednisone, 1–2 mg/kg q12h.
8. As an alternative to diazepam, consider the administration of clorazepate dipotassium, 0.5–1.0 mg/kg PO q12h.
9. Discharge the patient on either diazepam (0.1–1.0 mg/kg PO q8–12 h) or clorazepate dipotassium and prednisone for 3 weeks if SRTS is suspected.

CANINE SEIZURES

Diagnosis

History—The owner may observe generalized motor seizures (unconsciousness, recumbency, and major motor activity involving the entire body), hallucinations, pupil dilation, mastication, salivation, urination and defecation.

Mild generalized seizures may last several seconds, are characterized by decreased awareness, and mild bilateral motor activity without recumbency. Facial twitching may involve the ears, eyelids and whiskers. Shaking, salivation and urination may also be observed.

Partial seizures are infrequent in dogs, but may be characterized by a 'glazed look' and a lack of responsiveness, unilateral facial twitching, turning the head, or repetitive movements of one or both extremities on the same side, hallucinations, vocalization, frantic running, circling and biting.

The abnormal activity is usually followed by a postictal period of listlessness, confusion, pacing, thirst, hunger and sometimes sleepiness.

Status epilepticus is a period of sustained seizure activity lasting 30 minutes or longer, either because of serial seizures recurring at such a high frequency that the animal does not recover, or from an individual prolonged seizure. Status epilepticus is a life-threatening emergency requiring immediate treatment.

Physical exam—On initial presentation, the patient may appear normal, postictal, or be having seizures. If the patient is cyanotic or in respiratory distress, administer oxygen. If the patient is hyperthermic, initiate intravenous fluid therapy and cooling measures.

Laboratory evaluation—

1. Initially upon presentation, a critical patient should have a minimum database evaluated, including:
   A. PCV/TS
   B. Creatinine and BUN
   C. Blood glucose screen
   D. Serum calcium (ionized calcium is preferred)
   E. Blood or serum lactate level.
2. As time allows, further diagnostic parameters should be evaluated, including:
   A. CBC
   B. Complete serum biochemical profile, including ALT, SAP, BUN, creatinine, and electrolytes
   C. Blood gas analysis
   D. Consider performing an ethylene glycol test if the dog roams off the owner's property, or there is possible exposure to ethylene glycol from some other source.
   E. Additional testing may be indicated such as infectious disease titers or toxicology screens.

Differential diagnosis

Dogs less than 1 year of age or greater than 7 years of age, with an initial partial seizure, with seizures less than 4 weeks apart, or with a history of behavioral changes usually have an identifiable underlying cause including:

1. Rabies
2. Idiopathic epilepsy
3. Developmental abnormalities
4. Hydrocephalus
5. Meningoencephalitis (breed related, inflammatory, infectious, immune mediated, unknown etiology)
6. Canine distemper encephalitis
7. Toxoplasmosis
8. Cryptococcosis
9. Coccidioidomycosis
10. Rickettsial disease
11. Severe intestinal parasitism
12. Portosystemic shunt abnormalities
13. Central nervous system neoplasia
14. History of anoxia or cerebral trauma
15. Hypoglycemia (including neonatal and insulinoma)
16. Hypocalcemia
17. Hyperlipoproteinemia (especially in Schnauzers)
18. Tetanus
19. Toxicities (ethylene glycol, organophosphate, carbamates, strychnine, metaldehyde, lead, pyrethrin, pyrethroids, chlorinated hydrocarbons, black widow spider bite, brown recluse spider bite, toad poisoning, rattlesnake envenomation, tricyclic antidepressants, marijuana, ingestion of various plants, etc.).

Prognosis

The prognosis is variable depending on the underlying etiology.

Treatment

1. Inform the client of the diagnosis, prognosis and cost of the treatment.
2. Hospitalize the patient for observation and treatment.
3. Place an intravenous catheter, preferably in a cephalic vein. Avoid the jugular veins.
4. Obtain pretreatment blood samples. Do not use a serum separator tube as it will affect measurement of serum phenobarbital levels. If a serum separator tube is inadvertently used, decant the serum into a plain red top tube as soon as possible.
5. Control seizures with diazepam IV or pentobarbital IV as needed.
   A. Diazepam dosage = 0.7–3.0 mg/kg IV; wait 5 minutes for the full effect. May repeat. Diazepam can be administered per rectum at a dosage of 0.5–1.0 mg/kg if an intravenous catheter cannot be placed. General guidelines for diazepam dosages are:
      I. 5 kg dog—administer 2 mg IV
      II. 10 kg dog—administer 5 mg IV
      III. 20 kg dog—administer 10 mg IV.
   B. If diazepam is not sufficient, pentobarbital should be given slowly IV to effect (2–15 mg/kg).

C. Diazepam is indicated if an intracranial etiology is suspected, if two or more seizures have occurred or if one seizure episode lasts longer than 60 seconds. It is important to try to prevent additional seizures, as each seizure may increase the probability of the patient experiencing more seizures, lowering the brain's seizure threshold.

6. If diazepam or pentobarbital are not available or are ineffective, alternative therapies include:
   A. Midazolam, 0.07–0.2 mg/kg IV or IM, or 0.05–0.5 mg/kg/h IV CRI
   B. Propofol, 6 mg/kg IV, given as 1–2 mg/kg boluses to effect, followed by a propofol IV CRI, 0.1–0.2 mg/kg/min; **this is the preferred method of seizure control in patients with a history of or suspected diagnosis of hepatic disease**
   C. Thiopental, 10–20 mg/kg IV, given as 2–4 mg/kg boluses to effect.

7. At the same time, administer phenobarbital, 2–3 mg/kg IV. Repeat boluses may be administered 20 minutes apart, up to 16 mg/kg.
   A. The oral loading dosage for dogs not currently on phenobarbital is 6–8 mg/kg PO.
   B. The oral loading dosage for dogs currently on phenobarbital is 2–4 mg/kg PO.
   C. Another recommended treatment protocol for patients that are not currently on phenobarbital is to administer a loading dose using the following formula, the goal being to rapidly establish a therapeutic drug level of phenobarbital:

   $$\text{loading dose (total mg)} = \text{desired serum level (g/mL)} \times \text{body weight (kg)} \times 0.8 \, l/kg.$$

   D. For patients already on phenobarbital, obtain a serum sample (do not use a serum separator tube), and submit the serum sample to a reference lab for a STAT phenobarbital level. The therapeutic trough serum phenobarbital level is from 20 to 40 g/mL.
   E. For patients already on phenobarbital, administer phenobarbital at a dosage of 1 mg/kg for each g/mL that you wish to raise the patient's serum level. Slowly raise the serum phenobarbital level by increments of no more than 5 g/mL.

8. If phenobarbital is ineffective or contraindicated, bromide therapy may be administered as a primary or secondary medication to control seizures in dogs. Bromide is available in both the potassium and the sodium salts.
   A. Bromide may cause pneumonitis in cats and therefore should not be administered to cats.
   B. The starting dosage for potassium bromide is 20–30 mg/kg q24h with food. It may be administered either rectally or via orogastric tube if the patient is not able to swallow.
   C. The starting dosage for sodium bromide is 17–26 mg/kg q24h with food, a reduction of 15% because of the higher bromide concentration in the mixture.
   D. The loading dosage of potassium bromide to rapidly achieve target serum concentrations is 50 mg/kg every 6 hours for 2 days.

E. The serum concentration of bromide should be checked at 1 month and 3 months after starting daily maintenance dosing. The target range is 1–3 mg/mL when used as the only agent to control seizures, and 1–2 mg/mL when used concurrently with phenobarbital.

F. If the dog is fed a high-chloride diet, such as Eukanuba Response Formula FP®, Hill's h/d®, s/d® or i/d®, a dosage of 50–80 mg/kg PO q24h or 25–40 mg/kg PO q12h is recommended.

G. Reported side effects of bromide therapy include polyphagia, polyuria, polydipsia, weakness, ataxia, sedation, limb stiffness, vomiting, irritability, restlessness, pruritic skin rash, and a cough.

H. The signs of bromism (bromide toxicity) include inappropriate behavior, coma or stupor, ataxia, paraparesis or tetraparesis, dysphagia and megaesophagus.

9. Measure the patient's rectal temperature. Initiate cooling if the rectal temperature is greater than 39.5°C (103.1°F).

10. Administer oxygen if indicated.

11. Administer dextrose if the patient has hypoglycemia, 1 g/kg of 10% dextrose slow IV.

12. If the patient has hypocalcemia, administer 10% calcium gluconate, 0.5–1.5 mL/kg IV slowly over 5–10 minutes.

13. Administer IV fluids (balanced electrolyte solution or normal saline) at maintenance rates unless the patient is dehydrated. Use 0.9% NaCl if a diazepam CRI is anticipated.

14. If the seizure activity was prolonged or an underlying inflammatory etiology is suspected, consider the administration of a single dosage of dexamethasone sodium phosphate, 0.2–0.5 mg/kg IV.

15. If cerebral edema is suspected:
    A. Administer oxygen.
    B. Administer hypertonic saline, NaCl 7.5%, 4 mL/kg for dogs, 2 mL/kg for cats.
    C. Administer mannitol, 200–1000 mg/kg IV over 20 minutes.

16. If the seizures are refractory, administer either a diazepam CRI or pentobarbital CRI.
    A. Diazepam CRI
        I. Diazepam, 0.1–0.5 mg/kg/h in a 2.5% or 5% dextrose in 0.9% NaCl CRI IV.
        II. Decrease drip dosage rate by 50% every 6 hours for at least two decreases when weaning off.
        III. Continue to administer phenobarbital IV during the diazepam CRI period.
    B. Pentobarbital CRI
        I. After anesthesia from other agents has worn off, administer an initial bolus of pentobarbital at 2 mg/kg or higher slowly IV to effect.
        II. Following the bolus, begin a constant rate infusion of pentobarbital in a balanced electrolyte solution at 5 mg/kg/h IV.

III. Adjust to fit the needs of the individual patient, within the normal dosage range of 3–10 mg/kg/h.
IV. Continue at a constant level of anesthesia for 6 h then decrease the dosage by 1 mg/kg/h every 6 hours. The pentobarbital CRI should be administered for approximately 24 hours.
V. Continue to administer phenobarbital IV during the pentobarbital CRI period.

C. While administering a CRI of diazepam or pentobarbital, it is important to attend to the supportive care of the patient.
I. Provide adequate padding.
II. Turn the patient from side to side every 4 hours.
III. Monitor respiration, heart rate, temperature, blood pressure and oxygen saturation hourly.
IV. Place an endotracheal tube if the patient does not have a sufficient gag reflex.
V. Administer broad-spectrum antibiotics.
VI. Administer phenobarbital IV BID.
VII. Lubricate the eyes with a sterile ophthalmic ointment such as PuraLube.

D. If seizures are refractory and diazepam or pentobarbital is contraindicated, as in patients with hepatic encephalopathy of hepatotoxicity, maintain anesthesia with isoflurane.
I. Utilize a ventilator throughout the anesthetic period.
II. Monitor blood oxygenation with pulse oximetry hourly or arterial blood gas monitoring every 2–4 hours.

17. Pursue the diagnosis.
A. Rule out heart disease
B. Toxicity
C. Hypoglycemia
D. Allergic reaction
E. Eclampsia
F. Hepatic disease
G. Central nervous system disease
H. Infectious disease (distemper)
I. Treat for the specific condition as soon as a diagnosis is reached.

18. During recovery of suspected patients with epilepsy, begin oral phenobarbital administration to initiate maintenance blood levels.
A. Phenobarbital dosage = 2–5 mg/kg PO q8–12 h for dogs.
B. The above dosages may be doubled for the first 4 days of therapy to expedite achieving the therapeutic levels.

19. Additional maintenance medications for dogs
A. Zonisamide, 5 mg/kg PO q12h (dogs) as monotherapy, 5–10 mg/kg PO q24h when used in conjunction with other seizure control medications
B. Levetiracetam, 20 mg/kg PO q8h (dogs) as monotherapy or in conjunction with other medications
C. Gabapentin may be added to phenobarbital or bromide therapy, to improve seizure control. The starting dosage is 10 mg/kg PO every 8 hours.

Diagnosis

History—Generalized motor seizures (unconsciousness, recumbency and major motor activity involving the entire body) are often violent, with self-induced trauma such as contusions and biting of the tongue, hallucinations, piloerection, mastication, salivation, pupil dilation, and involuntary excretions.

Mild generalized seizures may last several seconds and are characterized by decreased awareness, mild bilateral motor activity without recumbency. Facial twitching may involve the ears, eyelids and whiskers. Shaking may also be observed.

Partial seizures may be characterized by a 'glazed look' and a lack of responsiveness, unilateral facial twitching, turning the head, or repetitive movements of one or both extremities on the same side, hallucinations, vocalization, frantic running, circling, self-chewing and biting.

The abnormal activity is usually followed by a postictal period of listlessness, confusion, pacing, thirst, hunger and sometimes sleepiness.

Status epilepticus is a period of sustained seizure activity lasting 30 minutes or longer, either because of serial seizures recurring at such a high frequency that the animal does not recover or from an individual prolonged seizure. Status epilepticus is a life-threatening emergency requiring immediate treatment.

Physical exam—Upon presentation, the patient may possibly appear normal, be postictal or may be having seizures.

Laboratory evaluation—

1. Initially, upon presentation, a critical patient should have a minimum database evaluated, including:
   A. PCV/TS
   B. Creatinine and BUN
   C. Blood glucose screen
   D. Serum calcium (ionized calcium is preferred).
2. As time allows, further diagnostic parameters should be evaluated, including:
   A. CBC
   B. Complete serum biochemical profile, including ALT, SAP, BUN, creatinine, and electrolytes
   C. Blood gas analysis
   D. Consider performing an ethylene glycol test if the cat roams outdoors or there is possible exposure to ethylene glycol from some other source.
   E. Serologic testing for FeLV, FIV, FIP and toxoplasmosis may be diagnostic.
   F. Additional testing may be indicated, such as infectious disease titers or toxicology screens.

Differential diagnosis

Primary idiopathic epilepsy is a rare diagnosis in cats.

1. Infectious diseases
   A. Toxoplasmosis
   B. Feline infectious peritonitis (FIP)
   C. Feline leukemia virus (FeLV)
   D. Feline immunodeficiency virus (FIV)
   E. Rabies
2. Meningoencephalitis of unknown origin
3. Feline cerebral ischemic encephalopathy
4. Meningiomas
5. Polycythemia vera with secondary hypoxic damage
6. Head trauma
7. Brain abscess
8. Developmental abnormalities
9. Primary idiopathic epilepsy
10. Hepatic encephalopathy
11. Hypoglycemia
12. Hypocalcemia
13. Toxicities (ethylene glycol, organophosphates, carbamates, strychnine, metaldehyde, lead, pyrethrins, pyrethroids, chlorinated hydrocarbons, black widow spider bite, brown recluse spider bite, toad poisoning, rattlesnake envenomation, tricyclic antidepressants, marijuana, ingestion of various plants, etc.)

Prognosis

The prognosis is variable depending on the cause. There is no correlation between the severity of the seizures and the clinical outcome.

Treatment

1. Inform the client of the diagnosis, prognosis and cost of the treatment.
2. Place an intravenous catheter.
3. Obtain pretreatment blood samples. Do not use a serum separator tube as it will affect measurement of serum phenobarbital levels. If a serum separator tube is inadvertently used, decant the serum into a plain red-top tube as soon as possible.
4. Control seizures with diazepam IV or pentobarbital IV as needed.
   A. Diazepam dosage = 0.5–3.0 mg/kg IV; wait 5 minutes for the full effect. May repeat diazepam administration if needed. Diazepam can be administered per rectum at a dosage of 0.5–1.0 mg/kg if an intravenous catheter cannot be placed. General dosage for diazepam is 2 mg IV for the average cat.
   B. If diazepam is not sufficient, pentobarbital should be given slowly IV to effect (2–4 mg/kg).
   C. Diazepam is indicated if an intracranial etiology is suspected, if two or more seizures have occurred or if one seizure episode lasts longer than 60 seconds.
5. At the same time, administer phenobarbital, 2.5 mg/kg IV. Repeat boluses may be administered 20 minutes apart, up to 16 mg/kg.

A. Another recommended treatment protocol for patients that are not currently on phenobarbital is to administer a loading dose using the following formula, the goal being to rapidly establish a therapeutic drug level of phenobarbital:

$$\text{loading dose (total mg)} = \text{desired serum level (g/mL)} \times \text{body weight (kg)} \times 0.8 \text{ L/kg.}$$

B. For patients already on phenobarbital, obtain serum sample (do not use a serum separator tube), and submit to a reference lab for a STAT phenobarbital level. The therapeutic trough serum phenobarbital level is from 10 to 30 g/mL.
C. For patients already on phenobarbital, administer phenobarbital at a dosage of 1 mg/kg for each g/mL that you wish to raise the patient's serum level. Slowly raise the serum phenobarbital level by increments of no more than 5 g/mL.

6. Obtain rectal temperature. Initiate cooling if temperature is greater than 39.5°C (103.1°F).
7. Administer oxygen if indicated.
8. Administer thiamine hydrochloride; 2 mg/kg IM or IV.
9. Administer dextrose if the blood glucose level is low, 1 g/kg of 10% dextrose slow IV.
10. Administer IV fluids (balanced electrolyte solution or normal saline) at maintenance rates unless the patient is dehydrated. If the patient is dehydrated or in shock, administer intravenous fluids at an increased and appropriate rate. Use 0.9% NaCl if a diazepam CRI is anticipated.
11. If the seizure activity was prolonged or you expect an underlying inflammatory etiology, consider the administration of a single dosage of dexamethasone sodium phosphate, 0.1 mg/kg IV or prednisolone sodium succinate, 1–3 mg/kg IV.
12. If cerebral edema is suspected:
   A. Administer oxygen.
   B. Administer hypertonic saline (NaCl 7.2%), 2–3 mL/kg IV.
   C. Administer mannitol, 100–500 mg/kg IV over 20 minutes.
13. If seizures are refractory, administer a diazepam CRI.
   A. Diazepam dosage = 0.1–0.5 mg/kg/h in a 2.5% or 5% dextrose in 0.9% NaCl CRI IV.
   B. Decrease drip dosage rate by 50% every 6 hours for at least two decreases when weaning off.
   C. Phenobarbital can be added to the diazepam infusion, if necessary, at the rate of 0.5–1.0 mg/kg/h.
   D. While administering a CRI of diazepam, it is important to attend to the supportive care of the patient.
      I. Provide adequate padding.
      II. Turn the patient from side to side every 4 hours.
      III. Monitor respiration, heart rate, temperature, blood pressure and oxygen saturation hourly.
      IV. Place an endotracheal tube.
      V. Administer broad-spectrum antibiotics.
      VI. Administer phenobarbital IV BID.

VII. Lubricate the eyes with a sterile ophthalmic ointment such as PuraLube.

Do not administer ophthalmic medication containing bacitracin, neomycin, or polymixin to cats as those medications have been linked to fatalities from anaphylactic reactions in cats.

E. If seizures are refractory and diazepam is contraindicated, as in patients with hepatic encephalopathy or hepatotoxicity, maintain anesthesia with isoflurane.

   I. Utilize a ventilator throughout the anesthetic period.

   II. Monitor blood oxygenation with pulse oximetry and $ETCO_2$ continuously, and arterial blood gas monitoring every 2 hours.

14. Pursue the diagnosis and treat for the specific condition as soon as a diagnosis is reached.
15. Hospitalize for observation.
16. During recovery of suspect epilepsy patients, begin oral phenobarbital administration to initiate maintenance blood levels.
    A. Phenobarbital dosage = 1.5–2.5 mg/kg PO q12h for cats
    B. Bromide should not be administered to cats as it may cause a fatal pneumonitis.
    C. Zonisamide, 5–10 mg/kg PO q24h, may be administered as an alternative.
    D. Levetiracetam, 20 mg/kg PO q8h, is effective in many cats when combined with phenobarbital.
    E. Diazepam should not be administered orally as maintenance medication owing to the risk of potentially fatal hepatic disease in cats.
17. Refer for a neurologic consultation and possible CT scan or MRI.

ALTERED MENTATION AND COMA

Definitions

1. Stuporous animals are laterally recumbent, respond slightly to painful stimuli and have some voluntary movements.
2. Comatose animals are completely nonresponsive to all external stimuli.

Diagnosis

History—Obtaining a thorough history is very important. Obtain information regarding a possibility of trauma, proper vaccinations, exposure to wildlife, previous behavioral abnormalities, seizures, exposure to drugs or toxins (barbiturates, sedatives, cyanide, ethylene glycol, organophosphates, marijuana, etc.), possibility of extreme heat exposure, history of previous illness, and thiamine content of the diet.
Physical exam—Immediately evaluate the patient's vital signs. Ensure an adequate airway. Evaluate the patient's respiration, cardiac rate and rhythm, mucous membrane color, body temperature, plus a thorough physical examination of all body systems.

Differential diagnosis

1. Head trauma
2. Hypoxia / anoxia

3. Drug or chemical intoxication
4. Viral encephalitis (rabies, distemper, FIP)
5. Fungal encephalitis
6. Hepatoencephalopathy
7. Uremic encephalopathy
8. Miscellaneous serum osmolality disturbances
9. Miscellaneous acid–base imbalances.
10. Hypoadrenocorticism (rare)
11. Granulomatous meningoencephalitis or meningoencephalitis of unknown etiology
12. Thiamine deficiency
13. Hydrocephalus
14. Heat stroke
15. Hypoglycemia
16. Hyperglycemia
17. Bacterial encephalitis
18. Protozoal encephalitis
19. Cerebral neoplasia
20. Postictal coma or stupor
21. Cerebrovascular disease

Prognosis

The prognosis is variable, depending upon the underlying etiology.

Treatment

1. Administer oxygen (establish patient airway if necessary).
   A. Intubation
   B. Nasal catheterization
   C. Oxygen cage
   D. Elizabethan collar hood
2. Inform the client of the diagnosis, prognosis and cost of the treatment.
3. Place an intravenous catheter.
4. Obtain pretreatment blood samples.
5. Check blood glucose, BUN, Creatinine, PCV/TP, WBC, sodium, potassium, calcium, ALT, and SAP in-house, as a minimum database.
6. Pursue the diagnosis; treat specifically as soon as diagnosis is obtained.
7. Administer symptomatic treatment until the diagnosis is reached, including intravenous fluids, antibiotics, etc. as indicated.
8. Perform gastric lavage and administer activated charcoal if toxicity is suspected.

ACUTE ULCERATIVE KERATITIS

Etiology

1. Mechanical trauma—clippers, bite wounds, cat scratches, self-inflicted by rubbing at head, eyelash diseases, foreign bodies, proptosis, eyelid paralysis, general anesthesia, entropion

2. Chemical trauma—acids and alkalies; yard and garden sprays, mace, soap, shampoos, detergents, exposure to heat and fumes from fires
3. Infectious—bacterial, mycotic, viral
4. Metabolic—keratoconjunctivitis sicca, hypoandrogenism, endothelial disease
5. Neurotropic—CN V sensory innervation failure
6. Immune mediated.

Diagnosis

History—The owner may notice that the pet is squinting its eye, rubbing at the eye or face, or may have an ocular discharge or discoloration to the cornea. The pet may have been exposed to plant material or bathed recently.

Physical exam—The physical abnormalities may include blepharospasms, photophobia, serous or purulent ocular discharge, conjunctivitis, corneal edema with a possibly clear center, corneal neovascularization and, possibly, signs of anterior uveitis. Carefully examine the eye and conjunctival tissues for the presence of foreign bodies.

Fluorescein stain is retained on areas where there is a loss of corneal integrity.

Prognosis

The prognosis is usually good.

Treatment

1. Inform the client of the diagnosis, prognosis and cost of the treatment.
2. Submit a corneal or conjunctival culture. Treat empirically pending culture results.
3. Administer topical medications.
   A. Antimicrobials
      I. Bacterial keratitis—perform a culture and sensitivity, initially start tobramycin, ofloxacin, ciprofloxacin or neomycin-polymyxin-bacitracin mixtures (in dogs only). **Bacitracin-neomycin-polymyxin or -gramicidin (in various combinations) in ophthalmic medications have been reported to cause fatal anaphylactic reactions in cats and therefore these medications should not be administered to a cat.**
      II. Viral keratitis—trifluorothymidine solution (Viroptic®), idoxuridine or vidarabine
      III. *Chlamydophila* keratitis—tetracycline, chloramphenicol
      IV. Mycotic—natamycin, miconazole, nystatin, fluconazole, econazole, clotrimazole or silver sulfadiazine
   B. Administer atropine 1% ophthalmic solution or ointment q6–8 h to relieve pain.
   C. For ulcers present for more than 5 days or rapidly progressive stromal ulcers, administer acetylcysteine or fresh serum obtained

from the patient. Debridement of loose corneal tissue may be necessary. Consider referral to an ophthalmologist.

D. Topical anti-inflammatory medications
  I. Nonsteroidal anti-inflammatories may be utilized, including flurbiprofen, suprofen, diclofenac and ketorolac.
  II. Corticosteroids should be avoided.

E. Muro 128® is a hypertonic saline, soothing ointment that reduces corneal edema.

4. Systemic medications.
  A. Antimicrobial medications
    I. Bacterial keratitis—systemic antibiotics are often helpful, including cephalosporin, enrofloxacin and ciprofloxacin.
    II. Viral keratitis—administer L-lysine, 500 mg PO q12h; interferon 30 IU/day for 7 days, then off for 7 days, repeat until clinical signs have resolved; other antiviral medications such as ganciclovir or penciclovir may be beneficial pending further investigation.
    III. Mycotic keratitis—administer systemic antifungal agents, including amphotericin B, ketoconazole, itraconazole, fluconazole.
  B. Anti-inflammatory medications
    I. Administer nonsteroidal anti-inflammatory agents, including carprofen, meloxicam and deracoxib.
    II. Systemic corticosteroids are not usually indicated for keratitis.

5. Consider the administration of analgesic medication, such as buprenorphine or tramadol.

6. Chemical keratitis
  A. Alkaline chemicals are severely erosive and destructive to the cornea.
    I. Immediately lavage the eye with large volumes (2 liters) of irrigating saline. This usually requires sedation or anesthesia.
    II. Administer systemic analgesics.
    III. Administer a specific antidote based on the advice from a poison control center.
    IV. Administer boric acid ophthalmic ointment to help neutralize weak alkaline compounds.
    V. Administer atropine if there is evidence of uveitis or corneal ulceration.
    VI. Administer topical ophthalmic antibiotics.
    VII. Administer acetylcysteine if there are stromal injuries.
    VIII. Do not administer topical corticosteroids.
  B. Acidic agents are precipitated by the corneal proteins and are less destructive to the cornea.
    I. Immediately lavage the eye with large volumes (2 liters) of irrigating saline. This usually requires sedation or anesthesia.
    II. Administer a specific antidote based on the advice from a poison control center.
    III. Administer atropine if there is evidence of uveitis or corneal ulceration.
    IV. Administer topical ophthalmic antibiotics.

V. Administer acetylcysteine if there are stromal injuries.

VI. Do not administer topical corticosteroids.

7. Provide corneal support and protection.

A. Elizabethan collar

B. Third-eyelid flap

C. Temporary tarsorrhaphy

D. Collagen shield

E. Extended-wear contact lens

F. Conjunctival flaps

G. Additional surgical procedures may be offered by an ophthalmologist.

8. Monitor closely for progression to a descemetocele, which requires a conjunctival graft or flap.

CORNEAL FOREIGN BODIES

Diagnosis

History—Prior to the injury the animal may have been hunting, traversing through tall plants, or may have strayed off of the owner's property. The pet may have had access to wood, glass or industrial refuse. There is usually an acute onset of extreme pain. The pet may be squinting, head-shy, lethargic and depressed.

Physical exam—The patient may present with blepharospasms, photophobia, epiphora, periorbital hemorrhage or ecchymosis, puncture wounds to the eyelids or face, facial fractures, corneal edema, miosis, iris prolapse, anterior synechia, severe hyphema, deformity of the globe and possibly blindness.

Visualization of the foreign body may require magnification and special imaging techniques such as MRI or CT.

Skull radiographs—May be helpful to determine the location of metallic foreign bodies.

Prognosis

The prognosis varies, depending on the type of foreign body, the placement of the foreign body, the duration and the severity of the injuries to the eye.

Treatment

1. Evaluate the patient for other injuries; stabilize the patient as necessary.

2. Inform the client of the diagnosis, prognosis and cost of the treatment.

3. Control periocular hemorrhage.

4. Removal of the foreign body is based upon the type of material and the location.

A. Plant debris, wood, steel, and iron are severely irritating.

B. Copper, bronze, and brass cause local abscesses.

C. Aluminum, lead, mercury, nickel, and zinc are moderately irritating.

D. Carbon, glass, gold, plaster, rubber, silver, stainless steel, and stone are inert and may be left in place if there is minimal anterior uveitis and the corneal wound has spontaneously healed.

E. Removal of corneal foreign bodies is usually best performed by ophthalmologists who are specially trained and equipped to perform limbal incisions and control intraocular hemorrhage.

5. Begin medical therapy while awaiting referral.
   A. Topical and systemic antibiotics
   B. Topical atropine
   C. Systemic anti-inflammatory agents
   D. Topical and systemic analgesics.

6. Apply an Elizabethan collar to reduce self-trauma.

ANTERIOR UVEITIS

Etiology

The etiologies of anterior uveitis include:

1. Trauma—including intraocular surgery
2. Inflammatory—deep keratitis, ulcerative keratitis
3. Infectious diseases—bacterial septicemia, brucellosis, canine distemper virus, ehrlichiosis, feline immunodeficiency virus, feline infectious peritonitis, feline leukemia virus, systemic fungal infections (aspergillosis, blastomycosis, coccidioidomycosis, cryptococcosis, histoplasmosis), infectious canine hepatitis (*Adenovirus*), heartworms, herpesvirus, hookworm migration, *Leishmania donovani*, leptospirosis, Lyme disease, mycobacteria, prototheca, pyometra, rabies, Rocky Mountain spotted fever, roundworm migration, *Streptococcus* spp., toxoplasmosis
4. Immune-mediated—ruptured lens, the uveodermatologic syndrome, coagulopathies, immune-mediated vasculitis
5. Neoplastic and paraneoplastic—ocular melanoma, adenocarcinoma, lymphosarcoma, fibrosarcoma, hyperviscosity syndrome
6. Idiopathic.

Diagnosis

History—The owner may observe squinting, increased tearing, and avoidance of sunlight. There may be a history of trauma, intraocular surgery, systemic disease or another health problem.

Physical exam—The patient may present with blepharospasms, increased lacrimation and photophobia. Enophthalmia secondary to ocular pain may be observed. The conjunctiva may appear hyperemic and there may be circumcorneal blood vessel injection. Chemosis may be present. Corneal edema, neovascularization and keratic precipitates may be present. The contents of the anterior chamber may be abnormal, including aqueous flare, fibrin clots, desquamated pigment epithelial cells, hyphema and hypopyon. The pupil may be miotic and the iris rough and swollen. Synechia may occur. Intraocular pressure may be low (hypotony). If the intraocular pressure is normal, consider that glaucoma may be developing as a secondary complication.

It is important to perform a thorough physical examination of all body systems to detect the presence of systemic infections and complicating factors.

Bilateral ocular involvement suggests systemic disease as the underlying etiology.

Laboratory findings—
1. Evaluate a CBC, serum biochemical profile and urinalysis in all affected patients.
2. Serologic testing and infectious disease titer assessment may be indicated.
3. Immune profile testing may be beneficial.
4. Thoracic and abdominal radiography may reveal evidence of systemic mycosis, other organ system involvement or disseminated neoplasia.
5. Ocular cytology, culture and aqueous fluid titers may be beneficial. Biopsy samples may be obtained and submitted for histopathology. These procedures should probably be performed by an ophthalmologic specialist rather than an emergency clinician.
6. Ocular sonography may reveal neoplasia of the iris or ciliary body, cataracts, lens luxation, clots or hemorrhage in the anterior chamber, penetrating foreign bodies, fungal masses, and other ocular lesions.

Differential diagnosis

The differential diagnosis includes acute conjunctivitis, acute glaucoma, episcleritis and ulcerative keratitis.

Prognosis

If anterior uveitis occurs owing to a fungal infections, the prognosis is poor. Other causes of anterior uveitis have a good prognosis, although the condition may become recurrent or relapsing. Complications including glaucoma, corneal scarring, synechia formation, cataracts and phthisis bulbi may occur.

Treatment

1. Inform the client of the diagnosis, prognosis and cost of the treatment.
2. Administer specific treatment to control the underlying etiology.
3. Administer anti-inflammatory medications.
   A. Corticosteroids are recommended for acute anterior uveitis.
      I. Systemic prednisolone or prednisone
      II. Topical prednisolone 1%, dexamethasone 0.1% or 0.05%, initially q2–3 h, then q6h
      III. Subconjunctival corticosteroids may be administered if systemic administration is not possible, the patient cannot be medicated on a regular basis, or if long-term systemic medication is contraindicated or cannot be administered.

B. Nonsteroidal anti-inflammatory medications may be administered when corticosteroids are contraindicated.
   I. Carprofen, 4 mg/kg q24h or 2 mg/kg q12h for dogs, 4 mg/kg SC or IV once for cats
   II. Meloxicam, 0.2 mg/kg PO, IV, SC initial dose then 0.1 mg/kg PO q24h for dogs, 0.1 mg/kg SC or PO once for cats
   III. Ketoprofen, 1–2 mg/kg IV, IM, SC q24h for maximum 3 days or 1 mg/kg PO q24h for maximum of 5 days in dogs, 0.5–2 mg/kg IV, IM, SC initial dose then 0.5–1 mg/kg PO q24h for a maximum of 5 days in cats
   IV. Aspirin, 10–15 mg/kg q12h PO for dogs, 10 mg/kg q48–72 hours PO in cats
   V. Flunixin meglumine (Banamine®), 0.25–0.5 mg/kg IV, may be administered as a single dose to dogs. A dosage of 0.11–0.22 mg/kg IV q24h for up to 3 days may be administered to a dog with severe ocular pain. Flunixin meglumine is particularly effective at controlling ocular pain.
   VI. Topical medications such as suprofen 1% (Profenal®), flurbiprofen 0.03% (Ocufen®), diclofenac 0.1% (Voltaren®) or ketorolac 0.5% may be administered q6h.
4. Immunosuppressive medications are indicated in combination with systemic prednisolone for refractory cases in the dog that requires long-term therapy.
   A. Azathioprine (Imuran®), 2.2 mg/kg PO q48h, then tapering the dose
   B. Cyclophosphamide (Cytoxan®), 50 mg/m² PO q24h × 4 days/week
5. The administration of a mydriatic agent may be beneficial.
   A. Atropine 1% q2–3h until the pupil starts to dilate, then q8h; atropine is contraindicated in glaucoma and should be used only on the hypotonic eye.
   B. Tropicamide may be used on a short term basis on the glaucomatous eye to achieve mydriasis.
   C. Phenylephrine 2.5–10% may be used on the glaucomatous eye.
   D. Epinephrine 1–2% may be used on the glaucomatous eye.
   E. A combination of phenylephrine 10% and atropine 1% may be mixed together and administered q1–2 h, or they may be alternated q1–2h.
6. Apply topical cyclosporine A, q6h.
7. Apply warm compresses to the periorbital area.
8. Avoid exposure to bright lights and sunlight.

HYPHEMA

Definition

Hyphema is hemorrhage into the anterior chamber of the eye.

Etiology

1. Trauma—including perforating wounds, severe blows to the head, choking

2. Infectious diseases (anterior uveitis)—FELV, FIP, toxoplasmosis, ehrlichiosis
3. Anterior uveal neoplasia
4. Congenital vascular abnormalities—collie eye syndrome
5. Chronic glaucoma—an unfavorable sign and usually associated with pain
6. Idiopathic—usually responds well to treatment
7. Post-cataract surgery—usually does not respond to treatment
8. Coagulopathy—immune-mediated thrombocytopenia, leukemia, DIC, clotting factor deficiencies, anticoagulant rodenticide toxicity
9. Hypertension.

Diagnosis

History—The patient may have a history of recent trauma, ocular surgery or exposure to anticoagulant rodenticide.

Physical exam—Evaluate the patient for signs of trauma or other signs of bleeding. Look for puncture wounds, cervical bruising, peripheral lymphadenopathy, petechiae or ecchymoses.

Perform a thorough ocular examination, including direct visualization, and direct and indirect ophthalmoscopy.

If the hemorrhage is fresh, bright-red blood will be visualized in the anterior chamber. Quite often, the clinician will be unable to evaluate the pupil, lens or retina owing to the hemorrhage.

Fluorescein stain the cornea to evaluate corneal integrity.

Laboratory evaluation—
1. Evaluate a CBC, including a platelet count.
2. Evaluate a complete serum biochemical profile.
3. Evaluate a coagulation profile.
4. Perform serologic testing for the infectious disease indigenous to the area.
5. Measure arterial blood pressure.
6. Measure intraocular pressure.

Ultrasonography (of the globe)—May be helpful. Intraocular neoplastic masses, abscesses, and other lesions may be diagnosed.

Prognosis

The prognosis is variable, depending on the underlying etiology. If the anterior chamber is entirely filled with darkened blood, 'eight-ball hemorrhage' following severe trauma, the prognosis is poor.

Treatment

Reference sources suggest treatment is both controversial and enigmatic. Consider the following:
1. Inform the client of the diagnosis, prognosis and cost of the treatment.
2. Sedate and allow cage rest.
3. Administer topical and systemic corticosteroid therapy (topical only if there are no corneal ulcers)—dexamethasone 0.1%, or prednisolone acetate 1%, q4–8h.

Neurologic and ocular emergencies

4. Pilocarpine 1% (topical)—facilitates drainage through the iridocorneal drainage angle. (**Caution: may predispose to complete posterior synechia.**)
5. Epinephrine 1% or 2% (topical)—may dilate the pupil and reduce hemorrhage. Reduces the risk of developing posterior synechiae.
6. Atropine 1% (topical)—stabilizes the blood–aqueous barrier; it is useful in the treatment of anterior uveitis, but also potentiates secondary glaucoma.
7. Combination therapy—use topical epinephrine for the first 24 hours followed by atropine.
8. Tissue plasminogen activator (t-PA), 25 g instilled intraocularly, will help dissolve clots and fibrin.
9. Remove the cause of bleeding.
    A. If coagulopathy, blood dyscrasia or underlying infectious etiology is suspected, draw pretreatment blood samples. Perform appropriate tests and treat the underlying etiology.
    B. Consider initiating treatment with vitamin K_1, if possible exposure to anticoagulant rodenticide has occurred.
    C. Check the patient's blood pressure and treat appropriately.
    D. Measure intraocular pressure; initiate treatment for glaucoma if appropriate.
10. Aspirin administration is contraindicated.
11. Inform the owners of the potential serious complications of hyphema, including:
    A. Posterior synechia
    B. Cataracts
    C. Glaucoma
    D. Blindness
    E. Phthisis bulbi.

PROPTOSED GLOBE

Diagnosis

History—The patient may have a history of a recent traumatic event, such as an attack by a larger dog, choking, automobile trauma, etc. *Physical exam*—Perform a thorough physical examination, including a neurologic examination. Look carefully for other signs of trauma. Perform a thorough ophthalmic exam and fluorescein staining of the cornea. The eyelids appear to be folded behind a globe that is too far forward. There may be extensive swelling, erythema and puncture wounds or abrasions periorbitally. Torn extraocular muscles may be observed. The eye may be blind.

Prognosis

The prognosis depends on the extent of the trauma.

1. The prognosis is better for those with a proptosis for less than 3 hours' duration, or with mild or partial proptosis.

2. If the duration is prolonged, the anterior chamber is filled with hyphema, there is avulsion of the optic nerve, the pupil is dilated or nearly normal, or there is severe facial trauma, the prognosis is guarded.
3. Even with severe injury and loss of vision, a cosmetic globe may be saved. Unless the extraocular muscles are so severely damaged that the globe is just dangling, do not remove the eye.
4. *Always* inform the client that vision cannot be evaluated adequately at this time.

Treatment

1. Thoroughly evaluate the extent of the other injuries.
2. Inform the client of the diagnosis, prognosis and cost of the treatment.
3. Stabilize the patient as needed (IV fluids, radiographs, thoracocentesis, etc.).
4. Administer systemic antibiotics (ampicillin, amoxicillin-clavulonate Clavamox®, trimethoprim-sulfa).
5. Administer flunixin meglumine (dogs only), 0.5 to 1 mg/kg IV **once** and not in conjunction with corticosteroids.
6. Administer a topical ophthalmic antibiotic, without steroids, to lubricate the eye
7. If the patient has a partially proptosed globe, attempt manual reduction without sedation. Gently lift up the superior and inferior palpebrae, pull dorsally and ventrally while pulling outward and sometimes the globe will slip back into proper position.
8. When the patient is stable, administer anesthesia and surgically replace or enucleate the globe.
   A. Administer inhalation anesthetics.
   B. Perform surgical reduction (Fig. 13.1).
      I. Apply an ophthalmic antibiotic to all exposed areas of the globe.
      II. Clip all long hair from the periorbital area.
      III. Flush the conjunctiva, globe and periorbital area with sterile saline.
      IV. Re-apply the ophthalmic antibiotic.
      V. Preplace three sutures in a horizontal mattress pattern or simple interrupted pattern in both the superior and inferior palpebrae, being careful to not go totally through the eyelids, so as to avoid corneal trauma.
      VI. Use 2-0 or 3-0 monofilament nonabsorbable suture on a cutting needle.
      VII. Avoid the use of stents, as they serve as a nidus for infection.
      VIII. Using a clean, flat surface such as a scalpel handle, or with digital pressure, gently push down on the globe as all of the sutures are pulled up. This will enable the globe to pop past the eyelids and return to normal position.

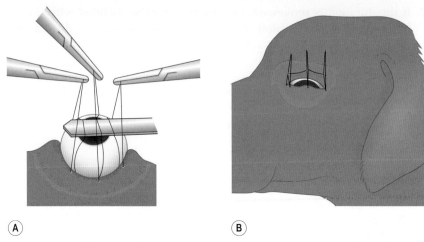

FIG 13.1 Surgical reduction of a proptosed globe. (A) Three or four simple interrupted sutures are pre-placed in the lid margins. Using a scalpel handle, apply gentle pressure down on the lubricated globe. (B) Assist reduction of the proptosis by pulling up on the sutures. Tie the suture knots to fix the globe in place once the reduction has been completed. The use of stents is not recommended.

IX. Tie the sutures to appose the eyelids, but allow for swelling. Do not tie too tightly.

9. Treat the patient's other wounds.

10. Send the patient home on systemic antibiotics and analgesics for 5–7 days. If the patient is manageable, have the owner administer ophthalmic antibiotic ointment q8–12 h at the nasal canthus. Do not dispense ophthalmic ointment if the patient is not easy to medicate.

11. Send the patient home with an Elizabethan collar, or show the owner how to make one. Have the patient wear the collar until the eyelid sutures are removed.

12. Leave the sutures in place for 1–3 weeks, until there is minimal tension against the eyelids.

ACUTE GLAUCOMA

Diagnosis

History—The patient may have a history of acute onset of ocular pain, blepharospasms, epiphora, corneal cloudiness and, possibly, blindness. Primary glaucoma occurs in many dog breeds and mixed-breed dogs, including the American and the English Cocker Spaniel, Beagle, Poodle, Basset Hound, Samoyed, Alaskan Malamute, Norwegian Elkhound, Siberian Husky, Shar Pei, Chow Chow, Smooth and Wire Hair Fox Terrier, Boston terrier, Great Dane and Bull Mastiff. Secondary glaucoma occurs in dogs and cats following chronic anterior uveitis, lens luxation, and intraocular neoplasia.

Physical exam—The physical abnormalities may include blepharospasms, conjunctival and episcleral hyperemia, buphthalmos, corneal edema, mydriatic and nonresponsive pupils; decreased menace response, and loss of vision may occur.

A fundic examination may not be able to be performed owing to severe corneal edema, but if possible the abnormalities observed may include cupping of the optic disc, corneal striae, lens luxation, retinal degeneration, optic nerve demyelination, and cataract formation. Measurement of intraocular pressure (IOP) indicates pressure usually between 45 and 70 mm Hg in acute glaucoma. Glaucoma is diagnosed when intraocular pressure is >30 mm Hg. Normal IOP is 15–25 mm Hg.

Prognosis

The prognosis is guarded to poor. Acute glaucoma is usually defined as <2 days' duration, whereas chronic glaucoma is defined as >5 days' duration. Vision may be preserved or regained if proper treatment is provided for acute glaucoma. Chronic glaucoma usually causes permanent blindness.

Treatment

1. Inform the client of the diagnosis, prognosis and cost of the treatment.
2. If IOP is between 25 mm Hg and 40 mm Hg, administer topical dorzolamide (Trusopt®), 2% q8–12h and oral methazolamide (Neptazene®), 5–10 mg/kg PO q8–12h or oral dichlorphenamide (Daranide®), 2–10 mg/kg PO q8–12h. These medications are carbonic anhydrase inhibitors that decrease the production of aqueous humor and thereby reduce IOP. Avoid the administration of these agents in cats.
   A. If IOP decreases below 25 mm Hg, continue the therapy and re-evaluate the patient in 3–5 days.
   B. If IOP remains over 25 mm Hg, follow the recommended therapy for IOP >40 mm Hg.
3. If IOP is >40 mm Hg, and the glaucoma appears to be chronic, administer topical dorzolamide (Trusopt®) and oral methazolamide (Neptazane®) or dichlorphenamide (Daranide®) as above, and add timolol maleate (Timoptic®), 0.5% or 0.25%, q12h. Timolol is a beta blocker that reduces the production of aqueous humor in dogs. It should not be administered to cats with feline asthma.
4. If IOP is >40 mm Hg and the glaucoma is acute, administer topical dorzolamide and oral dichlorphenamide (Daranide®) or methazolamide (Neptazane®) as above, and add mannitol, latanoprost (Xalatan®) and prednisone:
   A. Mannitol, 15–20% for IV administration: give 1–2 g/kg IV slowly over 15–20 minutes. Withhold water for 2–4 hours. Recheck IOP 6 hours after mannitol administration; if >25 mm Hg, give an additional dose of mannitol at 8 hours. If IOP remains >25 mm Hg, refer for emergency surgery.
   B. Latanoprost (Xalatan®) 0.005%, q12–24 h, is a prostaglandin analogue that decreases IOP in dogs by increasing outflow via the uveoscleral route. It is not normally recommended in cats. It should not be administered if the patient has a lens luxation or anterior uveitis.
   C. Prednisone 0.5 mg/kg PO q24h.

5. Administer an analgesic, such as tramadol or buprenorphine.
6. An alternative osmotic agent for mannitol is glycerin, 1–2 mL/kg PO q6–12 h (dilute with milk if emesis occurs).
7. Pilocarpine is a parasympathomimetic that reduces IOP by increasing aqueous humor outflow through the iridocorneal angle. The 1% solution is most commonly recommended: 1 drop q8h. It should be avoided when uveitis is present. Acute pain and redness may occur, requiring discontinuation of topical use.
8. Epinephrine is a sympathomimetic that increases the outflow of aqueous humor and decreases IOP. It is available as a 0.1% ophthalmic solution (Propine®), and can be used when desired to keep the pupil dilated in secondary glaucoma due to uveitis, or patients where pilocarpine is contraindicated.
9. Refer the patient to an ophthalmologist for additional therapy, or possibly surgery.

SUDDEN BLINDNESS

Acute blindness may be ocular, brainstem, cerebral or cortical in origin.

Diagnosis

History—A history of polyphagia, polydipsia and polyuria may been seen with pituitary neoplasia. The owner may comment that the pet has been bumping into walls, squinting, or that the eye has changed color. If the reason for seeking veterinary care is acute blindness, the condition is usually bilateral.

Physical exam—The patient may exhibit anterior uveitis, severe hyphema, severe keratitis, cataract, glaucoma, retinitis, papilledema or retinal detachment. Bilateral mydriasis with nonresponsive pupils may indicate optic neuritis.

Perform a complete neurologic examination.

Measure systemic arterial blood pressure. Measure intraocular pressure.

Laboratory evaluation—
1. Evaluate a CBC, including a platelet count.
2. Evaluate a complete serum biochemical profile.
3. Perform serologic testing for the infectious disease indigenous to the area.
4. Measure the serum lead level.

Differential diagnoses

1. Pituitary neoplasia
2. Optic neuritis
3. Lead poisoning
4. Lymphosarcoma
5. Cryptococcosis
6. Peracute canine distemper

7. Granulomatous meningoencephalitis
8. Anterior uveitis
9. Glaucoma
10. Retinal detachment, often secondary to systemic hypertension
11. Sudden acquired retinal degeneration (SARD)
12. Severe corneal edema
13. Severe hyphema.

Prognosis

The prognosis for regaining vision is guarded to poor.

Treatment

1. Inform the client of the diagnosis, prognosis and cost of the treatment.
2. Attempt to determine and treat the underlying cause.
3. Administer oral prednisolone, 1.0 mg/kg q12h, for the treatment of optic neuritis and SARD not associated with systemic hypertension.

REFERENCES/FURTHER READING

HEAD TRAUMA

Armitage-Chan, E.A., Wetmore, L.A., Chan, D.L., 2007. Anesthetic management of the head trauma patient. Journal of Veterinary Emergency and Critical Care 17 (1), 5–14.

Davis, D.P., 2008. Early ventilation in traumatic brain injury. Resuscitation 76, 333–340.

Fletcher, D.J., Dewey, C.W., 2009. Traumatic brain injury. In: Bonagura, J.D., Twedt, D.C. (Eds.), Kirk's Current Veterinary Therapy XIV. Saunders Elsevier, St Louis, pp. 33–37.

Fletcher, D.J., Syring, R.S., 2009. Traumatic brain injury. In: Silverstein, D.C., Hopper, K. (Eds.), Small Animal Critical Care Medicine. Elsevier, St Louis, pp. 658–662.

Heegaard, W., Biros, M., 2007. Traumatic brain injury. Emergency Medicine Clinics of North America 25, 655–678.

Kamel, H., Navi, B.B., Nakagawa, K., et al., 2011. Hypertonic saline versus mannitol for treatment of increased intracranial pressure: a meta-analysis of randomized clinical trials. Critical Care Medicine 39, 554–559.

Park, E., Bell, J.D., 2008. Traumatic brain injury: Can the consequences be stopped? Canadian Medical Association Journal 178 (9), 1163–1170.

Platt, S.R., Olby, N.J., 2004. Neurologic emergencies. In: Platt, S.R., Olby, N.J. (Eds.), BSAVA Manual of Canine and Feline Neurology, third ed. BSAVA, Gloucester, pp. 326–332.

Sande, A., West, C., 2010. Traumatic brain injury: a review of pathophysiology and management. Journal of Veterinary Emergency and Critical Care 20 (2), 177–190.

Timmons, S.D., 2010. Current trends in neurotrauma care. Critical Care Medicine 38 (Suppl), S431–S444.

ACUTE MYELOPATHIES

Besalti, O., Ozak, A., Pekcan, Z., et al., 2005. The role of extruded disk material in thoracolumbar intervertebral disk disease: A retrospective study in 40 dogs. Canadian Veterinary Journal 46, 814–820.

Boag, A.K., Otto, C.M., Drobatz, K.J., 2001. Complications of methylprednisolone sodium succinate therapy in Dachshunds with surgically treated intervertebral disc disease. Journal of Veterinary Emergency and Critical Care 11 (2), 105–110.

Brisson, B.A., 2010. Intervertebral disc disease in dogs. In: daCosta RC (guest ed), Spinal Diseases. The Veterinary Clinics of North America, Small Animal Practice 40 (5), 829–858.

Coates, J.R., 2004. Paraparesis. In: Platt, S.R., Olby, N.J. (Eds.), BSAVA Manual of Canine and Feline Neurology, third ed. BSAVA, Gloucester, pp. 237–261.

De Risio, L., Platt, S.R., 2010. Fibrocarilaginous embolic myelopathy in small animals. In: daCosta RC (guest ed), Spinal Diseases. The Veterinary Clinics of North America, Small Animal Practice 40 (5), 859–869.

Hillman, R.B., Kengeri, S.S., Waters, D.J., 2009. Reevaluation of predictive factors for complete recovery in dogs with nonambulatory tetraparesis secondary to cervical disk herniation. Journal of the American Animal Hospital Association 45, 155–163.

Joaquim, J.G.F., Luna, S.P.L., Brondani, J.T., et al., 2010. Comparison of decompressive surgery, electroacupuncture, and decompressive surgery followed by electroacupuncture for the treatment of dogs with intervertebral disk disease with long-standing severe neurologic deficits. Journal of the American Veterinary Medical Association 236, 1225–1229.

Johnson, K., Vite, C.H., 2009. Spinal cord injury. In: Silverstein, D.C., Hopper, K. (Eds.), Small Animal Critical Care Medicine. Elsevier, St Louis, pp. 419–423.

Mann, F.A., Wagner-Mann, C.C., Dunphy, E.D., et al., 2007. Recurrence rate of presumed thoracolumbar intervertebral disc disease in ambulatory dogs with spinal hyperpathia treated with anti-inflammatory drugs: 78 cases (1997–2000). Journal of Veterinary Emergency and Critical Care 17 (1), 53–60.

Marioni-Henry, K., 2010. Feline spinal cord diseases. In: daCosta RC (guest ed), Spinal Diseases. The Veterinary Clinics of North America, Small Animal Practice 40 (5), 1011–1028.

Marioni-Henry, K., Vite, C.H., Newton, A.L., et al., 2004. Prevalence of diseases of the spinal cord of cats. Journal of Veterinary Internal Medicine 18, 851–858.

Meintjes, E., Hosgood, G., Daniloff, J., 1996. Pharmaceutic treatment of acute spinal trauma. Compendium of Continuing Education 18 (6), 625–631.

Mikszewski, J.S., Van Winkle, T.J., Troxel, M.T., 2006. Fibrocartilaginous embolic myelopathy in five cats. Journal of the American Animal Hospital Association 42, 226–233.

Nesathurai, S., 1998. Steroids and spinal cord injury: revisiting the NASCIS 2 and NASCIS 3 trials [current opinion]. Journal of Trauma: Injury, Infection, and Critical Care 45 (6), 1088–1093.

Olby, N.J., 2004. Tetraparesis. In: Platt, S.R., Olby, N.J. (Eds.), BSAVA Manual of Canine and Feline Neurology, third ed. BSAVA, Gloucester, pp. 214–236.

Platt, S.R., 2004. Neck and back pain. In: Platt, S.R., Olby, N.J. (Eds.), BSAVA Manual of Canine and Feline Neurology, third ed. BSAVA, Gloucester, pp. 202–213.

Platt, S.R., Olby, N.J., 2004. Neurologic emergencies. In: Platt, S.R., Olby, N.J. (Eds.), BSAVA Manual of Canine and Feline Neurology, third ed. BSAVA, Gloucester, pp. 320–326.

Ruddle, T.L., Allen, D.A., Schertel, E.R., et al., 2006. Outcome and prognostic factors in nonambulatory Hansen type I intervertebral disc extrusions: 308 cases. Veterinary Comparative Orthopedic Traumatology 19, 29–34.

Rylander, H., Robles, J.C., 2007. Diagnosis and treatment of a chronic atlanto-occipital subluxation in a dog. Journal of the American Animal Hospital Association 43, 173–178.

Smarick, S.D., Rylander, H., Burkitt, J.M., et al., 2007. Treatment of traumatic cervical myelopathy with surgery, prolonged positive-pressure ventilation, and physical therapy in a dog. Journal of the Veterinary Medical Association 230, 370–374.

Taylor, S.M., 2009. Disorders of the spinal cord. In: Nelson, R.W., Couto, C.G. (Eds.), Small Animal Internal Medicine, fourth ed. Elsevier, Philadelphia, pp. 1065–1091.

LOWER MOTOR NEURON DISEASES

Abelson, A.L., Shelton, G.D., Whelan, M.F., et al., 2009. Use of mycophenolate mofetil as a rescue agent in the treatment of severe generalized myasthenia gravis in three dogs. Journal of Veterinary Emergency and Critical Care 19 (4), 369–374.

de Lahunta, A., Glass, E., 2009. Lower motor neuron: spinal nerve, general somatic efferent system. In: Delahunta, A. (Ed.), Veterinary Neuroanatomy and Clinical Neurology, third ed. Saunders Elsevier, St Louis, pp. 90–97.

Khorzad, R., Whelan, M., Sisson, A., et al., 2011. Myasthenia gravis in dogs with an emphasis on treatment and critical care management. Journal of Veterinary Emergency and Critical Care 21 (3), 193–208.

Olby, N.J., 2004. Tetraparesis. In: Platt, S.R., Olby, N.J. (Eds.), BSAVA Manual of Canine and Feline Neurology, third ed. BSAVA, Gloucester, pp. 230–234.

Shelton, G.D., 2009. Treatment of autoimmune myasthenia gravis. In: Bonagura, J.D., Twedt, D.C. (Eds.), Kirk's Current Veterinary Therapy XIV. Saunders Elsevier, St Louis, pp. 1108–1111.

Shelton, G.D., 2009. Treatment of myopathies and neuropathies. In: Bonagura, J.D., Twedt, D.C. (Eds.), Kirk's Current Veterinary Therapy XIV. Saunders Elsevier, St Louis, pp. 1111–1116.

Taylor, S.M., 2009. Disorders of the neuromuscular junction. In: Nelson, R.W., Couto, C.G. (Eds.), Small Animal Internal Medicine, fourth ed. Elsevier, Philadelphia, pp. 1101–1107.

Vite, C.H., Johnson, K., 2009. Lower motor neuron disease. In: Silverstein, D.C., Hopper, K. (Eds.), Small Animal Critical Care Medicine. Elsevier, St Louis, pp. 429–434.

VESTIBULAR DISORDERS

Bagley, R.S., 2009. Vestibular disease of dogs and cats. In: Bonagura, J.D., Twedt, D.C. (Eds.), Kirk's Current Veterinary Therapy XIV. Saunders Elsevier, St Louis, pp. 1097–1101.

Muñana, K.R., 2004. Head tilt and nystagmus. In: Platt, S.R., Olby, N.J. (Eds.), BSAVA Manual of Canine and Feline Neurology, third ed. BSAVA, Gloucester, pp. 155–171.

Platt, S.R., 2009. Vestibular disease. In: Silverstein, D.C., Hopper, K. (Eds.), Small Animal Critical Care Medicine. Elsevier, St Louis, pp. 442–447.

Rossmeisl, J.H., 2010. Vestibular disease in dogs and cats. In: Thomas WB (guest ed), Diseases of the Brain. The Veterinary Clinics of North America, Small Animal Practice 40 (1), 81–100.

Taylor, S.M., 2009. Head tilt. In: Nelson, R.W., Couto, C.G. (Eds.), Small Animal Internal Medicine, fourth ed. Elsevier, Philadelphia, pp. 1047–1053.

SHAKING AND TREMORS

Bagley, R.S. (guest ed), 1996. Intracranial Disease. The Veterinary Clinics of North America, Small Animal Practice 26 (4), 674–675.

Bagley, R.S., 2004. Tremor and involuntary movements. In: Platt, S.R., Olby, N.J. (Eds.), BSAVA Manual of Canine and Feline Neurology, third ed. BSAVA, Gloucester, pp. 189–201.

Wagner, S.O., Podell, M., Fenner, W.R., 1997. Generalized tremors in dogs: 24 cases (1984–1995). Journal of the American Veterinary Medical Association 211 (6), 731–734.

CANINE SEIZURES

Bagley, R.S. (guest ed), 1996. Intracranial Disease. The Veterinary Clinics of North America, Small Animal Practice 26 (4), 779–805.

Berendt, M., Gredal, H., Ersbøll, A.K., et al., 2007. Premature death, risk factors, and life patterns in dogs with epilepsy. Journal of Veterinary Internal Medicine 21, 754–759.

Chandler, K., 2006. Canine epilepsy: What can we learn from human seizure disorders? The Veterinary Journal 172, 207–217.

Dewey, C.W., 2009. New maintenance anticonvulsant therapies for dogs and cats. In: Bonagura, J.D., Twedt, D.C. (Eds.), Kirk's Current Veterinary Therapy XIV. Saunders Elsevier, St Louis, pp. 1066–1069.

Dewey, C.W., Cerda-Gonzalez, S., Levine, J.M., et al., 2009. Pregabalin as an adjunct to phenobarbital, potassium bromide, or a combination of phenobarbital and potassium bromide for treatment of dogs with suspected idiopathic epilepsy. Journal of the American Veterinary Medical Association 235, 1442–1449.

Moore, S.A., Muñana, K.R., Papich, M.G., et al., 2010. Levetiracetam pharmacokinetics in healthy dogs following oral administration of single and multiple doses. American Journal of Veterinary Research 71, 337–341.

Platt, S.R., Olby, N.J., 2004. Neurologic emergencies. In: Platt, S.R., Olby, N.J. (Eds.), BSAVA Manual of Canine and Feline Neurology, third ed. BSAVA, Gloucester, pp. 332–335.

Platt, S.R., Randell, S.C., Scott, K.C., et al., 2000. Comparison of plasma benzodiazepine concentrations following intranasal and intravenous administration of diazepam to dogs.

American Journal of Veterinary Research 61, 651–654.

Podell, M., 2004. Seizures. In: Platt, S.R., Olby, N.J. (Eds.), BSAVA Manual of Canine and Feline Neurology, third ed. BSAVA, Gloucester, pp. 97–112.

Podell, M., 2009. Treatment of status epilepticus. In: Bonagura, J.D., Twedt, D.C. (Eds.), Kirk's Current Veterinary Therapy XIV. Saunders Elsevier, St Louis, pp. 1062–1065.

Taylor, S.M., 2009. Seizures. In: Nelson, R.W., Couto, C.G. (Eds.), Small Animal Internal Medicine, fourth ed. Elsevier, Philadelphia, pp. 1036–1046.

Thomas, W.B., 2010. Idiopathic epilepsy in dogs and cats. In: Thomas WB (guest ed), Diseases of the Brain. The Veterinary Clinics of North America, Small Animal Practice 40 (1), 161–179.

Vernau, K.M., LeCouteur, R.A., 2009. Seizures and status epilepticus. In: Silverstein, D.C., Hopper, K. (Eds.), Small Animal Critical Care Medicine. Elsevier, St Louis, pp. 414–419.

Zimmermann, R., Hülsmeyer, V.I., Sauter-Louis, C., et al., 2009. Status epilepticus and epileptic seizures in dogs. Journal of Veterinary Internal Medicine 23, 970–976.

FELINE SEIZURES

Dewey, C.W., 2009. New maintenance anticonvulsant therapies for dogs and cats. In: Bonagura, J.D., Twedt, D.C. (Eds.), Kirk's Current Veterinary Therapy XIV. Saunders Elsevier, St Louis, pp. 1066–1069.

Podell, M., 2004. Seizures. In: Platt, S.R., Olby, N.J. (Eds.), BSAVA Manual of Canine and Feline Neurology, third ed. BSAVA, Gloucester, pp. 97–112.

Podell, M., 2009. Treatment of status epilepticus. In: Bonagura, J.D., Twedt, D.C. (Eds.), Kirk's Current Veterinary Therapy XIV. Saunders Elsevier, St Louis, pp. 1062–1065.

Schriefl, S., Steinberg, T.A., Matiasek, K., et al., 2008. Etiologic classification of seizures, signalment, clinical signs, and outcome in cats with seizure disorders: 91 cases (2000–2004). Journal of the American Veterinary Medical Association 233, 1591–1597.

Taylor, S.M., 2009. Seizures. In: Nelson, R.W., Couto, C.G. (Eds.), Small Animal Internal Medicine, fourth ed. Elsevier, Philadelphia, pp. 1036–1046.

Thomas, W.B., 2010. Idiopathic epilepsy in dogs and cats. In: Thomas WB (guest ed), Diseases of the Brain. The Veterinary Clinics of North America, Small Animal Practice 40 (1), 161–179.

Vernau, K.M., LeCouteur, R.A., 2009. Seizures and status epilepticus. In: Silverstein, D.C., Hopper, K. (Eds.), Small Animal Critical Care Medicine. Elsevier, St Louis, pp. 414–419.

ALTERED MENTATION OR COMA

Adamo, P.F., Rylander, H., Adams, W.M., 2007. Ciclosporin use in multi-drug therapy for meningoencephalomyelitis of unknown aetiology in dogs. Journal of Small Animal Practice 48, 486–496.

Bagley, R.S., 2004. Coma, stupor, and behavioral change. In: Platt, S.R., Olby, N.J. (Eds.), BSAVA Manual of Canine and Feline Neurology, third ed. BSAVA, Gloucester, pp. 113–132.

Coates, J.R., Barone, G., Dewey, C.W., et al., 2007. Procarbazine as adjunctive therapy for treatment of dogs with presumptive antemortem diagnosis of granulomatous meningoencephalomyelitis: 21 cases (1998–2004). Journal of Veterinary Internal Medicine 21, 100–106.

Daly, P., Drudy, D., Chalmers, W.S.K., et al., 2006. Greyhound meningoencephalitis: PCR-based detection methods highlight an absence of the most likely primary inducing agents. Veterinary Microbiology 118, 189–200.

Flegel, T., Boettcher, I.C., Matiasek, K., et al., 2011. Comparison of oral administration of lomustine and prednisolone or prednisolone alone as treatment for granulomatous meningoencephalomyelitis or necrotizing encephalitis in dogs. Journal of the American Veterinary Medical Association 238, 337–345.

Nghiem, P.P., Schatzberg, S.J., 2010. Conventional and molecular diagnostic testing for the acute neurologic patient. Journal of Veterinary Emergency and Critical Care 20 (1), 46–61.

Platt, S.R., 2009. Coma scales. In: Silverstein, D.C., Hopper, K. (Eds.), Small Animal Critical Care Medicine. Elsevier, St Louis, pp. 410–413.

Smith, P.M., Stalin, C.E., Shaw, D., et al., 2009. Comparison of two regimens for the treatment of meningoencephalomyelitis of unknown etiology. Journal of Veterinary Internal Medicine 23, 520–526.

Tarlow, J.M., Rudloff, E., Lichtenberger, M., et al., 2005. Emergency presentations of 4 dogs with suspected neurologic toxoplasmosis. Journal of Veterinary Emergency and Critical Care 15 (2), 119–127.

Walmsley, G.L., Herrtage, M.E., Dennis, R., et al., 2006. The relationship between clinical signs and brain herniation associated with rostrotentorial mass lesions in the dog. The Veterinary Journal 172, 258–264.

Windsor, R.C., Olby, N.J., 2007. Congenital portosystemic shunts in five mature dogs with neurological signs. Journal of the American Animal Hospital Association 43, 322–331.

Wong, M.A., Hopkins, A.L., Meeks, J.C., et al., 2010. Evaluation of treatment with a combination of azathioprine and prednisone in dogs with meningoencephalomyelitis of undetermined etiology: 40 cases (2000–2007). Journal of the American Veterinary Medical Association 237, 929–935.

Zarfoss, M., Schatzberg, S., Venator, K., et al., 2006. Combined cytosine arabinoside and prednisone therapy for meningoencephalitis of unknown aetiology in 10 dogs. Journal of Small Animal Practice 47, 588–595.

TETANUS

Adamantos, S., Boag, A., 2007. Thirteen cases of tetanus in dogs. Veterinary Record 161, 298–303.

Burkitt, J.M., Sturges, B.K., Jandrey, K.E., et al., 2007. Risk factors associated with outcome in dogs with tetanus: 38 cases (1987–2005). Journal of the American Veterinary Medical Association 230, 76–83.

Greene, C., 2006. Tetanus. In: Greene, C.E. (Ed.), Infectious Diseases of the Dog and Cat, third ed. Elsevier, Philadelphia, pp. 395–402.

Linnenbrink, T., McMichael, M., 2006. Tetanus: pathophysiology, clinical signs, diagnosis, and update on new treatment modalities. Journal of Veterinary Emergency and Critical Care 16 (3), 199–207.

Olby, N.J., 2004. Tetraparesis. In: Platt, S.R., Olby, N.J. (Eds.), BSAVA Manual of Canine and Feline Neurology, third ed. BSAVA, Gloucester, pp. 226–227.

Platt, S.R., 2009. Tetanus. In: Silverstein, D.C., Hopper, K. (Eds.), Small Animal Critical Care Medicine. Elsevier, St Louis, pp. 435–438.

Taylor, S.M., 2009. Involuntary alterations in muscle tone. In: Nelson, R.W., Couto, C.G. (Eds.), Small Animal Internal Medicine, fourth ed. Elsevier, Philadelphia, pp. 1115–1116.

ACUTE ULCERATIVE KERATITIS

Gelatt, K.N., 2000. Ulcerative keratitis. In: Gelatt, K.N. (Ed.), Essentials of Veterinary Ophthalmology. Lippincott Williams & Wilkins, Philadelphia, pp. 129–138.

Severin, G.A., 1995. Severin's Veterinary Ophthalmology Notes, third ed. Veterinary Ophthalmology Notes, Fort Collins, pp. 318–321.

Williams, D.L., Barrie, K., Evans, T.F., 2003. Corneal ulcers. In: Williams, D.L. (Ed.), Veterinary Ocular Emergencies. Butterworth Heinemann, Boston, pp. 37–54.

CORNEAL FOREIGN BODIES

Gelatt, K.N., 2000. Foreign bodies. In: Gelatt, K.N. (Ed.), Essentials of Veterinary Ophthalmology. Lippincott Williams & Wilkins, Philadelphia, p. 144.

Severin, G.A., 1995. Severin's Veterinary Ophthalmology Notes, third ed. Veterinary Ophthalmology Notes, Fort Collins, p. 348.

Williams, D.L., Barrie, K., Evans, T.F., 2003. Corneal foreign bodies. In: Williams, D.L. (Ed.), Veterinary Ocular Emergencies. Butterworth Heinemann, Boston, pp. 60–63.

ANTERIOR UVEITIS

Colitz, C.M.H., 2005. Feline uveitis: diagnosis and treatment. Clinical Techniques in Small Animal Practice 20, 117–120.

Gelatt, K.N., 2000. Anterior and posterior uveitis. In: Gelatt, K.N. (Ed.), Essentials of Veterinary Ophthalmology, Lippincott Williams & Wilkins, Philadelphia, pp. 316–323.

Gelatt, K.N., 2000. Uveal inflammations. In: Gelatt, K.N. (Ed.), Essentials of Veterinary Ophthalmology. Lippincott Williams & Wilkins, Philadelphia, pp. 201–215.

Powell, C.C., 2009. Anterior uveitis in dogs and cats. In: Bonagura, J.D., Twedt, D.C. (Eds.), Kirk's Current Veterinary Therapy XIV. Saunders Elsevier, St Louis, pp. 1200–1207.

Tolar, E.L., Hendrix, D.V.H., Rohrbach, B.W., et al., 2006. Evaluation of clinical characteristics and bacterial isolates in dogs with bacterial keratitis: 97 cases (1993–2003). Journal of the American Veterinary Medical Association 228, 80–85.

Williams, D.L., Barrie, K., Evans, T.F., 2003. Iris. In: Williams, D.L. (Ed.), Veterinary Ocular Emergencies. Butterworth Heinemann, Boston, pp. 64–69.

HYPHEMA

Gelatt, K.N., 2000. Hyphema. In: Gelatt, K.N. (Ed.), Essentials of Veterinary Ophthalmology, Lippincott Williams & Wilkins, Philadelphia, pp. 221–222.

Hendrix, E.V.H., 2009. Differential diagnosis of the red eye. In: Bonagura, J.D., Twedt, D.C. (Eds.), Kirk's Current Veterinary Therapy XIV. Saunders Elsevier, St Louis, pp. 1175–1178.

Severin, G.A., 1995. Severin's Veterinary Ophthalmology Notes, third ed. Veterinary Ophthalmology Notes, Fort Collins CO, pp. 353–355.

Sigler, R.L., Lorimer, D.W., 1989. Traumatic eye disease. Veterinary Focus: Focus on Ophthalmology 1 (3), 80–83.

Slatter, D.H., 1990. Fundamentals of Veterinary Ophthalmology, second ed. Veterinary Ophthalmology Notes, Fort Collins CO, p. 543.

PROPTOSED GLOBE

Cho, J., 2008. Surgery of the globe and orbit. Topics in Companion Animal Medicine 23 (1), 23–37.

Kirk, R.W., Bonagura, J.D. (Eds.), 1992. Current Veterinary Therapy XI. WB Saunders, Philadelphia, pp. 1084–1085.

Murtaugh, R.J., Kaplan, P.M., 1992. Veterinary Emergency and Critical Care Medicine. Mosby, St Louis, pp. 274–276.

Severin, G.A., 1995. Severin's Veterinary Ophthalmology Notes, third ed. Veterinary Ophthalmology Notes, Fort Collins CO, pp. 491–494.

Slatter, D.H., 1990. Fundamentals of Veterinary Ophthalmology, second ed. WB Saunders, Philadelphia, pp. 537–539.

ACUTE GLAUCOMA

Gelatt, K.N., 2000. The canine glaucomas. In: Gelatt, K.N. (Ed.), Essentials of Veterinary Ophthalmology. Lippincott Williams & Wilkins, Philadelphia, pp. 165–196.

Kural, E., Lindley, D., Krohne, S., 1995. Canine glaucoma—part II. Compendium of Continuing Education 17 (10), 1253–1262.

Miller, P.E., 2009. Feline glaucoma. In: Bonagura, J.D., Twedt, D.C. (Eds.), Kirk's Current Veterinary Therapy XIV. Saunders Elsevier, St Louis, pp. 1207–1214.

Moore, C.P. (guest ed), 2004. Ocular Therapeutics. The Veterinary Clinics of North America, Small Animal Practice 34 (3), XI–XII.

Sapienza, J.S., 2008. Surgical procedures for glaucoma: what the general practitioner needs to know. Topics in Companion Animal Medicine 23 (1), 38–45.

Severin, G.A., 1995. Severin's Veterinary Ophthalmology Notes, third ed. Veterinary Ophthalmology Notes, Fort Collins CO, pp. 453–464.

Van der Woerdt, A., 2001. The treatment of acute glaucoma in dogs and cats. Journal of Veterinary Emergency and Critical Care 11 (3), 199–205.

Ward, D.A., 2009. Ocular pharmacology. In: Bonagura, J.D., Twedt, D.C. (Eds.), Kirk's Current Veterinary Therapy XIV. Saunders Elsevier, St Louis, pp. 1145–1149.

Williams, D.L., Barrie, K., Evans, T.F., 2003. Glaucoma. In: Williams, D.L. (Ed.), Veterinary Ocular Emergencies. Butterworth Heinemann, Boston, pp. 70–74.

SUDDEN BLINDNESS

Ford, R.B., Mazzaferro, E.M. (Eds.), 1996. Kirk and Bistner's Handbook of Veterinary Procedures and Emergency Treatment, eighth ed. Saunders Elsevier, St Louis, pp. 440–442.

Hamilton, H.L., McLaughlin, S.A., 2009. Differential diagnosis of blindness. In: Bonagura, J.D., Twedt, D.C., (Eds.), Kirk's Current Veterinary Therapy XIV. Saunders Elsevier, St Louis, pp. 1163–1167.

Penderis, J., 2004. Disorders of eyes and vision. In: Platt, S.R., Olby, N.J. (Eds.), BSAVA Manual of Canine and Feline Neurology, third ed. BSAVA, Gloucester, pp. 140–143.

Williams, D.L., Barrie, K., Evans, T.F., 2002. Commonly presented conditions. In: Williams, D.L. (Ed.), Veterinary Ocular Emergencies. Butterworth Heinemann, Boston, pp. 18–20.

Williams, D.L., Barrie, K., Evans, T.F., 2003. Retina and vitreous. In: Williams, D.L. (Ed.), Veterinary Ocular Emergencies. Butterworth Heinemann, Boston, pp. 79–83.

Williams, D.L., Barrie, K., Evans, T.F., 2003. Optic nerve. In: Williams, D.L. (Ed.), Veterinary Ocular Emergencies. Butterworth Heinemann, Boston, pp. 84–85.

Neurologic and ocular emergencies

14

Toxicologic emergencies

ACETAMINOPHEN TOXICOSIS

Mode of action

Toxicity is due to an active metabolite that reduces hepatic and red blood cell glutathione concentrations leading to hepatic and erythrocyte damage. Dogs suffer more from hepatic necrosis. Cats develop more erythrocyte damage in the form of methemoglobinemia.

Conjugation to inactive glucuronide and sulfate metabolites is the primary route of elimination of acetaminophen. Glucuronyl transferase is required to conjugate acetaminophen to glucuronic acid. Glucuronyl transferase levels are lower in cats than in people and dogs. With acetaminophen toxicity, glutathione stores become depleted. The sulfate-conjugating mechanism is also less functional in cats. Because the other routes of metabolism are decreased, a much larger amount of acetaminophen must be acted upon by cytochrome p-450 system, which results in increased concentrations of N-acetyl p-benzoquinone imine (NAPQI). NAPQI causes inhibition of membrane ion-transporting systems, modification of cytoskeleton proteins and inhibition of the calmodulin-activated calcium (Ca) pump ATPase activity and the Na–K pump ATPase activity, resulting in cellular death.

Methemoglobin is a nonfunctional form of hemoglobin that results from the oxidation of the iron in hemoglobin from the ferrous to the ferric state. Heinz bodies form from the precipitation of damaged hemoglobin within the RBC. Both Heinz bodies and the damaged hemoglobin increase the osmotic fragility of RBCs and result in hemolytic anemia. The feline hemoglobin molecule has at least eight reactive sulfhydryl groups, compared with four in dogs and two in humans. The blood from affected animals appears darker and browner than normal.

Sources

Paracetamol, APAP and N-acetyl-p-aminophenol are other names for acetaminophen. Children's Tylenol® contains 80 mg of acetaminophen; Regular Strength Tylenol® contains 325 mg of acetaminophen; Extra Strength Tylenol®

contains 500 mg of acetaminophen. Numerous other human over-the-counter and prescription medications contain acetaminophen. Be sure to check the concentration in the specific product ingested.

Toxic dosages

Dogs = 200–600 mg/kg; however, an occasional dog will have problems with as low as 150 mg/kg. In dogs, methemoglobinemia is possible at high-dose exposures.
Cats = 50 mg/kg, although fatalities in cats have been reported with ingestion of 10 mg/kg.

Diagnosis

History—The owner may have administered a human over-the-counter medication or prescription medication containing acetaminophen, or the patient (usually canine) may have chewed a pill vial or swallowed tablets that had been dropped on the floor. Occasionally an owner is reluctant to admit they administered medication to their pet. If the patient exhibits the signs of acetaminophen toxicosis, treat accordingly.
Clinical signs—

Dogs
1. Depression that is progressive
2. Vomiting within hours of ingestion
3. Swelling of the feet and face
4. Abdominal pain
5. Dark, chocolate-colored urine and serum from methemoglobinemia
6. Transient keratoconjunctivitis sicca may occur
7. Death due to hepatic necrosis may occur within 2–5 days.

Cats
1. Effects develop within 1–2 hours of ingestion
2. Anorexia, salivation, vomiting
3. Hypothermia
4. Depression, weakness and coma may occur
5. Rapidly develop methemoglobinemia, life-threatening hemoglobinuria, resulting in brown or cyanotic mucous membranes, respiratory distress, and dark, chocolate-colored blood and urine
6. Swelling of the face and paws (Fig. 14.1)
7. Death due to hepatic necrosis occurs within 18–36 hours
   Laboratory findings—Methemoglobinemia, Heinz body anemia, elevated ALT, elevated SAP, elevated total and direct bilirubin. Blood gas evaluation may show a metabolic acidosis.

Prognosis

The prognosis is fair to guarded.

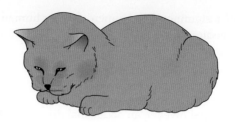

FIG 14.1 **Facial swelling of a cat with acetaminophen toxicity.** The paws will also often become swollen.

Treatment

1. Place the distressed cat in an oxygen cage immediately, provide supplemental oxygen and let it relax.
2. Inform the client of the diagnosis, prognosis and cost of the treatment.
3. If the patient is asymptomatic and presents less than 4 hours since exposure, attempt gastric decontamination with emesis or gastric lavage, followed by the administration of activated charcoal and a saline or osmotic cathartic.
   A. Induction of emesis in cats
      I. Administer xylazine, 0.44–1 mg/kg IM or SC (can reverse with yohimbine 0.1 mg/kg IM, SC, or IV slowly).
      II. Administer medetomidine, 10 µg/kg IM (can reverse with atipamezole (Antisedan®) 25 µg/kg IM).
      III. Hydrogen peroxide is very difficult to administer to cats and is no longer recommended.
   B. Induction of emesis in dogs
      I. Apomorphine 0.02–0.04 mg/kg IV or IM, or 1.5–6 mg dissolved and placed into the conjunctival fornix. If apomorphine was placed in the eye, after emesis, the patient's eye should be thoroughly lavaged with sterile saline. If excessive sedation occurs from apomorphine, the sedation may be reversed by the administration of naloxone (0.01–0.04 mg/kg IV, IM, SC) but this will not reverse the emetic effects.
      II. 3% hydrogen peroxide 1–5 mL/kg (0.5–2 mL/lb) PO; the maximum dose is 3 tablespoons (45 mL). If the patient does not vomit within 10 minutes, give 3% hydrogen peroxide 0.5 mL/kg (0.25 mL/lb) PO **once**.
   C. Gastric lavage
      I. Lightly anesthetize the patient.
      II. Administer oxygen and intravenous fluids to the patient while under anesthesia.
      III. Maintain anesthesia with the appropriate anesthetic as needed.
      IV. Intubate the patient with a cuffed endotracheal tube and inflate the cuff.
      V. Place the patient in lateral recumbency.

     VI. With the stomach tube held outside of the patient, alongside the patient, measure the distance from the tip of the nose to the last rib. Mark this distance on the stomach tube.

    VII. Lubricate the caudal end of the stomach tube with water-soluble jelly then pass the stomach tube gently into the stomach, passing the tube no farther than the marked distance on the tube.

   VIII. If desired, two stomach tubes may be utilized: a smaller ingress tube and a large egress tube.

    IX. Infuse warm (body-temperature) tap water, 5–10 mL/kg, through the tube (ingress tube if using two tubes) to moderately distend the stomach. For a small patient, use 0.9% NaCl for gastric lavage to avoid causing electrolyte shifts.

     X. Allow the fluid to drain from the stomach through the tube (egress tube if using two tubes).

    XI. Save samples of gastric contents, suspicious foreign material, seeds, etc. for possible toxicologic analysis.

   XII. The stomach tube may have to be manipulated, repositioned or flushed with fluid or air if the gastric contents do not flow freely through the tube.

  XIII. Turn the patient to the other side and continue to perform gastric lavage.

  XIV. Continue gastric lavage until the effluent is clear.

   XV. If using the two-tube method, crimp the end of one tube and remove it.

  XVI. Administer activated charcoal down the stomach tube.

 XVII. Crimp the end of the stomach tube and remove it.

XVIII. Monitor the patient during recovery from anesthesia, leaving the inflated cuffed endotracheal tube in place until the patient's swallowing reflex has returned.

D. Activated charcoal with sorbitol, 1–3 g/kg PO; repeat the administration of activated charcoal every 3–4 hours, due to enterohepatic recirculation. Administer sorbitol only once.

E. A single dose of an osmotic or saline cathartic should be administered along with activated charcoal. Alternative cathartics include:

     I. Sorbitol (70%), 2 g/kg (1–2 mL/kg) PO

    II. Magnesium sulfate (Epsom salt), 200 mg/kg for cats, 250–500 mg/kg for dogs. Mix magnesium sulfate with water, 5–10 mL/kg and administer PO

   III. Magnesium hydroxide (Milk of Magnesia®), 15–50 mL for cats, 10–150 mL for dogs, q6–12h PO as needed

   IV. Sodium sulfate, 200 mg/kg for cats, 250–500 mg/kg for dogs. Mix sodium sulfate with water, 5–10 mL/kg and administer PO.

4. Administer the antidote N-acetylcysteine (NAC) (Mucomyst®) IV or PO

  A. 280 mg/kg PO or IV loading dose, then 140 mg/kg PO or IV q4–6h for 3–7 treatments.

  B. For IV administration, dilute to a 5% concentration in 5% dextrose in water or sterile water, then administer slowly over 15–30 minutes.

Administer PO unless a bacteriostatic filter or a sterile solution of NAC is available.

C. The oral route may be preferred due to absorption of *N*-acetylcysteine from the gastrointestinal tract into the portal circulation where it is then presented in higher concentrations to the liver for detoxification. Activated charcoal inactivates the acetylcysteine if it is given PO. The administration of activated charcoal should be separated from the administration of oral *N*-acetylcysteine by 30–60 minutes.

5. Administer *S*-adenosyl-methionine (SAMe).
   A. Dogs: 40 mg/kg PO once followed by 20 mg/kg PO q24h for 9 days
   B. Cats: 180 mg PO q12h for 3 days then 90 mg PO q12h for 14 days

6. Administer vitamin C (ascorbic acid) 30 mg/kg PO or SC q6h or 20–30 mg/kg in the intravenous fluids q6h.

7. The administration of cimetidine is no longer recommended as it is thought to prolong the activity of the toxic metabolites.

8. Supportive therapy:

   A. Administer a balanced electrolyte crystalloid fluid IV.
   B. Oxygen administration is often beneficial.
   C. Administer RBCs or whole blood, if necessary. Be careful to avoid volume overload.
   D. The patient may require hospitalization for up to 72 hours.
   E. Cats stress and die easily due to severe methemoglobinemia; **handle carefully!**

ALBUTEROL

Mode of action

Severe hypokalemia develops secondary to the activation of cell membrane adenyl cyclase and cellular Na/K-ATPase. With higher plasma levels, both β_1 and β_2 receptors are activated, which result in tachycardia, peripheral vasodilation and hypotension.

Sources

Albuterol is a β_2-adrenergic receptor agonist, used in the treatment of bronchospasm in patients with respiratory diseases. It is available as oral, injectable or inhalant medication.

Toxic dosages

The toxic dose is unknown in dogs and cats, but in human pediatric patients it is 1 mg/kg. Adverse effects have been reported at therapeutic doses.

Diagnosis

History—Ingestion or inhalation of albuterol within 3–30 minutes of onset of clinical signs; delayed onset may occur if extended-release tablets were ingested. A family member may take albuterol.

Clinical signs—Dogs: panting, excessive thirst, vomiting, weakness, hyperactivity, agitation, muscle tremors, hindlimb paresis to generalized paresis to paraplegia, possibly paralysis of respiratory muscles, mydriasis, hyperthermia, polyuria, polydipsia, hypertension.
Laboratory findings—Abnormalities include hypokalemia, elevated creatine kinase activity, isosthenuria and high serum albuterol concentrations.
Electrocardiography—Ventricular and supraventricular arrhythmias, including atrioventricular block, sinus tachycardia, ventricular tachycardia, and ventricular premature contraction, may occur.

Prognosis

With appropriate medical care, the prognosis is good. If the patient has pre-existing cardiac disease, the prognosis is more guarded.

Treatment

1. Inform the client of the diagnosis, prognosis and cost of the treatment.
2. If the patient presents with no CNS or cardiac abnormalities and a history of recent ingestion, attempt gastric decontamination with emesis, unless the exposure was to a powder or liquid formulation or to a pressurized canister.
3. If the patient presents within 2 hours of exposure, gastric lavage may be beneficial.
4. Administer a single dose **of activated charcoal with sorbitol,** 1–3 g/kg PO.
5. Administer a balanced electrolyte crystalloid intravenous fluid IV, supplemented with potassium chloride as needed.
6. Monitor the serum potassium level every 4–6 hours.
7. Monitor blood pressure and ECG.
   A. For sinus tachyarrhythmias, administer propanolol (0.02 mg/kg IV slowly every 8 hours), esmolol (Brevibloc®) (0.1–0.5 mg/kg IV slowly then a CRI of 0.05–0.1 mg/kg/min IV), or diltiazem (Cardizem®) (0.1–0.2 mg/kg IV slowly then a CRI of 0.005–0.02 mg/kg/min IV).
   B. For ventricular arrhythmias, administer lidocaine (2 mg/kg slowly IV then 30–50 µg/kg/min IV CRI).
8. If the patient exhibits excessive agitation, administer diazepam, 0.2–0.5 mg/kg IV to effect.

AMITRAZ TOXICOSIS

Mode of action

Amitraz affects the peripheral α_1- and α_2-adrenergic receptor sites in the cardiovascular system and the α_2-adrenergic receptor sites in the CNS; thus it is an α_2-adrenergic receptor agonist. Toxic exposure can occur either through the oral or dermal route.

Sources

Amitraz is a pesticide found in Preventic® flea and tick collars, in pesticide products for cattle and pigs, and in external lotions and dip used to treat demodectic mange, which include Mitaban®. Mitaban® also contains xylene, which is also toxic.

Toxic dosages

The acute oral LD_{50} of Amitraz is 100 mg/kg for dogs, 400–800 mg/kg for guinea pigs, 515–938 mg/kg for rats, and greater than 1600 mg/kg for mice. **Amitraz should never be used on cats**.

Some dogs may exhibit transient clinical signs at dosages of 20 mg/kg. Chronic toxicity is not described.

Diagnosis

History—The animal may be receiving treatment for demodectic mange, or may have ingested a flea and tick collar. The owner may observe vomiting, polyuria, ataxia and depression that may progress to coma. The patient may seizure.

Clinical signs—The patient may have pale mucous membranes due to hypotension and peripheral vasoconstriction. Hypothermia may occur. The patient may present with depression, mydriasis, bradycardia, anorexia, vomiting, diarrhea, polyuria, ataxia, sedation, disorientation, vocalization, seizures or coma.

Laboratory findings—Hyperglycemia may be present. The CBC and complete serum biochemical profile are usually normal.

Differential diagnosis

Organophosphate toxicosis, carbamate toxicosis, pyrethrin or pyrethroid toxicosis, D-limonene toxicosis, rotenone toxicosis and methoprene toxicosis.

Prognosis

The prognosis is fair. Spontaneous recovery may occur in mildly affected animals.

Treatment

1. Inform the owner of the diagnosis, prognosis and the cost of treatment.
2. Ensure a patent airway. Intubate the patient if necessary.
3. Administer supplemental oxygen and ventilation if necessary.
4. Place an intravenous catheter. Administer a balanced electrolyte crystalloid fluid intravenously to maintain perfusion, hydration and diuresis.
5. In cases of dermal exposure, thoroughly wash the patient with warm, soapy water. Protective garments, including rubber gloves, should be worn while bathing the patient. Keep the patient warm.

6. If the patient is presented in an alert or mildly depressed state, induce emesis. Do not induce emesis if the toxic substance was Mitaban®, to avoid aspiration pneumonia that may occur following inhalation of xylene.
   A. Induction of emesis in dogs
      I. Administer apomorphine, 0.02–0.04 mg/kg IV or IM, or 1.5–6 mg dissolved and placed into the conjunctival fornix. If apomorphine was placed in the eye, after emesis, the patient's eye should be thoroughly lavaged with sterile saline. If excessive sedation occurs from apomorphine, the sedation may be reversed by the administration of naloxone (0.01–0.04 mg/kg IV, IM, SC), but this will not reverse the emetic effects.
      II. Administer 3% hydrogen peroxide, 0.5–2 mL/lb (1–5 mL/kg) PO, with a maximum dose of 3 tablespoons (45 mL). If the patient does not vomit within 10 minutes, give 3% hydrogen peroxide 0.5 mL/kg (0.25 mL/lb) PO **once**.
   B. Induction of emesis in cats
      I. Administer xylazine, 0.44–1 mg/kg IM or SC (can reverse with yohimbine 0.1 mg/kg IM, SC, or IV slowly).
      II. Administer medetomidine , 10 µg/kg IM (can reverse with atipamezole (Antisedan®) 25 µg/kg IM).
      III. Hydrogen peroxide is very difficult to administer to cats and is no longer recommended.
7. If the patient is sedate or comatose, attempt gastric decontamination with gastric lavage.
   A. Lightly anesthetize the patient.
   B. Administer oxygen and intravenous fluids to the patient while under anesthesia.
   C. Maintain anesthesia with the appropriate anesthetic as needed.
   D. Intubate the patient with a cuffed endotracheal tube and inflate the cuff.
   E. Place the patient in lateral recumbency.
   F. With a stomach tube held outside of the patient, alongside the patient, measure the distance from the tip of the nose to the last rib. Mark this distance on the stomach tube.
   G. Lubricate the caudal end of the stomach tube with water-soluble jelly, then pass the stomach tube gently into the stomach, passing the tube no farther than the marked distance on the tube.
   H. If desired, two stomach tubes may be utilized: a smaller ingress tube and a large egress tube.
   I. Infuse warm (body-temperature) tap water, 5–10 mL/kg, through the tube (ingress tube if using two tubes) to moderately distend the stomach.
   J. Allow the fluid to drain from the stomach through the tube (egress tube if using two tubes).
   K. Save samples of gastric contents, suspicious foreign material, seeds, etc. for possible toxicologic analysis.
   L. The stomach tube may have to be manipulated, repositioned, or flushed with fluid or air if the gastric contents do not flow freely through the tube.

M. Turn the patient over and continue to perform gastric lavage.

N. Continue gastric lavage until the effluent is clear.

O. If using the two-tube method, crimp the end of one tube and remove it.

P. Administer activated charcoal down the stomach tube.

Q. Crimp the end of the stomach tube and remove it.

R. Monitor the patient during recovery from anesthesia, leaving the inflated cuffed endotracheal tube in place until the patient's swallowing reflex has returned.

8. Administer activated charcoal, 2–5 g/kg (30–60 mL/10 lb) PO is usually administered in a slurry of 1 g to 5 mL water. Repeat the administration of activated charcoal q3–4h. Administer a cathartic only once.

9. A single dose of an osmotic or saline cathartic should be administered along with activated charcoal. Alternative cathartics include:

A. Sorbitol 70%, 2 g/kg (1–2 mL/kg) PO

B. Sodium sulfate, 200 mg/kg for cats, 250–500 mg/kg for dogs. Mix sodium sulfate with water, 5–10 mL/kg and administer PO.

10. Place an intravenous catheter.

11. Administer balanced electrolyte crystalloid fluids IV as necessary, depending on clinical signs, blood pressure and perfusion.

12. Administer an antidote.

A. Yohimbine—competitively displaces amitraz from the α_2-adrenergic receptors and reverses sedation, hypotension, bradycardia and gastrointestinal hypomotility.

   I. Dogs: 0.11 mg/kg slow IV

   II. Cats: 0.5 mg/kg slow IV

B. Atipamezole (Antisedan®)—an α_2-adrenergic receptor antagonist, at the dose of 50 mg/kg IM in the dog, repeated q3–4h as needed.

C. Atipamezole (Antisedan®), 50 mg/kg IM in the dog, followed by yohimbine, 0.1 mg/kg IM q6h.

13. Do not administer atropine, even if bradycardia occurs. Atropine may relieve some signs, worsen other signs, and may contribute to hypertension.

AMPHETAMINE TOXICOSIS

Mode of action

Amphetamines stimulate the release of norepinephrine. They act directly on both α_1- and β_1-adrenergic receptor sites. They also inhibit monoamine oxidase. The actions result in stimulation of the CNS.

Sources

Amphetamines are popular illegal drugs ('speed', 'bennies', 'uppers'). Other drug agents in this class include methamphetamines, phenmetrazine, mephentermine and various 'designer' amphetamines. Amphetamines have legitimate medical purposes in the treatment of obesity, narcolepsy and attention-deficit disorders.

Toxic dosages

The ingestion of methamphetamine 1.3 mg/kg has been fatal. The oral LD_{50} for mice and rats is 10–30 mg/kg.

Diagnosis

History—There may be a history of exposure.

Clinical signs—The patient may exhibit either pallor or hyperemic mucous membranes and skin, restlessness, hyperactivity, hyperthermia, hypertension or hypotension, tachypnea, tachycardia, dysrhythmias, ptyalism, mydriasis, muscle tremors, seizures, circulatory collapse and death.

Laboratory findings—
1. The complete serum biochemical profile may reveal hypoglycemia.
2. Blood gas evaluation may reveal a metabolic acidosis.
3. Chemical analysis of a urine sample may reveal the presence of amphetamines.

Differential diagnosis

Methylxanthine toxicosis, cocaine toxicosis, antihistamine toxicosis.

Prognosis

The prognosis varies with the substance ingested, the amount ingested and the severity of clinical signs at the time of presentation.

Treatment

1. Inform the client of the diagnosis, prognosis and the cost of treatment.
2. Ensure a patent airway. Intubate the patient if necessary.
3. Administer supplemental oxygen and ventilation if necessary.
4. Place an intravenous catheter. Administer a balanced electrolyte crystalloid fluid intravenously to maintain perfusion, hydration and diuresis.
5. Minimize external stimulation, lower the lights and avoid loud noises.
6. Administer diazepam or pentobarbital to control agitation or seizures.
   A. Diazepam 0.5–1 mg/kg IV in increments of 5–20 mg to effect
   B. Pentobarbital 2–30 mg/kg IV to effect
   C. If general anesthesia is required to control seizures, place a cuffed endotracheal tube and monitor the patient's respiration carefully. Monitor for aspiration also.
7. If the patient is presented within 60 minutes of ingestion, and is not having seizures or comatose, attempt decontamination by induction of emesis or gastric lavage.
   A. Induction of emesis in dogs
      I. Administer apomorphine 0.02–0.04 mg/kg IV or IM, or 1.5–6 mg dissolved and placed into the conjunctival fornix.
      If apomorphine was placed in the eye, after emesis, the patient's

eye should be thoroughly lavaged with sterile saline. If excessive sedation occurs from apomorphine, the sedation may be reversed by the administration of naloxone (0.01–0.04 mg/kg IV, IM, SC), but this will not reverse the emetic effects.

    II. Administer 3% hydrogen peroxide 1–5 mL/kg (0.5–2 mL/lb) PO, with a maximum dose of 3 tablespoons (45 mL). If the patient does not vomit within 10 minutes, give 3% hydrogen peroxide 0.25 mL/lb PO once.

B. Induction of emesis in cats

    I. Administer xylazine, 0.44–1 mg/kg IM or SC (can reverse with yohimbine 0.1 mg/kg IM, SC, or IV slowly).

    II. Administer medetomidine, 10 μg/kg IM (can reverse with atipamezole (Antisedan®) 25 μg/kg IM).

    III. Hydrogen peroxide is very difficult to administer to cats and is no longer recommended.

C. Gastric lavage

    I. Lightly anesthetize the patient.

    II. Administer oxygen and intravenous fluids to the patient while under anesthesia.

    III. Maintain anesthesia with the appropriate anesthetic as needed.

    IV. Intubate the patient with a cuffed endotracheal tube and inflate the cuff.

    V. Place the patient in lateral recumbency.

    VI. With a stomach tube held outside of the patient, alongside the patient, measure the distance from the tip of the nose to the last rib. Mark this distance on the stomach tube.

    VII. Lubricate the caudal end of the stomach tube with water-soluble jelly, then pass the stomach tube gently into the stomach, passing the tube no farther than the marked distance on the tube.

    VIII. If desired, two stomach tubes may be utilized: a smaller ingress tube and a large egress tube.

    IX. Infuse warm (body-temperature) tap water, 5–10 mL/kg, through the tube (ingress tube if using two tubes) to moderately distend the stomach.

    X. Allow the fluid to drain from the stomach through the tube (egress tube if using two tubes).

    XI. Save samples of gastric contents, suspicious foreign material, seeds, etc. for possible toxicologic analysis.

    XII. The stomach tube may have to be manipulated, repositioned or flushed with fluid or air if the gastric contents do not flow freely through the tube.

    XIII. Turn the patient over and continue to perform gastric lavage.

    XIV. Continue gastric lavage until the effluent is clear.

    XV. If using the two-tube method, crimp the end of one tube and remove it.

    XVI. Administer activated charcoal down the stomach tube.

XVII. Crimp the end of the stomach tube and remove it.

XVIII. Monitor the patient during recovery from anesthesia, leaving the inflated cuffed endotracheal tube in place until the patient's swallowing reflex has returned.

8. Activated charcoal, 2–5 g/kg (3–6 mL/lb) PO is usually administered in a slurry of 1 g to 5 mL water. Repeat the administration of activated charcoal q3–4h. Administer a cathartic only once.

9. **A single dose of an osmotic or saline cathartic should be administered along with activated charcoal.** Alternative cathartics include:

A. Sorbitol 70%, 2 g/kg (1–2 mL/kg) PO

B. Sodium sulfate, 200 mg/kg for cats, 250–500 mg/kg for dogs. Mix sodium sulfate with water, 5–10 mL/kg and administer PO.

10. Butyrophenones (dopamine agonists) and phenothiazines have been shown to be protective against the lethal effects of amphetamines. They oppose the amphetamine-induced hyperthermia, hypertension and seizures.

A. Administer chlorpromazine 1–2 mg/kg IV, IM q12h PRN or at the dose of 10–18 mg/kg for dogs that have ingested large quantities of amphetamine.

B. Haloperidol (a butyrophenone) 1 mg/kg IV.

11. If the patient is suspected of having increased intracranial pressure, furosemide or mannitol administration should be considered.

12. Control hyperthermia with intravenous fluid therapy, covering the patient with wet sheets or towels, or cold-water baths.

13. Monitor the ECG and treat severe arrhythmias as needed.

14. Administer ammonium chloride to acidify the urine and increase elimination of amphetamines.

A. Dogs: 100–200 mg/kg/day PO divided q8–12h

B. Cats: 20 mg/kg PO q12h

C. Ammonium chloride administration is contraindicated in the patient with acidemia, renal failure, or rhabdomyolysis and myoglobinuria.

ANTICOAGULANT RODENTICIDE TOXICOSIS

Mode of action

Anticoagulant rodenticides inhibit vitamin K_1 epoxide reductase, the enzyme responsible for recycling of vitamin K, which reduces production of vitamin-K-dependent coagulation factors (II, VII, IX and X), resulting in a shortage of these factors and an inability for coagulation to occur.

Sources

The sources of anticoagulant rodenticide toxicosis are divided for treatment purposes into three categories:

1. First-generation coumarins (warfarin, coumarin, etc.) (D-Con®, Warf 42®, RAX®, Dethmor®, Rosex®, Tox-Hid®, Prolin®, Frass-Ratron®, etc.)

A. Half life of about 14 hours. Toxicity depends on single dose versus repetitive exposure. Usually see clinical signs 4–5 days after exposure.

B. Toxic dose
    I. Dogs: warfarin LD_{50} = 20–50 mg/kg once, or 1–5 mg/kg/day for 5–15 days.
    II. Cats: warfarin LD_{50} = 5–30 mg/kg once, or 1 mg/kg/day for 5 days.

2. Second-generation coumarins (brodifacoum and bromadiolone) (Havoc®, Talon®, Contrac®, Maki®, Ratimus®, D-Con®, Mouse Prufe II®, etc.)

A. Half life of about 6 days. Secondary poisonings, in which a dog or cat consumes a poisoned rat or mouse, are a greater hazard than with first-generation products.

B. Toxic dose
    I. Dogs: brodifacoum LD_{50} = 0.25–2.5 mg/kg; bromadiolone = 11–15 mg/kg
    II. Cats: brodifacoum and bromadiolone LD_{50} = 25 mg/kg

3. Indandiones (diphacinone, chlorophacinone, valone, pindone, etc.) (Promar®, Diphacin®, Ramik®, Afnor®, Caid Drat®, Quick®, Raticide-Caid®, Ramucide®, Ratomet®, Raviac®, Pival®, PMP®, etc.)

A. Half life of 4–5 days.

B. The *toxic doses* vary depending on the specific agent involved.
    I. Dogs: diphacinone LD_{50} = 3–7.5 mg/kg
    II. Cats: diphacinone LD_{50} = 15 mg/kg.

Diagnosis

History—The owner may observe or be suspicious of exposure to the toxin. The animal may have a history of being a hunter or roaming. The owner may observe lethargy, epistaxis, melena, bruising, acute blindness, seizures or dyspnea.

Clinical signs—The patient may present with depression, weakness, pallor, melena, epistaxis, hematemesis, hematuria, gingival bleeding, profuse bleeding from wounds, dyspnea, blindness, paresis or paralysis, or seizures. There may be prolonged bleeding from venipuncture sites. Hematomas may be observed. Hemorrhage into body cavities is common. Lameness, joint swelling and pain may be observed if periarticular or intraarticular hemorrhage occurs. The most common cause of acute death is hemorrhage into the pleural cavity, lung parenchyma, and mediastinal spaces.

Predisposing factors, which may exacerbate clinical signs, include the administration of medications (such as aspirin, phenylbutazone, sulfonamides and chloramphenicol), hepatic disease and renal disease.

Laboratory evaluation—
1. The in-house acute evaluation should include a PCV, TP, CBC, platelet estimate and coagulation screen (either PT +/– PTT or ACT).
A. If severe hemorrhaging has occurred, the patient may be anemic. The anemia will usually be nonregenerative if the condition is acute.

B. The platelet count is not usually affected, but may be decreased due to blood loss. It will usually be 50000 to 150000/μL.
C. Coagulation screen –ACT or PT +/– PTT.
   I. Evaluation of PT is the preferred lab test. The PT is the most sensitive due to the short half life of Factor VII and prolongs as early as 6–18 hours following intoxication. In patients with anticoagulant rodenticide intoxication, the PT may be prolonged 2–6 times normal.
   II. In cases of known anticoagulant rodenticide ingestion, evaluation of PTT is unnecessary if the PT is prolonged. PTT prolongation typically occurs 36–48 hours following intoxication.
   III. If PTT evaluation is not available, assessment of the ACT may substitute. In patients with anticoagulant rodenticide intoxication the ACT may be prolonged to >150 seconds, often 2–10 times longer than normal. The normal ACT in the dog is 60–110 seconds, normal in the cat is 50–75 seconds.
2. Additional lab evaluation
   A. A PIVKA assay (proteins inhibited by vitamin K antagonists) is no longer considered necessary and is not indicated if the PT is prolonged.
   B. Fibrinogen levels are usually normal.
   C. Fibrin degradation products (FDPs) are usually normal.
   D. D-dimers are usually negative.
   E. Assessment of a complete serum biochemical profile may be beneficial.
   F. Urinalysis.
   G. Fecal examination.
   H. Blood gas analysis.
   I. Chemical analysis of heparinized plasma may reveal the presence of an anticoagulant rodenticide. Draw a pretreatment sample of heparinized whole blood (**not hemolyzed**).
Separate the plasma and freeze, then submit for lab analysis.
Diagnostic imaging—Thoracic radiographs may illustrate pulmonary hemorrhage (multilobular alveolar infiltration), hemothorax signs of pleural effusion, including pleural fissures, retraction of lung lobes, loss of cardiac silhouette, or pericardial effusion (enlarged cardiac silhouette).

Thoracic ultrasound findings may include pleural or pericardial effusion. Abdominal ultrasound may reveal intraperitoneal effusion or hemorrhage into the gastrointestinal or urinary tracts. MR or CT may show hemorrhage into the cranial vault or other areas.

Differential diagnosis

Immune-mediated thrombocytopenia, immune-mediated hemolytic anemia, von Willebrand disease, inherited coagulopathies, hepatic disease, or disseminated intravascular coagulation (DIC).

Prognosis

The prognosis depends upon the toxic agent ingested, the amount of the toxic agent ingested, the length of time from ingestion to presentation for treatment, and the severity of the clinical signs upon presentation.

Treatment

1. Find the source of exposure. The toxic agent will significantly affect the length of treatment, prognosis and cost of treatment.
2. Inform the client of the diagnosis, prognosis and the cost of treatment.
3. If the toxic agent was ingested within 60 minutes of presentation, attempt decontamination by inducing emesis.
   A. Induction of emesis in cats
      I. Administer xylazine, 0.44–1 mg/kg IM or SC (can reverse with yohimbine 0.1 mg/kg IM, SC, or IV slowly).
      II. Administer medetomidine , 10 µg/kg IM (can reverse with atipamezole (Antisedan®) 25 µg/kg IM).
      III. Hydrogen peroxide is very difficult to administer to cats and is no longer recommended.
   B. Induction of emesis in dogs
      I. Administer apomorphine 0.02–0.04 mg/kg IV or IM, or 1.5–6 mg dissolved and placed into the conjunctival fornix. If apomorphine was placed in the eye, after emesis, the patient's eye should be thoroughly lavaged with sterile saline. If excessive sedation occurs from apomorphine, the sedation may be reversed by the administration of naloxone (0.01–0.04 mg/kg IV, IM, SC), but this will not reverse the emetic effects.
      II. 3% hydrogen peroxide 1–5 mL/kg (0.5–2 mL/lb) PO, with a maximum dose of 3 tablespoons (45 mL). If the patient does not vomit within 10 minutes, give 3% hydrogen peroxide 0.25 mL/lb PO **once**.
   C. **Activated charcoal**, 1–5 g/kg (30–60 mL/10 lb) PO, combined with sorbitol, is usually administered once.
4. Administer the antidote, vitamin K_1 (phytonadione).
   A. Vitamin K_1 is very effective. It is the antidote of choice and is available in parenteral and oral forms.
   B. Vitamin K_3 is far less effective and is contraindicated.
   C. Routes of administration of vitamin K_1
      I. The recommended routes of administration of vitamin K_1 are oral and subcutaneous (with a 25-gauge needle divided into multiple sites).
      II. Intramuscular administration of vitamin K_1 may result in excessive hemorrhage and is not recommended.
      III. Intravenous administration of vitamin K_1 may cause anaphylactic reactions and is not recommended.
      IV. The bioavailability of oral vitamin K_1 is increased by administration concurrent with the feeding of a small fatty meal, such as 1 teaspoon of canned dog food.

D. Dosage of vitamin K_1
  I. Initial loading dosage of 5 mg/kg PO or SC in several sites.
  II. Subsequent dosages of 5 mg/kg PO q24h or divided q12h for 3–4 weeks.
E. Re-evaluate the PT 36–48 hours after stopping treatment with vitamin K_1.
F. If the client is unwilling to run the PT test, treatment should be continued for a minimum of 4 weeks.

5. Provide a hazard-free environment to avoid injury, postpone surgical procedures and avoid unnecessary injections until the PT is normal.

6. Treat clinical signs as they occur. Dyspnea may occur from anemia or pulmonary or pleural hemorrhage.

A. Intrapulmonary hemorrhage
  I. Administer fresh or fresh frozen plasma, at least 9 mL/kg IV, warmed and given at the rate of 5–10 mL/kg/h. Administer plasma through a blood filter.
  II. Administer oxygen, with either an oxygen cage or an Elizabethan collar hood. Nasal catheterization may cause severe epistaxis.
  III. Do not administer furosemide or aminophylline. These medications inhibit platelet function.

B. Intrapleural hemorrhage, including mediastinal—treat with caution.
  I. There is a risk of reinitiating hemorrhage by performing thoracocentesis. It is advisable to perform thoracocentesis only when the ability of the lungs to expand or the cardiac function is severely compromised. Ideally, administer plasma first. Use a nontraumatic technique. Sedate the patient to reduce movement.
  II. Administer fresh or fresh frozen plasma, at least 9 mL/kg IV, warmed, and given at the rate of 5–10 mL/kg/h. Administer plasma through a blood filter.
  III. Administer oxygen, with either an oxygen cage or an Elizabethan collar hood. Nasal catheterization may cause severe epistaxis.
  IV. Do not administer furosemide, aminophylline, aspirin or other medications that inhibit platelet function.

C. Severe anemia
  I. Administer fresh or fresh frozen plasma, 10–20 mL/kg IV, first or simultaneously.
  II. Administer RBCs, 10–20 mL/kg IV, after plasma, or delayed until the majority of the plasma dose has been delivered.
  III. Ideally, a major cross match should be performed and the RBC should be warmed prior to administration; however, life-threatening situations may indicate rapid administration is needed. In these cases, 25–50 mL of room temperature 0.9% NaCl may be added to the bag of RBC to warm the unit. The patient should be monitored and treated for hypothermia.

D. Hypovolemic shock
  I. Administer intravenous fluids, using a balanced electrolyte crystalloid such as LRS or Normosol®-R.
  II. Administer fresh or fresh frozen plasma.

III. Administer RBCs if the patient is severely anemic, following the administration of plasma.

IV. Monitor cardiac, respiratory and renal function closely.

V. Avoid the administration of synthetic colloids such as Dextran or Hetastarch, owing to their potential detrimental effects on coagulation.

ANTIHISTAMINE AND DECONGESTANT TOXICOSIS

Mode of action

Antihistamines inhibit histamine at H_1 receptors in a reversible and competitive process. They exhibit considerable anticholinergic, antiemetic, antitussive and sedative characteristics.

Most decongestant medications are sympathomimetic amines. Some are α-adrenergic agonists, some also produce mild $β_1$-adrenergic effects, while others stimulate both α- and β-adrenergic receptors.

Sources

There is a wide range of medications, with numerous active ingredients, and a broad range of sensitivities. These medications include pseudoephedrine, phenylephrine, phenylpropanolamine, diphenhydramine, dimenhydrinate, clemastine, terfenadine, loratadine, meclizine, hydroxyzine and chlorpheniramine. The imidazoline decongestants (oxymetazoline (Afrin®), tetrahydrozoline (Visine®), naphthazoline and tolazoline) are usually in nasal decongestants and ophthalmic medications.

Toxic dosages

The therapeutic dose of pseudoephedrine is 1–2 mg/kg. Moderate to severe clinical signs occur following the ingestion of 5–6 mg/kg, and death has been reported following 10–12 mg/kg,

The effects in people usually last 4–6 hours.

The ingestion of other medications, including other sympathomimetic agents or MAO inhibitors, or caffeine, theobromine or nicotine, may exacerbate the clinical signs. Erythromycin, itraconazole, ketoconazole and underlying conditions such as cardiac disease, renal disease or hepatic disease may potentiate the effects of certain decongestants by interfering with their metabolism or enhancing the effects.

Diagnosis

History—The patient may have a history of, or possibility of, exposure to medication, or the owner may observed abnormal behavior.

Clinical signs—The clinical signs include hyperexcitability, hypersalivation, agitation, tremors, possible seizures, vomiting, mydriasis, dry oral mucous membranes, and tachycardia. On physical examination, additional findings include hyperthermia, decreased bowel sounds, hypertension (+/− reflex bradycardia), ventricular dysrhythmias, urinary retention, and cyanosis.

A symptom referred to as anticholinergic delirium or central anticholinergic syndrome may be observed. It is characterized by disorientation, ataxia, agitation, hyperactivity, hallucinations, hyperesthesia, psychosis, coma, seizures, respiratory failure and cardiovascular collapse.

A mild overdose causes sinus tachycardia, a dry mouth, fixed mydriatic pupils, urinary retention and ileus, whereas a major overdose causes the signs of CNS stimulation and can lead to death.

The imidazolines usually cause lethargy, bradycardia and hypotension.

Laboratory findings—
1. The hematocrit may be elevated due to dehydration.
2. Acid–base disorders are common.

ECG—Abnormalities include sinus tachycardia, ventricular dysrhythmias and bradycardia.

Differential diagnosis

Ingestion of stimulants such as amphetamines, cocaine, methylxanthine, or sedatives, opioids and tranquilizers.

Prognosis

The prognosis is usually good.

Treatment

1. Inform the client of the suspected diagnosis, prognosis and the cost of treatment.
2. Ensure a patent airway. Intubate the patient if necessary.
3. Administer supplemental oxygen and ventilation if necessary.
4. If the medication has been ingested within 30 minutes prior to presentation, and the patient is asymptomatic, attempt decontamination with emesis. If the substance ingested was a sustained-release medication, gastric lavage after 1 hour may still be beneficial.
   A. Do not attempt to induce emesis in cats with exposure to imidazolines. A fatal combination may occur. Hydrogen peroxide is very difficult to administer to cats and is no longer recommended.
   B. Induction of emesis in dogs (if the dog is asymptomatic)
      I. Administer apomorphine 0.02–0.04 mg/kg IV or IM, or 1.5–6 mg dissolved and placed into the conjunctival fornix. If apomorphine was placed in the eye, after emesis, the patient's eye should be thoroughly lavaged with sterile saline. If excessive sedation occurs from apomorphine, the sedation may be reversed by the administration of naloxone (0.01–0.04 mg/kg IV, IM, SC) but this will not reverse the emetic effects.
      II. Administer 3% hydrogen peroxide 1–5 mL/kg (0.5–2 mL/lb) PO, with a maximum dose of 3 tablespoons (45 mL). If the patient

does not vomit within 10 minutes, give 3% hydrogen peroxide 0.5 mL/kg (0.25 mL/lb) PO **once**.

5. Administer activated charcoal with sorbitol, 2–5 g/kg (3–6 mL/lb) PO is usually administered in a slurry of 1 g to 5 mL water. If the medication ingested is a sustained-release medication, administer additional doses of activated charcoal, 1–2 g/kg without a cathartic, every 3–4 hours for 24 hours.

6. Hospitalize the patient and administer supportive care for 18–24 hours, or 24–72 hours for sustained-release medications, or until the clinical signs have resolved. Treat appropriately for hyperthermia or hypothermia, if present. Monitor blood pressure.

7. Place an intravenous catheter. Administer a balanced electrolyte crystalloid fluid intravenously to maintain perfusion and hydration. More aggressive fluid therapy is usually needed to treat the hypotension associated with imidazoline medications.
   A. If hypotension fails to resolve with crystalloid therapy, administer Hetastarch, 5 mL/kg IV aliquots; repeat up to 4 times.
   B. The administration of a vasopressor such as dopamine, 5–20 μg/kg/min IV CRI, may be beneficial if hypotension continues to be refractory to therapy.

8. Urinary acidification may aid in the excretion of pseudoephedrine and phenylephrine in dogs.
   A. Ascorbic acid (vitamin C), 20–30 mg/kg SC, IM or IV q8h
   B. Ammonium chloride, 50 mg/kg, PO q6h

9. Minimize external stimulation, lower the lights and avoid loud noises.

10. Sedation of the patient may be indicated.
    A. Do not administer diazepam. Diazepam may promote aggression, hysteria and seizures in the hyperactive patient suffering from antihistamine or decongestant toxicosis.
    B. Administer acepromazine, which has α-adrenergic receptor-blocking effects. The dose of acepromazine is 0.05–0.1 mg/kg SC, IM or IV. Repeat the administration of acepromazine if needed, up to 1 mg/kg. Use caution if the patient is hypotensive.
    C. Chlorpromazine is an alternative, 0.5–1 mg/kg IV or IM repeated to effect, to a maximum dosage of 10 mg/kg.
    D. If acepromazine provides inadequate sedation, administer phenobarbital 2–4 mg/kg IV in dogs, 1–2 mg/kg IV in cats.

11. The administration of an α_2- adrenergic antagonist may be beneficial in the treatment of imidazoline intoxication.
    A. Atipamezole, 50 μg/kg IM
    B. Yohimbine, 0.1 mg/kg IV
    C. Due to the short half life of the antagonists, they will probably have to be re-administered several times during treatment.

12. Administer methocarbamol 44.4–100 mg/kg slow IV or PO to decrease muscle spasms.

13. Administer propranolol 0.02–0.04 mg/kg slow IV, or esmolol 0.25–0.5 mg/kg IV then 10–200 μg/kg/min CRI IV if the patient has excessive tachycardia.

14. Administer atropine 0.02–0.04 mg/kg IV or SC if the patient has excessive bradycardia. Avoid the administration of atropine to a hypertensive patient as it may exacerbate the hypertension.
15. Monitor blood gas values. Acid–base abnormalities are common.

ARSENIC TOXICOSIS

Mode of action

Arsenicals inhibit the sulfhydryl enzyme system, which is responsible for cellular respiration and fat and carbohydrate metabolism.

Sources

Inorganic: ant and / or roach poisons, herbicides, wood preservatives.
Organic: sodium caparsolate, filaricide.

Toxic dosages

1. Arsenic trioxide: $\frac{1}{10}$ to $\frac{1}{3}$ (or 10–33%) as toxic as sodium arsenite; toxic dose = 3–75 mg/kg for dogs, 15–50 mg/kg for cats
2. Sodium arsenite: toxic dose for dogs is 1–25 mg/kg, for cats <5 mg/kg
3. Sodium arsenate: toxic dose for dogs is 7–14 mg/kg.

Diagnosis

History—History of exposure.
Clinical signs—The patient will exhibit acute severe hemorrhagic gastroenteritis. The onset of clinical signs can occur with 30 minutes to several hours following exposure.
1. Vomiting is the most common clinical sign
2. Restlessness, hypersalivation, nausea, vomiting, progressive illness
3. Severe abdominal pain often with bloody diarrhea with mucosal tags
4. Muscle weakness, trembling, staggering, ataxia
5. Polyuria and proteinuria lead to anuric renal failure
6. Severe dehydration, hypovolemic shock, paralysis, coma, death occurs within hours or 3–5 days.

Laboratory findings—
1. Urine arsenic level of 2–100 ppm
2. Analysis of gastric contents, liver or kidney post mortem
3. A complete CBC and serum biochemical profile may show hemoconcentration due to dehydration and may reveal the organ systems involved
4. Blood gas analysis may reveal metabolic acidosis.

Differential diagnosis

1. Thallium toxicosis
2. Lead poisoning
3. Garbage toxemia

4. Hemorrhagic gastroenteritis
5. Parvovirus gastroenteritis.

Prognosis

The prognosis is grave unless treatment is started before the clinical signs are advanced.

Treatment

1. Inform the client of the diagnosis, prognosis and the cost of treatment.
2. Ensure a patent airway. Intubate the patient if necessary.
3. Administer supplemental oxygen and ventilation if necessary.
4. Place an intravenous catheter. Administer a balanced electrolyte crystalloid fluid intravenously to maintain perfusion and hydration.
5. Prevent further absorption.
    A. In cases of dermal exposure, brush or vacuum then thoroughly wash the patient with warm, soapy water. Protective garments, including rubber gloves, masks, face shields and other precautions, should be worn while bathing the patient. Keep the patient warm.
    B. Induce emesis if the patient is not vomiting and is presented within 2 hours of ingestion and if there are no contraindications.
        I. Induction of emesis in cats
            a. Administer xylazine, 0.44–1 mg/kg IM or SC (can reverse with yohimbine 0.1 mg/kg IM, SC or IV slowly).
            b. Administer medetomidine, 10 µg/kg IM (can reverse with atipamezole (Antisedan®) 25 µg/kg IM).
            c. Hydrogen peroxide is very difficult to administer to cats and is no longer recommended.
        II. Induction of emesis in dogs
            a. Administer apomorphine 0.02–0.04 mg/kg IV or IM, or 1.5–6 mg dissolved and placed into the conjunctival fornix. If apomorphine was placed in the eye, after emesis, the patient's eye should be thoroughly lavaged with sterile saline. If excessive sedation occurs from apomorphine, the sedation may be reversed by the administration of naloxone (0.01–0.04 mg/kg IV, IM, SC), but this will not reverse the emetic effects.
            b. Administer 3% hydrogen peroxide 1–5 mL/kg (0.5–2 mL/lb) PO, with a maximum dose of 3 tablespoons (45 mL). If the patient does not vomit within 10 minutes, give 3% hydrogen peroxide 0.5 mL/kg (0.25 mL/lb PO) *once*.
    C. Perform gastric lavage with warm water or sodium bicarbonate if the patient is presented within 4 hours of ingestion and the clinical signs are not severe. If the clinical signs of vomiting and diarrhea are severe, there is an increased risk of gastrointestinal perforation and gastric lavage is contraindicated.

I. Lightly anesthetize the patient.

II. Administer oxygen and intravenous fluids to the patient while under anesthesia.

III. Maintain anesthesia with the appropriate anesthetic as needed.

IV. Intubate the patient with a cuffed endotracheal tube and inflate the cuff.

V. Place the patient in lateral recumbency.

VI. With a stomach tube held outside of the patient, alongside the patient, measure the distance from the tip of the nose to the last rib. Mark this distance on the stomach tube.

VII. Lubricate the caudal end of the stomach tube with water-soluble jelly then pass the stomach tube gently into the stomach, passing the tube no farther than the marked distance on the tube.

VIII. If desired, two stomach tubes may be utilized: a smaller ingress tube and a large egress tube.

IX. Infuse warm (body-temperature) tap water, or sodium bicarbonate 5–10 mL/kg, through the tube (ingress tube if using two tubes) to moderately distend the stomach.

X. Allow the fluid to drain from the stomach through the tube (egress tube if using two tubes).

XI. Save samples of gastric contents, suspicious foreign material, seeds, etc. for possible toxicologic analysis.

XII. The stomach tube may have to be manipulated, repositioned or flushed with fluid or air if the gastric contents do not flow freely through the tube.

XIII. Turn the patient over and continue to perform gastric lavage.

XIV. Continue gastric lavage until the effluent is clear.

XV. If using the two-tube method, crimp the end of one tube and remove it.

XVI. Administer activated charcoal down the stomach tube.

XVII. Crimp the end of the stomach tube and remove it.

XVIII. Monitor the patient during recovery from anesthesia, leaving the inflated cuffed endotracheal tube in place until the patient's swallowing reflex has returned.

D. Activated charcoal, 2–5 g/kg (3–6 mL/ lb) PO is usually administered in a slurry of 1 g to 5 mL water. In arsenical toxicosis patients, repeat the administration of activated charcoal q3–4h.

E. A cathartic is not recommended due to the severe diarrhea that results from the toxicosis.

6. Administer an antidote. Options include dimercaprol (BAL), succimer (Chemet®) (DMSA, mesodimercaptosuccinic acid) and N-acetylcysteine.

A. Dimercaprol (BAL)

I. 3–4 mg/kg IM q8h until recovery.

II. Increase the dose to 6–7 mg/kg IM q8h on the first day of treatment of severe poisonings.

B. Succimer (Chemet®) (DMSA, mesodimercaptosuccinic acid)

I. 10 mg/kg PO q8h for 10 days, in dogs; there are no published doses for cats.

II. This is a new chelator with a greater specificity for arsenic and lead than calcium EDTA or penicillamine and has been more effective than dimercaprol when used in children.

C. N-acetylcysteine

   I. Dogs 280 mg/kg PO or IV loading dose, then 140 mg/kg PO or IV q4h for 3 days.

   II. Cats 140 mg/kg PO or IV loading dose, then 70 mg/kg q6h for 7 treatments.

   III. For IV administration dilute to a 5% concentration in 5% dextrose in water and administer slowly over 15–30 minutes.

7. Provide intensive supportive care.

A. Hospitalize the patient for observation and treatment.

B. Consider adding B vitamins to the intravenous fluids.

C. If the patient becomes anemic, administer RBCs.

D. Monitor for and treat renal failure, hepatic damage and electrolyte abnormalities.

E. Administer broad-spectrum antibiotics, owing to the gastrointestinal irritation.

F. Administer oral kaolin when emesis has stopped.

ASPIRIN TOXICOSIS

Mode of action

Aspirin toxicity is much more severe for cats than for dogs. Cats are deficient in glucuronyl transferase activity, which is necessary for the detoxification and excretion of aspirin. Toxicity results from the cat's inability to rapidly metabolize and excrete aspirin.

The toxic effects include bone marrow suppression, inhibited platelet aggregation, metabolic acidosis, toxic hepatitis, renal disease and gastric ulceration.

Sources

Children's aspirin or reduced strength aspirin contains 81 mg per tablet; regular aspirin contains 325 mg; extra-strength aspirin contains 500 mg. Pepto-Bismol® contains 300 mg salicylate per tablet, and 262 mg per 15 mL (per tablespoon). Numerous other products contain aspirin. Be sure to check in the *Physicians' Desk Reference* or on the product label.

Toxic dosages

Dogs = 50 mg/kg/day
Cats = 25 mg/kg/day.

Diagnosis

History—The patient may have a history of exposure.
Clinical signs—

Acute:
1. Usually develop within 4–6 hours
2. Depression, anorexia, hyperthermia
3. Vomiting, possibly hematemesis
4. Tachypnea
5. Acute renal failure
6. Weakness, ataxia, coma, death.

Chronic: repeated doses may lead to gastric ulcers and perforation, toxic hepatitis, and bone marrow suppression (clinically resulting in anemia).

Laboratory findings—
1. Blood levels of aspirin can be measured.
2. A ferric chloride test can be performed by a reference laboratory to assess the patient's plasma salicylate level.
3. Blood gas evaluation may reveal a metabolic acidosis or respiratory alkalosis.
4. A serum biochemical profile may reveal an elevated BUN and creatinine, elevated hepatic enzymes and electrolyte abnormalities.
5. Heinz body anemia may occur in cats.
6. Bleeding times may be prolonged secondary to thrombocytopathia.

Differential diagnosis

Other nonsteroidal anti-inflammatory drug toxicoses, acute renal failure.

Prognosis

If treatment is started before severe acidosis develops, the prognosis is favorable. If the patient is already dehydrated, comatose, with bone marrow suppression or toxic hepatitis, the prognosis is poor.

Treatment

1. Inform the client of the diagnosis, prognosis and the cost of treatment.
2. Ensure a patent airway. Intubate the patient if necessary.
3. Administer supplemental oxygen and ventilation if necessary. Pulmonary edema and hypoxemia may occur.
4. Place an intravenous catheter. Administer a balanced electrolyte crystalloid fluid intravenously to maintain perfusion, hydration and diuresis.
5. Decontamination will be of value up to 6–12 hours' post-ingestion. Do not induce emesis if the patient is vomiting upon presentation.
   A. Induction of emesis in cats
      I. Xylazine, 0.44–1 mg/kg IM or SC (can reverse with yohimbine 0.1 mg/kg IM, SC, or IV slowly).
      II. Medetomidine, 10 µg/kg IM (can reverse with atipamezole (Antisedan®) 25 µg/kg IM).
      III. Hydrogen peroxide is very difficult to administer to cats and is no longer recommended.

Toxicologic emergencies

B. Induction of emesis in dogs
   I. Administer apomorphine 0.02–0.04 mg/kg IV or IM, or 1.5–6 mg dissolved and placed into the conjunctival fornix. If apomorphine was placed in the eye, after emesis, the patient's eye should be thoroughly lavaged with sterile saline. If excessive sedation occurs from apomorphine, the sedation may be reversed by the administration of naloxone (0.01–0.04 mg/kg IV, IM, SC), but this will not reverse the emetic effects.
   II. Administer 3% hydrogen peroxide 1–5 mL/kg (0.5–2 mL/lb) PO, with a maximum dose of 3 tablespoons (45 mL). If the patient does not vomit within 10 minutes, give 3% hydrogen peroxide 0.5 mL/kg (0.25 mL/lb) PO *once*.

C. Gastric lavage
   I. Lightly anesthetize the patient.
   II. Administer oxygen and intravenous fluids to the patient while under anesthesia.
   III. Maintain anesthesia with the appropriate anesthetic as needed.
   IV. Intubate the patient with a cuffed endotracheal tube and inflate the cuff.
   V. Place the patient in lateral recumbency.
   VI. With a stomach tube held outside of the patient, alongside the patient, measure the distance from the tip of the nose to the last rib. Mark this distance on the stomach tube.
   VII. Lubricate the caudal end of the stomach tube with water-soluble jelly then pass the stomach tube gently into the stomach, passing the tube no farther than the marked distance on the tube.
   VIII. If desired, two stomach tubes may be utilized: a smaller ingress tube and a large egress tube.
   IX. Infuse warm (body-temperature) tap water, 5–10 mL/kg, through the tube (ingress tube if using two tubes) to moderately distend the stomach.
   X. Allow the fluid to drain from the stomach through the tube (egress tube if using two tubes).
   XI. Save samples of gastric contents, suspicious foreign material, seeds, etc. for possible toxicologic analysis.
   XII. The stomach tube may have to be manipulated, repositioned or flushed with fluid or air if the gastric contents do not flow freely through the tube.
   XIII. Turn the patient over and continue to perform gastric lavage.
   XIV. Continue gastric lavage until the effluent is clear.
   XV. If using the two-tube method, crimp the end of one tube and remove it.
   XVI. Administer activated charcoal down the stomach tube.
   XVII. Crimp the end of the stomach tube and remove it.
   XVIII. Monitor the patient during recovery from anesthesia, leaving the inflated cuffed endotracheal tube in place until the patient's swallowing reflex has returned.

D. Activated charcoal with sorbitol, 1–5 g/kg (3–6 mL/lb) PO. In aspirin toxicosis patients, repeat the administration of activated charcoal without sorbitol 1–2 g/kg PO q3–4h. Administer a cathartic only once.

6. Administer a balanced electrolyte crystalloid replacement fluid such as LRS or Normosol®-R intravenously. Administer at the rate of 2–3 times maintenance rates

   A. Administer the dehydration deficit over the first 4–6 hours.
   % dehydration × body weight in kg × 1000 = volume of fluid to be administered in mL.

   B. The CVP should not increase more than 5–7 cm H_2O. Higher increases indicate possible fluid overload.

   C. Other signs of overhydration include tachycardia, restlessness, shivering, chemosis, exophthalmos, dyspnea, tachypnea, increased bronchovesicular sounds, pulmonary crackles and edema, serous nasal discharge, decreased mentation, nausea, vomiting, diarrhea, ascites, polyuria and subcutaneous edema (particularly of the tarsal joints and intermandibular space).

   D. If overhydration occurs, slow or discontinue fluid administration. Administer diuretics and / or vasodilators and oxygen if indicated.

8. Periodically pass a urethral catheter to closely monitor urine output. Minimum urine output should be 1–2 mL/kg/h. An indwelling urinary catheter may be used, but strict aseptic technique and a closed collection system must be utilized.

9. Monitor the patient's body weight every 12 hours. Monitor the patient closely for signs of overhydration.

10. After rehydration, induce diuresis with:

    A. Mannitol (10% or 20%), 0.1–0.5 g/kg slow IV, if there are no contraindications (vasculitis, bleeding disorders, hyperosmolar syndrome, congestive heart failure, volume overload). If no response, the same dose may be repeated if diuresis does not occur within 30 minutes. Do not exceed a mannitol dose of 2 g/kg/day.

    B. Furosemide, 2 mg/kg IV q8h in dogs, 0.5–2 mg/kg IV q12–24h in cats:

       I. Repeat furosemide at twice this dose (4 mg/kg) if diuresis does not occur within 1 hour.

       II. Furosemide can also be administered as a constant rate infusion at the dose of 2–5 mg/kg/min CRI IV.

11. If diuresis cannot be induced, consider hemodialysis or peritoneal dialysis. Indications for peritoneal dialysis include:

    A. Exposure to dialyzable toxins

    B. Treatment of overhydration

    C. Severe persistent uremia, acidosis or hyperkalemia

    D. Oliguria / anuria.

12. Placement of a peritoneal dialysis catheter (see Fig. 14.2)

    A. Administer a general anesthetic, being cautious to avoid hypotension.

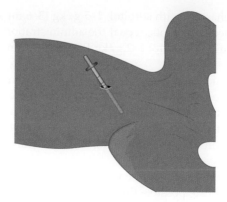

FIG 14.2 **Placement of a peritoneal dialysis catheter.** With the animal dorsal recumbent, make a 1 cm incision through the linea alba, 2–4 cm caudal to the umbilicus. Direct the catheter toward the pelvic inlet. Secure the catheter by suturing it to the abdominal wall, and utilize a 'Chinese finger-lock' suture to add stability. Cover the entry site with a sterile abdominal wrap.

B. Consider performing an omentectomy or partial omentectomy, to decrease omental plugging of the peritoneal dialysis catheter, particularly in the cat.

C. The surgeon *must* use sterile technique. Every junction of the peritoneal catheter set must be covered with a povidone-iodine wrap, which is changed daily.

D. Use a peritoneal dialysis catheter, a pediatric trocath, or for cats use a 14 GA Teflon IV catheter with additional side holes, placed all on the same side to preserve the integrity of the catheter.

E. Make a stab incision (1 cm) through the linea alba 2–4 cm caudal to the umbilicus.

F. Aim the catheter towards the pelvic inlet.

G. Secure the catheter by suturing to the abdominal wall, not just to skin. Use a purse-string suture at the entry site and a 'Chinese finger-lock' suture on the catheter to secure it in position.

H. Cover the entry site into the abdomen with a povidone-iodine patch and a sterile bandage.

I. Administer systemic broad-spectrum antibiotics. Administer an appropriate dose and at an appropriate frequency for a patient with ARF.

J. Use *warm* 1.5%, 4.0% or 7% dextrose dialysate solution, or LRS, or 0.9% NaCl. (The preferable solution, if commercial dialysate solution is not available, is 1.5% dextrose in LRS; it is made by adding 30 mL 50% dextrose to 1000 mL LRS.)

K. Add 250 units heparin/liter of dialysate.

L. Infuse 20–30 mL/kg IP.

M. Dwell time = 45 minutes.

N. Drainage time = 15 minutes.

O. Repeat continuously, or every 2 hours for until the BUN, creatinine and hydration status approaches normal values, then decrease the frequency of dialysis.

P. Flush the peritoneal catheter with heparinized saline after each infusion or drainage to diminish clogging of peritoneal catheter.

Q. Monitor the patient's CBC, TP, serum electrolytes, clotting parameters, urine (sediment and multilab stick) and the dialysate for signs of infection.

R. When peritoneal lavage is no longer necessary, sedate or anesthetize the patient, remove the peritoneal catheter, and close the abdominal incision with one to two sutures in the linea alba, then close the skin. Apply a sterile abdominal wrap.

13. Maintenance of the peritoneal dialysis catheter
    A. Sterility is very important.
    B. Wash hands thoroughly prior to handling the peritoneal dialysis catheter.
    C. Wear sterile gloves when handling the peritoneal dialysis catheter.
    D. Flush the catheter with heparinized saline after every installation and drainage.
    E. Wipe every connection and injection port with chlorhexidine or povidone-iodine solution every time prior to manipulation.
    F. Every junction of the peritoneal catheter set and every injection port must be covered with a sterile povidone-iodine wrap, which is changed daily.
    G. Cover the entry site into the abdomen with a povidone-iodine patch and a sterile bandage.
    H. Keep a clean, dry and sterile bandage on the abdomen, over the catheter entry site. Check the bandage, the entry site and change the bandage every 2 days.
    I. If at all possible, perform the installation and drainage of the peritoneal lavage fluid in the surgical suite to keep contamination to a minimum.

14. Control the patient's metabolic acidosis.
    A. Administer balanced electrolyte crystalloid fluids intravenously.
    B. Improve ventilation.
    C. Administer sodium bicarbonate only when the plasma bicarbonate level can be calculated reliably (or total P_{CO_2} measured) and the patient is determined to be severely acidotic (pH < 7.10, or HCO_3 <12 mEq/L).
        I. mEq HCO_3 needed = 0.3 × (kg body weight) × (desired total CO_2 mEq/l − measured total CO_2 mEq/L).
        II. Infuse half of the sodium bicarbonate amount needed over the first 3–4 hours, then re-evaluate and readjust the dose.
        III. Caution must be utilized while administering sodium bicarbonate. Possible complications that may result include: 'overshoot alkalosis', hypernatremia, intravascular volume overload, hypokalemia, hypocalcemia, tissue hypoxia, and paradoxical cerebrospinal fluid acidosis.

15. Administer gastric protectants such as misoprostol, 1–5 mcg/kg PO q8–12h (dogs only) or sucralfate, 250–1000 mg PO q6–8h in dogs and 250 mg PO q6–12h for cats.

16. Consider the administration of omeprazole to prevent ulcer formation, if no ulcers are suspected to have previously formed. The dose is 0.7 mg/kg q24h PO in dogs only.
17. Alkalinize the urine to increase urinary excretion. This is a side effect of sodium bicarbonate administration. The patient's blood gas status should be closely monitored and sodium bicarbonate should be cautiously administered as described above.

BACLOFEN INTOXICATION

Toxin

Baclofen is a derivative of the centrally acting inhibitory neurotransmitter gamma aminobutyric acid (GABA). It inhibits calcium influx by binding to $GABA_B$ receptors, which prevents the release of the excitatory neurotransmitters aspartate and glutamate. Baclofen may inhibit monosynaptic and polysynaptic reflexes on the spinal cord level.

Sources

Baclofen is a centrally acting muscle relaxant, used in the treatment of people with spinal cord injuries, spinal cord diseases and multiple sclerosis.

Toxic dosages

Dogs = clinical signs have been reported at ingestion of 1.3 mg/kg; death has occurred with the ingestion of more than 8 mg/kg.
Cats = unknown, but thought to be have increased sensitivity.

Diagnosis

History—Ingestion of medication.
Clinical signs—Dogs and cats exhibit agitation, vocalization, ataxia, disorientation, muscle weakness, respiratory depression and hypoventilation, cyanosis, bradycardia, hypertension, hypothermia, sedation, miotic pupils, coma. Aspiration pneumonia occurs commonly.
Laboratory findings—Monitor the patient for hypoxia with arterial blood gas analysis and pulse oximetry. Monitor end-tidal CO_2 for hypercapnia and hypoventilation.
Thoracic radiographs—These should be evaluated for aspiration pneumonia and pulmonary atelectasis periodically throughout the duration of hospitalization.

Prognosis

If the patient is presented quickly the prognosis is usually good, although 7 days of hospitalization and ventilator support may be required. If there is a delay in presentation for treatment, or the patient has seizures or aspiration pneumonia, the prognosis becomes guarded.

Treatment

1. Inform the client of the diagnosis, prognosis and cost of the treatment.
2. Treatment is symptomatic and supportive.
3. Ensure a patent airway. Intubate the patient if necessary.
4. Administer supplemental oxygen and ventilator support if necessary. In one report, ventilator support was necessary for 16 hours, during which hemodialysis was performed.
5. Place an intravenous catheter. Administer a balanced electrolyte crystalloid fluid intravenously to maintain perfusion and hydration and for dieresis, to enhance elimination.
6. Decontamination will be of value up to 1 hour post-ingestion.
   A. Induction of emesis is contraindicated if the patient exhibits neurologic disturbances.
   B. Following gastric lavage, activated charcoal with sorbitol should be administered via the orogastric tube.
7. For severe agitation and dysphoria, administer acepromazine (0.05–0.2 mg/kg IV, IM, SC q4–6h as needed), diazepam (0.1–0.25 mg/kg IV), or midazolam (0.1–0.5 mg/kg IV, IM to effect, as needed) followed by a constant rate infusion (CRI) of midazolam (0.3 mg/kg/h) may be beneficial.
8. If seizures develop, administer diazepam or propofol (1–8 mL/kg IV) to effect.
9. Atropine (0.02–0.04 mg/kg IV, IM, or SC), for bradycardia.
10. Administer intravenous fat emulsion (IFE), 20% emulsion, 1.5 mL/kg IV bolus then 0.25 mL/kg/min for 30–60 minutes IV. Repeat the initial bolus once or twice (maximum = <8 mg/kg/day.) IFE may help compartmentalize the baclofen into the lipid phase, leaving less free drug available to interact with tissues. It may improve cardiac performance and / or may increase intracellular calcium levels and improve myocardial function.
11. Administer cyproheptadine hydrochloride to decrease disorientation and vocalization.
    A. Dogs: 1.1 mg/kg PO or rectally q4–6h as needed
    B. Cats: 2–4 mg total cat dose q4–6h as needed.
12. Perform hemodialysis.
13. Monitor for aspiration pneumonia.

BATTERIES

Mode of action

Disc or button batteries can cause ingestion hazards. All batteries, including alkaline batteries such as a double A (AA) or triple A (AAA), are caustic. If they have been chewed and are leaking, they must be removed immediately. The electrical current that is generated by the battery's contact with esophageal wall cells and within the electrolyte-rich gastrointestinal fluids can cause tissue damage, ranging from ulcerations in the esophageal and gastric mucosa to tissue necrosis and perforation. Impaction of the battery and retention further complicate the injuries.

Batteries also contain toxic heavy metals, including mercury, zinc, nickel, lithium, silver and cadmium. Chelation therapy is sometimes needed for patients with mercury poisoning.

Diagnosis

History—A partially ingested battery or battery-containing item may be found, or the pet may be observed chewing on the battery or battery packaging.

Clinical signs—The patient may exhibit hypersalivation, nausea, erythema and ulceration of tongue, oral mucosa, laryngeal or pharyngeal area, blackened teeth, frequent swallowing, potential signs of gastrointestinal perforation or hemolysis. Abdominal pain, free abdominal fluid or an esophageal fistula may occur.

Laboratory findings—CBC may reveal hemolytic anemia, blood loss anemia, infection or inflammation.

Diagnostic imaging—Abdominal radiographs (or cervical or thoracic if the battery is in the esophagus) are indicated soon after ingestion and should not be delayed until a daytime veterinary hospital is open or available.

Prognosis

The prognosis varies with the severity of injury.

Treatment

1. Inform the client of the diagnosis, prognosis and cost of the treatment.
2. Every animal that has ingested or possibly ingested a battery of any kind should be brought in for emergency evaluation.
3. If the battery is in the esophagus, ideally it should be removed. Endoscopy may be helpful.
4. Do *not* induce emesis or perform gastric lavage.
5. Activated charcoal administration is not recommended.
6. Administer tepid water and rinse the oral cavity every 10–15 minutes for dilution.
7. If a disc battery is in the gastrointestinal tract or there is any sign of damage to a dry cell battery (carefully examine the radiographs) that may allow it to be leaking, or the patient has signs of mucosal hemorrhage or GI perforation, the battery should be removed. Skilled endoscopists may be able to evaluate the battery in the stomach and determine whether endoscopic removal would be safe, and then be able to safely perform such a task, protecting the esophagus. This would be hazardous for rookie endoscopists and should not be attempted by most emergency room (ER) doctors. Otherwise, gastrotomy and foreign-body removal are necessary.
8. If an ingested dry cell battery appears to be unharmed, abdominal radiographs should be repeated to track its progression through the gastrointestinal tract. Gastric protectants, fiber bulk laxatives, saline

cathartics, and enemas may be administered to encourage rapid passage of the battery.
9. If passage of the battery is delayed more than 36 hours, prompt removal is necessary.
10. Radiographs should be taken periodically to monitor for delayed retention and the patient should be monitored for deterioration.
11. Surgical removal of a damaged battery in the asymptomatic patient is also an option that should be offered to the client.
12. The clinical signs of pending gastrointestinal (GI) perforation include anorexia, tachypnea, fever, vomiting, abdominal hemorrhage, and black stools.
13. Gastric protectants should be administered.
    A. Famotidine (Pepcid®), 0.5–1 mg/kg IV or PO q12–24h
    B. Ranitidine (Zantac®), 0.5–2 mg/kg IV, PO q8h (dogs), 2.5 mg/kg IV q12h (cats) or 3.5 mg/kg PO q12h (cats)
    C. Omeprazole (Prilosec®)
        I. Dogs: 0.5–1.5 mg/kg PO q24h
        II. Cats: 0.5–1 mg/kg PO q24h
    D. Pantoprazole (Protonix®), 0.7–1 mg/kg IV q24h
    E. Sucralfate
        I. Dogs: 0.5–1 g PO q8h; can start with a loading dose 4× higher
        II. Cats: 0.25 g PO q8–12h
14. If signs of mercury toxicity are present, including ataxia, anorexia and central nervous system stimulation, chelation therapy with DMSA should be initiated.
    A. Administer succimer (*meso*-2,3-dimercaptosuccinic acid or DMSA) (Chemet®) 10 mg/kg PO q8h for 10 days.
    B. This is a newer chelator that appears to be more effective and less toxic than previously utilized chelators.

BETA BLOCKERS

Mode of action

Beta blockers block β-adrenergic receptors in the heart, eye, kidney, bronchial smooth muscle, etc. Beta blockade results in bradycardia, bronchospasms and hypotension. The effects are due to heart blocks (1st, 2nd or 3rd degree), prolongation of the PR and QT intervals and the QRS complex, myocardial depression, negative inotropic effects, hypotension, cardiogenic shock and hypoglycemia.

Sources

Beta blockers are found in medications used to treat glaucoma, anxiety, migraine headaches, tremors, hypertension and tachydysrhythmias.

Diagnosis

History—There may be a history of ingestion.
Clinical signs—Dogs and cats exhibit bradycardia, weakness, syncope, shock, altered mentation, seizures or coma.

Laboratory findings—Hypoglycemia is common.
ECG—May reveal numerous abnormalities (see mode of action).

Measurement of serum or urine beta-blocker concentration is not reflective of the clinical disease and is not readily available.

Differential diagnosis

Cardiac disease, sick sinus syndrome of Miniature Schnauzers, baclofen toxicosis, calcium channel blocker overdose, opiate toxicosis or other cardiovascular medication overdose.

Prognosis

The prognosis is guarded.

Treatment

1. Inform the client of the diagnosis, prognosis and cost of the treatment.
2. If the patient presents less than 1 hour since ingestion, attempt gastric decontamination with gastric lavage. Induction of emesis is not recommended.
   A. Gastric lavage
      I. Lightly anesthetize the patient.
      II. Administer oxygen and intravenous fluids to the patient while under anesthesia.
      III. Maintain anesthesia with the appropriate anesthetic as needed.
      IV. Intubate the patient with a cuffed endotracheal tube and inflate the cuff.
      V. Place the patient in lateral recumbency.
      VI. With a stomach tube held outside of the patient, alongside the patient, measure the distance from the tip of the nose to the last rib. Mark this distance on the stomach tube.
      VII. Lubricate the caudal end of the stomach tube with water-soluble jelly then pass the stomach tube gently into the stomach, passing the tube no farther than the marked distance on the tube.
      VIII. If desired, two stomach tubes may be utilized, a smaller ingress tube and a large egress tube.
      IX. Infuse warm (body-temperature) tap water, 5–10 mL/kg, through the tube (ingress tube if using two tubes) to moderately distend the stomach.
      X. Allow the fluid to drain from the stomach through the tube (egress tube if using two tubes).
      XI. Save samples of gastric contents, suspicious foreign material, seeds, etc. for possible toxicologic analysis.
      XII. The stomach tube may have to be manipulated, repositioned or flushed with fluid or air if the gastric contents do not flow freely through the tube.
      XIII. Turn the patient to the other side and continue to perform gastric lavage.

XIV. Continue gastric lavage until the effluent is clear.

XV. If using the two-tube method, crimp the end of one tube and remove it.

XVI. Administer activated charcoal down the stomach tube.

XVII. Crimp the end of the stomach tube and remove it.

XVIII. Monitor the patient during recovery from anesthesia, leaving the inflated cuffed endotracheal tube in place until the patient's swallowing reflex has returned.

B. Activated charcoal, 1–2 g/kg PO is usually administered in a slurry of 1 g to 5 mL water, once.

C. For patients with ingestion of sustained release or extended release preparations, consider whole bowel irrigated with polyethylene glycol (PEG) and electrolytes solution (GoLYTELY®).

3. Administer supportive therapy.

A. Intubation and positive pressure ventilator support may be needed.

B. Blood pressure monitoring

C. ECG monitoring

D. Blood gas and electrolyte monitoring

E. Renal function monitoring

F. Blood glucose monitoring

4. Place an intravenous catheter and administer crystalloid IV fluids.

5. Intravenous fat emulsion (IFE) therapy may be beneficial in the treatment of severe hypotension and dysrhythmias.

A. Administer IFE, 20% solution, 1.5 mL/kg IV bolus over 1 minute then continue with a CRI of 0.25 mL/kg/min for 30–60 minutes.

B. The IV bolus may be repeated in 3–5 minutes, up to a maximum dose of 3 mL/kg total.

C. If hypotension persists, increase the CRI rate up to 0.5 mL/kg/min.

D. The total maximum dose that should not be exceeded is 8 mL/kg.

6. Calcium gluconate 10%, 0.6 mL/kg IV, may be beneficial in the treatment of hypotension. Maintain the ionized calcium level at 1–2 times therapeutic levels (1.13–1.33 mmol/L).

7. Administer glucagon, 0.05–0.2 mg/kg slow IV bolus, followed by 0.1–0.15 mg/kg/h CRI IV, to increase myocardial inotropy.

8. High-dose insulin (HDI) therapy / glucose administration

A. Check the blood glucose.

B. If the blood glucose is <100 mg/dL for a dog, or 200 mg/dL for a cat, administer dextrose.

C. Administer regular insulin at 1 unit/kg IV bolus, then a CRI IV of 2 units/kg/h.

D. Every 10 minutes, as needed, increase the insulin CRI by 2 units/kg/h to10 units/kg maximum.

BLUE-GREEN ALGAE INTOXICATION

Toxin

Cyanobacteria intoxication is associated with ingestion of water with excessive growth of *Anabaena* spp., *Aphanizomenon* spp., *Oscillatoria* spp.,

Microcystis spp. or *Nodularia* spp. of cyanobacteria. The neurotoxins anatoxin-a and anatoxin-a$_s$ are produced by *Oscillatoria* spp. The hepatotoxin microcystin is produced by *Microcystis* spp. The hepatotoxin nodularin is produced by *Nodularia* spp.

Mode of action

The cyanobacteria are ingested with water and lysed in the acidic gastric environment, resulting in toxin release. The free toxins are rapidly absorbed from the small intestine. The hepatotoxins are transported to the liver via a bile acid transporter. The cytoskeleton of hepatocytes is altered by microcystins and nodularin. They inhibit serine / threonine protein phosphateses, which regulate the phosphorylation and dephosphorylation of regulatory intracellular proteins. They also induce cellular apoptosis.

The neurotoxin anatoxin-a causes rapid depolarization of neuronal nicotinic membranes, which leads to respiratory paralysis. The neurotoxin anatoxin-a$_s$ inhibits acetylcholinesterase in the peripheral nervous system, but does not cross the blood brain barrier.

Sources

'Blooms', which are a rapid increase in algae growth, occur in late summer and early fall, when the weather is warm and windy and there are increased nutrients in the water.

Toxic dosages

The LD$_{50}$ is unknown for dogs, but for mice is reported to be as follows, for each variety:

Microcytin-LR: oral exposure = 10.9 mg/kg; IP exposure = 50 µg/kg
Anatoxin-a: oral exposure = >5000 µg/kg; IP exposure = 200 µg/kg
Anatoxin-a$_s$: oral exposure unknown; IP exposure = 20 µg/kg.

Diagnosis

History—There may be a history of witnessed exposure to water, with or without algal bloom. Algae may be observed in vomit or on the haircoat. Other animals may be affected.

Clinical signs—The onset of clinical signs occurs within 1–4 hours following ingestion of contaminated water. Lethargy, vomiting, diarrhea, gastrointestinal atony, weakness and pallor are seen in patients with hepatoxicity. Death often occurs within 24 hours. Acute onset of muscle tremors, rigidity, lethargy, respiratory distress, convulsions and respiratory paralysis occurs in animals that ingest anatoxin-a. Death can occur within 30 minutes from the onset of clinical signs.

Increased salivation, urination, lacrimation and defecation, as well as tremors, dyspnea and seizures may be seen in animals that ingest anatoxin-a$_s$. Death can occur from respiratory arrest within 1 hour.

Laboratory findings—Hepatomegaly and elevated hepatic enzymes may be observed, due to intrahepatic hemorrhage. Histological examination of the liver reveals centrilobular to midzonal necrosis and hemorrhage.

A water sample taken from the area of greatest concentration of algae may be analyzed using a mouse bioassay, high-performance liquid chromatography (HPLC) / thin-layer chromatography (TLC) or gas chromatography-mass spectrometry (GC-MS).

A colorimetric assay may detect the presence of microcystin-LR in water.

Differential diagnosis

Aflatoxins, xylitol, cycad palms, amanitins and acetaminophen cause similar signs of hepatic failure. Mycotoxins, metaldehyde, methylxanthines, strychnine, amphetamines, ephedra, cyanide, oleander, organophosphate and carbamate intoxication cause similar signs.

Prognosis

The prognosis is poor to grave.

Treatment

1. Inform the client of the diagnosis, prognosis and cost of the treatment.
2. If the patient presents following recent exposure and is asymptomatic, attempt gastric decontamination by inducing emesis.
   A. Administer apomorphine 0.02–0.04 mg/kg IV or IM, or 1.5–6 mg dissolved and placed into the conjunctival fornix. If apomorphine was placed in the eye, after emesis, the patient's eye should be thoroughly lavaged with sterile saline. If excessive sedation occurs from apomorphine, the sedation may be reversed by the administration of naloxone (0.01–0.04 mg/kg IV, IM, SC), but this will not reverse the emetic effects.
   B. Administer 3% hydrogen peroxide 1–5 mL/kg (0.5–2 mL/lb) PO, with a maximum dose of 3 tablespoons (45 mL). If the patient does not vomit within 10 minutes, give 3% hydrogen peroxide 0.5 mL/kg (0.25 mL/lb) PO *once*.
3. Activated charcoal is questionable in efficacy.
4. The patient should be bathed if algae are on the hair coat. (Staff members should wear protective clothing.)
5. Administer supportive therapy.
6. Place an IV catheter and administer a balanced electrolyte crystalloid fluid IV. Shock boluses of 15–20 mL/kg IV may be needed initially.
7. Provide oxygen supplementation and mechanical ventilation if needed.
8. Administer frozen plasma or fresh frozen plasma, 10–20 mL/kg IV, if need to treat coagulation disorders.
9. Administer methocarbamol, 55–220 mg/kg IV, if needed to control muscle tremors.

10. If the patient develops seizures, administer diazepam, 2–5 mg/kg IV, or phenobarbital, 2–20 mg/kg IV.
11. Administer hepatoprotectants.
    A. SAMe, 18–20 mg/kg PO q24h
    B. Silymarin, 20–50 mg/kg PO q24h
12. Administer vitamin K_1, 1–5 mg/kg PO or SC q24h, if coagulation disorders occur.
13. Administer antiemetics if needed.
14. The administration of atropine, 0.02–0.04 mg/kg IV to effect, may be beneficial for patients with suspected anatoxin-a_s intoxication.

BORIC ACID/BORATES/BORON TOXICOSIS

Mode of action

Unknown, but acts as an irritant that is cytotoxic to all cells. Because borates are concentrated in the kidneys, the kidneys are usually the most severely damaged organ in toxicoses.

Sources

Ant and roach baits, flea products, herbicides, fertilizers, denture cleaners, contact lens solutions, antiseptics, disinfectants, cleaning compounds, mouthwash.

Toxic dosages

The oral LD_{50} in the rat is 2.7–4 g/kg. The lethal dose for oral boric acid ingestion in small mammals is 0.2–0.5 g/kg.

Diagnosis

History—History of exposure.
Clinical signs—Clinical signs include hypersalivation, vomiting, abdominal pain, diarrhea, depression, ataxia, hyperesthesia, muscle weakness, tremors, seizures, hematuria, oliguria, anuria, coma and death.
Laboratory findings—
1. Blood gas analysis reveals metabolic acidosis.
2. Urinalysis reveals renal tubular damage.
3. A serum biochemical profile may reveal hepatic enzyme elevation and an increased BUN and creatinine.
4. Boric acid may be detected in the urine.
5. Borate may be detected in blood; concentrations >50 mg/mL are diagnostic for borate toxicosis.

Differential diagnosis

The differential diagnosis includes intoxication with cholecalciferol, garbage, methylxanthines, mushrooms, organophosphates, pyrethrins or pyrethroids, rotenone and zinc.

Prognosis

The prognosis depends upon the severity of the clinical signs upon presentation and the amount of exposure.

Treatment

1. Inform the client of the diagnosis, prognosis and the cost of treatment.
2. Ensure a patent airway. Intubate the patient if necessary.
3. Administer supplemental oxygen and ventilation if necessary.
4. Place an intravenous catheter. Administer a balanced electrolyte crystalloid fluid intravenously to maintain perfusion, hydration and diuresis.
5. Decontamination will be of value up to 2 hours' post-ingestion.
   A. In cases of dermal exposure, thoroughly wash the patient with warm, soapy water. Protective garments, including rubber gloves, should be worm while bathing the patient. Keep the patient warm.
   B. Induction of emesis in cats
      I. Administer xylazine, 0.44–1 mg/kg IM or SC (can reverse with yohimbine 0.1 mg/kg IM, SC or IV slowly).
      II. Administer medetomidine, 10 µg/kg IM (can reverse with atipamezole (Antisedan®) 25 µg/kg IM).
      III. Hydrogen peroxide is very difficult to administer to cats and is no longer recommended.
   C. Induction of emesis in dogs
      I. Administer apomorphine 0.02–0.04 mg/kg IV or IM, or 1.5–6 mg dissolved and placed into the conjunctival fornix. If apomorphine was placed in the eye, after emesis, the patient's eye should be thoroughly lavaged with sterile saline. If excessive sedation occurs from apomorphine, the sedation may be reversed by the administration of naloxone (0.01–0.04 mg/kg IV, IM, SC), but this will not reverse the emetic effects.
      II. Administer 3% hydrogen peroxide1–5 mL/kg (0.5–2 mL/lb) PO, with a maximum dose of 3 tablespoons (45 mL). If the patient does not vomit within 10 minutes, give 3% hydrogen peroxide 0.5 mL/KG (0.25 mL/lb) PO *once*.
   D. Gastric lavage will be of value up to 2 hours' post-ingestion.
      I. Lightly anesthetize the patient.
      II. Administer oxygen and intravenous fluids to the patient while under anesthesia.
      III. Maintain anesthesia with the appropriate anesthetic as needed.
      IV. Intubate the patient with a cuffed endotracheal tube and inflate the cuff.
      V. Place the patient in lateral recumbency.
      VI. With a stomach tube held outside of the patient, alongside the patient, measure the distance from the tip of the nose to the last rib. Mark this distance on the stomach tube.
      VII. Lubricate the caudal end of the stomach tube with water-soluble jelly then pass the stomach tube gently into the

stomach, passing the tube no farther than the marked distance on the tube.

VIII. If desired, two stomach tubes may be utilized, a smaller ingress tube and a large egress tube.

IX. Infuse warm (body-temperature) tap water, 5–10 mL/kg, through the tube (ingress tube if using two tubes) to moderately distend the stomach.

X. Allow the fluid to drain from the stomach through the tube (egress tube if using two tubes).

XI. Save samples of gastric contents, suspicious foreign material, seeds, etc. for possible toxicologic analysis.

XII. The stomach tube may have to be manipulated, repositioned or flushed with fluid or air if the gastric contents do not flow freely through the tube.

XIII. Turn the patient to the other side and continue to perform gastric lavage.

XIV. Continue gastric lavage until the effluent is clear.

XV. If using the two-tube method, crimp the end of one tube and remove it.

XVI. Crimp the end of the stomach tube and remove it.

XVII. Monitor the patient during recovery from anesthesia, leaving the inflated cuffed endotracheal tube in place until the patient's swallowing reflex has returned.

E. Activated charcoal is usually not recommended due to the abnormally large volume needed to be effective.

F. A cathartic is usually not recommended due to the diarrhea that occurs from the toxicosis.

6. Administer a balanced electrolyte crystalloid replacement fluid such as LRS or Normosol®-R intravenously. Administer at the rate of 2–3 times maintenance rates.

A. If the patient presents in severe hypovolemic shock, administer fluids rapidly. In dogs, administer fluids at 70–90 mL/kg IV over the first hour. In cats, administer fluids at 30–40 mL/kg IV over the first hour.

B. If the patient presents in severe hypovolemic shock, is hypotensive, or is hypoproteinemic also consider the administration of Hetastarch (14–20 mL/kg IV) or plasma (10–30 mL/kg IV) in addition to the crystalloid fluids.

7. During the rehydration phase, monitor the CVP, PCV and TS frequently. Monitor for signs of overhydration.

8. Periodically pass a urethral catheter to closely monitor urine output. Minimum urine output should be 1–2 mL/kg/h. An indwelling urinary catheter may be used, but strict aseptic technique and a closed collection system must be utilized.

9. Monitor the patient's body weight every 12 hours. Monitor the patient closely for signs of overhydration.

10. After rehydration, induce diuresis with:

A. Mannitol (10% or 20%), 0.1–0.5 g/kg slow IV, if there are no contraindications (vasculitis, bleeding disorders, hyperosmolar syndrome, congestive heart failure, volume overload). If no response, the same dose may be repeated if urination does not occur within 30 minutes. Do not exceed a mannitol dose of 2 g/kg/day.

B. Hypertonic dextrose (10–20% solutions) may be used as an alternative to mannitol. Check the patient's blood glucose level first. Do not administer hypertonic dextrose if the patient is hyperglycemic. The dose of 10–20% dextrose is 25–50 mL/kg as an intermittent slow IV bolus over 1–2 hours, repeated q8–12h.

C. Furosemide, 2–6 mg/kg IV q8h in dogs, 0.5–2 mg/kg IV in cats:
  I. Repeat furosemide if urination does not occur within 1 hour.
  II. Furosemide can also be administered as a constant rate infusion at the dose of 2–5 mg/kg/min CRI IV.

D. Dopamine administration may be beneficial in dogs.
  I. To increase renal blood flow and urine volume, administer dopamine, 5–10 µg/kg/min in 0.9% NaCl CRI IV. Do not add dopamine to alkaline fluids.
  II. To enhance the likelihood of inducing diuresis, combine dopamine, at the rate of 5–10 µg/kg/min in 0.9% NaCl CRI IV with a furosemide drip at 0.25–1 mg/kg/h.

11. If urination cannot be induced, perform peritoneal dialysis or hemodialysis. Indications for dialysis include:
  A. Exposure to dialyzable toxins
  B. Treatment of overhydration
  C. Severe persistent uremia, acidosis or hyperkalemia
  D. Oliguria / anuria.

12. Control the patient's metabolic acidosis.
  A. Administer balanced electrolyte crystalloid fluids intravenously.
  B. Improve ventilation.
  C. Administer sodium bicarbonate only when the plasma bicarbonate level can be calculated reliably (or total P_{CO_2} measured) and the patient is determined to be severely acidotic (pH <7.10, or T_{CO_2} or HCO_3 <12 mEq/L).
    I. mEq HCO_3 needed $= 0.5 \times$ (kg body weight) $\times$ (desired total T_{CO_2} mEq/L – measured total CO_2 mEq/L).
    II. Infuse half of the sodium bicarbonate amount needed over the first 3–4 hours, then re-evaluate and readjust the dose.
    III. Caution must be utilized while administering sodium bicarbonate. Possible complications that may result include: 'overshoot alkalosis', hypernatremia, intravascular volume overload, hypokalemia, hypocalcemia, tissue hypoxia and paradoxical cerebrospinal fluid acidosis.

BREAD DOUGH

Toxin

Fermentation of yeast in bread dough causes the release of ethanol, and potential ethanol intoxication.

Mode of action

Ethanol intoxication, gastric foreign body obstruction, gastric dilatation and volvulus and gastric can possible occur. Ethanol metabolism results in severe metabolic acidosis.

Sources

Most cases occur due to the ingestion of large quantities of raw bread dough.

Toxic dosages

Dogs: blood ethanol levels = 2–4 mg/mL.

Diagnosis

History—Ingestion of 1–2 unbaked bread loaves or a pan of unbaked rolls.
Clinical signs—Dogs: behavioral changes, vocalization, ataxia, CNS depression, coma, gastric distention, vomiting or nonproductive attempts to vomit, gastric dilatation and volvulus, gastrointestinal obstruction, gastric rupture, weakness, muscle tremors, ataxia, blindness, seizures, urinary incontinence, respiratory depression, coma and death.
Laboratory findings—Hypoglycemia, metabolic acidosis, lactic acidosis. Abdominal radiographs may reveal gastric distension or gastric dilatation and volvulus.

Prognosis

The prognosis is excellent with prompt treatment.

Treatment

1. Inform the client of the diagnosis, prognosis and cost of the treatment.
2. If the patient presents soon after the ingestion and exhibits no clinical signs, attempt gastric decontamination with emesis, followed by cold-water gastric lavage, administration of activated charcoal and a saline or osmotic cathartic.
   A. Induction of emesis in dogs
      I. Administer apomorphine 0.02–0.04 mg/kg IV or IM, or 1.5–6 mg dissolved and placed into the conjunctival fornix. If apomorphine was placed in the eye, after emesis, the patient's eye should be thoroughly lavaged with sterile saline. If excessive sedation occurs from apomorphine, the sedation may be reversed by the administration of naloxone (0.01–0.04 mg/kg IV, IM, SC) but this will not reverse the emetic effects.
      II. Administer 3% hydrogen peroxide 1–5 mL/kg (0.5–2 mL/lb) PO, with a maximum dose of 3 tablespoons (45 mL). If the patient does not vomit within 10 minutes, give 3% hydrogen peroxide 0.5 mL/kg (0.25 mL/lb) PO *once*.
   B. If the patient is exhibiting nonproductive retching, the patient should be sedated and an orogastric tube should be passed to provide decompression.

C. Cold water should be administered via the orogastric tube and cold-water gastric lavage can be attempted.
3. Activated charcoal with sorbitol, 1–2 g/kg (3–6 mL/lb) PO may be administered *once*.
4. If the patient has life-threatening respiratory depression:
   A. For life-threatening respiratory depression or the patient in a coma, administer yohimbine, 0.1 mg/kg IV q2–3h, until the patient regains consciousness.
   B. Doxapram, 1–5 mg/kg IV, may be administered to treat respiratory depression.
   C. Mechanical ventilatory support is necessary for some patients.
5. Administer isotonic crystalloid intravenous fluids (LRS, Normosol®-R).
6. Provide supportive therapy.
   A. Cover the patient with warmed towels, utilize a Bair hugger, and / or administer warmed IV fluids if hypothermia develops.
   B. Monitor venous blood gases, anion gap, urine pH—metabolic acidosis commonly occurs. The administration of sodium bicarbonate should be considered in patients with a venous pH <7.1.
   C. Hypoglycemia commonly occurs, necessitating dextrose administration.

BROMETHALIN TOXICOSIS

Mode of action

Bromethalin decreases Na^+/K^+-ATPase activity by uncoupling oxidative phosphorylation. It is a potent diphenylamine neurotoxin. Clinical signs are related to CNS dysfunction. Respiratory paralysis is the usual cause of death.

Sources

Rodenticides, including Assault®, Trounce® and Vengeance®. It is usually dyed green and pelleted. It is often packeted to contain 300 pellets, each weighing an average of 140 mg. A packet usually contains 16–42.5 g of bait with a bromethalin concentration of 0.01%.

Toxic dosages

Dogs: 4.7 mg/kg (21.4 g of bait/lb).
Cats: 1.8 mg/kg (8.2 g of bait/lb).

Diagnosis

History—History of exposure.
Clinical signs—Acute signs of cerebral edema or posterior paralysis or paresis occur. Mild ingestion may cause Schiff – Sherrington posture, extensor rigidity, paresis, paralysis, miosis, anisocoria, depression,

anorexia, vomiting, tremors and death. Ingestion of large amounts of bromethalin may cause hyperexcitability, hyperreflexia of the hindlimbs, tremors, running fits, focal or generalized seizures and death.

Clinical signs may occur within 10–86 hours of exposure and may last for up to 12 days.

Laboratory findings—Bromethalin may be detected in gastric contents.

Differential diagnosis

Alcohol intoxication, botulism, ethylene glycol intoxication, rabies, polyradiculoneuritis, salt poisoning and tick paralysis.

Prognosis

The prognosis is guarded to grave, as death may occur following the ingestion of even a small amount of bromethalin.

Treatment

1. Inform the client of the diagnosis, prognosis and the cost of treatment.
2. Ensure a patent airway. Intubate the patient if necessary.
3. Administer supplemental oxygen and ventilation if necessary.
4. Place an intravenous catheter. Avoid the jugular veins. Administer a balanced electrolyte crystalloid fluid intravenously to maintain perfusion and, hydration.
5. Decontamination may be of value up to 4 hours' post-ingestion
   A. Induction of emesis in cats may be beneficial up to several hours after ingestion, in the asymptomatic patient.
      I. Administer xylazine, 0.44–1 mg/kg IM or SC (can reverse with yohimbine 0.1 mg/kg IM, SC, or IV slowly).
      II. Administer medetomidine, 10 µg/kg IM (can reverse with atipamezole (Antisedan®) 25 µg/kg IM).
      III. Hydrogen peroxide is very difficult to administer to cats and is no longer recommended.
   B. Induction of emesis in dogs may be beneficial up to several hours after ingestion, in the asymptomatic patient.
      I. Apomorphine 0.02–0.04 mg/kg IV or IM, or 1.5–6 mg dissolved and placed into the conjunctival fornix. If apomorphine was placed in the eye, after emesis, the patient's eye should be thoroughly lavaged with sterile saline. If excessive sedation occurs from apomorphine, the sedation may be reversed by the administration of naloxone (0.01–0.04 mg/kg IV, IM, SC) but this will not reverse the emetic effects.
      II. Administer 3% hydrogen peroxide 1–5 mL/kg (0.5–2 mL/lb) PO, with a maximum dose of 3 tablespoons (45 mL). If the patient does not vomit within 10 minutes, give 3% hydrogen peroxide 0.5 mL/kg (0.25 mL/lb) PO *once*.
   C. Gastric lavage may be beneficial if it is performed within 4 hours of exposure.

   I. Lightly anesthetize the patient.

   II. Administer oxygen and intravenous fluids to the patient while under anesthesia.

   III. Maintain anesthesia with the appropriate anesthetic as needed.

   IV. Intubate the patient with a cuffed endotracheal tube and inflate the cuff.

   V. Place the patient in lateral recumbency.

   VI. With a stomach tube held outside of the patient, alongside the patient, measure the distance from the tip of the nose to the last rib. Mark this distance on the stomach tube.

   VII. Lubricate the caudal end of the stomach tube with water-soluble jelly then pass the stomach tube gently into the stomach, passing the tube no farther than the marked distance on the tube.

   VIII. If desired, two stomach tubes may be utilized, a smaller ingress tube and a large egress tube.

   IX. Infuse warm (body-temperature) tap water, 5–10 mL/kg, through the tube (ingress tube if using two tubes) to moderately distend the stomach.

   X. Allow the fluid to drain from the stomach through the tube (egress tube if using two tubes).

   XI. Save samples of gastric contents, suspicious foreign material, seeds, etc for possible toxicologic analysis.

   XII. The stomach tube may have to be manipulated, repositioned or flushed with fluid or air if the gastric contents do not flow freely through the tube.

   XIII. Turn the patient to the other side and continue to perform gastric lavage.

   XIV. Continue gastric lavage until the effluent is clear.

   XV. If using the two-tube method, crimp the end of one tube and remove it.

   XVI. Administer activated charcoal down the stomach tube.

   XVII. Crimp the end of the stomach tube and remove it.

   XVIII. Monitor the patient during recovery from anesthesia, leaving the inflated cuffed endotracheal tube in place until the patient's swallowing reflex has returned.

D. Activated charcoal, 1–2 g/kg PO is usually administered in a slurry of 1 g to 5 mL water, once with sorbitol, 1–5 g/kg (3–6 mL/lb) PO. In bromethalin toxicosis patients, repeat the administration of activated charcoal without sorbitol q6–8h up to 24 hours after ingestion. Administer a cathartic only *once*.

E. Whole bowel irrigation with polyethylene glycol GoLYTELY® or CoLYTE® may also be beneficial.

6. Control seizures. If seizures occur, administer diazepam, 0.5–1.0 mg/kg IV, or phenobarbital, 2–4 mg/kg IV in dogs, 1–2 mg/kg IV in cats.

7. Treat hyperthermia if necessary.

8. Treat cerebral edema.

A. Hospitalize the patient for close observation and treatment. Elevate the front end of the patient by 30% and avoid pressure on the neck.

Position the head normally. Monitor temperature, pulse, and respiration. Avoid hyperthermia. Also monitor for arrhythmias, which may occur due to brainstem lesions.

B. Ventilate the patient with oxygen.

   I. Use an oxygen cage, a mask, or a hood made from an Elizabethan collar. Avoid applying pressure to the neck. Also avoid the use of a nasal catheter or nasal prongs as they may cause sneezing, which increases ICP.

   II. Administer humidified oxygen at 100 mL/kg/min. Monitor oxygen saturation with a pulse oximeter, maintain it at 90% or higher. If therapy is not able to maintain oxygen saturation, Pa_{CO_2} is >50 mm Hg, total CO_2 is above normal or the patient is apneic, mechanical ventilation is indicated

      a. If the patient requires mechanical ventilation and is stuporous or semi-comatose, administer 2% lidocaine, 0.75 mg/kg IV to the dog to prevent coughing during intubation. If the patient is a cat, spray the larynx with lidocaine (lidocaine may be toxic to cats).

      b. If the patient requires sedation for intubation, administer propofol or hydromorphone and diazepam or midazolam IV. Pentobarbital may be utilized at a constant rate infusion to prolong the sedative effect.

      c. Administer 2% lidocaine, 0.75 mg/kg IV in dogs, prior to extubation.

      d. Naloxone, 0.01–0.04 mg/kg IV, IM, SC, may be administered if narcotic-induced hypoventilation occurs.

C. Administer Hetastarch.

   I. Dogs: administer a 20 mL/kg IV bolus, followed by an additional 20 mL/kg IV over 4–6 hours daily as needed.

   II. Cats: administer a 10–15 mL/kg IV bolus, followed by an additional 10–15 mL/kg IV over 4–6 hours daily as needed.

   III. Reduce the crystalloid fluid volume administered by 40–60%.

D. Monitor the mean arterial blood pressure (MAP); it can be calculated from the systolic arterial pressure (SAP) and diastolic arterial pressure (DAP) as follows:

   I. $MAP = DAP + [(SAP - DAP) \div 3]$

   II. Maintain mean arterial blood pressure at 80–100 mm Hg, to maintain normal cerebral perfusion pressure. Maintain systolic pressure at 120–140 mm Hg.

   III. Avoid hypertension.

      a. Hypertension in dogs is defined as:
         i. Systolic pressure >180 mm Hg.
         ii. Diastolic pressure >120 mm Hg.
         iii. Mean arterial pressure >140 mm Hg.

      b. Hypertension in cats is defined as:
         i. Systolic pressure >160 mm Hg.
         ii. Diastolic pressure >95 mm Hg.
         iii. Mean arterial pressure >117 mm Hg.

      c. Reassess the neurological status for signs of increased ICP.

E. Administer furosemide, 1–2 mg/kg IV or IM q6–12h in dogs, 0.5–1.0 mg/kg IV or IM q6–12h in cats.
F. If an osmotic agent is required, administer mannitol, 0.1–0.5 mg/kg IV over 20 minutes.
  I. Administer furosemide, 1 mL/kg,15 minutes after the administration of mannitol.
  II. Repeat mannitol every 4 hours as needed.
  III. **Mannitol is contraindicated in a dehydrated patient or one with anuric renal failure, congestive heart failure, volume overload, hyperosmolar conditions and in patients with intracranial hemorrhage**.
  IV. In these patients, utilize furosemide, 1–2 mg/kg IV.

CALCIUM CHANNEL BLOCKER INTOXICATION

Toxin

Calcium.

Mode of action

Calcium-channel-blocking medications slow the influx of calcium into cells and inhibit calcium-dependent functions in cells. They cause decreased cardiac contractility, decreased cardiac rhythm conduction, and vasodilation.

Sources

There are several medications that contain calcium channel blockers, including verapamil, diltiazem, nifedipine and amlodipine.

Toxic dosages

Dosages greater than 0.7 mg/kg, or greater than two to three times the therapeutic dosage, have caused intoxication.

Diagnosis

History—There may be a history of ingestion.
Clinical signs—The clinical signs include nausea, vomiting, depression, bradycardia, disorientation and unconsciousness. Death may occur due to heart block.
Laboratory findings—High-performance liquid chromatography can quantify the serum concentration of the specific agent.
  Hypotension is usually present.
Electrocardiography—may reveal bradycardia, atrioventricular dissociation, first-degree, second-degree or complete heart block, accelerated idioventricular rhythms, junctional escape rhythms, and asystole.

Prognosis

The prognosis varies with the exposure and severity of clinical signs.

Treatment

1. Inform the client of the diagnosis, prognosis and cost of the treatment.
2. If the patient is asymptomatic and presents within 2 hours after exposure, attempt gastric decontamination with emesis or gastric lavage and administration of activated charcoal and a saline or osmotic cathartic.
   A. Induction of emesis in cats
      I. Administer xylazine, 0.44–1 mg/kg IM or SC (can reverse with yohimbine 0.1 mg/kg IM, SC, or IV slowly).
      II. Administer medetomidine, 10 µg/kg IM (can reverse with atipamezole (Antisedan®) 25 µg/kg IM).
      III. Hydrogen peroxide is very difficult to administer to cats and is no longer recommended.
   B. Induction of emesis in dogs
      I. Administer apomorphine 0.02–0.04 mg/kg IV or IM, or 1.5–6 mg dissolved and placed into the conjunctival fornix. If apomorphine was placed in the eye, after emesis, the patient's eye should be thoroughly lavaged with sterile saline. If excessive sedation occurs from apomorphine, the sedation may be reversed by the administration of naloxone (0.01–0.04 mg/kg IV, IM, SC), but this will not reverse the emetic effects.
      II. Administer 3% hydrogen peroxide 1–5 mL/kg (0.5–2 mL/lb) PO, with a maximum dose of 3 tablespoons (45 mL). If the patient does not vomit within 10 minutes, give 3% hydrogen peroxide 0.5 mL/kg (0.25 mL/lb) PO *once*.
   C. Gastric lavage may be beneficial for massive ingestion if it is performed within 2 hours of exposure.
      I. Lightly anesthetize the patient.
      II. Administer oxygen and intravenous fluids to the patient while under anesthesia.
      III. Maintain anesthesia with the appropriate anesthetic as needed.
      IV. Intubate the patient with a cuffed endotracheal tube and inflate the cuff.
      V. Place the patient in lateral recumbency.
      VI. With a stomach tube held outside of the patient, alongside the patient, measure the distance from the tip of the nose to the last rib. Mark this distance on the stomach tube.
      VII. Lubricate the caudal end of the stomach tube with water-soluble jelly then pass the stomach tube gently into the stomach, passing the tube no farther than the marked distance on the tube.
      VIII. If desired, two stomach tubes may be utilized, a smaller ingress tube and a large egress tube.

IX. Infuse warm (body-temperature) tap water, 5–10 mL/kg, through the tube (ingress tube if using two tubes) to moderately distend the stomach.

X. Allow the fluid to drain from the stomach through the tube (egress tube if using two tubes).

XI. Save samples of gastric contents, suspicious foreign material, seeds, etc. for possible toxicologic analysis.

XII. The stomach tube may have to be manipulated, repositioned or flushed with fluid or air if the gastric contents do not flow freely through the tube.

XIII. Turn the patient to the other side and continue to perform gastric lavage.

XIV. Continue gastric lavage until the effluent is clear.

XV. If using the two-tube method, crimp the end of one tube and remove it.

XVI. Administer activated charcoal down the stomach tube.

XVII. Crimp the end of the stomach tube and remove it.

XVIII. Monitor the patient during recovery from anesthesia, leaving the inflated cuffed endotracheal tube in place until the patient's swallowing reflex has returned.

D. If the patient is asymptomatic or has mild clinical signs with minimal risk for aspiration, activated charcoal with sorbitol, 1–5 g/kg (3–6 mL/lb) PO, should be administered. In cases of ingestion of sustained-release medications, the administration of activated charcoal should be repeated q3–4h. Administer a cathartic only once.

3. Ensure a patent airway and provide supplemental oxygenation if needed.

4. Placement of a central venous catheter will facilitate monitoring of central venous pressure, fluid therapy, frequent blood glucose level monitoring, and administration of dextrose 20% IV.

5. Administer intravenous crystalloid fluids to treat hypotension. Be careful to avoid fluid overload.

6. Administer the antidote, calcium (either calcium gluconate or calcium chloride).

A. Administer calcium gluconate 10%, 0.5–1.5 mL/kg IV slowly while monitoring the ECG closely for bradycardia.

B. Calcium chloride 10% has a higher calcium ion concentration (13.6 mEq compared with 4.5 mEq in 10 mL).

7. If hypotension is refractory to fluid therapy:

A. Administer Hetastarch 5 mL/kg IV boluses, to a maximum of 20 mL/kg.

B. Administer glucagon, 0.2–0.25 mg/kg IV bolus then 150 µg/kg/min CRI IV.

C. Administer isoproterenol 0.04–0.08 µg/kg/min IV CRI.

D. Administer a vasopressor such as dopamine, norepinephrine, and epinephrine.

8. The administration of a regular insulin IV CRI of 4 U/min in addition to the IV CRI of dextrose 20% may be beneficial to treat the hypoinsulinemia and hyperglycemia that commonly occurs.

Toxicologic emergencies

9. A temporary cardiac pacemaker may be needed in patients with severe bradycardic conduction disturbances that fail to respond to medical therapy.

CARBON MONOXIDE TOXICITY

Toxin

Carbon monoxide (CO) is an odorless, colorless gas that causes fatal hypoxia when inhaled in high concentrations.

Mode of action

The affinity of CO for hemoglobin is 260 times greater than that of oxygen. CO forms carboxyhemoglobin (COHb), which results in cellular hypoxia if present in high concentrations. COHb also impairs the release of oxygen at the tissue level, which shifts the oxyhemoglobin curve to the left. Brain damage, cardiac injury, delayed neurotoxicity and direct cytotoxicity occur.

Sources

Fires, smoke inhalation, car exhaust systems, generators and ventilatory failure may result in excessive levels of CO.

Toxic dosages

The amount of CO in the blood determines the carboxyhemoglobin level (brain damage may result if >40% and death may occur if >60%).

Diagnosis

History— The dog or cat may have a history of being in an enclosed space with inadequate ventilation or being in a fire.
Clinical signs—The patient may exhibit tachycardia, tachypnea, mental depression or obtundation or coma. Burns, other signs of smoke inhalation, or the smell of smoke on the haircoat may be present. Deafness may occur.
Laboratory findings—
1. Pulse oximetry will overestimate the saturated hemoglobin level.
2. A CBC, serum chemistry profile and urinalysis should be performed to evaluate the patient for organ dysfunction.
3. The COHb level should be measured on a co-oximeter. Check with a nearby human hospital if needed.
4. Arterial blood gas analysis of the partial pressure of oxygen in arterial blood (Pa_{O_2}) may be helpful.

Prognosis

If therapy is delayed and the blood COHb levels are very high, most patients do not survive. Rapid initiation of 100% oxygen therapy is essential.

Treatment

1. Inform the client of the diagnosis, prognosis and cost of the treatment.
2. Place an endotracheal tube (sedate the patient if necessary), and administer 100% oxygen for up to 18 hours, then decrease the oxygen concentration administered to <60%, if additional oxygen therapy is needed.
3. Provide supportive care.
   A. Place an intravenous catheter and maintain hydration with a balanced crystalloid fluid IV.
   B. Administer anticonvulsants if needed.
   C. Monitor the patient's temperature and support as needed.
   D. Treat burns as indicated.

CHOCOLATE AND CAFFEINE TOXICOSIS

Mode of action

Methylxanthine toxicosis causes increased cyclic AMP, increased catecholamines, competitive antagonists of cellular adenosine receptors, and increased calcium intracellularly leading to increased muscular contractility. Methylxanthines include caffeine, theobromine and theophylline.

Sources

Methylxanthines are found in caffeinated sodas, stimulants, coffee, tea and chocolate; the active ingredient in chocolate is theobromine (Table 14.1).

Table 14.2 shows the amounts of caffeine in common food products.

Toxic dosages (Tables 14.2 and 14.3)

Symptoms of toxicosis occur with ingestion of caffeine or theobromine at a dose of 15–20 mg/kg. Cardiotoxicity may occur in patients who ingest more than 50 mg/kg. Seizures may be observed in patients who ingest more than 60 mg/kg. The LD50 of caffeine and theobromine is 100–200 mg/kg. Milk chocolate contains 1.3–1.7 mg/kg (45–60 mg/oz), semi-sweet or dark chocolate contains 3.7–5.2 mg/kg (130–185 mg/oz) and unsweetened (baking) chocolate contains 11.3–12.8 mg/kg (400–450 mg/oz). The LD50 of caffeine and theobromine is 100–200 mg/kg.

Table 14.1 Theobromine concentrations (mg/oz)	
White chocolate	0.25–3
Milk chocolate	44–60
Dark chocolate	135–150
Unsweetened baker's chocolate	390–450
Cocoa powder	400–737
Cocoa beans	300–1500
Cocoa bean hulls	150–255
Cocoa mulch	56–900

Table 14.2 Caffeine concentrations in food products

Product	Concentration
Chocolate	2–40 mg/oz (0.06–1.1 mg/kg)
Tea	20–90 mg/5 oz cup (4–18 mg/oz; 135–608 mg/L)
Cola soft drinks	40–60 mg/8oz (5–7.5 mg/oz; 169–253 mg/L)
Coffee	
Decaffeinated	2–4 mg/5 oz cup (0.4–0.8 mg/oz; 13–27 mg/L)
Instant	30–90 mg/5 oz cup (6–18 mg/oz; 200–600 mg/L)
Drip	80–85 mg/5 oz cup (16–17 mg/oz; 540–574 mg/L)
Excedrin®	65 mg/tablet
Red Bull®	80 mg/8.3 oz (9.6 mg/oz; 324 mg/L)
OTC stimulants	200 mg/tablet
Coffee beans	280 570 mg/oz (8–16 mg/kg)

Table 14.3 Dangerous quantities of chocolate[1] in oz or kg of theobromine/kg of patient body weight

Dog's weight		Amount of milk chocolate		Amount of chocolate chips		Amount of unsweetened chocolate		Approximate amount of theobromine
(lb)	(kg)	(oz)	(kg)	(oz)	(kg)	(oz)	(kg)	(mg)
5	2.3	4	0.06	1.5	0.04	0.5	0.02	46
10	4.5	8	0.1	3.0	0.09	1.5	0.04	90
20	9.1	16	0.3	6.5	0.2	2.5	0.07	180
30	13.6	28	0.8	9.5	0.3	3.2	0.09	272
40	18.1	40	1.1	13.3	0.4	4.5	0.1	363
50	22.7	48	1.4	16.6	0.5	5.5	0.15	454
60	27.2	60	1.7	20.0	0.6	6.7	0.2	545
75	34.0	76	2.2	25.2	0.7	8.5	0.25	682

[1]**Warning:** These are approximate amounts only. Every animal has different sensitivity to chocolate. If the animal is exhibiting any clinical signs, has ingested a quantity near the approximated toxic amount or has a history of cardiac, hepatic, renal or seizure disorders recommend examination. There are significant amounts of caffeine contained within these products. Nestlé's® milk chocolate contains approximately 19 mg of caffeine per ounce while Hershey's® contains approximately 8 mg of caffeine per ounce. Caffeine is considered to enhance the clinical toxicity of chocolate.

Diagnosis

History—The patient may have a history of exposure to a methylxanthine.

Clinical signs—The clinical signs include vomiting, diarrhea, hyperactivity, restlessness, urination, ataxia, muscle tremors, tachycardia, bradycardia, arrhythmias, hyperthermia, seizures, coma and death. Clinical signs usually occur within 1–4 hours of ingestion. Secondary pancreatitis has been reported. Gastrointestinal obstruction may occur from ingestion of wrappers or if the chocolate congeals into a mass.

ECG abnormalities—Include tachycardia, ventricular dysrhythmias and bradycardia.

Differential diagnosis

Amphetamine toxicosis, antihistamine or decongestant toxicosis, cocaine toxicosis.

Prognosis

Patients usually recover with hospitalization and aggressive therapy. Methylxanthine toxicosis is occasionally fatal if a large amount is ingested and allowed to be absorbed.

Treatment

There is no specific antidote for methylxanthines.

1. Inform the client of the diagnosis, prognosis and the cost of treatment.
2. Ensure a patent airway. Intubate the patient if necessary.
3. Administer supplemental oxygen and ventilation if necessary.
4. Place an intravenous catheter. Administer a balanced electrolyte crystalloid fluid intravenously to maintain perfusion, hydration and diuresis.
5. Prevent further absorption. Induce emesis or perform gastric lavage if the patient is presented within 6 hours of ingestion.
   A. Induction of emesis in cats
      I. Administer xylazine, 0.44–1 mg/kg IM or SC (can reverse with yohimbine 0.1 mg/kg IM, SC, or IV slowly).
      II. Administer medetomidine, 10 µg/kg IM (can reverse with atipamezole (Antisedan®) 25 µg/kg IM).
      III. Hydrogen peroxide is very difficult to administer to cats and is no longer recommended.
   B. Induction of emesis in dogs
      I. Apomorphine 0.02–0.04 mg/kg IV or IM, or 1.5–6 mg dissolved and placed into the conjunctival fornix. If apomorphine was placed in the eye, after emesis, the patient's eye should be thoroughly lavaged with sterile saline. If excessive sedation occurs from apomorphine, the sedation may be reversed by the administration of naloxone (0.01–0.04 mg/kg IV, IM, SC), but this will not reverse the emetic effects.
      II. Administer 3% hydrogen peroxide 1–5 mL/kg (0.5–2 mL/lb) PO, with a maximum dose of 3 tablespoons (45 mL). If the patient does not vomit within 10 minutes, give 3% hydrogen peroxide 0.5 mL/kg (0.25 mL/lb) PO *once*.
   C. Gastric lavage
      I. Lightly anesthetize the patient.
      II. Administer oxygen and intravenous fluids to the patient while under anesthesia.
      III. Maintain anesthesia with the appropriate anesthetic as needed.
      IV. Intubate the patient with a cuffed endotracheal tube and inflate the cuff.
      V. Place the patient in lateral recumbency.

VI. With a stomach tube held outside of the patient, alongside the patient, measure the distance from the tip of the nose to the last rib. Mark this distance on the stomach tube.

VII. Lubricate the caudal end of the stomach tube with water-soluble jelly then pass the stomach tube gently into the stomach, passing the tube no farther than the marked distance on the tube.

VIII. If desired, two stomach tubes may be utilized, a smaller ingress tube and a large egress tube.

IX. Infuse warm (body-temperature) tap water, 5–10 mL/kg, through the tube (ingress tube if using two tubes) to moderately distend the stomach.

X. Allow the fluid to drain from the stomach through the tube (egress tube if using two tubes).

XI. Save samples of gastric contents, suspicious foreign material, seeds, etc. for possible toxicologic analysis.

XII. The stomach tube may have to be manipulated, repositioned or flushed with fluid or air if the gastric contents do not flow freely through the tube.

XIII. Turn the patient to the other side and continue to perform gastric lavage.

XIV. Continue gastric lavage until the effluent is clear.

XV. If using the two-tube method, crimp the end of one tube and remove it.

XVI. Administer activated charcoal down the stomach tube.

XVII. Crimp the end of the stomach tube and remove it.

XVIII. Monitor the patient during recovery from anesthesia, leaving the inflated cuffed endotracheal tube in place until the patient's swallowing reflex has returned.

D. Activated charcoal with sorbitol, 1–2 g/kg (3–6 mL/lb) PO once. In methylxanthine toxicosis patients, repeat the administration of activated charcoal without sorbitol q3–6h for 36 hours after ingestion. Administer a cathartic only once.

6. Sedation is necessary for some patients.
   A. Diazepam 0.5–2.0 mg/kg IV
   B. Pentobarbital 2–30 mg slow IV to effect as needed.

7. Monitor the patient's cardiovascular system function, ECG, blood pressure, oxygen saturation, and / or blood gases.
   A. If the patient has bradycardia, administer atropine 0.02 mg/kg IV.
   B. If the patient has PVCs, administer lidocaine.
      I. Dogs: 1–2 mg/kg IV bolus followed by 25–75 mg/kg/min IV infusion.
      II. Cats: 0.25–1 mg/kg IV bolus followed by 5–40 mg/kg/min IV infusion.
   C. If the patient has tachycardia, administer a beta blocker such as propranolol 0.02–0.06 mg/kg slow IV or metoprolol 0.5–1 mg/kg PO q8h in dogs, 12.5–25 mg/cat PO q8–12h.

8. Catheterize the urinary bladder to prevent re-absorption of methylxanthines from urine.

9. Do not administer erythromycin or corticosteroids as they decrease urinary excretion of methylxanthines.
10. Methylxanthines have a long half life and may require prolonged treatment (72 hours).
11. Insulin administration may be beneficial for caffeine toxicosis as insulin has been shown to be antagonistic to caffeine.
12. The administration of ranitidine, famotidine, and aluminum hydroxide (Amphojel®, Dialume®) or aluminum carbonate (Basalgel®) may neutralize the gastrointestinal irritation caused by caffeine toxicosis.
    A. Ranitidine (Zantac®), 0.5–2 mg/kg IV, PO q8h (dogs), 2.5 mg/kg IV q12h (cats) or 3.5 mg/kg PO q12h (cats)
    B. Famotidine (Pepcid®), 0.5–1 mg/kg IV or PO q12–24h
    C. Aluminum hydroxide (Amphojel®), 10–30 mg/kg PO q8h in dogs, 10–30 mL PO q12h in cats
    D. Aluminum carbonate (Basalgel®),10–30 mg/kg PO q8h
    E. Aluminum hydroxide (Dialume®), $\frac{1}{6}$–$\frac{1}{4}$ capsule PO.

CHOLECALCIFEROL TOXICOSIS

Mode of action

Cholecalciferol is metabolized to 25-hydroxyvitamin D in the liver, which is converted by the kidney to active 1,25-dihydroxyvitamin D (vitamin D_3). Vitamin D_3 promotes calcium retention. In toxic overdose levels this leads to lethal hypercalcemia and hemorrhage secondary to mineralization of blood vessels, renal tubules, stomach wall and lungs.

Sources

Several rodenticides contain cholecalciferol, including Ortho Mouse-B-Gone®, Rampage®, Rat-B-Gone®, Quintox®, etc.

Toxic dosages

Cholecalciferol is more potent than second-generation anticoagulants. One packet, one exposure is lethal. Clinical signs occur in dogs following ingestion of 0.5–3 mg/kg and lethal toxicosis is seen at 10–20 mg/kg. Cats are more sensitive to intoxication than dogs or rats.

Diagnosis

History—The patient may have a history of ingestion of a cholecalciferol-containing rodenticide. The owner may notice signs of acute renal failure, including vomiting, lethargy, anorexia, polydipsia, polyuria or anuria. The owner may observe hemorrhaging.
Clinical signs—The patient may appear depressed, lethargic and weak. Vomiting may lead to dehydration. Constipation, polyuria and polydipsia may occur. Renal failure may occur. Petechiation may be observed. Hematemesis and bloody diarrhea may be present. Shock, bradycardia and other cardiac dysrhythmias may occur. Muscle

twitching, seizures, stupor and death may occur. Clinical signs usually develop 12–36 hours after ingestion and worsen 24–36 hours after the onset of clinical disease.

Laboratory findings—

1. A serum biochemical profile may reveal hyperphosphatemia, hypercalcemia and azotemia
   A. Hyperphosphatemia may occur 12 hours prior to hypercalcemia and may be an early indicator of cholecalciferol intoxication.
   B. The serum calcium level may be greater than 12 mg/dL.
   C. As renal failure ensues, the BUN and creatinine levels rise.
   D. Analysis of renal tissue may reveal excessive levels of active 1,25-dihydroxy-vitamin D metabolites.
2. The hematocrit may be elevated due to dehydration.

Differential diagnosis

Acute renal failure, ethylene glycol intoxication, malignant lymphoma, anal fornix apocrine gland adenocarcinoma, metastatic bone tumors, multiple myeloma, osteomyelitis, primary hyperparathyroidism and hypoadrenocorticism.

Prognosis

The prognosis is guarded to poor. Death usually occurs within 2–5 days of the onset of clinical signs in acute cholecalciferol intoxication.

Treatment

1. Inform the client of the diagnosis, prognosis and the cost of treatment.
2. Hospitalize the patient for a few days, monitoring continuously, 24 hours per day.
3. Ensure a patent airway. Intubate the patient if necessary.
4. Administer supplemental oxygen and ventilation if necessary.
5. Place an intravenous catheter. Administer 0.9% NaCl intravenously to maintain perfusion, hydration and to promote diuresis and calciuresis. The initial fluid rate should be 120–180 mL/kg/day then 60–120 mL/kg/day depending on the size of the patient.
6. If the patient is presented within 4 hours of ingestion, attempt decontamination.
   A. Induction of emesis in dogs
      I. Administer apomorphine 0.02–0.04 mg/kg IV or IM, or 1.5–6 mg dissolved and placed into the conjunctival fornix. If apomorphine was placed in the eye, after emesis, the patient's eye should be thoroughly lavaged with sterile saline. If excessive sedation occurs from apomorphine, the sedation may be reversed by the administration of naloxone (0.01–0.04 mg/kg IV, IM, SC), but this will not reverse the emetic effects.

II. Administer 3% hydrogen peroxide 1–5 mL/kg (0.5–2 mL/lb) PO, with a maximum dose of 3 tablespoons (45 mL). If the patient does not vomit within 10 minutes, give 3% hydrogen peroxide 0.5 mL/kg (0.25 mL/lb) PO *once.*

B. Induction of emesis in cats

   I. Administer xylazine, 0.44–1 mg/kg IM or SC (can reverse with yohimbine 0.1 mg/kg IM, SC, or IV slowly).

  II. Administer medetomidine, 10 µg/kg IM (can reverse with atipamezole (Antisedan) 25 µg/kg IM).

 III. Hydrogen peroxide is very difficult to administer to cats and is no longer recommended.

C. Gastric lavage

      I. Lightly anesthetize the patient.

     II. Administer oxygen and intravenous fluids to the patient while under anesthesia.

   III. Maintain anesthesia with the appropriate anesthetic as needed.

   IV. Intubate the patient with a cuffed endotracheal tube and inflate the cuff.

    V. Place the patient in lateral recumbency.

   VI. With a stomach tube held outside of the patient, alongside the patient, measure the distance from the tip of the nose to the last rib. Mark this distance on the stomach tube.

  VII. Lubricate the caudal end of the stomach tube with water-soluble jelly then pass the stomach tube gently into the stomach, passing the tube no farther than the marked distance on the tube.

 VIII. If desired, two stomach tubes may be utilized, a smaller ingress tube and a large egress tube.

   IX. Infuse warm (body-temperature) tap water, 5–10 mL/kg, through the tube (ingress tube if using two tubes) to moderately distend the stomach.

    X. Allow the fluid to drain from the stomach through the tube (egress tube if using two tubes).

   XI. Save samples of gastric contents, suspicious foreign material, seeds, etc. for possible toxicologic analysis.

  XII. The stomach tube may have to be manipulated, repositioned or flushed with fluid or air if the gastric contents do not flow freely through the tube.

 XIII. Turn the patient to the other side and continue to perform gastric lavage.

 XIV. Continue gastric lavage until the effluent is clear.

  XV. If using the two-tube method, crimp the end of one tube and remove it.

 XVI. Administer activated charcoal down the stomach tube.

XVII. Crimp the end of the stomach tube and remove it.

XVIII. Monitor the patient during recovery from anesthesia, leaving the inflated cuffed endotracheal tube in place until the patient's swallowing reflex has returned.

7. Activated charcoal with sorbitol, 1–5 g/kg (3–6 mL/lb) PO is usually administered once. In cholecalciferol toxicosis patients, repeat the administration of activated charcoal q8h for 1–2 days. Administer a cathartic only *once*.
8. Administer furosemide 4–5 mg/kg IV q12h, then 2.5–4.5 mg/kg PO q6–12h for 2–4 weeks.
9. To promote calciuresis, administer prednisolone or prednisone 2–4 mg/kg SC or PO q12h for 2–4 weeks.
10. Monitor the BUN and creatinine after 24, 48 and 72 hours of therapy. Treat azotemia if detected.
11. Evaluate the serum calcium level q2–4h, especially after 24 hours of therapy.
12. Administer calcitonin (Calcimar®) 4–6 IU/kg SC q2–12h for severe hypercalcemia (calcium >18 mg/dL) in dogs and cats. If calcitonin is not effective, increase the dose to 10–20 IU/kg.
13. Administer an intestinal phosphate binder, aluminum hydroxide 10–30 mg/kg PO q8–12h if the patient has severe hyperphosphatemia.
14. Administer sodium bicarbonate cautiously if severe metabolic acidosis occurs.
15. Control seizures as necessary.
16. Treat hyperthermia if necessary.
17. Monitor the ECG for arrhythmias and treat accordingly.
18. Feed the patient a low-calcium diet for 4 weeks; avoid dairy products and calcium supplementation.
    A. Hill's prescription u/d®, w/d® or k/d® diets
    B. NF-Formula® (Purina CNM)
    C. Royal Canin Select Care Canine Modified Formula® (Innovative Veterinary Diets (IVD))
    D. Canine Low Protein® (Waltham Veterinary Diets)
19. To decrease skin conversion of sunlight to active vitamin D, decrease exposure to sunlight.

CITRUS OIL EXTRACT TOXICOSIS (LIMONENE AND LINALOOL TOXICOSIS)

Mode of action

D-Limonene and linalool are fragrant citrus oils with insecticidal properties. They are monoterpenoids, similar in structure to pulegones, which are derived from the limonene base structure. Pulegone is a toxic ketone that is metabolized by the hepatic cytochrome system and results in hepatic necrosis.

Sources

Citrus oil extracts, including D-limonene and linalool, are found in insecticidal sprays, dips, shampoos, insect repellents, food additives and fragrances.

Toxic dosages

Cats are more sensitive (five times more for D-limonene toxicosis) than dogs. The toxic dose for ingestion of D-limonene in dogs is 680 g/kg. If cats are treated with canine products at the concentration recommended for canines, the result may be fatal. Linalool exposure causes more severe clinical signs for a longer duration than D-limonene.

The toxic effects of citrus oil extracts may be potentiated by piperonyl butoxide, which is often contained in the same product.

Diagnosis

History—The patient may have a history of exposure. They usually will have a strong citrus smell to their skin.

Clinical signs—The patient may exhibit excessive salivation, depression, weakness, hypothermia, trembling, ataxia, falling, vasodilation, hypotension, and dermatitis that is especially severe in the scrotal and perineal areas. Death may occur.

Laboratory findings—Mass spectrometry or gas chromatography may detect the metabolites of limonene or linalool.

Differential diagnosis

Pyrethrin and pyrethroid toxicosis, organophosphate toxicosis, carbamate toxicosis.

Prognosis

The prognosis is usually good to excellent; however, deaths have occurred and are more common in cats.

Treatment

1. Inform the client of the diagnosis, prognosis and the cost of treatment.
2. Hospitalize the patient for a few days, monitoring continuously, 24 hours per day.
3. Ensure a patent airway. Intubate the patient if necessary.
4. Administer supplemental oxygen and ventilation if necessary.
5. In cases of dermal exposure, thoroughly wash the patient with warm water and a liquid dish washing detergent. Protective garments, including rubber gloves, should be worn while bathing the patient. Wash the patient repeatedly until the citrus odor has disappeared.
6. Keep the patient warm, by wrapping in towels, using heating pads, warmed rice bags, or other methods.
7. Place an intravenous catheter and administer warmed balanced electrolyte crystalloid replacement intravenous fluids such as Normosol®-R or LRS.
8. If the patient is presented within 4 hours of ingestion, attempt decontamination by performing gastric lavage.

A. Lightly anesthetize the patient.
B. Administer oxygen and intravenous fluids to the patient while under anesthesia.
C. Maintain anesthesia with the appropriate anesthetic as needed.
D. Intubate the patient with a cuffed endotracheal tube and inflate the cuff.
E. Place the patient in lateral recumbency.
F. With a stomach tube held outside of the patient, alongside the patient, measure the distance from the tip of the nose to the last rib. Mark this distance on the stomach tube.
G. Lubricate the caudal end of the stomach tube with water-soluble jelly then pass the stomach tube gently into the stomach, passing the tube no farther than the marked distance on the tube.
H. If desired, two stomach tubes may be utilized, a smaller ingress tube and a large egress tube.
I. Infuse warm (body-temperature) tap water, 5–10 mL/kg, through the tube (ingress tube if using two tubes) to moderately distend the stomach.
J. Allow the fluid to drain from the stomach through the tube (egress tube if using two tubes).
K. Save samples of gastric contents, suspicious foreign material, seeds, etc. for possible toxicologic analysis.
L. The stomach tube may have to be manipulated, repositioned or flushed with fluid or air if the gastric contents do not flow freely through the tube.
M. Turn the patient to the other side and continue to perform gastric lavage.
N. Continue gastric lavage until the effluent is clear.
O. If using the two-tube method, crimp the end of one tube and remove it.
P. Administer activated charcoal down the stomach tube.
Q. Crimp the end of the stomach tube and remove it.
R. Monitor the patient during recovery from anesthesia, leaving the inflated cuffed endotracheal tube in place until the patient's swallowing reflex has returned.

9. Activated charcoal, 0.5–1 g/kg PO (30–60 mL/10 lb) is usually administered in a slurry of 1 g to 5 mL water. In citrus oil extract ingestion toxicosis patients, repeat the administration of activated charcoal q8h for 1–2 days. Administer a cathartic only once.

10. A single dose of an osmotic or saline cathartic should be administered along with activated charcoal. Do not administer magnesium-containing cathartics. Alternative cathartics include:
   A. Sorbitol (70%), 2 g/kg (1–2 mL/kg) PO. (The sorbitol in activated charcoal preparations acts similarly to a saline cathartic.)
   B. Sodium sulfate, 200 mg/kg for cats, 250–500 mg/kg for dogs. Mix sodium sulfate with water, 5–10 mL/kg and administer PO.

11. Whole bowel irrigation with polyethylene glycol (PEG) electrolyte solution (CoLYTE® or GoLYTELY®) should be considered.

12. Do not administer atropine unless the patient develops severe bradycardia.

13. Provide symptomatic and supportive therapy, depending upon the individual patient's needs.

COCAINE INTOXICATION

Mode of action

Cocaine ingestion or inhalation leads to central nervous system stimulation by stimulation of, and blockade of the re-uptake of, presynaptic release of catecholamines, including norepinephrine and dopamine. Cocaine also blocks serotonin re-uptake. The local anesthetic effects are due to blockade of the membrane sodium channels. The neurologic signs are accompanied by sympathomimetic effects. Tachycardia, tachypnea, vasoconstriction, dysrhythmias, myocarditis, hyperthermia, hypertension, excitation, seizures, behavioral changes and sudden death may occur.

Sources

Cocaine is an illegal street drug with a high incidence of abuse. It may be sniffed (snorted) as a powder, smoked, injected or swallowed. It is available as a hydrochloride salt (coke, snow) or as the free-base form (crack, rock, free-base). It may be diluted with look-alikes, which can cause additional complications and side effects.

Toxic dosages

The oral LD_{50} for dogs is 24–40 mg/kg and for cats it is about 30 mg/kg.

Diagnosis

History—The patient may have a history of exposure to cocaine. Animals may gain exposure by eating a used tissue of a user. Oral absorption is excellent and ingestion is the most common route of exposure to pets.
Clinical signs—The patient may exhibit hypersalivation, vocalization, restlessness, mydriasis, hyperactivity, altered behavior, periods of depression, anxiety, delirium, muscle fasciculations, convulsions, tachycardia, tachypnea, ventricular dysrhythmias, hyperthermia, vomiting, nausea, diarrhea, abdominal pain, respiratory depression, pulmonary edema, cyanosis, coma, rhabdomyolysis, renal failure, respiratory arrest and cardiac arrest.

There have been reported cases of dogs force fed balloons or condoms containing cocaine, or cocaine packets having been surgically implanted into a dog's abdomen to smuggle cocaine. These gastrointestinal or abdominal packets require cautious surgical removal.
Laboratory findings—Analysis of blood or urine for the presence of cocaine metabolites may be performed. Urine is the preferred sample for submission. Hypoglycemia is common late in the course of toxicosis.

Differential diagnosis

Antihistamine or decongestant toxicosis, amphetamine toxicosis, methylxanthine toxicosis, marijuana intoxication.

Prognosis

The prognosis is fair to guarded.

Treatment

1. Inform the client of the diagnosis, prognosis and the cost of treatment.
2. Ensure a patent airway. Intubate the patient if necessary.
3. Administer supplemental oxygen and ventilation if necessary.
4. Place an intravenous catheter. Administer a balanced electrolyte crystalloid fluid intravenously to maintain perfusion, hydration and diuresis.
5. Administer diazepam, phenobarbital or pentobarbital if necessary to control seizures or hyperactivity.
   A. Diazepam 0.5–1 mg/kg IV in increments of 5–20 mg to effect
   B. Phenobarbital 2–4 mg/kg IV in dogs, 1–2 mg/kg IV in cats
   C. Pentobarbital 2–30 mg/kg slow IV to effect
6. Give the patient a cold-water bath if the patient is hyperthermic.
7. Evaluate the blood glucose level and administer dextrose intravenously if indicated.
8. Attempt decontamination by either inducing emesis or performing gastric lavage. Gastric lavage is the preferred method of decontamination because of the rapid rate of absorption of cocaine from the gastrointestinal tract.
   A. Induction of emesis in cats
      I. Administer xylazine, 0.44–1 mg/kg IM or SC (can reverse with yohimbine 0.1 mg/kg IM, SC, or IV slowly).
      II. Administer medetomidine, 10 µg/kg IM (can reverse with atipamezole (Antisedan®) 25 µg/kg IM).
      III. Hydrogen peroxide is very difficult to administer to cats and is no longer recommended.
   B. Induction of emesis in dogs
      I. Administer apomorphine 0.02–0.04 mg/kg IV or IM, or 1.5–6 mg dissolved and placed into the conjunctival fornix. If apomorphine was placed in the eye, after emesis, the patient's eye should be thoroughly lavaged with sterile saline. If excessive sedation occurs from apomorphine, the sedation may be reversed by the administration of naloxone (0.01–0.04 mg/kg IV, IM, SC), but this will not reverse the emetic effects.
      II. Administer 3% hydrogen peroxide 1–5 mL/kg (0.5–2 mL/lb) PO, with a maximum dose of 3 tablespoons (45 mL). If the patient does not vomit within 10 minutes, give 3% hydrogen peroxide 0.5 mL/kg (0.25 mL/lb) PO *once*.
   C. Gastric lavage
      I. Lightly anesthetize the patient.
      II. Administer oxygen and intravenous fluids to the patient while under anesthesia.
      III. Maintain anesthesia with the appropriate anesthetic as needed.
      IV. Intubate the patient with a cuffed endotracheal tube and inflate the cuff.

V. Place the patient in lateral recumbency.

VI. With a stomach tube held outside of the patient, alongside the patient, measure the distance from the tip of the nose to the last rib. Mark this distance on the stomach tube.

VII. Lubricate the caudal end of the stomach tube with water-soluble jelly then pass the stomach tube gently into the stomach, passing the tube no farther than the marked distance on the tube.

VIII. If desired, two stomach tubes may be utilized, a smaller ingress tube and a large egress tube.

IX. Infuse warm (body-temperature) tap water, 5–10 mL/kg, through the tube (ingress tube if using two tubes) to moderately distend the stomach.

X. Allow the fluid to drain from the stomach through the tube (egress tube if using two tubes).

XI. Save samples of gastric contents, suspicious foreign material, seeds, etc. for possible toxicologic analysis.

XII. The stomach tube may have to be manipulated, repositioned or flushed with fluid or air if the gastric contents do not flow freely through the tube.

XIII. Turn the patient to the other side and continue to perform gastric lavage.

XIV. Continue gastric lavage until the effluent is clear.

XV. If using the two-tube method, crimp the end of one tube and remove it.

XVI. Administer activated charcoal down the stomach tube.

XVII. Crimp the end of the stomach tube and remove it.

XVIII. Monitor the patient during recovery from anesthesia, leaving the inflated cuffed endotracheal tube in place until the patient's swallowing reflex has returned.

D. Activated charcoal, 2–5 g/kg (3–6 mL/lb) PO is usually administered in a slurry of 1 g to 5 mL water. In cocaine toxicosis patients, repeat the administration of activated charcoal q3–4h. Administer a cathartic only once.

E. A single dose of an osmotic or saline cathartic should be administered along with activated charcoal. Avoid magnesium cathartics if the patient is exhibiting signs of neurologic dysfunction. Alternative cathartics include:

I. Sorbitol (70%), 2 g/kg (1–2 mL/kg) PO

II. Sodium sulfate, 200 mg/kg for cats, 250–500 mg/kg for dogs. Mix sodium sulfate with water, 5–10 mL/kg and administer PO.

9. Hospitalize the patient for observation and continued therapy.

10. If the patient has swallowed balloons or condoms containing cocaine, surgical removal is recommended. If surgical removal is not an option, perform whole bowel irrigation using PEG electrolyte solution (GoLYTELY® or CoLYTE®).

11. If the patient is not having seizures, administer chlorpromazine, up to 15 mg/kg, which opposes many of the clinical signs of cocaine intoxication.
12. Administer propranolol 0.04–0.06 mg/kg or higher, slow IV to treat atrial or supraventricular tachycardia.
13. Avoid the administration of lidocaine, which may exacerbate cardiac conduction disturbances.
14. If the patient is presented comatose, consider the administration of naloxone, 0.01–0.04 mg/kg IV, IM, SC, since opiate narcotics are often combined with cocaine

N,N-DEITHYLTOLUAMIDE (DEET) TOXICOSIS

Mode of action

The mode of action is unknown.

Sources

Dog and cat flea collars, flea sprays, insect repellents (Off®, Deep Woods Off®, Cutters®, etc.). DEET is often combined with fenvalerate, a pyrethrin.

Toxic dosages

The toxic dose is unknown. Cats are more sensitive than dogs. Clinical signs are seen in dogs after exposure to 0.05 oz of 0.09% fenvalerate/9% DEET solution.

Diagnosis

History—History of exposure.
Clinical signs—Young female cats are particularly sensitive. Clinical signs include erythema, cutaneous blisters and necrosis, vomiting, tremors, central nervous system signs (excitation, ataxia and seizures), and death.
Laboratory findings—No characteristic laboratory abnormalities have been documented. The parent compound and its metabolites remain detectable in the serum for up to 2 weeks following exposure.

Differential diagnosis

Encephalopathy, organophosphate intoxication, pyrethrin intoxication, antihistamine and decongestant intoxication.

Prognosis

The prognosis is usually fair to good; however, fatalities may occur.

Treatment

1. Inform the client of the diagnosis, prognosis and the cost of treatment.
2. Ensure a patent airway. Intubate the patient if necessary.

3. Administer supplemental oxygen and ventilation if necessary.
4. Place an intravenous catheter. Administer a balanced electrolyte crystalloid fluid intravenously to maintain perfusion, hydration and diuresis.
5. Administer diazepam, phenobarbital or pentobarbital if necessary to control seizures or hyperactivity.
   A. Diazepam 0.5–1 mg/kg IV in increments of 5–20 mg to effect
   B. Phenobarbital 2–4 mg/kg IV in dogs, 1–2 mg/kg IV in cats
   C. Pentobarbital 2–30 mg/kg slow IV to effect
6. In cases of dermal exposure, thoroughly wash the patient with warm water and a liquid dish-washing detergent or mild shampoo. Protective garments, including rubber gloves, should be worn while bathing the patient. Keep the patient warm by wrapping the patient in a towel until dry to prevent chilling.
7. Attempt decontamination by performing gastric lavage. Induction of emesis is contraindicated.
   A. Lightly anesthetize the patient.
   B. Administer oxygen and intravenous fluids to the patient while under anesthesia.
   C. Maintain anesthesia with the appropriate anesthetic as needed.
   D. Intubate the patient with a cuffed endotracheal tube and inflate the cuff.
   E. Place the patient in lateral recumbency.
   F. With a stomach tube held outside of the patient, alongside the patient, measure the distance from the tip of the nose to the last rib. Mark this distance on the stomach tube.
   G. Lubricate the caudal end of the stomach tube with water-soluble jelly then pass the stomach tube gently into the stomach, passing the tube no farther than the marked distance on the tube.
   H. If desired, two stomach tubes may be utilized, a smaller ingress tube and a large egress tube.
   I. Infuse warm (body-temperature) tap water, 5–10 mL/kg, through the tube (ingress tube if using two tubes) to moderately distend the stomach.
   J. Allow the fluid to drain from the stomach through the tube (egress tube if using two tubes).
   K. Save samples of gastric contents, suspicious foreign material, seeds, etc. for possible toxicologic analysis.
   L. The stomach tube may have to be manipulated, repositioned or flushed with fluid or air if the gastric contents do not flow freely through the tube.
   M. Turn the patient to the other side and continue to perform gastric lavage.
   N. Continue gastric lavage until the effluent is clear.
   O. If using the two-tube method, crimp the end of one tube and remove it.
   P. Administer activated charcoal down the stomach tube.
   Q. Crimp the end of the stomach tube and remove it.

R. Monitor the patient during recovery from anesthesia, leaving the inflated cuffed endotracheal tube in place until the patient's swallowing reflex has returned.

8. Activated charcoal, 2–5 g/kg (3–6 mL/lb) PO is usually administered in a slurry of 1 g to 5 mL water. In DEET toxicosis patients, repeat the administration of activated charcoal q3–4h. Administer a cathartic only once.

9. A single dose of an osmotic or saline cathartic should be administered along with activated charcoal. Avoid magnesium cathartics if the patient is exhibiting signs of neurologic dysfunction. Alternative cathartics include:
   A. Sorbitol (70%), 2 g/kg (1–2 mL/kg) PO
   B. Sodium sulfate, 200 mg/kg for cats, 250—500 mg/kg for dogs. Mix sodium sulfate with water, 5–10 mL/kg and administer PO.

10. Whole bowel irrigation with PEG electrolyte solution (CoLYTE® or GoLYTELY®) should be considered.

11. Provide symptomatic and supportive therapy, depending upon the individual patient's needs.

ETHYLENE GLYCOL INTOXICATION

Mode of action

Ethylene glycol is metabolized to glycoaldehyde, glycolic acid, glyoxalic acid and oxalic acid, which cause severe metabolic acidosis and acute renal failure. Oxalic acid may combine with calcium to form calcium oxalate crystals, which precipitate in the renal tubules and in the microvasculature of other organ systems. The maximum blood concentration from a single ingestion occurs within 1–4 hours of ingestion. Within 16–24 hours of ingestion, nearly all of the ethylene glycol is metabolized or excreted.

Sources

Ethylene glycol is found in antifreeze, solvents, rust removers, film processing solutions and taxidermist preservative solutions.

Toxic dosages

Dogs: 4–6 mL/kg.
Cats: 1.5 mL/kg.

Diagnosis

History—The patient may have a history of exposure, or of being in area of possible exposure. The owner may state that the pet is walking like it is drunk, and may notice anorexia, lethargy, seizures or vomiting.
Clinical signs—There are three phases:
   Stage I—neurologic disease signs include mild depression, ataxia, knuckling, seizures, peripheral neuropathy, hyperexcitability, stupor, coma and death. Other clinical signs include anorexia, vomiting,

hypothermia, polyuria and polydipsia. Cats often present depressed with elevation of the third eyelids. Signs occur within 30 minutes to 12 hours' post-ingestion.

Stage II—cardiorespiratory disease signs, tachypnea and tachycardia, occur 12–24 hours post-ingestion.

Stage III—renal disease signs, which include severe depression, vomiting, diarrhea, dehydration, azotemia and oliguric renal failure, occur 24–72 hours post ingestion. Palpation of the abdomen may reveal enlarged and painful kidneys.

The fluid vomited by the patient who has ingested antifreeze may be bright green, or bright green gastric fluid may be observed during gastric lavage.

Laboratory findings—

1. Unexplained metabolic acidosis.
2. Increased anion gap (AG): AG (in mEq/L) = $(Na^+ + K^+) - (HCO_3 + Cl^-)$. The normal anion gap = 10–15 mEq/l.
3. Serum hyperosmolality.
4. Increased osmolal gap. When measured serum osmolality is compared with calculated serum osmolality the normal osmolal gap is <10 mOsm/kg, but with ethylene glycol intoxication the gap is increased. Calculated osmolality in mOsm/kg = $1.86 (Na^+ + K^+) + (glucose/18) + (BUN/2.8) + 9$.
5. Hyperglycemia.
6. Hypercalcemia or hypocalcemia.
7. Hyperphosphatemia (due to ingestion of ethylene glycol products containing high concentrations of a phosphate-containing rust inhibitor).
8. Increased BUN and creatinine.
9. Isosthenuria.
10. Calcium oxalate crystalluria (*45% accuracy, not 100%*) may be seen as early as 4–6 hours after ingestion.
11. Serum or urine ethylene glycol levels can be measured at some diagnostic labs.
12. The Ethylene Glycol In-House Detection Kit (EGT Test Kit, PRN Pharmacal, Inc., Penfornixola, FL 32504 USA) was discontinued in 2010.
    A. This kit detected blood concentrations of 500 ppm (50 mg/dL) or greater from exposure within 12 hours of testing. After 18 hours following ingestion, this test was not reliable and false negatives could occur.
    B. This kit was not sensitive enough to depend exclusively upon for diagnosis of ethylene glycol intoxication in cats. A negative result needed to be evaluated along with the clinical signs and history. If there was any chance the cat may have ingested ethylene glycol, ethanol therapy should be initiated immediately.
13. The Kacey Ethylene Glycol Kit provides an estimate of the blood ethylene glycol level. Concentrations of 20 mg/dL or greater may be detected. It does not measure metabolites of ethylene glycol, so it must be used soon after ingestion to prevent false negative results.

Abdominal ultrasonography—May reveal renal echogenicity of a much higher intensity than normal owing to the presence of ethylene glycol nephrosis. A pattern referred to as the 'halo sign' may be observed. This pattern is due to a greater than normal cortical and medullary echogenicity with persistence of areas of lesser echo intensity at the corticomedullary junction and central medullary regions.

1. After about 4 hours following ingestion of ethylene glycol, the renal cortical echogenicity may equal that of the splenic parenchyma and exceed the echogenicity of the liver.
2. Normally, renal echogenicity is less than that of the liver, which is less than that of the spleen.
3. When the patient is in stage III ethylene glycol toxicosis, with acute renal failure, the halo sign may be observed. The renal echogenicity at this stage is much greater than that of the liver and splenic parenchyma.
4. These ultrasonographic findings are not pathognomonic for ethylene glycol intoxication. Differential diagnoses include degenerative, infiltrative or inflammatory processes or nephrocalcinosis from another etiology.

Differential diagnosis

Acute renal failure from another cause, seizures must be differentiated from other causes.

Prognosis

The prognosis is grave if the patient is exhibiting *any* clinical signs and guarded if the patient is presented within 1–2 hours of ingestion. The prognosis is also affected by the quantity of ethylene glycol ingested. Massive toxin ingestion (over four times the LD_{50}), which is often consumed in malicious poisoning cases, carries a grave prognosis. Coma and death may occur within 12 hours. The antidote is easily overwhelmed and unable to inhibit enough ADH to be effective.

If the halo sign is observed during abdominal ultrasonography of patients with ethylene glycol intoxication, the prognosis is grave.

According to one clinical study, none of the dogs that were azotemic upon entry survived, whether treated with 4-MP or with ethanol.

Treatment

1. Inform the client of the diagnosis, prognosis and the cost of treatment.
2. Ensure a patent airway. Intubate the patient if necessary.
3. Administer supplemental oxygen and ventilation if necessary.
4. If the patient is presented within 1 hour of ingestion, attempt decontamination by inducing emesis or performing gastric lavage.
   A. Induction of emesis in cats
      I. Administer xylazine, 0.44–1 mg/kg IM or SC (can reverse with yohimbine 0.1 mg/kg IM, SC, or IV slowly).

    II. Administer medetomidine, 10 µg/kg IM (can reverse with atipamezole (Antisedan®) 25 µg/kg IM).

    III. Hydrogen peroxide is very difficult to administer to cats and is no longer recommended.

B. Induction of emesis in dogs

    I. Administer apomorphine 0.02–0.04 mg/kg IV or IM, or 1.5–6 mg dissolved and placed into the conjunctival fornix. If apomorphine was placed in the eye, after emesis, the patient's eye should be thoroughly lavaged with sterile saline. If excessive sedation occurs from apomorphine, the sedation may be reversed by the administration of naloxone (0.01–0.04 mg/kg IV, IM, SC) but this will not reverse the emetic effects.

    II. Administer 3% hydrogen peroxide 1–5 mL/kg (0.5–2 mL/lb) PO, with a maximum dose of 3 tablespoons (45 mL). If the patient does not vomit within 10 minutes, give 3% hydrogen peroxide 0.5 mL/kg (0.25 mL/lb) PO *once*.

C. Gastric lavage

    I. Lightly anesthetize the patient. Propofol, 4–6 mL/kg, IV, may be utilized.

    II. Administer oxygen and intravenous fluids to the patient while under anesthesia.

    III. Maintain anesthesia with the appropriate anesthetic as needed.

    IV. Intubate the patient with a cuffed endotracheal tube and inflate the cuff.

    V. Place the patient in lateral recumbency.

    VI. With a stomach tube held outside of the patient, alongside the patient, measure the distance from the tip of the nose to the last rib. Mark this distance on the stomach tube.

    VII. Lubricate the caudal end of the stomach tube with water-soluble jelly then pass the stomach tube gently into the stomach, passing the tube no farther than the marked distance on the tube.

    VIII. If desired, two stomach tubes may be utilized, a smaller ingress tube and a large egress tube.

    IX. Infuse warm (body-temperature) tap water, 5–10 mL/kg, through the tube (ingress tube if using two tubes) to moderately distend the stomach.

    X. Allow the fluid to drain from the stomach through the tube (egress tube if using two tubes).

    XI. Save samples of gastric contents, suspicious foreign material, seeds, etc. for possible toxicologic analysis.

    XII. The stomach tube may have to be manipulated, repositioned or flushed with fluid or air if the gastric contents do not flow freely through the tube.

    XIII. Turn the patient to the other side and continue to perform gastric lavage.

    XIV. Continue gastric lavage until the effluent is clear.

    XV. If using the two-tube method, crimp the end of one tube and remove it.

XVI. Crimp the end of the stomach tube and remove it.

XVII. Monitor the patient during recovery from anesthesia, leaving the inflated cuffed endotracheal tube in place until the patient's swallowing reflex has returned.

   D. Activated charcoal does not bind well with ethylene glycol and lacks efficacy. The administration of activated charcoal in the treatment of ethylene glycol ingestion is no longer recommended.

4. Place an intravenous catheter. Jugular catheterization is particularly useful as it will allow monitoring of central venous pressure.

5. Administer diazepam, phenobarbital or pentobarbital if necessary to control seizures or hyperactivity.

   A. Diazepam 0.5–1 mg/kg IV in increments of 5–20 mg to effect

   B. Phenobarbital 2–4 mg/kg IV in dogs, 1–2 mg/kg IV in cats

   C. Pentobarbital 2–30 mg/kg slow IV to effect.

6. Administer an antidote immediately: either 4-methylpyrazole or ethanol.

   A. Fomepizole (4-Methylpyrazole [4-MP]) therapy

      I. 4-MP is an alcohol dehydrogenase inhibitor that does not induce hyperosmolality, diuresis or CNS depression. It directly inhibits the alcohol dehydrogenase enzyme by forming a ternary complex with alcohol dehydrogenase and its coenzyme nicotinamide adenine dinucleotide (NAD).

      II. The administration of 4-MP is effective when given to a dog as late as 8 hours after ingestion of 10 mL/kg of antifreeze. Therapy should be initiated within 3 hours after ingestion by cats.

      III. Even if the dog is presented as late as 36 hours following ethylene glycol ingestion, the administration of 4-MP may be effective.

      IV. 4-MP will not contribute to CNS depression or serum osmolality.

      V. 4-MP is currently the treatment of choice for dogs and cats. If it is not available, or is cost prohibitive, ethanol therapy may be substituted.

      VI. The recommended dosages of 4-MP in dogs are:

         a. The recommended initial loading dose of 4-MP is 20 mg/kg IV.

         b. Administer 4-MP 15 mg/kg IV at 12 and 24 hours after initiation of therapy.

         c. Administer 4-MP 5 mg/kg IV at 36 hours after initiation of therapy.

         d. After 10–11 hours following the administration of the 36-hour dose of 4-MP, perform another ethylene glycol test on the dog. If the test is positive, continue to administer 4-MP 5 mg/kg every 12 hours for 2 treatments, then retest. Repeat until the test is negative.

         The recommended dosages of 4-MP in cats are:

         a. The recommended initial loading dose of 4-MP is 125 mg/kg IV.

     b. Administer 4-MP 31.25 mg/kg IV at 12, 24, and 36 hours after initiation of therapy.

     c. After 10–11 hours following the administration of the 36-hour dose of 4-MP, perform another ethylene glycol test on the cat. If the test is positive, continue to administer 31.25 mg/kg IV every 12 hours for 2 treatments, then retest. Repeat until the test is negative or the cat is euthanized.

  VII. If the test is negative, discontinue 4-MP therapy.

 VIII. The commercially available product is Antizol Vet®. A single 'Fomepizole Kit' contains one small vial of 1.5 g of 4-MP and a 30 mL bottle of sterile 0.9% NaCl. Once the two bottles are mixed together, the shelf life is 72 hours.

   IX. If the patient is a small dog that will not utilize an entire kit, or a large dog that requires more than one kit but less than two entire kits, portions of the 4-MP bottle may be utilized.

     a. The small vial containing 1.5 g of 4-MP is in a gel form that can be warmed by holding it in the hand until it liquefies. The total volume = 1.5 mL, which contains 1 g 4-MP/mL.

     b. If the dose needed is 300 mg of 4-MP, aspirate 0.3 mL of the liquid 4-MP concentrate and then dilute it with 0.9% NaCl, either from the kit or from the hospital shelf. The concentrated 4-MP must be diluted prior to administration. A standard concentration is 5% (50 mg/mL). To achieve this concentration, dilute the 0.3 mL 4-MP with 6 mL of 0.9% NaCl.

    X. If the substrates may be obtained, 4-MP may be prepared in the hospital.

     a. Add 5 g of 4-MP to 50 mL of polyethylene glycol 400 and 46 mL of bacteriostatic water to make 100 mL.

     b. Filter the solution through a 0.22 mm filter.

     c. The resulting concentration is 5% (50 mg 4-MP/mL).

     d. The solution should be protected from light and refrigerated.

     e. The shelf life of refrigerated 4-MP made from substrates in the hospital is 2 years.

   XI. The adverse clinical signs of 4-MP may include excessive salivation, gagging, tachypnea and trembling. Hepatotoxicity due to the pyrazole component is possible, but has not been reported.

B. Ethanol is a competitive substrate for ethylene glycol that has a higher affinity for alcohol dehydrogenase. However, treatment with ethanol may cause CNS depression, increases plasma hyperosmolality, enhances diuresis and is labor intensive

   I. Ethanol administration is most effective if initiated sooner than 4–8 hours after ingestion.

  II. Ethanol therapy is safe for both cats and dogs.

 III. Administer 7% ethanol; 7% ethanol = 70 mg/mL.

    a. **To make a 7% ethanol solution**
      Mix 140 mL 100 proof vodka with 1 liter 5% dextrose in 0.9% NaCl or in 1 liter Normosol®-R.

Toxicologic emergencies

b. Administer a loading dose of 7% ethanol, 600 mg/kg IV, followed by a maintenance dose of 7% ethanol, 100–200 mg/kg/h CRI IV.

  i. Loading dose = 600 mg/kg × 1 mL/70 mg = 8.6 mL/kg.
  ii. Maintenance dose = 100–200 mg/kg/h of 7% ethanol = 100 mg/kg × 1 mL/70 mg = 1.43 mL/kg/h CRI IV; or 200 mg/kg × 1 mL/70 mg = 2.86 mL/kg/h CRI IV.
  iii. The maintenance dose of 200 mg/kg/h CRI IV is recommended during peritoneal dialysis.
  iv. Continue the 7% ethanol IV at 100 mg/kg/h CRI for 10 hours after discontinuing peritoneal dialysis.

7. Administer 2.5% dextrose in 0.45% NaCl IV at a rate of 2–3 times maintenance, to maintain perfusion, hydration and diuresis.

  A. Administer the dehydration deficit over the first 4–6 hours; % dehydration × body weight in kg × 1000 = volume of fluid to be administered in mL.
  B. A fluid bolus of 20 mL/kg IV over 10 minutes may help assess the patient's response and the potential for fluid overload.
  C. If the patient presents in severe hypovolemic shock, administer fluids rapidly. In dogs, administer fluids at 70–90 mL/kg IV over the first hour. In cats, administer fluids at 30–40 mL/kg IV over the first hour.
  D. If the patient presents in severe hypovolemic shock, is hypotensive or is hypoproteinemic, also consider the administration of Hetastarch (14–20 mL/kg IV) or plasma (10–30 mL/kg IV) in addition to the crystalloid fluids.

9. During the rehydration phase of fluid therapy, monitor the CVP, PCV, TS, and body weight frequently.

  A. The CVP should not increase more than 5–7 cm H_2O. Higher increases indicate possible fluid overload.
  B. Other signs of overhydration include tachycardia, restlessness, shivering, chemosis, exophthalmos, dyspnea, tachypnea, increased bronchovesicular sounds, pulmonary crackles and edema, serous nasal discharge, decreased mentation, nausea, vomiting, diarrhea, ascites, polyuria and subcutaneous edema (particularly of the tarsal joints and intermandibular space).
  C. If overhydration occurs, slow or discontinue fluid administration. Administer diuretics and / or vasodilators and oxygen if indicated.

10. In cases of oliguric or anuric renal failure, it is best to have an indwelling urinary catheter from which urine production can be determined. It is also helpful to have an indwelling catheter in polyuric renal failure, but these cases can much more easily be managed without knowing exact urine production amounts. Minimum urine output should be 1–2 mL/kg/h after a patient is rehydrated. Strict aseptic technique and a closed collection system must be utilized.

11. Monitor the patient's body weight every 6–12 hours. Monitor the patient closely for signs of overhydration.

12. After rehydration, if urine output is insufficient, administer an IV fluid bolus of at least 5–10 mL/kg. If monitoring CVPs, attempt to increase the CVP by 5–7 cm H_2O with fluid boluses. If this does not improve urine production consider other agents:

A. Mannitol (10% or 20%), 0.1–0.5 g/kg administered IV over 10-15 minutes, if there are no contraindications (vasculitis, bleeding disorders, hyperosmolar syndrome, congestive heart failure, volume overload). If no increase in urine production within 30 minutes, the same dose may be repeated. Do not exceed a mannitol dose of 2 g/kg/day.

B. Hypertonic dextrose (10–20% solutions) may be used as an alternative to mannitol. Check the patient's blood glucose level first. Do not administer hypertonic dextrose if the patient is hyperglycemic. The dose of 10–20% dextrose is 25–50 mL/kg as an intermittent slow IV bolus over 1–2h, repeated q8–12h.

Mannitol and hypertonic dextrose may be more helpful in patients with renal tubular damage leading to filling of the renal tubules with debris that will be forced out by the osmotic effects of these drugs.

C. Furosemide is usually given as a bolus followed by a constant rate infusion. If the bolus (repeated 1–2 times total) does not lead to urine production then the CRI will not help either. Bolus dose = 1–6 mg/kg IV. Constant rate infusion is at the dose of 0.25–1 mg/kg/h CRI IV.

D. Dopamine administration may be beneficial in *dogs*.

I. To increase renal blood flow and urine volume, administer dopamine, 0.5–5 mcg/kg/min in 0.9% NaCl CRI IV. Do not add dopamine to alkaline fluids.

II. Does not help in cats due to reduced or absent dopaminergic receptors in cat kidneys.

E. Diltiazem has been shown in leptospirosis in *dogs* to have a positive effect. Diltiazem was administered 0.1–0.5 mg/kg IV over 30 minutes followed by 1–5 mcg/kg/min as a CRI to induce improved renal recovery in patients with leptospirosis. Diltiazem was added to patients' treatment regimens in addition to IV crystalloid fluid therapy, ampicillin, +/– furosemide and +/– dopamine.

13. If diuresis cannot be induced, perform peritoneal dialysis or hemodialysis. Indications for dialysis include:

A. Exposure to dialyzable toxins

B. Treatment of overhydration

C. Severe persistent uremia, acidosis or hyperkalemia

D. Oliguria / anuria.

14. Placement of a peritoneal dialysis catheter (Fig. 14.2)

A. Administer a general anesthetic, being cautious to avoid hypotension.

B. Consider performing an omentectomy or partial omentectomy, to decrease omental plugging of the peritoneal dialysis catheter, particularly in the cat.

C. The surgeon *must* use sterile technique. Every junction of the peritoneal catheter set must be covered with a povidone-iodine wrap, which is changed daily.

D. Use a peritoneal dialysis catheter, a pediatric trocath or, for cats, use a 14-GA Teflon IV catheter with additional side holes, placed all on the same side to preserve the integrity of the catheter.

E. Consider obtaining a renal biopsy at the time the peritoneal dialysis catheter is placed.

F. Make a stab incision (1 cm) through the linea alba 2–4 cm caudal to the umbilicus.

G. Aim the catheter towards the pelvic inlet.

H. Secure the catheter by suturing to the abdominal wall, not just to skin. Use a purse-string suture at the entry site and a 'Chinese finger-lock' suture on the catheter to secure it in position.

I. Cover the entry site into the abdomen with a povidone-iodine patch and a sterile bandage.

J. Administer broad-spectrum antibiotics. Administer an appropriate dose and at an appropriate frequency for a patient with ARF.

K. Use *warm* 1.5%, 4.0%, or 7% dextrose dialysate solution, or LRS, or 0.9% NaCl. (The preferable solution, if commercial dialysate solution is not available, is 1.5% dextrose in LRS; it is made by adding 30 mL 50% dextrose to 1000 mL LRS.)

L. Add 250 units heparin/liter of dialysate.

M. Infuse 20–30 mL/kg intraperitoneal (IP).

N. Dwell time = 45 minutes.

O. Drainage time = 15 minutes.

P. Repeat *continuously*, or every 2 hours until the BUN, creatinine and hydration status approach normal values, then decrease the frequency of dialysis.

Q. Flush the peritoneal catheter with 5–10 mL heparinized saline after each infusion or drainage to diminish clogging of peritoneal catheter.

R. Monitor the patient's CBC, TP, serum electrolytes, clotting parameters, body temperature, urine (sediment and dipstick) and the dialysate for signs of infection.

S. When peritoneal lavage is no longer necessary, sedate or anesthetize the patient, remove the peritoneal catheter and close the abdominal incision with one to two sutures in the linea alba, then close the skin. Apply a sterile abdominal wrap.

15. Maintenance of the peritoneal dialysis catheter

A. Sterility is *very important*.

B. Wash hands thoroughly prior to wearing sterile gloves when handling the peritoneal dialysis catheter.

C. Flush the catheter with heparinized saline after every installation and drainage.

D. Wipe every connection and injection port with chlorhexidine or povidone-iodine solution every time prior to manipulation.

E. Every junction of the peritoneal catheter set and every injection port must be covered with a sterile povidone-iodine wrap, which is changed daily. This is not always done any more, but it is not really wrong either.

F. Cover the entry site into the abdomen with a sterile bandage.

G. Keep a clean, dry and sterile bandage on the abdomen, over the catheter entry site. Check the bandage, the entry site and bandage every 12–24 hours. Change the bandage every 2 days.

H. If at all possible, perform the installation and drainage of the peritoneal lavage fluid in the surgical suite to keep contamination to a minimum.

16. If administering ethanol therapy, continue the 7% ethanol IV at 1.43 mL/kg/hr CRI IV for 10 hours after discontinuing peritoneal dialysis.

17. **Do not administer sodium bicarbonate** unless blood tests indicate a severe metabolic acidosis (HCO_3 <12 mEq/L, pH <7.10). To treat moderate metabolic acidosis, administer appropriate intravenous fluid therapy, intubate the patient, administer oxygen and improve ventilation.

A. 0.3–$0.5 \times$ body weight in kg $\times$ (24 – plasma bicarbonate level) = mEq of sodium bicarbonate needed.

B. Infuse half of the sodium bicarbonate amount needed over the first 3–4 hours, then re-evaluate and readjust the dose.

C. Caution must be utilized while administering sodium bicarbonate. Possible complications that may result include: 'overshoot alkalosis', hypernatremia, intravascular volume overload, hypokalemia, hypocalcemia, tissue hypoxia, and paradoxical cerebrospinal fluid acidosis.

18. If the client is unwilling or unable to hospitalize the patient, advise them to administer 40% alcohol (80 proof, which contains 40 g alcohol/100 mL) orally.

A. The oral dose of 40% alcohol (vodka, rum, etc.) is 2.25 mL/kg (1 mL/lb) PO q4h for 4 treatments.

B. Because dehydration is a common side effect, it is important to have drinking water available to the pet at all times and for the client to encourage drinking.

GARBAGE INTOXICATION (ENTEROTOXEMIA)

Mode of action

Altered gastrointestinal motility, altered gastrointestinal permeability and CNS signs occur due to endotoxin release from dead bacteria. Several different mechanisms and pathways are involved, the end result being a severe, life-threatening disease including many different syndromes such as DIC (disseminated intravascular coagulation), PTE (pulmonary thromboembolism), ARDS (acute respiratory distress syndrome), SIRS (systemic inflammatory response syndrome), MODS (multiple organ dysfunction syndrome), and death.

Penitrem A is a neurotoxin that affects nerves by increasing the resting potential, facilitating the transmission of impulses across motor end plates, and prolonging the duration of depolarization. Penitrem A may also act like strychnine in the spinal cord by inhibiting the effects of glycine.

Sources

The ingestion of decomposing carrion, garbage, spoiled food and compost is common by dogs. The common organisms implicated in food poisoning include *Escherichia coli*, *Staphylococcus*, *Streptococcus*, *Salmonella* spp., *Bacillus* spp., *Clostridium perfringens* and *Clostridium botulinum*.

Penitrem A occurs in moldy nuts (including peanuts, almonds and walnuts), moldy food, garbage and moldy grains.

Toxic dosages

The toxic doses are not established.

Diagnosis

History—The incidence of food poisoning increases during warmer months and around holidays. The owner may provide a history of the pet getting into the garbage or eating spoiled food. Some owners intentionally feed their dogs spoiled food, under the misguided opinion that it is safe.

Clinical signs—Clinical signs usually begin within 3 hours following ingestion. The signs include vomiting, diarrhea (which may become bloody), dehydration, fever and signs of endotoxic shock. The signs of endotoxic shock include depression, hypotension, collapse, either a rapid or a slow capillary refill time, hypothermia or hyperthermia, and oliguria.

The clinical signs of botulism include vomiting, hypersalivation, abdominal pain, dry eyes and hindlimb weakness. There is depression of the withdrawal, deep tendon, gag and pupillary reflexes.

The clinical signs of penitrem A intoxication include panting, restlessness, hypersalivation, incoordination, fine muscle tremors of the head and neck which progress to the entire body, tonic spasms (which appear similar to strychnine intoxication), hyperthermia, hypermetria, ataxia, opisthotonos, seizures, and death. The muscle spasms may be worsened by external stimuli similar to, but not as consistent as with strychnine intoxication.

Laboratory findings—
1. The CBC may reveal an early leukopenia and neutropenia followed by leukocytosis and neutrophilia with toxic neutrophils, and an increased hematocrit.
2. The platelet count may be decreased if the patient has DIC.
3. Hyperglycemia occurs early and hypoglycemia occurs late in the course of the disease.

4. Hepatic enzyme elevation may occur with sepsis.
5. Rhabdomyolysis may lead to acute renal failure.

Differential diagnosis

Garbage intoxication may resemble parvovirus gastroenteritis, gastrointestinal foreign body obstruction, gastric dilatation and volvulus, intestinal volvulus, intussusception, peritonitis and acute pancreatitis.

Botulism resembles myasthenia gravis, carbon monoxide poisoning, coral snake envenomation, algal intoxication, drug intoxication, polyradiculoneuritis, rabies, trauma and spinal cord disorders.

Penitrem A intoxication can appear similar to strychnine intoxication, boric acid intoxication, mushroom intoxication and eclampsia.

Prognosis

The prognosis varies with the substance ingested, the clinical signs and the duration of the illness by the time of presentation.

Treatment

1. Inform the client of the diagnosis, prognosis and the cost of treatment.
2. Ensure a patent airway. Intubate the patient if necessary.
3. Administer supplemental oxygen and ventilation if necessary.
4. Place an intravenous catheter. Administer a balanced electrolyte crystalloid fluid such as Normosol®-R or LRS intravenously to maintain perfusion, hydration and diuresis.
   A. If the patient is in shock, administer the fluids at the following rates:
      I. Dogs: 90–100 mL/kg first 1–2 hours
      II. Cats: 45–60 mL/kg first 1–2 hours
      III. After the first 1–2 hours, re-evaluate the patient's cardiovascular status. Generally decrease the rate to 20–40 mL/kg/h in dogs and 20–30 mL/kg/h in cats until the patient is stabilized. Continue at maintenance rates (1–2 mL/kg/h) when stable.
   B. If the patient is in severe shock, administer Hetastarch or Dextran 70, 20 mL/kg IV. An additional 20 mL/kg of Hetastarch may be administered over the next 6–8 hours if needed for continued shock.
   C. Consider the administration of plasma, 10–20 mL/kg IV, if the serum albumin is <2.0 g/dL and the patient exhibits signs of complications from hypoproteinemia.
   D. Control seizures or muscle spasms if necessary.
      I. Acepromazine may be used cautiously. The dose of acepromazine is 0.05–0.1 mg/kg IM. Repeat the administration of acepromazine q20–30 min until the patient calms down. Use caution if the patient is hypotensive.
      II. Administer diazepam 0.5–1 mg/kg IV in increments of 5–20 mg to effect.
      III. Administer phenobarbital 2–4 mg/kg IV in dogs, 1–2 mg/kg IV in cats.

IV. Administer pentobarbital 2–30 mg/kg slow IV to effect.

V. Administer methocarbamol to control muscle spasms. The dose of methocarbamol is 44.4–222 mg/kg slow IV in dogs, 44.4 mg/kg slow IV in cats.

6. Unless the patient has already purged its stomach by vomiting, attempt decontamination by performing *gastric lavage*. The administration of emetics is contraindicated since the disease process will result in excessive emesis, requiring antiemetic therapy.

   A. Lightly anesthetize the patient.

   B. Administer oxygen and intravenous fluids to the patient while under anesthesia.

   C. Maintain anesthesia with the appropriate anesthetic as needed.

   D. Intubate the patient with a cuffed endotracheal tube and inflate the cuff.

   E. Place the patient in lateral recumbency.

   F. With a stomach tube held outside of the patient, alongside the patient, measure the distance from the tip of the nose to the last rib. Mark this distance on the stomach tube.

   G. Lubricate the caudal end of the stomach tube with water-soluble jelly then pass the stomach tube gently into the stomach, passing the tube no farther than the marked distance on the tube.

   H. If desired, two stomach tubes may be utilized, a smaller ingress tube and a large egress tube.

   I. Infuse warm (body-temperature) tap water, 5–10 mL/kg, through the tube (ingress tube if using two tubes) to moderately distend the stomach.

   J. Allow the fluid to drain from the stomach through the tube (egress tube if using two tubes).

   K. Save samples of gastric contents, suspicious foreign material, seeds, etc. for possible toxicologic analysis.

   L. The stomach tube may have to be manipulated, repositioned or flushed with fluid or air if the gastric contents do not flow freely through the tube.

   M. Turn the patient to the other side and continue to perform gastric lavage.

   N. Continue gastric lavage until the effluent is clear.

   O. If using the two-tube method, crimp the end of one tube and remove it.

   P. Administer activated charcoal down the stomach tube.

   Q. Crimp the end of the stomach tube and remove it.

   R. Monitor the patient during recovery from anesthesia, leaving the inflated cuffed endotracheal tube in place until the patient's swallowing reflex has returned.

7. Activated charcoal, 2–5 g/kg (3–6 mL/lb) PO is usually administered in a slurry of 1 g to 5 mL water. In garbage intoxication (enterotoxemia) patients, repeat the administration of activated charcoal q2–4h. Monitor the serum sodium concentration frequently and avoid hypernatremia.

8. An osmotic or saline cathartic is usually not recommended because diarrhea is usually severe.
9. Hospitalize the patient for observation and continued therapy.
10. For maintenance therapy, administer intravenous crystalloid fluids at the rate of 60 mL/kg/24h for dogs and 40 mL/kg/24h for cats, plus the deficit plus losses.
11. Supplement potassium as indicated by the serum potassium level.
12. If the patient exhibits excessive, repeated vomiting, or nausea, administer antiemetics after volume replacement is achieved.
    A. Chlorpromazine, 0.05–0.1 mg/kg IV q4–6h as needed, 0.2–0.5 mg/kg SC, IM q6–8h, or 1 mg/kg diluted in 1 mL of 0.9% NaCl and administered rectally q8h via a plastic catheter. Avoid chlorpromazine if the patient is epileptic or is having seizures.
    B. Prochlorperazine, 0.25–0.5 mg/kg SC, IM q6–8h
    C. Ondansetron (Zofran®), 0.1–0.2 mg/kg IV q6–12h
    D. Dolasetron (Anzemet®), 0.6–1 mg/kg IV, SC or PO q24h
    E. Maropitant (Cerenia®), 1 mg/kg SC or 2 mg/kg PO q24h for up to 5 days
    F. Metoclopramide (Reglan®), 0.2–0.4 mg/kg SC or IM q8h or 0.01–0.02 mg/kg/h CRI IV. If the patient is on metoclopramide, it is very important to palpate the abdomen every 2–4 hours and closely monitor for intussusception. Avoid metoclopramide if a mechanical obstruction is suspected or if the patient has a history of seizures.
13. If hematemesis or signs of nausea (drooling, exaggerated swallowing motions) occur, administer:
    A. Famotidine (Pepcid®), 0.5–1 mg/kg IV q12h
    B. Ranitidine (Zantac®), 2 mg/kg IV or SC q8–12h in dogs or 2.5 mg/kg IV q12h in cats
    C. Omeprazole (Prilosec®)
       I. Dogs: 0.5–1.5 mg/kg PO q24h
       II. Cats: 0.5–1 mg/kg PO q24h
    D. Pantoprazole (Protonix®), 0.7–1 mg/kg IV q24h.
14. Administer broad-spectrum antibiotic therapy.
    A. Administer a combination of ampicillin (20–40 mg/kg q8h IV), or a first generation cephalosporin (cefazolin, 20 mg/kg q8h IV, or cephalothin, 20–30 mg/kg q6h IV), with a fluoroquinolone (enrofloxacin, 5–15 mg/kg IV, IM, SC q12h or 5–20 mg/kg q24h IV, ciprofloxacin, 5–15 mg/kg PO q12h or 10–20 mg/kg PO q24h in dogs, 5 mg/kg q24h in cats), with an aminoglycoside (amikacin, 3.5–5 mg/kg q8h IV or 10–15 mg/kg q24h IV, gentamicin, 6–9 mg/kg/24h IV or 2–3 mg/kg q8h IV, or tobramycin, 2–4 mg/kg q8h IV), or a third-generation cephalosporin (ceftizoxime 25–50 mg/kg IV, IM, SC q6–8h, cefotaxime 20–80 mg/kg IV, IM q6–8h) and metronidazole, 10 mg/kg IV CRI over 1 hour, q8–12h.
       I. Aminoglycosides are contraindicated in patients with suspected botulism.
       II. Aminoglycosides should be avoided in the presence of dehydration or azotemia as they may cause renal failure.

III. Aminoglycosides administered once every 24 hours are more effective and cause less renal toxicity.

IV. If furosemide is utilized, aminoglycosides should be discontinued, as the combination increases the risk of inducing iatrogenic renal failure.

V. When the patient is on aminoglycosides, urine sediment should be evaluated at least daily for casts and cellular debris.

VI. The penicillins have been combined with a β-lactamase inhibitor (ticarcillin-clavulanate (Timentin®, 30–50 mg/kg IV q6–8h), ampicillin-sublactam (Unasyn®, 50 mg/kg IV q6–8h), and piperacillin-tazobactam (Zosyn®, 50 mg/kg IV, IM q4–6h)) for increased efficacy.

B. Administer a combination of cefoxitin (40 mg/kg IV initially and continued at 20 mg/kg IV q6–8h in the dog and q8h in the cat) and metronidazole, 10 mg/kg IV CRI over 1 hour, q8–12h.

C. The antibiotics of choice for suspected botulism patients are penicillin G 20 000 U/kg IM q12h or sodium ampicillin 16 mg/kg IM or IV q6h.

15. Botulism antitoxin should be administered to patients with suspected botulism. Administer type A, B, C, and E antitoxins if available. Allergic reactions may occur from the antitoxins.

16. Additional medications useful in the treatment of botulism include:
A. Physostigmine (Antilirium®) 0.02 mg/kg, or neostigmine (Stiglyn®) 1–2 mg IM as needed (acetylcholinesterase inhibitors)
B. Atropine (to block the muscarinic effects) 0.02–0.04 mg/kg IV or SC if the patient has excessive bradycardia. Avoid the administration of atropine to a hypertensive patient as it may exacerbate the hypertension.

17. Consider the oral administration of barium in therapeutic doses; kaopectate, or bismuth subsalicylate may be beneficial.
A. Therapeutic barium sulfate, 0.5–1 mL/kg PO q12h
B. Kaopectate, 2–5 mL/kg PO q1–6h
C. Bismuth subsalicylate
I. Dogs: 0.25–2 mL/kg PO q6–8h
II. Cats: 0.25 mL/kg PO q6h

18. Provide symptomatic and supportive therapy for accompanying disease syndromes including DIC, ARDS, and PTE as indicated by the individual patient.

GLOW JEWELRY

Toxin

The toxic substance is dibutyl phthalate, which has a wide margin of safety.

Mode of action

The ingestion of dibutyl phthalate causes a severe adverse taste response, exhibited as agitation, severe hypersalivation, oropharyngeal discomfort, and emesis. Ocular exposure may cause copious lacrimation, stinging, conjunctivitis, conjunctival edema, and photophobia.

Dermal exposure in people may cause stinging, burning, redness and contact dermatitis.

Sources

Dibutyl phthalate is found in children's toys, emergency products, battery-free night-lights, etc. Some glow jewelry pieces contain small batteries or other luminescent chemicals not covered in this section.

Toxic dosages

Usually only a small amount is ingested, due to the extremely unpleasant taste.

Diagnosis

History—The pet may be observed chewing on the glow item or signs of destruction of an item may accompany the clinical signs in the pet.

Clinical signs—Immediately after exposure the patient may become agitated, and exhibit excessive hypersalivation and vomiting. To identify the product on the hair coat, take the patient into a darkened room. The contaminated areas may glow in the dark.

Prognosis

The prognosis is excellent.

Treatment

1. Inform the client of the diagnosis, prognosis and cost of the treatment.
2. Do *not* induce emesis.
3. Rinse the mouth several times with cool water.
4. Give the patient milk, liquid from a tuna fish can, chicken broth or other tasty treat to help get rid of the taste.
5. Remove dibutyl phthalate on the fur with a wet cloth or mild nonmedicated shampoo rinsed well to prevent re-exposure.
6. Administer supportive therapy as needed.
7. For patients with ocular exposure, lavage the eyes for 10–15 minutes with sterile saline. Evaluate the patient for corneal ulceration or keratitis.

GRAPES AND RAISINS TOXICITY

Toxin

The toxic principle is unknown. Many different species of grapes (*Vitis* spp.) throughout the world have been involved.

- Ochratoxin is a possibility.
- It is a possible inability to process flavonoids, tannins and excessive monosaccharides.

It appears to be an idiosyncratic reaction

Mode of action

Severe diffuse degeneration of the renal proximal tubules and acute renal failure occurs, resulting in death. Pancreatitis has also been reported.

Sources

Grapes or raisins.

Toxic dosages

There are no published cases of grape or raisin toxicity in cats. For dogs, the toxic amount is unknown. In one report, the amounts ingested were from 42 to 896 g (1.5–32 oz), with a median dosage of 19.6 g/kg (0.7 oz/kg), or as few as 4–5 grapes.

Due to the potentially fatal outcome, the APCC recommends that no amount of grapes or raisins be fed to a dog.

Diagnosis

History—There is a history of exposure or possible exposure within the 12 hours prior to the onset of clinical signs.

Clinical signs—The clinical signs include vomiting, diarrhea, lethargy, weakness, ataxia, abdominal pain and decreased urine output.

Laboratory findings—Increased serum BUN, creatinine, phosphorus, and electrolyte changes, isosthenuria, possible nephritic syndrome (increased cholesterol, azotemia, pathologic proteinuria, peripheral edema).

Run CBC to rule out pyelonephritis.

Run serum leptospirosis titers.

Run an ethylene glycol test (if there is any doubt, treat as for ethylene glycol intoxication, including the administration of 4-methylpyrazole).

Differential diagnosis

Ethylene glycol intoxication, NSAID ingestion, sepsis, heat stroke, pancreatitis, leptospirosis, pyelonephritis, vitamin D rodenticide intoxication, neoplasia, etc.

Prognosis

The prognosis is good to poor depending upon the clinical signs at presentation. In one study, 53% of 43 dogs survived, 35% of dogs were euthanized and 12% of dogs died.

Treatment

1. Inform the client of the diagnosis, prognosis and cost of the treatment.
2. Rapid gastric decontamination by inducing emesis should be performed, even in patients that are presented the following day after ingestion.
   A. Administer apomorphine 0.03 mg/kg IV, 0.04 mg/kg IM, or 1.5–6 mg dissolved and placed into the conjunctival fornix.
   B. Administer 3% hydrogen peroxide 1–2 mL/kg (0.5–1 mL/lb) PO, with a maximum dose of 2 tablespoons (30 mL). If the patient does not vomit within 15 minutes, give 3% hydrogen peroxide 0.5 mL/kg (0.25 mL/lb) PO *once*.
3. The benefits of activated charcoal administration are unknown and should be considered for each individual patient. The usually recommended dosage is 2–5 g/kg (3–6 mL/lb) PO.
4. There is no antidote. Administer 4-methylpyrazole if ethylene glycol intoxication is possible.
5. Treatment is supportive and symptomatic.
   A. Administer intravenous fluids (2.5% dextrose in 0.45% NaCl, LRS, Normosol®-R).
   B. Administer antiemetics as needed.
   C. Administer famotidine or other gastric protectants as needed.
   D. Administer antibiotics if the patient potentially has pyelonephritis or leptospirosis.
   E. Administer an oral phosphate binder if indicated.
   F. Monitor for hypertension and treat accordingly.
6. Dopamine, furosemide or mannitol may be indicated if urine output is insufficient.
7. Hemodialysis or peritoneal dialysis is indicated if the patient becomes oliguric, anuric, or if volume overload occurs.

HERB, VITAMIN AND NATURAL SUPPLEMENT TOXICOSIS

Definitions

- *Herb*—a plant used for medicinal purposes or for its olfactory or flavoring properties.
- *Homeopathic medications*—solutions containing extremely dilute concentrations of plant extracts that exhibit no significant pharmacologic action and present no toxicologic hazard.
- *Chinese patent medications*—herbs formulated into concentrated liquids such as tinctures, which use alcohol as a vehicle, pills or tablets. These products usually contain the greatest concentrations of herbal medications.
- *Raw herbs*—for consumption, they are consumed directly or dried and ground into powders.
- *Decoctions*—concentrated herbal extracts prepared in a small volume by boiling off the water in which raw herbs are steeped. These products also contain high concentrations of the active herbal constituents.
- *Herbal teas*—prepared by steeping raw herbs in hot or warm water.

These products are classified as dietary supplements rather than medications and are not regulated by the FDA.

Many herbal and natural products may be toxic to dogs and cats. Those reported include:

1. Aloe
   A. Ingestion of aloe may result in vomiting, diarrhea, nephritis and abdominal pain. Intoxication may also occur following grooming of topically applied aloe.
   B. The toxic principle is barbaloin, an anthraquinone glycoside contained in the leaf sap, which is metabolized to a sugar and an aglycone called emodin, which stimulates large bowel peristalsis.
   C. It is used topically to treat burns and is found in many shampoos, conditioners, lotions and skin products.
2. Chamomile
   A. Ingestion may result in vomiting and ataxia.
   B. The toxic principle is a volatile oil and anthemic acid derived from the botanical source *Anthemis flores* or *A. nobilis*.
   C. It is used as an antispasmodic, digestive aid and poultice.
3. Camphor
   A. Ingestion may result in vomiting, abdominal distress, muscle tremors, excitement, and seizures followed by CNS depression, apnea and coma.
   B. The toxic principle is an aromatic, volatile, terpene ketone derived from the wood of *Cinnamomum camphora*. It is also synthesized from turpentine oil.
   C. It is used as a topical antipruritic agent and rubefacient.
4. Cayenne pepper
   A. Ingestion may result in vomiting and diarrhea; topical applications are irritating to mucous membranes.
   B. The toxic principles are several volatile oils including capsaicin derived from the botanical source *Capsicum frutescens*.
   C. It is used as an external irritant and as a gastric stimulant.
5. Cinnamon oil
   A. Ingestion may result in vomiting and nausea; it is possibly nephrotoxic and neurotoxic.
   B. The toxic principle is an aromatic, volatile oil containing irritants such as cinnamaldehyde, which is derived from the bark of *Cinnamomum camphora*.
   C. It is used as an astringent in the treatment of flatulence and diarrhea.
6. Citrus oil extracts (see the section on Citrus oil extracts in this chapter)
7. Ephedra (Ma Huang)
   A. Ingestion may result in hypertension, hyperexcitability, mydriasis, restlessness, tachycardia, cardiac dysrhythmias, muscle tremors, seizures and death.
   B. The toxic principle is ephedrine, an alkaloid derived from the botanical source *Ephedra sinica*.

C. It is a stimulant used to treat nasal congestion, allergic disorders and bronchial asthma, and to promote weight loss.

8. Eucalyptus oil
   A. Ingestion may result in abdominal pain, bronchospasm, depression, vomiting, respiratory distress, respiratory depression, tachypnea, seizures and coma.
   B. The toxic principles are essential oil and tannins derived from the botanical source the *Eucalyptus globulus* and other species of tree in this genus.
   C. It is used as an antiseptic and as an antispasmodic stimulant agent in bronchitis, asthma, and respiratory disorders.
   D. Ingestion of 1 mL in humans has resulted in coma and 3.5 mL resulted in death.

9. Garlic
   A. Ingestion may result in anemia, allergic reactions, asthmatic attacks and contact dermatitis.
   B. The toxic principle is a volatile oil containing allyl disulfides such as allicin derived from the botanical source *Allium sativum* (garlic), a member of the onion family.
   C. It is used as a flavor enhancer in food, and is reported to have antiviral, bactericidal, fungicidal and insecticidal properties, to prolong bleeding and clotting times, to inhibit platelet aggregation, to increase fibrinolytic activity and to decrease serum lipid and cholesterol levels.

10. Ginseng
    A. Ingestion of extremely large amounts (more than 3 g daily in adult humans) may result in anxiety, diarrhea, restlessness, depression, dermatitis and hypertension.
    B. There are many active components in ginseng, but its pharmacologic action is thought to be due to triterpenoidal saponins called ginsenosides. The botanical source is ginseng, the common name for deciduous perennial plants of the genus *Panax*.
    C. It is used as a tonic to decrease fatigue, increase general strength, as an antihypertensive, an aphrodisiac and a mood elevator. Ginseng increases erythropoiesis, hemoglobin production, and iron absorption from the gastrointestinal tract, stimulates the central nervous system, increases blood pressure, increases heart rate, increases gastrointestinal motility, decreases serum glucose levels and decreases serum and liver cholesterol levels.

11. Lily-of-the-valley (see also 'Plant poisonings' section)
    A. Ingestion may result in cardiac arrhythmias, vomiting, nausea and diarrhea.
    B. The toxic principles are digitalis-like glycosides and irritant saponins derived from the botanical source *Convallaria majalis*.
    C. It is used as a diuretic and cardiotonic.

12. *Melaleuca* oil (tea tree oil)
    A. Dermal exposure may result in ataxia, nervousness, trembling, dehydration, hypothermia, ataxia, coma and death.

B. The toxic principle is a volatile oil that contains terpenes, sesquiterpenes, and hydrocarbons derived from the botanical source *Melaleuca alternifolia* (Australia tea tree).

C. It is used as a shampoo, for flea control and is an ingredient in many commercially available products.

13. Mistletoe

A. Ingestion may result in acute vomiting and diarrhea, ataxia, hyperesthesia, opisthotonos, seizures, coma and cardiovascular collapse.

B. The toxic principles are stimulant amines such as β-phenethylamine and tyramine derived from the botanical source the *Phoradendron* species.

C. It is used as a sedative, to induce labor and milk let-down, and in the treatment of high blood pressure.

14. Nux vomica

A. Ingestion may result in death.

B. The toxic principles are strychnine and brucine derived from the dried ripe seeds of the botanical source *Strychnos nuxvomica*.

C. It is used as an aid in digestive disturbances and as a treatment for feline leukemia.

D. The tincture is a 10% solution in 70% alcohol, the fluid extract is 1–1.2% strychnine and the dried powdered extract contains 7–7.7% strychnine. The approximate oral LD_{50} for dogs is 0.75 mg strychnine/kg and cats it is 2 mg strychnine/kg. The oral lethal dose of the 1% fluid extract for cats is 0.2 mL/kg.

15. Pennyroyal oil

A. Topical application of about 2000 mg/kg resulted in listlessness, vomiting, diarrhea, hemoptysis, epistaxis, seizures, hepatocellular necrosis and death in a dog. DIC has also been reported.

B. The volatile oil is derived from the botanical sources *Menta pulegium* and *Hedeoma pulegioides*. The toxic principle is pulegone, a ketone, which is bioactivated by the liver to menthofuran, which is a hepatotoxic metabolite.

C. It is used as a flea repellant, an abortifacient and to induce menstruation.

16. Pyrrolizidine alkaloids

A. Ingestion may result in hepatotoxicity and death.

B. Pyrrolizidine alkaloids are found in over 60 plants used medicinally, including comfrey (*Symphytum* spp.), coltsfoot (*Tussilago farfara*), borage (*Borago officinale*), *Eupatorium* spp., groundsel (*Senecio vulgaris*) and tansy ragwort (*Senecio jacobea*).

C. There are a wide variety of medicinal uses.

D. Toxicity in adult humans can result following ingestion of 85 mg of pyrrolizidine alkaloid.

17. Sassafras

A. Ingestion may result in mydriasis, vomiting, nausea, CNS depression and cardiovascular collapse.

B. The toxic principle is the volatile sassafras oil, which contains safrole, pinene, phenadrene, phenolics and D-camphor derived from the botanical source the *Sassafras albidum* tree.
C. It is used as an antiseptic, a diuretic, as a diaphoretic and to reduce flatulence.
D. Ingestion of 5 mL of the oil is toxic to the adult human. Cats are more sensitive than dogs, due to the presence of phenolics. A single tea bag may be toxic to a cat. Safrole is hepatotoxic, hepatocarcinogenic and an inhibitor of hepatic microsomal enzymes.

18. Senna
    A. Ingestion may result in abdominal pain, catharsis, vomiting and nausea.
    B. The toxic principles are anthraquinones derived from the botanical source *Cassia angustifolia*.
    C. It is used as a cathartic to relieve constipation.

19. Vitamin and mineral supplements
    A. Ingestion of multivitamin preparations may result in iron toxicosis, acute vitamin A toxicosis and / or acute vitamin D toxicosis.
    B. Iron toxicosis is further described later in the chapter.
    C. Vitamin A toxicosis can result from the ingestion of 5000–10 000 IU/ kg of vitamin A. Ingestion of topical ointments containing vitamin A can also be toxic.
    D. Vitamin D toxicosis in dogs can result from the ingestion of 64 000–460 000 IU/kg of vitamin D or from the ingestion of topical ointments containing vitamin D.

20. Oil of wintergreen
    A. Ingestion may result in nausea, vomiting, hematemesis, gastric ulceration, restlessness, seizures and coma in dogs; it may result in anorexia, depression, anemia, bone marrow hypoplasia, vomiting, emesis, toxic hepatitis, tachypnea and hyperthermia in cats.
    B. The toxic principle is a glycoside that releases methyl salicylate when it is hydrolyzed. The oil is derived from the botanical source *Gaultheria procumbens*.
    C. It is used as a topical aid to relieve muscle aches and pains.
    D. Clinical signs have been reported in dogs given 100–300 mg/kg/day orally for 4 weeks. Cats are much more sensitive, as with aspirin toxicosis.

21. Witch hazel
    A. Ingestion may result in constipation, vomiting and nausea; hepatotoxicity may occur if ingested in adequate amounts.
    B. The toxic principles are tannins derived from the botanical source *Hamamelis virginiana*.
    C. It is used as a mild astringent.

22. Wormwood
    A. Ingestion may result in vomiting, diarrhea, nausea, seizures and coma.
    B. The toxic principle is a volatile oil derived from the botanical source *Artemisia absinthium*.

C. It is used as a sedative, digestive aid and in the treatment of acute abdominal pain.

Diagnosis

History—A history of exposure to an herbal remedy or natural product is essential for diagnosis.
Clinical signs—Clinical findings vary with the substance involved.

Treatment

1. Inform the client of the diagnosis, prognosis and the cost of treatment.
2. Ensure a patent airway. Intubate the patient if necessary.
3. Administer supplemental oxygen and ventilation if necessary.
4. Place an intravenous catheter. Administer a balanced electrolyte crystalloid fluid intravenously to maintain perfusion, hydration and diuresis.
5. Administer diazepam, phenobarbital or pentobarbital if necessary to control seizures or hyperactivity.
   A. Diazepam 0.5–1 mg/kg IV in increments of 5–20 mg to effect
   B. Phenobarbital 2–4 mg/kg IV in dogs, 1–2 mg/kg IV in cats
   C. Pentobarbital 2–30 mg/kg slow IV to effect
6. In cases of dermal exposure, thoroughly wash the patient with warm water and a liquid dish-washing detergent or mild shampoo. Protective garments, including rubber gloves, should be worn while bathing the patient. Keep the patient warm by wrapping the patient in a towel until dry to prevent chilling.
7. In cases of ocular exposure, thoroughly flush the eyes with copious amounts of tepid tap water.
8. If the patient is presented within 2 hours of ingestion, attempt decontamination by inducing emesis or performing gastric lavage. Do not induce emesis if the patient is having seizures or if emesis is otherwise contraindicated.
   A. Induction of emesis in cats
      I. Administer xylazine, 0.44–1 mg/kg IM or SC (can reverse with yohimbine 0.1 mg/kg IM, SC, or IV slowly).
      II. Administer medetomidine, 10 µg/kg IM (can reverse with atipamezole (Antisedan®) 25 µg/kg IM).
      III. Hydrogen peroxide is very difficult to administer to cats and is no longer recommended.
   B. Induction of emesis in dogs
      I. Administer apomorphine 0.02–0.04 mg/kg IV or IM, or 1.5–6 mg dissolved and placed into the conjunctival fornix. If apomorphine was placed in the eye, after emesis, the patient's eye should be thoroughly lavaged with sterile saline. If excessive sedation occurs from apomorphine, the sedation may be reversed by the administration of naloxone (0.01–0.04 mg/kg IV, IM, SC) but this will not reverse the emetic effects.

II. Administer 3% hydrogen peroxide 1–5 mL/kg (0.5–2 mL/lb) PO, with a maximum dose of 3 tablespoons (45 mL). If the patient does not vomit within 10 minutes, give 3% hydrogen peroxide 0.5 mL/kg (0.25 mL/lb) PO *once*.

C. Gastric lavage

   I. Lightly anesthetize the patient.

   II. Administer oxygen and intravenous fluids to the patient while under anesthesia.

   III. Maintain anesthesia with the appropriate anesthetic as needed.

   IV. Intubate the patient with a cuffed endotracheal tube and inflate the cuff.

   V. Place the patient in lateral recumbency.

   VI. With a stomach tube held outside of the patient, alongside the patient, measure the distance from the tip of the nose to the last rib. Mark this distance on the stomach tube.

   VII. Lubricate the caudal end of the stomach tube with water-soluble jelly then pass the stomach tube gently into the stomach, passing the tube no farther than the marked distance on the tube.

   VIII. If desired, two stomach tubes may be utilized, a smaller ingress tube and a large egress tube.

   IX. Infuse warm (body temperature) tap water, 5–10 mL/kg, through the tube (ingress tube if using two tubes) to moderately distend the stomach.

   X. Allow the fluid to drain from the stomach through the tube (egress tube if using two tubes).

   XI. Save samples of gastric contents, suspicious foreign material, seeds, etc. for possible toxicologic analysis.

   XII. The stomach tube may have to be manipulated, repositioned or flushed with fluid or air if the gastric contents do not flow freely through the tube.

   XIII. Turn the patient to the other side and continue to perform gastric lavage.

   XIV. Continue gastric lavage until the effluent is clear.

   XV. If using the two-tube method, crimp the end of one tube and remove it.

   XVI. Administer activated charcoal down the stomach tube.

   XVII. Crimp the end of the stomach tube and remove it.

   XVIII. Monitor the patient during recovery from anesthesia, leaving the inflated cuffed endotracheal tube in place until the patient's swallowing reflex has returned.

D. Activated charcoal, 1–5 g/kg (3–6 mL/lb) PO is usually administered in a slurry of 1 g to 5 mL water. In herbal and natural product toxicosis patients, repeat the administration of activated charcoal q6–8h. Administer a cathartic only *once*.

E. A single dose of an osmotic or saline cathartic should be administered along with activated charcoal unless the patient has severe diarrhea. Do *not* administer magnesium-containing cathartics if the patient is exhibiting neurologic signs. Alternative cathartics include:

    I. Sorbitol (70%), 2 g/kg (1–2 mL/kg) PO

    II. Magnesium sulfate (Epsom salt), 200 mg/kg for cats, 250–500 mg/kg for dogs; mix magnesium sulfate with water, 5–10 mL/kg and administer PO.

    III. Magnesium hydroxide (Milk of Magnesia®), 15–50 mL for cats, 10–150 mL for dogs, q6–12h PO as needed

    IV. Sodium sulfate, 200 mg/kg for cats, 250–500 mg/kg for dogs; mix sodium sulfate with water, 5–10 mL/kg and administer PO.

9. Hospitalize the patient for symptomatic and supportive therapy.
10. If the toxic agent is cardiotoxic, monitor the ECG and treat cardiac dysrhythmias appropriately.
11. Administration of RBCs, whole blood, or a hemoglobin based oxygen carrier may be necessary if garlic-induced anemia or blood loss from pennyroyal oil intoxication is severe.
12. Treat symptomatically and supportively for hepatotoxicity if present.

HOUSEHOLD PRODUCT INTOXICATION

BLEACHES

1. Most household bleaches contain sodium hypochlorite, hypochlorite salts or compounds that form hypochlorite in aqueous solutions. The nonchlorine bleaches contain sodium peroxide, sodium perborate or enzymatic detergents.
2. Household bleaches are mild to moderate irritants. The incidence of gastrointestinal burns is low.

Diagnosis

Clinical signs—These include:
1. Hypersalivation
2. Abdominal pain
3. The hair coat may be bleached and smell like chlorine
4. Inhalation of fumes may appear as coughing, dyspnea and retching, resulting from pulmonary irritation
5. Vomiting
6. The oropharynx may appear irritated.

Treatment

1. Administer milk or water orally.
2. Wash the hair coat and skin with soap and rinse thoroughly.
3. Administer symptomatic care of dyspnea, vomiting and abdominal pain.

ACIDS

1. Many acids are found in products used in the home, including hydrochloric (muriatic) acid, sulfuric acid, nitric acid, and phosphoric acid.
2. Acids are found in numerous products, including pool chemicals, cleansers, toilet bowl cleaners, anti-rust compounds, gun barrel cleaning fluid, automobile batteries and soldering flux.

Diagnosis

Clinical signs—The clinical signs result from coagulation necrosis of contact tissues, such as the mouth, pharynx and gastric mucosa:
1. Necrotic lesions in the oral cavity
2. Laryngeal spasms
3. Laryngeal edema
4. Upper airway obstruction
5. Intense ocular pain and blepharospasms follow ocular exposure
6. Pulmonary edema
7. Shock
8. Emesis
9. Hematemesis.

Treatment

1. Ingestion
   A. Alkali antacids and carbonate preparations are contraindicated because of the possible presence of thermic burns, which may be produced by the resulting exothermic reaction.
   B. Emesis is contraindicated.
   C. In cases with minimal esophageal injury, the treatment of choice is gastric lavage and the oral administration of aluminum hydroxide preparations.
   D. Activated charcoal is ineffective.
   E. Intravenous fluid therapy and additional supportive care may be necessary.
   F. Endoscopy is indicated to determine the extent of the injuries.
   G. Corticosteroids are indicated to decrease constriction of circumferential lesions.
   H. Prophylactic antibiotics should be administered.
2. Dermal exposure
   A. Irrigate the skin with water for 10–20 minutes.
   B. Apply topical medications.
   C. Prevent additional self-trauma.
   D. Surgical debridement may be necessary in severe cases.
3. Ocular exposure
   A. Irrigate the eyes with isotonic-isothermic sterile saline solution for 30 minutes.
   B. Treat resulting lesions appropriately.

ALKALIS

1. Common household alkaline product ingredients include lye (sodium and potassium carbonate, sodium and potassium hydroxide, or potash), potassium permanganate and ammonium hydroxide.
2. Alkalis are found in drain cleaners, toilet bowl cleaners, ammonia, dishwasher detergents and 'button' alkali batteries.

Diagnosis

Clinical signs—These include:
1. Ptyalism
2. Irritated oral mucous membranes
3. Chest pain
4. Seizures
5. Rapid death
6. Keratitis from ocular exposure.

Treatment

1. Ingestion
   A. Induction of emesis and gastric lavage are contraindicated.
   B. Allow the patient no food or water until the extent of esophageal damage is determined.
   C. The administration of acids is contraindicated and can actually worsen the extent of the tissue damage.
   D. Immediate dilution with oral administration of milk or water is important.
2. Dermal contact
   A. Perform thorough rinsing of exposed skin for 10–20 minutes.
   B. Treat any skin lesions symptomatically.
   C. Prevent additional self-trauma.
   D. Severe lesions may require surgical debridement.
3. Ocular exposure
   A. Irrigate the eye with isotonic–isothermic sterile saline for 30 minutes.
   B. Treat ocular and periocular damage symptomatically.
   C. Petroleum-based ophthalmics are contraindicated.

DISINFECTANTS

PHENOL AND PHENOLIC COMPOUNDS

1. The oral toxic dose of phenol is about 0.5 g/kg, except in the cat, which is more sensitive.
2. Phenolic compounds are readily absorbed from dermal contact, inhalation or ingestion.
3. Concentrations above 1% cause dermal burns; concentrations above 5% cause oral burns.

Diagnosis

Clinical signs—These include:
1. Panting
2. Hyperactivity
3. Restlessness
4. Apprehension
5. Hypersalivation
6. Vomiting
7. Ataxia
8. Muscle fasciculations
9. Shock
10. Cardiac arrhythmias
11. Methemoglobinemia
12. Coma.

Treatment

1. Advise the client to administer milk or egg orally at home prior to immediate transport for emergency medical care.
2. If severe oral lesions are observed, emesis and gastric lavage are contraindicated. Administer activated charcoal and a saline cathartic.
3. Dermal exposure
   A. Apply polyethylene glycol or glycerol to the affected areas.
   B. Shampoo the patient with a liquid dishwasher detergent.
   C. Rinse thoroughly with water.
   D. The person treating the dermal exposure should wear heavy rubber gloves to avoid skin contact.
   E. Apply 0.5% sodium bicarbonate-soaked dressings to injured areas.
4. Ocular exposure
   A. Rinse eyes thoroughly with isotonic saline, for 20–30 minutes.
   B. Treat corneal erosions.
5. *N*-acetylcysteine administration (140 mg/kg IV loading dose, followed by 70 mg/kg PO q6h for 3 days) may help prevent hepatic and renal injuries.
6. Methemoglobinemia
   A. Dogs: methylene blue 4–8 mg/kg IV
   B. Dogs and cats: ascorbic acid 20–50 mg/kg PO or IV
   C. Oxygen administration.
7. Symptomatic treatment of shock, cardiopulmonary function, renal and hepatic function is essential.

PINE OIL DISINFECTANTS

1. The toxic dose is from 1 to 2.5 mL/kg body weight or less.
2. Cats, birds and certain reptiles appear to be more susceptible to toxicity following exposure.

Diagnosis

Clinical signs—These include:

1. Ingestion of these compounds causes irritation to oral mucous membranes, nausea, hypersalivation, vomiting, hematemesis and abdominal pain.
2. Ocular exposure causes epiphora, blepharospasms, conjunctivitis and photosensitivity.
3. Additional clinical signs include chemical pneumonitis, depression, ataxia, and hypotension. Acute renal failure and myoglobinuria may occur.

Treatment

1. Rapidly administer egg whites, milk or water orally.
2. Emesis and gastric lavage are contraindicated.
3. Administer activated charcoal and a saline cathartic orally.
4. Bathe the patient with soap and rinse thoroughly with water.
5. Administer symptomatic care and diuresis.
6. Methemoglobinemia
   A. Dogs: methylene blue 4–8 mg/kg IV
   B. Dogs and cats: ascorbic acid 20–50 mg/kg PO or IV
   C. Oxygen administration

ISOPROPANOL (ISOPROPYL ALCOHOL)

1. Isopropanol is found in skin lotions, hair tonics, after-shave lotions, cleaning solvents, window cleaners and sanitizers.
2. Isopropanol is a potent CNS depressant, approximately twice as toxic as ethanol.
3. Toxicity can result from inhalation of the vapors and from ingestion.

Diagnosis

Clinical signs—These include:

1. Distinctive odor to the hair coat
2. Emesis
3. Hematemesis
4. CNS depression that progresses into a coma
5. Cranial abdominal pain
6. Hypotensive shock
7. Retching.

Treatment

1. Administer emesis or gastric lavage within 2 hours of ingestion.
2. Administer mechanical ventilation if necessary to maintain ventilation.
3. Administer intravenous fluid therapy.

4. Correct acidosis.
5. Peritoneal dialysis for longer than 5 hours should be considered.

NAPHTHALENE

Sources

Naphthalene is found in toilet bowl deodorizers, moth balls, moth crystals and moth cakes.

Diagnosis

Clinical signs—The clinical signs include vomiting; an odor of moth balls from the patient's breath, mouth and vomitus; CNS stimulation including seizures; methemoglobinemia, anemia and hepatitis 3–5 days after ingestion.

Treatment

Treatment is symptomatic and supportive.

1. Ensure a patent airway. Intubate the patient if necessary.
2. Administer supplemental oxygen and ventilation if necessary.
3. **Do not induce emesis.**
4. **Do not perform gastric lavage** unless the patient is presented within 30–60 minutes following ingestion.
5. Administer activated charcoal and a saline cathartic once.
6. Place an intravenous catheter. Administer a balanced electrolyte crystalloid fluid intravenously to maintain hydration.
7. Administer diazepam, phenobarbital or pentobarbital if necessary to control seizures or hyperactivity.
   A. Diazepam 0.5–1 mg/kg IV in increments of 5–20 mg to effect
   B. Phenobarbital 2–4 mg/kg IV in dogs, 1–2 mg/kg IV in cats
   C. Pentobarbital 2–30 mg/kg slow IV to effect
8. Treat methemoglobinemia if present.

PARADICHLOROBENZENE

Sources

Paradichlorobenzene is found in diaper pails, toilet bowls, and restroom deodorizers and in moth balls, cakes and crystals.

Method of action

Paradichlorobenzene is an organochlorine insecticide that is metabolized to a hepatotoxic phenol.

Diagnosis

Clinical signs—The clinical signs include the odor of mothballs from the patient's mouth or vomitus, vomiting, CNS stimulation including seizures and possibly hepatitis.

Treatment

Treatment is symptomatic and supportive.

1. Ensure a patent airway. Intubate the patient if necessary.
2. Administer supplemental oxygen and ventilation if necessary.
3. **Do not induce emesis.**
4. Do not perform gastric lavage unless the patient is presented within 30–60 minutes following ingestion.
5. Administer activated charcoal and a saline cathartic once.
6. Place an intravenous catheter. Administer a balanced electrolyte crystalloid fluid intravenously to maintain hydration.
7. Administer diazepam, phenobarbital or pentobarbital if necessary to control seizures or hyperactivity.
    A. Diazepam 0.5–1 mg/kg IV in increments of 5–20 mg to effect
    B. Phenobarbital 2–4 mg/kg IV in dogs, 1–2 mg/kg IV in cats
    C. Pentobarbital 2–30 mg/kg slow IV to effect
8. Treat methemoglobinemia if present.

SOAPS AND DETERGENTS

SOAPS

1. The ingestion of true soaps is usually not toxic.
2. The ingestion of bar soaps usually causes vomiting and diarrhea associated with gastrointestinal irritation, but is not highly toxic. The treatment includes oral administration of milk or water and symptomatic treatment of vomiting and diarrhea.
3. Laundry soaps and homemade soaps may cause corrosive gastrointestinal lesions owing to their high free-alkali content.

NON-IONIC DETERGENTS

1. Examples are alkylethoxylate, alkylphenoxypolyethoxy ethanols and polyethylene glycol stearate.
2. They are found in hand dishwashing detergents, shampoos and some laundry detergents.
3. Ingestion most commonly results in vomiting and diarrhea.

Treatment

1. Rinse the eyes with water.
2. Thoroughly rinse the hair coat.
3. Administer milk or water orally.
4. Administer symptomatic treatment for vomiting and diarrhea.

ANIONIC DETERGENTS

1. Examples are alkylsodium sulfates, alkylsodium sulfonates, linear alkylbenzene lauryl sulfate and tetrapropylene benzene sulfonate.

2. They are found in laundry detergents, shampoos and electric dishwasher detergents.
3. The electric dishwasher detergents are the most toxic, but the rest are considered slightly to moderately toxic. Ingestion is usually not fatal.
4. They cause corrosive stomatitis, esophagitis, and gastritis, contact dermatitis and keratitis.

Treatment

1. Administer milk or water orally.
2. Administer symptomatic treatment for activated charcoal.
3. Rinse the eyes and hair coat.
4. Administer symptomatic treatment for vomiting, diarrhea and corrosive injuries.

CATIONIC DETERGENTS

1. Examples are benzalkonium chloride, benzethonium chloride, alkyldimethyl 3.4-dichlorobenzene and cetylpyridinium chloride.
2. They are found in fabric softeners, sanitizers and germicides.
3. They cause corrosive burns to the mouth, pharynx and esophagus.

Clinical signs—These are very similar to those of organophosphate toxicity, including:

1. Depression
2. Hypersalivation
3. Vomiting
4. Hematemesis
5. Muscle weakness and fasciculations
6. Seizures
7. Shock
8. Coma.

Treatment

1. Do not induce emesis if the concentration of the cationic detergent ingested is greater than 7.5%.
2. Administer egg whites, milk, or water orally.
3. Administer activated charcoal and a saline cathartic.
4. Rinse the skin and eyes following topical exposure.
5. Administer general symptomatic treatment of shock, vomiting, diarrhea and seizures.

HYDRAMETHYLNON INTOXICATION

Hydramethylnon is a hydrazone compound that is a slow-acting gastric insecticide, available as granules or as powder.

Mode of action

Hydramethylnon impairs the production of ATP by uncoupling oxidative phosphorylation in mitochondria. This results in reduced oxygen consumption and energy production by the mitochondria.

Sources

Hydramethylnon is a pesticide used to control ants (especially fire ants) and cockroaches. It is marketed under the names Amdro®, Blatex®, Cyaforce®, Cyclon®. Impact®, Matox®, Pyramdron®, Seige® and Wipeout®. Amdro contains 0.88% hydramethylnon. A cup of Amdro® contains about 2066 mg hydramethylnon.

Toxic dosages

The LD_{50} for dogs is 1131 mg/kg. An exposure of 113 mg/kg may cause clinical signs.

Diagnosis

History—The dog will usually have a history of exposure.
Clinical signs—The clinical signs include vomiting, diarrhea and hypothermia. The chemical is also an ocular irritant. Seizures and muscle tremors may occur following massive exposure in dogs. There have been very few reported fatalities.
Laboratory findings—Eosinopenia and leukopenia have been observed in dogs fed the LD_{50} dose daily for 7 days. There is no known hepatic or renal involvement. The chemical is not well absorbed from the gastrointestinal tract. Greater than 90% is excreted unchanged in the feces. Within 24 hours, 72% was eliminated. There is a rather long clearance time, with another 20% (total of 92%) being eliminated within 9 days.

Prognosis

The prognosis is usually good.

Treatment

1. Inform the client of the diagnosis, prognosis and cost of the treatment.
2. There is no known antidote. Treatment is symptomatic and supportive.
3. If the patient presents less than 4 hours since exposure, attempt gastric decontamination with emesis, gastric lavage, administration of activated charcoal and a saline or osmotic cathartic.
   A. Induction of emesis in cats
      I. Administer xylazine, 0.44–1 mg/kg IM or SC (can reverse with yohimbine 0.1 mg/kg IM, SC, or IV slowly).
      II. Administer medetomidine, 10 µg/kg IM (can reverse with atipamezole (Antisedan®) 25 µg/kg IM).

III. Hydrogen peroxide is very difficult to administer to cats and is no longer recommended.

B. Induction of emesis in dogs

    I. Administer apomorphine 0.02–0.04 mg/kg IV or IM, or 1.5–6 mg dissolved and placed into the conjunctival fornix. If apomorphine was placed in the eye, after emesis, the patient's eye should be thoroughly lavaged with sterile saline. If excessive sedation occurs from apomorphine, the sedation may be reversed by the administration of naloxone (0.01–0.04 mg/kg IV, IM, SC) but this will not reverse the emetic effects.

    II. Administer 3% hydrogen peroxide 1–5 mL/kg (0.5–2 mL/lb) PO, with a maximum dose of 3 tablespoons (45 mL). If the patient does not vomit within 10 minutes, give 3% hydrogen peroxide 0.5 mL/kg (0.25 mL/lb) PO *once*.

C. Gastric lavage

    I. Lightly anesthetize the patient. Propofol, 4–6 mL/kg, IV, may be utilized.

    II. Administer oxygen and intravenous fluids to the patient while under anesthesia.

    III. Maintain anesthesia with the appropriate anesthetic as needed.

    IV. Intubate the patient with a cuffed endotracheal tube and inflate the cuff.

    V. Place the patient in lateral recumbency.

    VI. With a stomach tube held outside of the patient, alongside the patient, measure the distance from the tip of the nose to the last rib. Mark this distance on the stomach tube.

    VII. Lubricate the caudal end of the stomach tube with water-soluble jelly then pass the stomach tube gently into the stomach, passing the tube no farther than the marked distance on the tube.

    VIII. If desired, two stomach tubes may be utilized, a smaller ingress tube and a large egress tube.

    IX. Infuse warm (body-temperature) tap water, 5–10 mL/kg, through the tube (ingress tube if using two tubes) to moderately distend the stomach.

    X. Allow the fluid to drain from the stomach through the tube (egress tube if using two tubes).

    XI. Save samples of gastric contents, suspicious foreign material, seeds, etc. for possible toxicologic analysis.

    XII. The stomach tube may have to be manipulated, repositioned or flushed with fluid or air if the gastric contents do not flow freely through the tube.

    XIII. Turn the patient to the other side and continue to perform gastric lavage.

    XIV. Continue gastric lavage until the effluent is clear.

    XV. If using the two-tube method, crimp the end of one tube and remove it.

    XVI. Administer activated charcoal down the stomach tube.

XVII. Crimp the end of the stomach tube and remove it.
XVIII. Monitor the patient during recovery from anesthesia, leaving the inflated cuffed endotracheal tube in place until the patient's swallowing reflex has returned.
D. Activated charcoal, 2–5 g/kg (3–6 mL/ lb) PO is usually administered in a slurry of 1 g per 5 mL water. In hydramethylnon toxicosis patients, repeat the administration of activated charcoal q3–4h. Administer a cathartic only once.
E. A single dose of an osmotic or saline cathartic should be administered along with activated charcoal. Alternative cathartics include:
  I. Sorbitol (70%), 2 g/kg (1–2 mL/kg) PO
  II. Magnesium sulfate (Epsom salt), 200 mg/kg for cats, 250–500 mg/kg for dogs; mix magnesium sulfate with water, 5–10 mL/kg and administer PO.
  III. Magnesium hydroxide (Milk of Magnesia®), 15–50 mL for cats, 10–150 mL for dogs, q6–12h PO as needed
  IV. Sodium sulfate, 200 mg/kg for cats, 250–500 mg/kg for dogs; mix sodium sulfate with water, 5–10 mL/kg and administer PO.
4. Administer intravenous fluids at maintenance rates or higher if indicated by shock or excessive fluid losses from vomiting and diarrhea. Diuresis is not indicated and has not been shown to be beneficial.
5. Administer anti-emetics as needed.
6. Control seizures if needed with diazepam, 0.5–1 mg/kg IV, or pentobarbital, 2–30 mg/kg slow IV.

HYDROCARBON TOXICITY

KEROSENE

Kerosene is absorbed percutaneously and from the gastrointestinal tract.

Clinical signs—The most common clinical signs include hypersalivation, vomiting, diarrhea, dyspnea, ataxia, tremors, seizures or coma. Kerosene is both cardiotoxic and nephrotoxic.

Treatment

1. Inform the client of the diagnosis, prognosis, and the cost of treatment.
2. Induction of emesis and gastric lavage are *contraindicated*.
3. Evaluate thoracic radiographs.
4. Monitor cardiac function.
5. Establish baseline hepatic enzymes and hematologic values.
6. Administer oxygen if the patient is hypoxic or comatose.
7. Bathe the patient with a mild detergent if percutaneous exposure.
8. Possible administration of short-acting corticosteroids.
9. Hospitalize the patient for a minimum of 24 hours.

GASOLINE

Clinical signs—The most common clinical signs include hypersalivation, vomiting, diarrhea, cardiac arrhythmias, hypothermia or hyperthermia, depression, hyperesthesia, ataxia, seizures and coma. If ocular exposure occurs, epiphora, keratitis, corneal edema and photophobia may be observed.

Treatment

1. Inform the client of the diagnosis, prognosis and the cost of treatment.
2. Administer supportive care.
3. Bathe the patient in mild detergent if dermal exposure.
4. Administer oxygen.
5. Induction of emesis is generally contraindicated.

HYMENOPTERA ENVENOMATION

The order Hymenoptera includes the following groups:

- Apoidea (bees)
- Vespoidea (wasps, hornets, yellow jackets)
- Formicidae (ants).

Honeybees can sting only once; they possess a barbed stinger that stays behind in the victim's skin after they sting. Wasp, hornet and yellow-jacket stingers are not barbed and each insect can deliver multiple venom-injecting stings without dying.

Most deaths from Hymenoptera stings are due to immediate hypersensitivity reactions causing anaphylaxis. These are not dose related; a single sting may be fatal. Respiratory obstruction is another example of a potentially lethal local reaction. Massive envenomation, as seen in swarm attacks, can cause the death of nonallergic victims.

Mode of action

Honeybee venom contains various toxic components (Box 14.1):

1. Mellitin, which acts as a detergent to disrupt cell membranes and liberate biogenic amines and potassium, causes hydrolysis of cell membranes, alteration of cellular permeability, histamine release, local pain, induction of catecholamine release, and intravascular hemolysis
2. Peptide 401 (mast cell degranulating peptide), which causes degranulation of mast cells, releasing histamine and vasoactive amines
3. Phospholipase A_2, which causes intravascular hemolysis and is the major allergenic component of bee venom
4. Hyaluronidase, also called 'spreading factor', which disrupts collagen, alters cell membranes, changes cell permeability, and is also allergenic
5. Vasoactive amines (histamine, dopamine), norepinephrine and other unidentified proteins

BOX 14.1   Comparison of Hymenoptera venoms

Apidae (bees) F
—Phospholipase A
—Hyaluronidase
—Mellitin
—Apamin

—Biogenic amines
—Acid phosphatase
—Minimine
—Peptide 401

Vespids (wasps, yellow jackets, hornets)
—Phospholipase A
—Hyaluronidase
—Antigen 5
—Kinins

—Biogenic amines
—Acid phosphatase
—Peptide 401

Formicides (fire ants)
—Phospholipase
—Hyaluronidase

—Biogenic amines
—Piperidines

6. Apamin, a neurotoxin that acts on the spinal cord
7. Adolapin, which inhibits prostaglandin synthetase and has anti-inflammatory actions.

Toxic dosages

The estimated lethal dose for most mammals is about 20 stings/kg. For the adult human, the estimated lethal dose is about 500 stings.

With each sting, the amount of venom injected is estimated to be:

1. Wasps: 17 µg
2. Africanized honeybees: 94 µg
3. European honeybees: 147 µg.

Diagnosis

History—There is usually a known exposure to massive envenomations. For individual stings, there may be no history of exposure. Most commonly the patient would have been outside.
Clinical signs—There are four primary reactions to Hymenoptera envenomation:
1. Local pain and swelling—due to vasoactive components
2. Larger, regional reaction, mediated by allergic mechanisms, involving parts of the body in continuity with the sting site
3. A systemic, anaphylactic response, characterized by urticaria, angioedema, nausea, vomiting, hypotension and dyspnea
   A. Occurs in individuals with specific IgE antibodies to allergenic components
   B. Develops within minutes of the sting
4. Skin rashes and serum sickness-like symptoms occurring within 3–14 days after envenomation.

Massive envenomations (many stings) cause fever, depression, hematemesis, hematochezia, melena, myoglobinuria, hemoglobinuria, and neurologic signs including facial paralysis, ataxia and seizures. Secondary immune-mediated hemolytic anemia may occur. DIC may develop. Acute renal failure may occur and death may result.

Laboratory findings—
1. CBC may show a stress leukogram. In patients with massive envenomation, leukocytosis and thrombocytopenia may be observed.
2. Patients that develop DIC may have thrombocytopenia and prolonged ACT, PT and PTT.
3. Hemolytic anemia may develop in patients with secondary IMHA.
4. Serum chemistry evaluation may show elevated BUN due to GI hemorrhage, dehydration (pre-renal azotemia) or acute renal failure. Creatinine may also be elevated. Elevation of creatinine phosphokinase and hepatic enzymes may occur in patients with massive envenomation.

Prognosis

Anaphylactic reactions may vary from mild to lethal. Massive envenomation of dogs is frequently fatal.

Treatment

1. Inform the client of the diagnosis, prognosis and cost of the treatment.
2. Treatment of local reactions may not be needed or may benefit from the application of cool water or ice compresses, topical camphor and menthol, or topical lidocaine.
3. Regional reactions and those involving multiple stings may benefit from the administration of dexamethasone sodium phosphate or prednisolone sodium succinate, followed by prednisolone orally.
   A. Intravenous fluids are beneficial in the treatment of hypotension, to correct hypovolemia, maintain renal perfusion and prevent vascular stasis.
   B. Broad-spectrum antibiotic administration may be beneficial in patients that develop secondary sepsis.
4. The treatment of anaphylaxis includes:
   A. Epinephrine 0.1–0.5 mL of 1:1000 SC immediately then repeated every 10–20 minutes as needed
   B. Intravenous fluids at shock volumes (90 mL/kg in the dog and 50–60 mL/kg in the cat) followed by aggressive fluid therapy
   C. Antihistamines (diphenhydramine, 1–4 mg/kg IV very slowly, IM, SC or PO)
   D. Glucocorticoids (prednisolone sodium succinate 10 mg/kg IV or dexamethasone sodium phosphate 1–2 mg/kg IV)
   E. Airway management including intubation if needed; albuterol or ipratropium via inhalation may provide bronchodilation
   F. Supplemental oxygen administration.
5. The patient should be hospitalized and monitored until it has recovered.

HYPERTONIC SODIUM PHOSPHATE (FLEET®) ENEMA INTOXICATION

Mode of action

The excessive amounts of sodium and phosphorus contained in the enema may be absorbed from the colon, resulting in hypernatremia, hyperphosphatemia, metabolic acidosis and increased serum osmolality.

Sources

Some Fleet® enemas contain sodium biphosphate and sodium phosphate equivalent to 2178 mEq sodium and 1756 mEq phosphorus.

Toxic dosages

Cats and dogs <11 kg (<25 lb) = 60 mL (2 fl oz).
Dogs >11 kg (>25 lb) = 120 mL (4 fl oz).

Diagnosis

History—The patient will have a history of exposure.
Clinical signs—The onset of signs occurs within 30–60 minutes after administration of the enema. Clinical signs include somnolence, vomiting, bloody diarrhea, tachycardia, cardiac dysrhythmias, weak pulse, hypothermia, ashen mucous membranes, ataxia, tetany or convulsions, and death.
Laboratory findings—Laboratory abnormalities include hyperglycemia, hypernatremia, hyperphosphatemia, hypocalcemia, hypomagnesemia, hypokalemia, metabolic acidosis and hyperosmolality.

Prognosis

The prognosis is variable.

Treatment

1. Inform the client of the diagnosis, prognosis and the cost of treatment.
2. Ensure a patent airway. Intubate the patient if necessary.
3. Administer supplemental oxygen and ventilation if necessary.
4. Place an intravenous catheter. Jugular catheterization is particularly useful as it will allow monitoring of central venous pressure. Administer isotonic crystalloids to maintain perfusion, and hydration.
5. Administer diazepam, phenobarbital or pentobarbital if necessary to control seizures or hyperactivity.
   A. Diazepam 0.5–1 mg/kg IV in increments of 5–20 mg to effect
   B. Phenobarbital 2–4 mg/kg IV in dogs, 1–2 mg/kg IV in cats
   C. Pentobarbital 2–30 mg/kg slow IV to effect

6. If the patient is hypokalemic add potassium chloride to the intravenous fluids.
7. If the patient has ionized hypocalcemia, calcium gluconate may be added to the intravenous fluids at a dose of 7–10 mEq/L. Higher doses may be administered in 0.9% NaCl, but should not be added to fluids containing lactate or acetate.
8. Administer 10% calcium gluconate (0.5–1.5 mL/kg) slow IV if tetany or other clinical signs exist. Monitor the patient's heart rate during administration. Stop or slow the infusion rate if bradycardia develops.
9. The administration of sodium bicarbonate is contraindicated.
10. The administration of insulin should be avoided.
11. The administration of mannitol may be necessary for treatment of cerebral edema.
12. If the patient has severe hypernatremia (>180 mEq Na/L), the serum sodium level must be lowered slowly to avoid cerebral edema. It is recommended to administer IV fluids with a sodium concentration about 10 mEq/L less than the patient's serum sodium level, with frequent monitoring and readjustment.

IRON TOXICOSIS

Mode of action

Excessive iron exerts a corrosive effect on the mucosa of the stomach and small intestine resulting in hemorrhagic gastroenteritis, necrosis, perforation and peritonitis. Also, excessive amounts of iron disrupt mitochondrial function and interfere with cellular respiration, which leads to lactic acidosis. Free iron also increases free-radical formation, which results in further cellular damage.

Sources

Rose fertilizer, multiple vitamin and mineral supplements. Many multivitamins contain 10–18 mg of elemental iron per tablet.

Toxic dosages

Rose fertilizer often contains iron at 5% concentration one teaspoon (5 mL) is toxic to a 9 kg (20 lb) dog. Ingestion of elemental iron in amounts exceeding 20–60 mg/kg are toxic, with ingestion of >100 mg/kg often being lethal.

Diagnosis

History—History of exposure.
Clinical signs—Clinical signs may not occur for 6–12 hours following ingestion. The nitrous component of rose fertilizer usually causes drowsiness, depression, gastrointestinal upset, vomiting, hematemesis and diarrhea that may become bloody. The nitrates in the fertilizer rarely lead to methemoglobinemia. The phosphorus / potash portions similarly cause gastrointestinal upset. The dog may appear to recover initially.

Signs of hepatic and renal failure occur within 12–24 or more hours. Iron passed in the urine will cause the urine to be dark. Dehydration, shock, acidosis, oliguria or anuria, tremors, coma, icterus, hemolytic anemia, hemoglobinemia, coagulopathy and death may occur.

Anaphylactic reactions from the injection of iron may result in cardiovascular collapse and death.

Laboratory findings—

1. Elevation of the serum iron level >350 mg/dL are indications for chelation therapy.
2. Urine may appear very dark due to the iron content and hemoglobinuria.
3. Hepatic enzymes and bilirubin levels may be elevated.
4. Azotemia, with elevations of BUN and serum creatinine levels, may be observed.
5. Metabolic acidosis may be present.
6. The hematocrit may be increased due to dehydration, decreased due to anemia and blood loss, or normal.

*Abdominal radiographs—*May reveal a radiodense ingesta pattern due to the ingestion of tablets or fertilizer.

Differential diagnosis

Arsenic intoxication, boric acid intoxication, garbage intoxication, mushroom intoxication and zinc intoxication.

Prognosis

The prognosis is variable.

Treatment

1. Inform the client of the diagnosis, prognosis and the cost of treatment.
2. Ensure a patent airway. Intubate the patient if necessary.
3. Administer supplemental oxygen and ventilation if necessary.
4. Place an intravenous catheter. Administer a balanced electrolyte crystalloid fluid intravenously to maintain perfusion, and hydration.
5. If the patient is experiencing anaphylaxis, administer epinephrine and antihistamines.
6. Decontamination will be of value up to 4 hours' post-ingestion.
   A. If the client calls on the telephone, advise them to give the patient egg, milk or water and to induce emesis.
   B. In cases of dermal exposure, thoroughly wash the patient with warm, soapy water. Protective garments, including rubber gloves, should be worn while bathing the patient. Keep the patient warm.
   C. Induction of emesis in cats
      I. Administer xylazine, 0.44–1 mg/kg IM or SC (can reverse with yohimbine 0.1 mg/kg IM, SC, or IV slowly).

II. Administer medetomidine, 10 µg/kg IM (can reverse with atipamezole (Antisedan®) 25 µg/kg IM).

III. Hydrogen peroxide is very difficult to administer to cats and is no longer recommended.

D. Induction of emesis in dogs

   I. Administer apomorphine 0.02–0.04 mg/kg IV or IM, or 1.5–6 mg dissolved and placed into the conjunctival fornix. If apomorphine was placed in the eye, after emesis, the patient's eye should be thoroughly lavaged with sterile saline. If excessive sedation occurs from apomorphine, the sedation may be reversed by the administration of naloxone (0.01–0.04 mg/kg IV, IM, SC) but this will not reverse the emetic effects.

   II. Administer 3% hydrogen peroxide 1–5 mL/kg (0.5–2 mL/lb) PO, with a maximum dose of 3 tablespoons (45 mL). If the patient does not vomit within 10 minutes, give 3% hydrogen peroxide 0.5 mL/kg (0.25 mL/lb) PO *once*.

E. Administer magnesium hydroxide (Milk of Magnesia®), 15–50 mL for cats, 10–150 mL for dogs, q6–12h PO as needed

F. Gastric lavage should be performed gently.

   I. Lightly anesthetize the patient.

   II. Administer oxygen and intravenous fluids to the patient while under anesthesia.

   III. Maintain anesthesia with the appropriate anesthetic as needed.

   IV. Intubate the patient with a cuffed endotracheal tube and inflate the cuff.

   V. Place the patient in lateral recumbency.

   VI. With a stomach tube held outside of the patient, alongside the patient, measure the distance from the tip of the nose to the last rib. Mark this distance on the stomach tube.

   VII. Lubricate the caudal end of the stomach tube with water-soluble jelly then pass the stomach tube gently into the stomach, passing the tube no farther than the marked distance on the tube.

   VIII. If desired, two stomach tubes may be utilized, a smaller ingress tube and a large egress tube.

   IX. Infuse warm (body-temperature) tap water, 5–10 mL/kg, through the tube (ingress tube if using two tubes) to moderately distend the stomach.

   X. Allow the fluid to drain from the stomach through the tube (egress tube if using two tubes).

   XI. Save samples of gastric contents, suspicious foreign material, seeds, etc. for possible toxicologic analysis.

   XII. The stomach tube may have to be manipulated, repositioned or flushed with fluid or air if the gastric contents do not flow freely through the tube.

   XIII. Turn the patient to the other side and continue to perform gastric lavage.

   XIV. Continue gastric lavage until the effluent is clear.

XV. If using the two-tube method, crimp the end of one tube and remove it.

XVI. Crimp the end of the stomach tube and remove it.

XVII. Monitor the patient during recovery from anesthesia, leaving the inflated cuffed endotracheal tube in place until the patient's swallowing reflex has returned.

G. **Activated charcoal is not effective**.

H. Repeat the **administration of magnesium hydroxide (Milk of Magnesia®)** following gastric lavage, 15–50 mL for cats, 10–150 mL for dogs, q6–12h PO as needed.

7. Administer Desferal® (deferoxamine) (or sodium EDTA if Desferal® is unavailable).

A. Two dosage recommendations are:

I. 15 mg/kg/h CRI.

II. 40 mg/kg slow IV q4–6h.

B. Deferoxamine is a more effective iron chelator than sodium EDTA.

C. When administering deferoxamine intravenously, hypotension can result. Administer slowly.

D. As a result of iron chelation with deferoxamine, the patient's urine will turn red to reddish-brown.

8. Vitamin C

A. Administer ascorbic acid (vitamin C) orally simultaneously with deferoxamine to enhance iron chelation.

B. **Do not administer vitamin C without deferoxamine** as it will increase iron absorption.

9. Monitor serum iron levels and continue therapy until the serum iron level is normal, which may take 2–3 days.

IVERMECTIN AND OTHER MACROLIDE ENDECTOCIDE TOXICOSIS

Mode of action

Ivermectin and other avermectins potentiate the action of GABA by stimulating the presynaptic release of GABA and increasing the binding of GABA to postsynaptic receptors. The result is neuromuscular blockade, which causes paralysis and death of vulnerable parasites.

Sources

Ivermectin is an antiparasitic agent; milbemycin is an avermectin and is also an antiparasitic agent.

Therapeutic dosages

1. Recommended therapeutic doses are:

A. Dogs: for the prevention of heartworm 6 mcg/kg PO once a month

B. Cats: for the prevention of heartworm 24 mcg/kg PO once a month

C. Puppies and kittens: for the treatment of *Sarcoptes scabei, Notoedres cati, Otodectes cynotis, Cheyletiella* spp., *Demodex canis, Pneumonyssus caninum, Ancylostoma caninum, Toxocara canis, Toxascaris leonina* and *Trichuris vulpis* 200 mcg/kg SC

D. Dogs: for the treatment of microfilaria of *Dirofilaria immitis* 50 mcg/kg.

Toxic dosages

2. Recognized toxic doses are:
   A. In puppies and kittens: >300 µg/kg SC.
   B. In cats: >500 µg/kg.
   C. The oral LD_{50} for most dogs is 80 000 µg/kg (80 mg/kg).
   D. Coma and death occurred in some dogs given 40 000–80 000 µg/kg (40–80 mg/kg).
   E. Dogs given doses of 5000 µg/kg (5 mg/kg) developed central nervous system signs including muscle tremors and ataxia.
   F. Dogs given doses of 2500 µg/kg (2.5 mg/kg) developed mydriasis.
   G. The highest single dose without effect was 2000 µg/kg (2 mg/kg).
3. Idiosyncratic toxicity in collies, Australian Shepherds, Old English Sheepdogs, Shetland Sheepdogs, other breeds and their crosses with MDR1 genetic mutation occurs at doses as low as 100 µg/kg (0.1 mg/kg). The increased sensitivity in these breeds is suspected to be due to the greater penetration of ivermectin across the blood–brain barrier.

Diagnosis

History—History of exposure.
Clinical signs—
1. General toxicosis—the clinical signs may develop with 4 hours of ingestion and include ataxia, aggression, behavior changes, bradycardia, cyanosis, depression, disorientation, dyspnea, head pressing or bobbing, hyperesthesia, hyperactivity, hyperthermia, mydriasis, muscle tremors, restlessness, seizures, tachycardia, vomiting, coma and death.
2. Idiosyncratic toxicosis—the clinical signs include ataxia, apparent blindness, behavior disturbances, depression, hypersalivation, mydriasis, muscle tremors, recumbency, coma and death.
Laboratory findings—Plasma, liver, fat and brain analysis may reveal the avermectin level. The CBC, serum biochemical profile, blood gas analysis and urinalysis are usually normal.

Prognosis

The prognosis varies with the species, breed and age of the patient, the product, the route of ingestion and the dose.

Treatment

1. Inform the client of the diagnosis, prognosis and the cost of treatment.
2. Ensure a patent airway. Intubate the patient if necessary.
3. Administer supplemental oxygen and ventilation if necessary.

Toxicologic emergencies

4. Place an intravenous catheter. Administer a balanced electrolyte crystalloid fluid intravenously to maintain perfusion, and hydration.
5. If the patient is experiencing anaphylaxis, administer epinephrine and antihistamines.
6. Administer phenobarbital or pentobarbital if necessary to control seizures or hyperactivity:
    A. Phenobarbital 2–4 mg/kg IV in dogs, 1–2 mg/kg IV in cats
    B. Pentobarbital 2–30 mg/kg slow IV to effect
    C. **Avoid diazepam and benzodiazepine tranquilizers, which also stimulate GABA receptors**.
7. If the patient is presented within 2 hours of ingestion, attempt decontamination by inducing emesis or performing gastric lavage. Do not induce emesis if the patient is having seizures or if emesis is otherwise contraindicated.
    A. Induction of emesis in cats
        I. Administer xylazine, 0.44–1 mg/kg IM or SC (can reverse with yohimbine 0.1 mg/kg IM, SC, or IV slowly).
        II. Administer medetomidine, 10 µg/kg IM (can reverse with atipamezole (Antisedan®) 25 µg/kg IM).
        III. Hydrogen peroxide is very difficult to administer to cats and is no longer recommended.
    B. Induction of emesis in dogs
        I. Apomorphine 0.02–0.04 mg/kg IV or IM, or 1.5–6 mg dissolved and placed into the conjunctival fornix. If apomorphine was placed in the eye, after emesis, the patient's eye should be thoroughly lavaged with sterile saline. If excessive sedation occurs from apomorphine, the sedation may be reversed by the administration of naloxone (0.01–0.04 mg/kg IV, IM, SC) but this will not reverse the emetic effects.
        II. Administer 3% hydrogen peroxide 1–5 mL/kg (0.5–2 mL/lb) PO, with a maximum dose of 3 tablespoons (45 mL). If the patient does not vomit within 10 minutes, give 3% hydrogen peroxide 0.5 mL/kg (0.25 mL/lb) PO *once*.
    C. Gastric lavage
        I. Lightly anesthetize the patient.
        II. Administer oxygen and intravenous fluids to the patient while under anesthesia.
        III. Maintain anesthesia with the appropriate anesthetic as needed.
        IV. Intubate the patient with a cuffed endotracheal tube and inflate the cuff.
        V. Place the patient in lateral recumbency.
        VI. With a stomach tube held outside of the patient, alongside the patient, measure the distance from the tip of the nose to the last rib. Mark this distance on the stomach tube.
        VII. Lubricate the caudal end of the stomach tube with water-soluble jelly then pass the stomach tube gently into the

stomach, passing the tube no farther than the marked distance on the tube.
VIII. If desired, two stomach tubes may be utilized, a smaller ingress tube and a large egress tube.
  IX. Infuse warm (body-temperature) tap water, 5–10 mL/kg, through the tube (ingress tube if using two tubes) to moderately distend the stomach.
   X. Allow the fluid to drain from the stomach through the tube (egress tube if using two tubes).
  XI. Save samples of gastric contents, suspicious foreign material, seeds, etc. for possible toxicologic analysis.
 XII. The stomach tube may have to be manipulated, repositioned or flushed with fluid or air if the gastric contents do not flow freely through the tube.
XIII. Turn the patient to the other side and continue to perform gastric lavage.
XIV. Continue gastric lavage until the effluent is clear.
 XV. If using the two-tube method, crimp the end of one tube and remove it.
XVI. Administer activated charcoal down the stomach tube.
XVII. Crimp the end of the stomach tube and remove it.
XVIII. Monitor the patient during recovery from anesthesia, leaving the inflated cuffed endotracheal tube in place until the patient's swallowing reflex has returned.

D. Activated charcoal, 1–5 g/kg (3–6 mL/lb) PO is usually administered in a slurry of 1 g per 5 mL water. In ivermectin toxicosis patients, repeat the administration of activated charcoal q3–4h. Administer a cathartic only once.

E. A single dose of an osmotic or saline cathartic should be administered along with activated charcoal unless the patient has severe diarrhea. Do not administer magnesium-containing cathartics if the patient is exhibiting neurologic signs. Alternative cathartics include:
   I. Sorbitol (70%), 2 g/kg (1–2 mL/kg) PO
  II. Magnesium sulfate (Epsom salt), 200 mg/kg for cats, 250–500 mg/kg for dogs; mix magnesium sulfate with water, 5–10 mL/kg and administer PO
 III. Magnesium hydroxide (Milk of Magnesia®), 15–50 mL for cats, 10–150 mL for dogs, q6–12h PO as needed
  IV. Sodium sulfate, 200 mg/kg for cats, 250–500 mg/kg for dogs. Mix sodium sulfate with water, 5–10 mL/kg and administer PO.

F. Administer an enema.

8. Hospitalize the patient for symptomatic and supportive therapy. The recovery period may be prolonged. There is one reported case of a dog recovering from a coma of 7 weeks duration.

9. If the patient has been severely poisoned, consider the administration of physostigmine (Antilirium®).
   A. Physostigmine 0.06 mg/kg, should be administered slow IV.
   B. The duration of action is short (30–90 minutes).

C. The administration of physostigmine may be repeated q12h for several days until recovery.
10. Picrotoxin may cause seizures and is not considered standard treatment.
11. If the patient has an acute anaphylactic reaction, administer epinephrine and antihistamines.
12. If the patient has severe bradycardia, administer atropine.

LEAD POISONING

Mode of action

Lead binds sulfhydryl groups and interferes with many sulfhydryl-containing enzymes. Lead may also compete with or replace zinc in other enzymes. The results on the interference with enzyme function include demyelination and decreased conduction velocity in the peripheral nervous system, interference with the action of γ-aminobutyric acid (GABA), with cholinergic function, with dopamine uptake, with heme synthesis and inhibition of the enzyme pyrimidine 5′-nucleotidase which results in increased erythrocyte fragility and basophilic stippling.

Sources

Lead containing paint, linoleum, tile, batteries, plumbing materials, putty, lead foil, solder, golf balls, certain roof coverings, lubricants, rug pads, acid (soft) drinking water from lead pipes or improperly glazed ceramic water bowls, lead weights, fishing sinkers, drapery weights, toys, newsprint, dyes, canned dog or cat foods, insulation, house dust, wine bottle cork foils, burnt lubricant oil, pool table chalk.

Diagnosis

History—History of exposure.
Clinical signs—These include:
1. Gastrointestinal signs: vomiting, abdominal pain, anorexia, occasionally diarrhea or constipation
2. Neurological signs: seizures, hysteria, behavior changes, ataxia, circling, compulsive pacing, chomping of the jaws, vocalizing, dementia, head pressing, muscle spasms, polyneuropathy, mydriasis and blindness.
Laboratory findings—
1. Analysis of 2 mL of whole heparinized blood from a lead free vial
   A. >60 mg lead/100 mL blood (0.6 ppm) is diagnostic.
   B. 30–50 mg/100 mL blood (0.3–0.5 ppm) indicates lead poisoning if associated with typical signs and hematologic findings.
   C. 5–25 mg/100 mL (0.05–0.25 ppm) is the normal baseline lead level.
2. Examination of a stained blood smear demonstrates large numbers of NRBCs (5–40/100 WBCs) without evidence of severe anemia (PCV <30%). Also anisocytosis, polychromasia, poikilocytosis, target cells, hypochromasia, and possibly basophilic stippling in RBCs may be observed.

3. Anemia may be found in some cases.
4. Urinalysis may be normal or renal casts may be observed. Urine lead levels >0.75 ppm indicate lead poisoning.

Abdominal radiographs—May reveal the presence of metallic foreign bodies in the gastrointestinal tract.

Differential diagnosis

1. Canine distemper
2. Epilepsy
3. Rabies
4. Intestinal parasitism
5. Hypoglycemia
6. Nonspecific gastrointestinal disturbance
7. Acute pancreatitis
8. Encephalitis
9. Vertebral problems
10. Other poisonings.

Prognosis

The prognosis is favorable in the majority of the cases that undergo chelation therapy. Continuous or uncontrolled seizures warrant an unfavorable prognosis.

Treatment

1. Inform the client of the diagnosis, prognosis and the cost of treatment.
2. Remove lead, if present, from the gastrointestinal tract.
    A. Administer warm water enemas.
    B. Induce emesis. Gastric lavage is not very successful.
        I. Induction of emesis in cats
            a. Administer xylazine, 0.44–1 mg/kg IM or SC (can reverse with yohimbine 0.1 mg/kg IM, SC, or IV slowly).
            b. Administer medetomidine, 10 μg/kg IM (can reverse with atipamezole (Antisedan®) 25 μg/kg IM).
            c. Hydrogen peroxide is very difficult to administer to cats and is no longer recommended.
        II. Induction of emesis in dogs
            a. Administer apomorphine 0.02–0.04 mg/kg IV or IM, or 1.5–6 mg dissolved and placed into the conjunctival fornix. If apomorphine was placed in the eye, after emesis, the patient's eye should be thoroughly lavaged with sterile saline. If excessive sedation occurs from apomorphine, the sedation may be reversed by the administration of naloxone (0.01–0.04 mg/kg IV, IM, SC) but this will not reverse the emetic effects.
            b. Administer 3% hydrogen peroxide 1–5 mL/kg (0.5–2 mL/lb) PO, with a maximum dose of 3 tablespoons (45 mL). If the

patient does not vomit within 10 minutes, give 3% hydrogen peroxide 0.5 mL/kg (0.25 mL/lb) PO *once*.
  C. Administration of activated charcoal is not recommended as it is not very useful.
  D. Administer a sodium or magnesium sulfate cathartic *once*:
    I. Sodium sulfate, 200 mg/kg for cats, 250–500 mg/kg for dogs; mix sodium sulfate with water, 5–10 mg/kg and administer PO.
    II. Magnesium sulfate (Epsom salt), 200 mg/kg for cats, 250–500 mg/kg for dogs; mix magnesium sulfate with water, 5–10 mL/kg and administer PO.
  E. Perform endoscopy or surgery to remove lead foreign bodies from the gastrointestinal tract.
3. Remove lead from blood and body tissues by administering a chelating agent.
  A. Administer calcium EDTA 25 mg/kg SC q6h or 50 mg/kg q12h for 2–5 days
    I. Prior to administration, dilute calcium EDTA to a concentration of 10 mg calcium EDTA/mL of 5% dextrose.
    II. Do not exceed 2 g/day in small animals.
  B. Administer penicillamine 33–55 mg/kg/day for 1 week, off 1 week, then repeat for 1 week. The daily dose can be divided and given at 6–8 hour intervals, on an empty stomach. Dissolving D-penicillamine in fruit juice may help improve palatability and mask the odor.
  C. The administration of dimercaprol (BAL) in combination with calcium EDTA is used in children, but seldom used in animals. It offers the advantages of removing lead directly from the RBC and excreting lead primarily via the bile.
    I. The dose of dimercaprol is 2.5 mg/kg IM q4h on days 1 and 2, q8h on day 3 and then q12h.
    II. If the case is acute and severe, administer 5 mg/kg IM q4h on day 1.
  D. Administer succimer (*meso*-2,3-dimercaptosuccinic acid or DMSA) (Chemet®) 10 mg/kg PO q8h for 10 days. This is a newer chelator that appears to be more effective and less toxic.
4. Supportive treatment
  A. Seizures are due to cerebral edema.
    I. Administer furosemide 1–5 mg/kg IV.
    II. Following the administration of furosemide, administer mannitol 100–1000 mg/kg IV over 15–30 minutes.
  B. Administer diazepam, phenobarbital or pentobarbital if necessary to control seizures or hyperactivity.
    I. Diazepam 0.5–1 mg/kg IV in increments of 5–20 mg to effect
    II. Phenobarbital 2–4 mg/kg IV in dogs, 1–2 mg/kg IV in cats
    III. Pentobarbital 2–30 mg/kg slow IV to effect
  C. Administer thiamine 1–2 mg/kg IM or 2 mg/kg PO q24h.
  D. Administer broad-spectrum antibiotics if the patient has severe hemorrhagic gastroenteritis.
  E. Continue chelator therapy until the blood lead levels have returned to the normal range.

Veterinarian's obligation

Animals may manifest signs of toxicity before humans when they are sharing the same environment. Warn the owners of lead poisoned pets, especially if there are small children in the family.

MACADAMIA NUTS

Toxin

The specific toxin is unknown.

Mode of action

The mode of action is unknown, but appears to involve neurotransmitters or neuromuscular junctions, motor neurons and muscle fibers.

Sources

Macadamia nuts come from *Macadamia tetraphylla* or *Macadamia intergrifolia* trees. The nuts contain sugars (4%) and oils (up to 80%).

Toxic dosages

Clinical signs are usually seen when ingestion exceeds 2 g/kg, but have been observed with 0.7 g/kg. There are approximately 12 nuts per ounce (0.5 nuts per gram).

Diagnosis

History—The dog will usually have a history of ingestion, or a chewed-up empty package of macadamia nuts or candy, cookies or other baked goods containing macadamia nuts may be found.
Clinical signs—Dogs usually exhibit weakness, especially of the hindlimbs. Depression, vomiting, ataxia and tremors may be seen. Hyperthermia, abdominal pain, lameness, pallor, recumbency and stiffness may occur.
Laboratory findings—Serum triglyceride levels, alkaline phosphatase and lipase may be elevated. Mild leukocytosis may be noted.

Prognosis

The prognosis is excellent. In most cases, the clinical signs resolve within 12–24 hours.

Treatment

1. Inform the client of the diagnosis, prognosis and cost of the treatment.
2. If the patient presents less than 4 hours since exposure, attempt gastric decontamination with emesis, especially for ingestion of >1 g/kg.

Toxicologic emergencies

3. Induction of emesis in dogs
   A. Apomorphine 0.02–0.04 mg/kg IV or IM, or 1.5–6 mg dissolved and placed into the conjunctival fornix. If apomorphine was placed in the eye, after emesis, the patient's eye should be thoroughly lavaged with sterile saline. If excessive sedation occurs from apomorphine, the sedation may be reversed by the administration of naloxone (0.01–0.04 mg/kg IV, IM, SC) but this will not reverse the emetic effects.
   B. Administer 3% hydrogen peroxide 1–5 mL/kg (0.5–2 mL/lb) PO, with a maximum dose of 3 tablespoons (45 mL). If the patient does not vomit within 10 minutes, give 3% hydrogen peroxide 0.5 mL/kg (0.25 mL/lb) PO *once*.
4. Administer activated charcoal with sorbitol, 1–5 g/kg (3–6 mL/lb) PO once.
5. Administer supportive therapy.
   A. Administer intravenous or SC fluids.
   B. Monitor for, and treat hyperthermia, if indicated.
   C. Administer antiemetics if needed.
   D. Encourage rest by confining the patient in a quiet environment.
6. If the macadamia nuts were covered with chocolate, or xylitol was used in the baked product, treat accordingly for the concurrent toxin.

MARIJUANA AND HASHISH TOXICOSIS

Mode of action

Tetrahydrocannabinol (THC) is the active ingredient. In the brain, THC interacts with all major neurotransmitters, including serotonin, dopamine, acetylcholine and norepinephrine. THC binds to specific receptors in the frontal cortex and cerebellum.

Sources

Marijuana is obtained from the hemp plant, *Cannabis sativa*. Marijuana is the dried leaves and flowers, and contains 1–5% THC. Hashish is the resin extracted from the hemp plant and contains 10% THC. Hash oil is a concentrated form of hashish, usually containing >50% THC. A capsular form is available for patients with glaucoma or undergoing chemotherapy.

Pets usually gain exposure through ingestion of leftover baked goods containing marijuana, from ingesting the butts of marijuana cigarettes or ingesting the dried leaves and flowers.

Toxic dosages

The lethal dose in dogs is >3 g/kg. Fatalities from ingestion are not common. The clinical signs occur at much lower doses.

Diagnosis

History—History of ingestion, if available. The client may be reluctant to provide an accurate history.

Clinical signs—The patient may exhibit mydriasis, ataxia, depression, hypothermia, bradycardia, rapidly changing signs, acute aggression, bizarre behavior, excessive salivation, vomiting, muscle tremors, hyperesthesia, disorientation, nystagmus and seizures. Hyperthermia and tachypnea occur in some patients.

Laboratory findings—THC can be detected in plasma or urine.

Differential diagnosis

The differential diagnoses include intoxications from amphetamines, antihistamines, cocaine, methylxanthines, tricyclic antidepressants, garbage intoxication, hallucinogenic mushrooms, other recreational drugs and plants, and black widow spider bites.

Prognosis

The prognosis is fair to good.

Treatment

1. Inform the client of the diagnosis, prognosis and the cost of treatment.
2. Ensure a patent airway. Intubate the patient if necessary.
3. Administer supplemental oxygen and ventilation if necessary
4. Administer diazepam, chlorpromazine, phenobarbital or pentobarbital if necessary to control seizures or hyperactivity.
   A. Diazepam 0.5–1 mg/kg IV in increments of 5–20 mg to effect
   B. Chlorpromazine 0.5–1 mg/kg IV as needed
   C. Phenobarbital 2–4 mg/kg IV in dogs, 1–2 mg/kg IV in cats
   D. Pentobarbital 2–30 mg/kg slow IV to effect
5. If ingestion occurred within 1 hour of presentation, attempt to induce emesis. Induction of emesis may not be effective owing to the antiemetic properties of THC. If the patient ingested a large amount of baked goods containing marijuana, consider gastric lavage.
   A. Induction of emesis in cats
      I. Administer xylazine, 0.44–1 mg/kg IM or SC (can reverse with yohimbine 0.1 mg/kg IM, SC, or IV slowly).
      II. Administer medetomidine, 10 µg/kg IM (can reverse with atipamezole (Antisedan®) 25 µg/kg IM).
      III. Hydrogen peroxide is very difficult to administer to cats and is no longer recommended.
   B. Induction of emesis in dogs
      I. Apomorphine 0.02–0.04 mg/kg IV or IM, or 1.5–6 mg dissolved and placed into the conjunctival fornix. If apomorphine was placed in the eye, after emesis, the patient's eye should be thoroughly lavaged with sterile saline. If excessive sedation occurs from apomorphine, the sedation may be reversed by the administration of naloxone (0.01–0.04 mg/kg IV, IM, SC) but this will not reverse the emetic effects.

II. Administer 3% hydrogen peroxide 1–5 mL/kg (0.5–2 mL/lb) PO, with a maximum dose of 3 tablespoons (45 mL). If the patient does not vomit within 10 minutes, give 3% hydrogen peroxide 0.5 mL/kg (0.25 mL/lb) PO *once*.

C. Gastric lavage

    I. Lightly anesthetize the patient.

    II. Administer oxygen and intravenous fluids to the patient while under anesthesia.

    III. Maintain anesthesia with the appropriate anesthetic as needed.

    IV. Intubate the patient with a cuffed endotracheal tube and inflate the cuff.

    V. Place the patient in lateral recumbency.

    VI. With a stomach tube held outside of the patient, alongside the patient, measure the distance from the tip of the nose to the last rib. Mark this distance on the stomach tube.

    VII. Lubricate the caudal end of the stomach tube with water-soluble jelly then pass the stomach tube gently into the stomach, passing the tube no farther than the marked distance on the tube.

    VIII. If desired, two stomach tubes may be utilized, a smaller ingress tube and a large egress tube.

    IX. Infuse warm (body-temperature) tap water, 5–10 mL/kg, through the tube (ingress tube if using two tubes) to moderately distend the stomach.

    X. Allow the fluid to drain from the stomach through the tube (egress tube if using two tubes).

    XI. Save samples of gastric contents, suspicious foreign material, seeds, etc. for possible toxicologic analysis.

    XII. The stomach tube may have to be manipulated, repositioned or flushed with fluid or air if the gastric contents do not flow freely through the tube.

    XIII. Turn the patient to the other side and continue to perform gastric lavage.

    XIV. Continue gastric lavage until the effluent is clear.

    XV. If using the two-tube method, crimp the end of one tube and remove it.

    XVI. Administer activated charcoal down the stomach tube.

    XVII. Crimp the end of the stomach tube and remove it.

    XVIII. Monitor the patient during recovery from anesthesia, leaving the inflated cuffed endotracheal tube in place until the patient's swallowing reflex has returned.

6. Administer activated charcoal with sorbitol, 1–5 g/kg (3–6 mL/lb) PO once.

7. Provide a quiet, darkened environment.

8. Hospitalize the patient for observation and provide supportive and symptomatic therapy for 18–24 hours.

9. If vomiting is persistent and severe, place an intravenous catheter and administer a balanced electrolyte crystalloid fluid intravenously to maintain hydration.

10. Administer antiemetic agents if vomiting continues.
    A. Maropitant, 1 mg/kg SC or 2 mg/kg PO q24h for up to 5 days
    B. Ondansetron, 0.1–0.2 mg/kg IV q8–12h
    C. Dolasetron, 0.6–1 mg/kg IV, SC or PO q24h
11. If the patient has respiratory depression, provide supplemental oxygen and administer doxapram 2.0–10.0 mg/kg slow IV.
12. If the patient is recumbent, turn the patient side to side every 4 hours.
13. Monitor body temperature and treat accordingly. Both hypothermia and hyperthermia may occur.

METALDEHYDE TOXICOSIS

Mode of action

The mode of action is unknown. Metabolic acidosis occurs as a result of the metabolism of acetaldehyde, which is the metabolite of metaldehyde, but acetaldehyde does not cause the clinical syndrome of toxicosis. Levels of GABA, serotonin and norepinephrine are reduced in patients with metaldehyde toxicosis, and lead to seizure activity.

Sources

Metaldehyde is found in snail, slug and rat poison. Exposure can occur through the ingestion of poisoned snails, slugs or rats. Metaldehyde is also found in some fuels used in small heaters.

Toxic dosages

The LD_{50} for dogs is 100 mg/kg and is suspected to be similar for cats. Clinical signs may occur at much lower doses.

Diagnosis

History—The owner may be able to provide a history of exposure.
Clinical signs—Signs appear within 30 minutes to 5 hours and include anxiety, hyperesthesia, ataxia, muscle fasciculations and tremors, nystagmus in cats, tachycardia, mydriasis may occur, salivation, and possibly vomiting and diarrhea. As the clinical course progresses, the patient may develop severe hyperthermia (possibly >108°F), severe metabolic acidosis, loss of consciousness, decreased respiration, cyanosis, continuous seizures and death may occur due to respiratory failure. Hepatic failure may occur 3–5 days following exposure.
Laboratory findings—
1. Urine, plasma, stomach contents and tissue samples may be analyzed to detect metaldehyde.
2. Blood gas analysis may reveal a severe metabolic acidosis.

Differential diagnosis

The differential diagnoses include intoxications from strychnine, organophosphates, carbamates, pyrethrins or pyrethroids and other toxicosis.

Prognosis

The prognosis is fair to guarded.

Treatment

1. Inform the client of the diagnosis, prognosis and the cost of treatment.
2. Ensure a patent airway. Intubate the patient if necessary.
3. Administer supplemental oxygen and ventilation if necessary.
4. Place an intravenous catheter. Administer a balanced electrolyte crystalloid fluid intravenously to maintain perfusion, hydration and diuresis.
5. Administer diazepam, phenobarbital, pentobarbital or propofol if necessary to control seizures or hyperactivity
   A. Diazepam 0.5–1 mg/kg IV in increments of 5–20 mg to effect
   B. Phenobarbital 2–4 mg/kg IV in dogs, 1–2 mg/kg IV in cats
   C. Pentobarbital 2–30 mg/kg slow IV to effect
   D. Propofol 2–6 mg/kg IV or as a CRI (0.1–0.6 mg/kg/min) IV if needed
6. Treat hyperthermia symptomatically.
7. Decontamination will be of value up to 2 hours' post-ingestion. Induce emesis or perform gastric lavage.
   A. Induction of emesis in cats
      I. Administer xylazine, 0.44–1 mg/kg IM or SC (can reverse with yohimbine 0.1 mg/kg IM, SC, or IV slowly).
      II. Administer medetomidine, 10 µg/kg IM (can reverse with atipamezole (Antisedan®) 25 µg/kg IM).
      III. Hydrogen peroxide is very difficult to administer to cats and is no longer recommended.
   B. Induction of emesis in dogs
      I. Administer apomorphine 0.02–0.04 mg/kg IV or IM, or 1.5–6 mg dissolved and placed into the conjunctival fornix. If apomorphine was placed in the eye, after emesis, the patient's eye should be thoroughly lavaged with sterile saline. If excessive sedation occurs from apomorphine, the sedation may be reversed by the administration of naloxone (0.01–0.04 mg/kg IV, IM, SC) but this will not reverse the emetic effects.
      II. Administer 3% hydrogen peroxide 1–5 mL/kg (0.5–2 mL/lb) PO, with a maximum dose of 3 tablespoons (45 mL). If the patient does not vomit within 10 minutes, give 3% hydrogen peroxide 0.5 mL/kg (0.25 mL/lb) PO *once*.
   C. Gastric lavage
      I. Lightly anesthetize the patient.
      II. Administer oxygen and intravenous fluids to the patient while under anesthesia.

III. Maintain anesthesia with the appropriate anesthetic as needed.

IV. Intubate the patient with a cuffed endotracheal tube and inflate the cuff.

V. Place the patient in lateral recumbency.

VI. With a stomach tube held outside of the patient, alongside the patient, measure the distance from the tip of the nose to the last rib. Mark this distance on the stomach tube.

VII. Lubricate the caudal end of the stomach tube with water-soluble jelly then pass the stomach tube gently into the stomach, passing the tube no farther than the marked distance on the tube.

VIII. If desired, two stomach tubes may be utilized, a smaller ingress tube and a large egress tube.

IX. Infuse warm (body-temperature) tap water, 5–10 mL/kg, through the tube (ingress tube if using two tubes) to moderately distend the stomach.

X. Allow the fluid to drain from the stomach through the tube (egress tube if using two tubes).

XI. Save samples of gastric contents, suspicious foreign material, seeds, etc. for possible toxicologic analysis.

XII. The stomach tube may have to be manipulated, repositioned or flushed with fluid or air if the gastric contents do not flow freely through the tube.

XIII. Turn the patient to the other side and continue to perform gastric lavage.

XIV. Continue gastric lavage until the effluent is clear.

XV. If using the two-tube method, crimp the end of one tube and remove it.

XVI. Administer activated charcoal down the stomach tube.

XVII. Crimp the end of the stomach tube and remove it.

XVIII. Monitor the patient during recovery from anesthesia, leaving the inflated cuffed endotracheal tube in place until the patient's swallowing reflex has returned.

D. Activated charcoal, 1–5 g/kg PO. The first dose should be combined with sorbitol 70%, 1–2 mL/kg PO. Repeat the administration of activated charcoal (without sorbitol) 0.5–2 g/kg PO every 4–8 hours.

8. To control muscle tremors :
   A. Administer diazepam 0.5–1 mg/kg IV in increments of 2.5–20 mg, or per rectum 1–4 mg/kg in increments of 5–20 mg, as needed. A diazepam CRI IV at 0.1–0.5 mg/kg/h may be beneficial.
   B. Administer methocarbamol IV as needed:
      I. Dogs: 55–220 mg/kg, give ½ of the dose IV slowly (<2 mL/min) then the remainder to effect if needed
      II. Cats: 55 mg/kg

9. For seizure control, if diazepam is not effective, administer:
   A. Pentobarbital 3–15 mg IV, repeated in 4–8 hours as needed

B. Propofol 6 mg/kg IV, 25% every 30 seconds, or 0.1–0.6 mg/kg/min CRI IV.

10. If the patient has a severe metabolic acidosis, pH <7.05, administer sodium bicarbonate IV.

    A. mEq HCO_3 needed $= 0.3 \times$ (kg body weight) $\times$ (desired total

$$CO_2 \text{ mEq/L} - \text{measured total } CO_2 \text{ mEq/L}).$$

    B. Infuse ¼–½ or 25–50% of the sodium bicarbonate amount needed over 30–60 minutes, then re-evaluate blood gas values and readjust the dose.

    C. Caution must be utilized while administering sodium bicarbonate. Possible complications that may result include: 'overshoot alkalosis', hypernatremia, intravascular volume overload, hypokalemia, hypocalcemia, tissue hypoxia and paradoxical cerebrospinal fluid acidosis.

11. Hospitalize the patient for monitoring and symptomatic and supportive therapy.

12. Administer antiemetics as needed.

13. Monitor hepatic enzymes as delayed hepatotoxicity may occur.

MISCELLANEOUS TOXICOSES

1. 5-Fluorouracil (5-FU)

    A. 5-Fluorouracil is an antimetabolite used in the treatment of superficial dermal neoplasia and for solar and actinic keratoses in people.

    B. It is found in topical creams and solutions such as Efudex® and Fluoroplex®.

    C. Animal toxicosis usually results following ingestion or dermal absorption of topical creams. The toxic oral dose is 6 mg/kg and the lethal oral dose is 43 mg/kg.

    D. The clinical signs include depression, hypersalivation, vomiting, bloody diarrhea, ataxia, tremors, hyperesthesia, hyperexcitability, seizures, pulmonary edema, respiratory failure, cardiac arrhythmias and cardiac failure. Death may occur within 6–16 hours.

    E. Treatment is symptomatic and supportive, including emetics, dermal decontamination, activated charcoal, anticonvulsants, gastrointestinal protectants, blood component therapy, and antiemetics.

2. Hexachlorophene

    A. Hexachlorophene is an antiseptic found in over-the-counter preparations including pHisoHex®.

    B. Hexachlorophene is particularly toxic to cats, owing to the cat's inability to conjugate glucuronic acid with phenolic compounds.

    C. Ingestion of 20 mg/kg daily in adult cats resulted in clinical signs in less than 14 days.

    D. The clinical signs result from severe myelin damage and secondary axonal degeneration.

    E. The clinical signs of intoxication include a gradual progressing degeneration of motor functions, starting in the hindquarters and

proceeding cranially. Hindlimb stiffness may progress to ataxia, hypermetria and weakness. Other signs include prostration, urinary retention, complete flaccid paralysis, mydriasis, hypothermia, CNS excitation, bradycardia, diarrhea, anorexia, salivation and death.
F. Treatment is symptomatic and supportive.
   I. Advise the owner to administer water, milk or egg whites orally prior to transporting the patient to the veterinary hospital.
   II. An attempt to decontaminate the skin should be made, but hexachlorophene is difficult to remove with water. Wash the patient with polyethylene glycol or glycerol then wash with dishwasher liquid and rinse thoroughly.
   III. The administration of an osmotic diuretic is beneficial.
   IV. The administration of prednisolone has not been beneficial.
   V. The administration of N-acetylcysteine (Mucomyst®) may be beneficial.
3. (2-methyl-4-chloro) phenoxyacetic acid (MCPA)
   A. MCPA is an herbicide. The commercial product also contains petroleum distillates, which may lead to aspiration pneumonia.
   B. Toxicosis occurs from either inhalation or ingestion.
   C. The petroleum distillates cause anemia, dizziness, weakness, weight loss, muscle fibrillations, myotonia and muscular weakness.
   D. Other clinical signs include vomiting, abdominal pain, anorexia, ataxia and generalized weakness.
   E. Chlorophenoxy acids are hematotoxic and cause aplastic anemia, agranulocytosis, thrombocytopenia and neutropenia.
   F. Laboratory findings include myoglobinuria, hemoglobinuria, anemia, thrombocytopenia, lymphopenia and neutropenia.
   G. Treatment is symptomatic and supportive.
      I. Induction of emesis is contraindicated owing to the presence of petroleum distillates.
      II. Administer activated charcoal orally.
      III. Administer 0.9% NaCI IV.
      IV. Administer warm-water enemas.
      V. Administer diazepam IV as needed for the muscle fibrillations.
      VI. Administer metoclopramide if antiemetic administration is necessary.
4. Metoclopramide
   A. Metoclopramide (Reglan®) is a dopaminergic agonist. It also sensitizes tissues to the effect of acetylcholine.
   B. Neurotoxicity may occur in patients given therapeutic levels.
   C. The clinical signs include slow to rapid twisting movements involving the face, neck, trunk or limbs. Other clinical signs include CNS depression, restlessness or nervousness.
   D. The treatment is symptomatic and supportive.
   E. The administration of diphenhydramine 4 mg/kg q8h may be beneficial.
   F. Within 2–3 days after stopping the administration of metoclopramide, the clinical signs usually resolve.

5. Metronidazole
  A. Metronidazole (Flagyl®) may cause neurotoxicity.
  B. The clinical signs usually occur with long term administration (7–12 days) following the initiation of metronidazole administration at high dosage rates (>66 mg/kg/day). It is recommended to administer a maximum daily dose of ≤50 mg/kg/day).
  C. Acute signs, within 4–6 days following the initiation of metronidazole administration, have been reported in dogs ingesting 250 mg/kg/day.
  D. The clinical signs include severe ataxia, stomatitis, glossitis, vertical or rotary nystagmus, opisthotonos, spasms of the lumbar and hindlimb muscles, seizures, head tilt, dorsiflexion of the tail, inability to walk, and death.
  E. Treatment is symptomatic and supportive.
  F. Within 1–2 weeks after stopping the administration of metronidazole, the clinical signs usually resolve.
6. Thallium intoxication
  A. Thallium may be found in some rodenticides and mole bait.
  B. The single-dose LD_{50} is 10–15 mg/kg.
  C. Thallium has an affinity for sulfhydryl groups of enzymes resulting in the inhibition of oxidative phosphorylation and decreased protein synthesis.
  D. The clinical signs of acute toxicosis usually develop within 12 hours to 4 days following ingestion. The clinical signs include acute onset of anorexia, abdominal pain, vomiting, diarrhea, hematochezia, hematemesis, dyspnea, lethargy, sialosis, stomatitis, mucopurulent ocular discharge, nervous signs and cardiovascular collapse.
  E. Signs of chronic exposure include erythema, dermatitis and alopecia.
  F. Thallium may be detected in urine or tissue samples.
  G. Differential diagnoses include parvovirus gastroenteritis, other viral gastroenteritis, acute hemorrhagic gastroenteritis, gastrointestinal foreign body, intussusception, acute necrotizing pancreatitis, metabolic diseases and other toxicoses (lead, arsenic, vitamin K anticoagulant rodenticides, brodifacoum, cholecalciferol and nonsteroidal anti-inflammatory agents).
  H. Treatment is controversial and often ineffective.
      I. The administration of prussian blue (potassium ferricyanoferrate (II) may be beneficial, but it is not approved for use in veterinary or human medicine and may contain contaminants and impurities.
      II. If prussian blue is not available, activated charcoal should be administered.
      III. Forced diuresis or hemodialysis may be beneficial in the long-term management of the patient.
      IV. Place an intravenous catheter. Administer a balanced electrolyte crystalloid fluid intravenously to maintain perfusion, hydration and diuresis.
      V. The administration of warm water enemas is recommended.
      VI. Administration of broad-spectrum antibiotics is recommended.

VII. **Avoid the administration of potassium chloride,** which may increase the release of intracellular thallium into the bloodstream and exacerbate the toxicosis.

MUSHROOM TOXICOSIS

Mode of action

The mode of action varies with the toxin contained in the species of mushroom ingested.

- Ibotenic acid, indoles and muscimol cause CNS effects including hallucinations, hyperactivity and coma.
- Some mushrooms contain toxins that cause autonomic nervous system signs, usually muscarinic signs.
- Gyromitrin is hydrolyzed to monomethylhydrazine (which is used as rocket fuel) and other metabolites that are hepatotoxic.
- Some mushrooms contain amantine, phalloidin or other complex polypeptides or cyclopeptides and cause cellular injury and death, which lead to cardiac, hepatic and renal damage and the death of the patient.
- Psilocybin and psilocyn in the *Psilocybe* spp. cause hallucinations, agitation and drowsiness.

Sources

Mushrooms grow in the wild in most areas of the world. The toxic species include *Amanita phalloides* (death angel), *A. virosa* (destroying angel), *A. muscaria* (fly agaric), *Boletus* spp., *Chlorophyllum molybdites* (backyard mushrooms), *Clitocybe* spp., *Cortinarius* spp., *Galerena* spp., *Gyromitra spp.* (false morels), *Inocybe* spp. and *Psilocybe cubensis* ('magic mushroom').

Toxic dosages

A child may be killed by ingesting the cap of one *Amanita* mushroom. The toxic dose varies with the species of mushroom.

Diagnosis

History—The owner may be able to provide a history of exposure.
Clinical signs—The clinical signs usually occur within 6–8 hours following ingestion and may include abdominal pain, ataxia, coma, depression, diarrhea, DIC, hallucinations, hyperthermia, muscarinic signs (lacrimation, urination, salivation and defecation), nausea, seizures, vomiting, circulatory collapse, acute hepatic failure, acute renal failure, and death.
Laboratory findings—
1. Severe hypoglycemia may be present.
2. The PCV and TP may be elevated owing to dehydration.
3. Hepatic enzyme elevation may be observed.
4. BUN and creatinine levels may elevate.

5. Thrombocytopenia and prolongation of the PT, PTT and ACT may occur in patients with DIC.
6. Evaluate the blood gas and electrolyte values.
7. Analysis of refrigerated stomach contents may reveal the presence of mushroom spores.

Differential diagnosis

The differential diagnoses include acute allergic reaction, garbage intoxication, boric acid intoxication, methylxanthine intoxication, organophosphate intoxication, pyrethrin or pyrethroid intoxication, rotenone intoxication and zinc intoxication.

Prognosis

The prognosis varies with the species ingested, the toxic effects and the amount ingested.

Treatment

1. Inform the client of the diagnosis, prognosis and the cost of treatment.
2. Ensure a patent airway. Intubate the patient if necessary.
3. Administer supplemental oxygen and ventilation if necessary.
4. Place an intravenous catheter. Administer a balanced electrolyte crystalloid fluid intravenously to maintain perfusion, hydration and diuresis.
5. Administer diazepam, phenobarbital or pentobarbital if necessary to control seizures or hyperactivity.
   A. Diazepam 0.5–1 mg/kg IV in increments of 5–20 mg to effect
   B. Phenobarbital 2–4 mg/kg IV in dogs, 1–2 mg/kg IV in cats
   C. Pentobarbital 2–30 mg/kg slow IV to effect
6. Treat hyperthermia symptomatically.
7. Decontamination will be of value up to 2 hours' post-ingestion. Induce emesis or perform gastric lavage if vomiting has not occurred.
   A. Induction of emesis in cats
      I. Administer xylazine, 0.44–1 mg/kg IM or SC (can reverse with yohimbine 0.1 mg/kg IM, SC, or IV slowly).
      II. Administer medetomidine, 10 μg/kg IM (can reverse with atipamezole (Antisedan®) 25 μg/kg IM).
      III. Hydrogen peroxide is very difficult to administer to cats and is no longer recommended.
   B. Induction of emesis in dogs
      I. Administer apomorphine 0.02–0.04 mg/kg IV or IM, or 1.5–6 mg dissolved and placed into the conjunctival fornix. If apomorphine was placed in the eye, after emesis, the patient's eye should be thoroughly lavaged with sterile saline. If excessive sedation occurs from apomorphine, the sedation may be reversed by the administration of naloxone

(0.01–0.04 mg/kg IV, IM, SC) but this will not reverse the emetic effects.

II. Administer 3% hydrogen peroxide 1–5 mL/kg (0.5–2 mL/lb) PO, with a maximum dose of 3 tablespoons (45 mL). If the patient does not vomit within 10 minutes, give 3% hydrogen peroxide 0.5 mL/kg (0.25 mL/lb) PO *once*.

C. Gastric lavage

    I. Lightly anesthetize the patient.

    II. Administer oxygen and intravenous fluids to the patient while under anesthesia.

    III. Maintain anesthesia with the appropriate anesthetic as needed.

    IV. Intubate the patient with a cuffed endotracheal tube and inflate the cuff.

    V. Place the patient in lateral recumbency.

    VI. With a stomach tube held outside of the patient, alongside the patient, measure the distance from the tip of the nose to the last rib. Mark this distance on the stomach tube.

    VII. Lubricate the caudal end of the stomach tube with water-soluble jelly then pass the stomach tube gently into the stomach, passing the tube no farther than the marked distance on the tube.

    VIII. If desired, two stomach tubes may be utilized, a smaller ingress tube and a large egress tube.

    IX. Infuse warm (body-temperature) tap water, 5–10 mL/kg, through the tube (ingress tube if using two tubes) to moderately distend the stomach.

    X. Lavaging with milk or sodium bicarbonate may aid in decreasing absorption.

    XI. Allow the fluid to drain from the stomach through the tube (egress tube if using two tubes).

    XII. Save samples of gastric contents, suspicious foreign material, seeds, etc. for possible toxicologic analysis.

    XIII. The stomach tube may have to be manipulated, repositioned or flushed with fluid or air if the gastric contents do not flow freely through the tube.

    XIV. Turn the patient to the other side and continue to perform gastric lavage.

    XV. Continue gastric lavage until the effluent is clear.

    XVI. If using the two-tube method, crimp the end of one tube and remove it.

    XVII. Administer activated charcoal down the stomach tube.

    XVIII. Crimp the end of the stomach tube and remove it.

    XIX. Monitor the patient during recovery from anesthesia, leaving the inflated cuffed endotracheal tube in place until the patient's swallowing reflex has returned.

D. Activated charcoal, 2–5 g/kg (3–6 mL/lb) PO is usually administered in a slurry of 1 g to 5 mL water. In mushroom toxicosis patients, repeat the administration of activated charcoal q4–6h. Administer a saline cathartic only *once*.

E. A single dose of an osmotic or saline cathartic should be administered along with activated charcoal. Do not administer magnesium-containing cathartics if the patient is exhibiting neurologic signs. Alternative cathartics include:

    I. Sorbitol (70%), 2 g/kg (1–2 mL/kg) PO

    II. Sodium sulfate, 200 mg/kg for cats, 250–500 mg/kg for dogs; mix sodium sulfate with water, 5–10 mL/kg and administer PO.

F. Whole bowel irrigation should be considered.

8. Hospitalize the patient and provide symptomatic and supportive treatment.
9. Monitor blood glucose levels.
10. Monitor hepatic and renal function.
11. Administer lactulose to reduce the ammonia level in the intestinal tract.
12. Anticipate DIC and treat aggressively with plasma or platelet administration, as indicated by the needs of the individual patient.
13. Treat hepatic and renal dysfunction as indicated. Administer hepatic protective agents.

    A. *N*-acetylcysteine (NAC), 50 mg/kg diluted to a 5% concentration in 5% dextrose in water or sterile water, then administer slowly over 15–30 minutes. Administer PO unless a bacteriostatic filter or a sterile solution of NAC is available.

    B. SAM-e, 18–20 mg/kg PO q24h

    C. Silymarin, 20–50 mg/kg PO q24h

14. Nutritional support may be beneficial.

NICOTINE INTOXICATION

Toxin

Nicotine is a dose-dependent, rapid-onset nicotinic ganglion depolarizer.

Mode of action

Nicotine causes depolarization and stimulation of nicotinic receptors in autonomic ganglia and neuromuscular junctions, the central nervous system, spinal cord and adrenal medulla. High-dose intoxication causes persistent ganglion and neuromuscular junction depolarization and blockade, followed by progressive and pervasive nervous system depression.

Sources

Nicotine is found in cigars, cigarettes, cigarette butts (which can also cause intestinal obstruction), nicotine patches, nicotine gum, chewing tobacco, nasal sprays, inhalers and electronic cigarettes. Xylitol is often found in some nicotine gums (see the Xylitol toxin section, below). If the nicotine product was obtained from a purse or bag, inquire about other concurrent potential toxin ingestions, such as medications or chocolate.

Toxic dosage

The oral LD$_{50}$ for dogs = 9–12 mg/kg.

Diagnosis

History—Ingestion is often witnessed, or chewed nicotine-containing products or wrappers may be found. Compatible clinical signs may be observed, and nicotine-containing products may be observed in the feces or vomitus.

Clinical signs—The patient may present with hyperexcitability, hypersalivation, vomiting, diarrhea, agitation, ataxia, tremors, mydriasis, tachypnea, tachycardia, hypertension, reflex bradycardia, depression or seizures.

Laboratory findings—Serum, gastric contents and urine may be evaluated for nicotine, but the level is rarely helpful for treatment.

ECG—Tachyarrhythmias, including atrial fibrillation and ventricular tachyarrhythmias, are commonly observed.

Differential diagnosis

Sepsis, hepatic disease, primary cardiac or neurologic disease, severe hypoglycemia, other toxicities (caffeine, methylxanthines, amphetamines, cocaine, ephedra / Ma Huang, organophosphates, carbamates, phenylpropanolamine, pyrethrins / pyrethroids, tremorgenic mycotoxins, strychnine and xylitol).

Prognosis

The prognosis depends upon the dose ingested. For low-dose ingestions the prognosis is excellent, but for high-dose ingestions the prognosis is poor unless treatment is started and the patient is stabilized within 4 hours after ingestion.

Treatment

1. Inform the client of the diagnosis, prognosis and cost of the treatment.
2. If the patient presents following recent ingestion with no clinical signs, induce emesis unless the patient is already vomiting.
   A. Induction of emesis in dogs
      I. Administer apomorphine 0.02–0.04 mg/kg IV or IM, or 1.5–6 mg dissolved and placed into the conjunctival fornix. If apomorphine was placed in the eye, after emesis, the patient's eye should be thoroughly lavaged with sterile saline. If excessive sedation occurs from apomorphine, the sedation may be reversed by the administration of naloxone (0.01–0.04 mg/kg IV, IM, SC) but this will not reverse the emetic effects.
      II. Administer 3% hydrogen peroxide 1–5 mL/kg (0.5–2 mL/lb) PO, with a maximum dose of 3 tablespoons (45 mL). If the patient does not vomit within 10 minutes, give 3% hydrogen peroxide 0.5 mL/kg (0.25 mL/lb) PO *once*.

B. Administer activated charcoal with sorbitol, 1–5 g/kg (3–6 mL/lb) PO once, unless the product ingested is sustained-release. In that case, administering multiple doses of activated charcoal without sorbitol (1–2 g/kg PO) may be repeated every 4 hours for 18–24 hours.

C. If the ingested product was a transdermal patch, and emesis is ineffective, remove the patch from the gastrointestinal tract with endoscopy or surgery to decrease absorption.

3. Administer supportive therapy.

4. Place an IV catheter and administer intravenous fluids (LRS, Normosol®-R) for the treatment of hypotension, to maintain hydration and to increase the rate of elimination.

5. Urine acidification may also enhance the elimination rate.

6. Administer an antiemetic, if needed.
   A. Maropitant, 1 mg/kg SC or 2 mg/kg PO q24h for up to 5 days
   B. Ondansetron, 0.1–0.2 mg/kg SC, IM, or IV q6–12h
   C. Dolasetron, 0.6–1 mg/kg IV, SC or PO q24h

7. Provide cardiovascular support as needed.
   A. For bradycardia, administer atropine, 0.02–0.04 mg/kg IV or IM.
   B. For tachycardia or hypertension, administer beta blockers such as propanolol, 0.02–0.06 mg/kg IV.

8. For sedation, administer acepromazine, 0.05–0.1 mg/kg SC, IM, or IV as needed.

9. For seizures, administer diazepam, 0.5–1 mg/kg IV, or phenobarbital, 2–10 mg IV, as needed.

10. Do *not* administer antacids as absorption increases when the gastric contents are alkalinized.

NONSTEROIDAL ANTI-INFLAMMATORY DRUG (NSAID) TOXICOSIS

Mode of action

The nonsteroidal anti-inflammatory drugs (NSAIDs) are a group of drugs with chemical differences but similar effects. They exhibit their analgesic, antipyretic and anti-inflammatory effects by direct inhibition of cyclo-oxygenase (COX) inhibitors (prostaglandin endoperoxidase synthase and prostaglandin synthetase). NSAIDs compete with the substrate arachaidonic acid for the active sites of the COX inhibitor enzymes. The inhibition of the COX enzyme is reversible except for that by aspirin. NSAIDs decrease the production of thromboxane and prostaglandins. NSAIDs differ from gluco-corticoids because glucocorticoids inhibit phospholipase, which is higher up the inflammatory cascade.

There are three isoforms of COX:

1. Constitutive COX-1—expressed in most tissue, involved in physiological functions
2. Inducible COX-2—rapidly induced at the site of inflammation, results in the production of pro-inflammatory prostaglandins, activation of the inflammatory cascade, which leads to SIRS and DIC.

3. COX-3—a splice variant of COX-1 that is involved in central control of pain.

NSAIDs are weak acids. They are well absorbed and rapidly absorbed following oral administration. They are primarily confined to plasma and ECF because they are largely ionized at physiological pH. They are lipid soluble, which enhances their penetration of cell membranes. NSAIDs are drawn to the acidic pH of inflamed tissue. They are highly protein bound, often 99% bound to albumin. Only the unbound portion is pharmacologically active.

Volume of distribution is often <10% of body weight. Many undergo enterohepatic re-circulation in the dog. Some NSAIDs that undergo renal excretion in the human are excreted in the feces in dogs, which may explain the gastrointestinal sensitivities of dogs compared with humans. The lipid-soluble drug must be metabolized to a water-soluble form for excretion. Phase I metabolism is catalyzed by enzymes within the endoplasmic reticulum of hepatocytes. Phase 2 metabolism also occurs within hepatocytes, where a large molecule (glucuronic acid, glutathione or sulfate) is added to the metabolite or to the parent compound. This 'inactivates' the drug, it becomes more water soluble, and may then be readily excreted in the urine.

The lipoxygenase (LOX) enzymes are also inhibited by NSAIDs, which further helps decrease inflammation. Medications that inhibit both COX and LOX are called 'dual inhibitors' and appear to have increased efficacy and fewer adverse gastrointestinal side effects.

Sources

Nonsteroidal anti-inflammatory medications are commonly used by people and therefore readily accessible to dogs and cats. There are also several different veterinary medications for dogs. The common medications involved in toxicosis of pets include ibuprofen, aspirin, acetaminophen, naproxen, carprofen, deracoxib and meloxicam.

Contraindications

Contraindications to NSAID administration include:

1. Renal insufficiency
2. Hepatic disease
3. Gastric ulceration
4. Gastrointestinal disease
5. Dehydration
6. Congestive heart failure
7. Thrombocytopenia, thrombocytopathia
8. Von Willebrand disease
9. Concurrent use of corticosteroids or other NSAIDs
10. Shock or trauma patients, immediately upon presentation
11. Asthma
12. Other pulmonary diseases
13. Head trauma
14. Epistaxis

15. Hypotension
16. Diuretic therapy.

Factors predisposing to the side effects include:

1. Patient age
2. High doses of NSAIDs
3. Decreased renal function / renal disease
4. Gastrointestinal disease
5. Dehydration or hypovolemia
6. Cardiac disease
7. Spinal injury
8. Hypotension, stress, severe trauma
9. Surgery, anesthesia
10. Other medications being administered including:
    A. Corticosteroids—increase the risk of GI ulceration and renal toxicity
    B. Heparin—increase the risk of bleeding
    C. Aminoglycosides—increase the risk of renal toxicity
    D. Digoxin—increase the risk of digoxin toxicity
    E. Oral anticoagulants—increase the anticoagulant effect
    F. Cisplatin—increase the risk of cisplatin toxicity
    G. Methotrexate—increase the risk of methotrexate toxicity
    H. Diuretics—decrease the response to diuretics
    I. ACE inhibitors—decrease the response to these medications
    J. Beta blockers—decrease the antihypertensive effect.

Toxic dosages

Dogs are predisposed to the toxic effects of NSAIDs (when compared with humans) because of the longer plasma half lives, higher gastrointestinal absorption rates, and higher plasma drug concentrations. Cats are more sensitive than dogs. The combination of two or more NSAIDs, or one NSAID combined with a corticosteroid, increases the occurrence and severity of adverse reactions.

Hepatic metabolism and renal excretion of NSAIDs may be altered by co-administration of medications, dietary supplements, or additives that increase (phenobarbital) or decrease (cimetidine, chloramphenicol) hepatic enzyme activity.

1. Aspirin and acetaminophen are covered in their own chapters.
2. Carprofen (Rimadyl®)
   A. Carprofen-associated hepatic toxicosis appears to be an idiosyncratic reaction.
   B. The clinical signs of hepatic toxicosis usually occur between 5 and 30 days after initiation of carprofen administration.
   C. The recommended dose of carprofen for dogs is 2.2 mg/kg (1 mg/lb) q12h PO, IM, SC, IV. For post-operative pain, carprofen may be administered once at the dose of 4.4 mg/kg IV, IM or SC followed by 2.2 mg/kg q12h IV, IM, SC or PO.

D. Although it is not approved in cats, the recommended dose of carprofen for cats is 4 mg/kg SC once.

E. The half life in dogs is 8 hours.

F. The mortality rate of carprofen-associated hepatic toxicosis is about 50%.

3. Deracoxib (Deramaxx®)

A. The recommended clinical dose for dogs is 1–4 mg/kg PO q24h.

B. It is not approved in cats.

4. Firocoxib (Previcox®)

A. The recommended dose for dogs is 5 mg/kg PO q24h.

B. It is not approved in cats.

5. Ibuprofen has a narrow margin of safety in pets. It should **never be recommended** for at-home use.

A. Ingestion of >50–125 mg/kg in dogs and >50 mg/kg in cats causes severe vomiting; gastric ulceration occurs within 1–4 hours.

B. Ingestion of >175 mg/kg in dogs and cats results in renal damage, and acute renal failure within 1–5 days.

C. Ingestion of >400 mg/kg in dogs may result in ataxia, altered mentation and seizures.

D. Sudden death may occur with ingestion of >600 mg/kg in dogs and cats.

E. The majority of the over-the-counter preparations of ibuprofen contain 200 mg ibuprofen per tablet.

6. Indomethacin

A. The toxic dose in dogs is 1 mg/kg.

B. Indomethacin is highly ulcerogenic and should not be administered to dogs or cats.

7. Ketoprofen (Anafen®, Orudis-KT®, Actron®, Ketofen®)

A. Ketoprofen appears to be a safe analgesic for dogs and cats if used short term.

B. The recommended dose for dogs is 0.5–2 mg/kg IV, IM, SC or PO initially then 0.5–1 mg/kg/day. For antipyretic activity, administer 0.25–0.5 mg/kg.

C. The recommended dose for cats is 0.5–2 mg/kg SC or PO, once. For antipyretic activity, administer 0.25–0.5 mg/kg.

D. The half life in cats and dogs is 2–3 hours.

E. An over-the-counter preparation contains 12.5 mg ketoprofen per tablet.

F. The prescription strengths are 25, 50 and 75 mg tablets.

G. The LD_{50} for dogs is 2000 mg/kg.

8. Ketorolac (Toradol®) and etodolac (EtoGesic®)

A. Ketorolac is available as a 10 mg tablet and as injectable.

I. The recommended dose for cats is 0.25 mg/kg IM, IV, SC q8–12h for 1–2 treatments.

II. The recommended dose for dogs is 0.3–0.5 mg/kg IM, IV, SC, PO q8–12h for 1–2 treatments.

III. Ketorolac should be used for a maximum of 3 days.

IV. The plasma half life in dogs is about 6 hours.

B. EtoGesic® is available in 150 and 300 mg tablets, for use in dogs only.
   I. The recommended dose of Etodolac for dogs is 5–15 mg/kg PO q24h.
   II. Ingestion of ≥40 mg/kg/day in dogs results in gastrointestinal ulceration, emesis, fecal occult blood and weight loss.
   III. Ingestion of ≥80 mg/kg/day in dogs results in severe gastrointestinal ulceration, anorexia, emesis, pallor, renal tubular nephrosis and death.
   IV. The plasma half life in dogs is about 7.5 hours.

9. Meloxicam (Metacam®)
  A. The recommended dose for dogs is 0.2 mg/kg PO, IV or SC once, then 0.1 mg/kg PO q24h.
  B. The recommended dose for cats is 0.2–0.3 mg/kg SC once. This may be followed by the administration of 0.05 mg/kg PO q24h for up to 4 days.

10. Naproxen (Aleve®, Naprosyn®)
  A. Naproxen is about 10 times more potent cyclo-oxygenase inhibitor than aspirin.
  B. The half life in dogs is 74 hours.
  C. The recommended dose for dogs is 2 mg/kg PO q48h.
  D. The dose of 5 mg/kg/day may cause gastrointestinal ulceration.
  E. The dose of >25 mg/kg/day causes renal failure in dogs.
  F. An over-the-counter preparation contains 200 mg naproxen per tablet.
  G. The prescription strengths are 250, 375 and 500 mg tablets.

11. Phenylbutazone (Butazolidin®)
  A. Phenylbutazone may cause hepatopathy, nephropathy, bleeding disorders and irreversible bone marrow suppression.
  B. Phenylbutazone administration is no longer recommended for dogs and was never recommended for cats. The previously recommended dose for dogs was 13 mg/kg (5.85 mg/lb) PO q8h for 48 hours then as needed. The maximum dose for an individual dog should not exceed 800 mg. There are now many alternatives that are safer for dogs.
  C. The toxic dose in dogs is 100 mg/kg q12h for 10 days.
  D. In cats the dose of 44 mg/kg q24h for 14 days has been lethal.

12. Piroxicam (Feldene®)
  A. Piroxicam is available in 10 and 20 mg capsules.
  B. Piroxicam should not be used in cats.
  C. The recommended dose in dogs is 0.3 mg/kg PO daily for 2 treatments, then every 48 hours.
  D. Misoprostol 2–5 mcg/kg PO q8h should be administered to dogs receiving piroxicam.

13. Tepoxalin (Zubrin®)
  A. The recommended dose for dogs is 20 mg/kg PO once, then 10 mg/kg PO q24h.
  B. It is not recommended for cats.

Diagnosis

History—History of exposure. Question the owner regarding all concurrent medications the patient is on, particularly other NSAIDs, arthritis treatments or glucocorticoid medications.

Clinical signs—The clinical signs of acute ingestion include anorexia, vomiting, diarrhea, abdominal pain, hematochezia, melena, icterus, ascites, depression, lethargy, stupor, ataxia, polyuria, polydipsia, pallor and collapse. If gastrointestinal perforation has occurred, the patient may present in shock, have hypothermia or hyperthermia, abdominal pain, and signs of sepsis (brick red mucous membranes, tachycardia, weak and thready femoral pulses or bounding femoral pulses).

The pathologic changes include:

1. Gastrointestinal tract—decreased appetite, emesis, hematemesis, abdominal pain, diarrhea, melena, superficial erosions, ulceration, hemorrhage, perforation, inflammation, stricture, protein-losing enteropathy
2. Renal—decreased renal blood flow, decreased GFR, sodium and fluid retention, hyperkalemia, azotemia, acute renal insufficiency, renal papillary necrosis
3. Hepatic—elevation of hepatic enzymes, jaundice
4. Hemostatic system—decreased platelet aggregation, prolonged bleeding time
5. Hematopoietic system—bone-marrow depression, aplastic anemia, hemolytic anemia, thrombocytopenia, thrombocytopathia, neutropenia, pancytopenia, methemoglobinemia
6. Central nervous system—behavioral changes, depression, seizures, coma
7. Immune system—allergic reactions, possible link to acute necrotizing fasciitis caused by β- hemolytic streptococcal infection.

Laboratory findings—

1. CBC, reticulocyte count—may show anemia.
2. Serum chemistry panel—hepatic enzyme elevation (ALT, AST, ALP, and total bilirubin) may be observed, particularly from carprofen toxicosis; BUN and creatinine levels may be elevated; hypoproteinemia and hypoalbuminemia may be present. Electrolyte abnormalities may be noted.
3. Urinalysis—may show isosthenuria, glucosuria and proteinuria.
4. Coagulation profile—with platelet count and bleeding times; TEG may be useful.
5. Blood gas evaluation—may reveal metabolic acidosis.
6. Fecal occult blood—false positive may occur if red meat was ingested within 3 days prior to testing.
7. Serum NSAID concentrations.

Diagnostic imaging—

Abdominal radiography—may reveal poor visualization of serosal surfaces of abdominal organs, free gas in the peritoneal cavity, and / or intestinal ileus.

Abdominal ultrasound—may reveal thickening of the gastric wall, loss of normal five-layer architecture of the gastric wall, disruption of the mucosa by crater formation and accumulation of gas bubbles, possible accumulation of peritoneal fluid.

Additional diagnostic procedures—

Endoscopy—most sensitive and specific test to detect gastrointestinal ulceration but some ulcers may be difficult to visualize, perforation is possible and usually repair cannot be achieved via endoscopy.

Exploratory laparotomy may be necessary.

Differential diagnosis

Acute renal failure, hepatic failure, gastroenteritis, ulcerative gastroenteritis.

Prognosis

The prognosis depends on the species of the patient, the NSAID ingested, the amount ingested and the duration of exposure.

Treatment

1. Inform the client of the diagnosis, prognosis and the cost of treatment.
2. Ensure a patent airway. Intubate the patient if necessary.
3. Administer supplemental oxygen and ventilation if necessary.
4. Place an intravenous catheter. Jugular catheterization is particularly useful as it will allow monitoring of central venous pressure. Administer a balanced electrolyte crystalloid fluid intravenously to maintain perfusion, hydration and diuresis.
5. Decontamination is most successful within 30 minutes of ingestion, but may be of value up to 6 hours' post-ingestion. Induce emesis if the patient is asymptomatic.
   A. Induction of emesis in cats
      I. Administer xylazine, 0.44–1 mg/kg IM or SC (can reverse with yohimbine 0.1 mg/kg IM, SC, or IV slowly).
      II. Administer medetomidine, 10 μg/kg IM (can reverse with atipamezole (Antisedan®) 25 μg/kg IM).
      III. Hydrogen peroxide is very difficult to administer to cats and is no longer recommended.
   B. Induction of emesis in dogs
      I. Apomorphine 0.02–0.04 mg/kg IV or IM, or 1.5–6 mg dissolved and placed into the conjunctival fornix. If apomorphine was placed in the eye, after emesis, the patient's eye should be thoroughly lavaged with sterile saline. If excessive sedation occurs from apomorphine, the sedation may be reversed by the administration of naloxone (0.01–0.04 mg/kg IV, IM, SC) but this will not reverse the emetic effects.
      II. Administer 3% hydrogen peroxide 1–5 mL/kg (0.5–2 mL/lb) PO, with a maximum dose of 3 tablespoons (45 mL). If the patient

does not vomit within 10 minutes, give 3% hydrogen peroxide 0.5 mL/kg (0.25 mL/lb) PO *once*.

C. Gastric lavage

    I. Lightly anesthetize the patient.

    II. Administer oxygen and intravenous fluids to the patient while under anesthesia.

    III. Maintain anesthesia with the appropriate anesthetic as needed.

    IV. Intubate the patient with a cuffed endotracheal tube and inflate the cuff.

    V. Place the patient in lateral recumbency.

    VI. With a stomach tube held outside of the patient, alongside the patient, measure the distance from the tip of the nose to the last rib. Mark this distance on the stomach tube.

    VII. Lubricate the caudal end of the stomach tube with water-soluble jelly then pass the stomach tube gently into the stomach, passing the tube no farther than the marked distance on the tube.

    VIII. If desired, two stomach tubes may be utilized, a smaller ingress tube and a large egress tube.

    IX. Infuse warm (body-temperature) tap water, 5–10 mL/kg, through the tube (ingress tube if using two tubes) to moderately distend the stomach.

    X. Allow the fluid to drain from the stomach through the tube (egress tube if using two tubes).

    XI. Save samples of gastric contents, suspicious foreign material, seeds, etc. for possible toxicologic analysis.

    XII. The stomach tube may have to be manipulated, repositioned or flushed with fluid or air if the gastric contents do not flow freely through the tube.

    XIII. Turn the patient to the other side and continue to perform gastric lavage.

    XIV. Continue gastric lavage until the effluent is clear.

    XV. If using the two-tube method, crimp the end of one tube and remove it.

    XVI. Administer activated charcoal down the stomach tube.

    XVII. Crimp the end of the stomach tube and remove it.

    XVIII. Monitor the patient during recovery from anesthesia, leaving the inflated cuffed endotracheal tube in place until the patient's swallowing reflex has returned.

D. Administer activated charcoal with sorbitol, 1–4 g/kg (3–6 mL/lb) PO once. In NSAID toxicosis patients, repeat the administration of activated charcoal without sorbitol, 1 g/kg PO, q4–6h. Administer a cathartic only *once*.

6. Hospitalize the patient for symptomatic and supportive therapy.

7. Administer an antiemetic as indicated.

A. Ondansetron (Zofran®), 0.1–1 mg/kg IV or PO q24h

B. Dolasetron (Anzemet®), 0.6–1 mg/kg IV, SC or PO q24h

C. Maropitant (Cerenia®), 1 mg/kg SC or 2 mg/kg PO q24h for up to 5 days

D. Metoclopramide (Reglan®), 0.2–0.5 mg/kg SC, IM, or PO q6h, 1–2 mg/kg/day as an CRI IV, or 0.01–0.02 mg/kg/h CRI IV

E. Chlorpromazine (Thorazine®), 0.5 mg/kg IV, IM, or SC q6–8h

F. Prochlorperazine (Compazine®), 0.1–0.5 mg/kg IM or SC q6–8h

8. Administer an H_2-receptor antagonist to treat gastrointestinal irritation.

A. Ranitidine (Zantac®), 0.5–2 mg/kg IV, PO q8h (dogs), 2.5 mg/kg IV q12h (cats) or 3.5 mg/kg PO q12h (cats)

B. Famotidine (Pepcid®), 0.5–1 mg/kg IV or PO q12–24h. Famotidine has been proven to reduce the cumulative incidence of both gastric and duodenal ulcers whereas cimetidine and ranitidine did not.

C. Do *not* administer cimetidine.

I. Cimetidine slows the clearance of some NSAIDs by inhibiting hepatic enzyme metabolism.

II. Cimetidine and ranitidine decrease gastric blood flow.

III. Cimetidine undergoes primarily renal excretion and the dosage should be decreased in patients with impaired renal function.

9. Omeprazole should be administered.

A. Omeprazole is a proton pump inhibitor that profoundly suppresses gastric acid secretion, protects against duodenal damage, and speeds healing of NSAID-induced gastric ulcers.

B. Dogs: 0.5–1.5 mg/kg PO q24h

C. Cats: 0.5–1 mg/kg PO q24h

10. Administer a gastroprotective medication.

A. Sucralfate protects ulcers from gastric acid and pepsin by forming a complex with exposed proteins on the ulcer surface. It may induce prostaglandin-mediated cytoprotection. It also adsorbs pepsin, bile acids and can interfere with the absorption of oral medications.

I. Dogs: 0.5–1 g PO q8h; can start with a loading dose 4× higher

II. Cats: 0.25 g PO q8–12h

B. Misoprostol is a prostaglandin PGE_1 analogue that has been shown to prevent the development of NSAID-induced gastric and duodenal ulcers and to reduce the risk of their complications. It is the appropriate medication for prophylaxis in at-risk patients requiring NSAID therapy.

I. Dogs: 0.7–5 mcg/kg PO q8h

II. Cats: not recommended

III. Misoprostol may cause abortions in the patient and pregnant women.

11. Monitor renal function closely.

12. Discontinue the administration of all potentially nephrotoxic drugs.

13. If gastrointestinal perforation is suspected:

A. Perform abdominal ultrasound and obtain aspirates of free intra-abdominal effusion.

B. Perform abdominocentesis.

C. Administer broad-spectrum antibiotics.

D. Administer supportive therapy to prepare the patient for exploratory laparotomy.
E. Perform an exploratory laparotomy
    I. Correct any lesions observed.
    II. Perform thorough gastric lavage with voluminous quantities of sterile saline.

14. Administer intravenous fluids, usually at the rate of 2–3 times maintenance rates. Use 0.9% NaCl, LRS, Normosol®-R, or use 2.5% dextrose in 0.45% NaCl if the patient is hypernatremic.
    A. Administer the dehydration deficit over the first 4–6 hours.
    % dehydration × body weight in kg × 1000 = volume of fluid to be administered in mL.
    B. A fluid bolus of 20 mL/kg IV over 10 minutes may help assess the patient's response and the potential for fluid overload.

15. If the patient presents in severe hypovolemic shock, administer fluids rapidly. In dogs, administer fluids at 70–90 mL/kg IV over the first hour. In cats, administer fluids at 30–40 mL/kg IV over the first hour.

16. If the patient presents in severe hypovolemic shock, is hypotensive, or is hypoproteinemic, also consider the administration of Hetastarch (14–20 mL/kg IV) or plasma (10–30 mL/kg IV) in addition to the crystalloid fluids.

17. During the rehydration phase, monitor the CVP, PCV, TS and body weight frequently.
    A. The CVP should not increase more than 5–7 cm H_2O. Higher increases indicate possible fluid overload.
    B. Other signs of overhydration include tachycardia, restlessness, shivering, chemosis, exophthalmos, dyspnea, tachypnea, increased bronchovesicular sounds, pulmonary crackles and edema, serous nasal discharge, decreased mentation, nausea, vomiting, diarrhea, ascites, polyuria and subcutaneous edema (particularly of the tarsal joints and intermandibular space).
    C. If overhydration occurs, slow or discontinue fluid administration. Administer diuretics and / or vasodilators and oxygen if indicated.

18. Periodically pass a urethral catheter to closely monitor urine output. Minimum urine output should be 1–2 mL/kg/h. An indwelling urinary catheter may be used, but strict aseptic technique and a closed collection system must be utilized.

19. Monitor the patient's body weight every 12 hours. Monitor the patient closely for signs of overhydration.

20. If urine output is insufficient, after rehydration, attempt to increase urine output with:
    A. Mannitol (20%), 250–500 mg/kg slow IV over 5–10 minutes, if there are no contraindications (vasculitis, bleeding disorders, hyperosmolar syndrome, congestive heart failure, volume overload). If urination does not occur within 30 minutes, the same dose may be repeated. Do not exceed a mannitol dose of 2 g/kg/day.
    B. Hypertonic dextrose (10–20% solutions) may be used as an alternative to mannitol. Check the patient's blood glucose level first. Do not administer hypertonic dextrose if the patient is

hyperglycemic. The dose of 10–20% dextrose is 25–50 mL/kg as an intermittent slow IV bolus over 1–2 hours, repeated q8–12h.
C. Furosemide, 1–2 mg/kg IV in dogs, 0.5–2 mg/kg IV in cats, q12–24h:
    I. Repeat furosemide at twice this dose (4 mg/kg) if diuresis does not occur within 1 hour.
    II. The dose may be increased to 6 mg/kg in dogs if diuresis fails to occur. If this dose is fails, switch to an alternative diuretic, and perform hemodialysis, peritoneal dialysis or a kidney transplant.
    III. Furosemide can also be administered as a constant rate infusion at the dose of 0.1–1 mg/kg/h CRI IV.
D. Dopamine administration may be beneficial in dogs but not cats.
    I. To increase renal blood flow and urine volume, administer dopamine, 0.5–3 µg/kg/min in 0.9% NaCl, D$_5$W or LRS, IV. Do not add dopamine to alkaline fluids. Protect the fluids and fluid line from light.
    II. To enhance the likelihood of inducing diuresis combine dopamine, at the rate of 2–3 mg/kg/min in 0.9% NaCl CRI IV, with a furosemide drip at 0.25–1 mg/kg/h CRI IV.
21. If diuresis cannot be induced, perform peritoneal dialysis, hemodialysis or a kidney transplant.
22. Supplement intravenous fluids with additional potassium as indicated by frequent monitoring of the serum potassium level (see Table 14.4).
23. If hyperphosphatemia is present, it may adversely affect the appetite. Administer an oral phosphate-binding agent such as aluminum hydroxide, 10–30 mg/kg PO q8h if vomiting is controlled. Magnesium-containing products are contraindicated in patients with renal insufficiency.
24. Monitor blood gases and correct acid–base abnormalities as needed. Administer sodium bicarbonate *only* if *measured* serum bicarbonate is 12 mEq/L or less or with arterial pH <7.1.
25. For maintenance fluid therapy after rehydration, use balanced electrolyte solutions such as LRS or Normosol®-R. Monitor the patient's serum sodium level. If hypernatremia develops, change the patient to Normosol®-M or other low-sodium maintenance IV fluid.

Table 14.4 *Suggested potassium¹ maximum infusion rate*

Estimated potassium losses	(mEq/L)	(mL/kg/h)
Maintenance (serum level = 3.6–5.0)	20	25
Mild (serum level = 3.1–3.5)	30	17
Moderate (serum level = 2.6–3.0)	40	12
Severe (serum level = 2.1–2.5)	60	8
Life threatening (serum level <2.0)	80	6

¹Potassium supplementation should not exceed 0.5 mEq/kg/h.

26. Administer fluids at a volume to match urine volume and other losses, including insensible losses (20 mL/kg/day) and continuing losses (from vomiting or diarrhea).
    A. Replace urine output losses over 6–8 hours.
    B. Replace continuing losses from vomiting and diarrhea over 24 hours.
    C. Monitor the serum sodium level.
27. Xylocaine (Lidocaine) Viscous solution®, 2–10 mL, may be applied orally prior to feeding to decrease the discomfort of oral ulcerations.
28. Eventually, the fluid needs decrease, usually after 5–6 days of profound diuresis and intravenous fluid therapy. Signs that the fluid volume should be decreased include:
    A. The patient is feeling better and showing interest in eating and drinking.
    B. The vomiting and diarrhea have been controlled.
    C. There have been significant decreases in the blood urea nitrogen (BUN) and phosphorus concentrations.
29. To taper the intravenous fluid administration volume, decrease the maintenance fluids administered by 25% per day. Return to prior volume administration for at least 48 hours if the PCV, TP, BUN, and / or creatinine levels increase, or if the patient loses weight.
30. If the patient experiences seizures, administer diazepam 0.5–1.5 mg/kg IV.

ORGANOPHOSPHATE AND CARBAMATE TOXICOSIS

Mode of action

These toxins bind with acetylcholinesterase (AChE) enzymes, inhibiting the catabolism of acetylcholine at the neurotransmitter junctions, which results in accumulation of acetylcholine and increased parasympathetic activity, causing over-stimulation of the end organ of cholinergic nerve synapses and at neuromuscular junctions. This may be delayed with some compounds.

Organophosphates have a higher affinity for the AChE enzyme sites than do carbamates, and are often referred to as 'irreversible' inhibitors, whereas carbamates are referred to as 'reversible' inhibitors.

Stability of the OP–AChE enzyme bond is enhanced through 'aging', which is caused by the loss of one of the alkyl groups.

Sources

Organophosphates are used as insecticides, fungicides, herbicides, systemic parasiticidal agents, sprays, dips, topical medications, flea collars and 'nerve gases'. They are the active ingredients in a very long list of compounds

Organophosphates include chlorfenvinphos (Dermaton® Dip), chlorpyrifos (Dursban®), coumaphos, cythioate (Proban®), diazinon, dichlorvos, dioxathion, disulfoton, fenthion (ProSpot®), malathion, parathion, phosdrin, ronnel, trichlorfon and vaponna.

Carbamates include aldicarb, bendiocarb, carbaryl (Sevin®), carbofuran, dimetilan, isolan, methiocarb, methomyl, mexacarbate, oxamyl and propoxur.

Toxic dosages

Cats have an increased sensitivity to organophosphates due to the extreme sensitivity of the pseudocholinesterase in their blood to inhibition by organophosphates.

The toxicity varies among the compounds involved, the species of the patient, the amount of exposure, acute versus chronic exposure, and the ingestion of potentiating medications or substances.

Diagnosis

History—History of exposure. Animals may be exposed via the oral, dermal or inhalation routes.
Clinical signs—
1. The onset of clinical signs is usually a few minutes to 12 hours after exposure.
2. The delayed onset of signs (19 days after exposure) has been reported.
3. The duration from the onset of clinical signs to death may be a few minutes to several hours.
4. The clinical signs are often referred to by the mnemonic SLUD or SLUDGE:
   Salivation, **L**acrimation, **U**rination, **D**efecation, **G**I distress, **E**mesis.
5. The clinical signs may also be divided into muscarinic signs and nicotinic signs.
   Muscarinic signs (DUMBELS): **D**iarrhea, **U**rination, **M**iosis, **B**radycardia / bronchospasm / bronchorrhea, **E**mesis, **L**acrimation, **S**alivation / secretion / sweating.
   Nicotinic signs (days of the week): **M**ydriasis, **T**achycardia, **W**eakness, **H**ypertension / hyperglycemia, **F**asciculations.
6. There is a syndrome in cats, following exposure to chlorpyrifos, called 'intermediate syndrome' that occurs several days after exposure and is associated with persistently low blood AChE activity. The patient exhibits muscular weakness, anorexia and depression.
7. There also is a delayed neuropathy syndrome ('Ginger Jake' paralysis) in dogs that occurs 1 week to 1 month after ingestion. It is associated with inhibition of a neurotoxic esterase, not to inhibition of AChE. Sensation deficits or pain leads to weakness and ataxia, the patient develops paralysis that changes from flaccid to spastic. Recovery is usually slow and incomplete.
Laboratory findings—
1. Reduced whole blood cholinesterase activity may be detected with organophosphate toxicosis.
   A. Brain cholinesterase levels may not correlate with blood cholinesterase levels in cases of severe acute exposures and death.

B. Brain cholinesterase levels also may not correlate with blood cholinesterase levels if the toxic substance involved does not readily cross the blood–brain barrier.

C. The severity of exposure cannot be assessed by measurement of blood cholinesterase levels.

2. Carbamates are transient cholinesterase inhibitors. Cholinesterase may be spontaneously reactivated, making measurement of whole blood cholinesterase activity levels at a single point in time unimportant.

3. Analysis of stomach contents may be beneficial.

4. Analysis of hair and skin samples may be beneficial in patients with dermal exposure.

5. Organophosphate metabolites may be found in the patient's urine. An atropine trial may be beneficial, but does not provide an absolute diagnosis

A. Administer atropine 0.02–0.04 mg/kg IV.

B. If the patient develops mydriasis, tachycardia and a dry mouth (the signs of atropinization), it is unlikely that the pet has an organophosphate or carbamate toxicosis.

Differential diagnosis

Strychnine toxicosis, pyrethrin or pyrethroid toxicosis, metaldehyde toxicosis.

Prognosis

The prognosis is guarded to poor depending upon the severity of the signs.

Treatment

1. Inform the client of the diagnosis, prognosis and the cost of treatment.

2. Ensure a patent airway. Intubate the patient if necessary.

3. Administer supplemental oxygen and ventilation if necessary.

4. Place an intravenous catheter. Administer a balanced electrolyte crystalloid fluid intravenously to maintain perfusion and hydration.

5. Administer the antidote atropine, 0.25–1 mg/kg, which can control the muscarinic signs but not the nicotinic signs.

A. Give ¼ of the dose IV, the remainder IM or SC.

B. Repeated administration, every 2–4 hours, may be necessary.

C. Monitor the effectiveness of atropinization by monitoring the reversal of excessive salivation, not by assessment of pupil size.

D. Decrease the dose of atropine or discontinue administration if the patient develops hyperthermia, tachycardia, severe behavioral changes or gastrointestinal stasis.

E. If the patient is exhibiting cyanosis or signs of respiratory distress, administer oxygen prior to the administration of atropine.

6. Administer diazepam, phenobarbital or pentobarbital if necessary to control seizures or hyperactivity.

A. One study reported that diazepam may stimulate muscarinic signs in patients with chlorpyrifos toxicosis through an unknown mechanism.

B. Administer diazepam 0.5–1 mg/kg IV in increments of 5–20 mg to effect.

C. Administer phenobarbital 2–4 mg/kg IV in dogs, 1–2 mg/kg IV in cats.

D. Administer pentobarbital 2–30 mg/kg slow IV to effect.

7. In patients with dermal exposure, thoroughly wash the patient with warm, soapy water.

A. Protective garments, including rubber gloves, should be worn while bathing the patient.

B. Keep the patient warm.

C. If the patient has long hair, consider clipping the patient.

8. In patients with oral exposure, if the patient is asymptomatic and the toxin is not in a petroleum-based carrier, induce emesis or perform gastric lavage. Decontamination may be of value up to 4 hours post-ingestion.

9. Activated charcoal, with or without sorbitol, 2–5 g/kg (3–6 mL/lb) PO is usually administered *once*.

10. If the patient is exhibiting nicotinic signs, administer diphenhydramine 1–4 mg/kg SC or IM q8h. Start with the lower dose.

11. If the patient exhibits signs of severe organophosphate toxicosis, administer pralidoxime chloride (2-PAM, Protopam®).

A. Pralidoxime is an enzyme reactivator that acts on the organophosphate––cholinesterase complex to free cholinesterase and restore normal function. The enzyme reactivator acts at the site of the newly formed, but not aged, enzyme–organophosphate complex.

B. Pralidoxime is **not recommended for administration to patients with carbamate toxicosis**. (Pralidoxime may exacerbate the action of carbamates.)

C. The recommended dose of pralidoxime is 10–20 mg/kg SC or slow IV over 1–2 hours, q8–12h if necessary. Start with the lower dose.

D. Slow IV administration of pralidoxime is necessary to avoid tachycardia, neuromuscular blockade, muscle rigidity, laryngospasm and death that may accompany rapid IV administration.

E. A constant rate infusion of pralidoxime, 10–20 mg/kg/h IV, has been utilized in human patients with severe organophosphate toxicosis.

F. Pralidoxime therapy is usually most effective if started within 24 hours following exposure, before the bond 'ages', but may still be effective if administered within 48 hours.

G. In some patients with chronic organophosphate toxicosis, pralidoxime administration has been necessary for as long as 2 weeks.

12. Hospitalize the patient and provide supportive therapy.

13. Administer antiemetics as needed.

14. Administer gastric protectants if needed.

15. Treat hyperthermia symptomatically.

16. Avoid exposure of the patient to another cholinesterase inhibitor for 4–6 weeks. The patient may also have increased sensitivity to pyrethrin and pyrethroid toxicosis during this time period.
17. Avoid the administration of medications that interfere with AChE activity including morphine, physostigmine, phenothiazine tranquilizers, pyridostigmine, neostigmine, succinylcholine, aminoglycoside antibiotics, inhalation anesthetics, clindamycin, lincomycin, magnesium, polymyxin A and B, procaine and theophylline.

PAINTBALLS

Toxin

Paintballs contain sodium and glycerol. They also contain propylene glycol, which may result in a positive antifreeze test. When in doubt, treat the patient for antifreeze intoxication, in addition to hypernatremia.

Mode of action

Hypernatremia and serum hyperosmolality.

Sources

Paintballs.

Toxic dosages

Unknown, 5–10 paintballs have caused illness in a 30 kg dog.

Diagnosis

History—Recent ingestion or comparable signs in a patient with paint on its face, forelimbs or in the vomitus.
Clinical signs—The common clinical signs include tachycardia, weakness, hyperactivity, vomiting, diarrhea, polyuria, polydipsia, ataxia, tremors, hyperthermia, blindness, seizures and coma.
Laboratory findings—
1. Hypernatremia, hyperproteinemia due to dehydration
2. Elevated PCV
3. An ethylene glycol test kit may show a false-positive result (if there is any doubt, treat for ethylene glycol intoxication). The serum glycerol level may be measured.

Prognosis

With therapy, the prognosis is usually good.

Treatment

1. Inform the client of the diagnosis, prognosis and cost of the treatment.
2. Since the most common presenting sign is vomiting or disorientation and ataxia, induction of emesis is not recommended. If the patient

presents following recent exposure and is not exhibiting clinical signs, attempted induction of emesis may be considered.

3. Activated charcoal is contraindicated as it may contribute to hypernatremia.
4. A saline or osmotic cathartic should *not* be administered.
5. Hospitalize the patient and provide symptomatic and supportive therapy.
6. Oxygen administration and possible ventilator support may be needed for the obtunded or comatose patient.
7. Place an IV catheter.
8. Administer intravenous fluids with the intent of replacing water lost from the body and/or diluting the sodium.
   A. Calculate the water deficit = weight (kg) × [(patient current Na divided by normal Na) – 1].
   B. Usually shortened to water deficit = weight (kg) × [(patient current Na divided by 140) – 1].
   C. Water deficit is in *liters*.
   D. Determine the time frame over which to replace the water deficit. This is usually dependent upon the chronicity of the hypernatremia.
      I. If there is acute development of hypernatremia (i.e. <6–12 hours), replace the water deficit over 6–12 hours. Add the water deficit replacement per hour to the patient's maintenance fluids for that hour.
      II. If there is a more chronic or unknown time frame for development of hypernatremia, replace the water deficit more slowly, often over 24–48 hours.
         a. Recheck the sodium concentration every 4–6 hours and try to lower the sodium at a rate of no more than 0.5 mEq/L/h.
         b. Try to avoid causing edema of the brain by replacing fluid too fast. With chronic hypernatremia, the brain forms idiogenic osmoles within brain cells that will draw water into the cells and cause edema. Slow replacement of fluid will allow the body to break down the idiogenic osmoles to protect brain cells.
   E. Recheck the serum sodium concentrations regularly during treatment (every 4–12 hours depending on the case). Chronic hypernatremia requires more frequent rechecks.
   F. Fluid chosen for the patient should have less sodium than the serum sodium.
      I. In acute cases, fluids containing large amounts of water are the best options to quickly reduce serum sodium. Examples would include 5% dextrose in water or hypotonic saline (0.45% saline).
      II. In chronic cases, fluids with higher sodium content are used to more slowly reduce the serum sodium. Examples would include 0.9% saline, Normosol®-R, Plasma-Lyte® or LRS.
9. Administer diazepam as needed for seizures.

AZALEAS AND RHODODENDRONS

Toxin

The toxic principles are the diterpenoid compounds known as grayanotoxin glycosides.

Mode of action

Grayanotoxins bind to and produce a modified opening of sodium channels of ventricular muscle fibers in dogs. This delays repolarization resulting in overly excited cell membranes from the continued depolarization.

Sources

Grayanotoxins and its various derivatives are present in the nectar and all portions of azaleas and rhododendrons. These wild flowering plants grow naturally in the Eastern and Western United States' mountains, from Northern hemisphere into the Southern hemisphere and South-east Asia. Azaleas are also used as household ornamental plants.

Toxic dosages

Dogs and cats = unknown.

Diagnosis

History—The patient may be observed chewing on the plant.
Clinical signs—The clinical signs include anorexia, abdominal pain, bruxism, hypersalivation, vomiting, diarrhea or constipation, tachycardia or bradycardia, weakness, hypotension, difficulty breathing, CNS depression, coma, collapse, tremors, seizures and death.
Laboratory findings—The serum chemistry changes noted with azalea or rhododendron intoxication are usually non-specific. The presence of grayanotoxins in serum, urine, and stomach contents may be determined with chromatographic methods. Grayanotoxins may be identified in body fluids.

Prognosis

With appropriate timely treatment, the prognosis is good.

Treatment

1. Inform the owner of the diagnosis, prognosis and cost of treatment.
2. If vomiting has not already occurred, attempt gastric decontamination with emesis and the administration of activated charcoal.

A. Induction of emesis in cats
  I. Administer xylazine, 0.44–1 mg/kg IM or SC (can reverse with yohimbine 0.1 mg/kg IM, SC, or IV slowly).
  II. Administer medetomidine, 10 µg/kg IM (can reverse with atipamezole (Antisedan®) 25 µg/kg IM).
  III. Hydrogen peroxide is very difficult to administer to cats and is no longer recommended.
B. Induction of emesis in dogs
  I. Apomorphine 0.02–0.04 mg/kg IV or IM, or 1.5–6 mg dissolved and placed into the conjunctival fornix. If apomorphine was placed in the eye, after emesis, the patient's eye should be thoroughly lavaged with sterile saline. If excessive sedation occurs from apomorphine, the sedation may be reversed by the administration of naloxone (0.01–0.04 mg/kg IV, IM, SC) but this will not reverse the emetic effects.
  II. Administer 3% hydrogen peroxide 1–5 mL/kg (0.5–2 mL/lb) PO, with a maximum dose of 3 tablespoons (45 mL). If the patient does not vomit within 10 minutes, give 3% hydrogen peroxide 0.5 mL/kg (0.25 mL/lb) PO *once*.
C. Administer activated charcoal with sorbitol, 2–5 g/kg (3–6 mL/lb) PO.
3. Hospitalize the patient for symptomatic therapy and monitoring.
4. Place an IV catheter and administer a balanced electrolyte crystalloid IV fluid (LRS, Normosol®-R, Plasma-Lyte®, etc.).
5. Monitor the electrocardiogram (ECG) for arrhythmias.
6. Monitor blood pressure.
7. If bradycardia develops, administer atropine, 0.02–0.04 mg/kg IV.
8. Administer vasopressors, such as dopamine or norepinephrine, if hypotension persists with IV fluid therapy.
9. Administer diazepam or other anticonvulsant for seizures.
10. Administer antiemetics if vomiting continues or is severe.
11. Administer gastric protectants.

CHINABERRY (*MELIA AZEDARACH*)

Toxin

The toxins in chinaberries are tetranortriterpenes, known as meliatoxins.

Mode of action

The mode of action is unknown.

Sources

Chinaberry trees are native to Asia, but are grown throughout the tropical regions and temperate zones of the world. The flowers are fragrant, making it an attractive tree in gardens. The berries contain the toxins.

Toxic dosages

The toxic dose is unknown.

Diagnosis

History—There may be a chewed plant or witnessed exposure.
Clinical signs—Clinical signs of poisoning in dogs develop within hours and are characteristic of gastrointestinal and CNS disturbances, including anorexia, vomiting, diarrhea, weakness, ataxia, paralysis and seizures. Sudden death may occur in acute poisoning cases.

Despite treatment, the toxicosis may be fatal, with death within 36 hours after the onset of clinical signs.
Laboratory findings—Necropsy of an affected dog revealed severe renal congestion, moderate hepatic congestion and a moderate amount of serosanguineous fluid in the abdominal cavity.

Prognosis

The prognosis varies with the toxicity of the berries, the amount ingested and the severity of the clinical signs.

Treatment

1. Inform the client of the diagnosis, prognosis and cost of the treatment.
2. If the patient presents soon after ingestion of the berries and is asymptomatic, attempt gastric decontamination with emesis and administer activated charcoal.
   A. Induction of emesis in cats
      I. Administer xylazine, 0.44–1 mg/kg IM or SC (can reverse with yohimbine 0.1 mg/kg IM, SC, or IV slowly).
      II. Administer medetomidine, 10 µg/kg IM (can reverse with atipamezole (Antisedan®) 25 µg/kg IM).
      III. Hydrogen peroxide is very difficult to administer to cats and is no longer recommended.
   B. Induction of emesis in dogs
      I. Apomorphine 0.02–0.04 mg/kg IV or IM, or 1.5–6 mg dissolved and placed into the conjunctival fornix. If apomorphine was placed in the eye, after emesis, the patient's eye should be thoroughly lavaged with sterile saline. If excessive sedation occurs from apomorphine, the sedation may be reversed by the administration of naloxone (0.01–0.04 mg/kg IV, IM, SC) but this will not reverse the emetic effects.
      II. Administer 3% hydrogen peroxide 1–5 mL/kg (0.5–2 mL/lb) PO, with a maximum dose of 3 tablespoons (45 mL). If the patient does not vomit within 10 minutes, give 3% hydrogen peroxide 0.5 mL/kg (0.25 mL/lb) PO *once*.
   C. Administer activated charcoal with sorbitol, 2–5 g/kg (3–6 mL/lb) PO once.

3. Hospitalize the patient and provide supportive therapy.
4. Place an IV catheter and administer a balanced electrolyte crystalloid fluid IV.
5. Administer antiemetics as needed.
6. Administer gastrointestinal protectants as needed.
7. Administer diazepam or other anticonvulsant medication if needed to control seizures.

KALANCHOE

Toxin

The toxic principles are cardiac glycosides, hellebrigenin 3-acetate and two other cardiotoxic bufadienolides.

Mode of action

Cardiac glycosides inhibit the sodium–potassium ATPase in myocytes, thus allowing potassium to leak out of the cell, and keeping calcium and sodium trapped in the cell.

Sources

The toxic compounds are located in all parts of the plant, with the highest concentration in the flowers.

Different species of this genus have varying levels of toxicity, although all are considered toxic.

Toxic dosages

The toxic amount is unknown.

Diagnosis

History—There may be a chewed plant or witnessed exposure.
Clinical signs—The toxins affect the GI, cardiovascular and neuromuscular systems. Acute clinical signs include anorexia, hypersalivation, polyuria, depression and diarrhea. Cardiac abnormalities such as bradycardia and AV block, and respiratory distress, may develop 1–2 days following ingestion. The cervical region may be noticeably weak. Weakness can progress to paresis, ataxia, paralysis, collapse and death within 4–5 days after exposure. In severe cases, death may occur within hours.
Laboratory findings—Changes in serum chemistry may include hyperglycemia, increased blood carbon dioxide levels, and increased blood urea nitrogen and creatinine secondary to mild renal disease or dehydration.

Prognosis

The prognosis varies with the amount ingested.

Treatment

1. Inform the client of the diagnosis, prognosis and cost of the treatment.
2. If the patient presents less than 4 hours since exposure, attempt gastric decontamination with emesis, gastric lavage, administration of activated charcoal and a saline or osmotic cathartic.
   A. Induction of emesis in cats
      I. Administer xylazine, 0.44–1 mg/kg IM or SC (can reverse with yohimbine 0.1 mg/kg IM, SC, or IV slowly).
      II. Administer medetomidine, 10 µg/kg IM (can reverse with atipamezole (Antisedan®) 25 µg/kg IM).
      III. Hydrogen peroxide is very difficult to administer to cats and is no longer recommended.
   B. Induction of emesis in dogs
      I. Apomorphine 0.02–0.04 mg/kg IV or IM, or 1.5–6 mg dissolved and placed into the conjunctival fornix. If apomorphine was placed in the eye, after emesis, the patient's eye should be thoroughly lavaged with sterile saline. If excessive sedation occurs from apomorphine, the sedation may be reversed by the administration of naloxone (0.01–0.04 mg/kg IV, IM, SC), but this will not reverse the emetic effects.
      II. Administer 3% hydrogen peroxide 1–5 mL/kg (0.5–2 mL/lb) PO, with a maximum dose of 3 tablespoons (45 mL). If the patient does not vomit within 10 minutes, give 3% hydrogen peroxide 0.5 mL/kg (0.25 mL/lb) PO *once*.
   C. Administer activated charcoal with sorbitol, 2–5 g/kg (3–6 mL/lb) PO. Repeat the administration of activated charcoal q4–6h. Administer a cathartic only once.
3. Hospitalize the patient and provide supportive therapy.
4. Place an IV catheter and administer a balanced electrolyte crystalloid fluid IV.
5. Monitor the patient's cardiac rhythm with an ECG and treat abnormalities as needed.

LILY

1. *Lilium* species and *Hemerocallis* species of lilies are toxic to cats. They can all cause kidney failure in cats. Examples of toxic lilies include the stargazer lily (*Lilium* spp.), tiger lily (*Lilium* spp.), Japanese show lily (*L. hybridum*), rubrum lily (*L. rubrum*), Easter lily (*L. longiflorum*) and day lily (*Hemerocallis* spp).
2. The peace lily (*Spathiphyllum* spp.), calla lily and lily-of-the-valley (*Convallaria majalis*) are not considered true lilies and, while they are able to make cats ill in other ways, they do not usually cause kidney failure. Cats should not be allowed to ingest these plants either.
3. The precise toxin is still unknown.
4. All parts of the lily plant are poisonous, even the pollen and the vase water which contained cut flowers.

Clinical signs—

1. Within 2–4 hours following ingestion, the cat may develop depression and start vomiting.
2. The cat then may appear to improve.
3. About 24–72 hours following ingestion, the cat will rapidly deteriorate. Vomiting, lethargy and anorexia were the most common initial clinical signs reported by cat owners. These signs developed between 1 and 5 days following ingestion.

Laboratory findings—

1. Serum chemistry abnormalities include elevated BUN, elevated creatinine, hyperphosphatemia and hyperkalemia.
2. The serum creatinine level increases disproportionately to the elevation of BUN (creatinine levels as high as 44 mg/dL have been reported).
3. Urinalysis may reveal epithelial casts, proteinuria and glucosuria within 18 hours of ingestion.

Differential diagnosis

Ethylene glycol intoxication, other acute nephrotoxicosis.

Prognosis

If the patient is not exhibiting clinical signs at the time of presentation, the prognosis is good to guarded, with aggressive therapy. If the patient is exhibiting clinical signs, the prognosis deteriorates to guarded to poor.

Treatment

1. Immediate decontamination is recommended.
   A. At home, an owner may attempt to administer hydrogen peroxide 3%, 1.5 mL/kg PO.
   B. Administer xylazine, 0.44–1 mg/kg IM or SC (can reverse with yohimbine, 0.1 mg/kg IM, SC, or IV slowly).
   C. Administer medetomidine, 10 µg/kg IM (can reverse with atipamezole (Antisedan®), 25 µg/kg IM.
2. Administer activated charcoal with or without sorbitol, 1–5 mL/kg PO. Repeat the administration of plain activated charcoal in 6–8 hours. Administer sorbitol only *once*.
3. Inform the owner of the diagnosis, prognosis and cost of treatment.
4. Hospitalize the patient for intravenous fluid therapy and monitoring.
5. Place an IV catheter and administer a balanced electrolyte crystalloid fluid IV for 60 hours.
6. Monitor body weight every 8 hours.
7. Monitor mentation, respiratory rate and pattern, and urine output.
8. After 48 hours of IV fluid therapy, recheck the BUN, creatinine and electrolytes. Supplement electrolytes as needed.
9. Continue IV fluid therapy for another 12–24 hours.

10. Recheck the BUN, creatinine, and electrolytes again. If the BUN and creatinine are normal, or near normal, wean the patient off IV fluids over the next 12 hours.
11. Recheck the BUN, creatinine and electrolytes again. If abnormal, continue fluid therapy. If normal, the patient may be discharged from the hospital.
12. Ideally, recheck the BUN, creatinine and electrolytes again 24–48 hours after stopping fluid therapy. If the BUN and creatinine have increased, resume IV fluid therapy.
13. If the patient develops renal failure, peritoneal dialysis, hemodialysis, continuous renal replacement therapy or a kidney transplant may be indicated.

CALLA LILY (*CALLA PALUSTRIS*)

Usually causes stomatitis and / or pharyngitis due to irritation from the oxalate crystals in the plants. Treatment is supportive.

Toxin

Oxalate crystals in the stems and leaves cause contact dermatitis and stomatitis.

Sources

The calla lily (*Calla palustris*) is not a true lily. Other names include white arum, water arum and water dragon. The plant is native to wetlands in Asia, Europe and North America. It is a popular plant for gardens, households and displays.

Toxic dosages

The toxic dosage is unknown.

Diagnosis

History—There may be a chewed plant or witnessed exposure.
Clinical signs—The clinical signs include hypersalivation, stomatitis, anorexia and vomiting. Conjunctivitis may occur in cases of ocular exposure.

Prognosis

The prognosis is good as the condition is usually self-limiting and resolves within a few days.

Treatment

1. Inform the owner of the diagnosis, prognosis and cost of treatment.
2. A mixture of lidocaine, diphenhydramine and sucralfate may be applied to oral mucous membranes to decrease discomfort.

3. If hypersalivation is severe, dehydration may occur. Fluid therapy may be needed.
4. If vomiting is severe, administer an antiemetic.

LILY-OF-THE-VALLEY (*CONVALLARIA MAJALIS*)

1. This is one of the most toxic cardiac glycoside-containing plants.
2. The cardiac glycosides in lily-of-the-valley include convallarin, convallamarin and convallatoxin.
3. These toxins cause reversible inhibition of the sodium–potassium–ATPase pump, which causes enhanced cardiac contraction, increased cardiac automaticity with conduction delays, partial to complete AV block, delayed after depolarizations, bradyarrhythmias, ventricular premature contractions, and tachyarrhythmias.

Diagnosis

Clinical signs—The most common clinical signs include vomiting, lethargy and cardiac arrhythmias.

Differential diagnosis

Digitalis ingestion, *Bufo* spp. toad intoxication, ingestion of other cardiac glycoside-containing plants (foxglove, oleander, dogbane, kalanchoe).

Treatment

1. Inform the client of the diagnosis, prognosis and cost of treatment.
2. If the patient is asymptomatic at the time of presentation, attempt gastric decontamination with emesis and activated charcoal.
    A. Induction of emesis in cats
        I. Administer xylazine, 0.44–1 mg/kg IM or SC (can reverse with yohimbine 0.1 mg/kg IM, SC, or IV slowly).
        II. Administer medetomidine, 10 µg/kg IM (can reverse with atipamezole (Antisedan®) 25 µg/kg IM).
        III. Hydrogen peroxide is very difficult to administer to cats and is no longer recommended.
    B. Induction of emesis in dogs
        I. Apomorphine 0.02–0.04 mg/kg IV or IM, or 1.5–6 mg dissolved and placed into the conjunctival fornix. If apomorphine was placed in the eye, after emesis, the patient's eye should be thoroughly lavaged with sterile saline. If excessive sedation occurs from apomorphine, the sedation may be reversed by the administration of naloxone (0.01–0.04 mg/kg IV, IM, SC) but this will not reverse the emetic effects.
        II. Administer 3% hydrogen peroxide 1–5 mL/kg (0.5–2 mL/lb) PO, with a maximum dose of 3 tablespoons (45 mL). If the patient does not vomit within 10 minutes, give 3% hydrogen peroxide 0.5 mL/kg (0.25 mL/lb) PO *once*.
        III. Administer activated charcoal with sorbitol, 1–5 g/kg PO, *once*.

3. Monitor the ECG.
   A. Administer atropine for bradycardia, propanolol for excessive symptomatic tachycardia.
   B. Consider transthoracic pacing if needed.
4. Consider the administration of ovine-derived digoxin antibody Fab fragments (Digibind®), 38–76 mg or more as needed.
5. Place an IV catheter. Administer IV fluids if indicated.
6. Administer an antiemetic such as maropitant or dolasetron if indicated.

OLEANDER

Toxin

The toxins in oleanders are steroidal cardiac glycosides known as glycosidic cardenolides. These compounds are structurally similar to digitalis and include oleandrin, nerine and some other glucosides.

Mode of action

The glycosidic cardenolides inhibit the sodium–potassium ATPase by inducing a conformational change in the enzyme, allowing potassium out of the cell, and preventing active transport of sodium.

Sources

Oleander grows outdoors in warmer regions of North America and is native to Asia and the Mediterranean. It is grown as a shrub, in hedges, and as ornamental plants. Dogs and cats are exposed by ingesting fresh or dried parts of the plant. Although the plant is reportedly unpalatable, hungry or bored animals will eat them. Different parts of the plant contain different concentrations of assorted cardenolides, with all parts containing enough toxin to cause clinical signs. Animals have become ill by drinking water in which oleander leaves floated.

Toxic dosages

The toxic dose is unknown.

Diagnosis

History—There may be a chewed plant or witnessed exposure.
Clinical signs—The clinical signs of oleander toxicosis include mydriasis, pale mucous membranes, weak and irregular pulse, hypersalivation, vomiting and diarrhea with or without blood, CNS depression, muscle tremors, collapse and coma. Cardiac abnormalities may include bradycardia, tachycardia, AV block, or various arrhythmias because of increased sympathetic tone, leading to sinus arrest.
Laboratory findings—Hyperkalemia is a common abnormality. The exposure can be confirmed by the presence of oleandrin in the stomach contents or other body fluids.

Prognosis

The prognosis varies with the amount ingested.

Treatment

1. Inform the client of the diagnosis, prognosis and cost of the treatment.
2. If the patient presents less than 4 hours since exposure, attempt gastric decontamination with emesis and administration of activated charcoal with sorbitol.
   A. Induction of emesis in cats
      I. Administer xylazine, 0.44–1 mg/kg IM or SC (can reverse with yohimbine 0.1 mg/kg IM, SC, or IV slowly).
      II. Administer medetomidine, 10 µg/kg IM (can reverse with atipamezole (Antisedan®) 25 µg/kg IM).
      III. Hydrogen peroxide is very difficult to administer to cats and is no longer recommended.
   B. Induction of emesis in dogs
      I. Apomorphine 0.02–0.04 mg/kg IV or IM, or 1.5–6 mg dissolved and placed into the conjunctival fornix. If apomorphine was placed in the eye, after emesis, the patient's eye should be thoroughly lavaged with sterile saline. If excessive sedation occurs from apomorphine, the sedation may be reversed by the administration of naloxone (0.01–0.04 mg/kg IV, IM, SC) but this will not reverse the emetic effects.
      II. Administer 3% hydrogen peroxide 1–5 mL/kg (0.5–2 mL/lb) PO, with a maximum dose of 3 tablespoons (45 mL). If the patient does not vomit within 10 minutes, give 3% hydrogen peroxide 0.5 mL/kg (0.25 mL/lb) PO *once*.
   C. If the patient ingested a large number of leaves, a surgical gastrotomy and physical emptying of the stomach is the quickest and most effective method to decontaminate the patient.
   D. Administer activated charcoal with sorbitol, 2–5 g/kg (3–6 mL/lb) PO *once*. Repeat the administration of activated charcoal without sorbitol q4–6h. Administer a cathartic only once.
3. Hospitalize the patient and provide supportive therapy.
4. Place an IV catheter and administer a balanced electrolyte crystalloid fluid IV.
5. Monitor the patient's cardiac rhythm with an ECG and treat arrhythmias symptomatically.
6. Digoxin-specific antibody fragments (Digibind®) may help to reverse cardiotoxic effects of the glycosides.
7. Administer atropine or propanolol as needed for cardiac arrhythmias.
8. Treat hyperkalemia or hypokalemia, if indicated.

SAGO PALM (CYCAD SPECIES OF PALM TREES)

Toxin

The toxins believed to be responsible for toxicosis are the azoglycosides cycasin and methylazomethanol, a neurotoxic amino acid (β-*N*-methylamino-L-alanine), and an unidentified high-molecular-weight compound.

Mode of action

The glucose molecule on cycasin is hydrolyzed by the gut bacterial enzyme β-glycosidase, yielding sugars and methylazomethanol. This compound then alkylates DNA and RNA, causing hepatotoxic, teratogenic, carcinogenic and gastrointestinal effects.

Sources

Seeds contain the highest concentrations, but all parts of the plant contain toxins.

Toxic dose

For the average size dog, ingestion of as few as 1–2 seeds may be lethal.

Diagnosis

History—There may be a chewed plant or witnessed exposure.
Clinical signs—The clinical signs occur within 24 hours following ingestion. These signs include hypersalivation, vomiting, diarrhea or constipation, hematemesis, hematochezia, melena and abdominal pain. Within 2–4 days, the signs include icterus, ascites, ecchymosis, weakness, ataxia, dull mentation, seizures, coma and death.
Laboratory evaluation—Serum chemistry changes include elevations in conjugated bilirubin, alanine aminotransferase, alkaline phosphatase, creatinine and possibly BUN. Hypoproteinemia is common. Hematology reveals an elevated white blood cell count, and thrombocytopenia. Increases in prothrombin time and partial prothromboblastin time can be observed. Urinalysis results can show glucosuria, bilirubinuria and hematuria.

Differential diagnosis

Xylitol ingestion, anticoagulant rodenticide intoxication, toxic mushroom ingestion, other hepatotoxins.

Prognosis

The prognosis is guarded to poor, with a mortality rate up to 33%.

Treatment

1. Inform the client of the diagnosis, prognosis and cost of treatment.
2. If the patient presents less than 2 hours following ingestion and is asymptomatic, induce emesis.
3. Administer activated charcoal with sorbitol once.
4. Hospitalize the patient for continued therapy and monitoring.
5. Place an IV catheter and administer IV fluids based on the patient's needs. Supplement with potassium or dextrose if needed.

6. Administer liver protectants:
    A. *N*-acetylcysteine, 50 mg/kg IV over 1 hour, diluted 1:4 with 0.9% NaCl; repeat every 6 hours for 2 days
    B. *S*-adenosyl L-methionine (SAMe), 18–20 mg/kg PO q24h
    C. Silybin, 20–50 mg/kg PO q24h.
7. Administer anti-emetics as indicated.
8. Administer gastrointestinal protectants.
9. Provide generalized supportive therapy.
10. If hepatic failure causes hepatic encephalopathy, administer lactulose and antibiotics.
11. Patients that develop coagulopathy may need supplemental vitamin K_1, plasma administration or blood transfusions.
12. Administer diazepam or other anticonvulsants to control seizures.

PLAY DOUGH (HOMEMADE)

Sources

Homemade play dough is used in crafts and as children's toys.

Toxic dosages

Approximately 3 tablespoons of homemade playdough is toxic to a 12 kg dog.

Diagnosis

History— The dog may be observed chewing on items made from homemade play dough or items may be missing or chewed.
Clinical signs—Dogs: Clinical signs are observed within 3 hours of ingestion. The most common clinical signs include polydipsia, polyuria, vomiting, ataxia, tremors, seizures and hyperthermia.
Laboratory findings—Hypernatremia, metabolic acidosis, lipemia, increased cholesterol.

Prognosis

The prognosis is poor if serum sodium >180 mEq/L.

Treatment

1. Inform the client of the diagnosis, prognosis and cost of the treatment.
2. If the patient presents less than 1 hour since exposure, attempt gastric decontamination with emesis.
    A. Induction of emesis in cats
        I. Administer xylazine, 0.44–1 mg/kg IM or SC (can reverse with yohimbine 0.1 mg/kg IM, SC, or IV slowly).
        II. Administer medetomidine, 10 µg/kg IM (can reverse with atipamezole (Antisedan®) 25 µg/kg IM).

III. Hydrogen peroxide is very difficult to administer to cats and is no longer recommended.
  B. Induction of emesis in dogs
    I. Apomorphine 0.02–0.04 mg/kg IV or IM, or 1.5–6 mg dissolved and placed into the conjunctival fornix. If apomorphine was placed in the eye, after emesis, the patient's eye should be thoroughly lavaged with sterile saline. If excessive sedation occurs from apomorphine, the sedation may be reversed by the administration of naloxone (0.01–0.04 mg/kg IV, IM, SC), but this will not reverse the emetic effects.
    II. Administer 3% hydrogen peroxide 1–5 mL/kg (0.5–2 mL/lb) PO, with a maximum dose of 3 tablespoons (45 mL). If the patient does not vomit within 10 minutes, give 3% hydrogen peroxide 0.5 mL/kg (0.25 mL/lb) PO *once*.
  C. Do *not* administer activated charcoal (may exacerbate hypernatremia).
  D. A saline or osmotic cathartic should not be administered.
3. Hospitalize the patient and provide symptomatic and supportive therapy.
4. Oxygen administration and possible ventilator support may be needed for the obtunded or comatose patient.
5. Place an IV catheter.
6. Administer intravenous fluids with the intent of replacing water lost from the body and / or diluting the sodium.
  A. Calculate the water deficit = weight (kg) × [(patient current Na/ normal Na) − 1].
  B. Usually shortened to water deficit = weight (kg) × [(patient current Na/140) −1].
  C. Water deficit is in *liters*.
  D. Determine the time frame over which to replace the water deficit. This is usually dependent upon the chronicity of the hypernatremia.
    I. If there is acute development of hypernatremia (i.e. <6–12 hours), replace the water deficit over 6–12 hours. Add the water deficit replacement per hour to the patient's maintenance fluids for that hour.
    II. If there is more chronic or unknown time frame for development of hypernatremia, replace the water deficit more slowly, often over 24–48 hours.
      a. Recheck the sodium concentration every 4–6 hours and try to lower the sodium at a rate of no more than 0.5 mEq/L/h.
      b. Try to avoid causing edema of the brain by replacing fluid too fast. With chronic hypernatremia, the brain forms idiogenic osmoles within brain cells that will draw water into the cells and cause edema. Slow replacement of fluid will allow the body to break down the idiogenic osmoles to protect brain cells.
  E. Recheck the serum sodium concentrations regularly during treatment (every 4–12 hours depending on the case). Chronic hypernatremia requires more frequency of rechecks.

F. Fluid chosen for the patient should have less sodium than the serum sodium.

   I. In acute cases, fluids containing large amounts of water are the best options to quickly reduce serum sodium. Examples would include 5% dextrose in water or hypotonic saline (0.45% saline).

   II. In chronic cases, fluids with higher sodium contents are used to more slowly reduce the serum sodium. Examples would include 0.9% saline, Normosol®-R, Plasma-Lyte® or LRS.

   III. The sodium concentration can be increased by adding hypertonic saline to a sodium concentration 10 mEq/L less than the patient's serum sodium concentration.

   IV. The patient's serum sodium concentration should be decreased less than 12 mEq/L over 24 hours, or no faster than 0.5 mEq/L/hr.

   V. Recheck the serum sodium concentration every 4 hours, and readjust the IV fluid sodium concentration until normal values are achieved.

7. Administer diazepam as needed for seizures.

POTPOURRI OIL

Toxin

Potpourri oils contain detergents and various essential oils.

Mode of action

The detergents cause tissue destruction and the essential oils may cause hepatic necrosis.

Sources

Potpourri oil is a household fragrance that is commonly placed in a bowl over a candle or heat source (simmer pot) to distribute the smell throughout the home. Cats may get it on their fur if exposed to a spill or they may lick the product.

Toxic dosages

The exact toxic dosage is unknown, but as little as 2–3 licks or dermal or ocular exposure may cause severe ulceration.

Diagnosis

History— There is usually a history of exposure or ingestion.
Clinical signs—Dogs and cats exhibit vomiting, diarrhea, hypersalivation, hypotension, dyspnea secondary to pulmonary edema, oral and esophageal mucosal irritation, dermal irritation, corneal or ocular injury and CNS depression.
Laboratory findings—Ingestion of potpourri oil may cause elevation of hepatic enzymes, prolonged PT and PTT.

Prognosis

The prognosis is good with supportive care, unless esophageal damage has occurred.

Treatment

1. Inform the client of the diagnosis, prognosis and cost of the treatment.
2. Do not induce emesis.
3. Administer milk or water orally, for dilution.
4. Do not administer activated charcoal.
5. For dermal exposure, bathe the patient in Dawn® hand dishwashing liquid or other nonmedicated shampoo.
6. Hospitalize the patient.
7. Place an IV catheter and start IV fluids.
8. Administer sucralfate 0.25 g/cat PO q8–12h.
9. Administer buprenorphine or another opioid for analgesia.
10. Administer an antiemetic as needed.
    A. Ondansetron, 0.1–0.2 mg/kg IV q8–12h
    B. Maropitant, 1 mg/kg SC q24h
    C. Metoclopramide, 1–2 mg/kg/day as a CRI IV
11. Administer a hepatoprotectant.
    A. SAMe, 18–20 mg/kg PO q24h
    B. Silymarin, 20–50 mg/kg PO q24h
    C. N-acetylcysteine, 50 mg/kg IV or PO every 6 hours for 24 hours. Dilute N-acetylcysteine to a 5% solution in 0.9% NaCl; administer IV slowly over 30 minutes.
12. Rinse the eyes thoroughly with sterile saline following ocular exposure. Then administer tobramycin or gentamicin sulfate ophthalmic ointment. Do not administer bacitracin neomycin polymyxin ophthalmic medication to cats.
13. Coagulopathies should be treated with fresh frozen plasma.
14. Endoscopy of the upper gastrointestinal tract will help to evaluate the extent of the damage.
15. Placement of a gastrotomy tube may be needed if anorexia persists or esophageal lesions are severe.
16. Offer soft food to avoid damage.
17. Esophageal strictures may occur, requiring additional therapy.

PYRETHRIN AND PYRETHROID TOXICOSIS

Mode of action

Pyrethrin and pyrethroid insecticides are thought to act by increasing normal nerve membrane sodium ion conduction.

Sources

Pyrethrins and pyrethroids are insecticides used in flea control and as premises sprays. They are found in shampoos, foams, dips, sprays and topical medications. Two classes of pyrethroids are recognized based on the clinical signs produced in the acutely poisoned animals:

1. **Type I** poisoning syndrome is produced by pyrethroids, which lack an alpha cyano group (e.g. permethrin, premethrin). Ataxia, hyperexcitability, seizures and tremors characterize the type I syndrome.
2. **Type II** signs are produced by compounds with an alpha cyano group (e.g. fenvalerate, deltamethrin, cypermethrin). The alpha cyano group enhances both the insecticidal properties as well as the mammalian toxicity. Clinical signs observed in the type II syndrome are believed to result from inhibition of gamma aminobutyric acid (GABA), an inhibitor of nerve impulse transmission. The clinical signs include incoordination, seizures, profuse salivation and coarse, whole body tremors.

The most frequent brand names of these products include Adams®, Hartz®, Mycodex®, Paramist, Raid® and Zodiac®. Hartz Blockade® contains fenvalerate, a type II pyrethroid, and the topical insect repellent, DEET (N, N-dimethyl-m-toluamide). It is probable that DEET serves as a carrier for the rapid absorption of fenvalerate in the topically exposed animal. Fenvalerate is considered to be one of the more toxic pyrethroids.

Toxic dosages

Young female cats appear predisposed to the development of the most severe signs of DEET / fenvalerate toxicosis.

Type II pyrethroids are usually more toxic than type I pyrethroids.

The oral toxic dose of several common pyrethrins varies from 100 to 2000 mg/kg.

Diagnosis

History—The owner may provide a history of recent exposure and the development of the appropriate clinical signs.

Clinical signs—The most common are tremors, muscle fasciculations, disorientation, vocalization, ataxia, hyperactivity, opisthotonus, seizures, excessive salivation, anorexia, vomiting, increased moist lung sounds, severe dyspnea, depression and bradycardia.

Other reported signs include abdominal pain, aggression, skin irritation, hair loss, emaciation, stupor or coma, cardiac irregularities, panting, mydriasis or miosis, prominent lung sounds and coughing, dehydration and increased thirst, vocalizing, crying (especially in cats) and partial paralysis (especially in dogs). Cats may also exhibit ear flicking, contractions of the superficial cutaneous muscles and shaking of their paws.

Young cats tend to have subnormal temperatures in addition to the other clinical signs.

Laboratory findings—
1. Hypoproteinemia
2. Increased BUN and creatinine, increased ALT, and hyperkalemia
3. Isosthenuria, hematuria, proteinuria, ketonuria and bilirubinuria

Differential diagnosis

Organophosphate toxicosis, carbamate toxicosis, metaldehyde toxicosis.

Prognosis

The prognosis is usually fair to good.

Treatment

1. Inform the client of the diagnosis, prognosis, and the cost of treatment.
2. Ensure a patent airway. Intubate the patient if necessary.
3. Administer supplemental oxygen and ventilation if necessary.
4. Place an intravenous catheter. Administer a balanced electrolyte crystalloid fluid intravenously to maintain perfusion, hydration and diuresis.
5. Decontamination
   A. In cases of dermal exposure, thoroughly wash the patient with warm, soapy water and shampoo or dishwashing liquid soap.
      I. Protective garments, including rubber gloves, should be worn while bathing the patient.
      II. Keep the patient warm by wrapping the patient in a towel until dry to prevent chilling.
   B. In cases of ingestion, if the patient is presented within 2 hours post-ingestion and shows no clinical signs, **and the ingested product does not contain petroleum distillates**, induce emesis or perform gastric lavage followed by activated charcoal and sodium sulfate or sorbitol cathartic administration if there was oral exposure.
      I. Induction of emesis in cats
         a. Administer xylazine, 0.44–1 mg/kg IM or SC (can reverse with yohimbine 0.1 mg/kg IM, SC, or IV slowly).
         b. Administer medetomidine, 10 µg/kg IM (can reverse with atipamezole (Antisedan®) 25 µg/kg IM).
         c. Hydrogen peroxide is very difficult to administer to cats and is no longer recommended.
      II. Induction of emesis in dogs
         a. Apomorphine 0.02–0.04 mg/kg IV or IM, or 1.5–6 mg dissolved and placed into the conjunctival fornix. If apomorphine was placed in the eye, after emesis, the patient's eye should be thoroughly lavaged with sterile saline. If excessive sedation occurs from apomorphine, the sedation may be reversed by the administration of naloxone (0.01–0.04 mg/kg IV, IM, SC) but this will not reverse the emetic effects.
         b. Administer 3% hydrogen peroxide 1–5 mL/kg (0.5–2 mL/lb) PO, with a maximum dose of 3 tablespoons (45 mL). If the patient does not vomit within 10 minutes, give 3% hydrogen peroxide 0.5 mL/kg (0.25 mL/lb) PO *once*.
      III. Gastric lavage
         a. Lightly anesthetize the patient.

b. Administer oxygen and intravenous fluids to the patient while under anesthesia.
c. Maintain anesthesia with the appropriate anesthetic as needed.
d. Intubate the patient with a cuffed endotracheal tube and inflate the cuff.
e. Place the patient in lateral recumbency.
f. With a stomach tube held outside of the patient, alongside the patient, measure the distance from the tip of the nose to the last rib. Mark this distance on the stomach tube.
g. Lubricate the caudal end of the stomach tube with water-soluble jelly then pass the stomach tube gently into the stomach, passing the tube no farther than the marked distance on the tube.
h. If desired, two stomach tubes may be utilized, a smaller ingress tube and a large egress tube.
i. Infuse warm (body-temperature) tap water, 5–10 mL/kg, through the tube (ingress tube if using two tubes) to moderately distend the stomach.
j. Allow the fluid to drain from the stomach through the tube (egress tube if using two tubes).
k. Save samples of gastric contents, suspicious foreign material, seeds, etc. for possible toxicologic analysis.
l. The stomach tube may have to be manipulated, repositioned or flushed with fluid or air if the gastric contents do not flow freely through the tube.
m. Turn the patient to the other side and continue to perform gastric lavage.
n. Continue gastric lavage until the effluent is clear.
o. If using the two-tube method, crimp the end of one tube and remove it.
p. Administer activated charcoal down the stomach tube.
q. Crimp the end of the stomach tube and remove it.
r. Monitor the patient during recovery from anesthesia, leaving the inflated cuffed endotracheal tube in place until the patient's swallowing reflex has returned.
V. Activated charcoal with sorbitol, 1–5 g/kg (3–6 mL/lb) PO is usually administered once. In pyrethrin or pyrethroid toxicosis patients, repeat the administration of activated charcoal q6h for 24 hours. Only *one* dose of the cathartic, should be administered.
6. Administer atropine 0.02–0.04 mg/kg IV, IM or SC. It is not an antidote but may alleviate some clinical signs.
7. Hospitalize the patient and provide symptomatic and supportive care.
8. The administration of methocarbamol (Robaxin®) 40–50 mg/kg, may be useful in controlling excessive muscle activity.
9. Administer diazepam, phenobarbital or pentobarbital if necessary to control seizures or hyperactivity.
   A. Diazepam 0.5–1 mg/kg IV in increments of 5–20 mg to effect
   B. Phenobarbital 2–4 mg/kg IV in dogs, 1–2 mg/kg IV in cats
   C. Pentobarbital 2–30 mg/kg slow IV to effect
10. Avoid the administration of acepromazine and other phenothiazines.

Toxin

Ricin and abrin are water-soluble lectins (proteins with an affinity for sugar molecules) and are destroyed by moist heat. The lectins are composed of two glycoprotein chains; one facilitates endocytosis and the other inhibits protein synthesis and causes cell death.

Mode of action

Once inside the cell, some of the toxin is transported through the Golgi network to the endoplasmic reticulum. There, the A-chain depurinates 28S ribosomal ribonucleic acid (rRNA) by removal of a specific adenine residue. This stops protein synthesis and causes cellular death.

Calcium uptake by the sarcoplasmic reticulum is decreased and sodium–calcium exchange is increased, resulting in abnormal calcium homeostasis and adverse effects on the cardiovascular system.

Intestinal absorption of nutrients is diminished.

Sources

Ricin is from castor beans and abrin is from precatory beans. All parts of the plant are toxic, but the seeds contain higher amounts of lectins.

Release of the phytotoxins may require chewing or piercing of the seed coat.

Toxic dosages

Lethal doses of ricin range from 0.025 µg given intraperitoneally in mice to 1 mg/kg orally in humans.

Less than one crushed precatory bean may kill a human. Inhalation of the toxin is also potentially fatal.

Diagnosis

History—Clinical signs may develop within 6 hours of castor bean ingestion in dogs. All dogs in one study show signs within 42 hours. The duration of clinical signs in dogs is 1.5–5.5 days. Most exposed people die within 24–48 hours.

Clinical signs—Dogs and cats may exhibit the following signs:
1. Gastrointestinal irritation, vomiting, diarrhea and abdominal pain may progress to hemorrhagic gastroenteritis from the disruption of normal microvilli in the jejunum.
2. Hepatic damage occurs.
3. Vascular endothelial injury occurs.
4. Myocardial necrosis and cardiac hemorrhage are often found at necropsy.
5. A respiratory form of intoxication may also occur, resulting in pulmonary edema, dyspnea and death.

Laboratory findings—A CBC and biochemistry panel may be helpful. Hepatic and renal values may not increase until 12–24 hours following lectin ingestion.

Prognosis

No specific antidote exists.

Treatment

1. Prevention of exposure of clients and colleagues is essential.
2. This is a reportable toxin. Notify the police immediately.
3. Inform the client of the diagnosis, prognosis and cost of the treatment.
4. If the patient presents less than 4 hours since exposure, attempt gastric decontamination with emesis or gastric lavage, followed by the administration of activated charcoal with sorbitol, *once*.
   A. Induction of emesis in cats
      I. Administer xylazine, 0.44–1 mg/kg IM or SC (can reverse with yohimbine 0.1 mg/kg IM, SC, or IV slowly).
      II. Administer medetomidine, 10 µg/kg IM (can reverse with atipamezole (Antisedan®) 25 µg/kg IM).
      III. Hydrogen peroxide is very difficult to administer to cats and is no longer recommended.
   B. Induction of emesis in dogs
      I. Apomorphine 0.02–0.04 mg/kg IV or IM, or 1.5–6 mg dissolved and placed into the conjunctival fornix. If apomorphine was placed in the eye, after emesis, the patient's eye should be thoroughly lavaged with sterile saline. If excessive sedation occurs from apomorphine, the sedation may be reversed by the administration of naloxone (0.01–0.04 mg/kg IV, IM, SC), but this will not reverse the emetic effects.
      II. Administer 3% hydrogen peroxide 1–5 mL/kg (0.5–2 mL/lb) PO, with a maximum dose of 3 tablespoons (45 mL). If the patient does not vomit within 10 minutes, give 3% hydrogen peroxide 0.5 mL/kg (0.25 mL/lb) PO *once*.
   C. Gastric lavage
      I. Lightly anesthetize the patient.
      II. Administer oxygen and intravenous fluids to the patient while under anesthesia.
      III. Maintain anesthesia with the appropriate anesthetic as needed.
      IV. Intubate the patient with a cuffed endotracheal tube and inflate the cuff.
      V. Place the patient in lateral recumbency.
      VI. With a stomach tube held outside of the patient, alongside the patient, measure the distance from the tip of the nose to the last rib. Mark this distance on the stomach tube.

VII. Lubricate the caudal end of the stomach tube with water-soluble jelly then pass the stomach tube gently into the stomach, passing the tube no farther than the marked distance on the tube.

VIII. If desired, two stomach tubes may be utilized, a smaller ingress tube and a large egress tube.

IX. Infuse warm (body-temperature) tap water, 5–10 mL/kg, through the tube (ingress tube if using two tubes) to moderately distend the stomach.

X. Allow the fluid to drain from the stomach through the tube (egress tube if using two tubes).

XI. Save samples of gastric contents, suspicious foreign material, seeds, etc. for possible toxicologic analysis.

XII. The stomach tube may have to be manipulated, repositioned or flushed with fluid or air if the gastric contents do not flow freely through the tube.

XIII. Turn the patient to the other side and continue to perform gastric lavage.

XIV. Continue gastric lavage until the effluent is clear.

XV. If using the two-tube method, crimp the end of one tube and remove it.

XVI. Administer activated charcoal down the stomach tube.

XVII. Crimp the end of the stomach tube and remove it.

XVIII. Monitor the patient during recovery from anesthesia, leaving the inflated cuffed endotracheal tube in place until the patient's swallowing reflex has returned.

D. Activated charcoal with sorbitol, 2–5 g/kg (3–6 mL/lb) PO is usually administered once. In ricin or abrin toxicosis patients, repeat the administration of activated charcoal q3–4h. Administer a cathartic only *once*.

5. Hospitalize the patient for supportive therapy. There is no antidote.
6. Oxygen supplementation is often beneficial.
7. Place an IV catheter and administer a balanced electrolyte crystalloid fluid IV. Acute renal failure may occur.
8. Administer sucralfate and omeprazole or other gastric protectants.
9. Administer lactulose if hepatic failure occurs.
10. Administer *N*-acetylcysteine or SAMe, or other hepatic protectants.
11. Provide dietary support as for hepatic disease.
12. Administer analgesics if indicated.
13. The administration of dexamethasone may inhibit lipid peroxidation and delay death.

ROTENONE TOXICOSIS

Mode of action

Rotenone inhibits electron transfer between flavoprotein and ubiquinone by forming a complex with reduced nicotinamide adenine dinucleotide (NADH) dehydrogenase. By binding to the mitotic spindle apparatus, it inhibits mitosis.

Sources

Rotenone is prepared from extracts from the *Derris* plant root. It is used as an insecticide. It is found in sprays, powders, dips and topical medication.

Toxic dosages

The acute oral LD_{50} for dogs is 300 mg/kg, and is less for cats, birds and fish.

Diagnosis

History—History of exposure.
Clinical signs—The patient may exhibit vomiting, lethargy, depression, ataxia, muscle tremors, seizures, respiratory failure and death.
Laboratory findings—
1. Hypoglycemia may be present.
2. Analysis of blood, urine, feces or vomitus may confirm exposure.

Differential diagnosis

Organophosphate toxicosis, carbamate toxicosis, pyrethrin or pyrethroid toxicosis.

Prognosis

The prognosis is usually good.

Treatment

1. Inform the client of the diagnosis, prognosis and the cost of treatment.
2. Ensure a patent airway. Intubate the patient if necessary.
3. Administer supplemental oxygen and ventilation if necessary.
4. Place an intravenous catheter. Administer a balanced electrolyte crystalloid fluid intravenously to maintain perfusion, hydration and diuresis.
5. Administer diazepam, phenobarbital or pentobarbital if necessary to control seizures or hyperactivity.
   A. Diazepam 0.5–1 mg/kg IV in increments of 5–20 mg to effect
   B. Phenobarbital 2–4 mg/kg IV in dogs, 1–2 mg/kg IV in cats
   C. Pentobarbital 2–30 mg/kg slow IV to effect
6. In cases of dermal exposure, thoroughly wash the patient with warm, soapy water.
   A. Protective garments, including rubber gloves, should be worn while bathing the patient.
   B. Keep the patient warm by wrapping the patient in a towel until dry to prevent chilling.
7. Attempt decontamination by either inducing emesis or performing gastric lavage.
   A. Induction of emesis in cats
      I. Administer xylazine, 0.44–1 mg/kg IM or SC (can reverse with yohimbine 0.1 mg/kg IM, SC, or IV slowly).

II. Administer medetomidine, 10 µg/kg IM (can reverse with atipamezole (Antisedan®) 25 µg/kg IM).

III. Hydrogen peroxide is very difficult to administer to cats and is no longer recommended.

B. Induction of emesis in dogs

   I. Apomorphine 0.02–0.04 mg/kg IV or IM, or 1.5–6 mg dissolved and placed into the conjunctival fornix. If apomorphine was placed in the eye, after emesis, the patient's eye should be thoroughly lavaged with sterile saline. If excessive sedation occurs from apomorphine, the sedation may be reversed by the administration of naloxone (0.01–0.04 mg/kg IV, IM, SC) but this will not reverse the emetic effects.

   II. Administer 3% hydrogen peroxide 1–5 mL/kg (0.5–2 mL/lb) PO, with a maximum dose of 3 tablespoons (45 mL). If the patient does not vomit within 10 minutes,
give 3% hydrogen peroxide 0.5 mL/kg (0.25 mL/lb) PO *once*.

C. Gastric lavage

   I. Lightly anesthetize the patient.

   II. Administer oxygen and intravenous fluids to the patient while under anesthesia.

   III. Maintain anesthesia with the appropriate anesthetic as needed.

   IV. Intubate the patient with a cuffed endotracheal tube and inflate the cuff.

   V. Place the patient in lateral recumbency.

   VI. With a stomach tube held outside of the patient, alongside the patient, measure the distance from the tip of the nose to the last rib. Mark this distance on the stomach tube.

   VII. Lubricate the caudal end of the stomach tube with water-soluble jelly then pass the stomach tube gently into the stomach, passing the tube no farther than the marked distance on the tube.

   VIII. If desired, two stomach tubes may be utilized, a smaller ingress tube and a large egress tube.

   IX. Infuse warm (body-temperature) tap water, 5–10 mL/kg, through the tube (ingress tube if using two tubes) to moderately distend the stomach.

   X. Allow the fluid to drain from the stomach through the tube (egress tube if using two tubes).

   XI. Save samples of gastric contents, suspicious foreign material, seeds, etc. for possible toxicologic analysis.

   XII. The stomach tube may have to be manipulated, repositioned or flushed with fluid or air if the gastric contents do not flow freely through the tube.

   XIII. Turn the patient to the other side and continue to perform gastric lavage.

XIV. Continue gastric lavage until the effluent is clear.

XV. If using the two-tube method, crimp the end of one tube and remove it.

XVI. Administer activated charcoal down the stomach tube.

XVII. Crimp the end of the stomach tube and remove it.

XVIII. Monitor the patient during recovery from anesthesia, leaving the inflated cuffed endotracheal tube in place until the patient's swallowing reflex has returned.

D. Activated charcoal, 2–5 g/kg (3–6 mL/lb) PO is usually administered in a slurry of 1 g to 5 mL water. In rotenone toxicosis patients, repeat the administration of activated charcoal q4–6h.

E. A single dose of an osmotic or saline cathartic should be administered along with activated charcoal. Avoid magnesium cathartics if the patient is exhibiting signs of neurologic dysfunction. Alternative cathartics include:

I. Sorbitol (70%), 2 g/kg (1–2 mL/kg) PO

II. Magnesium sulfate (Epsom salt), 200 mg/kg for cats, 250–500 mg/kg for dogs; mix magnesium sulfate with water, 5–10 mL/kg and administer PO

III. Magnesium hydroxide (Milk of Magnesia®), 15–50 mL for cats, 10–150 mL for dogs, q6–12h PO as needed

IV. Sodium sulfate, 200 mg/kg for cats, 250–500 mg/kg for dogs; mix sodium sulfate with water, 5–10 mL/kg and administer PO.

8. Hospitalize the patient and provide symptomatic and supportive care.

9. The administration of methocarbamol (Robaxin®) 40–50 mg/kg, may be useful in controlling excessive muscle activity.

10. Avoid the administration of acepromazine and other phenothiazines.

SCORPION STINGS

Mode of action

Scorpion venom contains digestive enzymes, hyaluronidase, phospholipase and a neurotoxin that alters sodium-channel flow. The result of action of the neurotoxin is stimulation of the autonomic nervous system and neuromuscular junctions.

Sources

The scorpion (Fig. 14.3) is an arthropod found all over the world, primarily in dry and arid regions. The species of importance in the United States is *Centruroides sculpturatus* Ewing (also known as *Centruroides exilicauda*), which is found in Arizona, Mexico, New Mexico, Texas, southern Nevada and California.

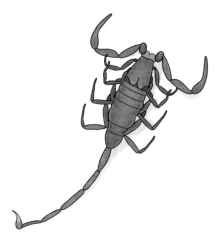

FIG 14.3 Scorpion. The distinctive characteristics of a scorpion include a pair of enlarged chelae (pincers), an elongated abdomen, four pairs of legs, a telson (tail) with a terminal bulbous segment called the vesicle and a stinger with a little tubercle or tooth at the tip.

Diagnosis

History—History of exposure; identify the scorpion.
Clinical signs—The patient may exhibit localized pain, dysphagia, nervousness, behavioral abnormalities, dyspnea, opisthotonic spasms, excessive salivation, gastric distention, mydriasis, nystagmus, blindness, lacrimation, micturition, defecation, piloerection, hypertension, cardiac and / or respiratory arrest.

Differential diagnosis

Organophosphate toxicosis, carbamate toxicosis, idiopathic epilepsy, pyrethrin or pyrethroid toxicosis.

Prognosis

The prognosis is variable.

Treatment

1. Inform the client of the diagnosis, prognosis and the cost of treatment.
2. Ensure a patient airway. Intubate the patient if necessary. The patient may experience pharyngeal spasms.
3. Administer supplemental oxygen and ventilation if necessary.
4. Administer dexamethasone sodium phosphate IV (0.5–1 mg/kg).
5. Provide analgesia. NSAIDs, narcotics and tramadol are alternatives and may be combined.
6. Place an intravenous catheter. Intravenous fluid therapy is not often needed. Assess the needs of the individual patient. Administer a

balanced electrolyte crystalloid fluid intravenously if needed to maintain perfusion, hydration and diuresis.

7. Administer diazepam, phenobarbital or pentobarbital if necessary to control seizures or hyperactivity.
   A. Diazepam 0.5–1 mg/kg IV in increments of 5–20 mg to effect
   B. Phenobarbital 2–4 mg/kg IV in dogs, 1–2 mg/kg IV in cats
   C. Pentobarbital 2–30 mg/kg slow IV to effect
8. Administer specific scorpion antivenom if available, especially indicated for ferrets.
   A. Administer IV at a very slow rate for 5 minutes. If well tolerated, increase the rate so that the infusion is completed within 15–30 minutes.
   B. A second vial may be administered if severe clinical signs persist longer than 1 hour following administration of the first vial.
9. ECG monitoring may be necessary in severe envenomations.
10. Hypertension may be treated with acepromazine, 0.05 mg/kg SC, IM, or IV unless it is severe, in which case, nitroprusside, enalapril, or hydralazine may be needed.
11. Administer methocarbamol (150 mg/kg) slow IV or 10% calcium gluconate (5–10 mL IV) followed by diazepam (2.5–20 mg IV) q4–6h for muscle spasms.

SEROTONIN SYNDROME

Toxin

Serotonin is a CNS neurotransmitter that regulates smooth muscle function and promotes platelet aggregation.

Mode of action

The various compounds work in different ways, all of which result in an increased amount of serotonin at the neuromuscular junctions.

1. L-tryptophan enhances serotonin synthesis.
2. SSRIs inhibit serotonin uptake.
3. MAOIs increase serotonin release and inhibit serotonin metabolism.
4. Amphetamines and cocaine increase serotonin release and inhibit serotonin uptake.
5. LSD and buspirone act as serotonin agonists.

Sources

There are several different medications and compounds that act as serotonin, norepinephrine and dopamine re-uptake inhibitors. These include:

- Selective serotonin reuptake inhibitors (SSRIs)
- Monoamine oxidase inhibitors (MAOIs)—including selegiline (used in the treatment of cognitive dysfunction and Cushing syndrome in dogs)
- Tricyclic antidepressants (TCAs)
- Lysergic acid diethylamide (LSD)

- Dextromethorphan
- L-Tryptophan
- Buspirone
- Amphetamines
- Cocaine
- St John's wort.

Toxic dosages

Toxicity varies with the individual toxin ingested.

Diagnosis

History—There usually is a history of exposure, or high suspicion based upon the clinical signs and possible access to SSRI medications.
Clinical signs—Clinical signs are usually observed within 1–8 hours of ingestion, but may be delayed with extended-release formulations. The signs include mydriasis, vomiting, tachypnea, tachycardia, ataxia and agitation. The signs of intoxication are referred to as 'serotonin syndrome', and include ataxia, disorientation, hyperesthesia, tremors, seizures, weakness, depression, blindness, hypersalivation, vocalization, abdominal pain, hyperthermia, vomiting, diarrhea, bloat, tachycardia, coma and death.
Laboratory findings—There are no specific abnormalities.

Prognosis

The prognosis is usually good with treatment.

Treatment

1. Inform the client of the diagnosis, prognosis and cost of the treatment.
2. If the patient presents less than 4 hours since exposure, attempt gastric decontamination with emesis, followed by the administration of activated charcoal.
   A. Induction of emesis in cats
      I. Administer xylazine, 0.44–1 mg/kg IM or SC (can reverse with yohimbine 0.1 mg/kg IM, SC, or IV slowly).
      II. Administer medetomidine, 10 µg/kg IM (can reverse with atipamezole (Antisedan®)] 25 µg/kg IM).
      III. Hydrogen peroxide is very difficult to administer to cats and is no longer recommended.
   B. Induction of emesis in dogs
      I. Apomorphine 0.02–0.04 mg/kg IV or IM, or 1.5–6 mg dissolved and placed into the conjunctival fornix. If apomorphine was placed in the eye, after emesis, the patient's eye should be thoroughly lavaged with sterile saline. If excessive sedation occurs from apomorphine, the sedation may be reversed by the administration of naloxone (0.01–0.04 mg/kg IV, IM, SC) but this will not reverse the emetic effects.

II. Administer 3% hydrogen peroxide 1–5 mL/kg (0.5–2 mL/lb) PO, with a maximum dose of 3 tablespoons (45 mL). If the patient does not vomit within 10 minutes, give 3% hydrogen peroxide 0.5 mL/kg (0.25 mL/lb) PO *once*.

C. Activated charcoal with sorbitol, 2–5 g/kg (3–6 mL/lb) PO should be administered once, then the administration of activated charcoal without sorbitol should be repeated q4–6h. Only *one* dose of sorbitol should be administered.

3. Treatment involves symptomatic and supportive therapy.
4. Hospitalize the patient.
5. Place an IV catheter and administer a balanced electrolyte crystalloid fluid IV.
6. The patient's thermoregulation may be altered, so provide external cooling or warming, as needed.
7. Agitation can be treated with acepromazine or chlorpromazine
8. If seizures occur, administer diazepam or barbiturates.
9. Administer cyproheptadine PO or per rectum, every 4–6 hours as needed.
   A. Dogs: 1.1 mg/kg
   B. Cats: 2–4 mg total dose per cat
10. Monitor blood pressure and heart rate. Propanolol has some serotonin antagonist activity but is rarely needed.

SNAKEBITE ENVENOMATION

Mode of action

1. Elapidae (coral snake) venom contains polypeptides and acetylcholinesterase.
   A. Small polypeptides that act by binding postsynaptically at the neuromuscular junction are the neurotoxic components.
   B. A postsynaptic, nondepolarizing blockade of the neuromuscular junctions similar to the effects of curare occurs.
   C. The proteolytic enzyme components of North American coral snake venom usually cause no or minimal tissue edema.
   D. Hemolysis occurs as a result of a phospholipase A_2 reaction with lecithin in the red blood cell membrane, which causes increased cell membrane permeability and hemolysis.
2. Crotalidae (rattlesnake, copperhead and cottonmouth) venom is designed to immobilize, kill and digest prey.

   A. Immobilization is usually not achieved by causing neuromuscular blockade, but rather by producing hypovolemic shock, induced by lethal polypeptide components of Crotalidae venom. The polypeptides damage endothelial cells in the victim, allowing plasma to exude, blood to extravasate into surrounding tissues, and third-spacing to occur, leading to hypovolemic shock.
   B. Digestion occurs owing to the release of numerous proteolytic and other enzymes, including hyaluronidase and phospholipase A_2,

which allow the snake to swallow its food whole, without mastication. The polypeptide-induced third-spacing also allows the digestive enzymes of the snake's venom to reach the tissues.

C. The Mojave rattlesnake with venom A is the exception. Venom A is a toxin that immobilizes prey by neuromuscular blockade. Venom A (also referred to as Mojave toxin) consists of a basic phospholipase A_2 subunit and an acidic peptide subunit.

D. Some Mojave rattlesnakes have venom B and lack Mojave toxin (venom A). These snakes immobilize prey by inducing hypovolemic shock. These Mojave rattlesnakes live primarily in the areas surrounding and between Phoenix and Tucson, Arizona.

E. The cardiovascular system, particularly the endothelial cells, is the primary toxic target of most Crotalidae venoms. The polypeptides damage endothelial cells, while hemorrhagic metalloproteinases destroy vascular basement membranes and perivascular extracellular matrices, leading to extravasation of erythrocytes. Clinically, this appears as hemorrhage into envenomated areas of the body.

F. A DIC-like syndrome is produced through fibrinogenolysis by thrombin-like, enzymatic venom glycoproteins. These glycoproteins do not activate factor XIII as thrombin does in true DIC. Thus, heparin and blood products are not beneficial in the treatment of venom induced DIC-like coagulopathies and may be detrimental.

G. Certain species of crotalids may produce characteristic coagulopathies in their victims. For instance, timber rattlesnake venom contains a protease (crotalocytin) that causes platelet aggregation and the southern Pacific rattlesnake causes significant thrombocytopenia, but not hypofibrinogenemia.

H. Thrombocytopenia is a common effect of crotalid envenomation. Thrombocytopenia occurs due to the consumption of platelets at the envenomation site. Endothelial cell and basement membrane damage results in platelet aggregation.

I. Kininogenases in rattlesnake venom cause activation of factor XII in the intrinsic blood coagulation pathway and act on plasma globulins to form bradykinins, which are potent vasodilators. Bradykinins may stimulate endogenous phospholipase A_2, which results in increased prostaglandin synthesis via stimulation of the arachidonic cascade.

Sources

There are five families of venomous snakes in the world, three of which are indigenous to North America:

1. Colubridae, (the boomslang), *Dispholidus typus*, are found in central and southern Africa.
2. Crotalidae, including the *Crotalus* (rattlesnakes), *Agkistrodon* (copperhead, cottonmouth, Malayan pit viper and mamushi), *Bothrops* (fer-de-lance, jararaca and barba amarilla) *Lachesis* (bushmaster) and *Trimeresurus* (habu) genera, are found throughout the world. Crotalidae are often referred to as 'pit vipers'.

3. Elapidae, including the *Micrurus* (coral snakes), *Bungarus* (kraits), *Dendroaspis* (mambas), *Ophiophagus* (king cobras) and *Naja* (cobras); coral snakes can be identified by the saying 'Red on yellow, kill a fellow. Red on black, venom lack.' (The red stripes on a coral snake are next to the yellow stripes).

4. Hydrophidae, including the *Astroria, Enhydrina, Hydrophis, Laticauda* and *Pelamis* genera (sea snakes and sea kraits), are found in the Pacific and Indian oceans.

5. Viperidae, including the *Vipera* (asp, Russell's, European and long-nosed vipers) and *Bitis*, (puff adder and African gaboon vipers), are found in Europe, Asia, South-east Asia, India and Africa.

The important venomous snakes indigenous to North America are listed in Table 14.5.

Table 14.5 *Some venomous snakes indigenous to North America*

Family/genus	Species	Subspecies	Common name	Location
Elapidae				
Micrurus	fulvius	fulvius	Eastern coral snake	Southeast USA
	fulvius	tenere	Texas coral snake	South central USA
	euryxanthus		Arizona or Sonoran coral snake	Southwest USA
Crotalidae				
Agkistrodon	contortrix	contortrix	Southern copperhead	VA to TX
	contortrix	mokeson	Northern copperhead	MA to VA
	piscivorus	piscivorus	Eastern cottonmouth	VA to TX
	piscivorus	conanti	Florida cottonmouth	FL
Crotalus	scutulatus	scutulatus	Mojave rattlesnake	Southwest USA
	atrox		Western diamondback	Southwest USA
	cerastes		Sidewinder	Southwest USA
	lepidus		Rock rattlesnake	Southwest USA
	mitchelli		Speckled rattlesnake	Southwest USA
	molussus		Black-tailed rattlesnake	Southwest USA
	pricei		Twin-spotted rattlesnake	Southwest USA
	tigris		Tiger rattlesnake	AZ
	viridis	abyssus	Grand Canyon rattlesnake	Grand Canyon, AZ
	viridis	cerebrus	Arizona black rattlesnake	AZ
	viridis	nuntius	Hopi rattlesnake	AZ
	willardi		Ridge-nosed rattlesnake	AZ, NM
	ruber		Red diamond rattlesnake	CA
	viridis	helleri	Southern Pacific rattlesnake	CA
	viridis	lutosus	Great Basin rattlesnake	Western USA
	viridis	concolor	Midget faded rattlesnake	CO, UT
	viridis	oreganus	Northern Pacific rattlesnake	Northwest USA
	viridis	viridis	Prairie rattlesnake	Rocky Mountains USA
	horridus		Timber rattlesnake	North and eastern USA
	adamanteus		Eastern diamondback	Southeast USA
Sistrurus	catenatus		Massasauga	Midwest to Southwest USA
	miliarius		Pygmy rattlesnake	Southeast USA

Toxic dosages

The toxicity of envenomation varies, depending upon the species of snake and the amount of venom injected. Colubridae envenomation, although not usually lethal to an adult human, may be lethal to a dog or cat or other small animal.

Diagnosis

History—History of exposure or location (usually remote). Determine where, when and under what conditions the bite occurred. Establish the time and sequence of manifestations. Question the owner regarding the patient's history of concomitant drug use and of allergies. Obtain a complete description of any and all first aid that has been administered, and by whom.

Clinical signs—

1. Elapidae—fang marks may not be observed. Hypersalivation, nausea, vomiting and weakness may be observed. Neurotoxic effects predominate, including local paresthesia, ataxia, drowsiness, bulbar paralysis, muscle fasciculations, quadriplegia with decreased spinal reflexes in all four limbs, acute flaccid ascending paralysis and seizures. The patient may exhibit hemolysis, hemoglobinuria, anemia, hypothermia, dysphagia, dyspnea, aspiration pneumonia, and death occurs due to respiratory failure. The clinical signs of envenomation may appear within 7 hours following the bite or may be delayed as much as 48 hours.

2. Crotalidae—the major clinical problems are local tissue destruction due to the digestive enzymes in the venom, edema due to exudation of plasma, hemorrhage due to destruction of the microvasculature, shock due to hypovolemia, and neuromuscular blockade in some victims.

   One, two or several small puncture wounds may be observed. Occasionally, the wounds cannot be found. The patient may exhibit excessive bleeding, erythema, petechiation, ecchymosis, extremely painful swelling, edema, lymphangitis, weakness, nausea, vomiting, hypotension, coagulopathies, hemoglobinuria, myoglobinuria, cardiovascular and hypovolemic shock, cardiac arrhythmias, neurologic signs including muscular weakness, muscle fasciculations, paresis, paralysis, seizures and death. Delayed signs include myonecrosis and tissue sloughing.

   The clinical signs of Crotalidae envenomation may occur within 30–60 minutes or may be delayed in onset for 24–72 hours following the bite. With minimal or no envenomation (dry bites) there are few or no local signs, no systemic signs, and normal laboratory findings. However, due to the possible delayed onset of clinical signs, these patients should be monitored very closely, in the hospital, for changes indicating a declining condition. The incidence of dry bites reported in published literature varies from 10 to 25%.

   Some envenomations by Mojave rattlesnakes have been life threatening with only slight tissue swelling and no pain.

Laboratory findings—

1. Perform a CBC including a platelet count. Hemoconcentration and hemolysis may occur.
2. Evaluate a blood smear for the presence of echinocytes (Fig. 14.4).
   A. Echinocytes are red blood cells with spikes on their outer membranes due to crenation of the red blood cells.
   B. Echinocytes appear in some dogs within 24 hours after envenomation by crotalidae.
   C. Within 48–72 hours after envenomation, they are usually absent.
   D. Be aware that echinocytes may not appear until after severe clinical signs of envenomation have occurred and may not appear in all envenomated patients.
   E. Treatment of envenomation should not be based upon the presence or absence of echinocytes.
   F. To evaluate the patient's blood for echinocytes, place a drop of saline and a drop of the patient's blood on a slide. Examine the slide under a microscope.
3. Coagulation profile including PT, PTT or ACT, FDPs, D-dimers and TEG if available.
   A. In-house lab analyzers are available for analysis of PT and PTT.
   B. Evaluate an activated coagulation time (ACT).
      I. The normal ACT for a dog is 60–120 seconds, for a cat it is 50–75 seconds.
      II. In acute DIC, there is a slight to moderate prolongation in ACT (120–200 seconds in dogs, 75–120 seconds in cats).
      III. In end-stage DIC, there is marked prolongation of ACT (>200 seconds in dogs, >120 seconds in cats).
      IV. Procedure—the ACT tubes should be warmed to 37°C prior to and during the test procedure. Two tubes should be used; 2 mL of blood are taken by clean venipuncture with rapid aspiration from a large vein, directly into the first tube with a Vacutainer® system, or quickly transferred from a syringe into the first tube and discarded. Without removing the

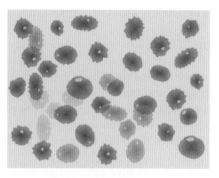

FIG 14.4   Echinocytes.

needle from the vein, additional blood is placed into the second tube and the test is performed. The time interval from injection of 2 mL of blood into the ACT tube until the first visible appearance of clot formation is determined to be the ACT.

4. Evaluate a urinalysis.
   A. Hemoglobinuria or myoglobinuria may be present.
   B. Renal tubular casts may be observed.
5. Evaluate a serum biochemical profile, including BUN, creatinine and serum electrolytes.
   A. Both hypokalemia and hyperkalemia are common findings.
   B. Creatinine kinase levels may be increased.
   C. Serum BUN and creatinine levels may be increased in patients with azotemia.
6. Blood gas evaluation may reveal a metabolic acidosis.

Differential diagnosis

Distinguish between bites from venomous and nonvenomous snakes, other animal bites, an acute allergic reaction with angioedema, plant thorn injury, tick paralysis, botulism, acute polyneuritis, DIC due to other causes, and other coagulopathies.

Prognosis

The prognosis varies with the species of snake involved, amount of venom injected and location of the bite wound.

Treatment

Treatment of Elapidae envenomation—
1. Advise the telephone caller to immobilize the affected limb if a patient was bitten on an extremity, to restrict the patient's activity (carry it if possible) and to come to the veterinary facility immediately.
   A. Advise the caller *not* to apply a tourniquet or ice and *not* to administer medication.
   B. While en route, they should elevate the affected limb if possible, to keep it at heart level.
   C. It is not necessary to capture the snake, but is helpful if they can determine whether it is a nonvenomous or a venomous species.
2. Inform the client of the diagnosis, prognosis and the cost of treatment.
3. Treat the patient, not the snake, the venom, or the known or suspected venom constituents.
4. Ensure a patent airway. Intubate the patient if necessary.
5. Administer supplemental oxygen and ventilation if necessary.
6. Obtain pretreatment blood and urine samples.
7. Place an intravenous catheter. Administer a balanced electrolyte crystalloid fluid intravenously to maintain perfusion, and hydration.

8. Administer diazepam, phenobarbital or pentobarbital if necessary to control seizures or hyperactivity.
    A. Diazepam 0.5–1 mg/kg IV in increments of 5–20 mg to effect
    B. Phenobarbital 2–4 mg/kg IV in dogs, 1–2 mg/kg IV in cats
    C. Pentobarbital 2–30 mg/kg slow IV to effect.
9. Evaluate the status of preadmission treatment.
    A. If a tourniquet or tight band has inadvertently been placed, apply a less constricting band proximal to the tourniquet, start a balanced electrolyte crystalloid fluid IV, then remove the tourniquet *slowly*.
    B. Determine if any medications have been given or if there is a history of allergies.
10. Clip and clean any visible wound(s).
11. If a wounds are present administer broad-spectrum antibiotics, such as cephalosporins and metronidazole or amoxicillin-clavulanate.
12. Loosely immobilize the affected body-part in a functional position if possible.
13. Consider administering antivenin before the onset of neurotoxic signs occurs.
14. If the decision is to administer antivenin to the patient, perform a skin test with antivenin prior to the administration of antihistamines or antivenin.
    A. Follow the package insert directions.
    B. Have all of the equipment and medications required to treat anaphylactic and anaphylactoid reactions available.
15. Following the skin test, administer diphenhydramine (2–4 mg/kg IV) for its sedative action and as pretreatment against possible allergic responses to antivenin.
16. Administer antivenom, *Micrurus fulvius*, equine origin for Eastern coral snake (*M. fulvius fulvius*) or Texas coral snake (*M. fulvius tenere*) envenomations, but not for Arizona or Sonoran coral snake (*M. euryxanthus*) envenomations.
    A. This antivenom is of equine origin.
    B. It may cause true anaphylaxis (type I hypersensitivity), anaphylactoid reactions and serum sickness (type III hypersensitivity).
17. After reconstitution, dilute antivenom in 10–100 mL of IV crystalloid fluid (adjust the volume for smaller patients).
    A. Antivenom may be swirled when reconstituted but should not be shaken, as it will denature and become foamy; warming antivenom to body temperature aids in speeding reconstitution.
    B. Antivenom can also be reconstituted by placing it on a blood vial rocker that gently rocks back and forth.
    C. Start the infusion of antivenom IV at a slow rate, increasing the rate after the first 10 minutes, if no reaction occurs.
    D. The initial dosage should be two vials. Smaller body-weight patients often require additional vials.
    E. Reduce the volume of diluent (crystalloids) in smaller patients (due to possible fluid overload).

F. Attempt to administer the total dose within 1–2 hours of beginning treatment.

G. The earlier the administration of antivenom the more effective it will be, therefore the lower the total dosage required.

18. Evaluation of whether additional antivenom should be administered should include evaluation of the patient's clinical signs and laboratory findings. Useful parameters in determining that additional antivenin is *not* needed include:

A. Stabilization of the cardiovascular system, including normalization of blood pressure and pulse rate

B. A cessation of muscle fasciculations

C. General improvement of the patient's condition.

19. Monitor the medial surface of the pinna for onset of hyperemia as anaphylactoid reactions to rapid infusion of foreign protein can occur.

20. If a reaction occurs immediately discontinue the antivenin infusion.

A. Administer diphenhydramine 1–4 mg/kg slow IV.

B. Some patients require the administration of epinephrine and corticosteroids.

C. Monitor the patient's blood pressure.

D. Wait 10 minutes then restart the infusion of antivenin at a slower rate.

21. If the allergic reaction recurs, stop antivenom, begin a crystalloid infusion and seek consultation. A simultaneous infusion of intravenous epinephrine, titrated to effect, may be beneficial.

22. A new, experimental, elapid, bovine-derived fragment antibody (Fab) antivenin has been developed.

A. It contains antivenom to the venom of *Micrurus fulvius* (Eastern coral snake).

B. This new antivenom reportedly is very effective, but is not commercially available at the time of publication.

23. Consider the administration of corticosteroids. Corticosteroid administration to victims of snakebite envenomation is controversial and usually not recommended as therapy for Elapidae envenomation.

24. The administration of atropine may be beneficial in reversing signs of cholinesterase activity from envenomation.

Treatment of Crotalidae envenomation—

1. Advise the telephone caller to immobilize the affected limb if a patient was bitten on an extremity, to restrict the patient's activity (carry it if possible) and to come to the veterinary facility immediately.

A. Advise the caller *not* to apply a tourniquet or ice and *not* to administer medication.

B. While en route, they should elevate the affected limb if possible, to keep it at heart level.

C. It is not necessary to capture the snake, but is helpful if they can determine whether it is a nonvenomous or a venomous species.

2. Inform the client of the diagnosis, prognosis and the cost of treatment.
3. Treat the patient, not the snake, the venom, or the known or suspected venom constituents.
4. If the patient is a dog that was previously vaccinated with the 'rattlesnake vaccine', the dog will still need the same treatment as an unvaccinated dog.
5. Ensure a patent airway. Intubate the patient if necessary.
6. Administer supplemental oxygen and ventilation if necessary.
7. If the swelling is on the head or neck, remove the collar and prepare to perform an emergency tracheostomy, if necessary.
8. Obtain pretreatment blood and urine samples. Do not perform cystocentesis if the patient may have a coagulopathy.
9. Place an intravenous catheter. Administer a balanced electrolyte crystalloid fluid intravenously to maintain perfusion, and hydration.
10. If the patient is presented in a state of severe hypovolemic shock, administer Hetastarch.
    A. The dose for dogs is 20 mL/kg IV bolus over 10 minutes, then 14–20 mL/kg IV infusion, as indicated by the clinical signs.
    B. The dose for cats is 5 mL/kg bolus IV over 10 minutes, then 5–10 mL/kg IV infusion, as indicated. Cats must be closely monitored for signs of volume overload.
11. If the patient is in shock and has signs of a coagulopathy, additional units of antivenom may be necessary.
    A. If defibrination has occurred, blood component therapy may be ineffective.
    B. Circulating venom will continue to destroy transfused platelets, red blood cells and coagulation factors.
12. If the patient is not in shock but has a prolonged ACT, or PTT, administer intravenous crystalloid fluids but avoid the administration of Hetastarch or heparin. Antivenom therapy may combat the possible coagulopathy.
13. Crotalid, thrombin-like enzymes are not inhibited by antithrombin III (heparin cofactor), making heparin ineffective for the therapy of crotalid venom-induced coagulopathies.
14. Administer diazepam, phenobarbital or pentobarbital if necessary to control seizures or hyperactivity. Avoid the use of phenothiazines, such as acepromazine, which may cause hypotension.
    A. Diazepam 0.5–1 mg/kg IV in increments of 5–20 mg to effect
    B. Phenobarbital 2–4 mg/kg IV in dogs, 1–2 mg/kg IV in cats
    C. Pentobarbital 2–30 mg/kg slow IV to effect.
15. Evaluate the status of preadmission treatment.
    A. If a tourniquet or tight band has inadvertently been placed, apply a less constricting band proximal to tourniquet, start a balanced electrolyte crystalloid fluid IV, then remove the tourniquet *slowly*.
    B. Determine if any medications had been administered or if there is a history of allergies.

16. Clip and clean the wound(s) if the patient will allow.
17. Antibiotic administration is unnecessary for the majority of snakebite victims. If the patient has an underlying immunosuppressive disorder, concurrent infection or the snakebite wounds are on the feet, extensive or severely necrotic, administer broad-spectrum antibiotics, such as metronidazole combined with cephalosporins or amoxicillin clavulanate. Aminoglycosides and ciprofloxacin are contraindicated owing to the possible occurrence of acute renal failure.
18. Loosely immobilize the affected body part in a functional position if possible.
19. Because the bites of Crotalidae are quite painful, the administration of analgesics is recommended.
    A. Initially, during hospitalization, do not administer NSAIDs, due to their renal and anticoagulant effects. Once the patient has improved and renal failure and coagulopathies are not at risk of development, an NSAID may be administered. Quite often, this starts at the time of discharge from the hospital.
    B. Antivenom decreases the painfulness of the bite wound. An additional vial of antivenom may be beneficial to the patient with severe pain.
    C. Commonly used analgesics include:
       I. Hydromorphone
          a. Dog: 0.05–0.2 mg/kg IV, IM, or SC q2–6h; 0.0125–0.05 mg/kg/h IV CRI
          b. Cat: 0.05–0.2 mg/kg IV, IM, or SC q2–6h
       II. Fentanyl
          a. Dog: 2–10 µg/kg IV to effect, followed by 1–10 µg/kg/h IV CRI
          b. Cat: 1–5 µg/kg/h to effect, followed by 1–5 µg/kg/h IV CRI
       III. Morphine
          a. Dog: 0.5–1 mg/kg IM, SC; 0.05–0.1 mg/kg IV
          b. Cat: 0.005–0.2 mg/kg IM, SC
       IV. Buprenorphine
          a. Dog: 0.005–0.02 mg/kg IV, IM q4–8h; 2–4 µg/kg/h IV CRI; 0.12 mg/kg OTM
          b. Cat: 0.005–0.01 mg/kg IV, IM q4–8h; 1–3 µg/kg/h IV CRI; 0.02 mg/kg OTM.
20. Following the skin test, and / or prior to the administration of antivenin, consider the administration of diphenhydramine (2–4 mg/kg IV) for its sedative action and as pretreatment against possible allergic responses to antivenin.
21. Administer antivenom. There are currently three different types of Crotalidae antivenoms possibly available to veterinarians in the United States.
    A. Antivenin®, distributed by Wyeth and Fort Dodge, a polyvalent Crotalidae antivenom, which contains antivenin to *Crotalus adamanteus* (Eastern diamondback rattlesnake), *C. atrox* (Western

diamondback rattlesnake), *C. durissus terrificus* (South American or tropical rattlesnake) and *Bothrops atrox* (fer-de-lance)

    I. This antivenin is able to neutralize venom from all North, South, and Central American crotalids.

    II. This antivenin is of equine origin and may cause true anaphylaxis (type I hypersensitivity), anaphylactoid reactions and serum sickness (type III hypersensitivity).

    III. If the culprit of the venomous snakebite was a copperhead, antivenin is usually not necessary; however, the patient should be monitored closely.

    IV. Antivenin administration is usually necessary, or at least beneficial, in the treatment of Eastern diamondback, cottonmouth, and water moccasin envenomation cases, and in the treatment of patients envenomated by all Crotalidae in the western United States.

B. CroFab®, a polyvalent, crotalid, ovine-derived fragment antibody (Fab) antivenom which is highly purified

    I. CroFab® contains antivenom to *Crotalus atrox* (Western diamondback rattlesnake), *C. adamanteus* (Eastern diamondback rattlesnake), *C. scutulatus scutulatus* (Mojave rattlesnake with venom A) and *Agkistrodon piscivorus piscivorus* (Eastern cottonmouth).

    II. CroFab® also contains fewer protein molecules, which decreases the risk of anaphylaxis.

    III. The smaller, fragment antibodies in CroFab® have an increased clearance rate. Occasionally, the administration of antivenom may need to be repeated in several hours.

    IV. CroFab® has become the primary antivenom administered to human Crotalidae envenomation victims in the United States.

C. Antivypmin® is another fragment antibody antivenom that has been developed in Mexico and can be imported to the United States with the appropriate documentation.

    I. In clinical trials, Antivypmin® appears to be very effective, with minimal or no side effects.

    II. Antivypmin® has shown to improve patient comfort and provide analgesia much more effectively than the other antivenoms.

    III. Antivypmin® requires little to no dilution and may be delivered slowly intravenously.

22. Ideally, antivenin should be administered within 2–4 hours of the bite. The effectiveness decreases after 8 hours and decreases even further after 12 hours. The use of antivenin after 30 hours may be limited to the reversal of a coagulopathy or thrombocytopenia. Antivenin administration has been reported to be beneficial up to 60 hours after envenomation.

23. Reconstitution of antivenom

A. Antivenom may be swirled while it is being reconstituted, but it should not be shaken as the proteins will denature and the product will become foamy.

B. Warming the antivenom and diluent to body temperature by placing the vials in pockets or on the body aids in speeding reconstitution.

C. Antivenom can also be reconstituted by placing it on a blood vial rocker that gently rocks back and forth.

24. After reconstitution, dilute antivenin (Crotalidae) polyvalent in a crystalloid IV fluid, in a volume that can safely be administered to the patient within 1 hour.

A. For cats and small dogs, 25 mL of fluids are used.

B. For medium dogs, 100 mL of fluids may be used.

C. For large dogs, 250 mL of crystalloid solution may be used.

25. Start the infusion of Antivenin IV at a slow rate, increasing the rate after the first 10 minutes, if no reaction occurs.

A. The initial dose should be one to two vials. Smaller body-weight patients and wounds on the digits often require additional vials.

B. Attempt to administer the total dose within 1–2 hours of beginning treatment.

C. The earlier the administration of antivenom the more effective it will be, therefore the lower is the total dose required.

26. Monitor the medial surface of the pinna for onset of hyperemia as anaphylactoid reactions to rapid infusion of foreign protein can occur.

27. If an anaphylactic or anaphylactoid reaction occurs immediately discontinue the antivenin infusion.

A. Administer diphenhydramine 1–2 mg/kg slow IV.

B. Consider the administration of cimetidine (Tagamet®), 5–10 mg/kg IV or IM q8–12h.

C. Some patients require the administration of epinephrine and corticosteroids.

D. Monitor the patient's blood pressure.

E. Wait 10 minutes then restart infusion of antivenin at a slower rate.

F. If allergic reaction recurs, stop antivenin, begin a crystalloid infusion, and seek consultation.

G. A simultaneous infusion of intravenous epinephrine, titrated to effect, may be beneficial.

28. Evaluation of whether additional antivenin should be administered should include evaluation of the patient's clinical signs, including increasing swelling, severity of pain and laboratory findings, especially PTT prolongation and thrombocytopenia.

A. Measure the circumference of the involved part at, below and above the bite site (Fig. 14.5).

B. Record measurements every 15 minutes before and during antivenin administration and every 1–2 hours thereafter to document swelling and edema.

C. Perform serial physical and neurologic examinations. Repeat evaluation of the PTT and platelet estimates.

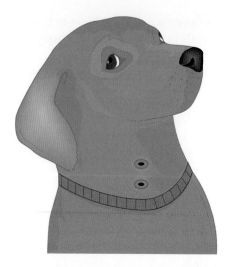

FIG 14.5 **Measuring the diameter of the location of a snakebite wound.** The diameter of the location of a snakebite wound should be noted in the medical record upon entry and measurements should be repeated to assist in patient monitoring.

    D. Useful parameters in determining additional antivenin is not needed include :
- I. Stabilization of the cardiovascular system, including normalization of blood pressure and pulse rate
- II. An increase in the platelet count or normalization of the PTT
- III. A cessation of muscle fasciculations
- IV. Swelling stabilizes, fails to increase, and may decrease
- V. The patient's pain appears to subside
- VI. General improvement of the patient's condition.

29. After the administration of antivenom, all patients should be hospitalized and observed for a minimum of 24 hours. Sometimes financial restraints prevent this from happening. In these cases, it is essential to advise the owner what they should monitor for and what to do when problems occur.

30. Corticosteroid administration to victims of snakebite envenomation is controversial and currently is *not* recommended.

31. Monitor the patient's urine output and renal function. Minimum urine output should be 1–2 mL/kg/h.

32. Monitor the patient's cardiovascular function, including the ECG for cardiac arrhythmias.

33. Reevaluate the patient's platelet count q2–6h initially, until it stabilizes.

34. Advise the client to monitor the patient for the signs of serum sickness. The average onset is 1 week after antivenom administration. The clinical signs include fever, malaise, myalgia, arthralgia, urticaria, lymphadenopathy, vasculitis, glomerulonephritis and neuritis. The condition is self-limiting and treatment involves administering a combination of antihistamines and glucocorticoids.

GENERAL RECOMMENDATIONS

1. Hospitalize and observe all patients for minimum of 12 hours, (24–48 hours for Elapidae bites) even when there are no clinical signs.
2. Do *not* leave the patient unattended (especially during antivenin administration).
3. Do *not* delay immediate and vigorous treatment if indicated.
4. Do *not* use ice or other cold applications.
5. Do *not* apply a tourniquet.
6. Parenteral fluids are usually adequate for hypotension. Vasopressors should be used only as shortterm agents in the presence of shock.
7. Do *not* administer heparin to treat Crotalidae venom-induced coagulopathies.
8. Excisional therapy is *not* recommended.
9. Do *not* explore wounds surgically to assess their severity.
10. Do *not* perform a fasciotomy unless there is objective evidence of true compartment syndrome, in which case a surgical consultation should be obtained. Despite the usual presence of severe edema and swelling in Crotalidae bites, vascular compromise or compartment syndrome is rarely documented.

SPIDER BITE ENVENOMATION

BLACK WIDOW SPIDERS (*LATRODECTUS* SPR) (FIG. 14.6)

Mode of action

Latrodectus spp. release α-latrotoxin, a neurotoxin that causes an increase of calcium ions at presynaptic nerve processes, enhancing depolarization. The ion-exchange channels are locked open, and acetylcholine and norepinephrine release are promoted.

Diagnosis

History—History of exposure.

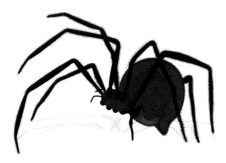

FIG 14.6   Black widow spider. The adult female is shiny black, about 1.5 cm long, and has a bright red hourglass-shaped marking on the ventral abdomen. Males resemble immature females: they are much smaller and patterned with red, brown and cream.

Clinical signs—
1. Local signs of black widow envenomation
   A. Small puncture wounds may be observed.
   B. A target lesion (a darkened necrotic area surrounded by a pale ring of ischemic tissue on an erythematous area) may be observed.
   C. In general, local tissue signs are absent and swelling is uncommon.
   D. Immediately after the bite, the area is intensely painful.
2. Systemic signs
   A. Regional numbness followed by hyperesthesia
   B. Tenderness in adjacent lymph nodes
   C. Progressive regional muscle pain
   D. Muscle fasciculations
   E. Cramping of large muscle masses (chest, abdomen, lumbar area, etc.)
   F. Abdominal muscle rigidity without tenderness
   G. Obvious restlessness, writhing, muscle spasms
   H. Seizures
   I. Hypertension and tachycardia
   J. Ascending motor paralysis (early and marked in cats)
   K. Excessive salivation
   L. Death may occur due to cardiovascular or respiratory collapse
   Cats are more sensitive to *Latrodectus* bites than are dogs. The clinical signs cats exhibit include hypersalivation, restlessness, severe pain, paralysis and death.
   Laboratory evaluation—There are usually no noted abnormalities.

Prognosis

The prognosis is variable. The prognosis is usually good in dogs and guarded in cats.

Treatment

1. First aid is essentially of no value. Do *not* apply constricting bands or tourniquets.
2. Inform the client of the diagnosis, prognosis and the cost of treatment.
3. Ensure a patent airway. Intubate the patient if necessary.
4. Administer supplemental oxygen and ventilation if necessary.
5. Obtain pretreatment blood and urine samples.
6. Place an intravenous catheter. Administer a balanced electrolyte crystalloid fluid intravenously to maintain perfusion, and hydration.
7. Administer diazepam, phenobarbital or pentobarbital if necessary to control seizures or hyperactivity.
   A. Diazepam 0.5–1 mg/kg IV in increments of 5–20 mg to effect
   B. Phenobarbital 2–4 mg/kg IV in dogs, 1–2 mg/kg IV in cats
   C. Pentobarbital 2–30 mg/kg slow IV to effect
8. Evaluate the status of preadmission treatment.
9. Administer diphenhydramine 1–2 mg/kg SC, IM, IV.

10. Consider the administration of Lyovac Antivenin® (Merke/Sharpe/ Dohme) in severely affected patients. Administer one vial slow IV.
11. If antivenin is not available, or the patient experiences severe muscle cramping or fasciculations, administer 10% calcium gluconate (0.5–1.5 mL/kg IV).
12. Administer methocarbamol for muscle cramping.
    A. Dogs: 44.4–222.2 mg/kg IV or PO as needed
    B. Cats: 22.2–44.4 mg/kg IV or PO as needed
13. Calcium may not be effective or may need to be repeated. Along with muscle relaxants, calcium will not decrease cardiovascular effects.
14. Control the patient's pain.
    A. Hydromorphone
        I. Dogs: 0.05–0.2 mg/kg IV, IM, or SC q2–6h; 0.0125–0.05 mg/kg/h IV CRI
        II. Cats: 0.05–0.2 mg/kg IV, IM, or SC q2–6h
    B. Fentanyl
        I. Dogs: 2–10 µg/kg IV to effect, followed by 1–10 µg/kg/h IV CRI
        II. Cats: 1–5 µg/kg/h to effect, followed by 1–5 µg/kg/h IV CRI
    C. Morphine
        I. Dogs: 0.5–1 mg/kg IM, SC; 0.05–0.1 mg/kg IV
        II. Cats: 0.005–0.2 mg/kg IM, SC
    D. Buprenorphine
        I. Dogs: 0.005–0.02 mg/kg IV, IM q4–8h; 2–4 µg/kg/h IV CRI; 0.12 mg/kg OTM
        II. Cats: 0.005–0.01 mg/kg IV, IM q4–8h; 1–3 µg/kg/h IV CRI; 0.02 mg/kg OTM
15. Monitor the patient closely for up to 72 hours.

BROWN SPIDERS (*LOXOSCELES* SPP.) (FIG. 14.7)

Mode of action

Loxosceles spp. spiders produce a toxin that contains at least eight proteins, including hemolysins, hyaluronidase and proteases. The toxin damages endothelial cell membranes, resulting in capillary thrombi formation, disseminated intravascular coagulation and tissue necrosis.

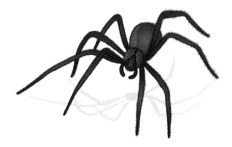

FIG 14.7 **Brown recluse spider.** The adult's body is about 9 mm long and has a leg span of 25 mm. They are tan to brown and have a violin-shaped darker marking on the cephalothorax, with the neck of the violin pointed at the abdomen. There are only three pairs of eyes on the cephalothorax, whereas most spiders have four pairs.

Diagnosis

History—History of exposure.

Clinical signs—

1. Local signs of brown spider envenomation
   A. Pain usually develops within 2–6 hours.
   B. There is localized erythema.
   C. A bleb or blister develops within 12 hours.
   D. The bleb or blister develops into a 'bulls eye' lesion, with a dark necrotic center, surrounded by a white ischemic ring on an erythematous area.
   E. An eschar may form.
   F. Focal ulceration may be evident by 7–14 days.
   G. The ulceration may enlarge and become indolent.
   H. Healing is slow.
2. Systemic manifestations
   A. The onset of systemic signs may be delayed 2–3 days post-envenomation, or may occur suddenly (this is particularly true of the hemolytic anemia).
   B. All reported cases of death due to *Loxosceles* spp. manifested systemic clinical signs.
   C. Fever.
   D. Arthralgia.
   E. Weakness.
   F. Emesis.
   G. Seizures.
   H. Of particular importance is the possible development of hemolysis, anemia, hemoglobinuria and thrombocytopenia.
   I. Secondary renal and hepatic involvement are possible sequelae.

Laboratory evaluation—

1. Hemolysis may result in hemolytic serum and anemia.
2. Hemoglobinuria may be present.

Prognosis

The prognosis is variable and is usually fair to good.

Treatment

1. Recommended first aid
   A. Application of cold compresses may be of some value.
   B. Application of heat is contraindicated.
2. Inform the client of the diagnosis, prognosis and the cost of treatment.
3. Ensure a patent airway. Intubate the patient if necessary.
4. Administer supplemental oxygen and ventilation if necessary.
5. Obtain pretreatment blood and urine samples.
6. Place an intravenous catheter. Administer a balanced electrolyte crystalloid fluid intravenously to maintain perfusion, hydration and diuresis.

7. Administer diazepam, phenobarbital or pentobarbital if necessary to control seizures or hyperactivity.
   A. Diazepam 0.5–1 mg/kg IV in increments of 5–20 mg to effect
   B. Phenobarbital 2–4 mg/kg IV in dogs, 1–2 mg/kg IV in cats
   C. Pentobarbital 2–30 mg/kg slow IV to effect
8. Evaluate the status of pre-admission treatment.
9. If hyperbaric oxygen is available, administer at 2 atmospheres q12h for 3 days.
10. Consider performing early surgical excision (before an ulcer forms).
11. It may be necessary to perform late surgical excision (6 weeks post-bite).
12. Corticosteroids, although ineffective for cutaneous lesions, may be of value in the treatment of venom-induced hemolysis.
13. Administer broad-spectrum antibiotics.
14. The administration of RBC, whole blood or a hemoglobin-based oxygen carrier may be needed in patients with severe hemolysis.
15. Pruritus may be controlled with antihistamines.
16. Treat renal and hepatic signs empirically.

STRYCHNINE TOXICOSIS

Mode of action

Strychnine reversibly and competitively antagonizes glycine, which is an inhibitory neurotransmitter found in the spinal cord and brain. The Renshaw cells in the reflex arc in the spinal cord and medulla are the neurons that mediate inhibitory influences between the motor neurons of antagonistic muscle groups. The Renshaw cells release glycine, which is antagonized by strychnine. This causes uninhibited simultaneous contraction of the antagonistic muscle groups, which results in muscle injury, hyperthermia and rhabdomyolysis. Mild to severe muscle spasms occur. Extreme hyperextension of the limbs and body dominated by the extensor muscle groups is observed. Full tetanic convulsion may then occur. Respiratory muscle failure results in death.

Sources

Strychnine is a pesticide used to eliminate coyotes, gophers, moles, rats, ground squirrels and other potential pests.

Toxic dosages

The oral LD_{50} in dogs is 0.5–1.2 mg/kg. The oral LD_{50} in cats is 2 mg/kg.

Diagnosis

History—History of exposure or running unsupervised.
Clinical signs—The onset of clinical signs is usually within 15 minutes to 2 hours following ingestion of a lethal dose of strychnine. The patient may exhibit anxiety, restlessness, tonic-clonic seizures, extreme muscle

rigidity, and hypersensitivity to touch and noise. The posture may resemble a 'saw-horse' stance with extensor rigidity. *Risus sardonicus* (the 'sardonic grin') may result from contraction of the facial muscles. Dyspnea, apnea, respiratory failure and death may occur. Gastric contents often contain milo or canary seed with turquoise blue coating. *Laboratory findings—*

1. Analysis of gastric contents or urine may confirm exposure.
2. Metabolic acidosis may be present.
3. The creatinine phosphokinase level may be elevated.
4. The patient may have myoglobinuria.

Differential diagnosis

Chlorinated hydrocarbon toxicosis, metaldehyde toxicosis, organophosphate or carbamate toxicosis, penitrem A toxicosis, sodium fluoroacetate (1080) toxicosis, tetanus toxin, zinc phosphide toxicosis and other seizure disorders.

Prognosis

The prognosis is guarded to good.

Treatment

1. Inform the client of the diagnosis, prognosis and the cost of treatment.
2. Ensure a patent airway. Intubate the patient if necessary.
3. Administer supplemental oxygen and ventilation if necessary.
4. Place an intravenous catheter. Administer a balanced electrolyte crystalloid fluid intravenously to maintain perfusion, hydration and diuresis.
5. Administer diazepam, phenobarbital or pentobarbital if necessary to control seizures or hyperactivity.
   A. Diazepam 0.5–1 mg/kg IV in increments of 5–20 mg to effect
   B. Phenobarbital 2–4 mg/kg IV in dogs, 1–2 mg/kg IV in cats
   C. Pentobarbital 2–30 mg/kg slow IV to effect
   D. If needed, administer inhalant anesthesia. The seizures must be controlled.
6. Decontamination will be of value up to 2 hours' post-ingestion. If the patient is alert and not having seizures, with no clinical signs, induce emesis; otherwise sedate the patient and perform gastric lavage.
   A. Induction of emesis in cats
      I. Administer xylazine, 0.44–1 mg/kg IM or SC (can reverse with yohimbine 0.1 mg/kg IM, SC, or IV slowly).
      II. Administer medetomidine, 10 µg/kg IM (can reverse with atipamezole (Antisedan®) 25 µg/kg IM).
      III. Hydrogen peroxide is very difficult to administer to cats and is no longer recommended.
   B. Induction of emesis in dogs
      I. Apomorphine 0.02–0.04 mg/kg IV or IM, or 1.5–6 mg dissolved and placed into the conjunctival fornix. If apomorphine was placed in the eye, after emesis, the patient's eye should be

thoroughly lavaged with sterile saline. If excessive sedation occurs from apomorphine, the sedation may be reversed by the administration of naloxone (0.01–0.04 mg/kg IV, IM, SC) but this will not reverse the emetic effects.

II. Administer 3% hydrogen peroxide 1–5 mL/kg (0.5–2 mL/lb) PO, with a maximum dose of 3 tablespoons (45 mL). If the patient does not vomit within 10 minutes, give 3% hydrogen peroxide 0.5 mL/kg (0.25 mL/lb) PO *once*.

C. Gastric lavage

I. Lightly anesthetize the patient.

II. Administer oxygen and intravenous fluids to the patient while under anesthesia.

III. Maintain anesthesia with the appropriate anesthetic as needed.

IV. Intubate the patient with a cuffed endotracheal tube and inflate the cuff.

V. Place the patient in lateral recumbency.

VI. With a stomach tube held outside of the patient, alongside the patient, measure the distance from the tip of the nose to the last rib. Mark this distance on the stomach tube.

VII. Lubricate the caudal end of the stomach tube with water-soluble jelly then pass the stomach tube gently into the stomach, passing the tube no farther than the marked distance on the tube.

VIII. If desired, two stomach tubes may be utilized, a smaller ingress tube and a large egress tube.

IX. Infuse warm (body-temperature) tap water, 5–10 mL/kg, through the tube (ingress tube if using two tubes) to moderately distend the stomach.

X. Consider using potassium permanganate (1:5000) or tannic acid solution (1–2%) as the lavage solution.

XI. Allow the fluid to drain from the stomach through the tube (egress tube if using two tubes).

XII. Save samples of gastric contents, suspicious foreign material, seeds, etc. for possible toxicologic analysis. Save gastric content samples, refrigerated and frozen, in case legal action is pursued.

XIII. The stomach tube may have to be manipulated, repositioned or flushed with fluid or air if the gastric contents do not flow freely through the tube.

XIV. Turn the patient to the other side and continue to perform gastric lavage.

XV. Continue gastric lavage until the effluent is clear.

XVI. If using the two-tube method, crimp the end of one tube and remove it.

XVII. Administer activated charcoal down the stomach tube.

XVIII. Crimp the end of the stomach tube and remove it.

XIX. Monitor the patient during recovery from anesthesia, leaving the inflated cuffed endotracheal tube in place until the patient's swallowing reflex has returned.

D. Activated charcoal with sorbitol, 2–5 g/kg (3–6 mL/lb) PO is usually administered once. In strychnine toxicosis patients, repeat the administration of activated charcoal q3–4h. Sorbitol, the cathartic should only be administered *once*. Monitor the patient's serum sodium concentration if activated charcoal is administered this frequently, as hypernatremia and hyperosmolality may occur.

7. Hospitalize the patient and provide symptomatic and supportive care. Hospitalization for 48–72 hours is usually necessary.
8. Treat hyperthermia symptomatically.
9. Monitor renal function electrolytes, and blood gases.
10. If the patient does not have a metabolic acidosis, acidification of the urine by the administration of ammonium chloride may enhance urinary excretion.
11. Administer muscle relaxants.
    A. Glyceryl guaiacolate 110 mg/kg as needed
    B. Methocarbamol 150 mg/kg initially followed by 90 mg/kg as needed.
12. Respiratory function should be closely monitored and supported if necessary.
    A. Supplemental oxygen administration may be needed.
    B. Mechanical ventilation may be needed by some patients.
13. Acid–base imbalances should be treated.
14. Avoid stimulation by sound or light. Keep the patient sedated and in a quiet, darkened room.
15. The administration of ketamine or morphine is contraindicated.

TOAD POISONING

Mode of action

Toads produce toxins in the parotid glands that contain cardioactive glycosides (bufotoxins and bufagenins); bufotenins, serotonin, dopamine, epinephrine and norepinephrine and 5-hydroxytryptamine may also be found in toad toxins. The toad toxins are absorbed through the oral mucous membranes and cause excessive stimulation, ventricular fibrillation and hypertension.

Sources

Bufo marinus (cane or marine toad) is found in Florida and Hawaii. *B. alvarius* (Colorado river toad) is found in the Southwest desert.

Toxic dosages

B. marinus toxicosis has a higher mortality rate than *B. alvarius*. Exposure to one toad may be lethal.

Diagnosis

History—History of exposure or acute onset of compatible signs in an endemic area.

Clinical signs—Within 15 minutes of exposure, the patient may exhibit slight to profuse ptyalism, hyperemic mucous membranes, pawing at the mouth, head shaking, cyanosis, tachypnea, vomiting or retching, depression, disorientation, apparent blindness, nystagmus, hyperthermia, weakness, ataxia, collapse, arrhythmias, seizures, coma and death.

Laboratory findings—

1. Evaluation of a CBC may reveal an elevated PCV and leukopenia.
2. Evaluation of the serum biochemical profile may reveal an elevated BUN, hyperglycemia, hypercalcemia and hyperkalemia.

Electrocardiogram—May reveal various cardiac arrhythmias including sinus bradycardia, atrioventricular block, sinus tachycardia, ventricular tachycardia and ventricular fibrillation.

Blood pressure—Measurement of the patient's blood pressure may reveal hypertension.

Differential diagnosis

Heat stroke, acute allergic reaction, other intoxication (theobromine, anticholinesterase insecticides, metaldehyde, amphetamine, oleander or other cardiogenic-glycoside-containing plant ingestion).

Prognosis

The prognosis is good to guarded.

Treatment

1. Advise the owner who telephones the clinic to carefully flush the patient's mouth with a slow-moving stream of water from a garden hose or tap pointed towards the nose before bringing the patient in for medical care.
2. Inform the client of the diagnosis, prognosis and the cost of treatment.
3. Ensure a patent airway. Intubate the patient if necessary.
4. Administer supplemental oxygen and ventilation if necessary.
5. Administer diazepam, phenobarbital or propofol if necessary to control seizures or hyperactivity.
   A. Diazepam 0.5–1 mg/kg IV in increments of 5–20 mg to effect
   B. Phenobarbital 2–4 mg/kg IV in dogs, 1–2 mg/kg IV in cats
   C. Propofol 4–6 mg/kg slow IV to effect
6. Lavage the oral cavity with copious quantities of water for at least 5 minutes. If the patient is exhibiting clinical signs, sedation and endotracheal intubation is indicated to facilitate oral cavity lavage.
7. Place an intravenous catheter. Administer a balanced electrolyte crystalloid fluid intravenously to maintain perfusion, and hydration. Administer a shock dose of fluids (90 mL/kg for dogs, 60 mL/kg for cats) divided into ⅓ to ½ boluses, if the patient is in shock.
8. If the toad was ingested, emesis is indicated. If clinical signs are present, other methods of oral decontamination should be utilized,

including endoscopic retrieval, surgical removal, or multiple dose administration of activated charcoal.

9. Administer corticosteroids to decrease oral irritation.
   A. Dexamethasone sodium phosphate, 0.5–1 mg/kg IV
   B. Prednisolone sodium succinate (Solu Delta Cortef®), 4–10 mg/kg slow IV
   C. Methylprednisolone sodium succinate, 5–15 mg/kg IV
10. Hospitalize the patient for monitoring and treatment.
11. Treatment of arrhythmias
   A. Bradycardia <50 beats/min: atropine 0.02 mg/kg IV
   B. Prolonged sinus tachycardia (>30 minutes at >180 beats per minute (dogs)): propanolol 0.02–0.05 mg/kg slow IV or esmolol (0.1–0.5 mg/kg IV then 50–200 µg/kg/min IV CRI)
   C. Ventricular tachycardia in dogs may be treated with lidocaine, 2–4 mg IV bolus, or 25–100 µg/kg/min IV CRI.
12. The administration of acepromazine IM or SC may be beneficial if the patient is restless or hyperactive.
13. To decrease the development of severe dysrhythmias, the administration of atropine should be reserved for those patients with severe bradycardia.
14. The administration of digoxin immune Fab may be beneficial for patients with neurologic signs, severe arrhythmias, or severe hyperkalemia.
15. Treat hyperthermia symptomatically if indicated.

TRICYCLIC ANTIDEPRESSANT (TCA) TOXICOSIS

Mode of action

Tricyclic antidepressants (TCA) inhibit the membrane pump mechanism responsible for the uptake of norepinephrine and serotonin in adrenergic, dopaminergic and serotonergic receptors on neurons. They also acts as antagonists at muscarinic cholinergic, α_1-adrenergic, H_1- and H_2-histaminergic receptor sites.

Sources

TCAs are increasing in popularity as antidepressants with sedative effects. They include amitriptyline, amoxapine, desipramine, doxepin, imipramine, nortriptyline, protriptyline and trimipramine. The brand names of TCAs include Ascendin®, Elavil®, Endep®, Etrafon®, Limbitrol®, Triavil®, Ludiomol®, Norpramin®, Pamelor®, Sinequan®, Tofranil®, Triavil® and Vivactil®.

Toxic dosages

The therapeutic dose is usually 2–4 mg/kg. Ingestion of 15–20 mg/kg is potentially lethal.

Diagnosis

History—History of ingestion or possible exposure to medications.
Clinical signs—The primary signs of toxicity are:
1. Seizures or status epilepticus
2. Cyclic comas
3. Fatal arrhythmias—including bradycardia, tachycardia, prolongation of the QRS complex, ventricular tachycardia, ventricular fibrillation.

Additional signs may include temporary confusion, visual hallucinations, drowsiness, ataxia, disorientation, weakness, tremors, agitation, aggression, hyperactive reflexes, muscle rigidity, hyperthermia, hyperexcitability, depression, hypothermia, tachycardia, congestive heart failure, mydriasis, severe hypotension, shock, vomiting, diarrhea, paralytic ileus, constipation, lingual edema, facial edema, rash, urticaria, polyuria, pulmonary edema, cardiac arrest and death.

Laboratory findings—Monitor the patient's blood gas status. Acidosis is common and enhances cardiotoxicity.
ECG evaluation—May reveal abnormalities including bradycardia, tachycardia, prolongation of the QRS complex, ventricular tachycardia and ventricular fibrillation.

Differential diagnosis

The differential diagnoses include intoxication from citrus oil, DEET, lead, marijuana, penitrem A (garbage intoxication), pyrethrin or pyrethroids, and zinc phosphide.

Prognosis

The prognosis is variable.

Treatment

1. Inform the client of the diagnosis, prognosis and the cost of treatment.
2. Ensure a patent airway. Intubate the patient if necessary.
3. Administer supplemental oxygen and ventilation if necessary.
4. Place an intravenous catheter. Administer a balanced electrolyte crystalloid fluid intravenously to maintain perfusion, hydration, and to treat metabolic acidosis. Monitor for exacerbation of any pulmonary edema that may be present.
5. Administer diazepam, phenobarbital or pentobarbital if necessary to control seizures or hyperactivity.
   A. Diazepam 0.5–1 mg/kg IV in increments of 5–20 mg to effect
   B. Phenobarbital 2–4 mg/kg IV in dogs, 1–2 mg/kg IV in cats
   C. Pentobarbital 2–30 mg/kg slow IV to effect
6. Decontamination will be of value up to 2 hours' post-ingestion. Due to the rapid onset of seizures, **do not induce emesis**. Perform gastric lavage.

A. Lightly anesthetize the patient.
B. Administer oxygen and intravenous fluids to the patient while under anesthesia.
C. Maintain anesthesia with the appropriate anesthetic as needed.
D. Intubate the patient with a cuffed endotracheal tube and inflate the cuff.
E. Place the patient in lateral recumbency.
F. With a stomach tube held outside of the patient, alongside the patient, measure the distance from the tip of the nose to the last rib. Mark this distance on the stomach tube.
G. Lubricate the caudal end of the stomach tube with water-soluble jelly then pass the stomach tube gently into the stomach, passing the tube no farther than the marked distance on the tube.
H. If desired, two stomach tubes may be utilized, a smaller ingress tube and a large egress tube.
I. Infuse warm (body-temperature) tap water, 5–10 mL/kg, through the tube (ingress tube if using two tubes) to moderately distend the stomach.
J. Allow the fluid to drain from the stomach through the tube (egress tube if using two tubes).
K. Save samples of gastric contents, suspicious foreign material, seeds, etc. for possible toxicologic analysis.
L. The stomach tube may have to be manipulated, repositioned or flushed with fluid or air if the gastric contents do not flow freely through the tube.
M. Turn the patient to the other side and continue to perform gastric lavage.
N. Continue gastric lavage until the effluent is clear.
O. If using the two-tube method, crimp the end of one tube and remove it.
P. Administer activated charcoal down the stomach tube.
Q. Crimp the end of the stomach tube and remove it.
R. Monitor the patient during recovery from anesthesia, leaving the inflated cuffed endotracheal tube in place until the patient's swallowing reflex has returned.

7. Administer activated charcoal, 2–5 g/kg (3–6 mL/lb) PO is usually administered in a slurry of 1 g to 5 mL water. In TCA toxicosis patients, repeat the administration of activated charcoal q4–6h for 24–48 hours.

8. A single dose of an osmotic or saline cathartic should be administered along with activated charcoal. The saline cathartic of choice is sodium sulfate. Magnesium sulfate is contraindicated. Alternative cathartics include:
A. Sorbitol (70%), 2 g/kg (1–2 mL/kg) PO
B. Sodium sulfate, 200 mg/kg for cats, 250–500 mg/kg for dogs. Mix sodium sulfate with water, 5–10 mL/kg and administer PO.

9. Always hospitalize and observe the patient for a minimum of 12 hours, providing symptomatic and supportive therapy.

10. ECG and close monitoring of cardiac function should be performed for 5 days. One of the first visual changes is a prolongation of the QRS complex.
11. Alkalinize the patient's blood (check urine pH) to increase excretion.
    A. Monitor the patient's blood gas status.
    B. If the patient is acidotic, administer sodium bicarbonate 1–3 mEq/kg IV injection over a period of 15–30 minutes.
    C. Repeat sodium bicarbonate administration every 40 minutes initially to maintain the plasma pH at 7.45–7.55.
    D. Do *not* administer sodium bicarbonate as a constant IV infusion, it is not effective.
12. Regulate the patient's body temperature as needed.
13. Administer physostigmine salicylate (Antilirium®) if arrhythmias, seizures, or coma develop.
    A. Dogs: 0.5–1 mg slow IV or 0.5–3 mg IM
    B. Cats: 0.25–0.5 mg slow IV or IM
14. Administer lidocaine, propranolol, neostigmine or pyridostigmine if cardiac arrhythmias occur. Administer digitalis if cardiac failure occurs.
    Do not administer dopamine, isoproterenol, quinidine, procainamide or disopyramide. They are contraindicated!
15. Monitor the patient's blood pressure. If the patient develops severe hypotension while on adequate intravenous fluid therapy, consider the administration of norepinephrine or phenylephrine.

XYLITOL TOXIN

Xylitol is a 5-carbon sugar alcohol used as a substitute for sugar, most often in foods for diabetics and low-carbohydrate dieters.

Mode of action

Xylitol stimulates insulin secretion from the pancreas. Hepatic necrosis and DIC occur via unknown mechanisms, possibly by depletion of hepatocellular ADP, ATP and inorganic phosphorus.

Sources

Xylitol is found in baked goods, desserts, toothpastes, other oral care products, sugar-free gums and candies; it can be purchased in bulk for baking.

Interpretation of chewing gum labels
• If the label reads 'contains less than 2% xylitol', use 38 mg xylitol per stick or piece of gum for calculations.
• If xylitol is the first ingredient, use 2 g xylitol per stick.
• If xylitol is the second, third or greater ingredient listed, and the package does not contain the phrase 'contains less than 2% xylitol', use 220 mg xylitol per stick of gum for calculating the ingested dose.

Toxic dosages

Ingestion of 100 mg/kg has been reported to cause hypoglycemia. Hepatic necrosis was reported following ingestion of 500 mg/kg.

Differential diagnosis

1. Other toxicosis including acetaminophen, sago palm, *Amanita spp.* mushrooms, aflatoxins, blue-green algae, anticoagulant rodenticides, or iron
2. Acute hepatitis, Leptospirosis, toxoplasmosis, mycotic infections, infectious canine hepatitis
3. Neoplasia, microvascular dysplasia, portosystemic shunt, hepatic cirrhosis
4. Heat stroke or trauma.

Diagnosis

History— Often the owner observed ingestion or found chewed-up wrappers.

Clinical signs—Weakness, depression, tremors, ataxia, collapse and seizures may occur within 10–60 minutes following ingestion. Vomiting, diarrhea, icterus, melena, petechiation, ecchymosis, hepatic encephalopathy, and diffuse hemorrhage may be observed 9–72 hours' post-ingestion.

Laboratory findings—Hypoglycemia, hypokalemia, elevated liver enzymes (ALT, ALP, GGT and hyperbilirubinemia) , mild neutrophilic leukocytosis and hemoconcentration, prolonged ACT, PTT, PT, increased D-dimer or FDP, and thrombocytopenia

Diagnostic imaging— The liver size may be normal to increased. The liver echogenicity may be normal to hypoechoic, or mottled due to hepatic necrosis.

Prognosis

If the clinical signs are restricted to hypoglycemia, the long-term prognosis is good. The prognosis is fair to guarded for patients with hepatic necrosis.

Treatment

1. Inform the client of the diagnosis, prognosis and cost of the treatment.
2. If the patient presents less than 6 hours after ingestion, attempt gastric decontamination with emesis unless the patient exhibits clinical signs of hypoglycemia. Induction of emesis after this time may be beneficial in cases of large ingestion.
   A. Induction of emesis in cats
      I. Administer xylazine, 0.44–1 mg/kg IM or SC (can reverse with yohimbine 0.1 mg/kg IM, SC, or IV slowly).
      II. Administer medetomidine, 10 μg/kg IM (can reverse with atipamezole (Antisedan®) 25 μg/kg IM).

III. Hydrogen peroxide is very difficult to administer to cats and is no longer recommended.

B. Induction of emesis in dogs

   I. Apomorphine 0.02–0.04 mg/kg IV or IM, or 1.5–6 mg dissolved and placed into the conjunctival fornix. If apomorphine was placed in the eye, after emesis, the patient's eye should be thoroughly lavaged with sterile saline. If excessive sedation occurs from apomorphine, the sedation may be reversed by the administration of naloxone (0.01–0.04 mg/kg IV, IM, SC) but this will not reverse the emetic effects.

   II. Administer 3% hydrogen peroxide 1–5 mL/kg (0.5–2 mL/lb) PO, with a maximum dose of 3 tablespoons (45 mL). If the patient does not vomit within 10 minutes, give 3% hydrogen peroxide 0.5 mL/kg (0.25 mL/lb) PO *once*.

C. Gastric lavage

   I. Lightly anesthetize the patient.

   II. Administer oxygen and intravenous fluids to the patient while under anesthesia.

   III. Maintain anesthesia with the appropriate anesthetic as needed.

   IV. Intubate the patient with a cuffed endotracheal tube and inflate the cuff.

   V. Place the patient in lateral recumbency.

   VI. With a stomach tube held outside of the patient, alongside the patient, measure the distance from the tip of the nose to the last rib. Mark this distance on the stomach tube.

   VII. Lubricate the caudal end of the stomach tube with water-soluble jelly then pass the stomach tube gently into the stomach, passing the tube no farther than the marked distance on the tube.

   VIII. If desired, two stomach tubes may be utilized, a smaller ingress tube and a large egress tube.

   IX. Infuse warm (body-temperature) tap water, 5–10 mL/kg, through the tube (ingress tube if using two tubes) to moderately distend the stomach.

   X. Allow the fluid to drain from the stomach through the tube (egress tube if using two tubes).

   XI. Save samples of gastric contents, suspicious foreign material, seeds, etc. for possible toxicologic analysis.

   XII. The stomach tube may have to be manipulated, repositioned or flushed with fluid or air if the gastric contents do not flow freely through the tube.

   XIII. Turn the patient to the other side and continue to perform gastric lavage.

   XIV. Continue gastric lavage until the effluent is clear.

   XV. If using the two-tube method, crimp the end of one tube and remove it.

   XVI. Crimp the end of the stomach tube and remove it.

XVII. Monitor the patient during recovery from anesthesia, leaving the inflated cuffed endotracheal tube in place until the patient's swallowing reflex has returned.

D. The administration of activated charcoal is not recommended.

3. Place an IV catheter and administer intravenous fluids supplemented with Dextrose 2.5% to 5%.

4. Monitor blood glucose levels frequently,

5. If the patient is hypoglycemic (blood glucose <60 mg/dL), administer 50% dextrose diluted to 25% with an equal volume of sterile saline, 0.5–1.5 mL/kg IV over 1–2 minutes. Then start the patient on a dextrose 2.5% to 5% CRI in IV fluids.

6. Feed the patient small, frequent meals to avoid hypoglycemia if the patient is not vomiting.

7. Administer antiemetics and GI protectants as indicated for the individual patient.

8. Administer fresh frozen plasma if the patient has coagulopathy or DIC.

9. Administer medications to support hepatic function.

   A. *N*-acetylcystine, 50 mg/kg IV or PO every 6 hours for 24 hours. Dilute *N*-acetylcysteine to a 5% solution in 0.9% NaCl, administer IV slowly over 30 minutes.

   B. S-adenosylmethionine (SAM-e), 18–20 mg/kg PO q24h

   C. Silymarin (milk thistle), 20–50 mg/kg PO q24h

   D. Vitamins C and E

   E. Vitamin K_1.

ZINC TOXICOSIS

Mode of action

Zinc toxicosis causes acute hemolysis by an unknown mode of action. The anemia is usually a result of intravascular hemolysis, possibly due to oxidative mechanisms.

Sources

Ingestion of numerous substances can cause zinc toxicity in dogs, cats, birds and ferrets, but the most commonly encountered in practice are coins (pennies made since 1983), zinc oxide skin preparations, and hardware items. Other sources of zinc include calamine lotion, suppositories, shampoos, Desenex®, fertilizers, paint, nails and galvanized metal objects.

Toxic dosages

Ingestion of zinc in doses of 0.7–1 g/kg may result in clinical signs of toxicity. Subacute zinc toxicosis may occur following the ingestion of up to five pennies.

Diagnosis

History—History of exposure.

Clinical signs—The patient may exhibit depression, anorexia, vomiting, lethargy, diarrhea and abdominal pain. Hemolytic anemia with hemoglobinuria and icterus may occur, as may acute renal failure.

Laboratory findings—

1. Hemolytic anemia
2. Inflammatory leukogram
3. Elevated hepatic and pancreatic enzymes
4. Azotemia, including increased BUN and serum creatinine levels
5. Hyperphosphatemia
6. Granular urinary casts
7. Increased levels of zinc in serum, plasma, urine and tissue specimens. Special blood collection tubes and syringes are required for collection of serum or plasma samples to be submitted for analysis of zinc levels.

Abdominal radiographs—May reveal radiodense foreign bodies suggestive of metal in the gastrointestinal tract.

Differential diagnosis

The differential diagnoses include intoxications from boric acid, garbage, mushrooms and rotenone IMHA or IHA, and acute renal failure from various other causes.

Prognosis

The prognosis is variable.

Treatment

1. Inform the client of the diagnosis, prognosis and the cost of treatment.
2. Ensure a patent airway. Intubate the patient if necessary.
3. Administer supplemental oxygen and ventilation if necessary.
4. Place an intravenous catheter. Administer a balanced electrolyte crystalloid fluid intravenously to maintain perfusion, hydration and diuresis.
5. Decontamination by induction of emesis will be of value up to 2 hours post-ingestion of the toxin. Gastric lavage is usually nonproductive.
   A. Induction of emesis in cats
       I. Administer xylazine, 0.44–1 mg/kg IM or SC (can reverse with yohimbine 0.1 mg/kg IM, SC, or IV slowly).
       II. Administer medetomidine, 10 μg/kg IM (can reverse with atipamezole (Antisedan®) 25 μg/kg IM).
       III. Hydrogen peroxide is very difficult to administer to cats and is no longer recommended.
   B. Induction of emesis in dogs
       I. Apomorphine 0.02–0.04 mg/kg IV or IM, or 1.5–6 mg dissolved and placed into the conjunctival fornix. If apomorphine was placed in the eye, after emesis, the patient's eye should be

thoroughly lavaged with sterile saline. If excessive sedation occurs from apomorphine, the sedation may be reversed by the administration of naloxone (0.01–0.04 mg/kg IV, IM, SC) but this will not reverse the emetic effects.

   II. Administer 3% hydrogen peroxide 1–5 mL/kg (0.5–2 mL/lb) PO, with a maximum dose of 3 tablespoons (45 mL). If the patient does not vomit within 10 minutes, give 3% hydrogen peroxide 0.5 mL/kg (0.25 mL/lb) PO *once*.

  C. Perform endoscopy and remove the gastric foreign body if possible.

6. Provide supportive treatment of vomiting and diarrhea, including intravenous fluid therapy, antiemetics and gastric protectants if indicated.
7. Blood component therapy or administration of a hemoglobin based oxygen carrier may be necessary.
8. Administer calcium disodium EDTA.
  A. Administer calcium EDTA 25 mg/kg SC q4h or 50 mg/kg q12h for 2–5 days.
  B. Prior to administration, dilute calcium EDTA to a concentration of 10 mg calcium EDTA/mL of 5% dextrose.
  C. Do not exceed 2 g/day in small animals.
9. After administering calcium EDTA for 24–48 hours, if the gastrointestinal foreign body has not been eliminated or removed then cautiously perform gastrointestinal surgery and remove the foreign body.
10. Following surgery, continue calcium EDTA administration or administer penicillamine for 1–3 more days post-operatively.
11. The recommended dose of penicillamine is 33–55 mg/kg/day PO for 1 week, off for 1 week, then repeat for 1 week. The daily dose can be divided and given at 6–8-hour intervals on an empty stomach. Dissolving D-penicillamine in fruit juice may help improve palatability and mask the odor.
12. Monitor urine output and renal function. The minimum urine output should be 1–2 mL/kg/h.

ZINC PHOSPHIDE TOXICOSIS

Mode of action

Following ingestion, when zinc phosphide reacts with gastric acid, the protoplasmic poison phosgene is released. Phosgene gas has the odor of garlic or rotten fish. Phosgene gas may damage capillary endothelium and erythrocyte membranes within the kidneys, liver and lungs. The damaged capillary endothelium results in increased vascular permeability and cardiovascular collapse. There may be direct myocardial effects. Phosgene also blocks cytochrome C oxidase, inhibiting oxidative phosphorylation, resulting in cell death. Gastric gas is rapidly produced, causing gastrointestinal irritation, abdominal distention, vomiting, hypoglycemia, shock and death.

Sources

Zinc phosphide is a rodenticide, formulated as meals, pellets or strips. Similar products with the same mode of action include aluminum or magnesium phosphide. Some commercial products include Acme Mole and Gopher Killer®, Gopha Rid®, Kikrat®, Mous-Con®, Mr. Rat Guard®, Phosvin®, Phosyin®, Rumetan®, True Grit Gopher Rid® and Zinc Tox®.

Toxic dosages

The lethal dose is 20–50 mg/kg. Toxicity can occur at levels below that which produces the odor. Toxicity can occur following ingestion or inhalation.

Diagnosis

History—The owner may provide a history of exposure.
Clinical signs—Within 4 hours following exposure, the patient may exhibit anorexia, lethargy, abdominal distention, weakness, salivation and vomiting. The clinical signs may progress to pulmonary edema, hypotension, shock, recumbency, generalized muscle tremors, hyperesthesia, seizures, cardiac arrhythmias and conduction disturbances, tachypnea, cyanosis and death.
Laboratory findings—
1. Evaluation of a serum biochemical profile may reveal hypoglycemia.
2. Hypocalcemia, hypophosphatemia and hyperphosphatemia have been observed.
3. Thrombocytopenia and methemoglobinemia may occur.
4. Blood gas evaluation may reveal acidosis.
5. Analysis of stomach contents, gastric lavage washings, or vomitus that is collected immediately into airtight containers and frozen may reveal increased levels of zinc, magnesium or aluminum.

Differential diagnosis

The differential diagnoses include intoxications from citrus oil, DEET, penitrem A (garbage intoxication), marijuana, pyrethrins, pyrethroids, and tricyclic antidepressants.

Prognosis

The prognosis is variable, but is usually guarded.

Treatment

1. Inform the client of the diagnosis, prognosis and the cost of treatment.
2. Ensure a patent airway. Intubate the patient if necessary.

3. Administer supplemental oxygen and ventilation if necessary.
4. Place an intravenous catheter. Administer a balanced electrolyte crystalloid fluid intravenously to maintain perfusion, hydration and diuresis.
5. Supplement the intravenous fluids with 5% dextrose.
6. Decontamination may be beneficial and should be performed in a well-ventilated area, preferably outside. If the patient is not vomiting, induce emesis, otherwise sedate the patient and perform gastric lavage.
   A. Induction of emesis in cats
      I. Administer xylazine, 0.44–1 mg/kg IM or SC (can reverse with yohimbine 0.1 mg/kg IM, SC, or IV slowly).
      II. Administer medetomidine, 10 µg/kg IM (can reverse with atipamezole (Antisedan®) 25 µg/kg IM).
      III. Hydrogen peroxide is very difficult to administer to cats and is no longer recommended.
   B. Induction of emesis in dogs
      I. Apomorphine 0.02–0.04 mg/kg IV or IM, or 1.5–6 mg dissolved and placed into the conjunctival fornix. If apomorphine was placed in the eye, after emesis, the patient's eye should be thoroughly lavaged with sterile saline. If excessive sedation occurs from apomorphine, the sedation may be reversed by the administration of naloxone (0.01–0.04 mg/kg IV, IM, SC) but this will not reverse the emetic effects.
      II. Administer 3% hydrogen peroxide 1–5 mL/kg (0.5–2 mL/lb) PO, with a maximum dose of 3 tablespoons (45 mL). If the patient does not vomit within 10 minutes, give 3% hydrogen peroxide 0.5 mL/kg (0.25 mL/lb) PO *once*.
   C. Gastric lavage
      I. Lightly anesthetize the patient.
      II. Administer oxygen and intravenous fluids to the patient while under anesthesia.
      III. Maintain anesthesia with the appropriate anesthetic as needed.
      IV. Intubate the patient with a cuffed endotracheal tube and inflate the cuff.
      V. Place the patient in lateral recumbency.
      VI. With a stomach tube held outside of the patient, alongside the patient, measure the distance from the tip of the nose to the last rib. Mark this distance on the stomach tube.
      VII. Lubricate the caudal end of the stomach tube with water-soluble jelly then pass the stomach tube gently into the stomach, passing the tube no farther than the marked distance on the tube.
      VIII. If desired, two stomach tubes may be utilized: a smaller ingress tube and a large egress tube.
      IX. Evacuate gas from the stomach.

    X. Infuse warm (body-temperature) tap water, 5–10 mL/kg, through the tube (ingress tube if using two tubes) to moderately distend the stomach.

    XI. Consider using sodium bicarbonate or 1:1000 potassium permanganate as the lavage solution.

    XII. Allow the fluid to drain from the stomach through the tube (egress tube if using two tubes).

    XIII. Save samples of gastric contents, suspicious foreign material, seeds, etc. for possible toxicologic analysis.

    XIV. The stomach tube may have to be manipulated, repositioned or flushed with fluid or air if the gastric contents do not flow freely through the tube.

    XV. Turn the patient to the other side and continue to perform gastric lavage.

    XVI. Continue gastric lavage until the effluent is clear.

    XVII. If using the two-tube method, crimp the end of one tube and remove it.

    XVIII. Administer activated charcoal down the stomach tube.

    XIX. Crimp the end of the stomach tube and remove it.

    XX. Monitor the patient during recovery from anesthesia, leaving the inflated cuffed endotracheal tube in place until the patient's swallowing reflex has returned.

  D. Administer one dose of activated charcoal with sorbitol, 2–5 g/kg (3–6 mL/lb) PO.

7. Hospitalize the patient and provide symptomatic and supportive care. Hospitalization for at least 48 hours is usually necessary.

8. Administer medication to decrease gastric acid production.
   A. Famotidine (Pepcid®), 0.5–1 mg/kg IV, PO q12h
   B. Ranitidine (Zantac®)
   - Dogs: 2–5 mg/kg IV, SC, PO q8–q12h
   - Cats: 2.5 mg/kg IV, PO q12h
   C. Cimetidine (Tagamet®), 5–10 mg/kg IV, IM, PO q6–8h
   D. Omeprazole (Prilosec®), dogs only, 0.7–2 mg/kg PO q24h. If the dog weighs >20 kg, administer 20 mg PO q24h. If the dog weighs <20 kg, administer 10 mg PO q24h.

9. If blood gas evaluation reveals a severe metabolic acidosis, administer sodium bicarbonate.
   A. $0.3 - 0.5 \times$ body weight in kg $\times (24 - $ plasma bicarbonate level$) = $ mEq of sodium bicarbonate needed.
   B. Infuse half of the sodium bicarbonate amount needed over the first 3–4 hours, then re-evaluate and readjust the dose.
   C. Caution must be utilized while administering sodium bicarbonate. Possible complications that may result include: 'overshoot alkalosis', hypernatremia, intravascular volume overload, hypokalemia, hypocalcemia, tissue hypoxia, and paradoxical cerebrospinal fluid acidosis.

10. Monitor the serum calcium and electrolyte levels.
11. Monitor renal and hepatic function.
12. Monitor the ECG and cardiac function.

ACETAMINOPHEN

Alwood, A.J., 2009. Acetaminophen. In: Silverstein, D.C., Hopper, K. (Eds.), Small Animal Critical Care Medicine. Elsevier, St Louis, pp. 334–337.

Aronson, L.R., Drobatz, K., 1996. Acetaminophen toxicosis in 17 cats. Journal of Veterinary Emergency and Critical Care 6 (2), 65–69.

Babski, D.M., Koenig, A., 2009. Acetaminophen. In: Osweiler, G.D., Hovda, L.R., Brutlag, A G., et al. (Eds.), Blackwell's Five-Minute Veterinary Consult Clinical Companion Small Animal Toxicology. Wiley-Blackwell, Ames, pp. 263–269.

Campbell, A., 2000. Paracetamol. In: Campbell, A., Chapman, M. (Eds.), Handbook of Poisoning in Dogs and Cats. Blackwell Science, Malden, pp. 31–38.

Campbell, A., 2000. Paracetamol. In: Campbell, A., Chapman, M. (Eds.), Handbook of Poisoning in Dogs and Cats. Blackwell Science, Malden, pp. 205–212.

Cope, R.B., White, K.S., More, E., et al., 2006. Exposure-to-treatment interval and clinical severity in canine poisoning: a retrospective analysis at a Portland Veterinary Emergency Center. Journal of Veterinary Pharmacology and Therapeutics 29, 233–236.

Fitzgerald, K.T., Bronstein, A.C., Flood, A.A., 2006. 'Over-the-counter' drug toxicities in companion animals. Clinical Techniques in Small Animal Practice 21, 215–226.

Mariani, C.L., Fulton, R.B., 2001. Atypical reaction to acetaminophen intoxication in a dog. Journal of Veterinary Emergency and Critical Care 11 (2), 123–126.

Meadows, I., Gwaltney-Brant, S., 2006. The 10 most common toxicoses in dogs. Veterinary Medicine March, 142–148.

Richardson, J.A., 2000. Management of acetaminophen and ibuprofen toxicoses in dogs and cats. Journal of Veterinary Emergency and Critical Care 10, 285–291.

Roder, J.D., 2004. Acetaminophen. In: Plumlee, K.H. (Ed.), Clinical Veterinary Toxicology. Mosby, St Louis, p. 284.

Sellon, R.K., 2006. Acetaminophen. In: Peterson, M.E., Talcott, P.A. (Eds.), Small Animal Toxicology, second ed. Saunders Elsevier, St Louis, pp. 550–558.

Wallace, K.P., Center, S.A., Hickford, F.H., et al., 2002. S-adenosyl-L-methionine (SAMe) for the treatment of acetaminophen toxicity in a dog. Journal of the American Animal Hospital Association 38, 246–254.

ALBUTEROL

Babski, D.M., Brainard, B.M., 2009. Albuterol. In: Osweiler, G.D., Hovda, L.R., Brutlag, A.G., et al. (Eds.), Blackwell's Five-Minute Veterinary Consult Clinical Companion Small Animal Toxicology. Wiley-Blackwell, Ames, pp. 119–124.

McCown, J.L., Lechner, E.S., Cooke, K.L., 2008. Suspected albuterol toxicosis in a dog. Journal of the American Veterinary Medical Association 232, 1168–1171.

Rosendale, M., 2004. Bronchodilators. In: Plumlee, K.H. (Ed.), Clinical Veterinary Toxicology. Mosby, St Louis, pp. 305–307.

AMITRAZ

Gruber, N.M., 2009. Amitraz. In: Osweiler, G.D., Hovda, L.R., Brutlag, A.G., et al. (Eds.), Blackwell's Five-Minute Veterinary Consult Clinical Companion Small Animal Toxicology. Wiley-Blackwell, Ames, pp. 613–619.

Gwaltney-Brant, S., 2004. Amitraz. In: Plumlee, K.H. (Ed.), Clinical Veterinary Toxicology. Mosby, St Louis, pp. 177–178.

Richardson, J.A., 2006. Amitraz. In: Peterson, M.E., Talcott, P.A. (Eds.), Small Animal Toxicology, second ed. Saunders Elsevier, St Louis, pp. 559–562.

AMPHETAMINES

Albretsen, J.C., 2002. Oral medications. In: Poppenga, R.H., Volmer, P.A. (Eds.), Toxicology, Veterinary Clinics of North America, Small Animal Practice, vol 32, no 2. Saunders, Philadelphia, pp. 425–427.

Drotar, T.K., 2009. Methamphetamine. In: Osweiler, G.D., Hovda, L.R., Brutlag, A.G., et al. (Eds.), Blackwell's Five-Minute Veterinary Consult Clinical

Companion Small Animal Toxicology. Wiley-Blackwell, Ames, pp. 230–236.

Volmer, P.A., 2006. Amphetamines. In: Peterson, M.E., Talcott, P.A. (Eds.), Small Animal Toxicology, second ed. Saunders Elsevier, St Louis, pp. 276–280.

Wismer, T., 2009. Amphetamines. In: Osweiler, G.D., Hovda, L.R., Brutlag, A.G., et al. (Eds.), Blackwell's Five-Minute Veterinary Consult Clinical Companion Small Animal Toxicology. Wiley-Blackwell, Ames, pp. 125–130.

ANTICOAGULANT RODENTICIDES

Brown, A.J., Waddell, L.S., 2009. Rodenticides. In: Silverstein, D.C., Hopper, K. (Eds.), Small Animal Critical Care Medicine. Elsevier, St Louis, pp. 346–350.

Hansen, N., Beck, C., 2003. Bilateral hydronephrosis secondary to anticoagulant rodenticide intoxication in a dog. Journal of Veterinary Emergency and Critical Care 13 (2), 103–107.

Luiz, J.A., Heseltine, J., 2008. Five common toxins ingested by dogs and cats. Compendium for the Continuing Education of the Practicing Veterinarian 30 (11), 578–588.

Meadows, I., Gwaltney-Brant, S., 2006. The 10 most common toxicoses in dogs. Veterinary Medicine March, 142–148.

Means, C., 2004. Anticoagulant rodenticides. In: Plumlee, K.H. (Ed.), Clinical Veterinary Toxicology. Mosby, St Louis, pp. 444–446.

Munday, J.S., Thompson, L.J., 2003. Brodifacoum toxicosis in two neonatal puppies. Veterinary Pathology 40, 216–219.

Murphy, M., 2009. Anticoagulants. In: Osweiler, G.D., Hovda, L.R., Brutlag, A.G., et al. (Eds.), Blackwell's Five-Minute Veterinary Consult Clinical Companion Small Animal Toxicology. Wiley-Blackwell, Ames, pp. 759–768.

Murphy, M.J., 2002. Rodenticides. In: Toxicology, Veterinary Clinics of North America, Small Animal Practice, vol 32, no 2. Saunders, Philadelphia, pp. 469–475.

Murphy, M.J., Talcott, P.A., 2006. Anticoagulant rodenticides. In: Peterson, M.E., Talcott, P.A. (Eds.), Small Animal Toxicology, second ed. Saunders Elsevier, St Louis, pp. 563–577.

Pachtinger, G.E., Otto, C.M., Syring, R.S., 2008. Incidence of prolonged prothrombin time in dogs following gastrointestinal decontamination for acute anticoagulant rodenticide ingestion. Journal of Veterinary Emergency and Critical Care 18 (3), 285–291.

ANTIHISTAMINES AND DECONGESTANTS

Albretsen, J.C., 2002. Oral medications. In: Poppenga, R.H., Volmer, P.A. (Eds.), Toxicology, Veterinary Clinics of North America, Small Animal Practice, vol 32, no 2. Saunders, Philadelphia, pp. 433–434.

Campbell, A., 2000. Terfenadine. In: Campbell, A., Chapman, M. (Eds.), Handbook of Poisoning in Dogs and Cats. Blackwell Science, Malden, pp. 247–249.

Fitzgerald, K.T., Bronstein, A.C., Flood, A.A., 2006. 'Over-the-counter' drug toxicities in companion animals. Clinical Techniques in Small Animal Practice 21, 215–226.

Gruber, N.M., 2009. Imidazoline decongestants. In: Osweiler, G.D., Hovda, L.R., Brutlag, A.G., et al. (Eds.), Blackwell's Five-Minute Veterinary Consult Clinical Companion Small Animal Toxicology. Wiley-Blackwell, Ames, pp. 300–305.

Gwaltney-Brant, S., 2004. Antihistamines. In: Plumlee, K.H. (Ed.), Clinical Veterinary Toxicology. Mosby, St Louis, pp. 291–293.

Meadows, I., Gwaltney-Brant, S., 2006. The 10 most common toxicoses in dogs. Veterinary Medicine March, 142–148.

Mean, C., 2004. Decongestants. In: Plumlee, K.H. (Ed.), Clinical Veterinary Toxicology. Mosby, St Louis, pp. 309–310.

Murphy, L., 2001. Antihistamine toxicosis. Veterinary Medicine Oct, 752–765.

Sioris, K.M., 2009. Decongestants. In: Osweiler, G.D., Hovda, L.R., Brutlag, A.G., et al. (Eds.), Blackwell's Five-Minute Veterinary Consult Clinical Companion Small Animal Toxicology. Wiley-Blackwell, Ames, pp. 285–291.

ARSENIC

Ensley, S., 2004. Arsenic. In: Plumlee, K.H. (Ed.), Clinical Veterinary Toxicology. Mosby, St Louis, pp. 193–195.

Gfeller, R.W., Messonnier, S.P., 1998. Handbook of Small Animal Toxicology and Poisonings. Mosby, Philadelphia, pp. 85–89.

Kirk, R.W. (Ed.), 1989. Current Veterinary Therapy X. WB Saunders, Philadelphia, pp. 159–161.

Murtaugh, R.J., Kaplan, P.M., 1992. Veterinary Emergency and Critical Care Medicine. Mosby, St Louis, pp. 441–442.

Osweiler, G.D., 1996. Toxicology. Williams & Wilkins, Philadelphia, pp. 181–185.

Osweiler, G.D., Carson, T.L., Buck, W.B., et al., 1985. Clinical and Diagnostic Veterinary Toxicology, third ed. Kendall/Hunt Publishing, Dubuque, pp. 72–86.

Pigott, D.C., Liebelt, E.L., 2007. Arsenic and arsine. In: Shannon, M.W., Borron, S.W., Burns, M.J. (Eds.), Haddad and Winchester's Clinical Management of Poisoning and Drug Overdose, fourth ed. Saunders Elsevier, Philadelphia, pp. 1147–1156.

ASPIRIN

Alwood, A.J., 2009. Salicylates. In: Silverstein, D.C., Hopper, K. (Eds.), Small Animal Critical Care Medicine. Elsevier, St Louis, pp. 338–341.

Fitzgerald, K.T., Bronstein, A.C., Flood, A.A., 2006. 'Over-the-counter' drug toxicities in companion animals. Clinical Techniques in Small Animal Practice 21, 215–226.

Kaplan, M.I., Smarick, S., 2009. Aspirin. In: Osweiler, G.D., Hovda, L.R., Brutlag, A.G., et al. (Eds.), Blackwell's Five-Minute Veterinary Consult Clinical Companion Small Animal Toxicology. Wiley-Blackwell, Ames, pp. 277–284.

Talcott, P.A., 2006. Nonsteroidal antiinflammatories. In: Peterson, M.E., Talcott, P.A. (Eds.), Small Animal Toxicology, second ed. Saunders Elsevier, St Louis, pp. 902–933.

BACLOFEN

Albretsen, J.C., 2002. Oral medications. In: Poppenga, R.H., Volmer, P.A. (Eds.), Toxicology, Veterinary Clinics of North America, Small Animal Practice, vol 32, no 2. Saunders, Philadelphia, pp. 436–439.

Campbell, A., 2000. Baclofen. In: Campbell, A., Chapman, M. (Eds.), Handbook of Poisoning in Dogs and Cats. Blackwell Science, Malden, pp. 74–76.

Gwaltney-Brant, S., 2004. Muscle relaxants. In: Plumlee, K.H. (Ed.), Clinical Veterinary Toxicology. Mosby, St Louis, pp. 326–330.

Malouin, A., Boller, M., 2009. Sedatives, muscle relaxants, and opioids toxicity. In: Silverstein, D.C., Hopper, K. (Eds.), Small Animal Critical Care Medicine. Elsevier, St Louis, pp. 350–356.

Quandt, J., 2009. Baclofen. In: Osweiler, G.D., Hovda, L.R., Brutlag, A.G., et al. (Eds.), Blackwell's Five-Minute Veterinary Consult Clinical Companion Small Animal Toxicology. Wiley-Blackwell, Ames, pp. 142–147.

Scott, N.E., Francey, T., Jandrey, K., 2007. Baclofen intoxication in a dog successfully treated with hemodialysis and hemoperfusion coupled with intensive supportive care. Journal of Veterinary Emergency and Critical Care 17 (2), 191–196.

Torre, D.M., Labato, M.A., Rossi, T., et al., 2008. Treatment of a dog with severe baclofen intoxication using hemodialysis and mechanical ventilation. Journal of Veterinary Emergency and Critical Care 18 (3), 312–318.

BATTERIES

Angle, C., 2009. Batteries. In: Osweiler, G.D., Hovda, L.R., Brutlag, A.G., et al. (Eds.), Blackwell's Five-Minute Veterinary Consult Clinical Companion Small Animal Toxicology. Wiley-Blackwell, Ames, pp. 560–567.

Campbell, A., 2000. Batteries. In: Campbell, A., Chapman, M. (Eds.), Handbook of Poisoning in Dogs and Cats. Blackwell Science, Malden, pp. 77–79.

Gwaltney-Brant, S., 2004. Batteries. In: Plumlee, K.H. (Ed.), Clinical Veterinary Toxicology. Mosby, St Louis, pp. 140–142.

Oehme, F.W., Kore, A.M., 2006. Miscellaneous indoor toxicants. In: Peterson, M.E., Talcott, P.A. (Eds.), Small Animal Toxicology, second ed. Saunders Elsevier, St Louis, pp. 223–243.

BETA BLOCKERS

Engebretsen, K.M., Syring, R.S., 2009. Beta-blockers. In: Osweiler, G.D., Hovda, L.R., Brutlag, A.G., et al. (Eds.), Blackwell's Five-Minute Veterinary Consult Clinical Companion Small Animal Toxicology. Wiley-Blackwell, Ames, pp. 155–163.

Malouin, A., King, L.G., 2009. Calcium channel and beta-blocker drug overdose. In: Silverstein, D.C., Hopper, K. (Eds.), Small Animal Critical Care Medicine. Elsevier, St Louis, pp. 357–362.

BLUE-GREEN ALGAE

Campbell, A., 2000. Blue-green algae / cyanobacteria. In: Campbell, A., Chapman, M. (Eds.), Handbook of Poisoning in Dogs and Cats. Blackwell Science, Malden, pp. 80–85.

Hooser, S.B., Talcott, P.A., 2006. Cyanobacteria. In: Peterson, M.E., Talcott, P.A. (Eds.), Small Animal Toxicology, second ed. Saunders Elsevier, St Louis, pp. 685–689.

Puschner, B., Hoff, B., Tor, E.R., 2008. Diagnosis of anatoxin-a poisoning in dogs from North America. Journal of Veterinary Diagnostic Investigation 20, 89–92.

Roder, J.D., 2004. Blue-green algae. In: Plumlee, K.H. (Ed.), Clinical Veterinary Toxicology. Mosby, St Louis, pp. 100–101.

Roegner, A., Puschner, B., 2009. Blue-green algae. In: Osweiler, G.D., Hovda, L.R., Brutlag, A.G., et al. (Eds.), Blackwell's Five-Minute Veterinary Consult Clinical Companion Small Animal Toxicology. Wiley-Blackwell, Ames, pp. 687–695.

BORIC ACID/BORATES

Campbell, A., 2000. Borax. In: Campbell, A., Chapman, M. (Eds.), Handbook of Poisoning in Dogs and Cats. Blackwell Science, Malden, pp. 86–88.

Gfeller, R.W., Messonnier, S.P., 1998. Handbook of Small Animal Toxicology and Poisonings. Mosby, Philadelphia, pp. 99–101.

Osweiler, G.D., 1996. Toxicology. Williams & Wilkins, Philadelphia, pp. 248–249.

Welch, S., 2004. Boric acid. In: Plumlee, K.H. (Ed.), Clinical Veterinary Toxicology. Mosby, St Louis, pp. 143–145.

Young-Jin, S., Pinkert, H., 2007. Baby powder, borates, and camphor. In: Shannon, M.W., Borron, S.W., Burns, M.J. (Eds.), Haddad and Winchester's Clinical Management of Poisoning and Drug Overdose, fourth ed. Saunders Elsevier, Philadelphia, pp. 1417–1419.

BREAD DOUGH

Means, C., 2003. Bread dough toxicosis. Journal of Veterinary Emergency and Critical Care 13 (1), 39–41.

Powell, L.L., 2009. Bread dough. In: Osweiler, G.D., Hovda, L.R., Brutlag, A.G., et al. (Eds.), Blackwell's Five-Minute Veterinary Consult Clinical Companion Small Animal Toxicology. Wiley-Blackwell, Ames, pp. 411–415.

BROMETHALIN

Adams, C.M., Hovda, L.R., 2009. Bromethalin. In: Osweiler, G.D., Hovda, L.R., Brutlag, A.G., et al. (Eds.), Blackwell's Five-Minute Veterinary Consult Clinical Companion Small Animal Toxicology. Wiley-Blackwell, Ames, pp. 769–774.

Brown, A.J., Waddell, L.S., 2009. Rodenticides. In: Silverstein, D.C., Hopper, K. (Eds.), Small Animal Critical Care Medicine. Elsevier, St Louis, pp. 346–350.

Dorman, D., 2004. Bromethalin. In: Plumlee, K.H. (Ed.), Clinical Veterinary Toxicology. Mosby, St Louis, pp. 446–448.

Dorman, D.C., 2006. Bromethalin. In: Peterson, M.E., Talcott, P.A. (Eds.), Small Animal Toxicology, second ed. Saunders Elsevier, St Louis, pp. 609–618.

Dorman, D.C., Simon, J., Harlin, K.A., et al., 1990. Diagnosis of bromethalin toxicosis in the dog. Journal of Veterinary Diagnostic Investigation 2, 123–128.

Dunayer, E., 2003. Bromethalin: the other rodenticide. Veterinary Medicine Sept, 732–736.

Meadows, I., Gwaltney-Brant, S., 2006. The 10 most common toxicoses in dogs. Veterinary Medicine March, 142–148.

Murphy, M.J., 2002. Rodenticides. In: Toxicology, Veterinary Clinics of North America, Small Animal Practice, vol 32, no 2. Saunders, Philadelphia, pp. 475–476.

CALCIUM CHANNEL BLOCKERS

Albretsen, J.C., 2002. Oral medications. In: Poppenga, R.H., Volmer, P.A. (Eds.), Toxicology, Veterinary Clinics of North America, Small Animal Practice, vol 32, no 2. Saunders, Philadelphia, pp. 434–436.

Costello, M., Syring, R.S., 2008. Calcium channel blocker toxicity. Journal of Veterinary Emergency and Critical Care 18 (1), 54–60.

Malouin, A., King, L.G., 2009. Calcium channel and beta-blocker drug overdose. In: Silverstein, D.C., Hopper, K. (Eds.), Small Animal Critical Care Medicine. Elsevier, St Louis, pp. 357–362.

Roder, J.D., 2004. Calcium channel blocking agents. In: Plumlee, K.H. (Ed.), Clinical

Veterinary Toxicology. Mosby, St Louis, pp. 308–309.

Syring, R.S., Engebretsen, K.M., 2009. Calcium channel blockers. In: Osweiler, G.D., Hovda, L.R., Brutlag, A.G., et al. (Eds.), Blackwell's Five-Minute Veterinary Consult Clinical Companion Small Animal Toxicology. Wiley-Blackwell, Ames, pp. 170–178.

CARBON MONOXIDE

Berent, A.C., Todd, J., Sergeeff, J., et al., 2005. Carbon monoxide toxicity: a case series. Journal of Veterinary Emergency and Critical Care 15 (2), 128–135.

Carson, T.L., 2004. Carbon monoxide. In: Plumlee, K.H. (Ed.), Clinical Veterinary Toxicology. Mosby, St Louis, pp. 159–161.

Fitzgerald, K.T., 2006. Carbon monoxide. In: Peterson, M.E., Talcott, P.A. (Eds.), Small Animal Toxicology, second ed. Saunders Elsevier, St Louis, pp. 619–628.

Kent, M., Creevy, K.E., deLahunta, A., 2010. Clinical and neuropathological findings of acute carbon monoxide toxicity in Chihuahuas following smoke inhalation. Journal of the American Animal Hospital Association 46, 259–264.

Powell, L.L., 2009. Carbon monoxide. In: Osweiler, G.D., Hovda, L.R., Brutlag, A.G., et al. (Eds.), Blackwell's Five-Minute Veterinary Consult Clinical Companion Small Animal Toxicology. Wiley-Blackwell, Ames, pp. 801–804.

Rahilly, L., Mandell, D.C., 2009. Carbon monoxide. In: Silverstein, D.C., Hopper, K. (Eds.), Small Animal Critical Care Medicine. Elsevier, St Louis, pp. 369–373.

Weaver, L.K., 2009. Carbon monoxide poisoning. New England Journal of Medicine 360, 1217–1225.

CHOCOLATE AND CAFFEINE

Albretsen, J.C., 2004. Methylxanthines. In: Plumlee, K.H. (Ed.), Clinical Veterinary Toxicology. Mosby, St Louis, pp. 322–326.

Campbell, A., 2000. Chocolate / theobromine. In: Campbell, A., Chapman, M. (Eds.), Handbook of Poisoning in Dogs and Cats. Blackwell Science, Malden, pp. 106–110.

Carson, T.L., 2006. Methylxanthines. In: Peterson, M.E., Talcott, P.A. (Eds.), Small Animal Toxicology, second ed. Saunders Elsevier, St Louis, pp. 845–852.

Craft, E.K., Powell, L.L., 2009. Chocolate and caffeine. In: Osweiler, G.D., Hovda, L.R., Brutlag, A.G., et al. (Eds.), Blackwell's Five-Minute Veterinary Consult Clinical Companion Small Animal Toxicology. Wiley-Blackwell, Ames, pp. 421–428.

Luiz, J.A., Heseltine, J., 2008. Five common toxins ingested by dogs and cats. Compendium for the Continuing Education of the Practicing Veterinarian 30 (11), 578–588.

Meadows, I., Gwaltney-Brant, S., 2006. The 10 most common toxicoses in dogs. Veterinary Medicine March, 142–148.

CHOLECALCIFEROL

Adams, C.M., 2009. Cholecalciferol. In: Osweiler, G.D., Hovda, L.R., Brutlag, A.G., et al. (Eds.), Blackwell's Five-Minute Veterinary Consult Clinical Companion Small Animal Toxicology. Wiley-Blackwell, Ames, pp. 775–780.

Brown, A.J., Waddell, L.S., 2009. Rodenticides. In: Silverstein, D.C., Hopper, K. (Eds.), Small Animal Critical Care Medicine. Elsevier, St Louis, pp. 346–350.

Campbell, A., 2000. Calciferol / vitamin D_3 and cholecalciferol / vitamin D_3. In: Campbell, A., Chapman, M. (Eds.), Handbook of Poisoning in Dogs and Cats. Blackwell Science, Malden, pp. 89–96.

Meadows, I., Gwaltney-Brant, S., 2006. The 10 most common toxicoses in dogs. Veterinary Medicine March, 142–148.

Morrow, C.K., Volmer, P.A., 2004. Cholecalciferol. In: Plumlee, K.H. (Ed.), Clinical Veterinary Toxicology. Mosby, St Louis, pp. 448–451.

Murphy, M.J., 2002. Rodenticides. In: Toxicology, Veterinary Clinics of North America, Small Animal Practice, vol 32, no 2. Saunders, Philadelphia, pp. 476–478.

Rumbeiha, W.K., 2006. Cholecalciferol. In: Peterson, M.E., Talcott, P.A. (Eds.), Small Animal Toxicology, second ed. Saunders Elsevier, St Louis, pp. 629–642.

Rumbeiha, W.K., Braselton, W.E., Nachreiner, R.F., et al., 2000. The postmortem diagnosis of cholecalciferol toxicosis: a novel approach and differentiation from ethylene glycol toxicosis. Journal of Veterinary Diagnostic Investigation 12, 426–432.

CITRUS OIL

Gfeller, R.W., Messonnier, S.P., 1998. Handbook of Small Animal Toxicology and Poisonings. Mosby, Philadelphia, pp. 172–173.

Murtaugh, R.J., Kaplan, P.M., 1992. Veterinary Emergency and Critical Care Medicine. Mosby, St Louis, p. 437.

Osweiler, G.D., 1996. Toxicology. Williams & Wilkins, Philadelphia, pp. 246–247.

Plumlee, K.H., 2006. Citrus oils. In: Peterson, M.E., Talcott, P.A. (Eds.), Small Animal Toxicology, second ed. Saunders Elsevier, St Louis, pp. 664–667.

COCAINE

Albertson, T.E., Chan, A., Tharratt, R.S., 2007. Cocaine. In: Shannon, M.W., Borron, S.W., Burns, M.J. (Eds.), Haddad and Winchester's Clinical Management of Poisoning and Drug Overdose, fourth ed. Saunders Elsevier, Philadelphia, pp. 755–772.

Bischoff, K., Kang, H.G., 2009. Cocaine. In: Osweiler, G.D., Hovda, L.R., Brutlag, A.G., et al. (Eds.), Blackwell's Five-Minute Veterinary Consult Clinical Companion Small Animal Toxicology. Wiley-Blackwell, Ames, pp. 212–217.

Brown, A.J., Mandell, D.C., 2009. Illicit drugs. In: Silverstein, D.C., Hopper, K. (Eds.), Small Animal Critical Care Medicine. Elsevier, St Louis, pp. 342–345.

Volmer, P.A., 2006. Cocaine. In: Peterson, M.E., Talcott, P.A. (Eds.), Small Animal Toxicology, second ed. Saunders Elsevier, St Louis, pp. 287–290.

N,N-DIETHYLTOLUAMIDE (DEET)

Borron, S.W., 2007. DEET. In: Shannon, M.W., Borron, S.W., Burns, M.J. (Eds.), Haddad and Winchester's Clinical Management of Poisoning and Drug Overdose, fourth ed. Saunders Elsevier, Philadelphia, pp. 1191–1192.

Dorman, D., 2004. Diethyltoluamide. In: Plumlee, K.H. (Ed.), Clinical Veterinary Toxicology. Mosby, St Louis, pp. 180–182.

Gfeller, R.W., Messonnier, S.P., 1998. Handbook of Small Animal Toxicology and Poisonings. Mosby, Philadelphia, pp. 124–125.

Murphy, M.J., 1994. Toxin exposures in dogs and cats: pesticides and biotoxins. Journal of the American Veterinary Medical Association 205 (3), 414–421.

Murtaugh, R.J., Kaplan, P.M., 1992. Veterinary Emergency and Critical Care Medicine. Mosby, St Louis, p. 437.

Osweiler, G.D., 1996. Toxicology. Williams & Wilkins, Philadelphia, pp. 248–249.

Plumlee, K.H., 2006. DEET. In: Peterson, M.E., Talcott, P.A. (Eds.), Small Animal Toxicology, second ed. Saunders Elsevier, St Louis, pp. 690–692.

ETHYLENE GLYCOL

Adams, C.M., Thrall, M.A., 2009. Ethylene glycol. In: Osweiler, G.D., Hovda, L.R., Brutlag, A.G., et al. (Eds.), Blackwell's Five-Minute Veterinary Consult Clinical Companion Small Animal Toxicology. Wiley-Blackwell, Ames, pp. 68–77.

Bates, N., Campbell, A., 2000. Ethylene glycol. In: Campbell, A., Chapman, M. (Eds.), Handbook of Poisoning in Dogs and Cats. Blackwell Science, Malden, pp. 22–26.

Brent, J., 2009. Fomepizole for ethylene glycol and methanol poisoning. New England Journal of Medicine 360, 2216–2223.

Campbell, A., 2000. Ethylene glycol. In: Campbell, A., Chapman, M. (Eds.), Handbook of Poisoning in Dogs and Cats. Blackwell Science, Malden, pp. 127–132.

Connally, H.E., Thrall, M.A., Hamar, D.W., 2010. Safety and efficacy of high-dose fomepizole compared with ethanol as therapy for ethylene glycol intoxication in cats. Journal of Veterinary Emergency and Critical Care 20 (2), 191–206.

Dalefield, R., 2004. Ethylene glycol. In: Plumlee, K.H. (Ed.), Clinical Veterinary Toxicology. Mosby, St Louis, pp. 150–154.

Doty, R.L., Dziewit, J.A., Marshall, D.A., 2006. Antifreeze ingestion by dogs and rats: influence of stimulus concentration. Canadian Veterinary Journal 47, 363–365.

Jacobsen, D., McMartin, K.E., 1997. Antidotes for methanol and ethylene glycol poisoning. Clinical Toxicology 35 (2), 127–143.

Krenzelok, E.P., 2002. New developments in the therapy of intoxications. Toxicology Letters 127, 299–305.

Luiz, J.A., Heseltine, J., 2008. Five common toxins ingested by dogs and cats. Compendium for the Continuing Education of the Practicing Veterinarian 30 (11), 578–588.

Rollings, C., 2009. Ethylene glycol. In: Silverstein, D.C., Hopper, K. (Eds.),

Small Animal Critical Care Medicine. Elsevier, St Louis, pp. 330–334.

Tart, K.M., Powell, L.L., 2011. 4-Methylpyrazole as a treatment in naturally occurring ethylene glycol intoxication in cats. Journal of Veterinary Emergency and Critical Care 21 (3), 268–272.

Thrall, M.A., Connally, H.E., Grauer, G.F., et al., 2006. Ethylene glycol. In: Peterson, M.E., Talcott, P.A. (Eds.), Small Animal Toxicology, second ed. Saunders Elsevier, St Louis, pp. 702–726.

GARBAGE INTOXICATION (ENTEROTOXEMIA)

Adams, C.M., Bischoff, K., 2009. Mycotoxins—aflatoxin. In: Osweiler, G.D., Hovda, L.R., Brutlag, A.G., et al. (Eds.), Blackwell's Five-Minute Veterinary Consult Clinical Companion Small Animal Toxicology. Wiley-Blackwell, Ames, pp. 445–450.

Dereszynski, D.M., Center, S.A., Randolph, J.F., 2008. Clinical and clinicopathologic features of dogs that consumed foodborne hepatotoxic aflatoxins: 72 cases (2005–2006). Journal of the American Veterinary Medical Association 232, 1329–1337.

Klatt, C.A., Hooser, S.B., 2009. Mycotoxins—tremorgenic. In: Osweiler, G.D., Hovda, L.R., Brutlag, A.G., et al. (Eds.), Blackwell's Five-Minute Veterinary Consult Clinical Companion Small Animal Toxicology. Wiley-Blackwell, Ames, pp. 451–456.

Meerdink, G.L., 2004. Aflatoxins. In: Plumlee, K.H. (Ed.), Clinical Veterinary Toxicology. Mosby, St Louis, pp. 231–235.

Newman, S.J., Smith, J.R., Stenske, K.A., 2007. Aflatoxicosis in nine dogs after exposure to contaminated commercial dog food. Journal of Veterinary Diagnostic Investigation 19, 168–175.

Pfohl-Leszkowicz, A., Manderville, R.A., Ochratoxin, A., 2007. an overview on toxicity and carcinogenicity in animals and humans. Molecular Nutrition and Food Research 51, 61–99.

Puschner, B., March 2002. Mycotoxins. In: Toxicology, Veterinary Clinics of North America, Small Animal Practice, vol 32, no 2. Saunders, Philadelphia, pp. 409–419.

Puschner, B., Penitrem, A., 2004. Roquefortine. In: Plumlee, K.H. (Ed.),

Clinical Veterinary Toxicology. Mosby, St Louis, pp. 258–259.

GLOW JEWELRY

Hovda, T.K., Lee, J.A., 2009. Glow jewelry. In: Osweiler, G.D., Hovda, L.R., Brutlag, A.G., et al. (Eds.), Blackwell's Five-Minute Veterinary Consult Clinical Companion Small Animal Toxicology. Wiley-Blackwell, Ames, pp. 673–678.

Oehme, F.W., Kore, A.M., 2006. Miscellaneous indoor toxicants. In: Peterson, M.E., Talcott, P.A. (Eds.), Small Animal Toxicology, second ed. Saunders Elsevier, St Louis, pp. 223–243.

GRAPES AND RAISINS

Craft, E.M., Lee, J.A., 2009. Grapes and raisins. In: Osweiler, G.D., Hovda, L.R., Brutlag, A.G., et al. (Eds.), Blackwell's Five-Minute Veterinary Consult Clinical Companion Small Animal Toxicology. Wiley-Blackwell, Ames, pp. 429–435.

Eubig, P.A., Brady, M.A., Gwaltney-Brant, S.M., et al., 2005. Acute renal failure in dogs after the ingestion of grapes or raisins: a retrospective evaluation of 43 dogs (1992–2002). Journal of Veterinary Internal Medicine 19, 663–674.

Knight, A.P., 2006. Vitis. In: Knight, A.P. (Ed.), A Guide to Poisonous House and Garden Plants. Teton NewMedia, Jackson, pp. 280–281.

Mazzaferro, E.M., Eubig, P.A., Hackett, T.B., et al., 2004. Acute renal failure associated with raisin or grape ingestion in 4 dogs. Journal of Veterinary Emergency and Critical Care 14 (3), 203–212.

Morrow, C.M.K., Valli, V.E., Volmer, P.A., 2005. Canine renal pathology associated with grape or raisin ingestion: 10 cases. Journal of Veterinary Diagnostic Investigation 17, 223–231.

Mostrom, M.S., 2006. Grapes and raisins. In: Peterson, M.E., Talcott, P.A. (Eds.), Small Animal Toxicology, second ed. Saunders Elsevier, St Louis, pp. 727–731.

HERB, VITAMIN AND NATURAL SUPPLEMENTS

Bischoff, K., Guale, F., 1998. Australian tea tree (Melaleuca alternifolia) oil poisoning in three purebred cats. Journal of Veterinary Diagnostic Investigations 10, 208–210.

Cohen, S.L., Brutlag, A.G., 2009. Tree oil / melaleuca oil. In: Osweiler, G.D., Hovda, L.R., Brutlag, A.G., et al. (Eds.),

Blackwell's Five-Minute Veterinary Consult Clinical Companion Small Animal Toxicology. Wiley-Blackwell, Ames, pp. 534–540.

Fitzgerald, K.T., Bronstein, A.C., Flood, A.A., 2006. 'Over-the-counter' drug toxicities in companion animals. Clinical Techniques in Small Animal Practice 21, 215–226.

Gfeller, R.W., Messonnier, S.P., 1998. Handbook of Small Animal Toxicology and Poisonings. Mosby, Philadelphia, pp. 241–244.

Kirk, R.W. (Ed.), 1986. Current Veterinary Therapy IX. WB Saunders, Philadelphia, pp. 212–215.

Means, C., 2002. Selected herbal hazards. In: Toxicology, Veterinary Clinics of North America, Small Animal Practice, vol 32, no 2. Saunders, Philadelphia, pp. 367–382.

Means, C., 2009. Ephedra / Ma Huang. In: Osweiler, G.D., Hovda, L.R., Brutlag, A.G., et al. (Eds.), Blackwell's Five-Minute Veterinary Consult Clinical Companion Small Animal Toxicology. Wiley-Blackwell, Ames, pp. 521–526.

Poppenga, R.H., 2006. Hazards associated with the use of herbal and other natural products. In: Peterson, M.E., Talcott, P.A. (Eds.), Small Animal Toxicology, second ed. Saunders Elsevier, St Louis, pp. 312–344.

Poppenga, R.H., 2009. Essential oils / potpourri. In: Osweiler, G.D., Hovda, L.R., Brutlag, A.G., et al. (Eds.), Blackwell's Five-Minute Veterinary Consult Clinical Companion Small Animal Toxicology. Wiley-Blackwell, Ames, pp. 527–533.

HOUSEHOLD PRODUCTS

Beasley, V.R. (guest ed), 1990. The Veterinary Clinics of North America, Small Animal Practice: Toxicology of Selected Pesticides, Drugs and Chemicals 20 (2), 525–536.

Coppock, R.W., Mostrom, M.S., Lillie, L.E., 1989. Toxicology of detergents, bleaches, antiseptics, and disinfectants. In: Kirk, R.W. (Ed.), Current Veterinary Therapy X. WB Saunders, Philadelphia, pp. 162–171.

Osweiler, G.D., Carson, T.L., Buck, W.B., et al., 1985. Clinical and Diagnostic Veterinary Toxicology, third ed. Kendall / Hunt Publishing, Dubuque, pp. 381–393.

BLEACH

Meadows, I., Gwaltney-Brant, S., 2006. The 10 most common toxicoses in dogs. Veterinary Medicine March, 142–148.

Oehme, F.W., Kore, A.M., 2006. Miscellaneous indoor toxicants. In: Peterson, M.E., Talcott, P.A. (Eds.), Small Animal Toxicology, second ed. Saunders Elsevier, St Louis, pp. 223–243.

Richardson, J., 2004. Bleaches. In: Plumlee, K.H. (Ed.), Clinical Veterinary Toxicology. Mosby, St Louis, pp. 142–143.

CORROSIVES

Brutlag, A.G., 2009. Acids. In: Osweiler, G.D., Hovda, L.R., Brutlag, A.G., et al. (Eds.), Blackwell's Five-Minute Veterinary Consult Clinical Companion Small Animal Toxicology. Wiley-Blackwell, Ames, pp. 543–550.

Brutlag, A.G., 2009. Alkalis. In: Osweiler, G.D., Hovda, L.R., Brutlag, A.G., et al. (Eds.), Blackwell's Five-Minute Veterinary Consult Clinical Companion Small Animal Toxicology. Wiley-Blackwell, Ames, pp. 551–559.

Oehme, F.W., Kore, A.M., 2006. Miscellaneous indoor toxicants. In: Peterson, M.E., Talcott, P.A. (Eds.), Small Animal Toxicology, second ed. Saunders Elsevier, St Louis, pp. 223–243.

Richardson, J., 2004. Acids and alkali. In: Plumlee, K.H. (Ed.), Clinical Veterinary Toxicology. Mosby, St Louis, pp. 139–140.

DISINFECTANTS

Phenols

Angle, A., Brutlag, A.G., 2009. Phenols / pine oils. In: Osweiler, G.D., Hovda, L.R., Brutlag, A.G., et al. (Eds.), Blackwell's Five-Minute Veterinary Consult Clinical Companion Small Animal Toxicology. Wiley-Blackwell, Ames, pp. 591–600.

Oehme, F.W., Kore, A.M., 2006. Miscellaneous Indoor Toxicants. In: Peterson, M.E., Talcott, P.A. (Eds.), Small Animal Toxicology, second ed. Saunders Elsevier, St Louis, pp. 223–243.

Wismer, T., 2004. Phenols. In: Plumlee, K.H. (Ed.), Clinical Veterinary Toxicology. Mosby, St Louis, pp. 164–167.

Pine oil disinfectants

Angle, A., Brutlag, A.G., 2009. Phenols / pine oils. In: Osweiler, G.D., Hovda, L.R., Brutlag, A.G., et al. (Eds.),

Blackwell's Five-Minute Veterinary Consult Clinical Companion Small Animal Toxicology. Wiley-Blackwell, Ames, pp. 591–600.

Wismer, T., 2004. Pine oils. In: Plumlee, K.H. (Ed.), Clinical Veterinary Toxicology. Mosby, St Louis, pp. 167–168.

ISOPROPANOL

Sivilotti, M.L., 2007. Isopropanol. In: Shannon, M.W., Borron, S.W., Burns, M.J. (Eds.), Haddad and Winchester's Clinical Management of Poisoning and Drug Overdose, fourth ed. Saunders Elsevier, Philadelphia, pp. 623–624.

NAPHTHALENE

Bischoff, K., 2004. Naphthalene. In: Plumlee, K.H. (Ed.), Clinical Veterinary Toxicology. Mosby, St Louis, pp. 163–164.

Cohen, S.L., Brutlag, A.G., 2009. Mothballs. In: Osweiler, G.D., Hovda, L.R., Brutlag, A.G., et al. (Eds.), Blackwell's Five-Minute Veterinary Consult Clinical Companion Small Animal Toxicology. Wiley-Blackwell, Ames, pp. 574–580.

Oehme, F.W., Kore, A.M., 2006. Miscellaneous indoor toxicants. In: Peterson, M.E., Talcott, P.A. (Eds.), Small Animal Toxicology, second ed. Saunders Elsevier, St Louis, pp. 223–243.

PARADICHLOROBENZENE

Cohen, S.L., Brutlag, A.G., 2009. Mothballs. In: Osweiler, G.D., Hovda, L.R., Brutlag, A.G., et al. (Eds.), Blackwell's Five-Minute Veterinary Consult Clinical Companion Small Animal Toxicology. Wiley-Blackwell, Ames, pp. 574–580.

SOAPS AND DETERGENTS

Oehme, F.W., Kore, A.M., 2006. Miscellaneous indoor toxicants. In: Peterson, M.E., Talcott, P.A. (Eds.), Small Animal Toxicology, second ed. Saunders Elsevier, St Louis, pp. 223–243.

Richardson, J., 2004. Detergents. In: Plumlee, K.H. (Ed.), Clinical Veterinary Toxicology. Mosby, St Louis, pp. 145–146.

Sioris, L.J., Haak, L.E., 2009. Soaps, detergents, fabric softeners, enzymatic cleaners, and deodorizers. In: Osweiler, G.D., Hovda, L.R., Brutlag, A.G., et al. (Eds.), Blackwell's Five-Minute Veterinary Consult Clinical Companion

Small Animal Toxicology. Wiley-Blackwell, Ames, pp. 601–609.

HYDRAMETHYLNON

Wismer, T., 2004. Hydramethylnon. In: Plumlee, K.H. (Ed.), Clinical Veterinary Toxicology. Mosby, St Louis, pp. 185–186.

HYDROCARBONS

Campbell, A., 2000. Petroleum distillates / white spirit / kerosene. In: Campbell, A., Chapman, M. (Eds.), Handbook of Poisoning in Dogs and Cats. Blackwell Science, Malden, pp. 52–54.

LeMaster, S.H., 2009. Hydrocarbon. In: Osweiler, G.D., Hovda, L.R., Brutlag, A.G., et al. (Eds.), Blackwell's Five-Minute Veterinary Consult Clinical Companion Small Animal Toxicology. Wiley-Blackwell, Ames, pp. 96–102.

Lewander, W.J., Aleguas, A., 2007. Petroleum distillates and plant hydrocarbons. In: Shannon, M.W., Borron, S.W., Burns, M.J. (Eds.), Haddad and Winchester's Clinical Management of Poisoning and Drug Overdose, fourth ed. Saunders Elsevier, Philadelphia, pp. 1343–1346.

Meadows, I., Gwaltney-Brant, S., 2006. The 10 most common toxicoses in dogs. Veterinary Medicine March, 142–148.

Mirkin, D.B., 2007. Benzene and related aromatic hydrocarbons. In: Shannon, M.W., Borron, S.W., Burns, M.J. (Eds.), Haddad and Winchester's Clinical Management of Poisoning and Drug Overdose, fourth ed. Saunders Elsevier, Philadelphia, pp. 1363–1376.

Palmer, R.B., Phillips, S.D., 2007. Chlorinated hydrocarbons. In: Shannon, M.W., Borron, S.W., Burns, M.J. (Eds.), Haddad and Winchester's Clinical Management of Poisoning and Drug Overdose, fourth ed. Saunders Elsevier, Philadelphia, pp. 1347–1361.

Raisbeck, M.F., Dailey, R.N., 2006. Petroleum hydrocarbons. In: Peterson, M.E., Talcott, P.A. (Eds.), Small Animal Toxicology, second ed. Saunders Elsevier, St Louis, pp. 986–995.

Young, B.C., Strom, A.C., Prittie, J.E., 2007. Toxic pneumonitis caused by inhalation of hydrocarbon waterproofing spray in two dogs. Journal of the American Veterinary Medical Association 231, 74–78.

HYMENOPTERA ENVENOMATION

Adams, C.M., 2009. Wasps, hornets, bees. In: Osweiler, G.D., Hovda, L.R., Brutlag, A.G., et al. (Eds.), Blackwell's Five-Minute Veterinary Consult Clinical Companion Small Animal Toxicology. Wiley-Blackwell, Ames, pp. 404–408.

Campbell, A., 2000. Hymenoptera. In: Campbell, A., Chapman, M. (Eds.), Handbook of Poisoning in Dogs and Cats. Blackwell Science, Malden, pp. 145–147.

Fitzgerald, K.T., Flood, A.A., 2006. Hymenoptera stings. Clinical Techniques in Small Animal Practice 21, 194–204.

Fitzgerald, K.T., Vera, R., 2006. Hymenoptera. In: Peterson, M.E., Talcott, P.A. (Eds.), Small Animal Toxicology, second ed. Saunders Elsevier, St Louis, pp. 744–767.

Oliveira, E.C., Pedroso, P.M., Meirelles, A.E., et al., 2007. Pathological findings in dogs after multiple Africanized bee stings, Toxicon 49, 1214–1218.

Thomas, J.D., Thomas, K.E., Kazzi, Z.N., 2007. Hymenoptera. In: Shannon, M.W., Borron, S.W., Burns, M.J. (Eds.), Haddad and Winchester's Clinical Management of Poisoning and Drug Overdose, fourth ed. Saunders Elsevier, Philadelphia, pp. 447–451.

Waddell, L.S., Drobatz, K.J., 1999. Massive envenomation by Vespula spp. in two dogs. Journal of Veterinary Emergency and Critical Care 9 (2), 67–71.

HYPERTONIC SODIUM PHOSPHATE ENEMA

Gfeller, R.W., Messonnier, S.P., 1998. Handbook of Small Animal Toxicology and Poisonings. Mosby, Philadelphia, pp. 241–244.

Kirk, R.W. (Ed.), 1986. Current Veterinary Therapy IX. WB Saunders, Philadelphia, pp. 212–215.

Roder, J.D., 2004. Hypertonic phosphate enema. In: Plumlee, K.H. (Ed.), Clinical Veterinary Toxicology. Mosby, St Louis, p. 319.

IRON

Albretsen, J.C., 2004. Iron. In: Plumlee, K.H. (Ed.), Clinical Veterinary Toxicology. Mosby, St Louis, pp. 202–204.

Campbell, A., 2000. Iron and iron salts. In: Campbell, A., Chapman, M. (Eds.), Handbook of Poisoning in Dogs and Cats. Blackwell Science, Malden, pp. 163–166.

Hall, J.O., 2006. Iron. In: Peterson, M.E., Talcott, P.A. (Eds.), Small Animal Toxicology, second ed. Saunders Elsevier, St Louis, pp. 777–784.

Hall, J.O., 2009. Iron. In: Osweiler, G.D., Hovda, L.R., Brutlag, A.G., et al. (Eds.), Blackwell's Five-Minute Veterinary Consult Clinical Companion Small Animal Toxicology. Wiley-Blackwell, Ames, pp. 647–656.

Marshall, J.L., Lee, J.A., 2009. Fertilizers. In: Osweiler, G.D., Hovda, L.R., Brutlag, A.G., et al. (Eds.), Blackwell's Five-Minute Veterinary Consult Clinical Companion Small Animal Toxicology. Wiley-Blackwell, Ames, pp. 495–498.

IVERMECTIN AND OTHER MACROLIDE ENDECTOCIDES

Campbell, A., 2000. Ivermectin. In: Campbell, A., Chapman, M. (Eds.), Handbook of Poisoning in Dogs and Cats. Blackwell Science, Malden, pp. 27–30, 167–173.

Clarke, D.L., Lee, J.A., 2009. Ivermectin / milbemycin / moxidectin. In: Osweiler, G.D., Hovda, L.R., Brutlag, A.G., et al. (Eds.), Blackwell's Five-Minute Veterinary Consult Clinical Companion Small Animal Toxicology. Wiley-Blackwell, Ames, pp. 332–342.

Gallagher, A.E., Grant, D.C., Noftsinger, M.N., 2008. Coma and respiratory failure due tomoxidectin intoxication in a dog. Journal of Veterinary Emergency and Critical Care 18 (1), 81–85.

Mealey, K.L., 2006. Ivermectin: macrolide antiparasitic agents. In: Peterson, M.E., Talcott, P.A. (Eds.), Small Animal Toxicology, second ed. Saunders Elsevier, St Louis, pp. 785–794.

Merola, V., Khan, S., Gwaltney-Brant, S., 2009. Ivermectin toxicosis in dogs: a retrospective study. Journal of the American Animal Hospital Association 45, 106–111.

Roder, J.D., 2004. Macrolide endectocides. In: Plumlee, K.H. (Ed.), Clinical Veterinary Toxicology. Mosby, St Louis, pp. 303–304.

Scott, N.E., 2009. Ivermectin toxicity. In: Silverstein, D.C., Hopper, K. (Eds.), Small Animal Critical Care Medicine. Elsevier, St Louis, pp. 392–394.

LEAD

Casteel, S.W., 2006. Lead. In: Peterson, M.E., Talcott, P.A. (Eds.), Small Animal Toxicology, second ed. Saunders Elsevier, St Louis, pp. 795–805.

Gwaltney-Brant, S., 2004. Lead. In: Plumlee, K.H. (Ed.), Clinical Veterinary Toxicology. Mosby, St Louis, pp. 204–210.

Knight, T.E., Kumar, M.S.A., 2003. Lead toxicosis in cats—a review. Journal of Feline Medicine and Surgery 5, 249–255.

Knight, T.E., Kent, M., Junk, J.E., 2001. Succimer for treatment of lead toxicosis in two cats. Journal of the American Veterinary Medical Association 218 (12, June 15), 1946–1948.

Miller, S., Bauk, T.J., 1992. Lead toxicosis in a group of cats. Journal of Veterinary Diagnosis and Investigation 4, 362–363.

Poppenga, R.H., 2009. Lead. In: Osweiler, G.D., Hovda, L.R., Brutlag, A.G., et al. (Eds.), Blackwell's Five-Minute Veterinary Consult Clinical Companion Small Animal Toxicology. Wiley-Blackwell, Ames, pp. 657–663.

MACADAMIA NUTS

Gwaltney-Brant, S.M., 2006. Macadamia nuts. In: Peterson, M.E., Talcott, P.A. (Eds.), Small Animal Toxicology, second ed. Saunders Elsevier, St Louis, pp. 817–821.

Knight, A.P., 2006. Macadamia. In: Knight, A.P. (Ed.), A Guide to Poisonous House and Garden Plants. Teton NewMedia, Jackson, pp. 181–182.

Liu, T.Y.D., Lee, J.A., 2009. Macadamia nuts. In: Osweiler, G.D., Hovda, L.R., Brutlag, A.G., et al. (Eds.), Blackwell's Five-Minute Veterinary Consult Clinical Companion Small Animal Toxicology. Wiley-Blackwell, Ames, pp. 441–444.

Plumlee, K.H., 2002. Plant hazards. In: Toxicology, Veterinary Clinics of North America, Small Animal Practice, vol 32, no 2. Saunders, Philadelphia, pp. 383–384.

Plumlee, K.H., 2004. Macadamia nuts. In: Plumlee, K.H. (Ed.), Clinical Veterinary Toxicology. Mosby, St Louis, pp. 435–436.

MARIJUANA

Brown, A.J., Mandell, D.C., 2009. Illicit drugs. In: Silverstein, D.C., Hopper, K. (Eds.), Small Animal Critical Care Medicine. Elsevier, St Louis, pp. 342–345.

Campbell, A., 2000. Cannabis / marihuana / hashish. In: Campbell, A., Chapman, M. (Eds.), Handbook of Poisoning in Dogs and Cats. Blackwell Science, Malden, pp. 97–100.

Klatt, C.A., 2009. Marijuana. In: Osweiler, G.D., Hovda, L.R., Brutlag, A.G., et al. (Eds.), Blackwell's Five-Minute Veterinary Consult Clinical Companion Small Animal Toxicology. Wiley-Blackwell, Ames, pp. 224–229.

Knight, A.P., 2006. Cannabis sativa. In: Knight, A.P. (Ed.), A Guide to Poisonous House and Garden Plants. Teton NewMedia, Jackson, pp. 61–62.

Luiz, J.A., Heseltine, J., 2008. Five common toxins ingested by dogs and cats. Compendium for the Continuing Education of the Practicing Veterinarian 30 (11), 578–588.

Volmer, P.A., 2006. Marijuana. In: Peterson, M.E., Talcott, P.A. (Eds.), Small Animal Toxicology, second ed. Saunders Elsevier, St Louis, pp. 293–299.

METALDEHYDE

Campbell, A., 2000. Metaldehyde. In: Campbell, A., Chapman, M. (Eds.), Handbook of Poisoning in Dogs and Cats. Blackwell Science, Malden, pp. 181–185.

Dolder, L.K., 2003. Metaldehyde toxicosis. Veterinary Medicine March, 213–215.

Firth, A.M., 1992. Part 2 Treatment of snail bait toxicity in dogs: retrospective study of 56 cases. Journal of Veterinary Emergency and Critical Care 2 (1), 31–36.

Firth, A.M., 1992. Part 1 Treatment of snail bait toxicity in dogs: literature review. Journal of Veterinary Emergency and Critical Care 2 (1), 25–30.

Luiz, J.A., Heseltine, J., 2008. Five common toxins ingested by dogs and cats. Compendium for the Continuing Education of the Practicing Veterinarian 30 (11), 578–588.

Richardson, J.A., Welch, S.L., Gwaltney-Brant, S.M., et al., 2003. Metaldehyde toxicosis in dogs, Compendium for Continuing Education of the Practicing Veterinarian 25 (5), 376–380.

Plumlee, K.H., 2009. Metaldehyde snail and slug bait. In: Osweiler, G.D., Hovda, L.R., Brutlag, A.G., et al. (Eds.), Blackwell's Five-Minute Veterinary Consult Clinical Companion Small

Animal Toxicology. Wiley-Blackwell, Ames, pp. 620–627.

Puschner, B., 2006. Metaldehyde. In: Peterson, M.E., Talcott, P.A. (Eds.), Small Animal Toxicology, second ed. Saunders Elsevier, St Louis, pp. 830–839.

Talcott, P.A., 2004. Metaldehyde. In: Plumlee, K.H. (Ed.), Clinical Veterinary Toxicology. Mosby, St Louis, pp. 182–183.

MISCELLANEOUS TOXINS
5-FLUOROURACIL (5-FU)

Powell, L.L., 2009. 5-Fluorouracil. In: Osweiler, G.D., Hovda, L.R., Brutlag, A.G., et al. (Eds.), Blackwell's Five-Minute Veterinary Consult Clinical Companion Small Animal Toxicology. Wiley-Blackwell, Ames, pp. 113–118.

Roberts, J., Powell, L.L., 2001. Accidental 5-fluorouracil exposure in a Dog. Journal of Veterinary Emergency and Critical Care 11 (4), 281–286.

Roder, J.D., 2004. Antineoplastics. In: Plumlee, K.H. (Ed.), Clinical Veterinary Toxicology. Mosby, St Louis, pp. 299–300.

Welch, S.L., March 2002. Oral toxicity of topical preparations. In: Toxicology, Veterinary Clinics of North America, Small Animal Practice, vol 32, no 2. Saunders, Philadelphia, pp. 445–446.

HEXACHLOROPHENE

Bradberry, S.M., Watt, B.E., Proudfoot, A.T., et al., 2000. Mechanisms of toxicity, clinical features, and management of acute chlorophenoxy herbicide poisoning: a review. Journal of Toxicology, Clinical Toxicology 38 (2), 111–122.

Thompson, J.P., Senior, D.F., Pinson, D.M., et al., 1987. Neurotoxicosis associated with the use of hexachlorophene in a cat. Journal of the American Veterinary Medical Association 190 (10), 1311–1312.

(2-METHYL-4-CHLORO)PHENOXYACETIC ACID (MCPA)

Bradberry, S.M., Proudfoot, A.T., Vale, J.A., 2007. Chlorophenoxy herbicides. In: Shannon, M.W., Borron, S.W., Burns, M.J. (Eds.), Haddad and Winchester's Clinical Management of Poisoning and Drug Overdose, fourth ed. Saunders Elsevier, Philadelphia, pp. 1200–1202.

Harrington, M.L., Moore, M.O., Talcott, P.A., et al., 1996. Suspected herbicide toxicosis in a dog. Journal of the American Veterinary Medical Association 209 (12), 2085–2087.

METOCLOPRAMIDE

Plumb, D.C., 2008. Plumb's Veterinary Drug Handbook, sixth ed. Blackwell Publishing, Ames, pp. 606–607.

METRONIDAZOLE

Dow, S.W., LeCouteur, R.A., Poss, M.L., et al., 1989. Central nervous system toxicosis associated with metronidazole treatment of dogs: five cases (1984–1987). Journal of the American Veterinary Medical Association 195 (3), 365–368.

Evans, J., Levesque, D., Knowles, K., et al., 2003. Diazepam as a treatment for metronidazole toxicosis in dogs: a retrospective study of 21 cases. Journal of Veterinary Internal Medicine 17, 304–310.

Olson, E.J., Morales, S.C., McVey, A.S., et al., 2005. Putative metronidazole neurotoxicosis in a cat. Veterinary Pathology 42, 665–669.

Plumb, D.C., 2008. Plumb's Veterinary Drug Handbook, sixth ed. Blackwell Publishing, Ames, pp. 610–611.

THALLIUM

Dorman, D.C., 1990. Toxicology of selected pesticides, drugs, and chemicals. Anticoagulant, cholecalciferol, and bromethalin-based rodenticides. Veterinary Clinics of North America Small Animal Practice 20 (2), 339–352.

Hall, A.H., Shannon, M.W., 2007. Other heavy metals. In: Shannon, M.W., Borron, S.W., Burns, M.J. (Eds.), Haddad and Winchester's Clinical Management of Poisoning and Drug Overdose, fourth ed. Saunders Elsevier, Philadelphia, pp. 1165–1166.

Ruhr, L.P., Andries, J.K., 1985. Thallium intoxication in a dog. Journal of the American Veterinary Medical Association 186 (5), 498–499.

Volmer, P.A., Merola, V., Osborne, T., et al., 2006. Thallium toxicosis in a Pit Bull Terrier. Journal of Veterinary Diagnosis and Investigation 18, 134–137.

Waters, C.B., Hawkins, E.C., Knapp, D.W., 1992. Acute thallium toxicosis in a dog. Journal of the American Veterinary Medical Association 201 (6), 883–885.

MUSHROOMS

Rossmeisl, J.H., Higgins, M.A., Blodgett, D.J., et al., 2006. Amanita muscaria toxicosis in two dogs. Journal of Veterinary Emergency and Critical Care 16 (3), 208–214.

Puschner, B., 2009. Mushrooms. In: Osweiler, G.D., Hovda, L.R., Brutlag, A.G., et al. (Eds.), Blackwell's Five-Minute Veterinary Consult Clinical Companion Small Animal Toxicology. Wiley-Blackwell, Ames, pp. 711–719.

Puschner, B., Rose, H.H., Filigenzi, M.S., 2007. Diagnosis of Amanita toxicosis in a dog with acute hepatic necrosis. Journal of Veterinary Diagnosis and Investigation 19, 312–317.

Spoerke, D., 2006. Mushrooms. In: Peterson, M.E., Talcott, P.A. (Eds.), Small Animal Toxicology, second ed. Saunders Elsevier, St Louis, pp. 860–887.

Tegzes, J.H., Puschner, B., 2002. Toxic mushrooms. In: Toxicology, Veterinary Clinics of North America, Small Animal Practice, vol 32, no 2. Saunders, Philadelphia, pp. 397–407.

NICOTINE

Knight, A.P., 2006. Nicotiana. In: Knight, A.P. (Ed.), A Guide to Poisonous House and Garden Plants. Teton NewMedia, Jackson, pp. 200–201.

Plumlee, K.H., 2006. Nicotine. In: Peterson, M.E., Talcott, P.A. (Eds.), Small Animal Toxicology, second ed. Saunders Elsevier, St Louis, pp. 898–901.

Renken, C.L., Brutlag, A.G., Koenig, A., 2009. Nicotine / tobacco. In: Osweiler, G.D., Hovda, L.R., Brutlag, A.G., et al. (Eds.), Blackwell's Five-Minute Veterinary Consult Clinical Companion Small Animal Toxicology. Wiley-Blackwell, Ames, pp. 306–312

NON-STEROIDAL ANTI-INFLAMMATORY DRUGS

Albretsen, J.C., 2002. Oral medications. In: Poppenga, R.H., Volmer, P.A. (Eds.), Toxicology, Veterinary Clinics of North America, Small Animal Practice, vol 32, no 2. Saunders, Philadelphia, pp. 427–433.

Campbell, A., 2000. Diclofenac sodium. In: Campbell, A., Chapman, M. (Eds.), Handbook of Poisoning in Dogs and Cats. Blackwell Science, Malden, pp. 119–125.

Campbell, A., 2000. Ibuprofen. In: Campbell, A., Chapman, M. (Eds.), Handbook of Poisoning in Dogs and Cats. Blackwell Science, Malden, pp. 148–155.

Campbell, A., 2000. Indomethacin. In: Campbell, A., Chapman, M. (Eds.), Handbook of Poisoning in Dogs and Cats. Blackwell Science, Malden, pp. 156–162.

Campbell, A., 2000. Naproxen. In: Campbell, A., Chapman, M. (Eds.), Handbook of Poisoning in Dogs and Cats. Blackwell Science, Malden, pp. 192–198.

Fitzgerald, K.T., Bronstein, A.C., Flood, A.A., 2006. 'Over-the-counter' drug toxicities in companion animals. Clinical Techniques in Small Animal Practice 21, 215–226.

Mensching, D., Volmer, P., 2009. Managing acute carprofen toxicosis in dogs and cats. Veterinary Medicine July, 325–333.

Peterson, K.L., 2009. Veterinary NSAIDs. In: Osweiler, G.D., Hovda, L.R., Brutlag, A.G., et al. (Eds.), Blackwell's Five-Minute Veterinary Consult Clinical Companion Small Animal Toxicology. Wiley-Blackwell, Ames, pp. 354–361.

Roder, J.D., 2004. Analgesics. In: Plumlee, K.H. (Ed.), Clinical Veterinary Toxicology. Mosby, St Louis, pp. 282–284.

Syring, R.S., 2009. Human NSAIDs. In: Osweiler, G.D., Hovda, L.R., Brutlag, A.G., et al. (Eds.), Blackwell's Five-Minute Veterinary Consult Clinical Companion Small Animal Toxicology. Wiley-Blackwell, Ames, pp. 292–299.

Talcott, P.A., 2006. Nonsteroidal antiinflammatories. In: Peterson, M.E., Talcott, P.A. (Eds.), Small Animal Toxicology, second ed. Saunders Elsevier, St Louis, pp. 902–933.

ORGANOPHOSPHATES AND CARBAMATES

Bates, N.A., 2000. Carbamate insecticides. In: Campbell, A., Chapman, M. (Eds.), Handbook of Poisoning in Dogs and Cats. Blackwell Science, Malden, pp. 101–105.

Bates, N., Campbell, A., 2000. Organophosphate insecticides. In: Campbell, A., Chapman, M. (Eds.), Handbook of Poisoning in Dogs and Cats. Blackwell Science, Malden, pp. 199–204.

Blodgett, D.J., 2006. Organophosphates and carbamates. In: Peterson, M.E., Talcott, P.A. (Eds.), Small Animal Toxicology, second ed. Saunders Elsevier, St Louis, pp. 941–955.

Corfield, G.S., Connor, L.M., Swindells, K.L., et al., 2008. Intussusception following methiocarb toxicity in three dogs. Journal of Veterinary Emergency Critical Care 18 (1), 68–74.

Gualtieri, J., 2009. Organophosphate and carbamate insecticides. In: Osweiler, G.D., Hovda, L.R., Brutlag, A.G., et al. (Eds.), Blackwell's Five-Minute Veterinary Consult Clinical Companion Small Animal Toxicology. Wiley-Blackwell, Ames, pp. 628–635.

Hopper, K., Aldrich, J., Haskins, S.C., 2002. The recognition and treatment of the intermediate syndrome of organophosphate poisoning in a dog. Journal of Veterinary Emergency and Critical Care 12 (2), 99–103.

Meerdink, G.L., 2004. Anticholinesterase insecticides. In: Plumlee, K.H. (Ed.), Clinical Veterinary Toxicology. Mosby, St Louis, pp. 178–180.

PAINTBALLS

Clarke, D.L., Lee, J.A., 2009. Paintballs. In: Osweiler, G.D., Hovda, L.R., Brutlag, A.G., et al. (Eds.), Blackwell's Five-Minute Veterinary Consult Clinical Companion Small Animal Toxicology. Wiley-Blackwell, Ames, pp. 581–590.

Gray, S.L., Lee, J.A., 2009. Salt. In: Osweiler, G.D., Hovda, L.R., Brutlag, A.G., et al. (Eds.), Blackwell's Five-Minute Veterinary Consult Clinical Companion Small Animal Toxicology. Wiley-Blackwell, Ames, pp. 461–469.

King, J.B., Grant, D.C., 2007. Paintball intoxication in a pug. Journal of Veterinary Emergency and Critical Care 17 (3), 290–293.

Oehme, F.W., Kore, A.M., 2006. Miscellaneous indoor toxicants. In: Peterson, M.E., Talcott, P.A. (Eds.), Small Animal Toxicology, second ed. Saunders Elsevier, St Louis, pp. 223–243.

Tegzes, J.H., 2006. Sodium. In: Peterson, M.E., Talcott, P.A. (Eds.), Small Animal Toxicology, second ed. Saunders Elsevier, St Louis, pp. 1049–1054.

PLANT POISONINGS

Barr, A.C., 2006. Household and garden plants. In: Peterson, M.E., Talcott, P.A. (Eds.), Small Animal Toxicology, second ed. Saunders Elsevier, St Louis, pp. 345–410.

Milewski, L.M., Khan, S.A., 2006. An overview of potentially life-threatening poisonous plants in dogs and cats.

Journal of Veterinary Emergency and Critical Care 16 (1), 25–33.

AZALEAS AND RHODODENDRONS

Butler, J., 2000. Rhododendron and related plant species. In: Campbell, A., Chapman, M. (Eds.), Handbook of Poisoning in Dogs and Cats. Blackwell Science, Malden, pp. 231–233.

Cargill, E., Hovda, L.R., 2009. Rhododendrons / azaleas. In: Osweiler, G.D., Hovda, L.R., Brutlag, A.G., et al. (Eds.), Blackwell's Five-Minute Veterinary Consult Clinical Companion Small Animal Toxicology. Wiley-Blackwell, Ames, pp. 737–742.

Knight, A.P., 2006. Rhododendron. In: Knight, A.P. (Ed.), A Guide to Poisonous House and Garden Plants. Teton NewMedia, Jackson, pp. 235–237.

Milewski, L.M., Khan, S.A., 2006. An overview of potentially life-threatening poisonous plants in dogs and cats. Journal of Veterinary Emergency and Critical Care 16 (1), 25–33.

Plumlee, K.H., 2002. Plant hazards. In: Toxicology, Veterinary Clinics of North America, Small Animal Practice, vol 32, no 2. Saunders, Philadelphia, p. 388.

Puschner, B., 2004. Grayanotoxins. In: Plumlee, K.H. (Ed.), Clinical Veterinary Toxicology. Mosby, St Louis, pp. 412–415.

CHINABERRIES

Hare, W.R., 2004. Meliatoxins. In: Plumlee, K.H. (Ed.), Clinical Veterinary Toxicology. Mosby, St Louis, pp. 415–416.

Knight, A.P., 2006. Melia azedarach. In: Knight, A.P. (Ed.), A Guide to Poisonous House and Garden Plants. Teton NewMedia, Jackson, pp. 184–185.

Plumlee, K.H., March 2002. Plant hazards. In: Toxicology, Veterinary Clinics of North America, Small Animal Practice, vol 32, no 2. Saunders, Philadelphia, pp. 387–388.

KALANCHOE

Galey, F.D., 2004. Cardiac glycosides. In: Plumlee, K.H. (Ed.), Clinical Veterinary Toxicology. Mosby, St Louis, pp. 386–388.

Gwaltney-Brant, S.M., 2006. Kalanchoe. In: Peterson, M.E., Talcott, P.A. (Eds.), Small Animal Toxicology, second ed. Saunders Elsevier, St Louis, pp. 652–655.

Knight, A.P., 2006. Kalanchoe. In: Knight, A.P. (Ed.), A Guide to Poisonous House and Garden Plants. Teton NewMedia, Jackson, pp. 159–161.

Milewski, L.M., Khan, S.A., 2006. An overview of potentially life-threatening poisonous plants in dogs and cats. Journal of Veterinary Emergency and Critical Care 16 (1), 25–33.

Plumlee, K.H., March 2002. Plant hazards. In: Toxicology, Veterinary Clinics of North America, Small Animal Practice, vol 32, no 2. Saunders, Philadelphia, pp. 391–392.

LILY

Berg, R.I.M., Francey, T., Segev, G., 2007. Resolution of acute kidney injury in a cat after lily (Lilium lancifolium) intoxication. Journal of Veterinary Internal Medicine 21, 857–859.

Brady, M.A., Janovitz, E.B., 2000. Nephrotoxicosis in a cat following ingestion of Asiatic hybrid lily (Lilium sp.). Journal of Veterinary Diagnosis and Investigation 12, 566–568.

Hall, J.O., 2004. Lily. In: Plumlee, K.H. (Ed.), Clinical Veterinary Toxicology. Mosby, St Louis, pp. 433–435.

Hall, J.O., 2006. Lilies. In: Peterson, M.E., Talcott, P.A. (Eds.), Small Animal Toxicology, second ed. Saunders Elsevier, St Louis, pp. 806–811.

Knight, A.P., 2006. Hemerocallis. In: Knight, A.P. (Ed.), A Guide to Poisonous House and Garden Plants. Teton NewMedia, Jackson, pp. 134–136.

Knight, A.P., 2006. Lilium. In: Knight, A.P. (Ed.), A Guide to Poisonous House and Garden Plants. Teton NewMedia, Jackson, pp. 174–176.

Langston, C.E., 2002. Acute renal failure caused by lily ingestion in six cats. Journal of the American Veterinary Medical Association 220 (1), 49–52.

Martinson, K.L., Hovda, L.R., 2009. Lilies. In: Osweiler, G.D., Hovda, L.R., Brutlag, A.G., et al. (Eds.), Blackwell's Five-Minute Veterinary Consult Clinical Companion Small Animal Toxicology. Wiley-Blackwell, Ames, pp. 705–710.

Milewski, L.M., Khan, S.A., 2006. An overview of potentially life-threatening poisonous plants in dogs and cats. Journal of Veterinary Emergency and Critical Care 16 (1), 25–33.

Plumlee, K.H., 2002. Plant hazards. In: Toxicology, Veterinary Clinics of North America, Small Animal Practice,

vol 32, no 2. Saunders, Philadelphia, pp. 390–391.

Rumbeiha, W.K., Francis, J.A., Fitzgerald, S.D., et al., 2004. A comprehensive study of Easter lily poisoning in cats. Journal of Veterinary Diagnosis and Investigation 16, 527–541.

Tefft, K.M., 2004. Lily nephrotoxicity in cats. Compendium for the Continuing Education of the Practicing Veterinarian 26, 149–156.

Calla lily

Hovda, L.R., Cargill, E., 2009. Oxalates—insoluble. In: Osweiler, G.D., Hovda, L.R., Brutlag, A.G., et al. (Eds.), Blackwell's Five-Minute Veterinary Consult Clinical Companion Small Animal Toxicology. Wiley-Blackwell, Ames, pp. 720–729.

Knight, A.P., 2006. Zantedeschia. In: Knight, A.P. (Ed.), A Guide to Poisonous House and Garden Plants. Teton NewMedia, Jackson, pp. 288–290.

Lily-of-the-valley

Atkinson, K.J., Fine, D.M., Evans, T.J., et al., 2008. Suspected lily-of-the-valley (Convallaria majalis) toxicosis in a dog. Journal of Veterinary Emergency and Critical Care 18 (4), 399–403.

Cargill, E., Martinson, K.L., 2009. Cardiac glycosides. In: Osweiler, G.D., Hovda, L.R., Brutlag, A.G., et al. (Eds.), Blackwell's Five-Minute Veterinary Consult Clinical Companion Small Animal Toxicology. Wiley-Blackwell, Ames, pp. 696–704.

Knight, A.P., 2006. Convallaria majalis. In: Knight, A.P. (Ed.), A Guide to Poisonous House and Garden Plants. Teton NewMedia, Jackson, pp. 83–84.

Plumlee, K.H., March 2002. Plant hazards. In: Toxicology, Veterinary Clinics of North America, Small Animal Practice, vol 32, no 2. Saunders, Philadelphia, pp. 389–390.

OLEANDER

Cargill, E., Martinson, K.L., 2009. Cardiac glycosides. In: Osweiler, G.D., Hovda, L.R., Brutlag, A.G., et al. (Eds.), Blackwell's Five-Minute Veterinary Consult Clinical Companion Small Animal Toxicology. Wiley-Blackwell, Ames, pp. 696–704.

Galey, F.D., 2004. Cardiac glycosides. In: Plumlee, K.H. (Ed.), Clinical Veterinary

Toxicology. Mosby, St Louis, pp. 386–388.

Knight, A.P., 2006. Nerium oleander. In: Knight, A.P. (Ed.), A Guide to Poisonous House and Garden Plants. Teton NewMedia, Jackson, pp. 197–199.

Milewski, L.M., Khan, S.A., 2006. An overview of potentially life-threatening poisonous plants in dogs and cats. Journal of Veterinary Emergency and Critical Care 16 (1), 25–33.

Plumlee, K.H., 2002. Plant hazards. In: Toxicology, Veterinary Clinics of North America, Small Animal Practice, vol 32, no 2. Saunders, Philadelphia, pp. 389–390.

SAGO PALM

Albretsen, J.C., Khan, S.A., Richardson, J.A., 1988. Cycad palm toxicosis in dogs: 60 cases (1987–1997). Journal of the American Veterinary Medical Association 213 (1), 99–101.

Albretsen, J.C., 2004. Cycasin. In: Plumlee, K.H. (Ed.), Clinical Veterinary Toxicology. Mosby, St Louis, pp. 392–394.

Klatt, C.A., Gruber, N.M., 2009. Sago palm. In: Osweiler, G.D., Hovda, L.R., Brutlag, A.G., et al. (Eds.), Blackwell's Five-Minute Veterinary Consult Clinical Companion Small Animal Toxicology. Wiley-Blackwell, Ames, pp. 743–749.

Knight, A.P., 2006. Cycas. In: Knight, A.P. (Ed.), A Guide to Poisonous House and Garden Plants. Teton NewMedia, Jackson, pp. 93–95.

Milewski, L.M., Khan, S.A., 2006. An overview of potentially life-threatening poisonous plants in dogs and cats. Journal of Veterinary Emergency and Critical Care 16 (1), 25–33.

Plumlee, K.H., 2002. Plant hazards. In: Toxicology, Veterinary Clinics of North America, Small Animal Practice, vol 32, no 2. Saunders, Philadelphia, pp. 386–387.

PLAY DOUGH (HOMEMADE)

Barr, J.M., Khan, S.A., McCullough, S.M., et al., 2004. Hypernatremia secondary to homemade play dough ingestion in dogs: a review of 14 cases from 1998 to 2001. Journal of Veterinary Emergency and Critical Care 14 (3), 196–202.

Gray, S.L., Lee, J.A., 2009. Salt. In: Osweiler, G.D., Hovda, L.R., Brutlag, A.G., et al. (Eds.), Blackwell's Five-Minute Veterinary Consult Clinical Companion Small Animal Toxicology. Wiley-Blackwell, Ames, pp. 461–469.

Oehme, F.W., Kore, A.M., 2006. Miscellaneous indoor toxicants. In: Peterson, M.E., Talcott, P.A. (Eds.), Small Animal Toxicology, second ed. Saunders Elsevier, St Louis, pp. 223–243.

Pouzot, C., Descone-Junot, C., Loup, J., et al., 2007. Successful treatment of severe salt intoxication in a dog. Journal of Veterinary Emergency and Critical Care, 17 (3), 294–298.

Tegzes, J.H., 2006. Sodium. In: Peterson, M.E., Talcott, P.A. (Eds.), Small Animal Toxicology, second ed. Saunders Elsevier, St Louis, pp. 1049–1054.

POTPOURRI OIL

Means, C., 2004. Essential oils. In: Plumlee, K.H. (Ed.), Clinical Veterinary Toxicology. Mosby, St Louis, pp. 149–150.

Poppenga, R.H., 2009. Essential oils / potpourri. In: Osweiler, G.D., Hovda, L.R., Brutlag, A.G., et al. (Eds.), Blackwell's Five-Minute Veterinary Consult Clinical Companion Small Animal Toxicology. Wiley Blackwell, Ames, pp. 527–533.

Schildt, J.C., Jutkowitz, L.A., Beal, M.A., 2008. Potpourri oil toxicity in cats: 6 cases (2000–2007). Journal of Veterinary Emergency and Critical Care 18 (5), 511–516.

PYRETHRIN AND PYRETHROIDS

Bates, N., 2000. Pyrethrins and pyrethroids. In: Campbell, A., Chapman, M. (Eds.), Handbook of Poisoning in Dogs and Cats. Blackwell Science, Malden, pp. 42–46.

Boller, M., Silverstein, D.C., 2009. Pyrethrins. In: Silverstein, D.C., Hopper, K. (Eds.), Small Animal Critical Care Medicine. Elsevier, St Louis, pp. 394–398.

Gruber, N.M., 2009. Pyrethrins and pyrethroids. In: Osweiler, G.D., Hovda, L.R., Brutlag, A.G., et al. (Eds.), Blackwell's Five-Minute Veterinary Consult Clinical Companion Small Animal Toxicology. Wiley-Blackwell, Ames, pp. 636–643.

Hansen, S.R., 2006. Pyrethrins and pyrethroids. In: Peterson, M.E., Talcott, P.A. (Eds.), Small Animal Toxicology, second ed. Saunders Elsevier, St Louis, pp. 1002–1010.

Volmer, P.A., 2004. Pyrethrins and pyrethroids. In: Plumlee, K.H. (Ed.),

Clinical Veterinary Toxicology. Mosby, St Louis, pp. 188–190.

RICIN AND ABRIN

Albretsen, J.C., 2004. Lectins. In: Plumlee, K.H. (Ed.), Clinical Veterinary Toxicology. Mosby, St Louis, pp. 406–408.

Bailey, E.M., 2006. Ricin. In: Peterson, M.E., Talcott, P.A. (Eds.), Small Animal Toxicology, second ed. Saunders Elsevier, St Louis, pp. 1011–1016.

Knight, A.P., 2006. Ricinus communis. In: Knight, A.P. (Ed.), A Guide to Poisonous House and Garden Plants. Teton NewMedia, Jackson, pp. 237–239.

Milewski, L.M., Khan, S.A., 2006. An overview of potentially life-threatening poisonous plants in dogs and cats, Journal of Veterinary Emergency and Critical Care 16 (1), 25–33.

Mouser, P., Filigenzi, M.S., Puschner, B., et al., 2007. Fatal ricin toxicosis in a puppy confirmed by liquid chromatography / mass spectrometry when using ricinine as a marker. Journal of Veterinary Diagnosis and Investigation 19, 216–220.

Plumlee, K.H., 2002. Plant hazards. In: Toxicology, Veterinary Clinics of North America, Small Animal Practice, vol 32, no 2. Saunders, Philadelphia, pp. 388–389.

Roberts, L.M., Smith, D.C., 2004. Ricin: the endoplasmic reticulum connection. Toxicon 44, 469–472.

ROTENONE

Murtaugh, R.J., Kaplan, P.M., 1992. Veterinary Emergency and Critical Care Medicine. Mosby, St Louis, pp. 436–437.

Osweiler, G.D., 1996. Toxicology. Williams & Wilkins, Philadelphia, pp. 243–245.

Talcott, P.A., Dorman, D.C., 1997. Pesticide exposures in companion animals. Veterinary Medicine 97 (2), 167–181.

SCORPION STINGS

Adams, C.M., 2009. Scorpions. In: Osweiler, G.D., Hovda, L.R., Brutlag, A.G., et al. (Eds.), Blackwell's Five-Minute Veterinary Consult Clinical Companion Small Animal Toxicology. Wiley-Blackwell, Ames, pp. 398–403.

Boyer, L.V., Theodorou, A.A., Berg, R.A., et al., 2009. Antivenom for critically ill children with neurotoxicity from scorpion stings. New England Journal of Medicine 360, 2090–2098.

Thomas, J.D., Thomas, K.E., Kazzi, Z.N., 2007. Scorpions and stinging insects. In: Shannon, M.W., Borron, S.W., Burns, M.J. (Eds.), Haddad and Winchester's Clinical Management of Poisoning and Drug Overdose, fourth ed. Saunders Elsevier, Philadelphia, pp. 440–447.

SEROTONIN SYNDROME

Albretsen, J.C., 2002. Oral medications. In: Poppenga, R.H., Volmer, P.A. (Eds.), Toxicology, Veterinary Clinics of North America, Small Animal Practice, vol 32, no 2. Saunders, Philadelphia, pp. 422–423.

Campbell, A., 2000. Selective serotonin re-uptake inhibitor antidepressants. In: Campbell, A., Chapman, M. (Eds.), Handbook of Poisoning in Dogs and Cats. Blackwell Science, Malden, pp. 242–244.

Reineke, E.L., Drobatz, K.J., 2009. Serotonin syndrome. In: Silverstein, D.C., Hopper, K. (Eds.), Small Animal Critical Care Medicine. Elsevier, St Louis, pp. 384–387.

Sioris, K.M., 2009. Selective serotonin reuptake inhibitors (SSRIs). In: Osweiler, G.D., Hovda, L.R., Brutlag, A.G., et al. (Eds.), Blackwell's Five-Minute Veterinary Consult Clinical Companion Small Animal Toxicology. Wiley-Blackwell, Ames, pp. 195–201.

SNAKE BITE ENVENOMATION

Berdoulay, P., Schaer, M., Starr, J., 2005. Serum sickness in a dog associated with antivenin therapy for snake bite caused by Crotalus adamanteus. Journal of Veterinary Emergency and Critical Care 15 (3), 206–212.

Borron, S.W., Chase, P.B., Walter, F.G., 2007. Elapidae: North American and selected non-native species. In: Shannon, M.W., Borron, S.W., Burns, M.J. (Eds.), Haddad and Winchester's Clinical Management of Poisoning and Drug Overdose, fourth ed. Saunders Elsevier, Philadelphia, pp. 422–432.

Dart, R.C., Seifert, S.A., Boyer, L.V., et al., 2001. A randomized multicenter trial of Crotalinae polyvalent immune Fab (ovine) antivenom for the treatment for crotaline snakebite in the United States. Archives of Internal Medicine 161 (16), 2030–2036.

French, W.J., Hayes, W.K., Bush, S.P., et al., 2004. Mojave toxin in venom of Crotalus helleri (Southern Pacific rattlesnake): molecular and geographic characterization. Toxicon 44, 781–791.

Gold, B.S., Dart, R.C., Barish, R.A., 2002. Bites of venomous snakes. New England Journal of Medicine 347 (5), 347–356.

Habib, A.G., 2003. Tetanus complicating snakebite in northern Nigeria: clinical presentation and public health implications. Acta Tropica 85, 87–91.

Keyler, D.E., Peterson, M.E., 2009. Crotalids (pit vipers). In: Osweiler, G.D., Hovda, L.R., Brutlag, A.G., et al. (Eds.), Blackwell's Five-Minute Veterinary Consult Clinical Companion Small Animal Toxicology. Wiley-Blackwell, Ames, pp. 382–392.

Krenzelok, E.P., 2002. New developments in the therapy of intoxications. Toxicology Letters 127, 299–305.

Najman, L., Seshadri, R., 2007. Rattlesnake envenomation. Compendium for the Continuing Education of the Practicing Veterinarian 29 (3), 166–177.

Odeleye, A.A., Presley, A.E., Passwater, M.E., et al., 2004. Rattlesnake venom-induced thrombocytopenia. Annals of Clinical and Laboratory Science 34 (4), 467–470.

Offerman, S.R., Barry, J.D., Schneir, A., et al., 2003. Biphasic rattlesnake venom-induced thrombocytopenia. Journal of Emergency Medicine 24 (3), 289–293.

Peterson, M.E., 2004. Coral snakes. In: Plumlee, K.H. (Ed.), Clinical Veterinary Toxicology. Mosby, St Louis, pp. 104–105.

Peterson, M.E., 2004. Pit vipers. In: Plumlee, K.H. (Ed.), Clinical Veterinary Toxicology. Mosby, St Louis, pp. 106–111.

Peterson, M.E., 2006. Snake bite: pit vipers. Clinical Techniques in Small Animal Practice 21, 174–182.

Peterson, M.E., 2006. Snake bite: coral snakes. Clinical Techniques in Small Animal Practice 21, 183–186.

Peterson, M.E., 2006. Snake bite: North American pit vipers. In: Peterson, M.E., Talcott, P.A. (Eds.), Small Animal Toxicology, second ed. Saunders Elsevier, St Louis, pp. 1017–1038.

Peterson, M.E., 2006. Snake bite: coral snakes. In: Peterson, M.E., Talcott, P.A. (Eds.), Small Animal Toxicology, second ed. Saunders Elsevier, St Louis, pp. 1039–1048.

Peterson, M.E., Keyler, D.E., 2009. Elapids (coral snakes). In: Osweiler, G.D., Hovda, L.R., Brutlag, A.G., et al. (Eds.), Blackwell's Five-Minute Veterinary

Consult Clinical Companion Small Animal Toxicology. Wiley-Blackwell, Ames, pp. 393–397.

Peterson, M.E., 2009. Snake envenomation. In: Silverstein, D.C., Hopper, K. (Eds.), Small Animal Critical Care Medicine. Elsevier, St Louis, pp. 399–404.

Peterson, M.E., Matz, M., Seibold, K., et al., 2011. A randomized multicenter trial of Crotalidae polyvalent immune Fab antivenom for the treatment of rattlesnake envenomation in dogs. Journal of Veterinary Emergency and Critical Care 21 (4), 335–345.

Walter, F.G., Chase, P.B., Fenrandez, M.C., et al., 2007. North American Crotalinae envenomation. In: Shannon, M.W., Borron, S.W., Burns, M.J. (Eds.), Haddad and Winchester's Clinical Management of Poisoning and Drug Overdose, fourth ed. Saunders Elsevier, Philadelphia, pp. 399–422.

Walton, R.M., Brown, D.E., Hamar, D.W., et al., 1997. Mechanisms of echinocytosis induced by Crotalus atrox venom. Veterinary Pathology 34 (5), 442–449.

White, J., 2005. Snake venoms and coagulopathy. Toxicon 45, 951–967.

SPIDER BITE ENVENOMATION

da Silvaa, P.H., da Silveiraa, R.B., Appela, M.H., et al., 2004. Brown spiders and loxoscelism. Toxicon 44, 693–709.

Graudins, A., 2007. Spiders. In: Shannon, M.W., Borron, S.W., Burns, M.J. (Eds.), Haddad and Winchester's Clinical Management of Poisoning and Drug Overdose, fourth ed. Saunders Elsevier, Philadelphia, pp. 433–439.

Pace, L.B., Vetter, R.S., 2009. Brown recluse spider (Loxosceles reclusa) envenomation in small animals. Journal of Veterinary Emergency and Critical Care 19 (4), 329–336.

Peterson, M.E., McNally, J., 2006. Spider envenomation: black widow. In: Peterson, M.E., Talcott, P.A. (Eds.), Small Animal Toxicology, second ed. Saunders Elsevier, St Louis, pp. 1063–1069.

Peterson, M.E., McNally, J., 2006. Spider envenomation: brown recluse. In: Peterson, M.E., Talcott, P.A. (Eds.), Small Animal Toxicology, second ed. Saunders Elsevier, St Louis, pp. 1070–1075.

Peterson, M.E., 2009. Spider bite. In: Silverstein, D.C., Hopper, K. (Eds.), Small Animal Critical Care Medicine. Elsevier, St Louis, pp. 405–407.

Peterson, M.E., Adams, C.M., 2009. Black widow spiders. In: Osweiler, G.D., Hovda, L.R., Brutlag, A.G., et al. (Eds.), Blackwell's Five-Minute Veterinary Consult Clinical Companion Small Animal Toxicology. Wiley-Blackwell, Ames, pp. 365–369.

Peterson, M.E., Adams, C.M., 2009. Brown recluse spiders. In: Osweiler, G.D., Hovda, L.R., Brutlag, A.G., et al. (Eds.), Blackwell's Five-Minute Veterinary Consult Clinical Companion Small Animal Toxicology. Wiley-Blackwell, Ames, pp. 370–375.

Roder, J.D., 2004. Black widow. In: Plumlee, K.H. (Ed.), Clinical Veterinary Toxicology. Mosby, St Louis, pp. 111–112.

Roder, J.D., 2004. Brown recluse. In: Plumlee, K.H. (Ed.), Clinical Veterinary Toxicology. Mosby, St Louis, pp. 112–113.

Swanson, D.L., Vetter, R.S., 2005. Bites of brown recluse spiders and suspected necrotic arachnidism. New England Journal of Medicine 352, 700–707.

Twedt, D.C., Cuddon, P.A., Horn, T.W., 1999. Black widow spider envenomation in a cat. Journal of Veterinary Internal Medicine 12, 613–616.

STRYCHNINE

Hall, J.O., 2009. Strychnine. In: Osweiler, G.D., Hovda, L.R., Brutlag, A.G., et al. (Eds.), Blackwell's Five-Minute Veterinary Consult Clinical Companion Small Animal Toxicology. Wiley-Blackwell, Ames, pp. 791–797.

Murphy, M.J., 2002. Rodenticides. In: Toxicology, Veterinary Clinics of North America, Small Animal Practice, vol 32, no 2. Saunders, Philadelphia, pp. 478–479.

Talcott, P.A., 2004. Strychnine. In: Plumlee, K.H. (Ed.), Clinical Veterinary Toxicology. Mosby, St Louis, pp. 454–456.

Talcott, P.A., 2006. Strychnine. In: Peterson, M.E., Talcott, P.A. (Eds.), Small Animal Toxicology, second ed. Saunders Elsevier, St Louis, pp. 1076–1082.

TOAD POISONING

Eubig, P.A., 2011. Bufo species toxicosis: big toad, big problem. Veterinary Medicine Aug, 594–599.

Peterson, M.E., Roberts, B.K., 2006. Toads. In: Peterson, M.E., Talcott, P.A. (Eds.), Small Animal Toxicology, second ed. Saunders Elsevier, St Louis, pp. 1063–1069.

Peterson, M.E., Hovda, L.R., 2009. Bufo toads. In: Osweiler, G.D., Hovda, L.R., Brutlag, A.G., et al. (Eds.), Blackwell's Five-Minute Veterinary Consult Clinical Companion Small Animal Toxicology. Wiley-Blackwell, Ames, pp. 376–381.

Roberts, B.K., Aronsohn, M.G., Moses, B.L., et al., 2000. Bufo marinus intoxication in dogs: 94 cases (1997–1998). Journal of the American Veterinary Medical Association 216, 1941–1944.

Roder, J.D., 2004. Toads. In: Plumlee, K.H. (Ed.), Clinical Veterinary Toxicology. Mosby, St Louis, p. 113.

TRICYCLIC ANTIDEPRESSANTS

Campbell, A., 2000. Tricyclic antidepressants. In: Campbell, A., Chapman, M. (Eds.), Handbook of Poisoning in Dogs and Cats. Blackwell Science, Malden, pp. 250–253.

Fletcher, D.J., Murphy, L.A., 2009. Cyclic antidepressant drug overdose. In: Silverstein, D.C., Hopper, K. (Eds.), Small Animal Critical Care Medicine. Elsevier, St Louis, pp. 378–380.

Volmer, P.A., 2006. Tricyclic antidepressants. In: Peterson, M.E., Talcott, P.A. (Eds.), Small Animal Toxicology, second ed. Saunders Elsevier, St Louis, pp. 303–306.

XYLITOL

Dunayer, E.K., Gwaltney-Brant, S.M., 2006. Acute hepatic failure and coagulopathy associated with xylitol ingestion in eight dogs. Journal of the American Veterinary Medical Association, 229, 1113–1117.

Liu, T.Y.D., Lee, J.A., 2009. Xylitol. In: Osweiler, G.D., Hovda, L.R., Brutlag, A.G., et al. (Eds.), Blackwell's Five-Minute Veterinary Consult Clinical Companion Small Animal Toxicology. Wiley-Blackwell, Ames, pp. 470–475.

Oehme, F.W., Kore, A.M., 2006. Miscellaneous indoor toxicants. In: Peterson, M.E., Talcott, P.A. (Eds.), Small Animal Toxicology, second ed. Saunders Elsevier, St Louis, pp. 223–243.

Piscitelli, C.M., Dunayer, E.K., Aumann, M., 2010. Xylitol toxicity in dogs. Compendium for the Continuing Education of the Practicing Veterinarian 32, E1–E4.

Todd, J.M., Powell, L.L., 2007. Xylitol intoxication associated with fulminant hepatic failure in a dog. Journal of Veterinary Emergency and Critical Care 17 (3), 286–289.

ZINC

Cahill-Morasco, R., DePasquale, M.A.,
2002. Zinc Toxicosis in Small Animals,
Compendium for the Continuing
Education of the Practicing Veterinarian
24 (9), 712–720.

Dziwenka, M.M., Coppock, R., 2004. Zinc.
In: Plumlee, K.H. (Ed.), Clinical
Veterinary Toxicology. Mosby, St Louis,
pp. 221–226.

Gurnee, C.M., Drobatz, K.J., 2007. Zinc
intoxication in dogs: 19 cases
(1991–2003). Journal of the American
Veterinary Medical Association, 230,
1174–1179.

Meurs, K.M., Peterson, K.L., Talcott, P.A.,
2009. Zinc. In: Osweiler, G.D., Hovda,
L.R., Brutlag, A.G., et al. (Eds.),
Blackwell's Five-Minute Veterinary
Consult Clinical Companion Small
Animal Toxicology. Wiley-Blackwell,
Ames, pp. 664–670.

Talcott, P.A., 2006. Zinc. In: Peterson, M.E.,
Talcott, P.A. (Eds.), Small Animal
Toxicology, second ed. Saunders Elsevier,
St Louis, pp. 1094–1100.

ZINC PHOSPHIDE

Albretsen, J.C., 2004. Zinc phosphide. In:
Plumlee, K.H. (Ed.), Clinical Veterinary
Toxicology. Mosby, St Louis, pp.
456–458.

Gray, S., 2009. Phosphides. In: Osweiler,
G.D., Hovda, L.R., Brutlag, A.G., et al.
(Eds.), Blackwell's Five-Minute
Veterinary Consult Clinical Companion
Small Animal Toxicology. Wiley-
Blackwell, Ames, pp. 781–790.

Knight, M.W., 2006. Zinc Phosphide. In:
Peterson, M.E., Talcott, P.A. (Eds.),
Small Animal Toxicology, second ed.
Saunders Elsevier, St Louis,
pp. 1101–1118.

Murphy, M.J., 2002. Rodenticides. In:
Toxicology, Veterinary Clinics of North
America, Small Animal Practice, vol 32,
no 2. Saunders, Philadelphia,
pp. 479–480.

Emergencies in exotic species
Christoph Mans MED. VET.

AVIAN SPECIES

Avian cardiopulmonary resuscitation (CPR)

1. Clear airway, intubate and begin ventilating at the rate of one breath per 4–5 seconds.
2. If there is no heart beat or bradycardia, administer epinephrine (1:1000, 0.1–1 mL/kg) and atropine (0.2–0.5 mg/kg) IV, IO or intratracheally.
3. Administer a fluid bolus of 10–25 mL/kg IV or IO over 5–7 minutes.

Protocol for critically ill avian patients

1. Keep handling and stress at minimum.
2. Stop any obvious bleeding by application of a pressure bandage or by suturing. For bleeding of nails and beaks use hemostatic agents or cautery. If a bleeding disorder is suspected, administer vitamin K_1 (2 mg/kg IM).
3. Administer warmed subcutaneous fluids (30–50 mL/kg) in mildly to moderately dehydrated birds and intravenous fluids IV, or IO in moderate to severely dehydrated birds. Use balanced isotonic electrolyte solution (e.g. lactated Ringer's solution (LRS), Normosol®-R).
4. If an underlying bacterial infection is suspected, administer a broad-spectrum bactericidal antibiotic parenterally (enrofloxacin 20 mg/kg SC, IM).
5. Place the bird in an incubator warmed to 85–90°F (29–32°C), unless the bird has head trauma or hyperthermia. If the bird has head trauma or hyperthermia, the environment should be cooler: 75°F (24°C).
6. Administer oxygen if the bird is in shock or respiratory distress.
7. When stabilized and rehydrated, offer food or tube feed.

Avian sedation

1. Sedation increases the tolerance towards unpleasant or stressful procedures in birds. Perform sedation in birds which are in respiratory

distress, intolerant to handling or are difficult to restrain. Use sedation for diagnostic procedures such as radiographic positioning, coelomic ultrasound and coelomocentesis, or blood collection. If sedation is combined with analgesia or local anesthesia, then minor surgical procedures such as laceration repair or wound debridement may also be performed. Use sedation for bandage and e-collar application.
2. Midazolam is the most commonly used sedative in birds.
   A. In psittacines and passerines use 1–2 mg/kg of midazolam depending on the sedative level desired and on the patient.
   B. Administer midazolam either by intramuscular injection or by intranasal administration.
3. For deeper sedation or if analgesia is required, combine midazolam with butorphanol.
   A. In psittacines and passerines use 1–2 mg/kg of butorphanol in addition to midazolam, depending on the sedative level desired and on the patient.
   B. Administer butorphanol either by intramuscular injection or by intranasal (IN) administration.
4. Flumazenil (0.05–0.1 mg/kg) reverses the effects of midazolam. Reverse every bird before discharging it from the hospital. Do not reverse birds which had e-collars or bandages placed, or in those who seem to be distressed by the hospital environment.
   A. Flumazenil can be administered IM, IV or IN.
   B. Some birds require a second dose of flumazenil before complete recovery from sedation is achieved.
5. It is not necessary to reverse the effects of butorphanol if it was given in combination with midazolam. Reversal with flumazenil alone usually results in recovery from sedation.

Avian fluid therapy

1. The recommended fluid volume for subcutaneous administration is 30–50 mL/kg.
2. The daily maintenance fluid requirement in most birds is 60 mL/kg/day.
3. The fluid deficit may be estimated, based on dehydration and body weight: estimated dehydration (%) × body weight (g) = fluid deficit (mL).
For example: A moderately (10%) dehydrated cockatiel (body weight: 90 g) has a fluid deficit of 9 mL (10% × 90 g = 9 mL).
4. Administer half of the fluid deficit and the daily maintenance requirements during the first 12–24 hours of therapy. Administer the remaining half of the fluid deficit during the next 48 hours, along with the daily maintenance fluid requirement and the estimated volume of the ongoing fluid losses.
5. Only warmed (100–102°F (38–39°C)) fluids should be administered.
6. For SC fluid administration, use lactated Ringer's solution, Normosol®-R, or a similar balanced electrolyte isotonic crystalloid.

A. The recommended site for SC fluid administration in a bird is in the knee-fold area. Use alcohol to improve visualization and inject strictly subcutaneously.

B. Split the fluid volume to be administered between both knee folds if necessary.

7. IV or IO fluid boluses may be administered to birds in shock. The dose is 10–25 mL/kg administered slowly over 5–7 minutes.

8. For IV or IO fluid administration, dextrose may be added to the fluids if desired.

9. A spinal needle (22-gauge, 1.5-inch) or regular syringe needle may be placed into the distal ulna or proximal tibiotarsus.

10. IO catheterization of the distal ulna (Fig. 15.1):

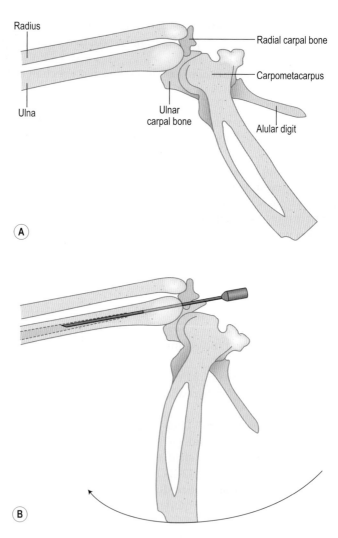

FIG 15.1 **Distal ulnar placement of an intraosseous catheter in an Amazon parrot.** *From Tully Jr, T.N., Dorrestein, G.M., Jones, A.K., 2009. Avian Medicine, second ed. WB Saunders; reprinted with permission from Elsevier.*

A. Surgically prep a site on the lateral side of the wing on the distal ulna.
B. While supporting the ulna with one hand, with the other hand introduce a needle into the distal ulna parallel to the diaphysis.
C. Remove the stylet and apply a prefilled adapter.
D. Flush the adapter and needle. Correct IO placement is confirmed by monitoring the ulnar vein running over the medial aspect of the elbow, while flushing the catheter. Alternatively, correct IO placement can be confirmed by aspirating blood or bone marrow. Incorrectly placed IO catheter will not reveal blood or bone marrow upon aspiration.
E. Secure the catheter with a bandage or tape.
F. Immobilize the wing with a figure-of-eight bandage (Fig. 15.2).

11. IO catheterization of the proximal tibiotarsus (Fig. 15.3):
A. Surgically prep a site on the proximal and cranial tibiotarsus, just distal to the stifle.
B. Holding the tibiotarsus in one hand, with the stifle flexed, introduce the needle into the cnemial crest (tibial crest) through the patellar tendon.

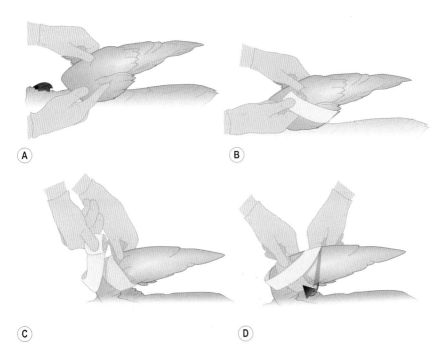

(A) (B)

(C) (D)

FIG 15.2 **A figure-of-eight bandage splint.** (A) The wing is held in its normal flexed position. (B) Gauze is wrapped around the ventral aspect of the humerus and brought over the dorsal aspect of the wing. (C) The gauze is then wrapped over the humero-radioulnar joint and around the carpus. (D) The gauze is then brought under the wing and wrapped back over the dorsum and under the humerus. From Altman, R.B., Clubb, S.L., Dorrestein, G.M., Quesenberry, K., 1997. Avian Medicine and Surgery. WB Saunders; reprinted with permission from Elsevier.

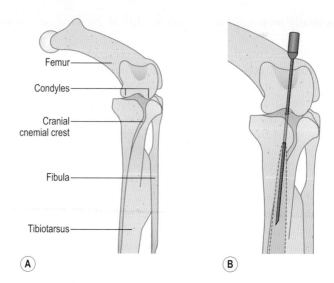

Femur —
Condyles —
Cranial — cnemial crest
Fibula —
Tibiotarsus —

A   B

FIG 15.3 **Schematic diagram of intraosseous catheter placed into the proximal tibiotarsus.** *From Tully Jr, T.N., Dorrestein, G.M., 2009. Jones, A.K., Avian Medicine, second ed. WB Saunders; reprinted with permission from Elsevier.*

C. Hold the needle parallel to the tibiotarsus as it is advanced into the medullary cavity up to the level of the needle hub

D. Remove the stylet and apply a prefilled adapter.

E. Flush the adapter and needle. Correct IO placement is confirmed by aspirating blood or bone marrow. Incorrectly placed IO catheter will not reveal blood or bone marrow upon aspiration.

F. Secure the catheter with a bandage or tape.

12. IV catheters are recommended in larger birds, such as waterfowl and other large nonpsittacine species. IV catheters are not recommended for psittacine birds, unless anesthetized or heavily sedated, because they are more difficult to place and maintain, and removal of the catheter by the bird may lead to possible fatal hemorrhage.

   The recommended catheter site for large birds is the medial tarsometatarsal vein, running on the medial aspect of the lower leg, distal to the hock joint. Catheters can also be placed into the ulnar (wing) veins, located at the medial aspect of the elbow or into the right jugular veins. However, the ulnar and jugular veins have a higher risk of complications, such as hematoma formation.

   Surgically prep the placement site:

   I. Place the IV catheter.

   II. Flush and cap the IV catheter.

   III. Secure leg catheters with a tape, and wing catheters with an adhesive transparent dressing (e.g. Tegaderm®) or with a butterfly tape sutured to the bird's skin. Secure a jugular catheter with surgical glue and with a butterfly tape sutured to the bird's skin.

   IV. Apply a figure-of-eight bandage for wing catheters, or a light bandage for jugular and leg catheters.

Avian nutritional support

1. Any anorexic bird should receive nutritional support, via gavage or tube feeding, in order to aid a successful recovery. Do not feed severely depressed or recumbent birds, moderately to severely dehydrated birds until they are rehydrated, birds with crop impaction or stasis, or birds that are regurgitating or seizuring. Avoid gaving birds prior to diagnostic procedures such as radiographs or blood collection.
2. In psittacines and passerines, a metal ball-tipped feeding cannula (gavage needle) is used to administer feeding formula directly into the crop. In bird species without a crop or poorly developed crop, a rubber feeding tube should be used and carefully advanced into the distal esophagus or proventriculus for food administration.
3. Use an easily digestible high-carbohydrate feeding formula. Hand-feeding formulas for baby birds or specifically designed recovery formulas are suitable. Feed only warm formula (100–102°F (38–39°C)).
4. Administer 30–50 mL/kg (3–5 mL/100 g) of feeding formula by crop gavage per feeding. For example a 90 g cockatiel should receive 3–4 mL; a 400 g African grey parrot should receive 10–20 mL. Feed the smaller volume initially, and increase the volume over subsequent feedings if bird is not regurgitating. Feed 2–4 meals a day, depending on the bird's condition and its metabolic state.
5. Carefully place a gavage needle into the crop (Fig. 15.4):
   A. Insert the gavage needle from the left oral commissure into the oral cavity.
   B. Carefully advance the tip over the base of the tongue towards the right side.
   C. Redirect the gavage needle towards the right side and caudally, into the oropharynx, avoiding the tracheal opening.
   D. Under minimal resistance advance the needle into the proximal esophagus. If resistance is encountered, ensure that the person restraining the bird is not compressing the esophagus and that the gavage needle is placed correctly.
   E. Advance the gavage needle into the crop, which is situated on the right side of the distal neck, overlying the thoracic inlet.
   F. Prior to administration of the feeding formula, confirm the correct placement of the gavage needle by palpation of the needle and the trachea as separate structures and by palpating the tip of the gavage needle through the crop wall.
   G. Administer the feeding formula in a steady fashion into the crop. Monitor for back-up of formula into the proximal esophagus and for regurgitation.
   H. Carefully remove the gavage needle and discontinue handling the bird, in order to avoid compression of the crop and regurgitation.

Avian emergencies

1. **Cat or dog bite wounds** – any cat or dog attack on a bird is an emergency, whether or not the skin appears broken. If open wounds are present, administer broad-spectrum antibiotics which provide coverage

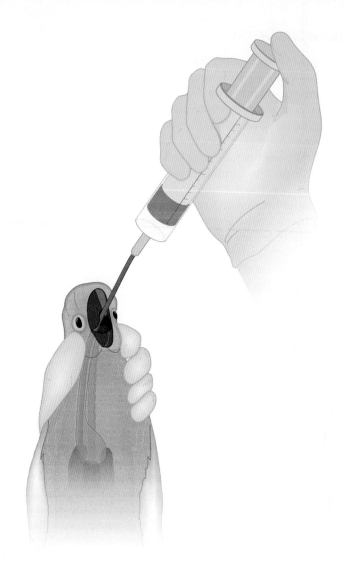

FIG 15.4   Insertion of a gavage needle into the crop of a bird.

for anaerobic bacteria (e.g. piperacillin 100–200 mg/kg IM q6–12h; or a combination of enrofloxacin (20 mg/kg IM, SC, PO q12h) with either azithromycin (40 mg/kg PO q24h) or metronidazole (20 mg/kg PO q12h)) for at least 5 days. Use long-acting ceftiofur (Excede®, 10 mg/kg IM q72h) in waterfowl. Clean and flush punctures and small wounds, leaving them open to drain and heal. Fresh, large lacerations should be flushed with diluted chlorhexidine solution or sterile saline and sutured partially closed.

2. **Broken blood feathers** – require careful pulling. Grasp the base of the feather shaft with a hemostat, and remove the feather from the follicle, by pulling firmly in the direction of the feather growth. Once the

feather is completely removed, bleeding will stop. Occasionally, placement of a suture or surgical glue is required to stop the hemorrhage. Do not apply hemostyptic agents, as they can cause tissue necrosis. If the hemorrhaging was severe and the bird is compromised, administer SC, IV or IO fluids and possibly a blood transfusion.

3. **Bleeding nails** – treatment at home includes: flour, pressure, super-glue, or hemostyptic products. Treatment in the hospital involves the application of hemostyptic products (e.g. ferric subsulfate, silver nitrogen stick), tissue glue or pressure bandage. Birds with substantial loss of the keratin sheath should be treated with a bandage initially.

4. **Severe blood loss** (estimated blood volume is 10 mL/100 g body weight); most birds can withstand up to 30% (3 mL/100 g) loss with minimal clinical complications.
   A. Stop the bleeding.
   B. Administer vitamin K_1 (2 mg/kg SC, IM) if a coagulopathy is suspected.
   C. Administer warmed intravenous fluids (LRS or Normosol®-R) IV, IO or SC if the bird is not in a critical condition.
   D. Place the bird in an incubator warmed to 85–90°F (29–32°C), unless the bird has head trauma or hyperthermia.
   E. Consider administration of whole blood if the PCV <20%.
      I. Approximately 1% (1 mL/100 g) of the donor bird's weight can be safely collected.
      II. Acid citrate dextrose (ACD) should be used as the anticoagulant at the dose of 0.15 mL ACD per milliliter of blood.
      III. The normal dose for whole blood administration is 10–20% of the calculated blood volume of the patient.
      IV. Blood volume is approximately 10% of a bird's body weight.
      V. Examples: an 80 g cockatiel should be given 0.8–1.6 mL of whole blood, while a 1000 g macaw should be given 10–20 mL of whole blood.
      VI. Although homologous transfusions are preferred, psittacines can usually receive a single transfusion from chickens, raptors, or pigeons. Heterologous blood transfusions are much shorter lived.
      VII. A quick partial cross match should be performed by mixing the recipient's plasma with the donor's erythrocytes. Agglutination or hemolysis indicates incompatibility.

5. Oil contamination of feathers
   A. Apply a water-based ophthalmic ointment into eyes for protection.
   B. Use cornstarch or sawdust as an adsorbent.
   C. Dissolve heavy oil with mineral oil.
   D. Remove light oils and mineral oil with a mild warm dishwashing detergent solution.
   E. Rinse with warm water.
   F. Dry with towels or blow dry.
   G. Provide supportive care.

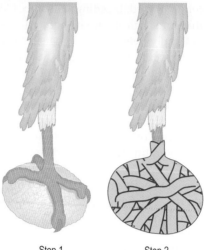

Step 1   Step 2

FIG 15.5 Ball bandage or snowshoe-type bandage. This splint is used for immobilization of the toes. Step 1 – a large ball of soft gauze is placed within the grasp of the foot. Step 2 – the toes are then bound to the ball by wrapping gauze over and around them. Tape is then placed over the gauze. *From Kirk, R.W., 1980. Current Veterinary Therapy VII. WB Saunders; reprinted with permission from Elsevier.*

6. Fractures
    A. Wrap wings in a figure-of-eight pattern if the fracture is distal to humerus (see Fig. 15.2). Add a body wrap to the figure-of-eight bandage if the humerus is fractured.
    B. For fractured or injured digits, use a ball bandage or a snowshoe-type bandage (Fig. 15.5).
    C. For tibiotarsal fractures use tape splints in birds <150 g (Fig. 15.6). The tape splint can serve as a definite treatment for closed fractures, and can remain in place until the fracture is healed. In larger birds use a Robert-Jones bandage or modified Ehmer-type sling to temporarily immobilize the fracture.
    D. Wrap femoral fractures against the body in birds <100 g.
    E. Provide supportive care and analgesia (butorphanol 1–3 mg/kg IM; meloxicam 0.5–1 mg/kg IM, PO) until fracture re-assessment or repair can be performed.
7. Head trauma
    A. Evaluate for bruising or fractures of the cranium, as well as trauma to the eyes, ears, beak, and oral cavity.
    B. Administer crystalloid fluids, ½–⅔ of the normally recommended volume.
    C. Place the bird in a dark, quiet area with an environmental temperature of 75°F (24°C).
    D. Consider the administration of mannitol (0.25–2 mg/kg slow IV, IO) if the bird does not respond to initial therapy or if a worsening neurologic status is suggestive of increased intracerebral edema (i.e. stupor to comatose).
    E. Do not administer corticosteroids.

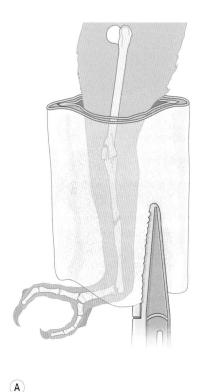
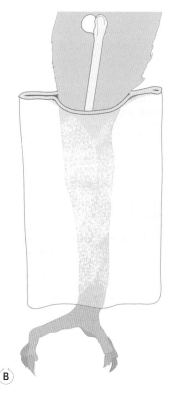

FIG 15.6 **Tape spint application for stabilization of tibiotarsal fractures.** (A) The tape is wrapped around the bird's leg using three to four layers while tension is applied to the leg to keep the fractured segments in apposition. The tibiotarsal-tarsometatarsal joint is flexed in the normal standing position for the species, and the tape is crimped with a needle holder or hemostat. (B) The tape is crimped as close as possible to the muscles surrounding the tibia. With proper angulation of the tibiotarsal–tarsometatarsal joint, the bird can perch in a normal standing position. From Altman, R.B., Clubb, S.L., Dorrestein, G.M., Quesenberry, K., 1997. Avian Medicine and Surgery. WB Saunders; reprinted with permission from Elsevier.

8. Beak trauma
   A. Stop any bleeding
   B. Clean the wounds and debride any loose keratin.
   C. Cover wounds with antimicrobial ointment (e.g. silver sulfadiazine).
   D. Provide supportive care and analgesia (butorphanol 1–3 mg/kg IM; meloxicam 0.5–1 mg/kg IM, PO), if indicated.
   E. Refer to a specialist for further evaluation and advanced beak repair methods if indicated.
9. Seizures
   A. The etiologies include trauma, vascular disease (e.g. hypertension, ischemia), lead poisoning, other intoxications, neoplasia, encephalitis, hepatic encephalopathy, hypocalcemia, hypoglycemia, heat stroke, yolk emboli formation, and idiopathic epilepsy.
   B. For diagnosis, consider CBC, biochemistry profile, blood lead level testing, and whole body radiographs.

C. Seizures in African grey parrots are often due to hypocalcemia. Evaluate ionized calcium levels if possible. Administer calcium gluconate 10–50 mg/kg IM or slow IV or IO (dilute 1:1 with saline or sterile water).

D. Rule out hypoglycemia. If hypoglycemic, administer dextrose (5–10% IV or IO).

E. Evaluate whole body radiographs for metallic GI foreign bodies. Administer calcium EDTA (100 mg/kg IM initial dose, then 40 mg/kg IM q12–24h) if the patient has lead poisoning.

F. Administer midazolam (0.5–3 mg/kg) IM, intranasally, IV or IO to stop ongoing seizures. Alternatively, administer diazepam (0.5–1 mg/kg) IV, IO or intranasally. IM administration of diazepam should be avoided, due to tissue irritation and delayed absorption.

G. Consider antiepileptic drugs for long-term management, after other possible causes for seizures have been ruled out. Phenobarbital may be administered for long-term therapy, but its clinical efficacy varies by species (e.g. not effective in African grey parrots). Use levetiracitam (30–50 mg/kg PO q12h) as an alternative to phenobarbital. Regularly evaluate therapeutic drug levels, and adjust dose and frequency of dosing accordingly.

H. Place the bird in an incubator warmed to 85–90°F (29–32°C), unless the bird has head trauma.

I. Remove all perches from the cage. Use soft bedding. Provide shallow food and water bowls, or spread the bird's food on the cage floor if necessary.

10. Respiratory distress

A. Dyspnea can be caused by various respiratory and nonrespiratory disorders. Any coelomic distention, effusion, organomegaly, obesity, or mass can lead to obliteration of the coelomic air sacs, resulting in dyspnea. Primary respiratory etiologies of dyspnea include: air sacculitis (fungal, bacterial), aspiration pneumonia, inhalation of toxins (e.g. smoke, fumes (e.g. Teflon®)), inhalation of foreign bodies leading to tracheal obstruction (e.g. seeds), tracheal strictures (i.e. post-intubation), and aspiration pneumonia (common in birds that are syringe fed). Tracheal mites are a common cause for dyspnea, common in canaries and other finches.

B. Administer oxygen in an oxygen cage until the bird is stabilized enough for diagnostic tests and definitive therapy.

C. Sedate the bird, if it is distressed or intolerant to manual restraint. Use midazolam (1–2 mg/kg) alone or in combination with butorphanol (1–2 mg/kg) IM or intranasally. Alternatively, administer isoflurane anesthesia. Oxygen mask administration of oxygen may be utilized during physical examination, specimen collection, and treatment.

D. Administer furosemide (2–4 mg/kg IM) if pulmonary edema is suspected.

E. Perform coelomocentesis as a diagnostic and therapeutic technique, if the coelom is fluid distended. Avoid iatrogenic trauma, by performing the centesis ultrasound guided if possible.

F. Administer antibiotics and antifungals if the diagnosis is open or cannot be established.
G. The recommended diagnostic procedures include:
   I. Whole body radiographs
   II. Coelomic ultrasound if coelomic distention is present or if underlying cardiac disease is suspected
   III. Cytology of coelomic fluid
   IV. CBC and plasma biochemistries (including bile acids)
   V. Endoscopy-guided examination or the respiratory tract, for visualization, biopsy, culture, lesion removal, and foreign-body removal
   VI. *Chlamydophila psittaci* testing (PCR from conjunctival–choanal–cloacal swab).
H. Air sac tube placement is indicated if a tracheal obstruction due to a foreign body, stricture or fungal granuloma is suspected. The left lateral approach is most commonly used.
   I. Place the bird in right lateral recumbency.
   II. The tube placement site is located caudal to the last rib.
   III. If possible, perform sterile preparation of the surgery site.
   IV. Make a small skin incision at the tube placement site.
   V. With curved hemostats or blunt scissors, bluntly dissect through the body wall and penetrate the air sac wall. Avoid iatrogenic damage of internal organs.
   VI. Insert a sterile, shortened endotracheal tube or modified, soft-rubber feeding tube of the same diameter, which would be used for endotracheal intubation, through the hole into the air sac.
   VII. Check the tube for patency.
   VIII. Place a butterfly of tape on the tube and suture the tube to the body wall.
   IX. Attach the breathing tube to an oxygen line or anesthetic machine.
   X. Place an e-collar, in order to prevent the bird to manipulate the air sac tube, after recovery from anesthesia.
   XI. Any bird that has had an air sac tube placed is at risk of developing air sacculitis, particularly if the tube is maintained for several days. Therefore limit duration of air sac tube maintenance and treat prophylactically with antibiotics and antifungals.

11. Smoke inhalation
   A. Administer oxygen and nebulize with saline in incubator.
   B. Sedate the bird, if it is distressed or intolerant to manual restraint. Use midazolam (1–2 mg/kg) alone or in combination with butorphanol (1–2 mg/kg) IM or intranasally.
   C. Administer bronchodilators:
      I. Terbutaline (0.1 mg/kg IM, PO or by nebulization (0.01 mg/kg with 9 mL of saline) q12–24h)
      II. Aminophylline (4–10 mg/kg IM, PO or by nebulization (3 mg/mL) q8–12h).

D. Administer nonsteroidal anti-inflammatory drugs – meloxicam (0.5 mg/kg q12h IM, PO).

E. Administer prophylactic antifungal and antibiotic medications.

12. Egg binding or dystocia

A. The etiologies include first-time egg laying, chronic egg laying, oviductal pathology, infection, malnutrition, malformed, oversized or broken eggs, obesity, or stress.

B. The clinical signs vary, based on size of bird and duration of egg binding. Anorexia, depression, a wide-based stance, straining, wagging of the tail, distended coelom, dyspnea, and possibly paralysis of the legs can be seen. Smaller birds (budgerigars, finches, canaries) are often in a more debilitated condition, and require a more aggressive therapy, compared with larger birds.

C. The egg may or may not be palpable.

D. Consider sedation for diagnostic and therapeutic procedures. Use midazolam (1–2 mg/kg) alone or in combination with butorphanol (1–2 mg/kg) IM or intranasally. Consider use of butorphanol (2–3 mg/kg IM) alone, in order to provide analgesia without sedation.

E. Whole body radiographs should always be performed. Standard lateral and ventrodorsal projections are preferred over a 'box shot', because of the greater diagnostic information obtained.

F. Perform a CBC and plasma biochemistries if possible, to rule out underlying or predisposing diseases and to evaluate for secondary complications, such as kidney failure, secondary to compression of the renal vessels and ureters by the retained egg.

G. Administer crystalloid replacement fluids SC, IV, IO as indicated.

H. Administer dextrose, or calcium, if indicated.

I. Administer butorphanol (2–3mg/kg IM) for analgesia.

J. Administer systemic antibiotics, if an underlying bacterial infection is suspected or damage to the oviduct or cloaca is suspected.

K. Place the bird in an incubator warmed to 85–90°F (29–32°C) and increase the humidity (place moist towels in the cage or incubator). Cover incubator with towels, in order to provide dark 'nest-box like' environment.

L. If no response to therapy occurs within several hours or the bird's condition is declining rapidly, and the egg is not located in the cloaca, apply prostaglandin E_2 (0.02–0.1 mg/kg topically) to the uterovaginal sphincter. Prostaglandin E_2 induces relaxation of the uterovaginal sphincter and induces oviductal contractions.

M. If the uterovaginal sphincter is relaxed and uterine adhesions are not suspected, and the egg is not too big, administer oxytocin (2–5 U/kg IM). Calcium should be administered parenterally (10–50 mg/kg IM, dilute 1:1) prior to oxytocin administration.

N. If there is no response to therapy, heavily sedate or anesthetize the bird and apply gentle, persistent pressure to the egg to move it ventrally and caudally into the cloaca. Avoid pushing the egg against the kidneys.

O. In larger birds, if the egg has not passed within 24 hours, perform ovocentesis. If the patient is a small bird, such as a finch or canary, more rapid and aggressive therapy is indicated within a few hours to prevent death.

    I. Heavily sedate or anesthetize the bird.

    II. Manipulate the egg to observe the tip through the uterine opening in the cloaca.

    III. Insert an 18- to 22-gauge needle into the egg and aspirate its contents.

    IV. Carefully collapse the egg by applying digital pressure; avoid placing pressure on the kidneys. Sharp edges or eggshell fragments can damage the uterine and cloacal mucosa.

    V. Remove all accessible eggshell fragments to decrease the incidence of salpingitis and oviductal lacerations.

P. If the egg is located in the cloaca (Fig. 15.7), perform a cloacotomy via a ventral midline incision. Do not cut through the cloacal sphincter. Remove the egg through the surgical incision. Close the cloacal wall with a continuous inverting suture pattern. Close the muscle layer and skin in a simple continuous suture pattern. The advantage of the cloacotomy over cloacocentesis is the reduced risk of iatrogenic trauma by shell fragments, and visualization of the egg during manipulation.

Q. If the uterus is ruptured or ectopic eggs are present, laparotomy is indicated. Refer to a specialist.

13. Cloacal prolapse

A. Cloacal tissues, cloacal masses, oviduct, intestines and/or phallus may be contained in a cloacal prolapse.

B. The etiologies include cloacitis, cloacal masses, enteritis, egg binding, trauma, infection, and neoplasia, or can be related to behavioral disorders in predominately male cockatoos that were hand reared.

C. The recommended diagnostic tests include:

    I. Whole body radiographs

    II. CBC and plasma biochemistry panel

    III. Fecal wet mount and flotation for parasitology

    IV. Diff quick stain of cloacal swab

    V. Cloacoscopy, including tissue biopsies if indicated.

D. Treatment

    I. Administer isoflurane anesthesia or perform sedation.

    II. Administer fluids SC, IV or IO.

    III. If the oviduct is prolapsed, examine it for an egg (Fig. 15.7A).

    IV. If an egg is present, follow the treatment recommendations for egg binding.

    V. If an egg is not present, continue to follow these recommendations.

    VI. To reduce the oviduct swelling and aid in controlling hemorrhage, apply 50% dextrose solution topically.

    VII. Rinse the prolapsed tissue with warm saline.

    VIII. After identification of the prolapsed tissue, apply sterile lubricating jelly.

    IX. With a lubricated sterile swab, replace the prolapsed tissues.

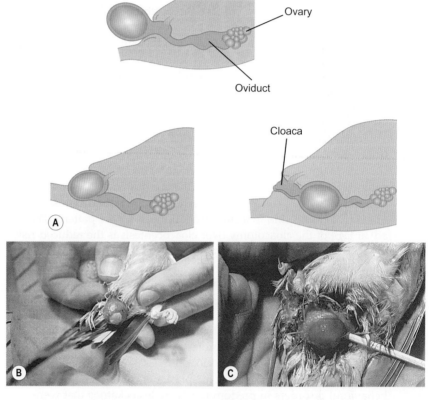

Ovary

Oviduct

Cloaca

(A)

(B)

(C)

FIG 15.7 **Egg binding.** (A). Three positions of egg binding. (Top) position 1: the egg is wrapped in the prolapsed oviduct, external to the cloacal opening. (Bottom left) position 2: the egg wrapped in the oviduct is retained in the cloaca and pelvic canal. (Bottom right) position 3: the egg is in the vagina, within the coelomic cavity, unable to pass the vaginal–cloacal orifice. (B) Egg-bound budgerigar (*Melopsittacus undulatus*) as seen in position 1. (C) The egg is in the pelvic canal and cloaca as seen in position 2. *From Altman, R.B., Clubb, S.L., Dorrestein, G.M., Quesenberry, K., 1997. Avian Medicine and Surgery. WB Saunders; reprinted with permission from Elsevier.*

    X. Place retention sutures (two simple transverse sutures) perpendicular to the vent. Stainless steel sutures are preferred.

    XI. Administer analgesics: butorphanol (2–3 mg/kg IM) and meloxicam (0.5 mg/kg IM, PO q12h).

    XII. Administer broad-spectrum antibiotics, if indicated.

    XIII. Identify and treat the underlying etiology. Recommend referral to a specialist.

14. Egg-related peritonitis

    A. Most commonly seen in cockatiels and budgerigars. Underlying etiologies include salpingitis, oviductal impaction, oviductal tumors, ruptured oviducts or previously performed surgical removal of the oviduct for treatment of reproductive disorders.

B. The clinical signs include anorexia, ascites, depression, dyspnea, weight loss and possibly coelomic distention. The process can be sterile or complicated by a bacterial infection, which results in more severe clinical signs and a poorer prognosis.

C. Perform whole body radiographs. Evaluate for presence of medullary deposition of calcium within the long bones (medullary bone, 'egg-laying bone') or calcified eggs.

D. Perform coelomocentesis as a diagnostic and therapeutic technique, if the coelom is fluid distended. Avoid iatrogenic trauma by performing the centesis ultrasound-guided if possible.

Obtained coelomic fluid may be clear to opaque, yellow, green or brown in color. Microscopically, it is comprised of inflammatory cells in a granular background, degenerative heterophils and, possibly, yolk or fat globules, or intracellular bacteria can be seen.

E. Treatment
   I. Provide supportive care.
   II. Administer meloxicam (0.5 mg/kg IM, PO q12h), if kidney function is normal.
   III. Administer antibiotic therapy based on culture and sensitivity results in case of septic peritonitis.
   IV. Administer leuprolide acetate, in order to suppress ovulation and ovarian activity temporarily (300–800 µg/kg IM). Duration of action of leuprolide is approximately 14–21 days in birds.

15. Regurgitation
   A. Underlying etiologies include: irritation or infections of the crop, crop stasis, lead intoxication, proventricular dilatation disease (PDD), foreign bodies in the crop, underlying organ disease (e.g. liver disease), chlamydophilosis, as well as goiter in budgerigars. It is important to differentiate these pathological causes for regurgitation from physiological regurgitation as part of courtship feeding behavior displayed predominately by male birds to either owners or toys (e.g. mirrors). Birds showing behavioral regurgitation are otherwise normal, and continue to eat and are alert and hydrated.
   B. Withhold food until the regurgitation is controlled.
   C. Administer crystalloid replacement fluids SC. In severe cases, administer fluids IV or IO.
   D. The recommended diagnostic tests include:
      I. Wet mount and Diff quick stain of a crop aspirate or wash
      II. Bacterial culture of crop aspirate or wash
      III. CBC and plasma biochemistries (including bile acids)
      IV. Whole body radiographs
      V. Measurement of blood lead and zinc levels.
   E. When the etiology is diagnosed, treat the underlying cause.
   F. Crop stasis leads to secondary bacterial overgrowth. Use ball-tipped gavage needle to empty the crop, lavage with warmed saline and

instill antimicrobials (amoxicillin / clavulanic acid 100–150 mg/kg PO q8h) and / or nystatin (100 000–300 000U/kg PO q8h).

16. Delayed crop emptying or crop stasis
    A. Any debilitating illness may cause crop stasis.
    B. The recommended diagnostic tests include:
        I. Wet mount and Diff quick stain of a crop aspirate
        II. Bacterial culture of the crop aspirate
        III. CBC and plasma biochemistries (including bile acids)
        IV. Whole body radiographs
        V. Blood lead and zinc levels
        VI. *Chlamydophila psittaci* testing.
    C. When the etiology is diagnosed, treat the underlying cause.
    D. Use a ball-tipped gavage needle to empty the crop; lavage with warmed saline. Massage the fluid and the material and then aspirate it from the crop.
    E. Instill antibiotics directly into the crop (amoxicillin / clavulanic acid 100–150 mg/kg PO q8h). Administer nystatin (100 000–300 000 U/kg PO q8h), if a large amount of yeast or budding yeast is seen on cytology of crop content.
    F. If the bird is debilitated, perform an ingluviotomy (crop incision) and evacuate the crop and administer broad-spectrum antibiotics parenterally.
    G. Administer crystalloid fluids SC, or IV/IO in cases of severe dehydration.
    H. When crop motility resumes, feed diluted hand-feeding formula and gradually increase the consistency to normal.
    I. Do not use prokinetic drugs such as metoclopramide.

17. Crop burns
    A. Administer antibiotics and antifungals.
    B. Feed the bird small volumes of food frequently, or use a proventricular feeding tube.
    C. Monitor the bird for 7–14 days, until the wound contracts and a fistula appears.
    D. After a fistula has formed, remove the scab from the crop burn and debride the necrotic skin and crop.
    E. Surgically close the wound.

18. Diarrhea
    A. Differentiate true diarrhea from polyuria. Polyuria is more common than diarrhea, but is often misidentified as diarrhea. Only if the fecal portion of the dropping is no longer formed should it be called diarrhea.
    B. The recommended diagnostic tests include:
        I. Wet mount and Diff quick stain of feces
        II. Fecal flotation
        III. Whole body radiographs
        IV. CBC and plasma biochemistry (including bile acids)
        V. Bacterial culture of feces or cloaca
        VI. Blood zinc levels.
    C. When the etiology is diagnosed, treat the underlying cause.

D. Administer crystalloid replacement fluids SC if the bird is dehydrated. Administer fluids IO or IV in cases of severe dehydration.

E. If the animal is depressed and sepsis is suspected, administer parenteral bactericidal broad Gram-negative spectrum antibiotics pending culture results (e.g. enrofloxacin 20 mg/kg IM, SC q12–24h, piperacillin 100–200 mg/kg IM q6–12h).

F. Identify and treat the underlying cause.

DRUG DOSAGES

Allopurinol: 10–30 mg/kg PO q12–24h

Aminophylline: 4–10 mg/kg IM, PO or by nebulization (3 mg/ mL), q8–12h

Amoxicillin / clavulanic acid: 100–150 mg/kg PO q8–12h

Amphotericin B: 1.5–4 mg/kg IO, IV q8h for 3–7 days; 1 mg/kg IT q8–12h; 0.5 mg/ mL for nebulization

Atropine: 0.1–0.5 mg/kg IT, IV, IO, IM (higher doses for CPR)

Azithromycin: 40 mg/kg PO q24–48h

Barium: 20 mL/kg PO

Butorphanol: 1–3 mg/kg IM, IN q2–4h

Calcium EDTA: 100 mg/kg IM initial dose, then 40 mg/kg IM q12–24h

Calcium gluconate: 10–50 mg/kg slowly IV to effect or IM, dilute prior to administration

Carnidazole (Spartix®): 20–30 mg/kg PO for 1–2 days

Cefotaxime: 75–100 mg/kg IM, IV q6–8h

Ceftazidime: 75v100 mg/kg IM, IV q4–8h

Ceftiofur sodium: 10 mg/kg IM q4–8h

Ceftiofur crystalline-free acid (Excede®): 10 mg/kg IM q72h (waterfowl)

Cephalexin: 100 mg/kg PO q8–12h

Ciprofloxacin: 10–20 mg/kg PO q12h

Clindamycin: 50–100 mg/kg PO, IM q12–14h

Clomipramine: 1–3 mg/kg PO q12–24h

Clotrimazole: 10 mg/ mL (1%) for nebulization or nasal flush

Dexamethasone sodium phosphate: 2–4 mg/kg IM, IV, q12–24h (avoid use if possible – immunosuppression and secondary fungal infections are likely; prophylactically prescribe antifungals)

Dextrose: 50–100 mg/kg IV slowly to effect

Diazepam: 0.5–1 mg/kg IN, IV, IO PRN

Diphenhydramine: 2–4 mg/kg PO q8–12h

Doxapram: 5–10 mg/kg IV, IM

Doxycycline: 35–40 mg/kg PO q24h (drug of choice for treatment of chlamydophilosis, may cause regurgitation, use lower dosages in macaws and lorikeets)

Enalapril: 1.25 mg/kg PO q12h

Enilconazole: 2–10 mg/ mL for nebulization or topical for fungal skin infections

Enrofloxacin: 10–25 mg/kg IM, SC, PO, IV q12–24h

Epinephrine (1:1000): 0.5–1 mL/kg IV, IO, IT, IM

Erythromycin: 60 mg/kg PO q12h

Fenbendazole: 10–50 mg/kg PO q24h for 5–10 days *(toxicity reported in pigeons and doves)*

Fluconazole: 2–5 mg/kg PO q24h *(use against yeasts, not for aspergillus spp., penetrates well into brain, CSF, and eyes)*

Fluoxetine: 2–3 mg/kg PO q12–24h

Furosemide: 2–4 mg/kg IM, IV, IO PO PRN

Gentamicin: 5 mg/ mL for nebulization 15–30 minutes q8h

Haloperidol: 0.1–0.2 mg/kg PO q12–24h

Hetastarch: 10–15 mL/kg IV

Iron dextran: 10 mg/kg IM; repeat in 7–10 days if needed

Isoxsuprine: 10 mg/kg PO q24h *(vasodilator, for treatment of ischemia)*

Itraconazole: 5–10 mg/kg PO q12h *(avoid use in African grey parrots or use lower dose of 5 mg/kg PO q24h; use lower doses for prophylaxis only)*

Ivermectin: 0.2–0.4 mg/kg IM, SC, PO; repeat in 10–14 days

Ketoconazole: 20–30 mg/kg PO q12h for 14–30 days *(narrow therapeutic margin, toxicity common, avoid use if possible)*

Leuprolide acetate (Lupron depot®): 300–800 µg/kg IM, q14–21d

Levetiracitam (Keppra®) 30–50 mg/kg PO q12h *(perform therapeutic blood levels)*

Levamisole: 20–40 mg/kg PO q10d

Mannitol: 0.25–0.5 mg/kg slow IV

Marbofloxacin 2.5–5 mg/kg PO q24h (psittacines), 10–15 mg/kg PO q12–24h (raptors)

Meloxicam 0.5–1 mg/kg PO, IM, IV q12–24h *(do not administer to dehydrated birds or if renal function is impaired)*

Metronidazole: 20–30 mg/kg PO q12h

Midazolam 1–2 mg/kg IM, IN, IV, IO PRN

Nystatin: 100000–300000 IU/kg PO q8–12h *(for yeast infections of the GI tract only, not systemically absorbed after PO administration)*

Oxytocin: 2–5 U/kg IM; may repeat in 30 minutes

Phenobarbital: 2–7 mg/kg or higher PO q12h *(monitor therapeutic blood levels; no therapeutic drug levels reached in African grey parrots after 17 mg/kg PO single dose)*

Piperacillin: 100–200 mg/kg IM, IV q6–12h

Praziquantel: 5–10 mg/kg PO, IM; repeat in 10–14 days if necessary

Prostaglandin E_2: 0.02–0.1mg/kg applied topically to uterovaginal sphincter

Pyrantel pamoate: 5–20 mg/kg PO; repeat in 10–14 days

Sulfadimethoxine: 25–50 mg/kg PO q24h

Terbinafine 20–30 mg/kg q24h PO

Terbutaline: 0.1 mg/kg IM, PO q12–24h, 0.01 mg/kg with 9 mL of saline

Theophylline 2 mg/kg PO q12h

Ticarcillin: 150–200 mg/kg IM, IV q2–4h

Trimethoprim-sulfamethoxazole: 15–30 mg/kg PO q12h

Vitamin A: 5000–20000 U/kg IM, PO

Vitamin K_1: 2–10 mg/kg SC, IM, PO

Voriconazole: 18 mg/kg PO q8h (Amazon parrots), q12h (African grey parrot).

CHINCHILLAS (*CHINCHILLA LANIGERA*)

Chinchillas are nocturnal and originate from the slopes of the Andes mountains of Argentina, Bolivia, Chile, and Peru. They are very active and require a lot of space. Multilevel housing is recommended, due to their enjoyment of jumping and climbing. They may be kept in pairs, colonies, or polygamous units. Daily access to a dust bath should be provided.

In the wild, they feed on grasses and shrubs. In captivity, the chinchilla's diet should consist mainly of good-quality grass hay, with 1–2 tablespoons per day of commercial chinchilla or rabbit pellets. Provide a calcium carbonate stone.

Adult average body weight = 400–800 g.

Average life span = 10 years, but they may live as long as 18 years.

Chinchillas are sexually mature at about 8 months of age and are seasonally polyestric. The main breeding season is between November and May. The estrus lasts 3–4 days, and the entire estrus cycle is 28–35 days. In females the vaginal opening is sealed by a membrane, except during estrus and during birth.

Gestation period = 105–118 days. Litter size = 1–6; average is 2. The newborns are precocious.

If there is insufficient mother's milk, the kits can be hand fed warm 50:50 evaporated milk / boiled water with dextrose added to make a 25% solution. Feed a few drops from an eyedropper every 2–3 hours in the first week, and then free choice every 8 hours until weaned. Chinchillas start eating solid food within 1 week of age and the weaning age is usually 6–8 weeks of age.

Heart rate = 100–150 beats/min.

Respiratory rate = 40–80 breaths/min.

Temperature = 98.6–100.4°F (37–38.0°C).

Normal blood values in chinchillas include:

PCV = 27–54%	Glucose = 109–193 mg/dL
TP = 3.8–5.6 g/dL	Phosphorus = 4–8 mg/dL
WBC = 5.4–15600/mL	Calcium = 5.6–12.1 mg/dL
BUN = 17–45 mg/dL	Potassium = 3.3–5.7 mEq/L
Creatinine = 0.4–1.3 mg/dL	Sodium = 142–166 mEq/L

Restraint—All restraint should be gentle to avoid fur 'slip', in which fur comes off in the handler's hand.

Sex determination—

- Males: A considerable distance (twice the distance of females) separates the penis from the anus. The testicles are in hemiscrotal sacs on each side lateral to the anus.
- Females: The anus is immediately caudal to the genital vaginal opening, which is sealed over unless the animal is in estrus or has underlying reproductive disease. Ventral to the vagina is a cone-shaped urethral papilla, on which the urethra ends, outside the vagina. There is one nipple in each lateral rib area and one in each inguinal area.

Sedation—

- Midazolam 0.5–1 mg/kg SC/IM.
- Midazolam 0.5 mg/kg + butorphanol (0.25 mg/kg) SC/IM.

Anesthesia—
- Dexmedetomidine 0.025 mg/kg + ketamine 5 mg/kg SC/IM.
- Isoflurane induction by mask after premedication.

Chinchilla fluid therapy

1. The daily maintenance fluid requirements are 60–100 mL/kg/day. For SC fluid administration, use LRS, Normosol®-R, or a similar balanced electrolyte isotonic crystalloid.
2. For IV or IO fluid administration, 5% dextrose may be added to the fluids if desired. Colloids and blood may also be administered IV or IO.
3. Only warmed (100–102°F (38–39°C)) fluids should be administered.
4. The shock fluid volume for chinchillas in 10–25 mL/kg IV or IO over 5–7 minutes.
5. Peripheral veins, including the cephalic, lateral saphenous, jugular and femoral veins, are usually accessible.
6. Intraosseous catheters may be placed through the trochanteric fossa into the femur or through the tibial crest into the tibia.
   A. Clip and surgically prepare the catheter site.
   B. Use either a spinal needle (20- or 22-gauge) or a syringe needle.
   C. The use of a stylet is highly recommended.
   D. Gently advance the needle through the bone into the marrow cavity with a gentle twisting motion.
   E. Aspirate until blood is visualized in the hub of the needle after removing the stylet.
   F. Flush the needle with heparinized saline.
   G. Suture tape tabs around the catheter to secure it to the skin.
   H. Administer intraosseous fluids.
   I. The catheter may be used for as long as 72 hours; then it should be removed.

CHINCHILLA NUTRITIONAL SUPPORT

1. Any anorexic or hyporexic chinchilla should receive nutritional support to minimize secondary gastrointestinal problems caused by reduced food intake (i.e. dysbacteriosis, constipation, tympany) and to avoid increased fat mobilization, which frequently leads to hepatic lipidosis and ketoacidosis.
2. Syringe feed with high-fiber diet for herbivores (e.g. Oxbow Critical Care for Herbivores®, 50–80 mL/kg PO q24h; divide in 4–5 feedings) or crushed and soaked pellets. Do not syringe feed an animal which is not swallowing.

COMMON DISEASES AND HEALTH PROBLEMS OF CHINCHILLAS

1. Gastrointestinal disease (diarrhea, constipation, rectal prolapse, tympany)
   A. Noninfectious causes (e.g. sudden change in diet, inappropriate oral antibiotic therapy) or infectious etiologies (parasites, bacteria) can be

found in chinchillas. Most infectious causes occur secondary to a noninfectious primary cause, which predisposes to dysbacteriosis leading to excessive replication of opportunistic pathogens such as *Giardia*. Gastrointestinal disorders include dysbacteriosis, enteritis, diarrhea, constipation, intussusception and rectal tissue prolapse, and tympany.

B. Diagnostic tests should include:
   I. Whole body radiographs
   II. Fecal wet mount and Diff quick stain
   III. Fecal flotation.

C. If the animal has diarrhea, perform fecal parasitology to rule out *Giardia duodenalis* or *Eimeria chinchillae*. Rule out dietary causes.
   I. Feed a high-quality grass-hay diet and administer fluids if the animal is dehydrated.
   II. Treat *Giardia* with metronidazole or fenbendazole. Treat *Eimeria* with sulfonamides (e.g. trimethoprim-sulfa drugs).
   III. Provide nutritional support, if the animal is anorexic.
   IV. Administer the appropriate antibiotic parenterally if severe bacterial enteritis is suspected and the risk of bacterial translocation and sepsis is high.

D. If the animal is not producing feces, rule out an intestinal intussusception. If the animal is constipated, small and irregular shaped fecal pellets in reduced numbers will be produced. Constipation is common in chinchillas, and is considered a secondary complication to many other etiologies, such as anorexia, dental disease, or systemic infections or organ disease. Identify the underlying cause and rehydrate the animal.

E. If constipation was diagnosed:
   I. Administer fluids subcutaneously initially (30–50 mL/kg SC), and then switch to oral fluids, in order to rehydrate the ingesta in the cecum and colon.
   II. Administer a critical care diet for herbivores by syringe (50–80 mL/kg/day, divide in 3–5 feedings per day).
   III. Diagnose and treat the primary underlying cause for constipation.

F. If a rectal tissue prolapse was diagnosed:
   I. Differentiate between rectal prolapse and intestinal prolapse secondary to an intussusception.
   II. Intussusceptions require immediate surgical correction. The prognosis is poor.
   III. Simple prolapse of the rectum can be treated as in other species. Identify and treat the underlying cause leading to rectal prolapse.
   IV. Provide additional symptomatic and supportive care based on the individual needs of the patient.

G. If tympany of the stomach and/or intestine was diagnosed:
   I. Administer shock rate fluids intravenously or intraosseously.
   II. Provide analgesia (buprenorphine (0.03–0.05 mg/kg SC, IM, IV).

III. Attempt decompression of the stomach if severely tympanic. Sedate the animal and use a lubricated large-diameter red rubber tube orally.

IV. Administer enrofloxacin (10 mg/kg IM, IV) owing to the usually concurrent or underlying dysbacteriosis.

V. The prognosis is poor if the animal is in shock, lateral recumbent or hypothermic.

2. Dental disease

A. Chinchillas have continuously growing cheek teeth and incisor teeth. Overgrowth and abnormal wear of the cheek teeth can lead to sharp edges or points, which cause lingual and particular buccal gingival ulceration.

B. The clinical signs include partial to complete anorexia, excessive drooling and wet fur around the chin, chest, and forepaws, weight loss, constipation, and poor fur condition.

C. Complete examination of the cheek teeth is only possible under general anesthesia and by the use of the mouth gag and cheek dilators. The use of an otoscope or ideally a rigid endoscope is highly recommended.

D. Complete evaluation and appropriate treatment of dental lesions in chinchillas is challenging, and even a severe dental lesion may be missed by an inexperienced person. Therefore consider referral to a specialist if one is unfamiliar with dental examination and treatments in chinchillas.

E. Use a low-speed dental drill with a diamond burr and soft tissue protector to remove dental spurs and shorten overgrown cheek teeth.

F. Chinchillas are commonly affected by periodontal disease as well as dental caries. Treatment includes debridement and cleaning of periodontal pockets and treatment with long-acting penicillin benzathine (40 000–60 000 IU/kg SC q5d) or another antibiotic with good anaerobic bacterial coverage.

G. Provide the appropriate supportive care as indicated:

I. Nutritional support if the animal is not eating

II. Fluid therapy (30–50 mL/kg SC bolus)

III. Analgesia (buprenorphine 0.03–0.05mg/kg SC), meloxicam (0.3–0.5 mg/kg SC, PO) if the animal is adequately hydrated and has a normal renal function.

H. Dental disease in chinchillas is progressive and a cure is usually not achieved. Recurrence of clinical signs is common and therefore regular dental treatment under general anesthesia need to be performed often for the rest of the animal's life.

3. Seizures and neurologic deficits

A. Hypocalcemia, hypoglycemia, hyperthermia, sepsis, cerebral nematodiasis, otitis media and interna and lead poisoning may cause seizures in chinchillas.

B. Administer midazolam, 0.5–1 mg/kg IM, IN or IV immediately.

C. Attempt to determine and treat the underlying etiology. Perform a biochemistry profile and a CBC to rule out extracranial causes.

D. Carefully evaluate the external ear canal and tympanic membranes. Perform a dorsoventral skull radiograph or CT scan of the head to rule out otitis media and interna. If otitis media was diagnosed, collect a sterile sample of the middle ear, through the dorsal wall of the tympanic bulla under anesthesia, prior to starting antibiotic therapy.

E. Sepsis is a common cause for neurologic deficits, depression and anorexia in chinchilla. Gram-negative aerobic bacteria such as *Pseudomonas aeruginosa*, *Escherichia coli* and others commonly cause systemic infections in chinchillas. Due to the advanced stage the chinchillas are usually presented in, the prognosis is poor. Treat empirically with broad-spectrum antibiotics with activity against these organisms (e.g. enrofloxacin 10 mg/kg SC, IM, IV). Administer any antibiotic parenterally, owing to impaired GI function. Provide supportive care.

F. Chinchillas affected by cerebrospinal nematodiasis with *Balisascaris procyonis* may exhibit ataxia, paralysis and torticollis. Raccoon feces contamination of hay, straw, or feed is the most common cause. Carefully review the husbandry history. There is no treatment.

G. Acute blindness and seizures may be due to lead poisoning.
  I. Measure the blood lead level. If the blood lead level is >25 mg/dL, the diagnosis is lead poisoning.
  II. Treatment includes the administration of calcium EDTA (30 mg/kg SC q12h) and symptomatic supportive therapy

4. Eye problems
  A. Chinchillas have a large and exposed corneal segment, possibly predisposing them to corneal trauma. They have only a rudimentary third eye lid.
  B. Conjunctivitis can be unilateral or bilateral. Infectious and noninfectious causes need to be distinguished.
    I. Common noninfectious causes are excessive dust bathing, inadequate cage ventilation or underlying nasolacrimal duct obstruction. These conditions can be complicated by secondary bacterial infections usually of the physiological conjunctival flora, which consist predominantly of Gram-positive bacteria.
    II. Primary bacterial conjunctivitis can be caused by *Pseudomonas aeruginosa*, as either a localized infection of the conjunctiva or part of a systemic infection. If the animal is active, eating and producing feces, then a localized infection is more likely. Animals that present with purulent conjunctivitis, and are depressed and anorexic, are more likely to suffer from a systemic pseudomonadal infection, and require aggressive and immediate therapy with empirically selected systemic antibiotics (i.e. enrofloxacin 10 mg/kg SC, IM, q12h; ceftazidime 30 mg/kg SC, IM, q8h) and supportive care in addition to treatment of the conjunctivitis.
    III. Collect a conjunctival swab for aerobic bacterial culture in all cases of purulent conjunctivitis.
    IV. Thoroughly lavage the conjunctival sac with physiological saline.
    V. Apply topical ophthalmic broad-spectrum antibiotics with coverage against possible pseudomonadal infections

(e.g. gentamicin, ciprofloxacin). Adjust antibiotic selection based on bacterial culture and sensitivity results. Avoid the use of ophthalmic ointments; use solutions instead.

VI. Carefully monitor the animal for changes in general condition, which could indicate a systemic disease process.

VII. Provide nutritional support if the animal is anorexic.

C. Corneal ulceration is often due to trauma from the cage interior or excessive dust bathing. Corneal ulcers frequently become secondarily infected by bacteria. Diagnosis is made by positive fluorescein dye uptake by corneal stroma. Treatment includes topical administration of antibiotics (e.g. gentamicin, ciprofloxacin). Treatment of complex or indolent ulcers is the same as in other species. Provide supportive care, if indicated.

D. Epiphora is characterized by bilateral or unilateral clear ocular discharge. The most common underlying cause is apical elongation of the reserve crowns of the maxillary cheek teeth, which leads to compression of the nasolacrimal ducts. Diagnosis is by skull radiography. Treatment includes topical and systemic application of nonsteroidal anti-inflammatory drugs. Since there is no specific treatment, recurrence is common.

5. Paraphimosis
   A. A fur ring may encircle the base of the glans penis, preventing retraction into the prepuce.
   B. Extreme penile swelling, urinary obstruction and vascular compromise to the penis may result.
   C. Lubricate and gently roll or cut off the fur ring.
   D. General anesthesia or sedation may be needed to facilitate the procedure.
   E. Do not force the glans penis back into the prepuce, if the presence of tissue swelling does not allow this. Keep the glans penis and everted preputial mucosa moist and clean by applying silver sulfadiazine cream or hydrogel. Do not use ointments containing bacitracin.

6. Heat stress
   A. Due to their natural environment of cool temperatures, high in the Andes mountains, chinchillas are highly susceptible to temperatures >80°F (27°C).
   B. The detrimental effects of high temperature worsen when accompanied by high humidity.
   C. Chinchillas with heat prostration will exhibit panting, hyperthermia, recumbency, cyanosis and death.
   D. Administer intravenous or intraosseous fluids and keep in a cool environment.

RECOMMENDED DRUG DOSAGES FOR CHINCHILLAS

Amoxicillin: Not recommended for oral administration
Ampicillin: Not recommended for oral administration
Atropine: 0.1–0.2 mg/kg IM or SC

Azithromycin: 30 mg/kg PO q24h
Buprenorphine: 0.03–0.05 mg/kg SC q8–12h
Butorphanol: 0.2–0.4 mg/kg SC q4h
Calcium disodium versenate (EDTA): 30 mg/kg SC q12h
Ceftazidime: 30 mg/kg IM, SC, IV, IO q8h
Cephalosporins: Not recommended for oral administration
Chloramphenicol palmitate: 30–50 mg/kg PO q8–12h
Clindamycin: Not recommended for oral administration
Dexamethasone: 0.5–2 mg/kg IV, IM, IP, SC
Dexmedetomidine 0.025 mg/kg + ketamine 5mg/kg SC/IM
Diazepam: 0.5–2 mg/kg IV
Doxycycline: 5 mg/kg PO q12h
Enrofloxacin: 10 mg/kg IM, SC, IV, PO q12–24h
Erythromycin: Not recommended for oral administration
Fenbendazole: 20–50 mg/kg PO q24h for 5 days
Furosemide: 2–4 mg/kg IM, SC, IV PO PRN
Gentamicin: Not recommended due to nephrotoxicity
Itraconazole 5–10 mg/kg PO q24h
Lincomycin: Not recommended for oral administration
Metronidazole: 20–30 mg/kg PO q12h *(may lead to anorexia dependent on formulation used)*
Midazolam: 0.5–1 mg/kg IM, SC, IV, IO
Nystatin: 100 000 U/kg PO q8h for 5 days
Oxytocin: 0.5–1 IU IM
Penicillin G benzathine: 40 000–60 000 IU/kg SC q5d.
Praziquantel: 6–10 mg/kg PO, SC; repeat in 10 days
Terbinafine: 10–30 mg/kg PO q24h
Trimethoprim-sulfa: 30 mg/kg PO q12h

FERRETS (MUSTELA PUTORIUS FURO)

There are two varieties: the fitch and the albino. Females are called jills, males are hobs, and babies are kits.

Adult body weight male = 1–2 kg; females 0.5–1 kg.

Average life span = 5–7 years.

Sexual maturity = 8–12 months (1st spring following birth). Estrus cycle = induced ovulators, seasonally polyestrus (March–September).

Gestation period = 39–44 days (average = 41); average litter size = 8. Ears and eyes open at 28–34 days of age, weaning is usually at 6–8 weeks.

Heart rate = 180–250 bpm.

Respiratory rate = 30–40 bpm.

Temperature = 100–104°F (37.8–40.0°C).

Normal blood values in ferrets include:

PCV = 36–48%
TP = 5.1–7.4 g/dL
WBC = 4300–10 700/mL
BUN = 10–45 mg/dL
Creatinine = 0.2–1 mg/dL
Glucose = 62–207 mg/dL

Phosphorus = 4–9 mg/dL
Calcium = 8–12 mg/dL
Potassium = 4.3–7.7 mEq/L
Sodium = 137–162 mEq/L
Bilirubin, total = <1 mg/dL
ALP = 9–120 U/L

ALT = 82–289 U/L   GGT = 0–5 U/L.
AST = 28–248 U/L

The jugular veins lie more laterally than those in a dog or cat. The ferret also lacks an appendix, cecum and teniae coli. The trachea is unusually long.

The male ferret has a 'J' shaped os penis, making urethral catheterization challenging.

Medications are usually administered at dosages used in cats, on a perkilogram basis. Intramuscular injections should be administered in the quadriceps muscle group, rather than the semimembranosus/semitendinosus, owing to the small muscle mass of the later group. Blood groups have not been demonstrated in ferrets, so cross matching is not necessary. A ferret should not be held off food for more than 6 hours without supplemental glucose administration.

Vaccinations are recommended against canine distemper (Purevax®, a live canary pox vector canine distemper vaccine, is the only distemper vaccine approved for ferrets) and rabies virus (inactivated, administered SC annually). Vaccine reaction can occur; consider premedication with diphenhydramine (2 mg/kg IM).

Diet—Ferrets are obligate carnivores and should be fed a high in fat (15–20%) and animal protein (30–35%) diet, with minimal carbohydrates or fiber. A whole prey diet is ideal, but most pet ferrets are fed a commercial dry ferret kibble diet.

Ferret nutritional support

1. Any anorexic or cachexic ferret should receive nutritional support unless a GI obstruction is suspected.
2. Feed a critical care diet formula for carnivores (e.g. Oxbow Critical Care for Carnivores® or Lafaber Emeraid Carnivore®) or a canned critical diet (e.g. Hill's a/d®).

Sedation— Midazolam 0.25 mg/kg *plus* butorphanol 0.25 mg/kg SC. Reverse with flumazenil 0.02 mg/kg *plus* naloxone 0.04 mg/kg SC. Moderate to deep sedation and rapid recovery are achieved with this protocol.

Anesthesia—

1. Premedicate with midazolam 0.25 mg/kg *plus* butorphanol 0.25 mg/kg SC.
2. Place IV catheter in cephalic vein.
3. Administer propofol 2–5 mg/kg IV for induction.
4. Perform endotracheal intubation using a 2–4 mm ET tube.
5. Maintain on isoflurane or sevoflurane.

Venipuncture in ferrets

1. Limited amounts of blood can be collected from the cephalic and lateral saphenous veins.
2. Larger blood samples can be collected from the jugular veins or from the cranial vena cava.

Intravenous catheter placement in ferrets

1. The cephalic, lateral saphenous, and jugular veins are usually accessible. The cephalic vein is recommended owing to ease of access and placement.
2. Use a 22- or 24-gauge catheter for the lateral saphenous or cephalic veins.
3. Sedation may be necessary unless the patient is debilitated.
4. It may be beneficial to puncture the skin at the placement site with a needle prior to attempting catheterization.
5. A 22-gauge, 8-inch (20 cm) through-the-needle catheter on a 19-gauge needle is recommended for jugular catheterization.
6. IO catheterization may be performed with a 20- or 22-gauge 1.5-inch (38 mm) spinal needle.
    A. The recommended sites for IO catheterization, in order of preference, include the femur, tibia and humerus.
    B. Anesthesia or deep sedation and a local anesthetic block should be administered.
    C. The technique is the same as that for a cat.
7. IV or IO catheters should be secured to the skin with tissue glue or butterfly tape tabs prior to applying a bandage.
8. Only small volumes of heparinized saline should be used when flushing any catheter in a ferret to avoid heparin overdosage.
9. Ferrets are prone to chew through IV lines and remove IV catheters. Incorporate a piece of syringe case in the bandage covering cephalic catheter site, to prevent damage. Keep ferret mildly sedated if necessary.
10. Daily maintenance fluid requirements are as in cats (60–70 mL/kg/day).

Urethral catheterization of the male ferret

1. Anesthesia or deep sedation is usually required.
2. Place the ferret in dorsal recumbency.
3. Aseptically prepare the prepuce.
4. The penile urethral opening lies on the ventral surface of the penis several millimeters proximal to the tip of the os.
5. The use of a surgical loupe or other magnification device will be beneficial.
6. The following catheters can be used for urethral catheterization:
    A. 3.0 or 3.5 Fr polytetrafluoroethylene urinary catheter (Slippery Sam Tomcat® urethral catheters, Smiths Medical, Norwell, KY)
    B. 3.5 Fr rubber feeding catheter
    C. A 20- or 22-gauge 8-inch (20 cm) jugular catheter with the stylet removed has been recommended as the urethral catheter.
7. If resistance is met during catheterization, the catheter may be flushed with sterile saline.
8. At the pelvic flexure, extreme caution should be used to avoid urethral perforation.
9. Secure the catheter to the skin by suturing tape butterflies to the skin.

10. Maintain the catheter on a closed collection system.
11. Prevent the ferret from removing the bandages or catheter, by maintaining sedation or placing an e-collar if necessary.

Ferret cardiopulmonary resuscitation

1. Use a 2.0–4.0 mm endotracheal tube to establish an airway.
2. Place the ferret in lateral recumbency.
3. Ventilate at a rate of 20–30 breaths/minute.
4. Be careful not to overinflate the lungs.
5. If cardiac arrest occurs, gently perform external cardiac massage at a rate of 100 compressions/minute.
6. Evaluate the cardiac rhythm with an ECG.
7. Monitor the strength and character of the femoral pulse frequently.
8. Place an intravenous catheter and administer isotonic crystalloids at a rate of 70 mL/kg/h IV.
9. If indicated, administer epinephrine: 0.02mg/kg IV, IO, IT.
10. If the heart is beating but bradycardic, administer atropine:
    A. 0.05 mg/kg IV or IO
    B. 0.10 mg/kg diluted with sterile water and delivered intratracheally.

COMMON DISEASES AND HEALTH PROBLEMS OF FERRETS

1. Gastrointestinal foreign bodies
   A. Common in ferrets less than 2 years of age, rubber, cloth, and latex objects are the most common GI foreign bodies. Trichobezoars are more common in older ferrets.
   B. Linear foreign bodies are uncommon.
   C. The ferret may resist abdominal palpation, grind its teeth, have a palpable fluid-dilated stomach or bowel, or may have a palpable foreign body.
   D. Vomiting is not common in ferrets with GI foreign bodies.
   E. Radiographic findings may include gaseous gastric distention, segmental ileus, and sometimes a visible foreign body or trichobezoar.
   F. Normal gastrointestinal tract transit time in the ferret is 2–3 hours, so a barium series is easily performed.
   G. If there are signs of GI obstruction, emergency surgery and removal of the foreign body are indicated.
   H. Perform a complete abdominal exploratory during the laparotomy.
   I. Gastrotomy incisions should be closed with 3-0 or 4-0 adsorbable monofilament sutures in a continuous or interrupted pattern.
   J. Enterotomy incisions should be closed with 4-0 or 5-0 adsorbable monofilament sutures in a simple interrupted pattern.
   K. Close the linea alba with a 3-0 or 4-0 absorbable suture.
   L. Flush the subcutis, then perform a subcuticular closure or place skin sutures with nonabsorbable suture.
   M. Offer water and food within as soon as the ferret is recovered from anesthesia.

2. Diarrhea
  A. The differential diagnoses for diarrhea in the ferret include:
    I. Dietary indiscretion
    II. GI foreign body or trichobezoar
    III. *Helicobacter mustelae* gastritis
    IV. *Clostridium* spp., *Campylobacter* spp. and *Salmonella* spp. are opportunistic pathogens in ferrets
    V. Viral infections: corona virus (epizootic catarrhal enteritis (ECE), common), rotavirus and influenza
    VI. GI parasitism (*Coccidia*, *Giardia*)
    VII. Eosinophilic gastroenteritis or other inflammatory bowel disease
    VIII. Proliferative bowel disease
    IX. Neoplasia (lymphoma most common)
    X. Metabolic diseases, including hepatic and renal disease.
  B. Diagnostic procedures indicated may include:
    I. Evaluation of the patient's PCV, TP, blood glucose and BUN immediately upon entry
    II. Evaluation of a CBC and serum biochemical profile
    III. Evaluation of a fecal sample wet mount, flotation and Diff quick stain
    IV. Abdominal survey radiographs
    V. Abdominal ultrasonography
    VI. Endoscopy and / or colonoscopy
    VII. Contrast GI radiographic studies.
    VIII. Fecal culture if *Salmonella* spp. are suspected.
  C. Treatment should be symptomatic and supportive until the diagnosis is reached, and then specific treatment should be directed at the underlying etiology.
    I. Maintain hydration. Intravenous or IO fluids are preferred.
    II. Correct electrolyte imbalances and maintain euglycemia.
    III. Provide nutritional support.
    IV. Administer antibiotics that treat salmonellosis and clostridial infections if frank blood or melena is observed in feces.
    V. Administer antiparasitics if fecal sample is positive for endoparasites.
  D. The treatment of *Helicobacter mustelae* gastritis includes:
    I. Protocol 1: Clarithromycin (50 mg/kg PO q24h) *plus* omeprazole (4 mg/kg PO q24h) for 2 weeks; preferred protocol
    II. Protocol 2: Clarithromycin (12.5 mg/kg q8h PO) *plus* ranitidine bismuth citrate (24 mg/kg POq12h) *or* ranitidine HCL (3.5 mg/kg PO q12h) for 2 weeks
    III. Protocol 3: Amoxicillin (10–20 mg/kg PO q12h) *plus* metronidazole 20 mg/kg PO q12h *plus* bismuth subsalicylate 17mg/kg PO q12h) for 2–4 weeks
    IV. Consider the administration of sucralfate 100 mg/kg PO q6h
    V. Administer fluid therapy, if dehydrated
    VI. Provide nutritional support.

3. Hypoglycemia
   A. Insulinoma (pancreatic islet cell neoplasia) is the most common cause of hypoglycemia in pet ferrets.
   B. The differential diagnoses include anorexia or starvation, hepatopathy or other metabolic disease, neoplasia and sepsis.
   C. Insulinoma is usually seen in ferrets between older than 2 years of age.
   D. The owner may report episodes of weakness or collapse with hypersalivation.
   E. If the animal is hypoglycemic on presentation the clinical signs include a dazed appearance, gagging, pawing at the mouth, depression, posterior weakness, paresis or ataxia. Seizures are rare.
   F. The blood glucose level is usually <60 mg/dL.
   G. The serum insulin concentration is elevated.
   H. Short-term resolution of clinical signs is frequently achieved by oral administration of dextrose, corn syrup, or honey.
   I. Treatment
      I. Depending on the ferret's condition, treat either as an inpatient or outpatient.
      II. Administer dextrose 50% by mouth. If no response, administer dextrose IV.
      III. Place an IV or IO catheter.
      IV. Administer 50% dextrose 0.5–2 mL slowly IV until a clinical response is achieved. Do not administer dextrose too rapidly.
      V. Administer intravenous fluids supplemented with 5% dextrose IV or IO.
      VI. If seizures occur, administer diazepam 1–2 mg IV to effect.
      VII. Medical management consists of:
         a. Prednisone 0.25–1 mg/kg PO q12–24h. Reduce or increase dose based on clinical response and blood glucose levels. Doses as high as 2 mg/kg q12h might be required in severe cases. Treatment with prednisone is life long.
         b. Diazoxide (Proglycem®) 5 mg/kg PO q12h gradually increased to 30 mg/kg as needed. The prednisone dose may often be decreased with the addition of diazoxide.
      VIII. Food should be available at all times. Encourage the ferret to eat a meat-based, high-protein ferret or feline diet. Avoid foods high in carbohydrates or sugar.
      IX. Surgical treatment should be considered for healthy ferrets <5 years of age. However, survival times are similar to medical treatment alone and surgical treatment is only palliative, in most cases, since complete excision is impossible owing to presence of micrometastasis.
4. Adrenal gland disease (alopecia, vulvar swelling, urinary blockage)
   A. Very common in desexed ferrets older than 3 years.
   B. Characterized by excessive sex steroid hormone, progesterone production by the adrenal glands owing to underlying adrenal hyperplasia or neoplasia (adenoma, adenocarcinoma). Increased cortisol release as seen in dogs with adrenal hyperplasia does not occur in most ferrets.

C. Clinical signs include alopecia (bilateral symmetric, starting at tail base), pruritus, behavioral changes, vulvar swelling in females, stranguria secondary to prostatomegaly and / or prostatic or paraurethral cysts in males.

D. Diagnoses is based on clinical signs and history. Abdominal ultrasound is strongly recommended to evaluate size and appearance of the adrenal glands.

E. Medical treatment includes administration of a long-acting GnRH-agonist (e.g. deslorelin acetate implant; leuprolide acetate depot injection), to suppress further sex hormone release from hyperplastic adrenal glands. If ultrasonography indicates that adrenal glands are neoplastic or no response to medical treatment is seen, adrenalectomy should be performed.

F. The prognosis is good in cases of adrenal hyperplasia, and in female ferrets. The prognosis is guarded in ferrets with prostatomegaly and stranguria.

G. For prevention of adrenal gland disease, treatment with deslorelin acetate implants has been recommended.

5. Urinary tract disorders (urolithiasis, prostatomegaly, urinary tract infections)
   A. Struvite urolithiasis occurs in both sexes.
   B. Urethral obstructions may occur in the males.
   C. Prostatic enlargement may be the most common cause of stranguria in male ferrets over 3 years of age, secondary to adrenal gland disease. Prostatic and paraurethral cysts secondary to adrenal gland disease are common too, and can lead to urethral obstruction and abdominal distention.
      I. Urethral catheterization or cystostomy tube placement is often necessary.
      II. Bacterial prostatitis is common and antibiotic therapy should be initiated pending urine bacterial culture and sensitivity. Prostatomegaly is treated by managing the underlying adrenal gland disease with GnRH-agonists, and adrenalectomy if indicated.
   D. Treatment of urolithiasis is the same as for cats (see Ch. 11).
   E. Recommended antibiotics for cystitis and prostatitis in ferrets include:
      I. Trimethoprim-sulfa 15–30 mg/kg PO q12h
      II. Enrofloxacin 5–20 mg/kg PO q12–24h
      III. Chloramphenicol 30–50 mg/kg PO q12h.
   F. Ferrets should not be fed diets containing plant protein, which will lead to alkaline urine and sterile struvite formation. Feed a high-quality ferret or cat diet, which will lead to acidification of the urine.

6. Canine distemper
   A. Fatality approaches 100%.
   B. The clinical signs include fever, anorexia, serous to mucopurulent oculonasal discharge, coughing, depression, diarrhea, rash under the chin and in the inguinal area, and hyperkeratotic foot pads. Secondary bacterial pneumonia can occur.

C. The CNS phase is exhibited by hyperexcitability, excess salivation, ataxia, muscular tremors, convulsions and coma.

D. Differentials for include influenza virus (ferrets are highly susceptible), rabies (CNS signs), and different causes that can lead to diarrhea.

E. Diagnosis is made by demonstrating viral inclusion, by fluorescent antibody test (IFA) in peripheral blood, conjunctival or other mucous membrane scrapings.

F. Treatment consists of hospitalization in an isolation room and symptomatic supportive care as recommended for dogs. However, the mortality rate of canine distemper infections in ferrets is up to 100% and therefore humane euthanasia should be considered, if the diagnosis has been made.

7. Human influenza virus

A. Ferrets are highly susceptible to human influenza virus type A and the source of infection is often the owner or other ferrets.

B. The initial clinical signs are similar to distemper and include listlessness, fever, anorexia, sneezing, epiphora, serous ocular discharge, rhinitis, and lethargy. Coughing may be noticed if secondary bacterial pneumonia has developed.

C. The disease may be fatal to neonatal ferrets, but it is usually mild and self-limiting in adult ferrets.

D. Recovery usually occurs in 5–7 days.

E. Treatment

   I. Maintain hydration.

   II. Provide nutritional support if the patient has anorexia.

   III. Provide symptomatic and supportive therapy.

   IV. Antihistamines, such as chlorpheniramine (1–2 mg/kg PO q8–12h) or diphenhydramine (0.5–2 mg/kg PO q8–12h), may reduce nasal discharge.

   V. Administer antibiotics only if a secondary bacterial infection is suspected.

   VI. Nebulization may be beneficial.

8. Dyspnea

A. The differential diagnoses include:

   I. Pleural effusion – cardiac disease, neoplasia, infection, heartworm disease, hypoproteinemia, metabolic disease

   II. Pulmonary edema – cardiac disease, electrical cord bite, hypoproteinemia, metabolic disease

   III. Anterior mediastinal mass (most often lymphoma)

   IV. Pneumonia

   V. Pneumothorax

   VI. Diaphragmatic hernia

   VII. Tracheal obstruction

   VIII. Metabolic disease (acidosis)

   IX. Profound weakness – anemia, circulatory collapse, hypoglycemia

   X. Pain or hyperthermia, which may cause signs of dyspnea.

B. Administer oxygen supplementation.

C. Obtain blood samples. Evaluate the CBC, blood glucose, TP, and serum biochemical profile.

D. Treat symptomatically and supportively until the definitive diagnosis is determined, then direct treatment specifically.

9. Cardiomyopathy
   A. Dilated cardiomyopathy is the most common form. Hypertrophic cardiomyopathy is also reported.
   B. It occurs most often in middle-to older-aged ferrets.
   C. The history often includes anorexia, lethargy, exercise intolerance, weight loss, periodic dyspnea, coughing and tachypnea.
   D. The clinical signs include hypothermia, hindlimb weakness, tachycardia, cardiac murmur, moist rales, and muffled heart and lung sounds.
   E. Radiographic findings include pleural effusion, pulmonary edema, an enlarged cardiac silhouette, ascites, splenomegaly, and hepatomegaly.
   F. Treatment of cardiomyopathy and congestive heart failure is similar to the treatment in cats (see Ch. 3):
      I. Furosemide, 2–4 mg/kg IV, IM initially, then PO, q8–12h. 1–2 mg/kg PO q8–12h long term, once stabilized
      II. 2% nitroglycerin ointment $\frac{1}{16}$ – $\frac{1}{8}$ inch (1.5–3 mm) applied to the skin or inner pinna q12–24h
      III. Enalapril, 0.25–0.5 mg/kg PO q48h; increase to q24h if tolerated
      IV. Benazepril 0.25–0.5 mg/kg POq24h
      V. Pimobendan 0.5 mg/kg PO q12h
      VI. Digoxin, 0.005–0.01 mg/kg PO q12–24h
      VII. Atenolol 6.25 mg/ferret PO q24h for treatment of supraventricular and ventricular arrhythmias. Monitor for side effects; titrate to effect.

10. Splenomegaly
    A. Splenomegaly is a common finding in healthy ferrets, and does not necessarily indicate an underlying disease process. The most common cause for splenomegaly is extramedullary erythropoesis.
    B. Splenomegaly can also be found in ferrets with severe anemia, splenic lymphoma, proliferative colitis and Aleutian disease.
    C. Splenomegaly in itself is not an indication for an exploratory laparotomy in an otherwise healthy ferret, but should be worked up diagnostically if the ferret is ill.

11. Ear mites (*Otodectes cynotis*)
    A. Infestation is common.
    B. Brown waxy ear debris is commonly observed, but head shaking and ear scratching are not usually observed.
    C. Ivermectin (0.2 mg/kg SC) or selamectin (10–18 mg/kg topically q21–28d) is effective.

RECOMMENDED DRUG DOSAGES FOR FERRETS

Amoxicillin: 10–30 mg/kg IM, SC, PO q12h
Amoxicillin-clavulanate: 12.5 mg/kg PO q12h
Atenolol: 3.125–6.25 mg/ferret PO q24h
Atropine: (cardiac arrest) 0.05 mg/kg IV or 0.10mg/kg intratracheally

Benazepril 0.25–0.5 mg/kg POq24h

Bismuth subsalicylate: 0.25–1 mL/kg PO q6–12h

Buprenorphine: 0.01–0.003 mg/kg IV, IM, SC q8–12h

Butorphanol: 0.1–0.5 mg/kg IV, IM, SC q6–12h *(highly sedative in ferrets)*

Cephalexin: 15–30 mg/kg PO q12h

Chloramphenicol: 30–50 mg/kg IM, SC, PO q12h

Chlorpheniramine: 1–2 mg/kg PO q8–12h

Cimetidine: 5–10 mg/kg IV, SC, IM, PO q8h

Clarithromycin: 12.5 mg/kg PO q8h *or* 50 mg/kg PO q24h *(drug of choice for treatment of Helicobacter gastritis)*

Deslorelin acetate: 4.7 mg slow release implant, q12 months

Dexamethasone: 0.5–2 mg/kg IM, IV

Dexamethasone sodium phosphate: 4–8 mg/kg IV, IM

Dextrose (50%): 0.5–2 mL IV; use 5% dextrose in crystalloid fluids for CRI

Diazepam: 1–2 mg/kg IV, IM

Diazoxide: 5–30 mg/kg PO q12h

Digoxin: 0.005–0.01 mg/kg PO q12–24h

Diltiazem: 1.5–7.5 g/kg PO q6–24h

Diphenhydramine: 0.5–2 mg/kg IM, IV, PO q8–12h

Doxycycline: 5–10 mg/kg PO 12h

Enalapril: 0.25–0.5 mg/kg PO q48h initially, q24h if tolerated *(monitor for hypotension)*

Enrofloxacin 5–20 mg/kg PO q12–24h

Erythromycin: 10 mg/kg PO q6h

Epinephrine: 0.02 mg/kg IV, IO, IT

Fenbendazole: 20 mg/kg PO q24h for 5 days

Furosemide: 1–4 mg/kg IV, IM, SC, PO q8–12h

Glycopyrrolate: 0.01–0.02 mg/kg SC, IM, IV

Insulin (NPH): 0.5–1 U/ferret SC q12h initially, adjusted to the needs of the individual

Insulin (Ultralente®): 1 U/ferret SC q24h initially adjusted to the needs of the individual

Ivermectin: 0.2–0.4 mg/kg (200–400 mg/kg) SC, PO

Ketamine + midazolam: 5–10 mg/kg (K) + 0.25–0.5 mg/kg (M) IM

Lactulose (15 mg/mL): 0.1–0.75 mL/kg PO q12h

Laxatone: 1–2 inch (25–50 mm) q8–12h PO

Leuprolide acetate (Lupron® 30 day depot): 100–300 µg/ferret IM q30d

Meloxicam: 0.2 mg/kg IM, SC, PO q24h

Metoclopramide: 0.2–1 mg/kg SC, PO q6–8h

Metronidazole: 15–30 mg/kg PO q12h

Naloxone: 0.02–0.04 mg/kg IV, IM, SC

Nitroglycerine (2% ointment): 1/8 inch applied to the skin or inner pinna q12–24h

Omeprazole: 4 mg/kg PO q24h

Oxymorphone: 0.05–0.2 mg/kg SC, IM, IV q2–6h

Oxytocin: 5–10 U IM, SC

Pimobendan: 0.5 mg/kg PO q12h

Prednisone / prednisolone: 0.25–2 mg/kg SC, PO q12–24h

Prednisolone sodium succinate: 25–40 mg/kg IV

Propofol: 2–5 mg/kg IV
Selamectin: 10–18 mg/kg topically q21–28d
Sucralfate: 25 mg/kg PO q6–12h
Sulfadimethoxine (Albon®): 50 mg/kg PO once, then 25 mg/kg PO q24h
for 9 days
Trimethoprim–sulfa 15–30 mg /kg PO q12h

FISH

Changes in their aquatic environment are the most common causes for presentation of pet fish to an emergency veterinary hospital. Because the owner cannot usually bring in the entire tank or pond, a thorough history must be obtained. The questions listed in Box 15.1 should be asked.

Rule out tank-mate aggression and poor water quality, which are the leading causes of acute mortality and morbidity in pet fish.

Diagnostic procedures

1. Water quality testing
   A. Temperature
   B. Ammonia level
   C. Nitrate level
   D. Nitrite level
   E. pH
   F. Dissolved oxygen
   G. Total alkalinity
   H. Copper level
   I. Chlorine level

BOX 15.1 Important questions for the client

1. How long have you been keeping pet fish?
2. What are the problems with the fish today?
3. When did you first notice these problems?
4. How long have you owned the sick fish and where did it come from?
5. Are there other fish in the same tank or pond with the sick fish and, if so, how are they doing?
6. What is the size (volume) of the pond or aquarium and how is it heated, filtered, lit and aerated?
7. Do you have a water test kit and, if so, how often do you test the water? What are your most current results?
8. What and how often do you feed your fish?
9. Have the fish already been treated? If so then by whom, and with what medications?
10. Is there a possibility that the fish were exposed either directly or indirectly to some type of toxin?

From Lewbart, G.A., 1995. Emergency pet fish medicine. In: Bonagura, J.D., Kirk, R.W. (Eds), Current Veterinary Therapy XII. WB Saunders, Philadelphia, pp. 1370, with permission from Elsevier.

2. Fecal parasitology
3. Cytology
    A. Skin scrapes should be performed under manual restraint, in order to avoid changes in the population of ectoparasites due to anesthetic drugs. Use a cover slip or back of a scalpel blade and collect samples of the surface mucus. Do not traumatize the skin and scales. Mix sample with a drop of tank water. Evaluate immediately under a microscope for particularly motile protozoa.
    B. Fin clips should be performed if lesions are present on the fins. Use iris scissor and collect a small sample of fin. Place directly on a glass slide with a drop of tank water and cover with a cover slip. Examine under the microscope for infectious organisms, such as bacteria or fungus.
    C. Gill clips may be performed under manual restrain or sedation. Use iris scissors to collect a small sample of gill filaments. Examine under the microscope for parasites, bacteria or fungus.
4. A blood sample for a blood smear evaluation, WBC, PCV/TP and blood culture may be obtained from fish >10 cm in length.
    A. Direct the needle at a 90° angle to the ventral margin of the thin lateral line on the fish caudal to the vent but cranial to the tail and caudal peduncle.
    B. Insert the needle until resistance is felt from the spinal column, then gently walk the needle ventrally until it slips into the venous sinus that is located just ventral to the spine.
5. Radiographs may reveal swim bladder disorders, gastrointestinal foreign bodies or gastrointestinal impactions.
    A. Place the fish in a plastic bag.
    B. Lay the fish directly on top of the cassette to obtain the lateral view.
    C. The easiest way to obtain a dorsoventral view is to rotate the radiographic machine and send a horizontal beam through the dorsoventral axis of the fish.
6. Biopsy and / or necropsy.
    Anesthesia—Fish may be restrained manually or tranquilized with tricaine methane sulfonate (MS-222, Finquel) 100–200 mg/L of water for induction and 50–100 mg/L of water for maintenance. 15–50 mg/L can be used for sedation. Make a 10 g/L stock solution and buffer with sodium bicarbonate (10 g/L). Alternatively anesthesia can be induced with clove oil (eugenol) diluted with 95% ethanol at a ratio of 1:9 (clove oil:ethanol). The stock solution of clove oil should contain 100 mg/mL. Concentrations of clove oil / ethanol of 40–120 mg/L of water are effective at tranquilizing freshwater and marine fish species. Recovery may be prolonged.

COMMON DISEASES AND HEALTH PROBLEMS OF FISH

1. Poor water quality
    A. This is the leading killer of pet fish.
    B. Freshwater tropical fish usually require a water temperature of 76–80°F (24–27°C).

C. Marine fish should be kept at water temperatures between 79 and 84°F (26–29°C).
D. The ideal pH for freshwater aquariums and ponds is between 6.5 and 7.5.
E. Marine fish should be kept in water with a pH between 7.5 and 8.5.
F. Every 7–10 days, 10% of the water should be changed.

2. Hypoxia
   A. Place the fish in a plastic bag containing 33% water by volume.
   B. Fill the rest of the bag with 100% oxygen from an anesthetic machine.
   C. Close the bag tightly.
   D. Keep the affected fish in the bag until they have resumed normal respiration and swimming behavior.

3. Elevated ammonia or nitrite levels
   A. The most common causes are tank or pond overloading (overcrowding), overfeeding, and inadequate filtration.
   B. Change 30–50% of the water with dechlorinated water q12–24h.
   C. Evaluate the filtration, biologic load, and feeding practices.
   D. Measure the pH level.

4. Abnormal pH
   A. Gradually change the water to bring pH back into the normal range (freshwater 6.5–7.5, marine 7.5–8.5).
   B. If the total alkalinity is low (<50 ppm), add crushed coral or dolomite.

5. Chlorine / chloramine toxicity
   A. Treat the water with a dechlorinating agent or move the fish to dechlorinated water.
   B. Put ice packs in the water to lower the temperature and increase the amount of dissolved oxygen in the water:
      I. Tropical fish may be lowered to 70°F
      II. Koi and goldfish may be lowered to 55°F.
   C. Bubble 100% oxygen into the water from an oxygen bottle.

6. Anorexia / starvation
   A. Evaluate for tank / pond-mate aggression.
   B. Tube feeding is possible.
   C. Use a/d, Iams recovery diet®, or add small amounts of water to flake or pelleted fish food.

7. External bacterial infections
   A. *Aeromonas* infections are the most common and cause deep ulcers on the body.
   B. Other signs may include a distended abdomen, ecchymoses and exophthalmus.
   C. Treatment includes systemic treatment with antibiotics.
   D. Apply silver sulfadiazine cream directly to the wound q12h.
   E. Keep the affected area out of the water for 30–60 seconds, to allow absorption of the medication while keeping the gills submerged.
   F. Add NaCl to the tank water to achieve a concentration of 3 g/L, in order to promote skin healing and as supportive care.

8. Systemic bacterial infections
   A. *Aeromonas hydrophila* complex are the most common bacterial pathogens of freshwater fish.
      I. Poor nutrition, transport, and environmental stresses, including crowding and temperature extremes, may predispose fish to developing motile aeromonad disease (MAD).
      II. The clinical signs include petechiation and ecchymosis, exophthalmia, engorged gill lamellae, abdominal distention, swelling around the vent, and skin and fin necrosis.
      III. Pathologically, hemorrhagic septicemia, and necrosis of the gastrointestinal tract, kidney, spleen and muscle result in death.
      IV. Treatment includes the administration of antibiotics and the correction of underlying husbandry problems.
      V. Add NaCl to the tank water to achieve a concentration of 3 mg/mL in order to promote skin healing and as supportive care.
   B. Tuberculosis (*Mycobacterium* spp.)
      I. Tuberculosis affects marine and freshwater fish.
      II. The clinical signs include fading colors, emaciation, anorexia, lethargy, edema, peritonitis, nodules in muscles, exophthalmos, skin and scale defects with ulceration and fin destruction.
      III. Treatment is usually ineffective and is not recommended owing to the zoonotic potential.
   C. Nocardiosis
      I. The clinical signs include opaque eyes, sloughing of scales, exophthalmia, anorexia, listlessness, fading colors, emaciation, fin and scale rot. It is very difficult to differentiate from tuberculosis.
      II. The infectious agent can be identified with immunofluorescence techniques or by culture.
      III. Infected animals are thought to be a reservoir of infection.
      IV. Treatment is not recommended.
9. Protozoal diseases
   A. *Ichthyophthirius multifilis* (ich) and *Cryptocaryon irritans* (saltwater ich) have an encysted stage that is resistant to chemotherapeutic treatment.
   B. Many protozoan infections in freshwater fish will respond to submersion of the freshwater fish into seawater (30–35 g/L) for 4–5 minutes.
   C. Alternatively add NaCl to the tank water to achieve a concentration of 3–5 g/L and increase the water temperature in order to speed up the parasite's life cycle and consequently improve the efficacy of antiparasitic treatments.
   D. Formalin 0.025 mg/L of tank water, for 12–24h q48h for three treatments. Change 50% of tank water on alternate days. Increase the water temperature.

RECOMMENDED DRUG DOSAGES FOR FISH

Amikacin: 5 mg/kg IM, IP q12–24h
Ampicillin: 10 mg/kg IM q24h

Clove oil: 95% ethanol (1:9), 100 mg/mL: 40–120 mg/L
Enrofloxacin: 5–10 mg/kg IM, IP, PO, q24h
Fenbendazole: 50 mg/kg PO q24h for 2 treatment, repeat q14d
Florfenicol: 25–50 mg/kg PO, IM q24h
Furosemide: 2–5 mg/kg IV, IP, IM, PO q12h
Gentamicin: 1–3.5 mg/kg IM q24–72h
Ivermectin: **Do not use**
Kanamycin: 20 mg/kg IP q72h for five treatments
Lidocaine: 1–2 mg/kg IV
Metronidazole: 25 mg/L tank water q24h for 3 consecutive days; 50 mg/kg PO q24h for 5 days
Oxytetracycline: 10–50 mg/kg IM, PO q24h
Praziquantel: 5–10 mg/L as a 3–6-hour bath; repeat in 7 days
Sulfadimethoxine: 50 mg/kg/day in feed for 5 days

GERBILS (*MERIONES UNGUICULATUS*)

Adult average body weight = males 65–100 g; females = 55–85 g.
  Average life span = 3–4 years.
  Sexually mature at 2–3 months of age.
  Gestation period = 24–26 days, litter size = 1–12; average is 4–6.
  Weaning at 21–28 days. Fertile at post-partum estrus.
  Heart rate = 250–500 bpm.
  Respiratory rate = 70–120 bpm.
  Temperature = 98.6–102.2°F (37–39°C).
  Normal blood values for gerbils include:

PCV = 35–45%	BUN = 17–31 mg/dL
TP = 4.3–12.0 g/dL	Glucose = 50–135 mg/dL
WBC = 7.500–11 000/mL	Calcium = 8–10 mg/dL

  Diet—Pelleted rodent diet that contains 18–20% protein. Gerbils are omnivorous, but predominately granivorous.
  Sedation—Midazolam 0.5–2 mg/kg IM, SC, IN. Add butorphanol (0.2–0.4 mg/kg) if deeper sedation is required.
  Anesthesia—Isoflurane or sevoflurane by mask or chamber.

Fluid therapy

Daily maintenance fluid requirements in gerbils are about 60–100 mL/kg/day.

Nutritional support

Any anorexic or emaciated gerbil should receive nutritional support. Syringe feed an omnivorous critical care formula or blended gerbil, hamster or rat pellets.

Caution: Penicillin, ampicillin, amoxicillin, cephalosporins, vancomycin, erythromycin, or clindamycin, administered orally, may cause severe dysbacteriosis, enterocolitis and death. Therefore do not administer these antibiotics orally.

Do not grasp a gerbil by the tail, distal to the base of the tail, as loss of the skin of the tail may easily occur.

COMMON DISEASES AND HEALTH PROBLEMS OF GERBILS

1. Tyzzer's disease (*Bacillus piliformis*)
   A. Tyzzer's disease is an acute, often fatal, hepatoenteric disease common in gerbils.
   B. The clinical signs include a rough hair coat, lethargy, watery diarrhea, and death.
   C. Treatment is often ineffective. Consider doxycycline, tetracycline or metronidazole and supportive care.
2. Salmonellosis (*Salmonella typhimurium*, *S. enteritidis*)
   A. The clinical signs include dehydration, diarrhea, weight loss and sudden death.
   B. Diagnosis is by isolation of the *Salmonella* by bacterial culture of fecal material.
   C. Treatment is not recommended due to the zoonotic potential from the development of a carrier state in surviving animals.
3. Dermatitis
   A. Etiologies include bite wounds (*Staphylococcus* spp. infections), ectoparasites including *Demodex*, nail abrasions, subcutaneous abscesses or neoplasia, and overcrowding.
   B. Irritation from Harderian gland porphyrins may cause alopecia and facial dermatitis.
   C. Treatment of demodex and other ectoparasites is with ivermectin or selamectin.
4. Geriatric diseases – common geriatric diseases in gerbils include cystic ovaries, chronic interstitial nephritis, spontaneous neoplasia, diabetes mellitus, hyperadrenocorticism and arteriosclerosis.
5. Seizures
   A. Many gerbils are suffering from spontaneous epileptiform seizures, which may be a form of catalepsy.
   B. Seizures may be precipitated by stressful stimuli.
   C. The frequency of the seizures tends to decrease with age.
   D. Anticonvulsant therapy is not recommended. Keep the animal in a dark and quiet environment and avoid stress.

RECOMMENDED DRUG DOSAGES FOR GERBILS

Amoxicillin: Not recommended for oral administration
Ampicillin: Not recommended for oral administration
Atropine sulfate: 0.2–0.4 mg/kg SC, IM
Buprenorphine: 0.05–0.1 mg/kg SC, IM q8–12h
Butorphanol: 0.2–0.4 mg/kg SC, IM q2–4h
Cephalosporins: Not recommended for oral administration
Clindamycin: Not recommended for oral administration
Chloramphenicol : 30–50 mg/kg q8h
Doxycycline: 5 mg/kg PO q12h

Enrofloxacin: 10–20 mg/kg IM, SC, PO q12–24h
Fenbendazole: 20–50 mg/kg PO q24h for 5 days
Furosemide: 2–4 mg/kg IM, SC, PO PRN
Itraconazole 5–10 mg/kg PO q24h
Ivermectin: 0.2–0.4 mg/kg SC, PO q7–14d *(administer 0.2 mg/kg PO q24h for demodicosis)*
Metronidazole: 10–20 mg/kg PO q12h
Midazolam: 0.5–2 mg/kg IM, SC, IN
Praziquantel: 6–10 mg/kg IM, SC, PO
Selamectin: 15–30 mg/kg topical q21–28d
Sulfadimethoxine (Albon®): 20–50 mg/kg PO q24h
Tetracycline: 450–540 mg/L water, add sucrose to increase palatability; 15–20 mg/kg PO q8–12h
Terbinafine: 10–30 mg/kg PO q24h
Trimethoprim-sulfa: 15–30 mg/kg IM, PO q12h

GUINEA PIGS (*CAVIA PORCELLUS*)

Guinea pigs, also known as cavies, are diurnal and originate from South America, where they have been domesticated for more than a thousand years. Currently, 13 different breeds are recognized in the United States. The male is called a boar; the female is a sow.

Diet—Guinea pigs should be fed predominately a good-quality grass hay, as well as commercial guinea pig pellets. Guinea pigs require a dietary source of vitamin C. Therefore offer fresh vegetables high in vitamin C daily (red and green peppers, cabbage, kale). Alternatively vitamin C can be added to the drinking water (0.4 g/L) daily.

Adult guinea pig males weigh 900–1200 g; females usually weigh 700–900 g.

Average life span = 5–6 years.
Sexual maturity occurs at 2–3 months. Estrous cycle = 15–17 days.
Gestation period = 60–70 days. Average litter size = 3–4.
Weaning occurs at 3 weeks of age, or at 180 g of body weight.
Heart rate = 230–380 beats/min.
Respiratory rate = 40–100 breaths/min.
Temperature = 99.0–103.1°F (37.2–39.5°C).
Normal blood values in guinea pigs include:

PCV = 35–45%
WBC = 7000–14 000/mL
BUN = 9–32 mg/dL
Creatinine = 0.6–2.2 mg/dL
Glucose = 60–125 mg/dL

Phosphorus = 4–8 mg/dL
Calcium = 9.6–12.4 mg/dL
Potassium = 4.5–8.8 mEq/L
Sodium = 130–150 mEq/L

Sex determination—Males have prominent scrotal pouches and large testes. The penis can be protruded from the prepuce.
Sedation—
• Midazolam 0.5–1 mg/kg SC/IM.
• Midazolam 0.5 mg/kg + butorphanol (0.25 mg/kg) SC/IM.

Anesthesia—Isoflurane or sevoflurane induction by mask or chamber after premedication.

Caution: Penicillin, ampicillin, amoxicillin, cephalosporins, vancomycin, erythromycin, or clindamycin, administered orally, may cause severe dysbacteriosis, enterocolitis and death. Therefore do not administer these antibiotics orally.

Guinea pig fluid therapy

1. The daily maintenance fluid requirements are 60–100 mL/kg/day. For SC fluid administration, use LRS, Normosol®-R, or a similar balanced electrolyte isotonic crystalloid.
2. For IV or IO fluid administration, 5% dextrose may be added to the fluids if desired. Colloids and blood may also be administered IV or IO.
3. Only warmed (100–102°F (38–39°C) fluids should be administered.
4. The shock fluid volume for guinea pigs is 10–25 mL/kg IV or IO over 5–7 minutes.
5. The cephalic veins are most suitable for intravenous catheter placement in guinea pigs. Sedate prior to catheter placement and use a 24- or 26-gauge catheter.
6. Intraosseous catheters may be placed through the trochanteric fossa into the femur or through the tibial crest into the tibia – the technique is performed identically to that in chinchillas.

Guinea pig nutritional support

1. Any anorexic or hyporexic guinea pig should receive nutritional support in order to minimize secondary gastrointestinal problems caused by reduced food intake (i.e. dysbacteriosis, diarrhea, tympany) and to avoid increased fat mobilization, which frequently leads to hepatic lipidosis.
2. Syringe feed with a high-fiber diet for herbivores (e.g. Oxbow Critical Care for Herbivores®, 50–80 mL/kg PO q24h; divide into 4–5 feedings) or crushed and soaked pellets. Do not syringe feed guinea pigs that are not swallowing.

COMMON DISEASES AND HEALTH PROBLEMS OF GUINEA PIGS

1. Gastrointestinal disease (diarrhea, tympany, gastric dilatation and volvulus (GDV))
   A. Guinea pigs are herbivorous hindgut fermenters. Noninfectious causes (e.g. sudden change in diet), inappropriate diet (e.g. high-starch food items, inappropriate oral antibiotic therapy) and less frequently infectious etiologies (parasites, bacteria) can be found in guinea pigs. Disruption of the normal gastrointestinal microflora (dysbacteriosis) occurs with most forms of gastrointestinal disease in guinea pigs, which leads to gastroenteritis, tympany of the stomach and intestine, diarrhea, endotoxemia, and in some cases bacterial translocation and sepsis. Both gastric and intestinal volvulus have been reported in guinea pigs.

B. Initial diagnostic tests should include:
   I. Whole body radiographs
   II. Fecal wet mount and Diff quick stain
   III. Fecal flotation.
C. If the animal has diarrhea, perform fecal parasitology to rule out *Eimeria caviae* and excessive numbers of motile protozoa (i.e. *Giardia, Trichomonas, Balantidium*). Rule out dental disease which can lead to diarrhea due to reduced food intake and selective intake of low-fiber food items.
   I. Feed a high-quality grass-hay diet and administer fluids if the animal is dehydrated.
   II. Treat excessive numbers of motile protozoa with metronidazole. Treat *Eimeria* with sulfonamides (e.g. trimethoprim-sulfa drugs).
   III. Provide nutritional support if the animal is anorexic.
   IV. Administer the appropriate antibiotic parenterally if severe bacterial enteritis is suspected and the risk of bacterial translocation and sepsis is likely.
   V. Treat dental disease.
D. If tympany was diagnosed:
   I. Consider that the stomach of guinea pigs always contains some gas. Do not misinterpret this as gastric tympany. The stomach is located in the left cranial abdomen.
   II. Rule out GDV. The stomach will be located in the right abdomen. Gastric tympany and dilatation frequently occurs without volvulus. If GDV was diagnosed, surgical correction might be attempted. Consider euthanasia, because the prognosis is poor.
   III. If the animal is in shock or hypovolemic, administer shock rate fluids intravenously or intraosseously.
   IV. Provide analgesia (buprenorphine 0.03–0.05 mg/kg SC, IM, IV).
   V. Attempt decompression of the stomach if tympanic and dilated. Sedate the animal and use a lubricated large-diameter red rubber tube orally.
   VI. Administer enrofloxacin (10 mg/kg IM, IV), owing to the usually concurrent or underlying dysbacteriosis.
   VII. The prognosis is poor if the animal is in shock, lateral recumbent or hypothermic.

2. Dental disease
  A. Guinea pigs have continuously growing cheek teeth and incisor teeth.
  B. The dental formula is: $2(I_1C_0P_1M_3) = 20$.
  C. The occlusal planes of the cheek teeth are oblique at about 30° to the horizontal plane.
  D. Vitamin C deficiency and inappropriate low-fiber diet may be underlying causes for the occurrence of dental disease in guinea pigs.
  E. The mandibular cheek teeth overgrow medially and commonly cause lingual entrapment.

F. Overgrowth and abnormal wear of the cheek teeth can lead to sharp edges or points, which cause lingual and buccal gingival ulceration.

G. The clinical signs include an apparent appetite but refusal to eat, eating of only soft fruit or vegetables, a sour mouth odor, stained or wet fur around the mouth, diarrhea, poor body condition and poor fur condition.

H. Complete examination of the oral cavity and cheek teeth is possible only under general anesthesia and by the use of the mouth gag and cheek dilators. The use of an otoscope or ideally a rigid endoscope is highly recommended. In guinea pigs the oral cavity always contains food particles, which should not be misinterpreted as food impaction.

I. Use a low-speed dental drill with a diamond burr and soft tissue protector to remove dental spurs and shorten overgrown cheek teeth under general anesthesia. Refer the patient to a specialist if unfamiliar with treatment of dental disease in guinea pigs.

J. Provide the appropriate supportive care as indicated:
   I. Nutritional support if the animal is not eating
   II. Fluid therapy (30–50 mL/kg SC bolus)
   III. Analgesia (buprenorphine 0.03–0.05 mg/kg SC, meloxicam 0.3–0.5 mg/kg SC, PO) if the animal is adequately hydrated and has a normal renal function.

K. Dental disease in guinea pigs can frequently only be managed, but not cured. Recurrence of clinical signs is common and therefore regular dental treatment under general anesthesia needs to be performed often for the rest of the animal's life.

3. Scurvy (hypovitaminosis C)
   A. The daily vitamin C requirement in guinea pigs is 15–25 mg/kg.
   B. The clinical signs may become apparent within 2 weeks of vitamin C deprivation in guinea pigs.
   C. The clinical signs include weakness, lethargy, anorexia, vocalization, enlarged limb joints and costochondral junctions, poor hair coats, oculonasal discharge, diarrhea and weight loss. Death may occur in 3–4 weeks, due to starvation or secondary infections.
   D. Treatment includes supplementation of ascorbic acid daily, in the water, food, or by parenteral injection (50–100 mg/kg body weight).
   E. Multivitamin drops should not be used due to the potential for toxic overdose with the other vitamins.
   F. Scurvy is prevented by providing guinea pigs with fresh, stabilized vitamin C daily, or supplementing the drinking water with 0.4 g vitamin C per liter. Fresh red or green peppers, cabbage and kale may be added to the diet.

4. Respiratory disease
   A. The guinea pig may be affected with an acute or chronic pneumonia. *Bordetella bronchiseptica* and *Streptococcus pneumoniae* are the two main bacterial pathogens. Transmission occurs via direct contact. Predisposing factors are stress, overcrowding, poor ventilation and cage sanitation.

B. Guinea pigs are obligate nasal breathers and upper respiratory tract disease can lead to significant dyspnea.

C. The clinical signs include sneezing, coughing, dyspnea, oculonasal discharge, depression, anorexia, weight loss and death. Torticollis and abortions may occur.

D. Differentials for respiratory tract disease in guinea pigs are cardiac disease, neoplasia, metabolic disease and sepsis. Perform diagnostics (thoracic radiographs, CT scan thorax, CBC, biochemistry) to establish diagnosis.

E. Prescribe antibiotics (e.g. trimethoprim-sulfa, enrofloxacin, or chloramphenicol).

F. Provide nutritional support if animal is anorexic.

G. Provide supportive care as indicated.

H. Ensure sufficient vitamin C intake.

5. Seizures and neurologic deficits

A. Hypocalcemia, hypoglycemia, hyperthermia, sepsis, otitis media and interna, and sarcoptic mange can cause seizures in guinea pigs.

B. Administer midazolam, 0.5–1 mg/kg IM, IN or IV if animal is seizuring.

C. Attempt to determine and treat the underlying etiology. Perform a biochemistry profile and a CBC to rule out extracranial causes.

Insulinoma causing hypoglycemia is common in guinea pigs. Differentials for hypoglycemia include liver disease, sepsis and starvation. Measure blood insulin levels to confirm diagnosis. Treat with dextrose infusions. Prognosis is guarded to poor.

D. Treatment similar to that in ferrets (see p. 720) with prednisone or diazoxide can be attempted.

E. Rule out sarcoptic mange, which can cause severe pruritus in guinea pigs and can lead to seizure-like episodes. Treat with ivermectin or selamectin.

F. Carefully evaluate the external ear canal and tympanic membranes. Perform a dorsoventral skull radiograph or CT scan of the head to rule out otitis media and interna. Treat with systemic antibiotics and provide supportive care. Prognosis is guarded.

G. Sepsis is a common cause for neurologic deficits, depression and anorexia in guinea pigs. Treat empirically with broad-spectrum antibiotics. Administer any antibiotic parenterally, due to impaired GI function. Provide intravenous fluids and supportive care. Prognosis is poor.

6. Cervical lymphadenitis

A. *Streptococcus zooepidemicus* is a commensal organism that can cause abscessation of lymph nodes, visceral organs, and abortions. Torticollis may be seen if the middle and inner ear is involved. In younger guinea pigs a systemic form with respiratory involvement resulting in oculonasal discharge, cyanosis, dyspnea as well as septicemia may be seen.

B. Confirm diagnosis by fine needle aspiration and cytology of enlarged cervical lymph nodes. Rule out lymphoma. Submit lymph node aspirate sample for aerobic bacterial culture.

C. Treatment
   I. Administer anesthesia.
   II. Perform surgical drainage of abscesses.
   III. Administer systemic antibiotics such as enrofloxacin, trimethoprim-sulfa, or chloramphenicol, based on culture and sensitivity results.

7. Pregnancy toxemia
  A. Pregnancy toxemia in guinea pigs often causes acute death within 24 hours.
  B. It is typically seen in stressed, heavily pregnant sows that are 56 or more days into gestation and carrying three or more fetuses.
  C. The clinical signs include acute death or anorexia, lethargy, dyspnea, and death within 2–5 days.
  D. Clinical pathology findings include hypoglycemia, hyperkalemia, hyponatremia, hypochloremia, elevated hepatic enzymes, hyperlipidemia, ketonemia, proteinuria, anemia, and thrombocytopenia.
  E. Treatment
   I. Administer fluids IV or IO.
   II. Administer intravenous dextrose.
   III. Administer systemic antibiotics.
  F. The prognosis is poor. Pregnancy toxemia is nearly 100% fatal, despite treatment.

8. Dystocia
  A. Dystocia occurs commonly in sows first bred after 6 months of age or extremely obese sows.
  B. Dystocia may result in excessive hemorrhage, exhaustion, toxemia and death.
  C. The optimal gestation is approximately 69 days.
  D. Treatment involves oxytocin injections (1–2 U/kg IM), vaginal delivery or a cesarean section.

RECOMMENDED DRUG DOSAGES FOR GUINEA PIGS

Amoxicillin: Not recommended for oral administration
Ampicillin: Not recommended for oral administration
Atropine: 0.1–0.2 mg/kg IM, SC
Buprenorphine: 0.03–0.05 mg/kg SC, IM q8–12h
Butorphanol: 0.2–0.4 mg/kg SC, IM q2–4h
Cephalosporins: Not recommended for oral administration
Chloramphenicol palmitate: 50 mg/kg PO q12h for 5–7d
Chloramphenicol sodium succinate: 30 mg/kg IM q12h for 5–7d
Clindamycin: Not recommended for oral administration
Doxycycline: 5 mg/kg PO q12h
Enrofloxacin: 10 mg/kg IM, SC, IV, PO q12–24h
Erythromycin: Not recommended for oral administration
Fenbendazole: 20–50 mg/kg PO q24h for 5 days
Furosemide: 2–4 mg/kg IM, SC, IV PO PRN
Gentamicin: Not recommended due to nephrotoxicity
Itraconazole 5–10 mg/kg PO q24h

Ivermectin: 0.2–0.5 mg/kg IM, SC, PO q7–14d
Metronidazole: 20–30 mg/kg IV, PO q12h
Midazolam: 0.5–1 mg/kg IM, SC, IV
Nystatin: 100 000 U/kg PO q8h for 5 days
Oxytocin: 1–2 U/kg IM
Praziquantel: 6–10 mg/kg IM, SC repeat in 10 days
Selamectin: 15–30 mg/kg topical q21–28d *(use 30 mg/kg for treatment of sarcoptic mange)*
Sulfadimethoxine (Albon): 25–50 mg/kg PO q24h for 10 days
Terbinafine: 10–30 mg/kg PO q24h
Tetracycline: 15–20 mg/kg PO q8–12h; 450–550 mg/L water PO
Trimethoprim-sulfa: 15–30 mg/kg PO q12h
Vitamin C: 50–100 mg/kg SC, IM, PO *(for treatment of deficiencies)*

HAMSTERS (*GOLDEN, MESOCRICETUS AURATUS, PHODOPUS SPP.*)

Syrian (golden) hamsters as well as dwarf hamsters are commonly kept as pets.
Average life span = 1.5–2 years.
 Gestation period = 15–18 days. Litter size is 4–12 pups. Weaning at 20–25 days. Do not handle the young during the first 7 days of life.
 Estrous cycle is 4 days; sexual maturity is reached at about 6–12 weeks of age.
 Weight = 85–150 g (Syrian hamster), 25–50 g (dwarf hamster).
 HR = 250–500 beats/min.
 Respiratory rate = 35–135 breaths/min.
 Temperature = 98–99°F (37–38°C).
 Normal blood values in hamsters include:

PCV = 31–57%	Glucose = 40–200 mg/dL
TP = 4.5–7.5 g/dL	Phosphorus = 3–8.4 mg/dL
WBC = 7000–10 000/mL	Calcium = 5.3–12 mg/dL
BUN = 12–26 mg/dL	Potassium = 3.9–5.5 mEq/L
Creatinine = 0.4–1 mg/dL	Sodium = 128–144 mEq/L

Diet—Pelleted rodent diet that contains 18–20% protein. Hamsters are omnivorous.
Sedation—Midazolam 0.5–2 mg/kg IM, SC, IN. Add butorphanol (0.2–0.4 mg/kg) if deeper sedation is required.
Anesthesia—Isoflurane or sevoflurane by mask or chamber.

Fluid therapy

Daily maintenance fluid requirements in hamsters are about 60–100 mL/kg/day.

Nutritional support

Any anorexic or emaciated hamster should receive nutritional support. Syringe feed an omnivorous critical care formula or blended hamster or rat pellets.

Caution: Penicillin, ampicillin, amoxicillin, cephalosporins, vancomycin, erythromycin, or clindamycin, administered orally, may cause severe dysbacteriosis, enterocolitis and death. Therefore do not administer these antibiotics orally.

COMMON DISEASES AND HEALTH PROBLEMS OF HAMSTERS

1. Enteritis (proliferative ileitis (wet tail), dysbacteriosis, diarrhea)
   A. Proliferative ileitis is caused by *Lawsonia intracellularis*, a gram-negative intracellular bacterial organism. Clinical signs include watery diarrhea, matting of the fur on the tail, hunched stance, irritability, dehydration and emaciation. This disease predominately affects young hamsters and stress, improper diet, change of diet, and overcrowding are predisposing factors. The prognosis is guarded.
      I. Treat with antibiotics effective against intracellular organisms (e.g. enrofloxacin, doxycycline).
      II. Provide supportive care in the form of nutritional support and SC fluids, if indicated.
   B. Tyzzer's disease is caused by *Clostridium piliforme*. Inappropriate oral antibiotic therapy will lead to dysbacteriosis and overgrowth of opportunistic pathogens, such as *Clostridium difficile* or *Escherichia coli*. *Salmonella typhimurium* and *S. enteritidis* can cause enteritis in hamsters. Clinical signs are similar and include diarrhea, perianal soiling, dehydration, emaciation and poor fur condition. Empirical treatment is often necessary. The prognosis is guarded to poor.
   C. Treatment for enteritis in hamsters includes supportive care.
      I. Administer subcutaneous fluids (3–5 mL/100 g). Daily maintenance requirement is 60–100 mL/kg/day.
      II. Provide nutritional support.
      III. Administer oral antibiotics. Administer doxycycline or metronidazole if clostridial overgrowth is suspected. Administer trimethoprim-sulfa if clostridial overgrowth is less likely.
      IV. Treatment of salmonellosis is not recommended due to the zoonotic potential from the development of a carrier state in surviving animals.
2. Cheek pouch prolapse
   A. Occurs secondary to impaction or infection of the cheek pouches. Animals will chew the prolapsed tissue, and cause further traumatization. Depending on the duration of the prolapse, the tissue might be necrotic.
   B. Anesthetize the hamster.
   C. Assess viability of tissue and evaluate for underlying disease (e.g. impaction, infection).
   D. If the prolapsed tissue is still viable, repositioning can be performed using a cotton-tipped applicator.
      I. Place a nonabsorbable percutaneous suture to keep the cheek pouch in its anatomically correct position. Remove suture in 10–14 days.

    II. Suture placement does not always prevent recurrence of prolapse. Reprolapse is common.

E. If the tissue is nonviable or the risk for recurrence of the cheek pouch prolapse is high, or has re-prolapsed, perform amputation of the cheek pouch.

F. Administer meloxicam (0.3–0.5 mg/kg SC, PO q24h).

G. Administer antibiotics if infection of the cheek pouch was diagnosed. Ensure good coverage against anaerobic bacteria (e.g. doxycycline, metronidazole).

H. Provide supportive care, if indicated.

3. Bacterial pneumonia

A. Bacterial pneumonia in hamsters may be caused by *Pasteurella pneumotropica*, *Streptococcus pneumoniae*, or other *Streptococcus* spp.

B. The clinical signs are depression, anorexia, oculonasal discharge and respiratory distress.

C. Treatment includes the administration of systemic antibiotics, fluid therapy and nebulization.

4. Abdominal distention

A. Abdominal distention is commonly seen in geriatric hamsters and can have a variety of underlying causes. Differentials include ascites secondary to cardiac or renal insufficiency, reproductive tract disease, neoplasia, or polycystic disease, which affects mainly the liver. Large space-occupying liver cysts are not uncommon in hamsters.

B. Under sedation or general anesthesia, perform abdominal ultrasound to further investigate the underlying causes for abdominal distention.

C. Aspirate fluid, if present, under ultrasound guidance. Fluid aspiration may be diagnostic and therapeutic in cases in which respiratory distress is caused by the abdominal distention.

D. Perform whole body radiographs if cardiac disease is suspected.

E. The prognosis for abdominal distention in hamsters, regardless of the underlying cause, is guarded to poor.

5. Ocular proptosis

A. The etiologies include trauma, molar abscessation, infection and excessive restraint.

B. The treatment is the same as for a dog, including a temporary tarsorrhaphy (see Ch. 13). Remove the sutures in 7–10 days.

C. Corticosteroids should not be administered.

D. Administer broad-spectrum antibiotics.

E. If enucleation is indicated, the subconjunctival technique should be performed and the Harderian gland should also be removed.

F. If excessive hemorrhage occurs during enucleation, the orbit may be packed with Gelfoam®.

6. Cardiomyopathy

A. The clinical signs include dyspnea, tachypnea, cyanosis, rales, tachycardia, poor peripheral pulses, ascites and pleural effusion.

B. Thoracic radiographs and echocardiography are useful.
C. Treatment
    I. Administer furosemide 2–4 mg/kg IM, SC, PO q4–6h.
    II. Administer an ACE inhibitor (e.g. enalapril 0.5–1 mg/kg PO q24h).
D. The prognosis is guarded.

RECOMMENDED DRUG DOSAGES FOR HAMSTERS

Amoxicillin: Not recommended for oral administration
Ampicillin: Not recommended for oral administration
Atropine sulfate: 0.2–0.4 mg/kg SC, IM
Buprenorphine: 0.05–0.1 mg/kg SC, IM q8–12h
Butorphanol: 0.2–0.4 mg/kg SC, IM q2–4h
Cephalosporins: Not recommended for oral administration
Clindamycin: Not recommended for oral administration
Chloramphenicol: 30–50 mg/kg q8h
Doxycycline: 5 mg/kg PO q12h
Enrofloxacin: 10–20 mg/kg IM, SC, PO q12–24h
Fenbendazole: 20–50 mg/kg PO q24h for 5 days
Furosemide: 2–4 mg/kg IM, SC, PO PRN
Itraconazole 5–10 mg/kg PO q24h
Ivermectin: 0.2–0.4 mg/kg SC, PO q7–14d (*administer 0.2 mg/kg PO q24h for demodicosis*)
Metronidazole: 10–20 mg/kg PO q12h
Midazolam: 0.5–2 mg/kg IM, SC, IN
Praziquantel: 6–10 mg/kg IM, SC, PO
Selamectin: 15–30 mg/kg topical q21–28d
Sulfadimethoxine (Albon®): 20–50 mg/kg PO q24h
Tetracycline: 450–540 mg/L water, add sucrose to increase palatability; 15–20 mg/kg PO q8–12h
Terbinafine: 10–30 mg/kg PO q24h
Trimethoprim-sulfa: 15–30 mg/kg IM, PO q12h

HEDGEHOGS (AFRICAN, *ATELERIX ALBIVENTRIS*)

Adult average body weight = males 400–600 g, females 250–400 g. Average life span = 3–6 years.

Sexual maturity = males 2–6 months, females 6–8 months. They are induced ovulators; there is no breeding season.

Gestation period = 32–37 days. Litter size = 1–7; average is 3–4. The newborns are born blind and deaf, with soft white spines. Weaning of the young is usually at 4–6 weeks of age.

Hedgehogs are nocturnal. They burrow and sleep most of the day and forage at twilight. They can swim and climb well. They do not need to hibernate and will not do so in captivity if they are kept well fed and warm. African hedgehogs should be kept at an enclosure temperature of 75–85°F (24–29°C).

Hedgehogs have a keen sense of hearing. They have a simple stomach and no cecum. GI transit time is 12–14 hours. Males have a prepuce, which is located on the ventral abdomen. The testes remain intra-abdominal. Females have 2–5 pairs of mammae and the vulva is a short distance from the rectal opening.

Heart rate = 180–280 bpm.

Respiratory rate = 25–50 bpm.

Rectal temperature = 97–99°F (36.1–37.2°C).

Normal blood values in hedgehogs include:

PCV = 36 ± 7%	Glucose = 89 ± 30 mg/dL
Total protein = 5.1–7.2 g/dL	Phosphorus = 5.3 ± 1.9 mg/dL
WBC = 11 000 ± 6000/mL	Calcium = 8.8 ± 1.4 mg/dL
BUN = 27 ± 9 mmol/L	Potassium = 4.9 ± 1 mEq/L
Creatinine = 0.4 ± 0.2 mg/dL	Sodium = 141 ± 9 mEq/L

Diet—In the wild, hedgehogs feed on insects, slugs, snails, worms, small vertebrates and fruit. In captivity, they should be fed a commercial dry hedgehog diet, or reduced calorie cat or dog food should be offered. In addition, a small amount of invertebrates, cottage cheese, canned dog or cat food, or boiled egg can be offered. Hedgehogs seem to have higher requirement for fiber in their diet than other carnivorous animals. Therefore a teaspoon of a vegetable and fruit mix should be offered daily. Do not feed seeds or nuts or hard foods such as carrots, as they frequently get lodged in the roof of the mouth.

Restraint—Pick up a hedgehog with light leather gloves and allow the hedgehog to relax and unroll. Placing the hedgehog in a glass or a transparent plastic container facilitates examination of the ventral aspect of the body. Anesthesia is often necessary to perform a complete examination or to perform clinical procedures.

Anesthesia—Isoflurane or sevoflurane is preferred. Premedication is often not feasible. Induction should be performed in a large anesthesia mask, which fits the entire hedgehog or in an induction chamber.

Intravenous injections and blood collection may be performed utilizing the lateral saphenous vein, cephalic vein, and jugular vein. Intramuscular injections may be administered in the thigh. Subcutaneous injections may be administered in the flank or back. Intraperitoneal injections may be given.

Fluid therapy

Daily maintenance fluid requirements in hedgehogs are about 60–100 mL/kg/day.

Nutritional support

Any anorexic or cachexic hedgehog should receive nutritional support, unless a GI obstruction is suspected. Feed a critical care diet formula for carnivores (e.g. Oxbow Critical Care for Carnivores® or Lafaber Emeraid Carnivore / Omnivore®) or a canned critical diet (e.g. Hill's a/d®)

1. Neoplasia
   A. Neoplasia is very common and should be considered as a differential in any sick hedgehog over 3 years of age.
   B. The clinical signs may include anorexia, weight loss, depression, pale mucous membranes, respiratory distress, etc.
   C. Neoplasia has been reported in all body systems.
   D. Treatment is empirical, surgical resection if indicated. No chemotherapy protocols have been published for hedgehogs.
2. Neurologic deficits ('wobbly hedgehog syndrome')
   A. 'Wobbly hedgehog syndrome' is a neurodegenerative disease of unknown etiology, which affects the brain and spinal cord of African hedgehogs. Up 10% of the captive population may be affected. Most animals are younger than 2 years, by the onset of the first clinical signs.
   B. Clinical signs include progressive paralysis, ataxia, seizures, muscle atrophy, and scoliosis.
   C. Differentials include intervertebral disc disease, toxins, hypothermia, neoplasia, vascular disease.
   D. There is no effective treatment for 'wobbly hedgehog syndrome'. Provide supportive and palliative care. The long-term prognosis is poor.
3. Respiratory diseases
   A. *Bordetella bronchiseptica* and *Pasteurella multocida* can cause rhinitis and bronchopneumonia in hedgehogs.
   B. Cardiac disease and neoplasia also cause respiratory distress in hedgehogs.
   C. The clinical signs may include dyspnea, tachypnea, sneezing, and nasal discharge.
   D. Diagnosis is made by thoracic radiographs or CT scan and echocardiography.
   E. Treat underlying cause:
      I. Administer oxygen as needed.
      II. Perform nebulization if indicated.
      III. Maintain hydration with the parenteral administration of fluids.
      IV. Administer broad-spectrum antibiotics if bacterial pneumonia is suspected:
         a. Amoxicillin / clavulanic acid: 12.5 mg/kg PO q12h
         b. Enrofloxacin: 5–10 mg/kg IM, SC, PO q12–24h
         c. Trimethoprim-sulfa: 30 mg/kg IM, PO q12h.
4. Cardiomyopathy
   A. Dilative cardiomyopathy is common in African hedgehogs.
   B. Clinical signs include dyspnea, tachypnea, tachycardia, heart murmur, depression, lethargy, anorexia, weight loss, and abdominal distention secondary to ascites.
   C. Differentials include primary respiratory tract disease (e.g. pneumonia), anemia, or neoplasia.
   D. Diagnosis is made by thoracic radiographs and echocardiography.
   E. Treatment of congestive heart failure is the same as in other species.

5. Dermatologic disorders
   A. Skin mites *(Caparinia tripolis)* are not uncommon in hedgehogs and in many cases a co-infection with dermatophytes is present.
   B. *Trichophyton* spp. and *Microsporum* spp. infections have been reported in hedgehogs.
   C. Clinical signs include quill loss leading to alopecia, white-brown skin crusts, and flaking of the skin.
   D. Diagnosis of skin mite infection is made by cytologic examination of samples collected by skin scraping and acetate tape.
   E. Treat skin mites with ivermectin (0.2–0.4 mg/kg SC, PO q10–14d) or selamectin (6–10 mg/kg topically q21–28d). Disinfect the environment and treat in-contact animals.
   F. Submit sample for a dermatophyte culture, while initiating symptomatic topical treatment with enilconazole (topical, 1:50 dilution, q72h). Disinfect the environment.
   G. If dermatophyte culture revealed growth, and response to topical antifungal and anti-parasitic treatment is not satisfactory, consider treatment with itraconazole (5–10 mg/kg PO q24h) or terbinafine (10–30 mg/kg PO q24h).
   H. Continue treatment with antifungals once two consecutive dermatophyte cultures 1 week apart have revealed no further growth.
6. Gastrointestinal diseases
   A. *Salmonella* and other bacteria may cause anorexia, diarrhea and weight loss.
      I. Submit fecal culture to confirm a tentative diagnosis of salmonellosis.
      II. Treatment includes fluid therapy and broad-spectrum antibiotics.
   B. Other causes of gastrointestinal disorders in hedgehogs include: periodontal disease, stomatitis, gastritis, enteritis, colitis, hepatic lipidosis and neoplasia of the gastrointestinal tract.
7. Obesity
   A. Obesity is a common problem in captive hedgehogs.
   B. Provide the proper diet.
   C. Do not allow free-choice foraging. Set out just enough food in the evening that the entire meal is eaten by morning. Only small snacks should be provided during the day.
   D. Encourage activity by providing a large enough enclosure and an exercise wheel, but avoid wire wheels or items in which the hedgehog may get a foot stuck.
8. Urethral obstruction
   A. Male hedgehogs may develop urethral obstructions secondary to crystalluria.
   B. If possible, relieve the urethral obstruction and administer fluid therapy; treat possible underlying cystitis.

RECOMMENDED DRUG DOSAGES FOR HEDGEHOGS

Amoxicillin: 15 mg/kg IM, SC, PO q12h
Amoxicillin / clavulanic acid: 12.5 mg/kg PO q12h

Ampicillin: 10 mg/kg IM q12h
Buprenorphine: 0.01–0.03 mg/kg IM, SC q8–12h
Butorphanol: 0.2–0.4 mg/kg SC q6–8h
Calcium gluconate: 10–50 mg/kg IM
Cephalexin: 25 mg/kg PO q12h
Chloramphenicol: 30 mg/kg IM q12h, 50mg/kg PO q12h
Clindamycin: 5.5–10 mg/kg PO q12h
Dexamethasone: 0.1–1.5 mg/kg IM for allergies or inflammation; up to 5 mg/kg for shock
Enalapril: 0.5 mg/kg PO q24h
Enrofloxacin: 5–10 mg/kg IM, SC, PO q12–24h
Erythromycin: 10 mg/kg IM, PO q12h
Furosemide: 2–4 mg/kg IM, SC, PO q8–12h or PRN
Fenbendazole: 20 mg/kg PO q12h for 5 days
Griseofulvin (microsize): 50 mg/kg/day PO divided q8–12h
Itraconazole: 5–10 mg/kg PO q12–24h
Ivermectin: 0.2–0.4 mg/kg PO, SC q10–14d
Meloxicam: 0.2 mg/kg IM, SC, PO q24h
Metronidazole: 20 mg/kg PO q12h
Midazolam: 0.25–1 mg/kg IM, SC
Penicillin G: 40000 IU/kg IM q24h
Praziquantel: 7 mg/kg PO, SC
Selamectin: 6–10 mg/kg topical q21–28d
Sulfadimethoxine (Albon®): 2–20 mg/day IM, SC, PO
Terbinafine: 10–30 mg/kg PO q24h
Tiletamine/zolazepam: 1–5 mg/kg IM
Trimethoprim-sulfa: 30 mg/kg IM, PO q12h

LIZARDS

Herbivorous lizards that are popular pets include the green iguanas, prehensile-tailed skink, *Corucia zebrata*, and spiny-tailed lizards, *Uromastyx* spp.

Popular omnivorous lizards include bearded dragons and skinks.

Popular insectivorous lizards include leopard geckos, chameleons, anoles, Chinese water dragons, and skinks.

The popular carnivorous lizards include the monitors, *Varanus* spp., and the tegus, *Tupinambis* spp.

Zoonotic diseases—salmonellosis.

Diet—Green iguanas in the wild feed on the leaves of vines and trees. They are hindgut fermenters and are able to digest high-fiber diets. Herbivorous lizards should never be fed products containing animal protein owing to the risk of developing kidney disease. Vitamin supplementation is not required in herbivorous lizards, and can lead to intoxications. Calcium should be supplemented and access to UVB light provided.

The insectivorous lizards should be fed a variety of captive-raised insects. Crickets should be 'gut-loaded' for at least 48 hours prior to feeding them to the lizard. Vitamin and mineral supplementation is also required.

Carnivorous lizards should be fed pre-killed whole prey, including mice, rats, rodents, chicks, and fish. Commercial canned complete diets for carnivorous reptiles are available. Muscle meat should not be fed, as it may cause severe nutritional deficiencies.

Sex determination—
1. Mature male iguanas have bilateral hemipenis bulges at the base of the tail, larger and more developed femoral pores on the ventral aspect of the thigh, taller dorsal spines, a larger dewlap, and larger operculum scales than females.
2. Male geckos also have prominent precloacal and femoral pores.
3. Male chameleons may have elaborate head ornamentation, including horns, crests and plates, which are absent in females.
4. Male lizards tend to be larger in size, and have brighter colors and bigger crests than females.
5. Endoscopic visualization of the gonads may be necessary in some species.

Clinical pathology

1. Reptilian blood should be handled in the same manner as avian blood.
2. EDTA should not be used for CBC samples.
3. Lithium heparin is the preferred anticoagulant.
4. Blood smears should be made as soon as the blood is drawn.

Venipuncture in lizards

1. The preferred site is the ventral tail vein (Fig. 15.8).
2. Place the lizard in dorsal recumbency, or in left sternal recumbency, with its tail hanging over the edge of a table.
3. Aseptically prepare the venipuncture site.
4. Insert a needle of the appropriate size for the patient at an angle between 45° and 90° to the axis of the tail on the ventral midline.
5. Advance the needle until the tip touches the ventral vertebral surface.
6. Withdraw the needle slightly while applying negative pressure.
7. A blood sample should then be obtained.

Fluid administration in lizards

1. Balanced electrolyte solutions (e.g. LRS, Normosol®-R) can be used.
2. Routes of administration include:
   A. Soaking in the appropriate liquid
   B. Subcutaneous injection
   C. Intravenous infusion
   D. Intraosseous infusion.
3. Soaking a lizard in the appropriate water encourages drinking and also rehydrates by absorption.
   A. The water should be lukewarm.
   B. The depth should be halfway up the lizard's back.

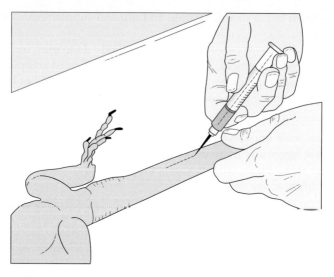

FIG 15.8 **Venipuncture of the ventral tail vein in an iguana.** *Adapted from Quesenberry, K., Hillyer, E.V., 1994. The Veterinary Clinics of North America, Small Animal Practice: Exotic Pet Medicine II 24 (1), 153–173, with permission from Elsevier.*

C. Soaking should last for 10–20 minutes.

D. The lizard should be monitored to prevent drowning.

4. Subcutaneous fluids – administer SC fluids in the lateral body wall, along the lateral skin fold if present.

5. Intravenous fluids may be administered through the ventral tail vein.

6. Intraosseous fluids may be administered through the proximal, medial, tibial crest.

A. Administer local or general anesthesia.

B. Sterile technique is necessary.

C. Use a 20- to 22-gauge needle or spinal needle.

7. The maintenance fluid requirement is 20–40 mL/kg/day.

Any drug injections should be administered in the cranial half of the body due to the presence of a renal and hepatic portal system, which significantly reduces systemic drug levels because the first-pass effect.

Keep isopropyl alcohol available when handling lizards. If a lizard bites someone and refuses to let go, a few drops of alcohol placed in the lizard's mouth will induce it to do so.

Sedation—

- Propofol 3–5 mg/kg IV.
- Dexmedetomidine (0.1 mg/kg SC, IM) *plus* midazolam (1 mg/kg SC, IM). Reverse with atipamezole (equal volume of dexmedetomidine, SC, IM) *and* flumazenil (0.05 mg/kg SC, IM).
- Dexmedetomidine (0.05–1 mg/kg SC, IM) *plus* midazolam (1 mg/kg SC, IM) *plus* ketamine (3 mg/kg SC, IM). Reverse with atipamezole (equal volume of dexmedetomidine, SC, IM) *and* flumazenil (0.05 mg/kg SC, IM). Deep sedation is usually achieved with this protocol. Suitable for endotracheal intubation.

Anesthesia—
- If the animal's size allows, administer propofol 5–15 mg/kg IV to effect, followed by endotracheal intubation and maintenance on isoflurane or sevoflurane for longer procedures.
- Small lizards are induced with isoflurane or sevoflurane in an induction chamber or zip-lock bag. Maintain anesthesia by delivering the anesthetic gas by face mask.

Surgical techniques

1. Scrub under the edges of scales when surgically preparing the skin.
2. Sterile, transparent, self-adhering drapes are recommended.
3. Incisions should be made between scale rows rather than through scales.
4. Absorbable monofilament suture (e.g. polydioxanone) is recommended for buried suture.
5. Skin incisions should be closed with nylon suture in a slightly everting horizontal mattress.
6. Sutures should be placed between scales rather than through them.
7. Skin sutures or staples should not be removed for 4 weeks.
8. A paramedian celiotomy incision should be made to avoid the ventral abdominal vein.
9. The most common indications for celiotomy include biopsy, egg retention, gastrointestinal foreign objects, and uroliths.

   Euthanasia—The standard euthanasia solutions may be administered via IC, IV, or intracoelomic injection.

COMMON DISEASES AND HEALTH PROBLEMS OF LIZARDS

1. Renal failure
   A. The clinical signs include anorexia, bloating, flaccid paresis, weight loss, and lethargy. Dyschezia, cloacal prolapse, and obstipation may occur.
   B. Palpation anterior to the pelvis or dorsal to the cloaca may reveal renomegaly.
   C. Measurement of urine specific gravity is not useful because reptiles do not concentrate their urine.
   D. BUN and creatinine are not useful parameters to evaluate renal function in reptiles.
   E. Late in renal disease, phosphorus and uric acid levels rise.
   F. The prognosis is grave to poor.
   G. Treatment includes fluid therapy, phosphorus restriction and dietary therapy.
   H. The administration of oral phosphate binders may be beneficial.
   I. Cystic uroliths are possibly a result of insufficient bladder emptying, due to chronic mild dehydration.
      I. Cystic uroliths can be removed by cystoscopy or by cystotomy.
      II. Stone analysis and bacterial culture should be performed.

2. Trauma
  A. Control bleeding with electrocautery, the application of light pressure, or vessel ligation.
  B. Administer sedation and scrub wounds with a dilute disinfectant.
  C. Flush the wounds with warm, sterile saline.
  D. Apply antibiotic cream (e.g. silver sulfadiazine) to the wounds or suture the wounds if they are severe.
  E. If the wounds are infected, delay closure until the infection is controlled.
  F. Horizontal mattress sutures or stents should be used, and the sutures should be removed after 4–6 weeks.
  G. Treatment of bite wounds from dogs, cats, rodents, etc. is the same as for other patients (see Ch. 5).
  H. Fractures can usually be managed with splints or cage rest, but internal fixation might be necessary.
  I. Lizard tails may break or develop avascular necrosis secondary to vascular injury.
    I. The tail will regrow.
    II. Bleeding may be controlled with silver nitrate sticks or cautery.
    III. If the tail is infected, surgical amputation should be performed and the wound closed.

3. Metabolic bone disease
  A. The etiologies include a lack of dietary calcium, lack of dietary vitamin D (not in herbivorous), improper calcium: phosphorus ratio, lack of ultraviolet light (only in herbivorous), and disease of the kidneys.
  B. The diagnosis is based on the history.
  C. Radiographs may be useful to evaluate the severity of the disease and to monitor the response to treatment.
  D. Plasma biochemistry should be performed (calcium, phosphorous, uric acid).
  E. Softening of the mandible is often the first clinical sign.
  F. Other clinical signs include a shortened mandible, symmetrical swelling of the mandible, firm swelling of any or all of the long leg bones, pathologic fractures, vertebral collapse, kyphosis, paralysis, lethargy, anorexia, muscle fasciculations, tremors and seizures.
  G. Treatment
    I. Improve husbandry, particularly diet, ultraviolet light, and provide a focal hot spot that is near 37°C.
    II. Administer calcium gluconate only if the animal is in an acute hypocalcemic crisis (10–50 mg/kg IM, SC, dilute 1:1).
    III. Administer calcium glubionate or calcium carbonate (10 mg/kg PO q12–24h).
    IV. Administer vitamin D_3 (400 IU/kg IM once). Provide exposure to artificial UV light or direct sunlight, if appropriate for the species.
    V. Soak the lizard in warm water for 10–20 minutes q12–24h.
    VI. Remove climbing branches to prevent fractures.
    VII. Handle affected lizards gently and only when necessary.

4. Dystocia
    A. If the lizard is not in obvious distress or prolapsed, dystocia management can be delayed overnight.
    B. Intervention should be considered if the gravid lizard refuses food for 3–4 weeks without laying eggs.
    C. Intervention should also be considered if a gravid lizard becomes weak, lethargic, loses muscle tone, oviposition is overdue, or there are abnormalities in the hematology or serum chemistry profile.
    D. Administer fluid therapy.
    E. Place the lizard in a warm, quiet environment.
    F. Lizards do not respond well to oxytocin administration.
    G. The recommended treatment is surgical removal of the eggs and ovariectomy or ovariosalpingectomy, to prevent recurrence of egg retention or dystocia.
5. Cloacal organ prolapse
    A. Cloacal tissues, cloacal masses, oviduct, intestines or hemipenises may be prolapsed.
    B. The etiologies include cloacitis, cloacal masses, enteritis (e.g. endoparasitism), dystocia, coelomitis.
    C. The recommended diagnostic tests include:
        I. Fecal wet mount and fecal flotation
        II. Fecal or cloacal swab cytology (Diff quick stain)
        III. Whole body radiographs
        IV. Coelomic ultrasound
        V. CBC and plasma biochemistry panel
        VI. Cloacoscopy and coeliotomy.
    D. Treatment
        I. Administer anesthesia or perform sedation.
        II. Administer fluids SC, IV or IO.
        III. Identify the cloacal tissue (oviduct vs intestine vs cloaca).
        IV. Reduce the swelling and control hemorrhage of the prolapsed cloacal tissue by applying 50% dextrose solution topically
        V. Rinse the prolapsed tissue with warm saline.
        VI. If necrotic tissue is present, surgical debridement or resection is necessary.
        VII. After identification of the prolapsed tissue, apply sterile lubricating jelly.
        VIII. With a lubricated sterile swab, replace the prolapsed tissues.
        IX. Place retention sutures (two simple transverse sutures) perpendicular to the vent. Do not place purse-string sutures.
        X. After initial stabilization, coeliotomy and ovariosalpingectomy is the treatment of choice for most cases of oviductal prolapse.
        XI. Administer analgesics: meloxicam (0.2 mg/kg IM q24h).
        XII. Administer broad-spectrum antibiotics, if indicated.
        XIII. Treat endoparasites, if indicated.
        XIV. Identify and treat the underlying etiology.

6. Infectious diseases
   A. Dermatitis
      I. The signs of dermatitis and pyoderma include a well-demarcated pale or dark discoloration of the skin, blisters filled with clear or bloody fluid, crusts, erythema and ulceration.
      II. Dermatitis usually occurs on the ventral aspect of the tail, feet and body.
      III. Differentials include thermal burns and rostral abrasions.
      IV. Treatment includes topical antibiotic ointments, injectable antibiotics based on bacterial culture and sensitivity, and correction of husbandry problems.
      V. Yellow-fungus disease is an often-fatal disorder in bearded dragons and green iguanas, which is caused by *Chrysosporium* anamorph of *Nannizziopsis vriesii* (CANV), a keratinophilic fungus. Biopsies are diagnostic. Treatment involves surgical debridement and long term systemic antifungal therapy. The prognosis is guarded to poor.
   B. Abscesses and granulomas
      I. These may be caused by bacterial infections, foreign bodies, fungal infections and metazoan parasites.
      II. Treatment includes administration of a local or general anesthetic, excision with the capsule intact or lancing, curettage or flushing, bacterial culture from the abscess lining, fluid therapy, and systemic antibiotic therapy.
   C. Diarrhea
      I. Diagnostic procedures should include fecal flotation and direct smear. Radiographs and plasma biochemical profile should be considered if endoparasites are not the underlying cause.
      II. Endoparasites are the most common cause of diarrhea in lizards. Coccidia are very common in bearded dragons.
      III. Treatment should address the underlying cause.

RECOMMENDED DRUG DOSAGES FOR LIZARDS

Amikacin: 5 mg/kg IM, then 2.5mg/kg q72h (only in patients which are hydrated and have normal renal function)
Atropine: 0.01–0.04 mg/kg IM, SC (bradycardia or preanesthetic); 0.5 mg/kg IM, IV, IT, IO (CPR)
Butorphanol: 0.4–1 mg/kg IM (sedation, does not provide analgesia)
Calcium glubionate: 10 mg/kg PO q12–24h
Calcium gluconate: 10–50 mg/kg IM, SC (dilute 1:1)
Ceftazidime: 20–40 mg/kg IM, SC q48–72h (q24h in chameleons)
Ciprofloxacin: 10 mg/kg PO q48h
Clindamycin: 5 mg/kg PO q12h
Diazepam: 0.5–2 mg/kg IV, IM, IN
Doxycycline: 5–10 mg/kg PO q24h
Enrofloxacin: 5–10 mg/kg IM, SC, PO q24h
Fenbendazole: 50 mg/kg PO q24h for 3–5 days

Furosemide: 2–5 mg/kg IM, IV, PO q12–24h
Gentamicin: 5 mg/mL in saline for nebulization for 15 minutes q8h
Ivermectin: 0.2 mg/kg IM, SC, PO repeat in 14 days **(do not use in skinks)**
Ketamine: 2.5–10 mg/kg IM (combine with midazolam and/or (dex-) medetomidine to achieve sedation)
Metronidazole: 50 mg/kg PO; repeat in 10–14 days
Morphine: 1.5–2 mg/kg IM, SC (analgesia, respiratory depression may occur)
Praziquantel: 8 mg/kg IM, SC, PO; repeat in 14 days
Propofol: 5–15 mg/kg IV, IO to effect
Pyrantel pamoate: 25 mg/kg PO q24h for 3 days
Sulfadimethoxine: 50 mg/kg PO q24h for 3–5 days, then q48h PRN
Toltazuril: 5–15 mg/kg PO q24h for 3 days
Vitamin A: 1000–5000 IU/kg IM, SC
Vitamin D_3: 400 IU/kg IM, PO
Vitamin K_1: 0.25–0.5 mg/kg IM

POT-BELLIED PIGS (VIETNAMESE)

A young female pig is called a gilt; the older female is a sow. The intact male pig is a boar; the castrated male is a barrow.

Average body weight = 35–90 kg. Average life span = 15–18 years. Sexual maturity = 3–4 months.

Pigs are polyestrous. Estrous cycles average 21 days. Estrus lasts 1–3 days. Gestation = 114 days average. Litter size = 4–15 piglets (6–8 average).

The following normal values are listed for the adult pig:

Heart rate = 70–80 beats/min
Respiratory rate = 13–18 breaths/min
Temperature = 99–102°F (37.2–38.9°C).

Normal blood values include:

PCV = 38.1–48.8%	Calcium = 10.2–12.2 mg/dL
TP = 6.3–9.4 g/dL	Phosphorus = 5–10.7 mg/dL
WBC = 5200–17900/mL	ALT = 23–83 U/L
Glucose = 68–155 mg/dL	ALP = 35–536 U/L
BUN = 10–47 mg/dL	AST <109 U/L
Creatinine = 0.4–1.1 mg/dL	GGT = 21–57 U/L
Albumin = 3.1–4.3 g/dL	Bilirubin, total <0.3 mg/dL

Venipuncture sites

The auricular ear veins and subcutaneous abdominal vein are accessible even without sedation or anesthesia. The jugular vein and anterior vena cava are commonly used, but are blind sticks and should be performed under anesthesia or sedation. The cephalic, lateral saphenous may also be used.

Anesthesia—
- Protocol 1: Medetomidine (0.04–0.07 mg/kg) + butorphanol (0.15–0.3 mg/kg) + midazolam (0.1–0.3 mg/kg) IM. Reverse with

atipamezole as well as flumazenil (1 mg/10–15 mg of midazolam IV, IM) if necessary. This is the preferred anesthetic protocol, with rapid induction and recovery.

- Protocol 2: Midazolam (0.1–0.3 mg/kg) + ketamine (5–10 mg/kg) – provides short-term anesthesia.
- Isoflurane or propofol is recommended for maintenance if necessary.
- For long procedures, or anesthesia of large, obese pigs, tracheal intubation is recommended.

Vaccinations—Those against *Erysipelothrix rhusiopathiae*, *Actinobacillus pleuropneumoniae* and leptospirosis are recommended for pet pigs. Tetanus vaccine should be considered if trauma is likely, or after trauma and surgery.

Regulatory guidelines—Pot-bellied pigs are subject to the same restrictions and testing policies as commercial swine. The veterinarian should contact the offices of their state veterinarians or USDA prior to issuing a health certificate for travel. Testing for pseudorabies and swine brucellosis may be necessary.

COMMON DISEASES AND HEALTH PROBLEMS OF POT-BELLIED PIGS

1. Dog bite wounds
   A. Assess the extent of the injuries.
   B. Administer fluid therapy.
   C. Administer parenteral antibiotics.
   D. Administer tetanus antitoxin 500–1500 IU/pig, if not currently on tetanus vaccine.
   E. Thoroughly clean and flush the wounds with an antiseptic solution.
   F. Anesthesia and debridement of deep wounds may be indicated.
2. Shock
   A. The causes include severe indigestion and bloating, being chased or bitten by dogs, or being hit by a car.
   B. The clinical signs include lateral recumbency, tachycardia, dyspnea, pale or cyanotic mucous membranes, extension of the legs, shaking and moaning.
   C. Treatment is the same as any other animal in shock.
3. Heat stroke or stress
   A. Adult pot-bellied pigs prefer an environmental temperature of 60–70°F (16–21°C).
   B. Pigs are unable to sweat.
   C. The clinical signs include weakness, tachypnea, tachycardia, and open-mouthed breathing.
   D. The prognosis is grave if open-mouthed breathing is present.
   E. Treatment includes intravenous fluid therapy and cooling of the patient.
4. Vomiting and diarrhea
   A. The causes include overeating, bacterial or viral diseases, foreign-body obstruction, dietary indiscretion, and gastric ulceration.

B. The clinical signs include moaning, refusal to stand, walking with an arched back, vomiting and diarrhea.
C. Pigs with gastric ulceration may exhibit hematemesis, melena, and anemia.
D. Administer fluid therapy.
E. The administration of metoclopramide may be beneficial, but should be avoided if a gastrointestinal obstruction is suspected.
F. Contrast radiography may be useful.
G. Rule out endoparasites.
H. If surgery is indicated, a ventral midline incision is recommended. The surgical procedure for a gastrotomy or enterotomy is the same as in the dog (see Ch. 9).
I. Treatment of gastric ulcerations includes the administration of H_2 blockers such as cimetidine or famotidine, omeprazole, antacids and antibiotics.

5. Poisoning
A. Emesis may be induced by administering hydrogen peroxide 1 mL/5kg PO or syrup of ipecac 7–15 mL PO.
B. Treatment is the same as for a dog.

RECOMMENDED DRUG DOSAGES FOR POT-BELLIED PIGS

(Most medications and dosages used to treat dogs in an emergency may also be used to treat pigs in an emergency.)

Acepromazine: 0.03–0.22 mg/kg IM
Aspirin: 10 mg/kg PO q6–8h
Atropine: 0.02–0.04 mg/kg IM or SC *(pre-anesthetic)*
Butorphanol: 0.1–0.3 mg/kg IM
Carprofen: 2.2 mg/kg q12h or 4.4 mg/kg q24h PO
Ceftiofur sodium (Naxel®): 2.2 mg/kg IM q24h
Ceftiofur crystalline-free acid (Excede®): 5 mg/kg IM q5–7d
Cephalexin: 30 mg/kg PO q8–12h
Dantrolene: 2–5 mg/kg IV *(treatment of malignant hyperthermia)*
Diazepam: 0.5–1.5 mg/kg IV
Enrofloxacin: 2.5–5 mg/kg IM, PO q24h **(prohibited in food-producing animals)**
Fenbendazole: 10 mg/kg PO q24h for 3 days
Florfenicol: 200 mg/kg IM, IV q6–8h or q12h if given PO
Hydrogen peroxide: 1 mL/5kg PO *(induction of emesis)*
Iron dextran: 50–100 mg/piglet IM
Ivermectin: 300 mg/kg IM, SC, PO
Ketoprofen: 1–3 mg/kg PO q24h
Lincomycin: 10 mg/kg IM q12–14h
Metronidazole: 20 mg/kg PO q12 **(prohibited in food-producing animals)**
Oxytocin: 10–20 IU IM
Penicillin G procaine: 20000–60000 U/kg IM q24h
Phenylbutazone: 0.5–1 mg/kg q24h
Prostaglandin F2α: 5 mg/animal IM

Pyrantel pamoate: 6.6 mg/kg PO
Syrup of ipecac: 7–15 mL PO
Tetanus antitoxin: 500–1500 IU/pig IM
Tetracycline: 10–20 mg/kg IM q24h
Tramadol: 2–4 mg/kg PO q6–24h
Trimethoprim-sulfa: 25–50 mg/kg PO q24h
Tylosin: 9 mg/kg IM q12–24h

RABBITS (ORYCTOLAGUS CUNICULUS)

Domestic rabbits originate from the European wild rabbit (*Oryctolagus cuniculus*) and are not related to the cotton-tailed rabbits found in the wild in North America. All information in this section pertains to domestic rabbits, not wild rabbits.

Although rabbits share many similarities in their anatomy and physiology with rodents, they are classified in different taxonomic orders (Lagomorpha vs Rodentia). Rabbits possess no foot pads, and have four maxillary incisor teeth.

Average life span = 5–10 years.
Adult body weight = 1–6 kg.
Heart rate = 130–300/min.
Respiratory rate = 35–60/min.
Temperature = 101.0–104°F (38.5–40°C).
Normal blood values in rabbits include:

PCV = 30–50%	Calcium = 8–14.8 mg/dL
TP = 5.4–7.5 g/dL	Potassium = 3.6–6.9 mEq/L
WBC = 65 000–12 000/mL	Sodium = 131–155 mEq/L
BUN = 13–30 mg/dL	ALP = 4–70 U/L
Creatinine = 0.5–2.5 mg/dL	ALT = 14–80 U/L
Glucose = 75–155 mg/dL	AST = 14–113 U/L
Phosphorus = 2.3–6.9 mg/dL	Bilirubin, total = 0–0.7 mg/dL.

Sexual maturity occurs at 4–10 months. Estrus cycle = induced ovulators, 9–13h after coitus. Gestation period = 30–32 days.

Rabbits are born altricial, with no fur and with closed eyes. Their eyes open after about 10 days. Neonatal rabbits are unable to thermoregulate on their own.

Average litter size = 4–10. Rabbits have four pairs of mammary glands. Does nurse their young only once a day for 3–5 minutes, during which time a young rabbit may drink up to 20% of this body weight. Weaning is at 4–6 weeks.

Mixture to feed orphaned rabbits—
1. Rabbit milk is higher in protein and lower in carbohydrates compared with most other mammals. Several rabbit milk replacer recipes have been published:
   A. Recipe 1: ½ cup evaporated milk, ½ cup water, 1 egg yolk and 1 tablespoon of corn syrup.
   B. Recipe 2: 1 part of Esbilac®, 1 part of Multi-Milk® (powder), 1.5 parts of water.

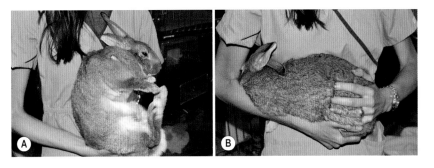

FIG 15.9   **Restraint and handling of rabbits.**

2. Feed three meals a day. Young rabbits up to day 10 completely depend on milk replacer.

Restraint—The back should be supported at all times, in order to avoid overextension, which leads to back injury. A rabbit is picked up by placing one hand underneath the thorax and the other hand underneath the hindlimbs and pelvis (Fig. 15.9). If the rabbit is nervous, tries to jump, or the handler is unfamiliar with handling and restraint of rabbits, perform physical examination and diagnostic procedures on the floor to avoid jumping off the exam table. Consider restraining a rabbit in a towel ('bunny burrito') for procedures that require access only to the head (e.g. syringe feeding, nasolacrimal duct flush, ear vein catheterization).

Sex determination—The anogenital distance is identical between males and females. Males have prominent hemiscrotal sacs and testicles. The glans penis can be manually protruded and the round urethral opening is visible in males. In females protrusion of the genital reveals a slit-like vulva.

Caution: Oral administration of penicillin, ampicillin, amoxicillin, cephalosporins, vancomycin, erythromycin or clindamycin may cause severe dysbacteriosis, enterocolitis and death. Therefore do not administer these antibiotics orally.

Many rabbits are not affected by atropine, owing to the presence of a serum atropinase. Use glycopyrrolate instead.

Sedation—
• Midazolam: 0.25–1 mg/kg IM, SC, IV
• Midazolam 0.5 mg/kg IM, SC *plus* butorphanol (0.25 mg/kg) or buprenorphine (0.03 mg/kg).

Anesthesia—
• Isoflurane or sevoflurane by mask or chamber, preferably after premedication with midazolam and butorphanol or buprenorphine. Rabbits are obligate nasal breathers, and therefore can be effectively maintained under inhalant anesthesia, with a face or nasal mask.
• Ketamine 10–15 mg/kg IM, *plus* medetomidine 0.1mg/kg IM, plus butorphanol 0.25 mg/kg IM.

Endotracheal intubation in the rabbit

1. Use an uncuffed 2–3 mm endotracheal tube (ET).
2. Place the rabbit in sternal recumbency.
3. Extend the head so that the trachea is perpendicular to the surface of the table.
4. Spray lidocaine topically on the larynx.
5. Advance the ET to the proximal larynx.
6. During inspiration, advance the ET into the trachea. Monitor for condensation of the ET tube during expiration.
7. The rabbit usually coughs during advancement of the ET into the trachea.
8. Auscult for breathing sounds from the ET tube.
9. Perform endoscopy-guided endotracheal intubation, if possible, in order to increase the chance of successful intubation and to decrease the risk of iatrogenic damage to the larynx.
10. Perform intranasal intubation if orotracheal intubation cannot be performed.

Diet—Rabbits are herbivorous hindgut fermenters. They should be fed predominately on high-quality (e.g. Timothy) grass hay and leafy greens. Avoid greens that are high in calcium (e.g. parsley) in order to reduce the risk of urolithiasis and 'bladder sludge'. Commercial rabbit pellets can be offered in limited amounts. Pregnant, nursing or growing animals should be fed pellets free choice, and alfalfa hay and pellets can be offered to these animals owing to the higher protein and calcium content.

Rabbit fluid therapy

1. The daily maintenance fluid requirements are 60–100 mL/kg/day.
2. For SC fluid administration, use LRS, Normosol®-R, or a similar balanced electrolyte isotonic crystalloid.
3. Administer fluids IV 2 × 3 times the maintenance rate IV if the animal is moderately dehydrated and showing signs of peripheral vasoconstriction.
4. If the animal is in hypovolemic shock, administer 60–90 mL/kg/h for the first 1–2 hours, then re-evaluate.
5. Alternatively an initial shock fluid bolus of 25 mL/kg can be given slowly over 5–7 minutes.
6. Alternatively administer crystalloid fluid bolus (30 mL/kg) plus Hetastarch bolus (5 mL/kg) if the animal is in hypovolemic shock.

Rabbit nutritional support

1. Any anorexic or hyporexic rabbit should receive nutritional support in order to minimize secondary gastrointestinal problems caused by reduced food intake (i.e. GI stasis, dysbacteriosis, tympany) and to avoid increased fat mobilization, which frequently leads to hepatic lipidosis.

2. Syringe feed with a high-fiber diet for herbivores (e.g. Oxbow Critical Care for Herbivores®, 50–80 mL/kg PO q24h; divide into 4–5 feedings) or crushed and soaked pellets. Do not syringe feed rabbits that are not swallowing.

Rabbit CPR

1. Use an uncuffed 1.5–2.5 mm endotracheal tube to establish an airway. Alternatively, perform nasotracheal intubation or use a tight-fitting nasal mask to ventilate.
2. Ventilate at a rate of 30–50 breaths/min.
3. Be careful not to overinflate the lungs.
4. Gently perform external cardiac massage at a rate of 100 compressions/min.
5. Evaluate the cardiac rhythm with an ECG.
6. Monitor the strength and character of the femoral pulse frequently.
7. Place an intravenous catheter and administer isotonic crystalloids bolus at a rate of 25 mL/kg slowly over 5–7 minutes IV.
8. If indicated, administer:
   A. Epinephrine 0.1–0.4 mg/kg IV or IO or intratracheally
   B. Atropine 0.1–0.5 mg/kg SC, IM, IV (may not be effective, or high doses may be required due to the presence of atropinase in many rabbits).

Intravenous catheter placement in the rabbit

1. The lateral marginal ear veins, saphenous, cephalic and jugular veins are usually accessible. Jugular veins can be difficult to access owing to the dewlap. The marginal ear vein catheters are preferred and easiest to maintain (Fig. 15.10).
2. Use a 22-, 24-, or 26-gauge catheter.
3. IO catheterization may be performed with a 20- or 22-gauge 1.5-inch (38 mm) spinal needle.

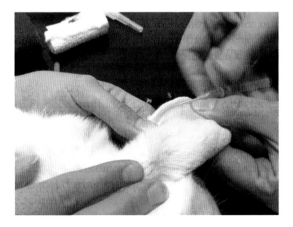

FIG 15.10 **Ear vein catheter placement.** From Varga, M. A Textbook of Rabbit Surgery (2014), Butterworth Heinemann. In press. With permission from Elsevier.

A. The recommended sites for IO catheterization, in order of preference, are the proximal femur and the proximal tibia.
B. Anesthesia or a local anesthetic block should be administered.
C. The technique is the same as that for a cat.
D. IV or IO catheters should be secured to the skin with tissue glue or butterfly tape tabs prior to applying a bandage.

Venipuncture in the rabbit

1. The available sites for venipuncture in the rabbit include the lateral saphenous vein, central ear artery, cephalic vein and jugular vein. The lateral saphenous veins are easiest to access to obtain diagnostic samples from. Jugular veins can be difficult to access owing to the dewlap.
2. The maximum blood volume to be removed is 1% of the body weight in grams.
3. Use small gauge hypodermic needles and small syringes. Rabbit veins are thin walled, and hematoma formation is common. Apply digital pressure and a pressure bandage after venipuncture.

COMMON DISEASES AND HEALTH PROBLEMS OF RABBITS

1. Anorexia and GI stasis
   A. Many causes can lead to anorexia and subsequently GI stasis in rabbits. Underlying causes include: stress, anxiety, pain (e.g. dental disease, spastic colic), hyperthermia, gastrointestinal disease (tympany, small intestinal obstruction, liver lobe torsion), urolithiasis, CNS disorders, neoplasia, metabolic disorders and systemic infections.
   B. History and physical examination are used to differentiate between an acute and a chronic problem. Perform appropriate diagnostic tests to establish a diagnosis including:
      I. Whole body radiographs
      II. Biochemistry profile, PCV / TP, CBC
      III. Abdominal ultrasound.
   C. Pending a definite diagnosis provide supportive care:
      I. Analgesia: buprenorphine 0.03–0.05 mg/kg SC, IM, IV
      II. Fluid therapy: 30–50 mL/kg SC bolus if rabbit is mildly dehydrated. Administer fluids IV 2×3 times the maintenance rate IV if the animal is moderately dehydrated. Maintenance rate is 60–100 mL/kg/day.
      III. Provide nutritional support if GI obstruction was ruled out. Do not syringe feed rabbits which do not swallow. Consider nasogastric or esophageal feeding tubes if indicated.
   D. Rule out dental disease by complete examination of the oral cavity in an anesthetized rabbit, if no other cause for anorexia and depression is found.
   E. Liver lobe torsion is common in rabbits. Anorexia, GI stasis, depression, pain upon palpation of the cranial abdomen and high activities of ALT, AST and ALP are suggestive. Confirm by

ultrasonography. Treatment is surgical. The prognosis is good if diagnosed timely.
   F. Many rabbits will respond to analgesia, fluid therapy and nutritional support if stress or a spastic colic were the underlying cause. Regularly re-evaluate the condition of the rabbit while it is hospitalized and adjust the diagnostic and treatment plans accordingly.
2. Gastric dilatation and intestinal obstruction
   A. Acute obstruction of the small intestine or pylorus by pellets of compressed hair (trichobezoars), insufficiently chewed food items or neoplasia is common in rabbits. Rabbits cannot vomit, and therefore intestinal or pyloric obstruction will lead to gastric dilatation, which is a life-threatening condition.
   B. The presenting complaint is usually very sudden onset of anorexia and depression, unwillingness to move, and lack of fecal output.
   C. Clinical findings include tense and painful abdomen, abdominal distention with a firm, enlarged stomach easily palpable in the left cranial abdomen, poor response to external stimulation, and hunched or stretched body position. Tachycardia or brachycardia, tachypnea, pale mucous membranes and cold ears on touch indicate hypovolemia, which might progress into shock if not corrected.
   D. Place an intravenous catheter in the marginal ear vein, cephalic or lateral saphenous vein and start aggressive fluid therapy if in shock (60–90 mL/kg/h for the first 1–2 hours, then re-evaluate). If no signs of shock, administer 2×3 the maintenance rate (which is 60–100 mL/kg/day).
   E. Administer buprenorphine (0.03–0.05 mg/kg SC,IM, IV) and sedate with midazolam (0.25–0.5 mg/kg).
   F. Radiographs are usually diagnostic, and show a fluid- or gas-distended stomach, gas-filled small intestinal loops and lack of gas in the cecum.
   G. Depending on the rabbit's condition and the client, surgical and medical options are available.
   H. Medical treatment should be attempted first if the animal is in a stable condition. Medical treatment includes administration of analgesia and intravenous fluid therapy as initiated already and decompression of the stomach.
   I. Under sedation, perform orogastric intubation, by inserting a large diameter red-rubber tube into the stomach. Decompression might be challenging, owing to clogging of the tube with hair or food material. If the procedure is too stressful for the rabbit or decompression is unsuccessful, abort the procedure.
   J. Administer ranitidine (2–5 mg/kg SC, IV q12h) to prevent gastric ulcers.
   K. Repeat radiographs after about 60–120 minutes, in order to monitor the response to treatment. If the small intestinal obstruction has resolved, gas will have passed in the cecum and the stomach will have reduced in size.

L. If the obstruction has not resolved, consider surgical exploration. If surgery is not an option then continue medical therapy and repeat radiographs if the animal's condition is stable. Consider humane euthanasia if the animal's condition is declining and surgery is not an option.

M. Surgical treatment carries a guarded to poor prognosis in most cases, due to intraoperative or post-surgical complications, including cardiac arrest or post-surgical ileus, particularly if surgical treatment was delayed and the animal's condition has deteriorated further. Clients need to be educated about guarded to poor prognosis of surgical exploration and treatment.

N. Surgical treatment includes removal of small intestinal foreign bodies by either milking them into the stomach and performing a gastrotomy, or milking them caudally into the cecum. If a foreign body was successfully milked in the cecum, typhlotomy is not necessary as the foreign body will pass unaided. Cases in which enterotomy was performed often have a poorer prognosis, and therefore an enterotomy should be avoided if possible. Minimize handling of the GI tract in order to limit the formation of adhesions and ileus post-surgically.

O. Post-surgical care includes fluid therapy, analgesia and H_2-blockers.

P. Consider metoclopramide by constant rate infusion (0.01–0.02 mg/kg/h) or IV as a bolus (0.5 mg/kg q6–8h).

Q. Consider treatment with cisapride (0.5 mg/kg PO q8–12h).

3. Diarrhea

A. Causes include *Bacillus piliformis* (Tyzzer's disease), *Salmonella* spp., *E. coli*, *Clostridium spiroforme*, *Campylobacter* spp., viruses, parasites (coccidiosis) and diet (sudden change in diet, inappropriate diet), and dental disease.

B. The clinical signs include diarrhea ranging from soft stool to profuse, liquid malodorous feces, lethargy, anorexia, dehydration, weight loss and sudden death.

C. If possible, determine the underlying cause; rule out endoparasites.

D. Treatment

  I. Administer supportive fluid therapy IV, IO, or SC.

  II. Administer broad-spectrum antimicrobials:

    a. Trimethoprim-sulfa 30 mg/kg IM, SC, PO q12h (also effective against *Coccidia* spp.)

    b. Enrofloxacin 10–20 mg/kg IV, IM, SC, PO q12–24h

    c. Metronidazole 20 mg/kg PO q12h (for treatment of clostridial overgrowth)

    d. Chloramphenicol 30–50 mg/kg PO q8–12h

    e. Nystatin: 100 000 U/kg PO q8h for 5 days (if large numbers of yeast are found on fecal cytology).

4. Dental disease

A. Rabbits have continuously growing cheek teeth and incisor teeth. Overgrowth and abnormal wear of the cheek teeth can lead to sharp edges or points, which cause trauma to the tongue and buccal mucosa. Overgrown incisor teeth can cause trauma to the lips and hard palate or prevent food intake. Abscesses due to periapical tooth infections are common in rabbits.

B. The clinical signs include partial to complete anorexia, drooling, staining of the fur around the mouth, weight loss, GI stasis, facial abscesses, exophthalmos, and nasal or ocular discharge.

C. Complete examination of the cheek teeth is possible only under general anesthesia and by the use of a mouth gag and cheek dilators. The use of an otoscope or ideally a rigid endoscope is highly recommended. Limited oral exams can be performed in conscious rabbits, but the absence of visible lesions does not rule out presence of dental disease, and any dental treatment needs to be performed under anesthesia. Therefore anesthesia cannot be avoided if dental disease is suspected.

D. Diagnostic imaging of the head is necessary to fully stage dental disease in rabbits. CT scans of the head are preferred to skull radiographs.

E. Consider referral to a specialist if one is unfamiliar with dental examination and treatments in rabbits.

F. Use a low-speed dental drill with a diamond burr and soft tissue protector to remove dental spurs and shorten overgrown cheek teeth.

G. Use a cutting disk or a high-speed dental burr to shorten overgrown incisor teeth. Incisor teeth need to be trimmed every 4–6 weeks Consider surgical extraction to achieve permanent resolution. Refer to a specialist.

H. Treatment of tooth-related abscesses in rabbits is complex and the prognosis is guarded. Most tooth-related abscesses are caused by mixed anaerobic–aerobic infections. Treatment with antibiotics with good coverage against anaerobic bacteria is critical, pending surgical treatment:

   I. Penicillin G procaine / benzathine 40000–60000 U/kg SC q5d

   II. Metronidazole 20 mg/kg PO q12h, combined with trimethoprim-sulfa or enrofloxacin.

I. Provide the appropriate supportive care as indicated:

   I. Nutritional support if the animal is not eating

   II. Fluid therapy (30–50 mL/kg SC bolus)

   III. Analgesia (buprenorphine 0.03–0.05 mg/kg SC), meloxicam (0.3–0.5 mg/kg SC, PO q12h) if the animal is adequately hydrated and has a normal renal function.

J. Dental disease in rabbits is often progressive and a cure is usually not achieved. Recurrence of clinical signs is common and therefore regular dental treatment under general anesthesia needs to be performed often for the rest of the animal's life.

5. Upper respiratory tract disease ('snuffles')

A. Upper respiratory disease is common in rabbits, and is often a multi-factorial chronic disease. *Pasteurella multocida* and *Bordetella bronchiseptica* are commensal organisms of the nasal cavities, but predisposing factors such as stress, poor air quality or low humidity can lead to overgrowth of these organisms and secondary bacterial rhinitis. Certain strains of *P. multocida* are highly pathogenic, and can cause pneumonia, abscesses and sepsis.

B. Clinical signs include usually bilateral mucopurulent nasal discharge, epiphora, conjunctivitis, wetting of inner forelimbs, and sneezing.

C. Differentials for rhinosinusitis include foreign bodies in the nasal cavities, dental disease with periapical infections, and less frequently fungal or mycobacterial infections or neoplasia. Perform a CT scan of the head and possibly rhinoscopy if a more complex underlying cause is suspected, or rhinitis is not responsive to initial therapeutic approach.

D. Initial treatment of upper respiratory tract disease involves:

   I. Rehydration of the nasal cavities by saline nebulization or nasal drops

   II. Administration of systemic antibiotics (trimethoprim-sulfa, enrofloxacin, chloramphenicol) if purulent discharge is present

   III. Supportive care, if indicated.

E. Identify and treat the underlying cause (e.g. low environmental humidity, dental disease).

F. The prognosis is fair to guarded for recurrence if the underlying cause is not identified and treated.

6. Dyspnea and tachypnea

A. Important differentials for dyspnea and tachypnea in rabbits are bacterial pneumonia, lung abscesses, thymoma, mediastinal lymphoma, congestive heart failure, pleural effusion (cardiac, neoplastic, septic) and metastasizing uterine adenocarcinoma (intact females). Upper respiratory tract disease can also lead to dyspnea because rabbits are obligate nasal breathers. Anemia, metabolic acidosis, pain, anxiety, stress or obesity can cause tachypnea.

B. History, physical examination and thoracic radiograph are usually diagnostic. Perform thoracic ultrasound or CT scan of the thorax if necessary. PCV / TP and biochemistry profile should be performed if no primary respiratory cause was found by diagnostic imaging.

C. Bacterial pneumonia can be caused by a variety of bacteria including *Staphylococcus aureus*, *P. multocida*, etc. Treatment includes systemic administration of antibiotics and supportive care.

D. Metastasizing uterine adenocarcinoma carries a poor prognosis and any treatment is only palliative. Euthanasia should be considered.

E. Congestive heart failure should be treated as in dogs and cats.

F. Pleural effusion should be aspirated if severe to improve respiration or for diagnostic reasons.

G. Mediastinal neoplasia (thymoma, lymphoma) have been successfully treated with radiation therapy or surgery.

H. While establishing a diagnosis, provide supportive care:

   I. Oxygen therapy if indicated

   II. Mild sedation if indicated (midazolam 0.25–0.5 mg/kg IM, SC)

   III. Fluid therapy and nutritional support if indicated.

7. Head tilt (vestibular disease)
   A. Head tilt, torticollis and vestibular signs are common in rabbits.
   B. The main differentials include bacterial otitis media and interna or an active infection with *Encephalitozoon cuniculi*. Less frequently toxoplasmosis, *Baylisascaris* spp. larvae, neoplasia or trauma is the underlying cause.
   C. Clinical signs include head tilt, torticollis, nystagmus, strabismus, conjunctivitis, corneal ulcers, ataxia, rolling or circling, seizure-like episodes and depression.
   D. Attempt to localize the lesion within the CNS (e.g. peripheral vs central vestibular). Carefully evaluate the external ear canals and rule out otitis externa, which can lead to head tilt without vestibular signs, due to pain.
   E. Diagnostic imaging of the head is used to rule out otitis media. CT scan is strongly recommended. Skull radiography is less sensitive, and acute otitis media might be missed.
   F. An initial diagnosis is made based on diagnostic imaging results, clinical signs and history. Rabbits with concurrent purulent nasal discharge are more likely to suffer from a bacterial infection (otitis media and interna, encephalitis).
   G. Treatment should focus on stabilizing the patient, and preventing self-injury.
      I. Keep the rabbit in a quiet and dark room.
      II. Administer midazolam (0.25–1 mg/kg) IM, SC, IV, PRN if the animal is rolling or seizuring.
      III. Administer fluids SC if the animal is dehydrated.
      IV. Administer nutritional support if the animal is unable to eat unaided.
      V. Administer antibiotics parenterally if a bacterial infection is suspected:
         a. Enrofloxacin 10–20 mg/kg SC, IV, IM q12–24h
         b. Trimethoprim-sulfa 30 mg/kg PO q12h
         c. Penicillin G procaine / benzathine 40 000–60 000 U/kg SC q5d
         d. Azithromycin 30 mg/kg PO q24h.
      VI. Administer meloxicam (0.3–0.5 mg/kg IM, SC, IV, PO q12h) if the animal is hydrated and has normal renal function.
      VII. Treatment with meclizine (12.5–25 mg/kg PO q8–12h) or metoclopramide (0.5 mg/kg SC, PO q6–8h) may lead to reduction of vestibular signs and control nausea.
   H. Urinary incontinence and fecal soiling is a common consequence and animals often remain recumbent. Therefore intensive nursing care is required.
   I. *E. cuniculi* IgG and IgM antibody titers can be measured. IgG titers can remain high for years after initial exposure, and demonstrate only previous exposure, not active infection. High IgM titers indicate either an acute infection or reactivation of a persistent dormant infection. If IgM is high and other causes have been ruled out, *E. cuniculi* is the likely cause of clinical signs. Treatment against

E. cuniculi should be performed only if IgM titers are high. Start empiric treatment while awaiting titer results:

Fenbendazole 20 mg/kg PO q24h for 21–28 days

J. The prognosis is guarded to poor, depending on the underlying cause. *E. cuniculi* cases often improve over time, although a head tilt might remain. Bacterial otitis media might require surgical therapy. The prognosis for other underlying causes is poor and most cases are diagnosed post-mortem.

8. Posterior paresis and paralysis

A. Rabbits that are allowed to kick during restraint, become excited in their cages, or are dropped, commonly fracture or luxate their lumbar spines.

B. Rarely is the trauma mild, with resulting spinal cord swelling and local inflammation that responds to medical therapy and cage rest.

   I. Administer meloxicam 0.5 mg/kg IV, IM, SC.

   II. The use of corticosteroids in rabbits should be avoided whenever possible, due to their immunosuppressive effects.

C. Usually the damage is severe, with radiographically visible or physically palpable vertebral canal damage, and associated spinal cord damage.

D. Although some patients with severe damage may recover to a certain degree, the prognosis is guarded to poor. If the client is unable to perform the required long-term nursing care, humane euthanasia should be discussed.

9. Eye disorders

A. Commonly seen disorders include bacterial conjunctivitis, nasolacrimal duct obstruction or infection, corneal ulceration, trichiasis, phacoclastic uveitis and exophthalmia.

B. Perform a Jones test (fluorescein dye to demonstrate patency of nasolacrimal duct). The dye will appear within a few seconds at the nostril after application on the eye. Evaluate dye uptake on cornea. Rule out foreign body in the conjunctival sac.

C. Conjunctivitis and corneal ulceration are treated as in dogs and cats. Do not use corticosteroid-containing formulations. Rule out nasolacrimal duct disease, trichiasis, exophthalmia and uveitis. Recommended topical antibiotics that provide coverage against commonly isolated bacteria include gentamicin, ciprofloxacin, ofloxacin and tetracycline / polymyxin B combinations.

D. Nasolacrimal infections usually ascend from the nasal cavity. Infection or dental disease (periapical infection or elongation) can lead to obstruction of the tear duct. If discharge is present from the nasolacrimal duct, submit for bacterial culture and sensitivity. Flush the nasolacrimal duct if blocked or infected.

   I. Restrain the rabbit or sedate if necessary.

   II. Apply topical anesthetic to the eye (e.g. proparacaine).

   III. Use a 22- to 24-gauge intravenous catheter attached to a 6–12 mL syringe.

   IV. Use sterile physiological saline.

    V. The opening of the nasolacrimal duct is slit-like and located medially in the lower conjunctival sac.

   VI. Hold the rabbit's nose lowered, so lavage fluid is not aspirated.

 VII. Carefully attempt to flush the duct; manipulate the position of the catheter if resistance is encountered.

VIII. Nasolacrimal duct rupture can occur if too much pressure is applied.

  IX. Repeat the nasolacrimal duct flush every 3–7 days, depending on the severity of infection.

   X. Prescribe topical and systemically nonsteroidal anti-inflammatory drugs if noninfectious causes of obstruction (i.e. dental disease) are present.

  XI. Prescribe topical antibiotics, and if infection is severe also systemic antibiotics.

 XII. Clinical signs recur if the cause of obstruction is noninfectious. Prognosis for cure of bacterial nasolacrimal duct infection is guarded.

E. Phacoclastic uveitis is caused by *E. cuniculi*, which replicates in the lens and causes cataracts, eventually leading to rupture of the lens capsule and leakage of lens protein, causing a severe pyogranulomatous inflammation. Clinical findings include a white mass protruding in the anterior chamber, uveitis (hyperemic iris, miosis, aqueous flare, low IOP) and conjunctivitis. Treatment includes treatment against *E. cuniculi* and topical nonsteroidal anti-inflammatory drugs (e.g. flurbiprofen). The use of topical corticosteroids should be limited to short periods, since immunosuppression due to systemic absorption is possible. Treatment of choice is surgical removal of the lens. Enucleation should be considered if the uveitis cannot be controlled with medical therapy.

F. Unilateral exophthalmia is most commonly caused by retrobulbar abscesses in rabbits, secondary to underlying periapical infection of the maxillary cheek teeth. Diagnosis is made by CT scan of the head or skull radiography. Treatment includes removal of the infected cheek teeth, establishing a drainage tract into the oral cavity, and systemic treatment with antibiotics. Periapical teeth infections are predominately caused by anaerobic bacteria or are mixed anaerobic–aerobic infections. Collect a sample for aerobic bacterial culture to rule out aerobic bacterial involvement. Treat with appropriate antibiotics. The prognosis is guarded. Referral to a specialist is recommended.

G. Bilateral exophthalmia is frequently caused by mediastinal neoplasia. Thoracic radiographs or thoracic CT scan and fine needle aspiration and/or biopsy are usually diagnostic. Radiation therapy is the treatment of choice for thymomas in rabbits.

RECOMMENDED DRUG DOSAGES FOR RABBITS

Atropine 0.1–0.5 mg/kg SC, IM, IV *(may not be effective, or high doses may be required owing to presence of atropinase in many rabbits)*

Azithromycin 30 mg/kg PO q24h
Buprenorphine: 0.03–0.05 mg/kg IM, SC, IV q8h
Butorphanol: 0.2–0.4 mg/kg IM, SC, IV q2–4h
Chloramphenicol 30–50 mg/kg PO q8–12h
Cisapride: 0.5 mg/kg PO q8–12h
Diazepam: 0.5–1 mg/kg IV
Doxycycline: 5 mg/kg PO q12h
Enalapril: 0.5 mg/kg PO q12–24h
Enrofloxacin: 10–20 mg/kg IM, SC, IV, PO q12–24h
Epinephrine 0.1–0.4 mg/kg IV, IO or intratracheal
Fenbendazole 20 mg/kg PO q24h for 21–28 days (for treatment of
E. cuniculi)
Florfenicol: 25–30 mg/kg PO, IM, SC, q8h
Flumazenil: 0.01–0.1 mg/kg IM, SC, IV
Furosemide: 2–5 mg/kg IV, IM, SC, PO q12h
Glycopyrrolate: 0.01–0.02 mg/kg IM, SC, IV
Itraconazole: 5–10 mg/kg PO q24h
Ivermectin: 0.2–0.4 mg/kg q7–10d
Marbofloxacin: 5 mg/kg PO q24h
Meclizine: 12.5–25 mg/kg PO q8–12h
Meloxicam: 0.3–0.5 mg/kg PO, SC, IM, IV, q12–24h
Metoclopramide: 0.5 mg/kg IV, SC, PO q6–8h *(administer as IV CRI for
treatment of ileus, SC and PO routes are for treatment of nausea)*
Metronidazole: 20 mg/kg PO q12h
Midazolam: 0.25–1 mg/kg IV, IM
Naloxone: 0.01–0.1 mg/kg IV, IM
Nystatin: 100 000 U/kg PO q8h for 5 days
Penicillin G procaine: 40 000–60 000 IU/kg SC, IM q24h
Penicillin G benzathine: 40 000–60 000 IU/kg SC, q5d
Pimobendan: 0.1–0.3 mg/kg PO q12–24h
Propofol: 7.5–15 mg/kg IV.
Pyrantel pamoate: 5–10 mg/kg PO.
Ranitidine: 2–5 mg/kg SC, IV q12h
Selamectin: 15–30 mg/kg topical q21–28d
Sulfadimethoxine (Albon®): 50 mg/kg PO first dose, then 25 mg/kg PO
q24h for 5–20 days
Terbinafine: 10–30 mg/kg PO q24h
Trimethoprim-sulfa: 30 mg/kg PO q12h

RATS (*RATTUS NORVEGICUS*)

Average life span = 1.5–2.5 years.

Estrus cycle = 4–5 days, continually polyestrous. Gestation period = 19–21 days. Average litter size = 4–14, weaning at 21–28 days.

Average weight = males 350–500 g, females 250–300 g.

Heart rate = 250–490 beats/min.

Respiratory rate = 70–115 breaths/min.

Temperature = 96.9–99.5°F (35.9–37.5°C).

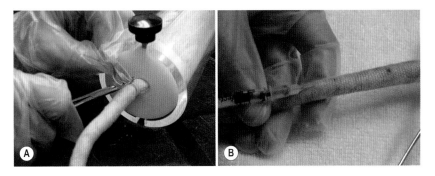

FIG 15.11 **Blood collection from the lateral tail vein in a rat.** *From Sheldon, C.C., Topel, V., Sonsthagen, T.F. 2006. Animal Restraint for Veterinary Professionals, Mosby; reprinted with permission from Elsevier.*

Normal blood values for rats include:

PCV = 35–45%   Glucose = 50–135 mg/dL
TP = 5.6–7.6 g/dL   Phosphorus = 6.5–12.2 mg/dL
WBC = 4700–9400/ mL   Calcium = 5.3–13 mg/dL
BUN = 15–21 mg/dL   Potassium = 5.6–7.4 mEq/L
Creatinine = 0.2–0.8 mg/dL   Sodium = 135–155 mEq/L

Diet—Pelleted rat diet that contains 14–16% protein. Rats are omnivorous.
Sedation—Midazolam 0.5–2 mg/kg IM, SC. Add butorphanol (0.2–0.4 mg/kg) or buprenorphine (0.05 mg/kg) if deeper sedation or analgesia is required.
Anesthesia—Isoflurane or sevoflurane by mask or chamber, preferably after premedication with midazolam and butorphanol or buprenorphine.

Fluid therapy

Daily maintenance fluid requirements in rats are about 60–100 mL/kg/day. Administer SC. Intravenous catheters can be placed in the lateral or dorsal tail veins (Fig. 15.11).

Nutritional support

Any anorexic or emaciated rat should receive nutritional support. Syringe feed an omnivorous critical care formula or blended rat pellets mixed with water.

COMMON DISEASES AND HEALTH PROBLEMS OF RATS

1. Respiratory disease
   A. Differentiate between acute and chronic respiratory disease in rats.
   B. *Streptococcus pneumoniae, Corynebacterium kutscheri, Mycoplasma pulmonis* and sialodacryoadenitis virus (SDV) (co-)infections are common in rats.

C. Multifactorial disorder, immune status, concurrent disease and husbandry are risk factors.

D. The clinical signs include nasal discharge, snuffling, porphyrin staining around the eyes (red tears), dyspnea, rough hair coat, torticollis and death.

E. Acute pneumonia can occur in young rats, and *S. pneumoniae and C. kutscheri* are often the predominate pathogens. Septicemia may develop. Treatment includes:
   I. Amoxicillin / clavulanic acid 15–20 mg/kg PO, SC q12h *(safe to use in rats orally)*
   II. Azithromycin 15–30 mg/kg PO q12h
   III. Doxycycline 5–10 mg/kg q12h
   IV. Oxygen therapy, saline nebulization and supportive care if indicated.

F. Chronic pneumonia is common in older rats with a history of respiratory problems in the past. Treatment for chronic pneumonia includes:
   I. Enrofloxacin 10–20 mg/kg PO q12–24h, plus doxycycline 5–10 mg/kg q12h
   II. Azithromycin 15–30 mg/kg PO q12h
   III. Tylosin 10 mg/kg PO q12h
   IV. Oxygen therapy, saline nebulization and supportive care if indicated.

G. In chronic cases the prognosis is guarded, due to the severity of the underlying lung pathology. Diagnostic imaging is recommended to evaluate the extent and severity of the lower respiratory tract disease. Treatment with antibiotics is often required long term in order to prevent reoccurrence of clinical signs. A cure is not achieved. Optimize husbandry and nutrition, and minimize stress.

2. Dermatologic disorders (mammary gland tumors, dermatitis, alopecia)

A. Alopecia may result from barbering, trauma, dermatophytes or ectoparasites.

B. Benign fibroadenomas of the mammary glands are the most common cause of subcutaneous masses. The mammary tissue in rats is widespread and mammary gland neoplasia can occur in many areas of the body. Surgical removal often results in local cure, but reoccurrence at other sites of the body is common. Ovariohysterectomy is recommended to reduce the chance of recurrence. Alternatively, a GnRH agonist can be administered (i.e. deslorelin acetate implant)

C. Bacterial infections may respond to amoxicillin / clavulanic acid, cephalexin or trimethoprim-sulfa drugs.

D. Itraconazole or terbinafine should be used for treatment of dermatophytosis.

E. Ivermectin or selamectin should be used for treatment of ectoparasites.

F. Prevent self-trauma or con-specific trauma. Apply an e-collar or separate the animal if necessary.

3. Neuromuscular disorders
   A. Bacterial infections, viral infections, neoplasia, poisoning, or trauma to the brain, ear or spinal cord may cause ataxia, paresis, seizures or torticollis.
   B. Pituitary adenomas are common in older rats. Central vestibular signs are seen. Treatment can be attempted with cabergoline, which may lead to temporarily reduction in size of the pituitary gland.

RECOMMENDED DRUG DOSAGES FOR RATS

Amoxicillin / clavulanic acid: 15–20 mg/kg PO q12h *(safe to use in rats orally)*
Atropine sulfate: 0.2–0.4 mg/kg SC, IM
Azithromycin: 15–30 mg/kg PO q24h
Deslorelin: 4.7 mg implant SC
Buprenorphine: 0.05–0.1 mg/kg SC, IM q8–12h
Butorphanol: 0.2–0.4 mg/kg SC, IM q2–4h
Cephalosporins: 15–30 mg/kg PO q8–12h
Clindamycin: **Not recommended for oral administration**
Chloramphenicol : 30–50 mg/kg q8h
Doxycycline: 5–10 mg/kg PO q12h
Enrofloxacin: 10–20 mg/kg IM, SC, PO q12–24h
Fenbendazole: 20–50 mg/kg PO q24h for 5 days
Furosemide: 2–4 mg/kg IM, SC, PO PRN
Itraconazole 5–10 mg/kg PO q24h
Ivermectin: 0.2–1 mg/kg SC, PO q7–14d *(administer 0.2 mg/kg PO q24h for demodicosis)*
Meloxicam: 0.5–1 mg/kg PO q12–24h *(use only in hydrated animals with normal kidney function)*
Metronidazole: 10–20 mg/kg PO q12h
Midazolam: 0.5–2 mg/kg IM, SC, IN
Praziquantel: 6–10 mg/kg IM, SC, PO
Selamectin: 15–30 mg/kg topical q21–28d.
Trimethoprim-sulfa: 15–30 mg/kg q12–24h
Tylosin (Tylan®): 10 mg/kg PO q12h

SNAKES

Sex determination—
1. Male snakes have two paired hemipenises, which lie invaginated in pouches in the ventral tail base just caudal to the cloaca.
2. A smooth blunt-tipped probe may be inserted into the lumen of the hemipenis. The male snake will probe relatively deeply compared with a female of the same species.

Clinical pathology

1. Reptilian blood should be handled in the same manner as avian blood.
2. EDTA should not be used for CBC samples.

3. Lithium heparin is the preferred anticoagulant.
4. Blood smears should be made as soon as the blood is drawn.
5. Normal blood values for snakes include:

PCV = 20–40%   Glucose = 60–100 mg/dL
TP = 4.6–8.0 mg/dL   Uric acid = 0–10 mg/dL
WBC = 6–12000/μL   ALT = 5–35 U/L
Calcium = 8–20 mg/dL   Sodium = 130–152 mEq/L
Phosphorus = 1–5 mg/dL   Potassium = 3.0–5.7 mEq/L

Venipuncture in snakes

1. The recommended blood collection site in most snakes is the ventral tail vein. In some species (e.g. ball pythons) it might be impossible to obtain a diagnostic blood sample from this site. Alternative blood collection technique is by cardiocentesis.
2. For collection from the ventral tail vein, use a 23–25-gauge needle attached to the appropriately sized syringe.
   A. Place the snake in dorsal recumbency with the tail flat.
   B. Thoroughly clean a point caudal to the vent in female snakes and caudal to the hemipenis in male snakes.
   C. Cranial to the selected venipuncture site, apply gentle pressure across the tail.
   D. Insert the needle at the midline, perpendicular to the skin, to the level of the vertebra.
   E. While applying a small amount of suction on the syringe, slowly withdraw the needle until blood flows into the syringe.
3. Cardiocentesis is controversial. The risk of hemopericardium and laceration of the atria and large vessels exists.
   A. Usually larger samples can be collected by this technique.
   B. Anesthesia is recommended for this technique.
   C. The minimal body weight is 300 g.
   D. Place the snake in dorsal recumbency.
   E. The heart is located about 15–20% caudal to the snout. Monitor the ventral scales for movement or use an ultrasonic Doppler probe to detect the heart.
   F. Visualize the heart beat, or palpate the heart beat to locate the heart.
   G. Stabilize the heart between the thumb and index finger placed cranially and caudally to the heart.
   H. Use a 22- to 28-gauge needle and an appropriately sized syringe to collect blood.
   I. Slowly advance the needle under a scute and into the heart.
   J. Withdraw blood.

Fluid administration in snakes

1. Balanced electrolyte solutions (e.g. LRS, Normosol®-R) can be used.
2. The fluids should be warmed prior to administration.
3. SC fluids may be administered laterally along the body wall. The amount that can be delivered is limited.

4. Intracoelomic fluids can be administered in the lower quadrant of the abdomen, just cranially to the cloaca.
5. The maintenance fluid requirement is 20–40 mL/kg/day.

Injections—
- IM injections should be administered in the approximately one-third of the body length caudal from the head and halfway between the dorsal midline and true lateral aspect of the body.
- Irritating substances should not be administered SC.

Sedation—
- Midazolam (1–2 mg/kg SC, IM) will cause mild sedation, but effects can be inconsistent. Reverse with flumazenil (0.05 mg/kg SC, IM).
- Ketamine (5–10 mg/kg SC, IM) will cause mild to moderate sedation. Combine with midazolam for improved sedation and better muscle relaxation.

Anesthesia—
- Isoflurane or sevoflurane delivered by induction chamber.
- Propofol (3–5 mg/kg IV ventral tail vein) for induction and short procedures.
- Perform endotracheal intubation and maintain on anesthetic gas. Perform IPPV 1–2 breaths per minute.

Surgical techniques

1. Scrub under the edges of scales when surgically preparing the skin.
2. Sterile, transparent, self-adhering drapes are recommended.
3. Incisions should be made between scale rows rather than through scales.
4. Absorbable monofilament suture (e.g. polydioxanone) is recommended for buried sutures.
5. Skin incisions should be closed with nylon suture in a slightly everting horizontal mattress.
6. A celiotomy incision should be performed between the 2nd and 3rd row of lateral scutes. Do not make an incision through the ventral scales.
7. Skin incisions should be closed with nylon suture in a slightly everting horizontal mattress.
8. Sutures should be placed between scales rather than through them.
9. Skin sutures or staples should stay in place for at least 4 weeks.

*Euthanasia—*The standard euthanasia solutions may be administered via IC, IV, or intracoelomic injection.
*Zoonotic diseases—*Salmonellosis.

COMMON DISEASES AND HEALTH PROBLEMS OF SNAKES

1. Trauma
   A. Control bleeding with electrocautery, the application of light pressure or vessel ligation.
   B. Administer anesthesia and scrub wounds with a dilute disinfectant.
   C. Flush the wounds with warm sterile saline.

D. Apply antibiotic cream to the wounds, or suture the wounds if they are severe.

E. If the wounds are infected, delay closure until the infection is controlled.

F. Horizontal mattress sutures or stents should be used and the sutures should be removed after 4–6 weeks.

G. Treatment of bite wounds from dogs, cats, rodents, etc. is the same as for other patients.

2. Burns

A. Burns may be caused by the use of inappropriate heat sources or if the snake is forced onto the heat source for an extended time period.

B. They are classified as full thickness, partial thickness, or superficial.

C. Full and partial thickness burns

I. The appearance is that of a white or dry black eschar.

II. Treatment includes wound cleaning, then topical application of silver sulfadiazine cream. Bandaging may be necessary, but is challenging in snakes.

II. Consider fluid therapy and the systemic administration of antibiotics.

IV. Dyscedysis may occur at the wound margins.

V. The snake usually needs assistance with shedding.

VI. The burns may take months to heal.

D. Superficial burns involving only the epidermis

I. The appearance is erythema and discoloration, with possible skin wrinkling.

II. Treatment includes cleansing, avoiding further skin trauma, and keeping the patient at its preferred optimal temperature zone (POTZ).

3. Anorexia and regurgitation

A. Regurgitation usually occurs secondary to an underlying disease.

B. Anorexia is usually due to behavior or environmental factor.

C. Bacterial, viral or fungal infections, parasitic infestations, neoplasia, and ingestion of foreign bodies may result in anorexia or regurgitation.

D. Cryptosporidiosis is a common cause for regurgitation in snakes. A mid-body swelling due to severe thickening of the stomach walls is commonly seen on physical examination. Gastric biopsy or lavage and cytology are usually diagnostic. There is no effective treatment for cryptosporidiosis, which would lead to eradication. Therefore the prognosis is guarded to poor.

E. Force-feeding is usually recommended if the snake has lost 10% of its body mass.

4. Pneumonia

A. Pneumonia in snakes is usually caused by secondary bacterial infections, as a result of poor husbandry. Ophidian paramyxovirus and inclusion body disease (see below) can lead to lower respiratory signs.

B. Clinical signs include open mouth breathing and discharge or bubbling from the glottis.

C. A tracheal wash for cytology and bacterial culture and sensitivity should be performed.

D. Treatment includes the correction of the husbandry conditions and treatment of the secondary bacterial infection:

   I. Systemic antibiotics such as ceftazidime (20–40 mg/kg SC, IM, q48–72h) or enrofloxacin (10 mg/kg IM q48h)

   II. Nebulization with saline, gentamicin (5 mg/mL for 15 min q8–12h) and / or N-acetyl-L-cysteine (22 mg/mL for 15 minutes q8–12h)

   III. Fluid therapy, if indicated.

5. Constipation

A. The causes of constipation in snakes include dried and frozen food, dehydration, impaction by rodent hair, viral infections, bacterial infections of the lower gastrointestinal tract, and neoplasia of the lower gastrointestinal tract.

B. Treatment includes oral administration of fluids and lactulose (0.5 mL/kg PO q24h).

C. Anesthesia and manual milking of the colon may be attempted. However, trauma may be caused to the rectum.

D. Identify and treat the underlying cause.

6. Dystocia

A. Egg retention occurs commonly in snakes.

B. The eggs may be seen in outline against the body wall or visualized on radiographs.

C. Oxytocin 1–10 IU/kg IM may be administered, with variable results.

D. Anesthesia may be administered, and manual removal by massaging the eggs from the oviduct may be attempted.

E. Salpingotomy may be necessary for egg removal.

7. Ocular infections

A. Infections of the spectacle and subspectacular space occur commonly in snakes.

B. These infections may be bilateral or unilateral.

C. Infections of the oral cavity may occur simultaneously.

D. Treatment includes the administration of topical and systemic antibiotics.

E. Treatment of infections of the spectacle may require removal of a portion of the spectacle for drainage and flushing.

8. Ophidian paramyxovirus (OMPV)

A. All snake species should be considered susceptible.

B. The clinical signs include anorexia, neurologic deficits, loss of muscle tone, nasal discharge, hemorrhagic discharge from the glottis, and regurgitation.

C. Diagnosis is by serial serology or histopathology.

D. No therapy exists. The prognosis is poor.

E. Quarantine of at least 3 months and serial OMPV serology are recommended.

9. Inclusion body disease (IBD)
   A. This viral infection affects predominately boas and pythons.
   B. The clinical signs include regurgitation, disorientation, head tilt, opisthotonos and death.
   C. Diagnosis can be made by histopathology of biopsy specimens (liver, esophagus, kidney), but the sensitivity is low, and a lack of characteristic eosinophilic intranuclear inclusion bodies does not rule out IBD.
   D. No treatment is available. Euthanasia of confirmed cases is recommended. Prognosis is poor.
   E. Quarantine of at least 3 months is strongly recommended.
10. Stomatitis ('mouth rot')
   A. This is a secondary bacterial infection that initially affects the oral mucosa but may progress to osteomyelitis of the skull. The primary cause is often immunosuppression due to poor husbandry or concurrent disease.
   B. Bacterial pneumonia and / or sepsis may occur.
   C. The most commonly involved bacteria are *Aeromonas*, *Pseudomonas*, *E. coli*, *Morganella*, *Proteus*, *Providencia* and *Salmonella* spp..
   D. The clinical signs include oral ulcerations with an accumulation of caseous material.
   E. To examine a snake's mouth, use a soft spatula, padded tongue depressor or plastic as a speculum inserted into the lateral aspect of the mouth and gently twist it to a transverse position.
   F. Full diagnostic work-up and thorough husbandry review are necessary to attempt to identify the primary underlying cause and treat it appropriately.
   G. Surgical debridement, systemic antibiotics and supportive care are indicated.
   H. Identify and treat the underlying cause.
   I. The prognosis is good to fair if the underlying cause can be identified and the infection has not affected the underlying bone.

RECOMMENDED DRUG DOSAGES FOR SNAKES

Amikacin: 5 mg/kg IM first dose, then 2.5 mg/kg IM q72h *(only in patients which are hydrated and have normal renal function)*
Atropine: 0.01–0.04 mg/kg IM, SC (bradycardia); 0.5 mg/kg IM, IV, IT (CPR)
Carbenicillin: 400 mg/kg IM q24h
Ceftazidime: 20–40 mg/kg IM, SC q48–72h
Ciprofloxacin: 11 mg/kg PO q48–72h
Clindamycin: 5 mg/kg PO q12h
Enrofloxacin: 10 mg/kg IM q48h
Fenbendazole: 50 mg/kg PO q24h for 3–5 days
Gentamicin: 5 mg/mL in saline for nebulization for 15 minutes q8h
Ivermectin: 0.2 mg/kg IM, SC, PO repeat in 14 days **(do not use in indigo snakes)**
Metronidazole: 50 mg/kg PO repeat in 10–14 days

Midazolam: 1–2 mg/kg IM
Piperacillin: 100 mg/kg q48h IM
Praziquantel: 8 mg/kg IM, SC, PO repeat in 14 days
Pyrantel pamoate: 25 mg/kg PO q24h for 3 days

SUGAR GLIDERS (*PETAURUS BREVICEPS*)

These are small nocturnal arboreal marsupials originating from New Guinea and the eastern coast of Australia. They are social and territorial animals living in colonies of 6–8 animals.

Adult average body weight = males 115–160 g, females 95–135 g.

Average life span = 4–7 years.

Sexual maturity = males 12–14 months, females 8–12 months. Seasonally polyestrus, estrus cycle = 29 days.

Gestation period = 15–17 days. Litter size = 1–4. Birth weight = 0.19 g. Pouch emergence after 50–74 days. Weaning age = 85–120 days.

Preferred environmental temperature = 81–88°F (27–31°C).

Diet—Free-ranging gliders feed on plant exudates (sap, gum, nectar, manna, honeydew), pollen, insect larvae, and arachnids during most of the year. The exact nutritional requirements have not been determined for captive sugar gliders and a variety of captive diets are propagated. Different recipes for captive sugar glider diets are available in the literature. The diet should include nectar, insects and other protein sources. Fruits and vegetables should be offered in limited amounts. Ensure sufficient protein and calcium intake. Avoid overfeeding, which will lead to obesity.

Heart rate = 200–300 bpm.

Respiratory rate = 16–40 bpm.

Cloacal temperature = 97.2 ± 0.7°F (36.2 ± 0.4°C).

Normal blood values in sugar gliders include:

PCV = 43–53%
Total protein = 5.1–6.1 g/dL
WBC = 5000–11 000/ mL
BUN = 18–24 mmol/L
Creatinine = 0.3–0.5 mg/dL

Glucose = 130–183 mg/dL
Phosphorus = 5.3 ± 1.9 mg/dL
Calcium = 6.9–8.4 mg/dL
Potassium = 3.3–5.9 mEq/L
Sodium = 135–145 mEq/L

Restraint—Sugar gliders can be restrained with the bare hands or with a light towel for a limited physical examination. Sedation or anesthesia is required for a complete physical exam and diagnostic procedures.

Anesthesia—Isoflurane or sevoflurane is preferred. Premedication is with midazolam (0.25–0.5 mg/kg SC) and buprenorphine (0.01–0.03 mg/kg SC) or butorphanol (0.1–0.5 mg/kg SC) should be considered. Induction should be performed in a large anesthesia mask that fits the entire sugar glider or in an induction chamber.

Venipuncture

This is challenging in sugar gliders and animals usually need to be anesthetized unless severely depressed. Due to the small body size of sugar gliders, only limited amounts of blood can be collected (<1% of BW). Use of 0.5–1 mL syringes and 25- to 28-gauge needles is recommended. Larger samples can be collected from the jugular veins. Smaller samples can be collected from the saphenous, femoral or ventral tail vein.

Fluid therapy

Daily maintenance fluid requirements in sugar gliders are about 60–100 mL/kg/day. Subcutaneous fluids should be administered between the shoulder blades. Avoid SC fluid administration laterally into the patagium.

Nutritional support

Any anorexic or cachexic sugar glider should receive nutritional support unless a GI obstruction is suspected. Consider feeding a critical care formula by syringe (e.g. Lafaber Emeraid Omnivore®).

COMMON DISEASES AND HEALTH PROBLEMS OF SUGAR GLIDERS

1. Lethargy, weakness, anorexia
   A. A variety of disorders can cause these unspecific signs, including nutritional deficiencies, hypothermia, metabolic disease, organ dysfunction, neoplasia or infection.
   B. Hypoglycemia and hypocalcemia can cause lethargy, depression and seizures. If a blood sample cannot be obtained, administer 50% dextrose orally and monitor the response to treatment. If hypocalcemia is suspected based on history and physical examination, administer calcium.
   C. A protein deficient diet can lead to hypoproteinemia, lethargy, muscle atrophy and anemia.
   D. Neoplasia and organ disease (chronic renal insufficiency, liver disease) is common in sugar gliders >4 years of age.
   E. Administer warmed subcutaneous fluids.
   F. Provide thermal support, if indicated.
   G. Perform whole body radiographs to evaluate for underlying disease.
   H. Attempt to identify and treat the underlying cause. The prognosis is guarded.
2. Diarrhea
   A. Enteritis and diarrhea can be caused by bacteria (e.g. *E. coli*, *Clostridium* spp.), endoparasites, and liver or kidney dysfunction, stress and an inappropriate diet.
   B. Perform fecal wet mount examination and fecal flotation to rule out endoparasites.
   C. Perform fecal cytology (Diff quick stain) to evaluate spore-forming bacteria.
   D. Attempt to rule out organ disease by whole body radiographs and plasma biochemistry.
   E. Administer subcutaneous fluids if dehydrated.

F. Administer nutritional support if cachexic or anorexic.

G. Administer appropriate antibiotics if bacterial enteritis is suspected.

3. Seizures
   A. Seizures can be caused by CNS trauma, hypoglycemia, hypocalcemia, bacterial meningitis, neoplasia, intoxications and parasites affecting the CNS (e.g. toxoplasmosis, *Balisascaris* larva).
   B. Rule out hypoglycemia and hypocalcemia, or treat empirically and monitor response to treatment.
   C. Attempt to rule out intoxications and CNS parasites by history.
   D. If the animal is seizuring at presentation, administer midazolam (0.5–1 mg/kg IM, SC, IN).
   E. Administer fluids and keep in quiet and warm environment.
   F. Administer parenteral antibiotics if a bacterial infection is suspected.
   G. Regularly reassess changes in neurologic status.

4. Self-mutilation
   A. Sugar gliders frequently self-mutilate, particular after surgical procedures, secondary to stress or inappropriate husbandry.
   B. Sugar gliders are highly social animals, and should never be housed alone. Deprivation of social interaction or other forms of stress can lead to self-mutilation.
   C. Genital self-mutilation in male sugar gliders has been suggested to be secondary to sexual frustration. Castration is recommended.
   D. To prevent further self-trauma the animal should be treated with an e-collar or sugar-glider vest, which prevents self-mutilation.
   E. Administer analgesics and nonsteroidal anti-inflammatory drugs if pain or trauma is suspected to be the underlying cause.
   F. Administer mild sedation (midazolam 0.25–0.5 mg/kg) if necessary.
   G. Ensure that the animal is eating sufficient amounts of food if an e-collar was placed or the animal is sedated. Starvation can lead to hypoglycemia and dehydration.
   H. Identify and correct the underlying cause (e.g. husbandry) in order to prevent recurrence.

5. Respiratory problems
   A. Tachypnea and / or dyspnea can be caused by a variety of disorders including pneumonia, pleural effusion, cardiac disease, anemia, neoplasia and abdominal distention.
   B. Perform whole body radiographs to evaluate the thorax.
   C. Congestive heart failure is treated as in other species. Administer diuretics in order to stabilize the patient and supplement with oxygen if necessary.
   D. If a bacterial pneumonia is suspected, administer systemic antibiotics and provide supportive care.
   E. The prognosis is guarded to poor.

6. Urinary disorders
   A. Cystitis and urolithiasis are frequently the underlying causes of animals presented for hematuria, stranguria or dysuria.
   B. Poor nutrition, abnormal urine marking behavior, chronic insufficient water intake, and inactivity have also been suggested as underlying causes.

C. Perform whole body radiographs to evaluate uroliths.
D. Perform urine analysis and urine culture if possible.
E. Administer systemic antibiotics for treatment of bacterial cystitis.
F. Cystic calculi require surgical removal.
G. Identify and correct the underlying cause.

RECOMMENDED DRUG DOSAGES FOR SUGAR GLIDERS

Amoxicillin: 30 mg/kg IM, SC, PO q12–24h
Amoxicillin/clavulanic acid: 12.5 mg/kg PO q12h
Buprenorphine: 0.01–0.03 mg/kg IM, SC q8–12h
Butorphanol: 0.1–0.5 mg/kg IM, SC q6–8h
Calcium glubionate: 150 mg/kg PO q24h
Calcium gluconate: 100 mg/kg SC (dilute 1:1)
Cephalexin: 30 mg/kg PO q12h
Enalapril: 0.5 mg/kg PO q24h
Enrofloxacin: 5 mg/kg IM, SC, PO q12–24h
Furosemide: 1–5 mg/kg IM, SC, PO q8–12h or PRN
Fenbendazole: 20–50 mg/kg PO q24h for 3–5d
Itraconazole: 5–10 mg/kg PO q12–24h
Ivermectin: 0.2 mg/kg PO, SC q10–14d
Meloxicam: 0.1–0.2 mg/kg IM, SC, PO q12–24h
Metronidazole: 25 mg/kg PO q12h
Midazolam: 0.25–1 mg/kg IM, SC
Penicillin G: 22000–25000 IU/kg SC q12–24h
Praziquantel: 7 mg/kg PO, SC
Selamectin: 6–18 mg/kg topical q21–28d
Trimethoprim-sulfa: 15 mg/kg PO q12h

TORTOISES AND TURTLES (*CHELONIA*)

Diet—Tortoises and turtles are herbivores or omnivores.
- North American Box turtles (omnivorous): 50% canned dog food, supplement with crickets, vegetables and some fruits.
- African spurred tortoise, leopard tortoise, Russian tortoise (herbivorous): tortoise pellets (hay-based), hay, grass, leafy greens and calcium carbonate supplementation. These species require a UV-B light or direct sunlight access for endogenous vitamin D synthesis.
- Red-eared slider and other freshwater turtles (omnivorous): 75% commercial turtle pellets, supplemented with leafy greens and feeder fish and worms.

Environment—The common box turtle should be housed at 23.9–28.1°C (75–82.5°F). Tortoises require a warm environment 77–95°F (25–35°C). It is essential to provide a temperature gradient within the enclosure. Exposure to natural sunlight or artificial UVB light is also essential.

Freshwater turtles may be either semi-aquatic or aquatic. All semi-aquatic turtles should be provided with a basking spot. Water quality is a very important aspect of freshwater turtle husbandry.

Physical exam—

1. Assess body weight and length of the carapace (dorsal shell). Evaluate the carapace, plastron (ventral shell), and integument for brightness of color and skin turgor over the dorsal aspect of the neck, brightness and position of the eye, and check for swelling in the tympanic membrane.
2. Assess the respiratory pattern by observing subtle forelimb movement, open-mouthed breathing, or wheezing. Auscultation of the heart and lungs is complicated by the presence of the shell and may be facilitated by placing a damp cloth between the head of the stethoscope and the carapace.
3. Observe locomotion and swimming (in aquatic species), and palpate all limbs.

Sedation—

- Dexmedetomidine (0.1 mg/kg SC, IM) *plus* midazolam (1 mg/kg SC, IM). Reverse with atipamezole (equal volume of dexmedetomidine, SC, IM) *and* flumazenil (0.05 mg/kg SC, IM, IN).
- Dexmedetomidine (0.1 mg/kg SC, IM) *plus* midazolam (1 mg/kg SC, IM) *plus* ketamine (2–5 mg/kg SC, IM). Reverse with atipamezole (equal volume of dexmedetomidine, SC, IM, IN) *and* flumazenil (0.05 mg/kg SC, IM, IN).
- Drugs can be mixed be administered in one syringe as a single injection.
- Subcutaneous injections result in a longer onset time, but allow for administration of larger volumes.

Anesthesia—Dexmedetomidine (0.1–0.15 mg/kg SC, IM) *plus* ketamine (10 mg/kg SC, IM). Add morphine (1.5 mg/kg SC, IM) *or* hydromorphone (0.5 mg/kg SC, IM) for analgesia. Reverse with atipamezole (equal volume of dexmedetomidine, SC, IM, IN). Administer naloxone (0.04 mg/kg SC, IM, IN) if recovery is slow.
Recommended protocols for general anesthesia are:

- Freshwater turtles: propofol 5–10 mg/kg IV, for induction and short procedures. Intubate and maintain on isoflurane or sevoflurane for longer procedures.
- Land tortoises: premedicate with drug protocols recommended for sedation. Intubate if possible, otherwise administer propofol IV. After intubation, maintain on isoflurane or sevoflurane for longer procedures.

Blood samples—Sedation might be necessary to perform venipuncture. The jugular vein is the recommended venipuncture site, as it has the least chance of lymph contamination and iatrogenic complications. In land tortoises >500 g the brachial plexus can also be used. The subcarapacial sinus and the dorsal tail vein should be avoided if possible, due to the high risk of lymph contamination and possible iatrogenic complications. Use lithium heparin as the anticoagulant.
Injections—IM injections should be given in the muscle mass of the forelimbs. SC injections should be given in between the neck and the forelimbs. IV injections can be performed in the jugular vein and in tortoises also in the brachial plexus.

Fluid therapy

Fluid therapy may be accomplished by numerous methods, depending upon the degree of dehydration.

1. Mildly dehydrated patients may be soaked in water 1–2 cm deep for 15–30 minutes.
2. Subcutaneous fluids can be administered in front of the hindlimbs (prefemoral fossae).
3. Intravenous fluids can be administered through the jugular vein. The volume administered should not exceed 5% of the body weight (20 mL/kg/day).
4. Balanced electrolyte solutions (e.g. LRS, Normosol®-R) can be used.
5. Daily maintenance fluid requirements in reptiles are 20–40 mL/kg/day. Do not overhydrate.

COMMON DISEASES AND HEALTH PROBLEMS OF TORTOISES AND TURTLES

1. Shell trauma and bite wounds
   A. Due to predator attack or other trauma. Any bite wound (soft tissue or shell) should be treated as an infected wound, regardless of time between presentation and the predator attack.
   B. Administer fluid therapy.
   C. Administer antibiotics, with good coverage against gram-negative and anaerobic bacteria (e.g. ceftazidime), if bite wounds are present. Adjust antibiotic selection based on bacterial culture and sensitivity results.
   D. Debride and remove devascularized bone fragments. Reassess viability of bone fragments daily.
   E. Lavage the affected area with sterile saline. Do allow lavage fluid to enter coelomic cavity of lungs.
   F. Stabilize shell fragments with screws and cerclage wire or similar methods. **Do not** cover shell fractures with polymethacrylate or epoxy.
   G. Treat shell fractures as open bone fractures.
   H. Fungal shell infection may develop. Treat topically and / or parenterally, if indicated.
   I. Cover all wounds with dressing and bandages. Use honey, sugar or antimicrobial hydrogels for the initial treatment of infected wounds. Use hydrogels or silver sulfadiazine once infection is eradicated and a healthy wound bed has formed.
   J. Consider placing an esophageal feeding tube to facilitate oral fluid therapy, nutritional support and drug administration.
   K. Provide analgesia.
   L. Provide the optimum temperature environment for the involved species.
   M. Avoid contact of the wounds and bandages with water. Do not soak animals if contact of the wounds with water cannot be avoided. Maintain hydration by administration fluids via an esophageal feeding tube.

2. Respiratory disease
   A. The etiologies include bacterial, fungal and mycoplasmal pathogens.
   B. Herpesviruses are involved in upper respiratory infections in certain tortoise species.
   C. The clinical signs include mucopurulent nasal and ocular discharges, open-mouthed breathing, anorexia, dyspnea and lethargy.
   D. Aquatic and semi-aquatic turtles may have difficulty swimming with a normal posture or difficulty in regulating buoyancy.
   E. Radiography (preferably a CT scan) and tracheal wash are helpful diagnostic tools.
   F. Treatment
      I. Nebulization with an antibiotic and saline. Nebulize with anti-fungals if indicated.
      II. Administration of a parenteral antibiotic based on culture and sensitivity results.
      III. Maintain hydration.
      IV. Keep the patient at its preferred optimal temperature range.
      V. Provide electrolyte replacement and nutritional support, if indicated.

3. Gastrointestinal disease
   A. Anorexia may be due to infectious diseases, metabolic diseases, parasitism, GI obstruction, inappropriate diet, environmental stress, or poor husbandry.
   B. The clinical signs include anorexia, dehydration, lethargy, weight loss, abnormal stool quality and quantity.
   C. Treatment varies depending on the underlying etiology.

4. Dystocia
   A. The clinical signs include anorexia, lethargy, hemorrhagic discharge from the cloaca, and a history of straining to pass eggs.
   B. Radiography is essential. Whole body CT scan is preferred, if available.
   C. Rule out any underlying disease and treat. Do not attempt to induce egg laying in a turtle or tortoise that is sick due to another disease process. Address the primary disease process first.
   D. If there is no radiographic evidence of obstructive dystocia, provide a nesting site (sand–soil mix).
   E. Be sure to maintain the patient at the preferred optimal temperature range.
   F. Administer calcium gluconate if hypocalcemia is suspected.
   G. If there is no response in cases of nonobstructive dystocia, oxytocin may be used cautiously. However, oxytocin can lead to ectopic eggs in the coelom or urinary bladder, which require (endo-) surgical removal.
   H. If there is radiographic evidence of fractured eggs or obstructive dystocia, egg removal should be considered. This requires coeliotomy or cloacoscopy. Refer to a specialist.

5. Cloacal organ prolapse
   A. Cloacal tissues, cloacal masses, oviduct, intestines or phallus may be prolapsed.

B. The etiologies include cloacitis, cloacal masses, enteritis (e.g. endoparasites), dystocia and coelomitis.

C. The recommended diagnostic tests include (not necessary for phallus prolapse):

  I. Fecal wet mount and fecal flotation
  II. Fecal or cloacal swab cytology (Diff quick stain)
  III. Whole body radiographs
  IV. Coelomic ultrasound
  V. CBC and plasma biochemistry panel
  VI. Cloacoscopy and coeliotomy.

D. Treatment

  I. Administer anesthesia or provide sedation.
  II. Amputation of the phallus is recommended because recurrent prolapse and secondary trauma are common.
  III. Identify the cloacal tissue (oviduct vs intestine vs cloaca)
  IV. To reduce the swelling and control hemorrhage of the prolapsed cloacal tissue, apply 50% dextrose solution topically.
  V. Rinse the prolapsed tissue with warm saline.
  VI. If necrotic tissue is present, surgical debridement or resection is necessary.
  VII. After identification of the prolapsed tissue, apply sterile lubricating jelly.
  VIII. Replace the prolapsed tissues.
  IX. Place retention sutures (two simple transverse sutures) perpendicular to the vent. Do not place purse-string sutures.
  X. After initial stabilization, coeliotomy and ovariosalpingectomy is the treatment of choice for most cases of oviductal prolapse.
  XI. Administer analgesics: meloxicam (0.2 mg/kg IM q24h).
  XII. Administer broad-spectrum antibiotics, if indicated.
  XIII. Treat endoparasites, if indicated.
  XIV. Identify and treat the underlying etiology.

RECOMMENDED DRUG DOSAGES FOR TORTOISES AND TURTLES

Acyclovir: 80 mg/kg PO q24h

Allopurinol: 10–20 mg/kg PO q24h

Amikacin: 5 mg/kg IM q48h *(only in patients that are hydrated and have normal renal function)*

Ampicillin: 20 mg/kg IM q24h

Atropine: 0.01–0.04 mg/kg IM, SC *(bradycardia or preanesthetic)*; 0.5 mg/kg IM, IV, IT, IO *(CPR)*

Buprenorphine: Not recommended as an analgesic, due to the lack of evidence of analgesic efficacy in turtles

Butorphanol: Not recommended as an analgesic, due to the lack of evidence of analgesic efficacy in turtles and tortoises

Calcium glubionate: 10 mg/kg PO q12–24h

Calcium gluconate: 50–100 mg/kg IM, SC (dilute 1:1)

Carbenicillin: 200–400 mg/kg IM q48h

Ceftazidime: 20–40 mg/kg IM, SC q48–72h

Chlortetracycline: 200 mg/kg PO q24h

Ciprofloxacin: 10 mg/kg PO q48h

Clindamycin: 5 mg/kg PO q24h

Enrofloxacin: 5–10 mg/kg IM q24–48h

Fenbendazole: 50 mg/kg PO q24h for 3–5 days

Furosemide: 2–5 mg/kg IM, SC, PO PRN

Gentamicin: 5 mg/mL by nebulization for 15–30 minutes q8–12h

Hydromorphone 0.5–1 mg/kg SC, IM

Ivermectin: **Do not use in tortoises and turtles**

Ketamine: 2–10 mg/kg IM, SC *(combine with midazolam and/or (dex-) medetomidine)*

Meloxicam: 0.2 mg/kg SC, IM q24–48h

Meperidine: 1–5 mg/kg IM q2–4h

Metronidazole: 50 mg/kg PO repeat in 10–14 days

Morphine: 1.5–2 mg/kg IM, SC *(analgesia, respiratory depression may occur)*

Oxytocin: 5–10 IU/kg body weight IM

Praziquantel: 8 mg/kg IM, SC, PO; repeat in 14 days

Propofol: 5–20 mg/kg IV, to effect

Pyrantel pamoate: 25 mg/kg PO q24h for 3 days

Vitamin A: 1000–5000 IU/kg IM, SC once (**do not use in herbivorous tortoises**; *for treatment of hypovitaminosis A in omnivorous turtles*)

Vitamin D$_3$: 400 IU/kg IM once

REFERENCES/FURTHER READING

AVIAN SPECIES

Bowles, H., Lichtenberger, M., Lennox, A., 2007. Emergency and critical care of pet birds. Veterinary Clinics of North America: Exotic Animal Practice 10 (2), 345–394.

Chavez, W., Echols, M.S., 2007. Bandaging, endoscopy, and surgery in the emergency avian patient. Veterinary Clinics of North America: Exotic Animal Practice 10 (2), 419–436.

de Matos, R., Morrisey, J.K., 2005. Emergency and critical care of small psittacines and passerines. Seminars in Avian and Exotic Pet Medicine 14 (2), 90–105.

Flammer, K., 2006. Antibiotic drug selection in companion birds. Journal of Exotic Pet Medicine 15 (3), 166–176.

Hawkins, M.G., Paul-Murphy, J., 2011. Avian analgesia. Veterinary Clinics of North America: Exotic Animal Practice 14 (1), 61–80.

Lennox, A.M., 2008. Intraosseous catheterization of exotic animals. Journal of Exotic Pet Medicine 17 (4), 300–306.

Orosz, S.E., Lichtenberger, M., 2011. Avian respiratory distress: etiology, diagnosis, and treatment. Veterinary Clinics of North America: Exotic Animal Practice 14 (2), 241–255.

CHINCHILLAS

Hawkins, M.G., Graham, J.E., 2007. Emergency and critical care of rodents. Veterinary Clinics of North America: Exotic Animal Practice 10 (2), 501–531.

Mans, C., Donnelly, T.M., 2012. Disease problems of chinchillas. In: Quesenberry, K.E., Carpenter, J.W. (Eds.), Ferrets, Rabbits and Rodents: Clinical Medicine and Surgery, third ed. WB Saunders, Philadelphia, pp. 311–325.

Mayer, J., Donnelly, T.M. (Eds.), 2012. Veterinary Clinical Advisor: Birds and Exotic Pets, first ed. Elsevier, St Louis.

Quesenberry, K.E., Donnelly, T.M., Mans, C., 2012. Biology, husbandry, and clinical techniques of guinea pigs and chinchillas. In: Quesenberry, K.E., Carpenter, J.W. (Eds.), Ferrets, Rabbits and Rodents: Clinical Medicine and

Surgery, third ed. WB Saunders, Philadelphia, pp. 279–294.

Yarto-Jaramillo, E., 2011. Respiratory system anatomy, physiology, and disease: guinea pigs and chinchillas. Veterinary Clinics of North America: Exotic Animal Practice 14 (2), 339–355.

FERRETS

Chen, S., 2010. Advanced diagnostic approaches and current medical management of insulinomas and adrenocortical disease in ferrets (*Mustela putorius* furo). Veterinary Clinics of North America: Exotic Animal Practice 13 (3), 439–452.

Mayer, J., Donnelly, T.M. (Eds.), 2012. Veterinary Clinical Advisor: Birds and Exotic Pets, first ed. Elsevier, St Louis.

Oglesbee, B.L., 2011. Blackwell's Five-Minute Veterinary Consult: Small Mammal, second ed. Wiley Blackwell, Chichester, Sussex.

Pollock, C., 2007. Emergency medicine of the ferret. Veterinary Clinics of North America: Exotic Animal Practice 10 (2), 463–500.

Quesenberry, K.E., Carpenter, J.W. (Eds.), 2012. Ferrets, Rabbits and Rodents: Clinical Medicine and Surgery, third ed. WB Saunders, Philadelphia.

Wagner, R.A., Finkler, M.R., Fecteau, K.A., et al., 2009. The treatment of adrenal cortical disease in ferrets with 4.7-mg deslorelin acetate implants. Journal of Exotic Pet Medicine 18 (2), 146–152.

FISH

Hadfield, C.A., Whitaker, B.R., Clayton, L.A., 2007. Emergency and critical care of fish. Veterinary Clinics of North America: Exotic Animal Practice 10 (2), 647–675.

Mayer, J., Donnelly, T.M. (Eds.), 2012. Veterinary Clinical Advisor: Birds and Exotic Pets, first ed. Elsevier, St Louis.

Roberts, H.E., Palmeiro, B., Weber III, E.S., 2009. Bacterial and parasitic diseases of pet fish. Veterinary Clinics of North America: Exotic Animal Practice 12 (3), 609–638.

Saint-Erne, N., 2010. Diagnostic Techniques and treatments for internal disorders of koi (*Cyprinus carpio*). Veterinary Clinics of North America: Exotic Animal Practice 13 (3), 333–347.

Sneddon, L.U., 2012. Clinical anesthesia and analgesia in fish. Journal of Exotic Pet Medicine 21 (1), 32–43.

GUINEA PIGS

Hawkins, M.G., Bishop, C.R., 2012. Disease problems of guinea pigs. In: Quesenberry, K.E., Carpenter, J.W. (Eds.), Ferrets, Rabbits and Rodents: Clinical Medicine and Surgery, third ed. WB Saunders, Philadelphia, pp. 295–310.

Mayer, J., Donnelly, T.M. (Eds.), 2012. Veterinary Clinical Advisor: Birds and Exotic Pets, first ed. Elsevier, St Louis.

Oglesbee, B.L., 2011. Blackwell's Five-Minute Veterinary Consult: Small Mammal, second ed. Wiley Blackwell, Chichester, Sussex.

Quesenberry, K.E., Donnelly, T.M., Mans, C., 2012. Biology, husbandry, and clinical techniques of guinea pigs and chinchillas. In: Quesenberry, K.E., Carpenter, J.W. (Eds.), Ferrets, Rabbits and Rodents: Clinical Medicine and Surgery, third ed. WB Saunders, Philadelphia, pp. 279–294.

Yarto-Jaramillo, E., 2011. Respiratory system anatomy, physiology, and disease: guinea pigs and chinchillas. Veterinary Clinics of North America: Exotic Animal Practice 14 (2), 339–355.

HEDGEHOGS

Dierenfeld, E.S., 2009. Feeding behavior and nutrition of the african pygmy hedgehog (*Atelerix albiventris*). Veterinary Clinics of North America: Exotic Animal Practice 12 (2), 335–337.

Ivey, E., Carpenter, J.W., 2012. African hedgehogs. In: Quesenberry, K.E., Carpenter, J.W. (Eds.), Ferrets, Rabbits and Rodents: Clinical Medicine and Surgery, third ed. WB Saunders, Philadelphia, pp. 411–427.

Johnson, D.H., 2011. Hedgehogs and sugar gliders: respiratory anatomy, physiology, and disease. Veterinary Clinics of North America: Exotic Animal Practice 14 (2), 267–285.

Mayer, J., Donnelly, T.M. (Eds.), 2012. Veterinary Clinical Advisor: Birds and Exotic Pets, first ed. Elsevier, St Louis.

LIZARDS

Girling, S.J., Raiti, P. (Eds.), 2004. BSAVA Manual of Reptiles, second ed. British Small Animal Veterinary Association, Quedgeley.

Klaphake, E., 2010. A fresh look at metabolic bone diseases in reptiles and amphibians. Veterinary Clinics of North

America: Exotic Animal Practice 13 (3), 375–392.

Martinez-Jimenez, D., Hernandez-Divers, S.J., 2007. Emergency care of reptiles. Veterinary Clinics of North America: Exotic Animal Practice 10 (2), 557–585.

Mayer, J., Donnelly, T.M. (Eds.), 2012. Veterinary Clinical Advisor: Birds and Exotic Pets, first ed. Elsevier, St Louis.

Schumacher, J., 2011. Respiratory medicine of reptiles. Veterinary Clinics of North America: Exotic Animal Practice 14 (2), 207–224.

Sladky, K.K., Mans, C., 2012. Clinical anesthesia in reptiles. Journal of Exotic Pet Medicine 21 (1), 17–31.

Sykes IV, J.M., 2010. Updates and practical approaches to reproductive disorders in reptiles. Veterinary Clinics of North America: Exotic Animal Practice 13 (3), 349–373.

POT-BELLIED PIGS

Bonagura, J.D., Kirk, R.W. (Eds.), 1995. Current Veterinary Therapy XII. WB Saunders, Philadelphia, pp. 1388–1392.

Quesenberry, K.E., Hillyer, E.V. (guest eds.), 1993. Veterinary Clinics of North America, Small Animal Practice: Exotic Pet Medicine I 23 (6), 1149–1177.

Rupley, A.E. (guest ed.), 1998. Veterinary Clinics of North America, Exotic Animal Practice: Critical Care 1 (1), 177–189.

RABBITS

Harcourt-Brown, F.M., 2007. The progressive syndrome of acquired dental disease in rabbits. Journal of Exotic Pet Medicine 16 (3), 146–157.

Harcourt-Brown, T.R., 2007. Management of acute gastric dilation in rabbits. Journal of Exotic Pet Medicine 16 (3), 168–174.

Johnson-Delaney, C.A., Orosz, S.E., 2011. Rabbit respiratory system: clinical anatomy, physiology and disease. Veterinary Clinics of North America: Exotic Animal Practice 14 (2), 257–266.

Lichtenberger, M., Lennox, A., 2010. Updates and advanced therapies for gastrointestinal stasis in rabbits. Veterinary Clinics of North America: Exotic Animal Practice 13 (3), 525–541.

Mayer, J., Donnelly, T.M. (Eds.), 2012. Veterinary Clinical Advisor: Birds and Exotic Pets, first ed. Elsevier, St Louis.

Oglesbee, B.L., 2011. Blackwell's Five-Minute Veterinary Consult: Small Mammal, second ed. Wiley Blackwell, Chichester, Sussex.

Quesenberry, K.E., Carpenter, J.W. (Eds.), 2012. Ferrets, Rabbits and Rodents: Clinical Medicine and Surgery, third ed. WB Saunders, Philadelphia.

Wagner, F., Fehr, M., 2007. Common ophthalmic problems in pet rabbits. Journal of Exotic Pet Medicine 16 (3), 158–167.

Wenger, S., 2012. Anesthesia and analgesia in rabbits and rodents. Journal of Exotic Pet Medicine 21 (1), 7–16.

RATS

Hawkins, M.G., Graham, J.E., 2007. Emergency and Critical Care of Rodents. Veterinary Clinics of North America: Exotic Animal Practice 10, 501–531.

Mayer, J., Donnelly, T.M. (Eds.), 2012. Veterinary Clinical Advisor: Birds and Exotic Pets, first ed. Elsevier, St Louis.

Oglesbee, B.L., 2011. Blackwell's Five-Minute Veterinary Consult: Small Mammal, second ed. Wiley Blackwell, Chichester, Sussex.

Quesenberry, K.E., Carpenter, J.W. (Eds.), 2012. Ferrets, Rabbits and Rodents: Clinical Medicine and Surgery, third ed. WB Saunders, Philadelphia.

Wenger, S., 2012. Anesthesia and Analgesia in Rabbits and Rodents. Journal of Exotic Pet Medicine 21, 7–16.

SNAKES

Girling, S.J., Raiti, P. (Eds.), 2004. BSAVA Manual of Reptiles, second ed. British Small Animal Veterinary Association, Quedgeley.

Martinez-Jimenez, D., Hernandez-Divers, S.J., 2007. Emergency care of reptiles. Veterinary Clinics of North America: Exotic Animal Practice 10 (2), 557–585.

Mayer, J., Donnelly, T.M. (Eds.), 2012. Veterinary Clinical Advisor: Birds and Exotic Pets, first ed. Elsevier, St Louis.

Schumacher, J., 2011. Respiratory medicine of reptiles. Veterinary Clinics of North America: Exotic Animal Practice 14 (2), 207–224.

Sladky, K.K., Mans, C., 2012. Clinical anesthesia in reptiles. Journal of Exotic Pet Medicine 21 (1), 17–31.

Sykes, I.V., J.M., 2010. Updates and practical approaches to reproductive disorders in reptiles. Veterinary Clinics of North America: Exotic Animal Practice 13 (3), 349–373.

SUGAR GLIDERS

Dierenfeld, E.S., 2009. Feeding behavior and nutrition of the sugar glider (*Petaurus breviceps*). Veterinary Clinics of North America: Exotic Animal Practice 12 (2), 209–215.

Lennox, A.M., 2007. Emergency and critical care procedures in sugar gliders (*Petaurus breviceps*), African hedgehogs (Atelerix albiventris), and prairie dogs (*Cynomys* spp). Veterinary Clinics of North America: Exotic Animal Practice 10 (2), 533–555.

Mayer, J., Donnelly, T.M. (Eds.), 2012. Veterinary Clinical Advisor: Birds and Exotic Pets, first ed. Elsevier, St Louis.

Ness, R.D., Johnson-Delaney, C.A., 2012. Sugar gliders. In: Quesenberry, K.E., Carpenter, J.W. (Eds.), Ferrets, Rabbits and Rodents: Clinical Medicine and Surgery, third ed. WB Saunders, Philadelphia, pp. 393–410.

TORTOISES AND TURTLES

Girling, S.J., Raiti, P. (Eds.), 2004. BSAVA Manual of Reptiles, second ed. British Small Animal Veterinary Association, Quedgeley.

Martinez-Jimenez, D., Hernandez-Divers, S.J., 2007. Emergency care of reptiles. Veterinary Clinics of North America: Exotic Animal Practice 10 (2), 557–585.

Mayer, J., Donnelly, T.M. (Eds.), 2012. Veterinary Clinical Advisor: Birds and Exotic Pets, first ed. Elsevier, St Louis.

Schumacher, J., 2011. Respiratory medicine of reptiles. Veterinary Clinics of North America: Exotic Animal Practice 14 (2), 207–224.

Sladky, K.K., Mans, C., 2012. Clinical anesthesia in reptiles. Journal of Exotic Pet Medicine 21 (1), 17–31.

Sykes, I.V., J.M., 2010. Updates and practical approaches to reproductive disorders in reptiles. Veterinary Clinics of North America: Exotic Animal Practice 13 (3), 349–373.

Appendices

I. ANALGESICS

Analgesic class	Analgesic	Canine dosage*	Feline dosage*
Opioid	Buprenorphine	0.005–0.02 mg/kg q4–8h IV, IM, SC	0.005–0.01 mg/kg q4–8h IV, IM, SC
		5–20 µg/kg IV, IM q4–8h	5–10 µg/kg IV, IM q4–8h
		2–4 µg/kg/h IV CRI (D)	1–3 µg/kg/h IV CRI (C)
		120 µg/kg OTM (D)	20 µg/kg OTM (C)
		0.12 mg/kg OTM (D)	0.02 mg/kg OTM q6–8h (C)
			SR: 0.12 mg/kg SC q12h (C)
	Butorphanol	0.1–0.4 mg/kg IV, IM, SC q1–2h (D)	
		0.05–0.2 mg/kg/h IV CRI (D)	
		0.5–2 mg/kg PO q6–8h (D)	
	Codeine	0.5–2 mg/kg PO q6–8h (D)	0.5–1 mg/kg PO q12h (C)
	Fentanyl	2–10 µg/kg IV to effect (D)	1–5 µg/kg IV to effect (C)
		1–10+ µg/kg/h IV CRI (D)	1–5 µg/kg/h IV CRI (C)
		0.001–0.01 mg/kg/h IV CRI (D)	0.001–0.005 mg/kg/h IV CRI (C)
		Or transdermally as follows:	

Fentanyl transdermal:

Body weight	Patch size	
<10 kg (20 lb)	25 µg/h	<5 kg: fold back the liner to expose ⅓–½ of a 25 µg/h patch
10–25 kg (20–50 lb)	50 µg/h	
25–40 kg (50–88 lb)	75 µg/h	>5 kg: fold back the liner to expose ⅔ of a 25 µg/h patch or use the full patch
>40 kg (>88 lb)	100 µg/h	

787

Continued

Analgesic class	Analgesic	Canine dosage*	Feline dosage*
	Hydromorphone	0.05–0.2 mg/kg IV, IM or SC q2–6h (D) 0.0125–0.05 mg/kg/h IV CRI (D) Premed 0.1 mg/kg with acepromazine 0.02–0.05 mg/kg IM (D)	0.02–0.1 mg/kg IV, IM or SC q2–6h (C) 0.0125–0.03 mg/kg/h IV CRI (C) Premed 0.08 mg/kg with acepromazine 0.02–0.05 mg/kg IM (C)
	Meperidine	2–5 mg/kg IM, SC q1–4h (B)	
	Methadone	0.1–0.5 mg/kg IV, IM, SC q2–4h (B)	
	Morphine	0.5–1 mg/kg IM, SC (D) 0.1 0.5 mg/kg IV q2–4h (D) 0.05–0.5 mg/kg/h (D) 0.1–0.3 mg/kg epidural q4–12h (D)	0.05–0.2 mg/kg IM, SC (C)
	Morphine sulfate sustained release	2–5 mg/kg PO q12h (D)	Not recommended
	Morphine sulfate tablets and oral liquid	1 mg/kg PO q4–6h (D)	Not recommended
	Oxycodone	0.1–0.3 mg/kg PO q6–12h (D)	Not recommended
	Oxymorphone	0.02–0.2 mg/kg/h IV q2–4h (D) 0.05–0.2 mg/kg IM, SC q2–6h (D) 0.05–0.3 mg/kg/h epidural (D)	0.02–0.1 mg/kg IV (C) 0.05–0.1 mg/kg IM, SC q2–4h (C)
	Tramadol	2–8 mg/kg q8 – 12h PO (D)	2–5 mg/kg q12h PO (C)
NSAIDs	Aspirin	10–20 mg/kg q8-12h PO (D)	1–25 mg/kg q72h PO (C)
	Carprofen	4 mg/kg q24h (D) 2 mg/kg q12h PO (D)	4 mg/kg SC or IV once (C)
	Deracoxib	3–4 mg/kg q24h PO (D)	Not recommended
	Etodolac	10–15 mg/kg q24h PO (D)	Not recommended
	Firocoxib	5 mg/kg q24h PO (D)	0.75–3 mg/kg PO once (C)
	Flunixin meglumine	1 g/kg PO or IM once (D)	Not recommended
	Ketoprofen	1–2 mg/kg IV, IM, SC q24h for maximum 3 days, 1 mg/kg PO q24h for maximum of 5 days (D)	0.5–2 mg/kg IV, IM, SC initial dose, then 0.5–1 mg/kg PO q24h for a maximum of 5 days (C)
	Ketorolac	0.3–0.5 IV, IM, PO q12h for 1–2 doses 5–10 mg/dog PO q24h for no more than 3 days (10 mg for dogs >30 kg)	Not recommended
	Meloxicam	0.2 mg/kg initial dose then 0.1 mg/kg q24h PO (D)	0.1 mg/kg SC or PO once (C)
	Naproxen	5 mg/kg initial dose then 2 mg/kg	Not recommended

Analgesic class	Analgesic	Canine dosage*	Feline dosage*
	Piroxicam	0.3 mg/kg q24–48h PO (B)	1 mg/cat PO q24h for max. 5 days
	Tepoxalin	10–20 mg/kg initial dose then 10 mg/kg q24h PO (D)	Not recommended
NMDA antagonists	Ketamine	0.2–0.6 mg/kg/h (B) 0.5 mg/kg IV (B) 2–10 µg/kg/min CRI IV (B)	
	Amantadine	3–5 mg/kg PO q24h (B)	
α₂-Adrenergic agonists	Dexmedetomidine	0.005–1.5 µg/kg/h (D)	0.1–1 µg/kg/h (C)
	Medetomidine	1–3 µg/kg/h (D)	0.5–2 µg/kg/h (C)
Miscellaneous	Gabapentin	3–10 mg/kg PO q8–12h (B)	
	Lidocaine	2–4 mg/kg/h (D)	Not recommended
	Pregabalin (Lyrica®)	2–4 mg/kg PO q8h (D)	1–2 mg/kg PO q12h (C)

*D = dog; C = cat; B = both; OTM = oral transmucosal; IV = intravenous; IM = intramuscular; IT = intratracheal; SC = subcutaneous; PO = per os; CRI = constant rate infusion.

II. BLOOD CROSSMATCHING

METHOD A (from KIRK, 1903, with permission of ELSEVIER)

1. Centrifuge samples at 3400 × g for 1 minute. Remove and retain plasma.
2. Wash RBCs three times in isotonic saline, re-suspend, centrifuge and discard supernatant, retaining the packed RBCs.
3. Prepare 2% RBC saline suspension: 0.02 mL washed packed RBCs plus 0.98 mL of 0.9% saline.
4. Major crossmatch: 2 drops donor red cell suspension, 2 drops recipient plasma.
5. Minor crossmatch: 2 drops recipient red cell suspension, 2 drops donor plasma.
6. Control: 2 drops recipient red cell suspension, 2 drops recipient plasma.
7. Incubate major, minor, and control at 25°C for 30 minutes.
8. Centrifuge all tubes at 3400 × g for 1 minute.
9. Positive test = agglutination.

METHOD B

1. Centrifuge heparinized or EDTA blood samples for 10 minutes at 3000 rpm.
2. Set up the following four slides:
   a. 1 drop donor plasma + 1 drop donor RBC suspension (0.2 mL RBCs + 4.8 mL 0.9% NaCl – control sample, should be no reaction).
   b. 1 drop recipient plasma + 1 drop recipient RBC suspension (0.2 mL RBCs + 4.8 mL 0.9% NaCl – control sample, should be no reaction).
   c. 1 drop donor plasma + 1 drop recipient RBC suspension (minor crossmatch).

d. 1 drop recipient plasma + 1 drop donor RBC suspension (major cross-match).
3. Rock each slide gently from side to side.
4. For 5–15 minutes, watch for agglutination reactions on slides 3 and 4.

III. BLOOD COMPONENT INDICATIONS

Table A Blood component indications

Component	Recommended for	Products delivered
Fresh whole blood	1. Anemia 2. Thrombocytopenia 3. Coagulopathy	Red cells, platelets, clotting factors, plasma protein
Stored whole blood	1. Anemia 2. Coagulopathy 3. Thrombocytopenia (if less than 72 hours old)	Red cells, plasma protein, some clotting factors, platelets (if less than 72 hours old)
Packed red cells	Anemia	Red cells, some plasma protein, some clotting factors, and platelets (if less than 72 hours old)
Platelet-rich plasma	Thrombocytopenia	Platelets, clotting factors, plasma protein
Fresh plasma	1. Hypovolemia 2. Hypoproteinemia 3. Coagulopathy	Clotting factors, plasma protein
Fresh-frozen plasma	1. Hypoproteinemia 2. Coagulopathy	Plasma protein, clotting factors
Stored or frozen plasma	1. Hypoproteinemia 2. Hypovolemia	Plasma protein, some clotting factors
Cryoprecipitate	1. von Willebrand disease 2. Hemophilia A	Factor VIII and fibrinogen

Adapted from Schaer, M. (ed.): The Veterinary Clinics of North America, Small Animal Practice: Fluid and Electrolyte Disorders, Vol. 19, No. 2, 1989.

Table B Recommended usage of blood and blood products in the treatment of emergency transfusion patients[1,2]

	FWB[3]	RBC	FFP	SP	PRP[4]	CRYO
Acute blood loss anemia (trauma)	2	1	—	—	—	—
Chronic blood loss or consumptive anemia (IMHA)	2	1	—	—	—	—
Coagulopathy with bleeding and anemia Acute blood loss anemia (trauma) Chronic blood loss or consumptive anemia (IMHA)	1	2 and	2	—	—	—
Anticoagulant rodenticide toxicity	3	—	1	—	—	2
Anticoagulant rodenticide toxicity with anemia	1	2 and	2	—	—	3
Thrombocytopenia with bleeding (Ehrlichia, ITP)	2	—	—	—	1	—
Thrombocytopathia with bleeding (NSAIDs)	2	—	—	—	1	—

Table B Recommended usage of blood and blood products in the treatment of emergency transfusion patients—cont'd

	FWB[3]	RBC	FFP	SP	PRP[4]	CRYO
DIC with decreased ATIII	—	—	1	—	—	2
DIC with acute anemia	2	1 and	1	—	—	3
Hypoalbuminemia	—	—	2	1	—	—
Hypofibrinogenemia	3	—	2	—	—	1
Dysfibrinogenemia	—	—	2	—	—	1
Prothrombin deficiency	3	—	2	1	—	—
Hemophilia A	3	—	2	—	—	1
Hemophilia B	3	—	2	1	—	—
Hemophilia C	3	—	2	1	—	—
Factor VII deficiency	3	—	2	1	—	—
Factor X deficiency	3	—	2	1	—	—
Factor XII deficiency	—	—	1	2	—	—
von Willebrand	3	—	2	—	—	1

[1]Packed red blood cells, fresh whole blood, or a hemoglobin-based oxygen carrier should be considered if severe hemorrhage has occurred.

[2]Some patients will have more than one problem at a time, such as anemia and hypoalbuminemia and should be carefully evaluated. More than one type of blood component may be needed in the individual patient.

[3]FWB = fresh whole blood, RBC = packed red blood cells, FFP = fresh frozen plasma, SP = stored plasma/cryofree plasma, PRP = platelet rich plasma, CRYO = cryoprecipitate. 1 = first choice, 2 = second choice, 3 = third choice.

[4]Because platelet-rich plasma is preferred but is not readily available, one unit of fresh whole blood may be substituted. However, one unit of fresh whole blood may only raise the platelet count 3000–5000, which may not make a significant difference.

IV. FLUID THERAPY

Table A Approximate daily energy and water requirements of dogs and cats based on body mass*

Body mass (kg)	Total energy (kcal) per day	Total water (ml) per hour
1	100	4.2
2	130	5.4
3	160	6.7
4	190	7.9
5	220	9.2
6	250	10.4
7	280	11.7
8	310	12.9
9	340	14.2
10	370	15.4
11	400	16.7
12	430	17.9
13	460	19.2
14	490	20.4
15	520	21.7
16	550	22.9
17	580	24.2
18	610	25.4
19	640	26.7
20	670	27.9
21	700	29.2

Continued

Table A   Approximate daily energy and water requirements of dogs and cats based on body mass—cont'd

Body mass (kg)	Total energy (kcal) per day	Total water (ml) per hour
22	730	30.4
23	760	31.7
24	790	32.9
25	820	34.2
26	850	35.4
27	880	36.7
28	910	37.9
29	940	39.2
30	970	40.4
35	1120	16.7
40	1270	52.9
45	1420	59.2
50	1570	65.4
55	1720	71.7
60	1870	77.9
65	2020	84.2
70	2170	90.4
75	2320	96.7
80	2470	102.9
85	2620	109.2
90	2770	115.4
95	2920	121.7
100	3070	127.9

*30 x BWkg + 70 =kcal/day=mL/day. Note: This formula will slightly underestimate the requirements for patients that are less than 2 kg and will slightly overestimate the requirements for patients greater than 70 kg.

From Ford, R.B. and Mazzaferro, E.M., Kirk and Bistner's Handbook of Veterinary Procedures and Emergency Treatment, 8th Ed. p 44, Saunders Elseveir 2006, with permission of Abbott Laboratories, Abbott Park, Illinois.

Table B   Estimating the degree of dehydration

Percentage dehydration	Physical examination findings
<5	History of vomiting or diarrhea, but no physical examination abnormalities
6–8	Mild to moderate degree of decreased skin turgor; dry oral mucous membranes
10–12	Marked degree of decreased skin turgor, dry mucous membranes, weak and rapid pulse, slow capillary refill time, moderate to marked mental depression.

From Schaer, M. (ed.): The Veterinary Clinics of North America, Small Animal Practice: Fluid and Electrolyte Disorders, Vol. 19, No. 2, 1989, with permission of Elsevier.

Table C   Components of fluid therapy

1. Hydration deficit (replacement requirement)
    a. Body weight (lb) × % dehydration as a decimal × 500* = deficit in milliliters.
    b. Body weight (kg) × % dehydration as a decimal = deficit in liters.
2. Maintenance requirement (40–60 mL/kg per day)
    a. Sensible losses (urine output): 27–40 mL/kg per day.
    b. Insensible losses (fecal, cutaneous, respiratory): 13–20 mL/kg per day.
3. Contemporary (ongoing) losses: examples are vomiting, diarrhea and polyuria.

*500 mL = 1 lb fluid

From Kirk, R. W. (ed.): Current Veterinary Therapy VIII. Philadelphia, W. B. Saunders, 1983, with permission of Elsevier.

V. GUIDELINES FOR POTASSIUM SUPPLEMENTATION

Estimated potassium losses	Suggested potassium (mEq/l)	Maximum infusion rate (ml/kg per hour)*
Maintenance (serum level = 3.6–5.0)	20	25
Mild (serum level = 3.1–3.5)	30	17
Moderate (serum level = 2.6–3.0)	40	12
Severe (serum level = 2.1–2.5)	60	8
Life threatening (serum level <2.0)	80	6

*Potassium supplementation should not exceed 0.5 mEq/kg per hour.

VI. INSULIN PREPARATIONS AVAILABLE

Type of insulin	Time required to take effect (h)*	Maximum action (h)	Duration of effect (h)
Regular (crystalline)	0.15–0.5	1–5	4–10
NPH	0.5–2	2–10	4–18
Lente	0.5–2	2–10	8–20
PZI	0.5–4	4–14	6–20
Ultra Lente	0.5–8	4–16	6–24
Glargine	1–2	2.5–9	10–16
Detemir	1–2.5	3.5–10	10–17

*After subcutaneous injection

VII. POISON CONTROL AGENCIES IN THE USA

1. ASPCA Animal Poison Control Center: 888-426-4435, www.aspca.org
2. Pet Poison Helpline: 800-213-6680, www.petpoisonhelpline.com
3. USA National Poison & Drug Information Center (human): 800–222–1222. Calls from each state are routed through this phone number.
4. National Pesticide Information Center 800-858-7378, www.npic@aca.orst.edu
5. For pet food recalls in the USA, www.fda.gov or www.aspca.org

VIII. POISONOUS PLANTS

ACONITE

A. *Aconitum* spp.
B. Poisonous part: entire plant, especially leaves and roots
C. Toxic principle: aconitine and related alkaloids
D. Toxic effects: stomatitis, vomiting, excessive salivation, altered vision, mydriasis, weakness, ataxia, cardiac arrhythmias
E. Treatment: induce emesis or perform gastric lavage, supportive

ALMOND

A. *Prunus amygdalus*
B. Poisonous part: kernel in the pit

C. Toxic principle: cyanogenetic glycosides (amygdalin) liberate hydrocyanic acid on hydrolysis
D. Toxic effects: vomiting, abdominal pain, lethargy, cyanosis, seizures, muscle flaccidity, incontinence, coma
E. Treatment: induce emesis or perform gastric lavage, administration of activated charcoal and cyanide antidote, supportive

ALOE

A. *Aloe* spp.
B. Poisonous part: sap
C. Toxic principle: barbaloin (an anthraquinone glycoside)
D. Toxic effects: diarrhea
E. Treatment: induce emesis or perform gastric lavage, supportive

ALOE VERA

A. *Aloe vera*
B. Poisonous part: foliage, sap
C. Toxic principle: saponins
D. Toxic effects: gastroenteritis, anorexia, depression, tremors
E. Treatment: symptomatic

AMARYLLIS

A. *Amaryllis spp.*
B. Poisonous part: entire plant
C. Toxic principle: lycorine
D. Toxic effects: gastroenteritis, excessive salivation, anorexia, depression, tremors
E. Treatment: symptomatic

AMARYLLIS HYBRID

A. *Amaryllis* spp.
B. Poisonous part: bulbs
C. Toxic principle: unidentified
D. Toxic effects: gastroenteritis
E. Treatment: symptomatic

AMERICAN HOLLY

A. *Ilex* spp.
B. Poisonous part: fruit
C. Toxic principle: saponins
D. Toxic effects: vomiting, diarrhea
E. Treatment: as for gastroenteritis, supportive

AMERICAN NIGHTSHADE

A. *Phytolacca americana*
B. Poisonous part: leaves and roots
C. Toxic principle: phytolaccatoxin and related triterpenoid glycosides
D. Toxic effects: vomiting, abdominal pain, diarrhea
E. Treatment: induce emesis or perform gastric lavage, supportive

AMERICAN YEW

A. *Taxus canadensus*
B. Poisonous part: entire plant
C. Toxic principle: taxine A and B, volatile oils
D. Toxic effects: gastroenteritis, tremors, seizures, difficulty breathing, acute heart failure, death
E. Treatment: symptomatic

ANGEL'S TRUMPET

A. *Datura arborea*
B. Poisonous part: foliage and seeds
C. Toxic principle: atropine, hyoscyamine, and hyoscine (scopolamine) (alkaloids)
D. Toxic effects: mydriasis, visual disturbances, cardiac arrhythmias, delirious behavior, seizures
E. Treatment: symptomatic

APPLE

A. *Malus sylvestris*
B. Poisonous part: stems, leaves, seeds
C. Toxic principle: cyanogenic glycosides
D. Toxic effects: mydriasis, brick red mucous membranes, difficulty breathing, panting, shock
E. Treatment: symptomatic

APPLE OF PERU

A. *Datura meteloides*
B. Poisonous part: foliage and seeds
C. Toxic principle: atropine, hyoscyamine, and hyoscine (scopolamine) (alkaloids)
D. Toxic effects: mydriasis, visual disturbances, cardiac arrhythmias, delirious behavior, seizures
E. Treatment: symptomatic

APPLE OF SODOM

A. *Solanum* spp.
B. Poisonous part: immature fruit

C. Toxic principle: solanine glycoalkaloids
D. Toxic effects: vomiting, diarrhea
E. Treatment: induce emesis or perform gastric lavage, supportive

APRICOT

A. *Prunus armeniaca*
B. Poisonous part: stems, leaves, seeds
C. Toxic principle: cyanogenetic glycosides (amygdalin) liberate hydrocyanic acid on hydrolysis
D. Toxic effects: mydriasis, brick red mucous membranes, difficulty breathing, panting, shock
E. Treatment: induce emesis or perform gastric lavage, administration of activated charcoal and cyanide antidote, supportive

ASPARAGUS FERN

A. *Asparagus densiflorus cv sprengeri*
B. Poisonous part: foliage and berries
C. Toxic principle: unidentified
D. Toxic effects: gastroenteritis, dermatitis
E. Treatment: symptomatic

AUTUMN CROCUS

A. *Colchicum autumnale*
B. Poisonous part: entire plant
C. Toxic principle: colchicines and other alkaloids
D. Toxic effects: stomatitis, gastroenteritis, hematemesis, diarrhea, shock, bone marrow suppression, multiple organ dysfunction, death
E. Treatment: symptomatic

AVOCADO

A. *Persea americana*
B. Poisonous part: entire plant (foliage, bark, fruit, seeds)
C. Toxic principle: persin
D. Toxic effects: gastroenteritis in dogs and cats, acute heart failure and death in birds
E. Treatment: symptomatic

AZALEA

A. *Rhododendron* spp.
B. Poisonous part: leaves and honey from the flower nectar
C. Toxic principle: grayanotoxins (andromedotoxins)
D. Toxic effects: stomatitis, vomiting, diarrhea, weakness, visual deficits, bradycardia, seizures, coma
E. Treatment: induce emesis or perform gastric lavage, monitor cardiac function, supportive

BABY'S BREATH

A. *Gypsophila elegans*
B. Poisonous part: foliage and flowers
C. Toxic principle: gyposenin
D. Toxic effects: gastroenteritis
E. Treatment: symptomatic

BARBADOS PRIDE

A. *Caesalpinia pulcherrima*
B. Poisonous part: bark, foliage, flowers, berries, seeds
C. Toxic principle: gastrointestinal irritants, tannins
D. Toxic effects: vomiting, diarrhea
E. Treatment: supportive as for gastroenteritis

BEGONIA

A. *Begonia spp.*
B. Poisonous part: foliage and flowers, the tubers are the most toxic
C. Toxic principle: insoluble calcium oxalates
D. Toxic effects: stomatitis, dysphagia, gastroenteritis
E. Treatment: symptomatic

BIRD OF PARADISE

A. *Poinciana gilliesii*
B. Poisonous part: bark, foliage, flowers, berries, seeds
C. Toxic principle: tannins
D. Toxic effects: severe stomatitis, vomiting, diarrhea, dysphagia, ataxia
E. Treatment: supportive as for gastroenteritis

BIRD'S EYE PRIMROSE

A. *Primula* spp.
B. Poisonous part: leaves and stems
C. Toxic principle: unknown
D. Toxic effects: stomatitis, vomiting, diarrhea, contact dermatitis
E. Treatment: induce emesis or perform gastric lavage, wash skin with soap and water, supportive

BITTERSWEET

A. *Celastrus scandens*
B. Poisonous part: all
C. Toxic principle: euonymin and sesquiterpene alkaloids
D. Toxic effects: vomiting, diarrhea, seizures
E. Treatment: induce emesis or perform gastric lavage, supportive

BLACK WALNUTS

A. *Juglans nigra*
B. Poisonous part: hulls and moldy nuts
C. Toxic principle: unknown
D. Toxic effects: gastroenteritis, seizures, tremors
E. Treatment: symptomatic

BLUE CARDINAL FLOWER

A. *Lobelia* spp.
B. Poisonous part: entire plant
C. Toxic principle: lobeline and related alkaloids
D. Toxic effects: vomiting, excitement, weakness, ataxia, tremors and seizures
E. Treatment: induce emesis or perform gastric lavage with 1:10000 potassium permanganate, control seizures, supportive

BUCKEYE

A. *Aesculus* spp.
B. Poisonous parts: nuts and twigs
C. Toxic principle: mixture of saponins known as aesculin
D. Toxic effects: severe vomiting, diarrhea
E. Treatment: supportive as for gastroenteritis

BULL NETTLES

A. *Laportea canadensis*
B. Poisonous part: hairs on leaves and stems
C. Toxic principle: histamine, acetylcholine, serotonin, formic acid
D. Toxic effects: excessive salivation, pawing at mouth, muscular weakness, tremors, vomiting, dyspnea, bradycardia
E. Treatment: atropine, removal of plant material from haircoat, analgesia

BUTTERCUP

A. *Ranunculus* spp.
B. Poisonous part: sap
C. Toxic principle: protoanemonin
D. Toxic effects: stomatitis, dermatitis, vomiting, abdominal pain, diarrhea, renal failure, incoordination, seizures
E. Treatment: induce emesis or perform gastric lavage, monitor renal function, supportive

CALLA LILY

A. *Zantedeschia aethiopica*
B. Poisonous part: leaves
C. Toxic principle: insoluble calcium oxalate

D. Toxic effects: oral, skin, and mucosal irritation, stomatitis and irritant dermatitis
E. Treatment: flush the skin, eyes, or mouth with cool liquids or demulcents.

CARDBOARD PALM

A. *Zamia furfuracea*
B. Poisonous part: foliage, seeds
C. Toxic principle: cycasin
D. Toxic effects: hemorrhagic gastroenteritis, coagulopathy, hepatic failure, death
E. Treatment: symptomatic

CARDINAL FLOWER

A. *Lobelia cardinalis*
B. Poisonous part: entire plant
C. Toxic principle: lobeline and related alkaloids
D. Toxic effects: vomiting, excitement, weakness, ataxia, tremors and seizures
E. Treatment: induce emesis or perform gastric lavage with 1:10 000 potassium permanganate, control seizures, supportive

CARNATION

A. *Dianthus caryophyllus*
B. Poisonous part: foliage and flowers
C. Toxic principle: unknown irritant
D. Toxic effects: gastroenteritis, dermatitis
E. Treatment: symptomatic

CAROLINA ALLSPICE

A. *Calycanthus* spp.
B. Poisonous part: seeds
C. Toxic principle: calycanthin and related alkaloids
D. Toxic effects: vomiting, ataxia, depression, convulsions, cardiac dysfunction
E. Treatment: induce emesis or perform gastric lavage, control convulsions, supportive

CAROLINA HORSE NETTLE

A. *Solanum* spp.
B. Poisonous part: immature fruit
C. Toxic principle: solanine glycoalkaloids
D. Toxic effects: vomiting, diarrhea
E. Treatment: induce emesis or perform gastric lavage, supportive

CASTOR BEAN

A. *Ricinus communis*
B. Poisonous part: seeds and foliage
C. Toxic principle: ricin
D. Toxic effects: delayed onset (12–48 hours post ingestion) of gastroenteritis, depression, fever, abdominal pain, hemorrhagic diarrhea, cardiac arrhythmias, seizures, coma, death
E. Treatment: induce emesis or perform gastric lavage, fluid therapy, symptomatic

CASTOR OIL PLANT

A. *Ricinus communis*
B. Poisonous part: seeds
C. Toxic principle: ricin
D. Toxic effects: delayed onset (18–24 hours post ingestion) of gastroenteritis, depression, fever, abdominal pain, hemorrhagic diarrhea, cardiac arrhythmias, seizures
E. Treatment: induce emesis or perform gastric lavage, fluid therapy, symptomatic

CHERRY

A. *Prunus* spp.
B. Poisonous part: kernel in the pit
C. Toxic principle: cyanogenetic glycosides (amygdalin) liberate hydrocyanic acid on hydrolysis
D. Toxic effects: brick red mucous membranes, vomiting, abdominal pain, lethargy, cyanosis, seizures, muscle flaccidity, incontinence, coma
E. Treatment: induce emesis or perform gastric lavage, administration of activated charcoal and cyanide antidote, supportive

CHINABERRY

A. *Melia azedarach*
B. Poisonous part: bark, flowers and fruit
C. Toxic principle: narcotic resinoid or alkaloid
D. Toxic effects: hypoventilation, respiratory depression, miosis, nausea, vomiting, depression, euphoria, coma, death.
E. Treatment: narcotic antagonists may be beneficial, symptomatic and supportive

CHINESE JADE

A. *Crassula arborescens*
B. Poisonous part: entire plant
C. Toxic principle: unknown
D. Toxic effects: gastroenteritis
E. Treatment: symptomatic

CHOKE CHERRY

A. *Prunus* spp.
B. Poisonous part: kernel in the pit
C. Toxic principle: cyanogenetic glycosides (amygdalin) liberate hydrocyanic acid on hydrolysis
D. Toxic effects: vomiting, abdominal pain, lethargy, brick red mucous membranes, cyanosis, seizures, muscle flaccidity, incontinence, coma
E. Treatment: induce emesis or perform gastric lavage, administration of activated charcoal and cyanide antidote, supportive

CHRYSANTHEMUM

A. *Chrysanthemum* spp.
B. Poisonous part: entire plant
C. Toxic principle: sesquiterpene, lactones, pyrethrins
D. Toxic effects: contact dermatitis, erythema, rash, pruritus, crusting and scaling, excessive salivation, gastroenteritis, ataxia
E. Treatment: prompt removal of irritant with running water, topical steroid

CLIMBING LILY

A. *Gloriosa superba*
B. Poisonous part: entire plant
C. Toxic principle: colchicine
D. Toxic effects: stomatitis, vomiting, abdominal pain, diarrhea, renal failure and hepatic failure, bone marrow suppression
E. Treatment: induce emesis or perform gastric lavage, fluid therapy, supportive

CORN PLANT

A. *Dracaena fragrans*
B. Poisonous part: foliage and flowers
C. Toxic principle: saponins
D. Toxic effects: mydriasis, excessive salivation, depression, anorexia, vomiting
E. Treatment: symptomatic

CRAB-EYES

A. *Abrus precatorius*
B. Poisonous part: chewed or broken seed
C. Toxic principle: abrin
D. Toxic effects: vomiting, diarrhea, potentially fatal
E. Treatment: induce emesis or perform gastric lavage, supportive

CROCUS

A. *Colchicum* spp.
B. Poisonous part: entire plant
C. Toxic principle: colchicine
D. Toxic effects: vomiting, abdominal pain, diarrhea, renal failure
E. Treatment: induce emesis or perform gastric lavage, fluid therapy, supportive

CROWFOOT

A. *Ranunculus* spp.
B. Poisonous part: sap
C. Toxic principle: protoanemonin
D. Toxic effects: stomatitis, dermatitis, vomiting, diarrhea, abdominal pain, renal failure, ataxia, seizures
E. Treatment: induce emesis or perform gastric lavage, monitor renal function, supportive

CYCLAMEN

A. *Cyclamen spp.*
B. Poisonous part: entire plant, especially the tubers
C. Toxic principle: terpenoid saponins
D. Toxic effects: arrhythmias, excessive salivation, gastroenteritis, seizures, death
E. Treatment: symptomatic

DAFFODIL

A. *Narcissus pseudonarcissus*
B. Poisonous part: bulbs, flowers, leaves
C. Toxic principle: galanthamine, lycorine, and narciclasine alkaloids
D. Toxic effects: vomiting, diarrhea, hypothermia, hypotension, bradycardia, seizures, collapse, death
E. Treatment: symptomatic, including atropine and IV fluid therapy

DAISY

A. *Chrysanthemum* spp.
B. Poisonous part: all parts
C. Toxic principle: sesquiterpene, lactones, pyrethrins
D. Toxic effects: contact dermatitis, erythema, rash, pruritus, crusting, scaling, gastroenteritis, ataxia
E. Treatment: prompt removal of irritant with running water, topical steroids

DAY LILY

A. *Hemerocallis spp.*
B. Poisonous part: entire plant

C. Toxic principle: unknown
D. Toxic effects: renal failure in cats
E. Treatment: emesis or gastric lavage, activated charcoal, IV fluids, symptomatic

DEVIL'S IVY

A. *Epipremnum aureum*
B. Poisonous part: entire plant
C. Toxic principle: calcium oxalate raphides and unidentified protein
D. Toxic effects: stomatitis and irritant dermatitis
E. Treatment: flush the skin, eyes or mouth

DESERT AZALEA (DESERT ROSE)

A. *Adenium obesum*
B. Poisonous part: entire plant
C. Toxic principle: digitalis-like glycosides
D. Toxic effects: anorexia, depression, gastroenteritis, arrhythmias, death
E. Treatment: symptomatic

DIFFENBACHIA

A. *Diffenbachia amoena*
B. Poisonous part: foliage and stems
C. Toxic principle: insoluble calcium oxalates, proteolytic enzyme
D. Toxic effects: stomatitis, pharyngitis, gastroenteritis
E. Treatment: symptomatic, flush the skin, eyes or mouth

DOG LAUREL

A. *Leucothoe davisiae*
B. Poisonous part: foliage
C. Toxic principle: grayanotoxins
D. Toxic effects: hypotension, depression, weakness, excessive salivation, collapse, coma, death
E. Treatment: symptomatic

DUMBCANE

A. *Diffenbachia* spp.
B. Poisonous part: foliage and stems
C. Toxic principle: insoluble calcium oxalate, proteolytic enzymes
D. Toxic effects: stomatitis and irritant dermatitis
E. Treatment: flush the skin, eyes or mouth

DWARF POINCIANA

A. *Caesalpinia* spp.
B. Poisonous part: seeds

C. Toxic principle: tannins
D. Toxic effects: vomiting, diarrhea, recovery usually in 24 hours
E. Treatment: supportive, as for gastroenteritis

EASTER LILY

A. *Lilium longiflorum*
B. Poisonous part: entire plant
C. Toxic principle: unknown
D. Toxic effects: toxic to cats, not dogs; anorexia, lethargy, vomiting, renal failure, death
E. Treatment: emesis or gastric lavage, activated charcoal, IV fluids, symptomatic

ELDERBERRY

A. *Sambucus* spp.
B. Poisonous part: entire plant
C. Toxic principle: cyanogenetic glycosides (especially in the leaves, stems, and roots), and an unidentified cathartic (mainly in the roots and bark)
D. Toxic effects: vomiting, abdominal pain, diarrhea
E. Treatment: induce emesis or perform gastric lavage, supportive

ELEPHANT'S EAR

A. *Alocasia* spp., *Caladium* spp. and *Colocasia* spp.
B. Poisonous parts: *Alocasia*, leaves and stems; *Caladium*, entire plant; *Colocasia*, leaves
C. Toxic principle: calcium oxalate raphides
D. Toxic effects: stomatitis and irritant dermatitis
E. Treatment: flush the skin, eyes or mouth

ENGLISH HOLLY

A. *Ilex aquifolium*
B. Poisonous part: leaves and berries
C. Toxic principle: saponins
D. Toxic effects: vomiting, diarrhea
E. Treatment: supportive, as for gastroenteritis

ENGLISH IVY

A. *Hedera helix*
B. Poisonous part: foliage and fruit
C. Toxic principle: hederagenin, a saponic glycoside
D. Toxic effects: gastroenteritis, may become comatose and die within 24–48h
E. Treatment: symptomatic

ENGLISH WALNUT

A. *Juglans regia*
B. Poisonous part: hulls
C. Toxic principle: unknown
D. Toxic effects: gastroenteritis, seizures
E. Treatment: symptomatic

EUCALYPTUS

A. *Eucalyptus* spp.
B. Poisonous part: entire plant
C. Toxic principle: eucalyptol
D. Toxic effects: excessive salivation, gastroenteritis, depression, weakness
E. Treatment: symptomatic

EUROPEAN MISTLETOE

A. *Viscum album*
B. Poisonous part: leaves and stems
C. Toxic principle: viscumin
D. Toxic effects: vomiting, abdominal pain, diarrhea
E. Treatment: induce emesis or perform gastric lavage, supportive

FEVERFEW

A. *Chrysanthemum* spp.
B. Poisonous part: sap
C. Toxic principle: sesquiterpene lactones in all parts except the pollen
D. Toxic effects: contact dermatitis, erythema, rash, pruritus, crusting and scaling
E. Treatment: prompt removal of irritant with running water, topical steroids

FIELD GARLIC

A. *Allium* spp.
B. Poisonous part: bulbs, bulbets, flowers, stems
C. Toxic principle: *n*-propyl sulfide, methyl disulfide and allyl disulfide
D. Toxic effects: vomiting, diarrhea, weakness, methemoglobinemia, hemolytic anemia, Heinz body anemia, hepatic damage
E. Treatment: induce emesis or perform gastric lavage, activated charcoal, supportive

FLAG

A. *Iris* spp.
B. Poisonous part: bulbs
C. Toxic principle: unidentified

D. Toxic effects: gastroenteritis
E. Treatment: symptomatic

FOXGLOVE (PURPLE)

A. *Digitalis purpurea*
B. Poisonous parts: whole plant, including smoke from burning and water in which the flowers have been placed
C. Toxic principle: cardioactive glycosides similar to digitalis
D. Toxic effects; vomiting, abdominal pain, diarrhea, cardiac arrhythmias
E. Treatment: induce emesis or perform gastric lavage, administration of activated charcoal and saline cathartics, control cardiac arrhythmias

GARDENIA

A. *Gardenia jasminoides*
B. Poisonous part: foliage and flowers
C. Toxic principle: genioposide, gardenoside
D. Toxic effects: urticaria, gastroenteritis
E. Treatment: symptomatic

GARLIC

A. *Allium* spp.
B. Poisonous part: bulbs, bulbets, flowers, stems
C. Toxic principle: *n*-propyl sulfide, methyl disulfide and allyl disulfide
D. Toxic effects: vomiting, diarrhea, weakness, methemoglobinemia, hemolytic anemia, Heinz body anemia, hepatic damage
E. Treatment: induce emesis or perform gastric lavage, activated charcoal, supportive

GEISHA GIRL

A. *Duranta erecta*
B. Poisonous part: fruit, leaves
C. Toxic principle: unknown pyridine alkaloid
D. Toxic effects: drowsiness, hyperanesthesia, vomiting, diarrhea, gastrointestinal hemorrhage, melena, tetanic seizures, swollen lips and eyelids
E. Treatment: symptomatic and supportive.

GERANIUM

A. *Pelargonium species*
B. Poisonous part: entire plant
C. Toxic principle: geraniol, linalool
D. Toxic effects: anorexia, depression, dermatitis, vomiting
E. Treatment: symptomatic and supportive.

GERMAN PRIMROSE

A. *Primula* spp.
B. Poisonous part: leaves and stems
C. Toxic principle: unknown
D. Toxic effects: stomatitis, vomiting, diarrhea, contact dermatitis
E. Treatment: induce emesis or perform gastric lavage, wash skin with soap and water, supportive

GLADIOLA

A. *Gladiolus species*
B. Poisonous part: entire plant, especially the bulbs
C. Toxic principle: unknown
D. Toxic effects: excessive salivation, lethargy, vomiting, diarrhea.
E. Treatment: symptomatic

GLORIOSA LILY

A. *Gloriosa* spp.
B. Poisonous part: entire plant
C. Toxic principle: colchicine
D. Toxic effects: stomatitis, vomiting, abdominal pain, diarrhea, renal failure
E. Treatment: induce emesis or perform gastric lavage, fluid therapy, supportive

GLORY LILY

A. *Gloriosa* spp.
B. Poisonous part: entire plant
C. Toxic principle: colchicine
D. Toxic effects: stomatitis, vomiting, abdominal pain, diarrhea, renal failure
E. Treatment: induce emesis or perform gastric lavage, fluid therapy, supportive

GRAPEFRUIT

A. *Citrus paradisii*
B. Poisonous part: entire plant
C. Toxic principle: psoralens and essential oils
D. Toxic effects: depression, gastroenteritis, photosensitivity
E. Treatment: symptomatic

HEAVENLY BAMBOO

A. *Nandina domestica*
B. Poisonous part: entire plant
C. Toxic principle: cyanogenic glycosides

D. Toxic effects: weakness, ataxia, seizures, coma, respiratory failure, death
E. Treatment: symptomatic

HEDGE PLANT

A. *Ligustrum vulgare* spp.
B. Poisonous part: entire plant
C. Toxic principle: syringin (ligustrin, an irritant glycoside), secoiridoid glycosides
D. Toxic effects: vomiting, abdominal pain, diarrhea
E. Treatment: induce emesis or perform gastric lavage, supportive as for gastroenteritis

HELLEBORE (CHRISTMAS ROSE)

A. *Hellebore niger*
B. Poisonous part: foliage and flowers
C. Toxic principle: bufodienolides, glycosides, veratin, protoanemonin
D. Toxic effects: depression, excessive salivation, gastroenteritis
E. Treatment: symptomatic

HOLLY

A. *Ilex* spp.
B. Poisonous part: fruit
C. Toxic principle: saponins
D. Toxic effects: vomiting, diarrhea
E. Treatment: as for gastroenteritis, supportive

HOPS

A. *Humulus lupulus*
B. Poisonous part: fruit
C. Toxic principle: unknown
D. Toxic effects (in dogs): panting, hyperthermia, seizures, death.
E. Treatment: symptomatic.

HYACINTH

A. *Hyacinthus orientalis*
B. Poisonous part: entire plant, especially the bulbs
C. Toxic principle: narcissus- like alkaloids
D. Toxic effects: dermatitis, gastroenteritis
E. Treatment: symptomatic

HYDRANGEA

A. *Hydrangea macrophylla*
B. Poisonous part: flower bud
C. Toxic principle: cyanogenetic glycoside (hydrangin)

D. Toxic effects: vomiting, abdominal pain, lethargy, cyanosis, seizures, muscle flaccidity, incontinence, coma
E. Treatment: induce emesis or perform gastric lavage, activated charcoal, cyanide antidote, supportive

INDIAN TOBACCO

A. *Lobelia* spp.
B. Poisonous part: entire plant
C. Toxic principle: lobeline and related alkaloids
D. Toxic effects: vomiting, excitement, weakness, ataxia, tremors and seizures
E. Treatment: induce emesis or perform gastric lavage with 1:10000 potassium permanganate, control seizures, supportive

IRIS

A. *Iris* spp.
B. Poisonous part: rhizomes
C. Toxic principle: zeorin, missourin and missouriensin (pentacylic terpenoids)
D. Toxic effects: excessive salivation, vomiting, diarrhea, abdominal pain
E. Treatment: as for gastroenteritis, supportive

JAMESTOWN WEED (JIMSON WEED)

A. *Datura stramonium*
B. Poisonous part: foliage and seeds
C. Toxic principle: atropine, hyoscyamine and hyoscine (scopolamine) alkaloids
D. Toxic effects: mydriasis, visual disturbances, cardiac arrhythmias, delirious behavior, seizures
E. Treatment: symptomatic

JAPANESE YEW

A. *Podocarpus macrophylla*
B. Poisonous part: foliage and flowers
C. Toxic principle: unknown
D. Toxic effects: gastroenteritis
E. Treatment: symptomatic

JEQUIRITY BEAN

A. *Abrus precatorius*
B. Poisonous part: chewed or broken seed
C. Toxic principle: abrin
D. Toxic effects: vomiting, diarrhea, potentially fatal
E. Treatment: induce emesis or perform gastric lavage, supportive

JERUSALEM CHERRY

A. *Solanum* spp.
B. Poisonous part: immature fruit
C. Toxic principle: solanine glycoalkaloids
D. Toxic effects: vomiting, diarrhea
E. Treatment: induce emesis or perform gastric lavage, supportive

JESSAMINE (YELLOW)

A. *Gelsemium sempervirens*
B. Poisonous part: entire plant
C. Toxic principle: gelsemicine and related alkaloids
D. Toxic effects: ataxia, altered vision, dry mouth, dysphagia, muscular weakness, seizures, respiratory failure
E. Treatment: induce emesis or perform gastric lavage, activated charcoal, control seizures, supportive

JONQUIL

A. *Narcissus pseudonarcissus*
B. Poisonous part: bulbs
C. Toxic principle: unidentified
D. Toxic effects: gastroenteritis
E. Treatment: symptomatic

KALANCHOE

A. *Kalanchoe tubiflora*
B. Poisonous part: entire plant
C. Toxic principle: bufodienolides
D. Toxic effects: gastroenteritis, arrhythmias
E. Treatment: symptomatic

KIDNEY BEAN TREE

A. *Wisteria* spp.
B. Poisonous part: entire plant
C. Toxic principle: unidentified glycoside, wistarine and lectin
D. Toxic effects: vomiting, abdominal pain, diarrhea
E. Treatment: induce emesis or perform gastric lavage, supportive

LANTANA

A. *Lantana camara*
B. Poisonous part: entire plant
C. Toxic principle: pentacyclic triterpenoids
D. Toxic effects: vomiting, diarrhea, abdominal pain, icterus, hepatic disease / failure
E. Treatment: induce emesis or perform gastric lavage, supportive

LILY

A. *Lilium* spp.
B. Poisonous part: entire plant
C. Toxic principle: unknown
D. Toxic effects: renal failure in cats
E. Treatment: induce emesis or perform gastric lavage, activated charcoal, IV fluids, supportive

LILY-OF-THE-VALLEY

A. *Convallaria majalis*
B. Poisonous parts: whole plant, including smoke from burning and water in which the flowers have been placed
C. Toxic principle: cardioactive glycosides similar to digitalis
D. Toxic effects: vomiting, abdominal pain, diarrhea, cardiac arrhythmias
E. Treatment: induce emesis or perform gastric lavage, administration of activated charcoal and saline cathartics, control cardiac arrhythmias

LOVAGE

A. *Ligustrum vulgare*
B. Poisonous part: entire plant
C. Toxic principle: syringin (ligustrin, an irritant glycoside), secoiridoid glycosides
D. Toxic effects: vomiting, abdominal pain, diarrhea
E. Treatment: induce emesis or perform gastric lavage, supportive, as for gastroenteritis

LOVE APPLE

A. *Solanum* spp.
B. Poisonous part: immature fruit
C. Toxic principle: solanine glycoalkaloids
D. Toxic effects: vomiting, diarrhea
E. Treatment: induce emesis or perform gastric lavage, supportive

LUPIN, LUPINE

A. *Lupinus* spp.
B. Poisonous part: entire plant
C. Toxic principle: lupinine and related alkaloids
D. Toxic effects: muscular weakness, paralysis, respiratory depression, seizures
E. Treatment: induce emesis or perform gastric lavage, control seizures, supportive

MACADAMIA NUT

A. *Macadamia integrifolia*
B. Poisonous part: entire plant

C. Toxic principle: unknown
D. Toxic effects: tachycardia, hyperthermia, depression, weakness, muscular stiffness, tremors, vomiting
E. Treatment: symptomatic

MANCHINEEL

A. *Hippomane mancinella*
B. Poisonous part: sap
C. Toxic principle: diterpenes
D. Toxic effects: stomatitis, vomiting, bloody diarrhea, dermatitis, keratoconjunctivitis
E. Treatment: induce emesis or perform gastric lavage, wash skin with soap and water, supportive

MARGUERITE

A. *Chrysanthemum* spp.
B. Poisonous part: sap
C. Toxic principle: sesquiterpene lactones in all parts except the pollen
D. Toxic effects: contact dermatitis, erythema, rash, pruritus, crusting, and scaling
E. Treatment: prompt removal of irritant with running water, topical steroids

MARIJUANA

A. *Cannabis sativa*
B. Poisonous part: leaves and stems
C. Toxic principle: tetrahydrocannabinol
D. Toxic effects; nervous system depression and derangement
E. Treatment: symptomatic, induce emesis or perform gastric lavage

MESCAL

A. *Lophophor williamsii*
B. Poisonous part: buttons
C. Toxic principle: mescaline
D. Toxic effects: gastroenteritis, mydriasis, blurred vision, dizziness, hallucinations, circulatory depression
E. Treatment: symptomatic

MISTLETOE

A. *Phoradendron* spp.
B. Poisonous part: entire plant
C. Toxic principle: phoratoxin
D. Toxic effects: vomiting, abdominal pain, diarrhea
E. Treatment: induce emesis or perform gastric lavage, supportive, as for gastroenteritis

MONKSHOOD

A. *Aconitum* spp.
B. Poisonous part: entire plant, especially leaves and roots
C. Toxic principle: aconitine and related alkaloids
D. Toxic effects: stomatitis, vomiting, salivation, altered vision, mydriasis, weakness, ataxia, cardiac arrhythmias
E. Treatment: induce emesis or perform gastric lavage, supportive

MOTHER IN LAW PLANT

A. *Kalanchoe tubiflora*
B. Poisonous part: all
C. Toxic principle: bufodienolides
D. Toxic effects: gastroenteritis, lethargy
E. Treatment: symptomatic

MOUNTAIN LAUREL

A. *Kalmia* spp.
B. Poisonous part: leaves and nectar
C. Toxic principle: grayanotoxins (andromedotoxins)
D. Toxic effects: stomatitis, salivation, vomiting, diarrhea, weakness, altered vision, bradycardia, seizures, coma
E. Treatment: induce emesis or perform gastric lavage, supportive

MUSHROOMS

A. Numerous species are toxic, particularly the *Amanita* spp.
B. Poisonous part: entire fungus
C. Toxic principle: varies
D. Toxic effects: gastroenteritis, neurological signs, hallucinations, hyperexcitability, coma, hepatotoxicity
E. Treatment: symptomatic, physostigmine (0.25–0.5 mg for cats, and 0.5–3 mg for dogs) for the neurological signs

NAKED LADY

A. *Brunsvigia rosea*
B. Poisonous part: bulbs
C. Toxic principle: unidentified
D. Toxic effects: gastroenteritis
E. Treatment: symptomatic

NETTLE SPURGE

A. *Cnidoscolus stimulosum*
B. Poisonous part: hairs on leaves and stems
C. Toxic principle: histamine, acetylcholine, serotonin, formic acid

D. Toxic effects: excessive salivation, pawing at mouth, muscular weakness, tremors, vomiting, dyspnea, bradycardia
E. Treatment: atropine, removal of plant material from haircoat, analgesia

NIGHTSHADE

A. *Solanum* spp.
B. Poisonous part: immature fruit
C. Toxic principle: solanine glycoalkaloids
D. Toxic effects: vomiting, diarrhea
E. Treatment: induce emesis or perform gastric lavage, supportive

NIPPLEFRUIT

A. *Solanum* spp.
B. Poisonous part: immature fruit
C. Toxic principle: solanine glycoalkaloids, saponins
D. Toxic effects: vomiting, diarrhea, excessive salivation, anorexia, depression, confusion, weakness, mydriasis
E. Treatment: induce emesis or perform gastric lavage, supportive

NORFOLK PINE

A. *Araucaria heterophylla*
B. Poisonous part: all
C. Toxic principle: unidentified
D. Toxic effects: gastroenteritis, depression
E. Treatment: symptomatic

OLEANDER

A. *Nerium oleander*
B. Poisonous parts: whole plant, including smoke from burning and water in which the flowers have been placed
C. Toxic principle: cardioactive glycosides similar to digitalis
D. Toxic effects; vomiting, abdominal pain, diarrhea, cardiac arrhythmias
E. Treatment: induce emesis or perform gastric lavage, administration of activated charcoal and saline cathartics, control cardiac arrhythmias

ONION

A. *Allium* spp.
B. Poisonous part: bulbs, bulbets, flowers, stems
C. Toxic principle: *n*-propyl sulfide, methyl disulfide and allyl disulfide
D. Toxic effects: vomiting, diarrhea, weakness, methemoglobinemia, hemolytic anemia, Heinz body anemia, hepatic damage
E. Treatment: induce emesis or gastric lavage, activated charcoal, supportive

ORANGE (CALAMONDIN)

A. *Citrus mitis*
B. Poisonous part: foliage and flowers
C. Toxic principle: essential oils and psoralens
D. Toxic effects: gastroenteritis, depression, photosensitivity
E. Treatment: symptomatic

PALMA CHRISTI

A. *Ricinus communis*
B. Poisonous part: seeds
C. Toxic principle: ricin
D. Toxic effects: delayed onset (18–24 hours post ingestion) of gastroenteritis, depression, fever, abdominal pain, hemorrhagic diarrhea, cardiac arrhythmias, seizures
E. Treatment: induce emesis or perform gastric lavage, fluid therapy, symptomatic

PEACH

A. *Prunus* spp.
B. Poisonous part: kernel in the pit
C. Toxic principle: cyanogenetic glycosides (amygdalin) liberate hydrocyanic acid on hydrolysis
D. Toxic effects: vomiting, abdominal pain, lethargy, cyanosis, seizures, muscle flaccidity, incontinence, coma
E. Treatment: induce emesis or perform gastric lavage, administration of activated charcoal and cyanide antidote, supportive

PENCIL CACTUS

A. *Euphorbia milii*
B. Poisonous part: entire plant
C. Toxic principle: irritant sap (latex)
D. Toxic effects: stomatitis, mild gastritis
E. Treatment: lavage mouth, symptomatic

PEYOTE

A. *Lophophor williamsii*
B. Poisonous part: buttons
C. Toxic principle: mescaline
D. Toxic effects: gastroenteritis, mydriasis, blurred vision, dizziness, hallucinations, circulatory depression
E. Treatment: symptomatic

PIERIS (LILY-OF-THE-VALLEY BUSH)

A. *Pieris japonica*
B. Poisonous part: foliage

C. Toxic principle: grayanotoxins
D. Toxic effects: excessive salivation, gastroenteritis, depression, weakness, hypotension, cardiovascular collapse, coma, death
E. Treatment: symptomatic

PHILODENDRON

A. *Philodendron* spp.
B. Poisonous part: leaves
C. Toxic principle: calcium oxalate raphides and unidentified protein
D. Toxic effects: stomatitis and irritant dermatitis
E. Treatment: flush the skin, eyes, or mouth

PLUM

A. *Prunus* spp.
B. Poisonous part: kernel in the pit
C. Toxic principle: cyanogenetic glycosides (amygdalin) liberate hydrocyanic acid on hydrolysis
D. Toxic effects: vomiting, abdominal pain, lethargy, cyanosis, seizures, muscle flaccidity, incontinence, coma
E. Treatment: induce emesis or perform gastric lavage, administration of activated charcoal and cyanide antidote, supportive

POINSETTIA

A. *Euphorbia pulcherrima*
B. Poisonous part: leaves and stems
C. Toxic principle: complex terpenes
D. Toxic effects: mild vomiting, diarrhea
E. Treatment: induce emesis or gastric lavage, supportive as for gastroenteritis

POISON HEMLOCK

A. *Conium maculatum*
B. Poisonous part: entire plant
C. Toxic principle: various alkaloids
D. Toxic effects: signs occur within minutes of ingestion and may include excessive salivation, abdominal pain, frequent urination and defecation, tachypnea, central nervous system excitation, muscle tremors, ataxia, weakness, muscular paralysis, death
E. Treatment: symptomatic.

POISON IVY

A. *Toxicodendron* spp.
B. Poisonous part: entire plant
C. Toxic principle: various unsaturated, long-chain, substituted catechols

D. Toxic effects: allergic contact dermatitis
E. Treatment: prompt removal with running water, topical steroids

POISON OAK

A. *Toxicodendron* spp.
B. Poisonous part: entire plant
C. Toxic principle: various unsaturated, long-chain, substituted catechols
D. Toxic effects: allergic contact dermatitis
E. Treatment: prompt removal with running water, topical steroids

POISON SUMAC

A. *Toxicodendron* spp.
B. Poisonous part: entire plant
C. Toxic principle: various unsaturated, long-chain, substituted catechols
D. Toxic effects: allergic contact dermatitis
E. Treatment: prompt removal with running water, topical steroids

POKE

A. *Phytolacca americana*
B. Poisonous part: leaves and roots
C. Toxic principle: phytolaccatoxin and related triterpenoid glycosides
D. Toxic effects: vomiting, abdominal pain, diarrhea
E. Treatment: induce emesis or perform gastric lavage, supportive

POKEWEED

A. *Phytolacca americana*
B. Poisonous part: leaves and roots
C. Toxic principle: phytolaccatoxin and related triterpenoid glycosides
D. Toxic effects: vomiting, abdominal pain, diarrhea
E. Treatment: induce emesis or perform gastric lavage, supportive

POTATO

A. *Solanum* spp.
B. Poisonous part: immature fruit
C. Toxic principle: solanine glycoalkaloids
D. Toxic effects: vomiting, diarrhea
E. Treatment: induce emesis or perform gastric lavage, supportive

POTHOS

A. *Epipremnum aureum*
B. Poisonous part: entire plant
C. Toxic principle: insoluble calcium oxalates and unidentified protein
D. Toxic effects: stomatitis and irritant dermatitis
E. Treatment: flush the skin, eyes or mouth

PRECATORY BEAN

A. *Abrus precatorius*
B. Poisonous part: chewed or broken seed
C. Toxic principle: abrin
D. Toxic effects: vomiting, diarrhea, potentially fatal
E. Treatment: induce emesis or perform gastric lavage, supportive

PRIM

A. *Ligustrum vulgare*
B. Poisonous part: entire plant
C. Toxic principle: syringin (ligustrin, an irritant glycoside), secoiridoid glycosides
D. Toxic effects: vomiting, abdominal pain, diarrhea
E. Treatment: induce emesis or gastric lavage, supportive as for gastroenteritis

PRIMULA

A. *Primula* spp.
B. Poisonous part: leaves and stems
C. Toxic principle: unknown
D. Toxic effects: stomatitis, vomiting, diarrhea, contact dermatitis
E. Treatment: emesis or gastric lavage, wash skin with soap and water, supportive

PRIVET

A. *Ligustrum vulgare*
B. Poisonous part: entire plant
C. Toxic principle: syringin (ligustrin, an irritant glycoside), secoiridoid glycosides
D. Toxic effects: vomiting, abdominal pain, diarrhea, ataxia
E. Treatment: induce emesis or gastric lavage, supportive as for gastroenteritis

RHODODENDRON

A. *Rhododendron* spp.
B. Poisonous part: leaves and honey from the flower nectar
C. Toxic principle: grayanotoxins (andromedotoxins)
D. Toxic effects: stomatitis, vomiting, diarrhea, weakness, visual deficits, bradycardia, seizures, coma
E. Treatment: emesis or gastric lavage, monitor cardiac function, supportive

ROSARY PEA

A. *Abrus precatorius*
B. Poisonous part: chewed or broken seed

C. Toxic principle: abrin
D. Toxic effects: vomiting, diarrhea, potentially fatal
E. Treatment: induce emesis or perform gastric lavage, supportive

SAGO PALM (FALSE)

A. *Cycas revoluta* and *Zamia* spp.
B. Poisonous part: entire plant
C. Toxic principle: azoxyglycosides (cycasin, neocycasins); β-methyldiamino-propanoic acid is found in the leaves and seeds; azoxyglycosides are metabolized to hepatotoxic and carcinogenic aglycone methylazoxymethanol
D. Toxic effects: emesis, hypersalivation, trembling, congestion of oral mucous membranes, abdominal tenderness, CNS depression, excessive water consumption; seizures, diarrhea and hemorrhagic enteritis may occur in severe cases
E. Treatment: if ingestion of one seed or more than one leaf has occurred, induce emesis, administer activated charcoal up to two or three times at 3–4-hour intervals, provide aggressive symptomatic and supportive therapy, with hospitalization and observation for at least 24 hours

SCHEFFLERA

A. *Brassaia actinophylla*
B. Poisonous part: foliage
C. Toxic principle: terpenoids, saponins, insoluble calcium oxalates
D. Toxic effects: gastroenteritis
E. Treatment: symptomatic

SLOE

A. *Prunus* spp.
B. Poisonous part: kernel in the pit
C. Toxic principle: cyanogenetic glycosides (amygdalin) liberate hydrocyanic acid on hydrolysis
D. Toxic effects: vomiting, abdominal pain, lethargy, cyanosis, seizures, muscle flaccidity, incontinence, coma
E. Treatment: induce emesis or perform gastric lavage, administration of activated charcoal and cyanide antidote, supportive

STAR POTATO VINE

A. *Solanum* spp.
B. Poisonous part: immature fruit
C. Toxic principle: solanine glycoalkaloids
D. Toxic effects: vomiting, diarrhea
E. Treatment: induce emesis or perform gastric lavage, supportive

STINGING NETTLE

A. *Urtica diocia*
B. Poisonous part: hairs on leaves and stems
C. Toxic principle: histamine, acetylcholine, serotonin, formic acid
D. Toxic effects: excessive salivation, pawing at mouth, muscular weakness, tremors, vomiting, dyspnea, bradycardia
E. Treatment: atropine, removal of plant material from haircoat, analgesia

THORN APPLE

A. *Datura metaloides*
B. Poisonous part: foliage and seeds
C. Toxic principle: atropine, hyoscyamine and hyoscine (scopolamine) alkaloids
D. Toxic effects: mydriasis, visual disturbances, cardiac arrhythmias, delirious behavior, seizures
E. Treatment: symptomatic

TOBACCO

A. *Nicotiana tobaccum*
B. Poisonous part: leaf
C. Toxic principle: nicotine
D. Toxic effects: gastroenteritis, shaking, muscle tremors, stilted gait, ataxia, weakness, prostration, dyspnea, paralysis, rapid death.
E. Treatment: symptomatic, assisted ventilation, gastric lavage

TRUMPET VINE

A. *Datura arborea*
B. Poisonous part: foliage and seeds
C. Toxic principle: atropine, hyoscyamine and hyoscine (scopolamine) alkaloids
D. Toxic effects: mydriasis, visual disturbances, cardiac arrhythmias, delirious behavior, seizures
E. Treatment: symptomatic

TULIP

A. *Tulipa* spp.
B. Poisonous part: bulbs
C. Toxic principle: unidentified
D. Toxic effects: gastroenteritis
E. Treatment: symptomatic

VINCA

A. *Vinca rosea*
B. Poisonous part: entire plant

C. Toxic principle: vinca alkaloids
D. Toxic effects: hypotension, depression, gastroenteritis, tremors, seizures, coma, death.
E. Treatment: symptomatic

WAHOO (BURNING BUSH, SPINDLE TREE)

A. *Euonymua atroprurea*
B. Poisonous part: foliage and flowers
C. Toxic principle: alkaloids, cardenolides
D. Toxic effects: gastroenteritis, abdominal pain, weakness, arrhythmias
E. Treatment: symptomatic

WATER HEMLOCK

A. *Cicuta maculata*
B. Poisonous part: entire plant
C. Toxic principle: cicutoxin
D. Toxic effects: mydriasis, diarrhea, extreme stomach pain, seizures, tremors, respiratory depression, and death
E. Treatment: symptomatic

WISTERIA/WISTARIA

A. *Wisteria* spp.
B. Poisonous part: entire plant
C. Toxic principle: unidentified glycoside, wistarine, and lectin
D. Toxic effects: vomiting, abdominal pain, diarrhea
E. Treatment: induce emesis or perform gastric lavage, supportive

WOLFSBANE

A. *Aconitum* spp.
B. Poisonous part: entire plant, especially leaves and roots
C. Toxic principle: aconitine and related alkaloids
D. Toxic effects: stomatitis, vomiting, excessive salivation, altered vision, mydriasis, weakness, ataxia, cardiac arrhythmias
E. Treatment: induce emesis or perform gastric lavage, supportive

YAUPON

A. *Ilex* spp.
B. Poisonous part: fruit
C. Toxic principle: saponins
D. Toxic effects: vomiting, diarrhea
E. Treatment: as for gastroenteritis, supportive

YEW

A. *Taxus* spp.

B. Poisonous parts: most of the plant, including the seeds but not the red aril

C. Toxic principle: taxine alkaloids

D. Toxic effects: ataxia, dry mouth initially, mydriasis, abdominal pain, vomiting, excessive salivation, cyanosis, weakness, coma, cardiac arrhythmias, cardiac or respiratory failure

E. Treatment: induce emesis or perform gastric lavage, administration of activated charcoal, monitor cardiac and respiratory function, supportive treatment

IX. RELATIVELY NONTOXIC INGESTIONS

abrasives
antacids
antibiotics
baby product cosmetics
ballpoint pen inks
bath oil (castor oil and perfume)
bathtub floating toys
birth control pills
body conditioners
bubble bath soaps (detergents)
calamine lotion
candles (beeswax or paraffin)
chalk (calcium carbonate)
cosmetics
crayons marked AP, CP
dehumidifying packets (silica or charcoal)
deodorants
deodorizers, spray
Elmer's Glue®
Etch-A-Sketch®
fabric softeners
glues and pastes
hair dyes, sprays, tonics
hand lotions and creams
hydrogen peroxide, 3% medicinal
incense
indelible markers
iodophil disinfectant
laxatives

lipstick
Magic Marker®
makeup (eye, liquid, facial)
matches
mineral oil
modeling clay
newspaper
pencil (graphite lead, coloring)
petroleum jelly (Vaseline®)
phenolphthalein laxatives (Ex-Lax®)
Play-Doh®
Polaroid® picture-coating fluid
porous tip marking pens
prussian blue (ferricyanide)putty
(less than 56 g)
shampoos (liquid)
shaving creams and lotions
soap and soap products
spackles
suntan preparations
saccharin
teething rings (water sterility)
thermometers (mercury)
toothpaste, with or without fluoride
vitamins
water colors (excluding aniline and gum cambogia)
zirconium oxide

APPENDICES

X. DRUGS WITH POTENTIAL ADVERSE EFFECTS DURING PREGNANCY

Drug	Effect
Acetaminophen	Methemoglobinemia
Acetazolamide	Fetal anomalies
ACTH	Fetal anomalies
Adriamycin	Embryotoxicity, neonatal malformations
Albendazole	Teratogenic and embryotoxic
Amikacin	Ototoxicity and nephrotoxicity
Amitraz	Congenital anomalies
Amphotericin B	Congenital anomalies
Androgens	Masculinization
Antineoplastics	Fetal death and anomalies
Asparaginase	Fetal death and anomalies
Aspirin	Embryotoxicity, pulmonary hypertension, bleeding problems
Aurothioglucose	Rash from milk ingestion
Azathioprine	Mutagenic and teratogenic
Bishydroxycoumarin	Fetal death and intrauterine bleeding
Boldenone undecylenate	Fetal anomalies
Butorphanol	Manufacturer's advice
Captopril	Embryotoxic
Chloramphenicol	Fetal death and anomalies
Chlorothiazide	Fetal anomalies, thrombocytopenia
Chlorpromazine	Neonatal hepatic necrosis
Cholinesterase Inhibitors (term)	Fetal death
Chorionic gonadotropin	Abortion (first trimester)
Cisplatin	Fetal death and anomalies
Ciprofloxacin	Articular cartilage defects
Cloprostenol sodium	Abortion
Corticosteroids	Cleft palate, premature labor and abortions
Cyclophosphamide	Fetal death and anomalies
Cytarabine	Teratogenic and embryotoxic
Dantrolene sodium	Manufacturer's advice
Diazepam	Congenital defects and CNS effects (first trimester)
Diethylstilbestrol	Fetal malformations of genitourinary system
Diazoxine	Fetal anomalies
Dinoprost	Abortion
DMSO	Fetal anomalies
Doxorubicin	Teratogenic and embryotoxic
Doxycycline	Bone and teeth malformations (first half of pregnancy)
EDTA	Fetal anomalies
Enrofloxacin	Articular cartilage defects
Estradiol	Fetal malformations, bone marrow depression
Estrogens	Feminization
Ethoxyzolamides	Fetal anomalies
Flucytosine	Fetal anomalies
Flunixin meglumine	Fetal anomalies
Gentamicin	Ototoxicity and nephrotoxicity
Glycerin	Manufacturer's advice
Glycopyrrolate	Manufacturer's advice
Gold salts	Fetal anomalies
Griseofulvin	Teratogenic
Indomethacin	Premature closure of ductus arteriosus
Iodides	Fetal goiter
Iodinated casein	Neonatal goiter

Continued

Drug	Effect
Iododeoxyuridine	Destruction of fetal islet cells
Isoniazid	Retarded psychomotor activity
Isoproterenol	Fetal tachycardia
Levamisole	No information available
Lithium salts	Fetal goiter
Kanamycin	Ototoxicity and nephrotoxicity
Ketoconazole	Abortion, teratogenic
Meclofenamic acid	Delay of parturition, possibly teratogenic
Medizine	Fetal anomalies
Medroxyprogesterone acetate	Fetal anomalies
Megestrol acetate	Fetal anomalies
Meperidine	Inhibits closure of ductus arteriosus
Mepivacaine	Fetal bradycardia
DL-Methionine	Methemoglobinemia and Heinz body anemia in cats
Methocarbamol	Manufacturer's advice
Methotrexate	Fetal anomalies
Methoxamine	Placental vasoconstriction, fetal hypoxia
Methylene blue	Heinz body anemia
Metronidazole	Teratogenic
Midazolam	Congenital defects, CNS effects (first trimester)
Misoprostol	Abortion
Mitotane	Manufacturer's advice
Nandrolone decanoate	Fetal anomalies
Naproxen	Manufacturer's advice
Neostigmine	Fetal death
Nitrofurantoin	Fetal hemolysis
Nitroprusside	Fetal cyanide toxicity
Oxytocin	Premature parturition
Penicillamine	Teratogenic
Pentazocine	Manufacturer's advice
Phenobarbital (high doses)	Neonatal hemorrhage
Phenylbutazone	Neonatal goiter and nephrosis
Phenylephrine	Placental constriction, fetal hypoxia
Phenytoin	Fetal anomalies
Primidone	Congenital defects, hepatitis
Prochlorperazine	Anomalies
Propranolol	Fetal bradycardia
Propylthiouracil	Neonatal goiter
Prostaglandins	Abortion
Quinine	Deafness and thrombocytopenia
Reserpine	Respiratory obstruction
Rifampin	Possible teratogen
Salicylates	Neonatal bleeding (near term)
Sodium selenite	Impaired fetal growth
Spironolactone	Manufacturer's advice, discontinue nursing
Streptomycin	Hearing loss and anomalies
Succinylcholine	Fetal death, neuromuscular blockade
Sulfasalazine	Neonatal kernicterus
Testosterone	Fetal anomalies
Tetracyclines	Impaired bone and tooth development (first half)
Thiacetarsamide	Hepatotoxic and nephrotoxic
Thiazides	Fetal death and thrombocytopenia
Thiopental	Fetal death
Tiletamine/zolazepam	Fetal death, possible teratogen
Tobramycin	Fetal anomalies
Trimeprazine tartrate	Fetal death, possible teratogen with prednisolone
Trimethoprim-sulfa	Increased fetal mortality

Drug	Effect
Valproic acid	Fetal anomalies
Vasopressin	May induce parturition
Vinblastine	Teratogenic and embryotoxic
Vincristine	Fetal anomalies
Vitamin A (large doses)	Anomalies
Vitamin D (large doses)	Hypercalcemia and mental retardation
Vitamin K (and analogs)	Hyperbilirubinemia
Warfarin	Intrauterine hemorrhage, embryotoxic
Yohimbine	Manufacturer's advice
Xylazine	Induction of premature parturition (especially in last trimester)

XI. DRUGS SAFE FOR USE DURING PREGNANCY

Acetylcysteine
Activated charcoal
Ammonium chloride
Amoxicillin
Ampicillin
Atropine
Bumetanide
Cephalexin
Cephaloridine
Cephalothin sodium
Chloramphenicol (latter half)
Chlorpheniramine
Chymotrypsin
Clindamycin
Clonazepam
Codeine
Colistin
Cromolyn
Dextromethorphan
Diazepam
Dichlorvos
Dicloxacillin
Diethylcarbamazine
Digoxin

Digitoxin
Dimethylhydramine
Diphenhydramine
Disophenol
Doxapram
Doxylamine
Enflurane
Ephedrine
Erythromycin
Ethrane
Furosemide
Gentamicin
Glycopyrrolate
Guaifenesin
Halothane
Heparin
Isoflurane
Ivermectin
Kanamycin
Ketamine
Lidocaine
Lincomycin
Mannitol
Mebendazole
Metaproterenol

Methenamine
Miconazole
Morphine
Niclosamide
Nitrous oxide
Penicillin
Pentobarbital
Phenobarbital
Pilocarpine
Piperazine
Polymyxin B
Pralidoxime
Primidone
Procaine
Pyrantel
Pyrilamine
Salbutamol
Tetracaine
Theophylline
Thiopental
Tiletamine
Triamterene
Urokinase

XII. DRUGS TO AVOID IN SEVERE RENAL FAILURE

Drug	Pharmacological class	Adverse signs
Methenamine mandelate	Urinary tract antiseptic	GI distress, crystalluria, systemic acidosis
Nalidixic acid[1]	Urinary tract antiseptic	Nausea, vomiting, nephrotoxicity, dermatotoxicity
Neomycin	Antibiotic	Renal failure, ototoxicity

Continued

Drug	Pharmacological class	Adverse signs
Nitrofurantoin	Urinary tract antiseptic	Polyneuritis, GI disturbances, rapid emergence of bacterial resistance, pulmonary infiltrates
Polymyxin B	Antibiotic	Renal failure, neurotoxicity
Tetracyclines (except doxycycline)	Antibiotics	Vomiting, diarrhea, renal sodium wasting, antianabolic effect
Thiacetarsamide	Antiparasitic (dirofilariasis)	Vomiting, anorexia, thromboembolism, hepatic failure

¹This drug is contraindicated in any dog or cat.

From Kirk RW (ed), Current Veterinary Therapy VIII, 1983, p 1038, with permission of Elsevier.

XIII. DRUGS REQUIRING DOSE REDUCTION IN PATIENTS WITH RENAL FAILURE

Drug	Dosage adjustment*	Adverse signs
Amikacin	Interval extension	Renal failure, ototoxicity, neuromuscular blockage
Amoxicillin	Half dose or double interval with severe renal failure	Anaphylaxis, neurotoxicity
Amphotericin B	Half dose in severe renal failure	Renal failure, hypokalemia
Ampicillin	Half dose or double interval with severe renal failure	Anaphylaxis, neurotoxicity
Azathioprine	Double interval in severe renal failure	Renal failure, bone marrow and immunosuppression
Bleomycin	Decrease dose	Dermatotoxicity, pulmonary fibrosis
Carbenicillin	Mild dose adjustment with severe renal failure	Anaphylaxis, neurotoxicity
Cephalosporins	Interval extension	Renal failure, anaphylaxis, may potentiate aminoglycoside nephrotoxicity
Cephalothin	Double interval with severe renal failure	Renal failure, anaphylaxis, may potentiate aminoglycoside nephrotoxicity
Cis-platinum	Increase interval	Renal failure
Cyclophosphamide	Double interval in severe renal failure	Vomiting, diarrhea, bone marrow depression, cystitis, hyponatremia
Digoxin	Decrease dose 50% for each 50 mg/dl elevation in BUN	Vomiting, weakness, arrhythmias
5-Fluorocytosine	Interval extension	Hepatic and bone marrow toxicity
Gentamicin	Interval extension	Renal failure, ototoxicity, neuromuscular blockade
Kanamycin	Interval extension	Renal failure, ototoxicity, neuromuscular blockade
Lincomycin	Triple interval in severe renal failure	Vomiting, diarrhea, enterocolotoxic reaction
Methicillin	Half dose or double interval with severe renal failure	Anaphylaxis, neurotoxicity, interstitial nephritis

Drug	Dosage adjustment*	Adverse signs
Methotrexate	Half dose in severe renal failure	Renal failure, bone marrow depression, vomiting
Methoxyflurane	Avoid in severe renal failure	Renal failure
Penicillin	Half dose or double interval with severe renal failure	Anaphylaxis, neurotoxicity
Phenobarbital	Double interval with severe renal failure	Excessive sedation
Primidone	Double or triple interval with severe renal failure	Excessive sedation
Procainamide	Double interval with severe renal failure	Hypotension, myocardial depression
Streptomycin	Double or triple interval with severe renal failure	Renal failure, ototoxicity, neuromuscular blockade
Sulfisoxazole	Double or triple interval	Renal failure
Ticarcillin	Half dose or double interval with severe renal failure	Anaphylaxis, neurotoxicity
Tetracycline	Decrease dose or lengthen interval with severe renal failure	Renal failure, gastroenteritis
Tobramycin	Interval extension	Renal failure, ototoxicity, neuromuscular blockade
Trimethoprim-Sulfamethoxazole	Avoid in severe renal failure	Vomiting, diarrhea
Vancomycin	Interval extension	Ototoxicity, possible nephrotoxicity

*Consult pharmacology or nephrology texts for proper interval extension.

XIV. COMMONLY USED FORMULAE

Osmolality (mOsmol/kg) = $2[Na (mEq/L) + K (mEq/L)] + [glucose (mg/dL)]/18 + [BUN (mg/dL)]/2.8$

Anion gap = $(Na + K) - (Cl + HCO_3)$ in mEq/L

Corrected reticulocyte percentage (CRP) = [reticulocyte percentage × (patient's HCT) / normal HCT]

Temperature conversion
   Celsius to Fahrenheit: $(°C) × (9/5) + 32 = °F$
   Fahrenheit to Celsius: $(°F − 32) (5/9) = °C$

Mean arterial pressure (MAP) = $DAP − 1/3 (SAP − DAP)$ or MAP = $[(SAP − DAP) ÷ 3] + DAP$
   DAP = diastolic arterial pressure   SAP = systolic arterial pressure

MPP = ADP − RAP (myocardial perfusion pressure = aortic diastolic pressure − right atrial pressure)

CPP = MAP − ICP (cranial perfusion pressure = mean arterial pressure − intracranial pressure

Ejection fraction = $[(EDV − ESV) ÷ EDV] × 100$
   EDV = end-diastolic volume   ESV = end-systolic volume

Fractional shortening = $[(EDD − ESD) ÷ EDD] × 100$
   EDD = end-diastolic diameter   ESD = end-systolic diameter

Alveolar–arterial oxygen difference (A—a gradient) = $P_{AO2} − Pa_{O2}$
   $PA_{O_2} = Fi_{O_2} (P_B − P_{H_2O}) − Pa_{CO_2}/RQ$
   PA_{O_2} = partial pressure of oxygen in alveolar air

Pa_{O_2} = partial pressure of oxygen in arterial air

Fi_{O_2} = inspired fraction of oxygen (in room air = 0.21 or 21%)

P_B = barometric pressure (760 mm Hg at sea level, decreases with increasing altitude)

P_{H_2O} = pressure of water (47 mm Hg at 37°C)

Pa_{CO_2} = partial pressure of carbon dioxide in arterial blood

RQ = respiratory quotient (ratio of CO_2 production to O_2 consumption; often the value 0.8 is used)

Short cut, if on room air at sea level = $150 - (Pa_{CO_2} / 0.8) - Pa_{O_2}$

Normal A–a gradient = <10 – 15.

>15 = compromised ability of the lungs to oxygenate blood

>30 = severely impaired gas exchange

Oxygen content of arterial blood (Ca_{O_2}) = $(1.34 \times Sa_{O_2} \times HgB) + (0.003 \times Pa_{O_2})$

Sa_{O_2} = oxygen saturation of arterial blood

$P:F$ ratio $(Pa_{O_2}:Fi_{O_2}$ ratio)

500 = normal

300–500 = mild pulmonary disease

200–300 = moderate pulmonary disease

<200 = severe pulmonary disease

Corrected chloride for dogs = measured [Cl] × 146 / measured [Na]

Corrected chloride for cats = measured [Cl] × 156 / measured [Na]

Free water deficit (L) = 0.6 × BW(kg) × [(145 ÷ patient's Na) – 1]

Sodium deficit (mEq/L) = 0.6 × BW(kg) × (desired Na – measured Na)

Fractional excretion of sodium (Fe_{Na}) = $[(U_{Na} \times P_{Cr}) \div (P_{Na} \times U_{Cr})] \times 100$

Urine sodium concentration (U_{Na}) Plasma creatinine concentration (P_{Cr})

Plasma sodium concentration (P_{Na}) Urine creatinine concentration (U_{Cr})

Kleiber–Brody equation

BER (kcal/day) = $70 \times (BWkg)^{0.75}$ (for patients <2 kg and >45 kg)

BER = (30 × BWkg) + 70 (for patients 2 to 45 kg)

BER = basal energy requirement

XV. CONSTANT RATE INFUSION FORMULAE

1. Drug dosage (mg/kg per minute) × BW (kg) × 0.36 = number of mg required for 6 hours.
2. Drug dosage (mg/kg per minute) × BW (kg) = number of mg to add to 250 mL base solution at a rate of 15 mL/h.

$$M = (D)(W)(V)/(R)(16.67) \quad \text{or} \quad R = (D)(W)(V)/(M)(16.67)$$

where M = number of mg of drug to add to base solution, D = dosage of drug in mg/kg per minute, W = body weight in kg, V = volume in ml of base solution, R = rate of delivery in ml/h, and 16.67 = conversion factor.

3. Dopamine or dobutamine CRI

$6 \times BW_{kg}$ = number of mg to add to 100 mL of 0.9% NaCl, which, when delivered at 1 mL/h IV = 1 µg/kg/min IV.

4. Epinephrine CRI $0.6 \times BW_{kg}$ = number of mg to add to 100 mL of 0.9% NaCl, which, when delivered at 1 mL/h IV = 0.1 µg/kg/min IV.

XVI. DRUGS COMMONLY ADMINISTERED BY CRI

Drug	Actions/indications	Dosage
Amrinone	Positive inotrope, systemic vasodilator	0.75 mg/kg IV bolus (slowly over 3–5 min) then 5–10 mg/kg/min
Atracurium	Induction of respiratory paralysis for controlled mechanical ventilation	0.2 mg/kg IV, then 3–8 mg/kg/min
Butorphanol	Analgesic	0.05–0.2 mg/kg/h IV
Buprenorphine	Analgesic	Dogs: 2–4 µg/kg/h IV Cats: 1–3 µg/kg/h IV
Deferoxamine	Iron chelator, iron toxicosis	15 mg/kg/h
Diazepam	Sedative, refractory seizures	0.1–0.5 mg/kg/h
Dobutamine	Positive inotrope, cardiogenic or septic shock	Dogs: 2–20 µg/kg/min Cats: 2–15 µg/kg/min
Dopamine	Dilates renal arteries, controversial	0.5–2 µg/kg/min (low dose)
Dopamine	Positive inotrope, cardiogenic or septic shock	3–10 µg/kg/min (moderate dose)
Dopamine	Pressor agent, increases BP, promotes peripheral vasoconstriction	11–20 µg/kg/min (high dose)
Epinephrine	Anaphylaxis, cardiac and BP support	0.1–1 µg/kg/min
Esmolol	Short-acting beta blocker, decreases tachycardia	25–200 mg/kg per minute following a 500 mg/kg loading dose (over 1 min)
Ethanol (7%)	Alcohol, ethylene glycol toxicosis	600 mg/kg IV bolus, then 100–200 mg/kg per hour
Fenoldopam	Increase renal blood flow	0.1–0.6 mg/kg/min IV CRI
Fentanyl	Analgesia, sedation, mechanical ventilation	Dogs: 2–10 µg/kg IV, then 1–10 µg/kg/h IV Cats: 1–5 µg/kg IV bolus, then 1–5 µg/kg/h IV
Furosemide	Diuretic	3–8 mg/kg per minute
Hydromorphone	Analgesic	Dogs: 0.0125–0.05 mg/kg/h IV Cats: 0.0125–0.03 mg/kg/h IV
Isoproterenol	Vasodilator, positive inotrope, bronchodilator	0.02–0.1 mg/kg per minute
Ketamine	Analgesic adjunct (combined with opioids, +/– lidocaine)	0.1–0.6 mg/kg/h; 2–10 µg/kg/min IV
Lidocaine	Ventricular antiarrhythmic	Dogs: 2–4 mg/kg IV bolus, then 25–80 mg/kg per minute Cats: 0.25 mg/kg IV bolus, then 10 mg/kg per minute
Methylprednisolone sodium succinate	Anti-inflammatory, spinal trauma	2.5 mg/kg/h for 24 h
Metoclopramide	Antiemetic	0.7–1.4 mg/kg per minute
Nitroprusside	Vasodilator, acute congestive heart failure	0.5–10 mg/kg per minute
Norepinephrine	Vasopressor, positive inotrope	0.05–1 µg/kg/min
Pentobarbital seizures	Sedative, refractory	3–10 mg/kg/h

Continued

Drug	Actions/indications	Dosage
Phenobarbital	Antiepileptic, refractory	Cats: 0.5–1 mg/kg/h, combined
seizures		with diazepam CRI
Phosphate (Na or K)	Elemental nutrient	0.01–0.03 mmol/kg per hour
Pralidoxime	Cholinesterase enzyme reactivator severe organophosphate toxicosis	10–20 mg/kg/h
Procainamide	Ventricular antiarrhythmic	Dogs: 2 mg/kg IV bolus, repeated to a maximum cumulative dose of 20 mg/kg, then 10–40 mg/kg/min
Propofol	Sedative	0.1–0.2 mg/kg/min;6–12 mg/kg/h
Tissue plasminogen activator	Thrombolytic, thromboembolism dissolution	4.2–16.5 mg/kg/min
Vasopressin	Vasopressor	0.5–2 mU/kg/min IV

XVII. METRIC CONVERSION CHART (APPROXIMATIONS)

When you know	Multiple by	To find
grain	60.0	milligram (mg)
milligram	1000	microgram (μg)
milligram	0.001	gram (g)
gram	0.035	ounce (oz)
gram	1000.0	milligram (mg)
gram	1,000,000	microgram (μg)
gram	0.001	kilogram (kg)
kilogram	2.21	pound (lb)
kilogram	1000.0	gram
ounce	28.35	gram
pound	16.0	ounce
pound	453.6	gram
pound	0.4536	kilogram
mg/kg	0.4536	mg/lb
mg/g	453.6	mg/lb
mg/kg	0.4536	mg/lb
mg/g	0.1	% (percentage)
mg/kg	0.0001	% (percentage)
g/kg	0.1	% (percentage)
parts per million (p.p.m.)	0.0001	% (percentage)
p.p.m.	1.0	mg/g
p.p.m.	1.0	mg/kg
p.p.m.	0.4536	mg/lb
kilocalorie/kg (kcal/kg)	0.4536	kcal/lb
kcal/lb	2.2046	kcal/kg
Mcal	1000	kcal
milliliter (mL)	0.20	teaspoon (tsp)
milliliter	0.06	tablespoon (tbs)
liter (l)	4.23	cup (c)
liter	2.12	pint (pt)
liter	1.06	quart (qt)
drop (gt)	0.06	milliliter
milliliter	15.0	drop (gt)
teaspoon	4.93	milliliter
tablespoon	14.78	milliliter
fluid ounce (fl oz)	29.57	milliliter

When you know	Multiple by	To find
cup	0.24	liter
pint	0.47	liter
quart	0.95	liter
inch (in)	2.54	centimeter (cm)
foot (ft)	30.48	centimeter
yard (yd)	91.44	centimeter

XVIII. BODY SURFACE AREA TABLE FOR DOGS AND CATS

Body surface area table for dogs

kg	m²	kg	m²
0.5	0.06	26.0	0.88
1.0	0.10	27.0	0.90
2.0	0.15	28.0	0.92
3.0	0.20	29.0	0.94
4.0	0.25	30.0	0.96
5.0	0.29	31.0	0.99
6.0	0.33	32.0	1.01
7.0	0.36	33.0	1.03
8.0	0.40	34.0	1.05
9.0	0.43	35.0	1.07
10.0	0.46	36.0	1.09
11.0	0.49	37.0	1.11
12.0	0.52	38.0	1.13
13.0	0.55	39.0	1.15
14.0	0.58	40.0	1.17
15.0	0.60	41.0	1.19
16.0	0.63	42.0	1.21
17.0	0.66	43.0	1.23
18.0	0.69	44.0	1.25
19.0	0.71	45.0	1.26
20.0	0.74	46.0	1.28
21.0	0.76	47.0	1.30
22.0	0.78	48.0	1.32
23.0	0.81	49.0	1.34
24.0	0.83	50.0	1.36
25.0	0.85		

Body surface area table for cats

kg	m²	kg	m²
0.5	0.06	5.5	0.29
1.0	0.10	6.0	0.31
1.5	0.12	6.5	0.33
2.0	0.15	7.0	0.34
2.5	0.17	7.5	0.36
3.0	0.20	8.0	0.38
3.5	0.22	8.5	0.39
4.0	0.24	9.0	0.41
4.5	0.26	9.5	0.42
5.0	0.28	10.0	0.44

From Ettinger SJ, Textbook of Veterinary Internal Medicine, Diseases of the Dog and Cat, 2nd edn, 1975, p 146, with permission from S.J. Ettinger and Elsevier.

Drug name	Dog	Cat
Abciximab	0.25 mg/kg IV then 0.125 µg/kg/min IV CRI	
Acepromazine	0.025–0.20 mg/kg IV, IM SC; maximum 3 mg; 0.55–2.2 mg/kg PO	0.05–0.10 mg/kg IV, IM, SC max. 1 mg; 0.8–2.2 mg/kg PO
Acetazolamide (Diamox®, Vetamox®)	Glaucoma: 5–10 mg/kg PO q8–12h	5 mg/kg PO q8–12h
Acetaminophen	10–15 mg/kg PO q8–12h	Not recommended
Acetaminophen with codeine (Tylenol 4®)	300 mg acetaminophen with 60 mg codeine; give 1–2 mg/kg of codeine PO q6–8h	Not recommended
Acetylcysteine (Mucomyst®)	Acetaminophen toxicity: 280 mg/kg PO IV, then 140 mg/kg q4h, for seven treatments.	Acetaminophen toxicity: 140 mg/kg PO, IV, then 70 mg/kg q6h, for seven treatments.
	Ocular: With artificial tears, dilute to 2% and apply topically q2h for max. of 48 h.	Same
	Antioxidant: 50 mg/kg diluted at least 1:1 slow IV over 1 hour, repeated every 6 hours for 24 hours	Same
Acetylpromazine	0.025–0.20 mg/kg IV, IM SC; maximum 3 mg; 0.55–2.2 mg/kg PO	0.05–0.10 mg/kg IV, IM, SC; max. 1 mg; 0.8–2.2 mg/kg PO
Acetylsalicylic acid (aspirin)	Anti-inflam.: 10–20 mg/kg PO q8–12h	Anti-inflam.: 1–25 mg/kg PO q72h;
	Antithrombotic: 0.5 mg/kg PO q12-24h	Antithrombotic: 5 mg/cat PO q72h
Actigall® (ursodeoxycholic acid)	5–7.5 mg/kg PO q12h or 10–15 mg/kg PO q24h	
Activase® (alteplase, tissue plasminogen activator; t-PA)	0.4–1 mg/kg/h IV CRI up to 10 hours (10 mg/kg)	0.25–1 mg/kg/h IV CRI up to 10 hours (10 mg/kg)
Activated charcoal	2–5 g/kg (6–12 mL/kg) PO q2–6h	Same
AcuTrim® (Dexatrim®, phenylpropanolamine)	1.5 mg/kg PO q8–12h	
Adequan® (polysulfated glycosaminoglycan)	2–5 mg/kg IM, SC, or intra-articular q3–6 days, up to eight injections	
Albendazole	25–50 mg/kg PO q12h × 3 days	Same
Albon® (sulfadimethoxine)	25–55 mg/kg PO, IV, IM q24h 55 mg/kg PO 1st day, then 27.5 mg/kg PO q24h for 14–20 days	Same
Albumin (canine)	4 mL/kg IV then 0.1–1.7 mL/kg/h IV; maximum 25 mL/kg/72 hours	Not recommended
Albumin (human)	2.5–5 mL/kg IV	Not recommended
Albuterol (Proventil®)	0.02–0.05 mg/kg PO q8–12h; nebulization of 0.5% solution in 4 mL saline 0.1 mL/5 kg	0.02–0.05 mg/kg PO q8–24h; 1 actuation (puff) of 90 mcg/m q 30minutes for 2–4h or q12h

Drug name	Dog	Cat
Alcohol (40%, 80 proof), see ethanol	2.25 mL/kg PO q4h for ethylene glycol toxicosis	Same
Aldactone® (spironolactone)	1–2 mg/kg PO q12h	
Aleve® (naproxen, Naprosyn®)	2–5 mg/kg PO once; then 1–2 mg/kg PO q48h	None
Alfaxalone	1–3 mg/kg IV	
Allopurinol	7–10 mg/kg q8h PO × 30 days then decrease to 10 mg/kg	9 mg/kg PO q24h; PO q24h
Alprazolam (Xanax®)	0.025–0.1 mg/kg PO q8h	0.0125–0.025 mg/kg PO q12h
Alternagel	1–3 mL small dog q6h; 5–10 mL large dog q6h;	1–3 mL q6h; 0.25–0.75 mL/5 kg
Aluminum hydroxide (Amphojel®) 10–30 mg/kg PO q8h; 0.5–1.5 mL/kg PO 68h	10–30 mL/cat PO q12h; 0.5–1.5 mL/kg PO q12h	
Aluminum magnesium hydroxide (Maalox®)	2–10 mL PO q2–4h	2–10 mL/cat PO q12–24h
Amantadine	3–5 mg/kg PO q24h	Same
Amikacin (Amiglyde-V®)	15–30 mg/kg IV, IM, SC q24h	10–15 mg/kg IV, IM, SC q24h
Aminophylline	5–10 mg/kg PO, IM, IV (very slowly) q8–12h	4–6 mg/kg PO, 2–4 mg/kg IV, IM, q8–12h
Aminopropazine (Jenotone®, Peritone®)	2 mg/kg SC or PO	Same
Amiodarone	5 mg/kg IV, IO over 10 minutes; repeat after 3–5 minutes if needed at 2.5 mg/kg IV, IO over 10 minutes	Same
Amitraz (Mitaban®)	10.6 mL in 9 IL water, dip q2 week for three treatments, let dry on	None
Amitriptyline	1–2 mg/kg PO q12– 24h or 2 mg/kg PO q24h	5–10 mg PO q24h
Amlodipine	0.2–0.4 mg/kg PO q12h; 0.25–0.5 mg/kg PO q24h	0.625–1.25 mg PO q24h
Ammonium chloride	100 mg/kg PO q12h	800 mg PO q24h or ¼ tsp on food q24h
Amoxicillin	6.6 20 mg/kg PO, IM, SC q8 12h	10–22 mg/kg PO, IM, SC q8–12h
Amoxicillin-clavulanate (Clavamox®, Augmentin®)	12.5–25 mg/kg PO q8–12h	62.5 mg PO q12h; 13.8 mg/kg PO q12h
Amphojel (aluminum hydroxide)	10–30 mg/kg PO q8h or 0.5–1.5 mL/kg PO q8h	10–30 mL/cat PO q12h; 0.5–1.5 mL/kg PO q12h
Amphotericin B (lipid complex diluted in dextrose 5% to 1 mg/mL and infused over 1–2 hours IV)	0.5–3 mg/kg IV three times per week for 9–12 treatments for a cumulative dosage of 8–10 mg/kg for blastomycosis or histoplasmosis; 12 mg/kg for some yeast and fungi; 24–30 mg coccidioidomycosis, aspergillosis, and other fungal infections	0.25– 1 mg/kg IV 3 days per week for a total of 12 treatments for cumulative dosage of 12 mg/kg for cryptococcosis
Ampicillin sodium	10–40 mg/kg PO, IV, IM, SC q6–8h	Same
Ampicillin-sulbactam (Unasyn®)	10–12 mg/kg IV, IM q8h	Same
Ampicillin trihydrate (Polyflex®)	6.5–10 mg/kg IM, SC q12h	Same

Continued

Drug name	Dog	Cat
Amrinone (Inocor®)	0.75–3 mg IV bolus over 3–5 min, then 50–100 mg/kg per min CRI IV	Same
Anadrol® (oxymetholone)	1–3 mg/kg q24h; or 1 mg/kg PO q12–24h	
Ancef® (cefazolin, Kefzol®)	10–30 mg/kg IM, IV q4–8h	Same
Antilirium® (physostigmine)	0.02–0.06 mg/kg slow IV q12h	Same
Antisedan® (atipamezole)	50 mg/kg IM q3–4h	
Antivenin crotalidae polyvalent	1–5 vials diluted, slow IV over 1–2 h; additional vials as needed	Same
Antivenin micrurus fulvius	Two or more vials, diluted, slow IV over 1–2 h	Same
Antizol-Vet® (fomepizole, 4-methylpyrazole, 4-MP)	Loading dose = 20 mg/kg IV, 15 mg/kg IV at 12 and 24 h, 5 mg/kg IV at 36 (48, and 60) hours after initiation of treatment	Loading dose = loading dose = 125 mg/kg IV, 31.25 mg/kg IV at 12 hours, 24 hours and 36 hours after initiation of treatment
Anzemet® (dolasetron mesylate)	0.6–1 mg/kg SC, IV, PO q24h	Same
Apomorphine	1.5–6 mg in conjunctival sac; 0.02–0.04 mg/kg IV, IM; 0.1 mg/kg SC	0.02–0.04 mg/kg IV, IM, SC
Apresoline® (hydralazine)	0.5–3 mg/kg PO q12h	0.5–0.8 mg/kg PO q8h; 2.5 mg/kg PO q12h
Aprindine	100 mg PO q12h	None
Aramine® (metaraminol bitartrate)	0.01–0.10 mg/kg slow IV; or 10 mg in 250 mL D5W IV to effect	Same
Arava® (Leflunomide)	4 mg/kg PO q24h	
Arginine		1 g/day PO
Anzemet® (dolasetron mesylate)	0.6–1 mg/kg SC, IV, PO q24h	Same
Arquel® (meclofenamic acid)	0.5–1 mg/kg PO q24–48h for maximum 5 days	None
Ascorbic acid (vitamin C)	100–500 mg/day (maintenance); or 100–500 mg q8h (urinary acidifier) Acetaminophen toxicosis: 30 mg/kg PO, SC q6h or 20–30 mg/kg in IV fluids q6h	125 mg/cat PO q6h
Aspirin (acetylsalicylic acid)	Anti-inflammatory: 10–20 mg/kg PO q8–12h Antithrombotic: 0.5 mg/kg PO q72h	Anti-inflammatory: 1–25 mg/kg PO q72h Antithrombotic: 5 mg/cat PO q12–24h
Atracurium besylate (Tracrium®)	0.2 mg/kg IV, then 3–8 mg/kg/min CRI IV	Same
Atenolol (Tenormin®)	0.25–1 mg/kg PO q12–24h	6.25–12.5 mg PO q12–24h
Atipamezole (Antisedan®)	0.1–0.2 mg/kg IV or IM	0.1–0.2 mg/kg IV or IM
Atovaquone (atavaquone)		13.5 mg/kg PO q8h
Atropine sulfate	CPR dosages: 0.04 mg/kg IV or 0.08–0.1 mg/kg intratracheal	Same
	Preanesthetic: 0.02–0.04 mg/kg SC, IM, IV	Same
	Organophosphate toxicity: 0.2–2.0 mg/kg IV, SC, IM. Give ¼ dose IV and remainder IM or SC as needed	Same

Drug name	Dog	Cat
	Antiarrhythmic: 0.02–0.04 mg/kg SC, IM, IV q4–6h	Same
	Emergency bronchodilator: 0.04 mg/kg SC, IM or 0.15 mg/kg IV	Same
Augmentin (Clavamox®, amoxicillin-clavulanate)	12.5–25 mg/kg PO q8–12h	13.8 mg/kg PO q12h; 62.5 mg PO q12h
Axid AR® (nizatidine)	2.5–5 mg/kg PO q24h	None
Azactam® (aztreonam)	30 mg/kg IV q6	
Azathioprine (Imuran®)	Immune hemolytic anemia: 2 mg/kg q24h	Same
	Immune thrombocytopenia: 50 mg/m^2 or 2 mg/kg PO q24h, taper to 0.5–1.0 mg/kg PO q48h	Same
	Chronic active hepatitis: 2–2.5 mg/kg PO q24h	
	Eosinophilic enteritis: 0.3–0.5 mg/kg PO q24–48h	Same
Azithromycin (Zithromax®)	5–10 mg/kg IV, PO q24h for 5 days	5 mg/kg IV, PO q24–48h for 5 days
Aztreonam (Azactam®)	30 mg/kg IV q6h	
Azulfidine® (sulfasalazine)	15–50 mg/kg PO divided q8h (maximum 4 g/day)	20–25 mg/kg PO q24h for maximum of 7 days
BAL (British anti-Lewisite, dimercaprol)	3–7 mg/kg IM q8h for 1–2 days, 3–4 mg/kg q8h the 3rd day until recovery	2.5–5 mg/kg IM q4h for 2 days, then q12h until recovery
Banamine® (flunixin meglumine)	0.5–1 mg/kg IV, IM, SC, PO q24h for up to 3 days	None
Barium sulfate	Contrast: 8 mL/kg PO	Same
	Therapeutic: 0.5–1 mL/kg PO q12h	Same
Basalgel® (aluminum carbonate)	10–30 mg/kg PO q8h	Same
Baytril® (enrofloxacin)	2.5–15 mg/kg PO, IV, IM, SC q12–24h 5–20 mg/kg q24h	Same
Benadryl® (diphenhydramine)	1–2 mg/kg IM, IV; 2–4 mg/kg PO q8h	5–50 mg/cat IM, IV q12h; 2–4 mg/kg PO q8h
Benazepril (Lotensin®)	0.25–0.5 mg/kg PO q12–24h	Same
Betamethasone	0.028–0.055 mL/kg IM once, 0.1–0.2 mg/kg PO q12–24h	None
Betapace® (sotalol)	0.5–5 mg/kg PO q12h	
Bethanechol (Urecholine®)	5–15 mg q8h PO	1.25–5 mg q8h PO
Bisacodyl (Dulcolax®)	5–15 mg/dog PO q24h	5 mg/cat PO q24h
Bismuth subsalicylate (Pepto Bismol®)	10–30 mL PO; 0.25–2 mL/kg PO q6–12h	0.25–0.5 mL/kg PO q12h for max. 3 days
Black widow antivenin (Lyovac®)	1 vial slow IV	Same
Blood	20 mL/kg IV or to effect	Same
Bonine (Meclizine®)	12.5–25 mg PO q24h	12.5 mg PO q24h
Bretylium tosylate	25–50 mg/kg IV	
Brevibloc® (esmolol)	0.05–0.1 mg/kg slow IV; 500 mg/kg IV over 1 min then 25–200 mg/kg per minute CRI IV	
Brewer's yeast	200 mg/kg/day	100 mg/kg per day

Continued

Drug name	Dog	Cat
Bromide (potassium)	Loading dose: 400 mg/kg per day divided q12h for 2–3 days; maintenance: 22–30 mg/kg/day with phenobarbital or 60 mg/kg per day as a single agent	Contraindicated
Bromide (sodium) (15% less than the potassium bromide dose)	Loading dose: 340 mg/kg per day divided q12h for 2–3 days; maintenance: 18–25 mg/kg/day with phenobarbital or 50 mg/kg per day as a single agent	Contraindicated
Bumetanide (Bumex®)	0.05–0.2 mg/kg PO or IV, as needed	Same
Bupivacaine hydrochloride (Marcaine®)	Epidural: 0.2–0.3 mL or 1 mL/3.5 kg ± morphine 0.1 mg/kg	
Buprenorphine	0.005–0.02 mg/kg q48h IV, IM, SC; 5–20 µg/kg IV, IM q4–8h; 2–4 µg/kg/h IV CRI (D); 120 µg/kg OTM (D); 0.12 mg/kg OTM (D)	0.005–0.01 mg/kg q48h IV, IM, SC; 5–10 µg/kg IV, IM q4–8h; 1–3 µg/kg/h IV CRI (C); 20 µg/kg OTM (C); 0.02 mg/kg OTM q6–8h (C)
Buprenorphine SR		0.12 mg/kg SC q12h (C)
Buspirone (BuSpar®)	2.5–15 mg/dog PO q8–12h; 1–2 mg/kg PO q8–12h	2.5–7.5 mg PO q8–12h; 0.5–1 mg/kg PO q8–12h; start at 2.5 mg/cat PO q12h
Butorphanol (Torbutrol®, Torbugesic®)	0.1–0.5 mg/kg IV q1–4h; 0.2–0.8 mg/kg SC, IM, PO q1–6h; or 0.55–1.1 mg/kg PO q6–12h 0.1 mg/kg/h CRI IV Cough suppressant: 0.05–0.12 mg/kg SC q6–12h or 0.5–1 mg/kg PO q8–12h	0.1–0.8 mg/kg IV, IM, SC q1–6h; 0.5–2 mg/kg PO q4–8h
Calcitonin salmon	4–6 IU/kg SC q8–12h	
Calcitriol (1,25-dihydroxy-vitamin D, Rocaltrol®)	1.5–60 ng/kg per day PO (0.0025–0.06 mg/kg/day PO)	Same
Calcium carbonate	1–4 g/day PO	Same
Calcium chloride (10%)	0.05–0.1 mL/kg IV	Same
Calcium EDTA (calcium sodium EDTA)	100 mg/kg diluted to 10 mg/mL in 5% dextrose and given SC in four divided doses; continue for 5 days	Same
Calcium gluconate (10%)	0.5–1.5 mL/kg IV, maximum 20 mL IV; administer slowly over 15–30 min. May repeat q6–8h. 500–700 mg/kg per day PO	0.2–0.5 mL/kg slow IV
Calcium lactate	400–600 mg/day PO in three or four divided doses	
Capoten® (captopril)	0.25–2 mg/kg PO q8–12h	2–6.25 mg PO q8h
Captan	0.2–0.25% solution topically, two or three times weekly	Same

Drug name	Dog	Cat
Captopril (Capoten®)	0.25–2 mg/kg PO q8–12h	2–6.25 mg PO q8h
Caricide® (Filaribits®, diethylcarbamazine)	Heartworm preventative: 6.6 mg/kg q24h PO	
Carafate® (sucralfate)	0.5–1 g PO q6–8h (34 mg/kg); loading dose of 3–6 g PO if severe GI hemorrhage	0.25 g/cat PO q8h
Carbenicillin (Geopen®)	10–50 mg/kg PO, IV, IM, q6–8h	Same
Cardizem® (diltiazem)	0.5–2 mg/kg PO q8–12h	1–2 mg/kg PO q8–12h or 7.5–15 mg/cat PO q8h
Cardoxin® (Lanoxin®, digoxin)	0.005–0.01 mg/kg PO q12h	0.0312 mg/kg PO q12–48h
L-Carnitine	110 mg/kg PO q12h	
Carprofen (Rimadyl®)	4 mg/kg IV, IM, SC once; 0.5–2.2 mg/kg PO q12h	4 mg/kg SC or IV once
Carvedilol (Coreg®)	0.5–1.5 mg/kg PO q12h, start with ¼–½ of a 3.125 mg tablet	
Castor oil	8–30 mL PO	4–10 mL PO
Cefaclor (Ceclor®)	6.6–13.3 mg/kg PO q8h	Same
Cefadroxil (Cefa Tabs®)	22 mg/kg q8–12h PO	22 mg/kg PO q12–24h
Cefadyl® (cephapirin, cefapirin)	10–30 mg/kg IM, IV q4–8h	Same
Cefazolin (Ancef®, Kefzol®)	10–30 mg/kg IM, IV q4–8h	Same
Cefixime (Suprax®)	10 mg/kg PO q12h; 5 mg/kg PO q12h for urinary tract infections	Same
Cefmetazole (Zefazone®)	15 mg/kg IV, IM, SC	Same
Cefotan® (cefotetan)	30 mg/kg IV q8h or SC q12h	Same
Cefotaxime (Claforan®)	30–80 mg/kg IM, IV q6–8h	Same
Cefotetan (Cefotan®)	30 mg/kg IV q8h or SC q12h	Same
Cefoxitin (Mefoxin®)	15–40 mg/kg IV, IM SC, q6–8h	Same
Cefovecin sodium (Convenia®)	8 mg/kg SC, repeat in 14 days if needed	Same
Cefpodoxime proxetil (Simplicef®)	5–10 mg/kg q24h PO for 5–28 days	5 mg/kg PO q12h; or 10 mg/kg PO q24h
Ceftiofur (Naxcel®)	2.2–4.4 mg/kg SC q12–24h	Same
Ceftazidime (Fortaz®)	4.4 mg/kg IV loading dose then 4 mg/kg/h CRI/IV	Same
Ceftizoxime (Ceftizox®)	25–50 mg/kg IV, IM, SC q6–8h	Same
Ceftriaxone (Rocephin®)	15–50 mg/kg IV, IM q24h	
Cephalexin (Keflex®)	10–30 mg/kg PO q6–12h	Same
Cephalothin sodium (Keflin®)	10–30 mg/kg q4–8h IM, IV	Same
Cephapirin (Cefadyl®)	10–30 mg/kg IM, IV q4–8h	Same
Cephradine (Velosef®)	10–25 mg/kg PO, IV, IM q6–8h	Same
Cephulac® (lactulose)	3–10 mL PO q8h; or 0.5–1 mL/kg PO q8–12h	1–3 mL PO q12–24h; 0.5–1 mL/kg PO q8–12h or 5–10 mL diluted 1:3 with water given per rectum
Cerenia® (maropitant)	1 mg/kg SC; 2 mg/kg PO q24h for up to 5 days	Same
Cestex® (episprantel)	5.5 mg/kg PO	2.75 mg/kg PO

Continued

Drug name	Dog	Cat
Charcoal (activated)	2–5 g/kg PO q2–6h (6–12 mL/kg PO)	Same
Chemet® (succimer, DMSA)	10 mg/kg PO q8h × 10 days	None
Chloramphenicol	30–50 mg/kg PO, IV, IM, SC q6–8h	30–50 mg/kg PO, IV, IM, SC q12h
Chlorothiazide (Diuril®)	10–40 mg/kg PO q12h	Same
Chlorpheniramine maleate	2–4 mg PO q8–12h; or 4–8 mg PO q12h	1–2 mg PO q8–12h
Chloramphenicol	30–50 mg/kg PO, IV, IM, SC q6–8h	30–50 mg/kg PO, IV, IM, SC q12h
Chlorpromazine (Thorazine®)	Antiemetic dose: 0.05–0.10 mg/kg IV q4–6h; or 0.20–0.50 mg/kg SC, IM q6–8h; or 1 mg/kg diluted in 1 mL 0.9% NaCl administered per rectum q8h Tranquilization: 0.8–2.2 mg/kg 0.5 mg/kg IM PO q8–12h	0.01–0.25 mg/kg IV q4h
Chlortetracycline	20–25 mg/kg PO q6–8h	Same
Cimetidine (Tagamet®)	5–10 mg/kg PO, IV, IM q6–8h	Same
Ciprofloxacin (Cipro®)	5–15 mg/kg PO q12h or 10–20 mg/kg PO q24h	5–15 mg/kg PO q12h
Cisapride (Propulsid®)	0.1–0.5 mg/kg PO q8–12h	1 mg/kg q8h; 1.5 mg/kg PO q12h; 2.5–5 mg/cat PO q8–12h
Claforan® (cefotaxime)	30–80 mg/kg IM, IV q6–8h	Same
Clavamox (Augmentin®, amoxicillin-clavulanate)	12.5–25 mg/kg PO q8–12h	13.8 mg/kg PO q12h; 62.5 mg PO q12h
Clemastine fumarate (Tavist-D®)	0.05 mg/kg PO q12h	0.1 mg/kg PO q12h
Clindamycin	5–15 mg/kg IV, IM, PO q8–12h	2–25 mg/kg IV, IM, PO, q8–12h
Clomipramine (Clomicalm®, Anafril®)	1–2 mg/kg PO q12h	1–5 mg/cat PO q12–24h
Clonazepam (Klonopin®)	1–10 mg PO q6–24h (0.5 mg/kg PO q8–12h)	0.5 mg/kg PO q8–12h
Clopidogrel (Plavix®)	1–5 mg/kg PO q24h	18.75 mg/cat PO q24h
Clorazepate dipotassium (Tranxene®)	0.5–2 mg/kg PO q12h	Same
Cloxacillin	10–40 mg/kg PO, IV, IM q6–8h	Same
Cod liver oil	0.5 mL/kg PO q24h	Same
Codeine	Analgesic: 0.5–2 mg/kg PO q4–8h Antitussive: 0.1–0.3 mg/kg, PO q6–8h	0.5–1 mg/kg PO q6–8h
Colchicine	0.01–0.03 mg/kg PO q12–24h	Same
Compazine® (prochlorperazine)	0.1–0.5 mg/kg IM, SC q6–8h	Same
Cortrosyn® (cosyntropin)	250 μg (0.25 mg) IV or IM; or 1 μg/kg IV or IM (blood samples drawn pre and 60 minutes post administration)	125 μg (0.125 mg) IV or IM (blood samples drawn pre and 30 minutes and 60 minutes post administration)
Cryoprecipitate	1 unit/10 kg IV	Same

Drug name	Dog	Cat
Cyclophosphamide (Cytoxan®, Neosar®)	200–300 mg/m² IV bolus once; 200 mg/m² PO divided over 4 days (50 mg/m²), stop for 3 days, repeat CBC and re-evaluate; 50 mg/m² PO q48h for 7 days, stop 3 days, repeat CBC and re-evaluate	6.25–12.5 mg/cat q24h × 4 days/wk
Cyclosporine	3–10 mg/kg PO q12–24h	4–10 mg/kg PO q12h
Cyproheptadine (Periactin®)	Antihistamine: 1.1 mg/kg PO q8–12h	Appetite stimulant: 1–2 mg PO q12h
Cytotec® (misoprostol)	0.7–5.0 mcg/kg PO q8h	Same
Dalteparin sodium (Fragmin®)	150 IU/kg SC q8h	150–180 U/kg SC q4–6h
Danazol (Danocrine®)	5–10 mg/kg PO q12h	Same
Dapsone	1.1–2 mg/kg PO q6–8h	Same, or 12.5–25 mg PO q12–24h
Daranide® (dichlorphenamide)	2–5 mg/kg PO q8–12h	
Daraprim® (pyrimethamine)	0.5–1.0 mg/kg PO q24h for 2 days, then 0.25 mg/kg PO q24h for 2 weeks	Same
Darbazine	0.14–0.2 mL/kg SC q12h	0.14–0.22 mg/kg SC q12h
Darbid (isopropamide)	2.5–5 mg PO q8–12h; 0.1–0.2 mg/kg PO q12h	0.07 mg/cat PO q12h
DDAVP (desmopressin acetate, deamino 8-D-arginine vasopressin)	2–4 drops intranasal or in conjunctival sac q12–24h; 1 mcg/kg SC for von Willebrand's 0.4 mcg/kg SC for factor VIII	Same
Deferoxamine (Desferal®)	25–50 mg/kg slow IV; 15 mg/kg/h CRI IV	None
Demerol® (meperidine)	2–5 mg/kg IM, SC q2–4h	2–5 mg/kg IM, SC q2–4h
Depakene® (valproic acid)	6–90 mg/kg per day PO	
Deracoxib (Deramaxx®)	3–4 mg/kg PO q24h	Not recommended
Desferal® (deferoxamine)	25–50 mg/kg slow IV; 15 mg/kg/h CRI IV	None
Desmopressin acetate (DDAVP, deamino 8-D-arginine vasopressin)	2–4 drops intranasal or in conjunctival sac q12–24h; 1 mcg/kg SC for von Willebrand's 0.4 mcg/kg SC for factor VIII	Same
Desoxycorticosterone pivalate (DOCP)	1.5–2.2 mg/kg IM	Same
Detemir® (insulin)	0.1–0.2 units/kg SC q12h	1 unit/cat SC q12h
Dexamethasone	0.02–1 mg/kg q24h IV, IM, SC, PO	Same
Dexamethasone sodium phosphate	0.5–1 mg/kg IV, IM, SC q12–24h	Same
Dexatrim® (AcuTrim®, phenylpropanolamine)	1.5 mg/kg PO q8–12h	
Dextran 70	14–20 mL/kg/day IV	Same
Dextromethorphan [Robitussin Pediatric® cough syrup (1.5 mg/mL), Vicks Formula 44® (2 mg/mL)]	1–2 mg/kg PO q6–8h	2 mg/kg PO q8h
Dextrose (25%)	0.25 mL/kg IV	Same
Diabeta® (glyburide)	0.2 mg/kg PO q24h	0.625 mg/cat PO q24h

Continued

Drug name	Dog	Cat
Dialume	$\frac{1}{4}$ to $\frac{1}{6}$ capsule	
Dialysate	20–30 mL/kg IP	Same
Diamox® (acetazolamide)	Glaucoma: 3.5–10 mg/kg IV, PO q8–12h	50 mg/kg IV once; 7 mg/kg PO q8–12h
Diazepam (Valium®)	Status epilepticus: 0.5–3 mg/kg IV or 2.5–20 mg intratracheal; 0.1–0.5 mg/kg/h CRI IV	Same
	Preanesthetic: 0.1 mg/kg IV	Same
	Restraint: 0.2–0.6 mg/kg IV per rectum or intranasal: 0.5–1 mg/kg	Same
	Behavior modification: 0.5–2.2 mg/kg PO PRN	Behavior modification: 1–2 mg PO q12h Appetite stimulation: 0.05–0.15 mg/kg IV q24–48h or 1.0 mg PO q24h
Diazepam/ketamine	Mix 50:50, give 1 mL/4.5–9 kg IV (0.2 mg/kg diazepam and 10 mg/kg ketamine)	Same
Diazoxide (Proglycem®)	5–13 mg/kg PO q8h; maximum 30 mg/kg q8h	Same
Dibenzyline® (phenoxybenzamine)	0.25–0.5 mg/kg PO q8–12h	2.5–5 mg PO q12–24h, gradually increase to 10 mg
Dichlorphenamide (Daranide®)	2–5 mg/kg PO q8–12h	1 mg/kg PO q8–12h
Dichlorvos®	11–33 mg/kg PO, repeat in 3 weeks	11 mg/kg PO
Dicloxacillin (Dicloxin®)	10–50 mg/kg q8h PO	Same
Didronel (etidronate disodium)	5–17 mg/kg PO, IV q8–12h	10 mg/kg PO, IV q24h
Diethylcarbamazine (Caricide®, Filaribits®)	Heartworm preventative: 6.6 mg/kg q24h PO	
Diethylstilbestrol (DES)	0.1–1.0 mg/day PO	0.05–0.10 mg/day (caution)
Difloxacin (Dicural®)	5–10 mg/kg q24h	Same
Diflucan® (fluconazole)	2.5–5 mg/kg PO q12h	50 mg/cat PO q12h
DiGel® (aluminum magnesium hydroxide)	2–10 mL PO q2–4h	2–10 mL/cat PO q12–24h
Digitoxin	0.013–0.033 mg/kg PO q8h	0.005–0.015 mg/kg PO q24h
Digoxin	0.005–0.01 mg/kg PO q12h	0.0312 mg/kg PO q12–48h
Dihydrocodenione	5 mg q8h PO	None
Dilantin (Phenytoin®)	15–40 mg/kg PO q8h	None
Diltiazem (Cardizem®)	0.5–2 mg/kg PO q8–12h	1–2 mg/kg PO q8–12h; or 7.5–15 mg/cat PO q8h
Dimenhydrinate (Dramamine®)	4–8 mg/kg PO q8–24h; 12.5–50 mg PO q8–24h; 6.25 mg in puppies 1–4 kg	12.5 mg PO q8–24h
Dimercaprol (BAL)	3–7 mg/kg IM q8h for 1–2 days, 3–4 mg/kg q8h the 3rd day until recovery	2.5–5 mg/kg IM q4h for 2 days, then q12h until recovery

Drug name	Dog	Cat
Dioctyl sodium sulfosuccinate (DSS)	25–100 mg PO q12–24h	25 mg PO q12–24h
Diphenhydramine (Benadryl®)	1–2 mg/kg IM, IV; 2–4 mg/kg PO q8h	5–50 mg/cat IM, IV q12h;
Diphenoxylate (Lomotil®)	2.5–10 mg PO; 0.05–0.2 PO q8–12h	None
Dipyrone (Novin®)	10–25 mg/kg SC, IM, IV; may repeat q8h	0.25 mL/cat or 0.06 mL/kg IM, SC, IV; max. of two doses, 8 h apart
Dithiazanine iodide		50 mg daily for 7–10 days
Di-Trim® (trimethoprim-sulfadiazine)	15–30 mg/kg PO, SC, q12–24h	30 mg/kg PO, SC q12–24h
Diuril® (chlorothiazide)	10–40 mg/kg PO q12h	Same
DMSA (meso-dimercapto-succinic acid, succimer, Chemet®)	10 mg/kg PO q8h × 10d	None
DMSO (dimethylsulfoxide)	250 mg/kg IV (10–25%), SC, PO, topical or intra-articular	
Dobutamine	2–20 µg/kg/min IV CRI	1–5 µg/kg/min IV CRI
DOCP (desoxycortisone pivalate)	1.5–2.2 mg/kg IM	Same
Dolasetron mesylate (Anzemet®)	0.6–1 mg/kg SC, IV, PO q24h	Same
Dopamine	5–10 µg/kg/min	
Doxapram (Dopram®)	2–10 mg/kg slow IV Neonate: 1–5 mg SC, IV, or sublingual	Same
Doxepin	0.5–1 mg/kg q12h	
Doxycycline	5–20 mg/kg PO or IV loading dose then 5–10 mg/kg q12h	2.5–15 mg/kg IV, PO q12h
Dramamine® (dimenhydrinate)	4–8 mg/kg PO q8–24h; 12.5–50 mg PO q8–24h; 6.25 mg in puppies weighing 1–4 kg	12.5 mg PO q8–12h
Droncit® (praziquantel)	<6.8 kg: 7.5 mg/kg PO; >6.0 kg: 5 mg/kg PO SC, IM; 2.7–4.5 kg: 6.3 mg/kg SC, IM; >5 kg: 5 mg/kg SC, IM	6.3 mg/kg PO, SC for cats <1.8 kg; 5 mg/kg PO, SC for cats >1.8 kg; 5 mg/kg IM, SC
Dulcolax® (bisacodyl)	5–15 mg/dog PO q24h	5 mg/cat PO q24h
Edrophonium chloride (Tensilon®)	0.11–0.22 mg/kg IV	2.5 mg/cat IV
Elavil® (amitriptyline)	2.2–4.4 mg/kg PO q24h; or 1–2 mg/kg PO q12h	5–10 mg PO q24h; or 2 mg/kg PO q24h
Enalapril	0.25–3 mg/kg PO q12–24h	0.25–0.5 mg/kg PO q24–48h
Enoxaparin sodium	0.8 – 1 mg/kg SC q6h	1 – 1.5 mg/kg SC q6h (Lovenox®)
Enrofloxacin (Baytril®)	2.5–15 mg/kg PO, IV, IM, SC q12–24h; or 5–20 mg/kg q24h	2.5 – 5 mg/kg PO, IV, IM, SC q12 – 24h
Ephedrine	5–15 mg PO q8–12h	2–5 mg PO q8–12h

Continued

Appendices

Drug name	Dog	Cat
Epinephrine (1 : 1000)	0.01 mg/kg IV, IO; 0.03–0.1 mg/kg IT. Repeat dose 0.1 mg/kg IV, IO, IT. Repeat every 3–5 min	Same
Epinephrine	0.1–1 µg/kg/min IV CRI Rapid bronchodilation: 0.1–0.5 mL of 1 : 1000 solution SC	Same
Episprantel (Cestex®)	5.5 mg/kg PO	2.75 mg/kg PO
Epogen® (erythropoietin)	50–100 mg/kg SC two to three times per week	Same
Erythromycin	10–20 mg/kg PO q8–12h	Same
Erythropoietin (Epogen®)	50–100 mg/kg SC two to three times per week	Same
Esmolol (Brevibloc®)	0.05–0.1 mg/kg slow IV; 500 mg/kg IV over 1 min, then 25–200 mg/kg/min CRI IV	
Esomeprazole	0.5 mg/kg IV q12 – 24h	
Ethanol (7%)	Ethylene glycol toxicity: 600 mg/kg IV loading dose, then 100–200 mg/kg per hour IV (1.43 mL/kg per hour IV)	Same
Ethanol (35%)	Severe pulmonary edema: dilute with sterile water, nebulize with oxygen	Same
Ethanol (40%, 80 proof)	2.25 mL/kg PO q4h for ethylene glycol toxicosis	Same
Etidronate disodium (Didronel®)	5–17 mg/kg PO, IV q8–12h	10 mg/kg PO, IV q24h
Etodolac (EtoGesic®)	5–15 mg/kg PO q24h	None
Etomidate	0.5 to 2.0 mg/kg IV	
Etretinate (Tegison®)	0.75–1 mg/kg PO q24h	2 mg/kg PO q24h
Famotidine (Pepcid®)	0.3–1 mg/kg IV, IM, PO q12–24h; 0.5–5 mg/kg PO q12–24h	Same
Feldene® (piroxicam)	0.3 mg/kg PO q24–48h	1 mg/cat PO q24h for max. 5 days
Fenbendazole (Panacur®)	50 mg/kg per day PO for 3 days; repeat in 3 weeks	50 mg/kg PO once
Fenoldopam (Corlopam®)	0.1–0.6 mg/kg/min IV CRI	Same
Fentanyl	2–10 µg/kg IV to effect (D); 1–10 + µg/kg/h IV CRI (D); 0.001–0.01 mg/kg/h IV CRI (D)	1–5 µg/kg IV to effect (C); 1–5 µg/kg/h IV CRI (C) 0.001–0.005 mg/kg/h IV CRI (C)

Or transdermally as follows:

body weight	patch size	
<10 kg (20 lb)	25 µg/h	<5 kg: fold back the liner to expose $\frac{1}{3} - \frac{1}{2}$ of a 25 µg/h patch
10–25 kg (20–50 lb)	50 µg/h	
25–40 kg (50–88 lb)	75 µg/h	>5 kg: fold back the liner to expose $\frac{2}{3}$ of a 25 µg/h patch or use the full patch
>40 kg (>88 lb)	100 µg/h	

Drug name	Dog	Cat
Ferrous sulfate	100–300 mg/kg PO q24h	50–100 mg PO q24h
Filaribits® (Caricide®, diethylcarbamazine)	Heartworm preventative: 6.6 mg/kg q24h PO	

Drug name	Dog	Cat
Firocoxib (Equioxx®, Previcox®)	5 mg/kg PO q24h	0.75–3 mg/kg PO once
Flagyl® (metronidazole)	10–15 mg/kg PO q12h; 7.5–10 mg/kg IV CRI over 1 h q8–12h; 15 mg/kg IV q12h	Liver/GI: 7.5 mg/kg PO; q8–12h Giardiasis: 10 mg/kg PO q12h × 5 days Gingivitis: 50 mg/kg PO q24h
Flatulex	>22.6 kg: 1 tablet PO q12h	
Florinef® acetate (fludrocortisone acetate)	0.2–0.8 mg PO q24h; 0.02 mg/kg PO q24h	0.1–0.2 mg PO q24h
Fluconazole (Diflucan®)	2.5–5 mg/kg PO q12h	50 mg/cat PO q12h
Fludrocortisone acetate (Florinef® acetate)	0.2–0.8 mg PO q24h; 0.02 mg/kg PO q24h	0.1–0.2 mg PO q24h
Flumazenil	0.02 mg/kg IV	Same
Flumethasone	0.06–0.25 mg PO, IV, IM, SC q24h	0.03–0.125 mg PO, IV, IM, SC q24h
Flunixin meglumine (Banamine®)	0.5–1 mg/kg IV, IM, SC, PO q24h for up to 3 days	None
Fluoxetine (Prozac®)	1–2 mg/kg PO q24h	None
Folic acid	5 mg/day PO	2.5 mg/day PO
Fomepizole (Antizol-Vet®, 4-methylpyrazole, 4-MP)	Loading dose = 20 mg/kg IV, 15 mg/kg IV at 12 and 24 h, 5 mg/kg IV at 36 (48, and 60) hours after initiation of treatment	Loading dose = 125 mg/kg IV, 31.25 mg/kg IV at 12 hours, 24 hours and 36 hours after initiation of treatment
Fortaz® (ceftazidime)	4.4 mg/kg IV loading dose then 4.0 mg/kg/h CRI IV	Same
Fresh frozen plasma	For coagulopathy: 10–15 mL/kg IV For hypoalbuminemia: 40 mL/kg IV	Same
Fresh whole blood	20–25 mL/kg IV	Same
Furosemide (Lasix®)	1–4 mg/kg IV, IM, PO q1–2h or q6–12h; 0.1–0.2 mg/kg/h CRI IV; 3–8 mg/kg/min CRI IV	0.5–4 mg/kg IV, IM, PO; q1–2h or q6–12h
Gabapentin	3–10 mg/kg PO q8-12h	Same
G-CSF (Neupogen®)	5–10 mg/kg SC, IV q24h	Same
Gentamicin (Gentocin®)	2–4 mg/kg IV, IM, SC q8h; or 6.6–9 mg/kg IV, IM q24h; injectable preparation PO: 2 mg/kg PO q8h	Same
Geopen® (carbenicillin)	10–50 mg/kg IV, IM, PO q6–8h	Same
Glargine (insulin, Lantus®)	0.25–0.5 units/kg SC q12h	1 unit/cat SC q12h
Glipizide (Glucatrol®)	2.5–5 mg PO q12h	Same
Glucagon	0.15 mg/kg IV bolus followed by CRI of 0.05–0.1 mg/kg IV	
Glyburide (Diabeta®)	0.2 mg/kg PO q24h	0.625 mg/cat PO q24h
Glycerin (50%)	1–2 mL/kg PO q6h	Same
Glycopyrrolate (Robinul V®)	Preanesthetic: 0.011 mg/kg IV, IM, SC 0.01–0.02 mg/kg IM, SC Bradycardia: 0.005–0.01 mg/kg IV, IM; 0.01–0.02 mg/kg SC q8–12h	0.011 mg/kg IM Bradycardia: 0.005–0.01 mg/kg SC q8–12h
Griseofulvin (microsized)	25–60 mg/kg PO q12h for 3–6 weeks	Same

Continued

Drug name	Dog	Cat
(ultramicrosized)	5–15 mg/kg PO q12–24h	
Guaifenesin (Organidin®)	0.05–0.1 mL/kg PO q6h; 1 mL/kg per hour CRI IV	Same
Haloperidol	1 mg/kg IV	
Heparin (UFH)	5–10 U/kg/h IV CRI; 200–300 U/kg SC q6 –8h	Same
Hespan® (hetastarch)	10–20 mL/kg IV, may repeat	10–15 ml/kg IV
Hetacillin	20–40 mg/kg PO q8h	Same
Hetastarch (Hespan®)	10–20 mL/kg IV, may repeat	10–15 ml/kg IV
Hismanal (astemizole)	0.2 mg/kg PO q24h-1 mg/kg PO q12h	
HIVIG (human intravenous Immunoglobulin)	0.5–1.5 g/kg IV over 6–12 h	
Hycodan® (Tussigon®, hydrocodone)	0.25–0.5 mg/kg PO q6–12h	2.5–5 mg/cat PO q8–12h
Hydralazine (Apresoline®)	0.5–3 mg/kg PO q12h	0.5–0.8 mg/kg PO q8h; 2.5 mg/kg PO q12h
Hydrochlorothiazide (HydroDiuril®)	1–4 mg/kg PO q12h	
Hydrocodone (Hycodan®, Tussigon®)	0.25–0.5 mg/kg PO q6–12h	2.5–5 mg/cat PO q8–12h
Hydrogen peroxide (3%)	1–2 mL/kg PO; max. dose of 2 tbsp (30 mL), repeat $\frac{1}{2}$ dose only once if no emesis within 15 minutes	Same
Hydromorphone	0.05–0.2 mg/kg IV, IM or SC q2–6h (D); 0.0125–0.05 mg/kg/h IV CRI (D); premed 0.1 mg/kg with acepromazine 0.02–0.05 mg/kg IM (B)	0.02–0.1 mg/kg IV, IM or SC q2–6h (C); 0.0125 – 0.03 mg/kg/h IV CRI (C); premed 0.08 mg/kg with acepromazine 0.02–0.05 mg/kg IM (B)
Hydroxyzine HCl	2.2 mg/kg PO q8h	6.6 mg/kg PO q8h
Hypertonic saline (7.5% NaCl)	4–5 mL/kg IV over 5–10 minutes	3–4 mL/kg IV over 5–10 minutes
Imidocarb	5 mg/kg IM once	Same
Imipenem (Primaxin®)	5 mg/kg CRI IV in IV fluids over 20–30 min q6h or 5–10 mg/kg q6–8h	Same
Imodium® (loperamide)	0.08–0.2 mg/kg PO q8–12h	0.08–0.16 mg/kg PO q12h
Imuran® (azathioprine)	Immune hemolytic anemia: 2 mg/kg q24h	Same
	Immune thrombocytopenia: 50 mg/ m² or 2 mg/kg PO q24h, taper to 0.5–1.0 mg/kg PO q48h	Same
	Chronic active hepatitis: 2–2.5 mg/ kg PO q24h	
	Eosinophilic enteritis: 0.3–0.5 mg/ kg PO q24–48h	Same
Inderal® (propranolol)	0.02–0.06 mg/kg IV over 5–10 min q8h; 0.2–1.0 mg/kg PO q8h	0.01–0.03 mg/kg IV; 2.5–5 mg PO q8–12h

Drug name	Dog	Cat
Inocor® (amrinone)	0.75–3 mg IV bolus over 3–5 min, then 50–100 mg/kg per minute CRI IV	Same
Insulin (regular crystalline)	2 U/kg in 250 mL at 5–10 mL/h CRI IV; 0.2 U/kg IM then 0.1–0.4 U/kg IM q4–6h; or 0.5 U/kg SC q6–8h; or 0.25 U/kg SC q4–6h	1.1 U/kg in 250 mL at 5–10 mL/h CRI IV; 0.1 U/kg IM q1h then 0.2 U/kg IM then 0.1 U/kg IM q1h then 0.1–0.4 U/kg IM q4–6h; or 0.5 U/kg SC q6–8h; or 0.25 U/kg SC q4–6h
Insulin (detemir, Levemir®)	0.1–0.2 U/kg SC q12h	1 unit/cat SC q12h
Insulin (glargine, Lantus®)	0.25–0.5 U/kg SC q12h	1 unit/cat SC q12h
Insulin (intermediate, Lente®, Humulin®, NPH)	0.4–0.5 U/kg SC q12–24h	0.2–0.5 U/kg SC q12h
Insulin (long-lasting, PZI, Ultralente®)	0.6–0.7 U/kg SC q24h in the morning	1–3 U SC q24h in the morning
Intralipid (10% fat emulsion)	0.44 mL/kg IV, maximum of 4 g/day	Same
Ipecac (syrup of)	1–2 mL/kg PO; may repeat once (not recommended)	3.3 mL/kg, diluted to 50% with water, given via orogastric or nasogastric tube (5–10 mL total) (not recommended)
Isopropamide (Darbid®)	2.5–5 mg PO q8–12h; 0.1–0.2 mg/kg PO q12h	0.07 mg/cat PO q12h
Isoproterenol (Isuprel®)	0.04–0.08 µg/kg/min IV CRI; 0.5 mL nebulized	Same Rapid bronchodilation: 0.1–0.2 mL of 1:5000 solution IM, SC
Isosorbide dinitrate (Isordil®)	0.22–1.1 mg/kg PO q8–12; 2.5–5 mg/animal PO q12h	Same
Itraconazole (Sporanox®)	5.0–10.0 mg/kg PO q12–24h; 2.5 mg/kg PO q12h–5 mg/kg PO q24h	5 mg/kg PO q12h
Ivermectin	Preventative: 6 mcg/kg PO q30 days; 200–250 mcg/kg SC in appropriate breeds	Preventative: 24 mcg/kg PO q30 days; 200–300 mcg/kg PO, SC
IVIG (human intravenous immunoglobulin)	0.5–1.5 g/kg IV over 6–12 hours	
Jenotone® (aminopropazine fumarate)	2 mg/kg IM, SC q12h	Same
Kanamycin	10 mg/kg PO q6h; 4–6 mg/kg IM, SC q6h	Same
Kaopectate	1–2 mL/kg q2–6h	Same
Keflex® (cephalexin)	10–30 mg/kg PO q6–12h	Same
Keflin® (cephalothin sodium)	10–30 mg/kg IV, IM q4–8h	Same
Kefzol® (cefazolin, Ancef®)	10–30 mg/kg IM, IV q4–8h	Same
Ketamine	Mix with diazepam 50:50 give 1 mL per 4.5–9 kg IV (0.2 mg/kg diazepam and 10 mg/kg ketamine)	Restraint: 11 mg/kg IM Sedation: 22–33 mg/kg IM, 2.2–4.4 mg/kg IV

Continued

Drug name	Dog	Cat
Ketoconazole	5–30 mg/kg PO with acid food q12–24h; Hyperadrenocorticism: 15 mg/kg PO q12h	5–10 mg/kg PO q24–48h
Ketoprofen	1–2 mg/kg IV initial dose; 1 mg/kg IV, IM, SC, PO q24h for a maximum of 5 days Antipyretic dose: 0.25–0.5 mg/kg IV, IM, SC, PO	1–2 mg/kg SC, IV, IM then 1 mg/kg PO, SC, IV IM q24h for a maximum of 5 days Antipyretic dose: 0.25–0.5 mg/kg SC
Ketorolac (Toradol®)	0.3–0.5 mg/kg IV, IM PO q12h for 1–2 doses; 5–10 mg/dog PO for no more than 3 days (10 mg for dogs >30 kg)	0.25 mg/kg IM q12h for 1–2 doses
Lactated Ringer's Solution (LRS)	40–60 mL/kg per day IV, SC, IO; shock dose = 90 mL/kg per hour IV	20–30 mL/kg per day IV, SC, IO; shock dose = 60 mL/kg per hour
Lactulose (Cephulac®)	3–10 mL PO q8h; or 0.5–1 mL/kg PO q8–12h	1–3 mL PO q12–24h; 0.5–1 mL/kg PO q8–12h; or 5–10 mL diluted 1:3 with water, given per rectum
Lanoxin® (Cardoxin®, digoxin)	0.005–0.01 mg/kg PO q12h	0.0312 mg/kg PO q12–48h
Lasix® (furosemide)	1–6 mg/kg IV, IM, PO q1–2h or q6–12h; 0.1–0.2 mg/kg/h CRI IV; 3–8 mg/kg/min CRI IV	0.5–4 mg/kg IV, IM, PO q1–2h or q6–12h
Leflunomide (Arava®)	4 mg/kg PO q24h	
Levarterenol® (norepinephrine)	0.01–0.04 mg/kg/min IV CRI	Same
Lidocaine	2–4 mg/kg IV or 4 mg/kg intratracheal 25–80 mg/kg per minute; CRI IV (maximum dose 8 mg/kg)	0.25–1 mg/kg slow IV; 10 mg/kg per minute CRI IV
Lincomycin	15–20 mg/kg q8–12h PO; 10 mg/kg q12h IV, IM	Same
Lisinopril	0.5 mg/kg PO q24h	
Lomotil® (diphenoxylate)	2.5–10 mg PO q6–12h	0.6–1.2 mg PO q8–12h
Loperamide (Imodium®)	0.08–0.2 mg/kg PO q8h	0.08–0.16 mg/kg PO q12h
Lopressor® (metoprolol)	0.5–1 mg/kg PO q8h	2.5–25 mg PO q8–12h
Losec® (omeprazole)	0.2–0.7 mg/kg PO q12h	None
Lotensin® (benazepril)	0.25–0.5 mg/kg PO q24h	Same
Lutalyse® (PGF$_2\alpha$)	0.1–0.25 mg/kg SC q24h for 5–7 days	0.1 mg/kg SC q24h for 5–7 days
Lyovac® (black widow antivenin)	1 vial slow IV	Same
Maalox® (aluminum magnesium hydroxide)	2–10 mL PO q2–4h	5–15 mL PO q8–12h
Magnesium hydroxide (Milk of Magnesia®)	Antacid: 5–30 mL PO Cathartic: 15–150 mL PO q6–12h	5–15 mL PO; 5–50 mL PO q6–12h
Magnesium sulfate (Epsom salts)	250–500 mg/kg PO	200 mg/kg PO
Magnesium sulfate	0.15–0.3 mEq/kg IV slowly over 10 minutes	Same

Drug name	Dog	Cat
Mandelamine® (methenamine mandelate)	10 mg/kg PO q6–12h to effect	Same
Mannitol	100–1000 mg/kg IV q6h	Same
Marcaine® (bupivacaine hydrochloride)	Epidural: 0.2–0.3 mL; or 1 mL/3.5 kg ± morphine 0.1 mg/kg	
Mazicon® (flumazenil)	0.02 mg/kg IV	Same
Mebendazole (Telmintic®)	22 mg/kg PO q24h for 3 days with food	Same
Meclizine (Bonine®)	12.5–25 mg PO q24h	12.5 mg PO q24h (4 mg/kg PO q24h)
Mefoxin® (cefoxitin)	15–40 mg/kg IV, IM q6–8h	Same
Meloxicam	0.2 mg/kg PO, SC loading dose, then 0.1 mg/kg q24h PO	0.1 mg/kg PO, SC once
Meperidine (Demerol®)	2–5 mg/kg IM, SC q1–4h	2–5 mg/kg IM, SC q1–4h
2-Mercaptaproprionylglycine	10–15 mg/kg PO q12h	
Meso-dimercaptosuccinic acid (succimer, Chemet®, DMSA)		10 mg/kg PO q8h × 10d
Metamucil	2–10 g q12–24h in wetted or liquid food	1–4 g q12–24h in food
Metaraminol bitartrate (Aramine®)	0.01–0.10 mg/kg slow IV; or 10 mg in 250 mL D5 W IV to effect	Same
Methadone	0.1–0.5 mg/kg IV, IM, SC q2–4h	Same
Methazolamide (Neptazane®)	2.5–5 mg/kg PO q8–12h	Same
Methenamine mandelate (Mandelamine®)	10–20 mg/kg PO q6–12h to effect	Same
Methicillin	25–40 mg/kg IM q6h	Same
DL-Methionine	0.2–1.0 g PO q8h	0.2–1.0 g PO q24h
Methocarbamol (Robaxin®)	44.4–222.2 mg/kg IV, PO; 44.4 mg/kg PO q8h first day then 22.2–44.4 mg/kg PO q8h	44.4 mg/kg PO, IV, IM then 22.2–44.4 mg/kg PO q8h
Methoxamine (Vasoxyl®)	1–2 mg IV or 0.01 mg/kg slow IV	None
Methylene blue	4–8 mg/kg IV	None
Methylprednisolone	1.0 mg/kg IM every 2 weeks	20 mg/cat IM once
Methylprednisolone sodium succinate (Solu Medrol®)	Spinal trauma: initial dose of 30 mg/kg IV followed by 10–12.5 mg/kg IV 2–3 h later, then 10–12.5 mg/kg IV 2–3 h later (4–6 h after presentation), then 6–9 h after presentation start a continuous IV infusion of 2.5 mg/kg per hour for 24 h	Same
Methylpyrazole (Antizol-vet®, fomepizole, 4-methylpyrazole, 4-MP)	Loading dose = 20 mg/kg IV; 15 mg/kg IV at 12 and 24 hours, 5 mg/kg IV at 36 (48, and 60) hours after initiation of treatment	Loading dose = 125 mg/kg IV; 31.25 mg/kg IV at 12 hours, 24 hours and 36 hours after initiation of treatment
Metoclopramide (Reglan®)	0.2–0.5 mg/kg PO, IV, IM, SC q6–8h; 1–2 mg/kg IV drip over 24 h (0.01–0.02 mg/kg/h CRI IV)	Same

Continued

Drug name	Dog	Cat
Metoprolol (Lopressor®)	0.5–1 mg/kg PO q8h	2.5–25 mg PO q8–12h
Metronidazole (Flagyl®)	10–15 mg/kg PO q12h for 5 days; 7.5–10 mg/kg IV CRI over 1 h q8–12h; 15 mg/kg IV q12h	Liver/GI: 7.5 mg/kg PO q8–12h Giardiasis: 10 mg/kg PO q12h × 5 days Gingivitis: 30 mg/kg PO q24h
Mexilitine (Mexitil®)	5–8 mg/kg PO q8–12h	
Midazolam (Versed®)	0.1–0.25 mg/kg IV, IM or 0.1–0.3 mg/kg/h CRI IV	Same
Milbemycin	Heartworm preventative: 0.5 mg/kg PO q30 days Demodicosis: 0.5–1 mg/kg per day PO for minimum of 90 days	Same
Milk thistle	3–7 mg/kg PO q8h	
Milrinone (Primacor®)	0.5–1.0 mg/kg PO q12h; 1–10 mg/kg per min CRI IV	None
Mineral oil	2–60 mL PO	2–10 mL PO
Minipress (prazosin)	0.25–2 mg PO q8–12h	0.25–1 mg PO q8–12h
Minocycline	5–25 mg/kg PO q12–24h	
Misoprostol (Cytotec®)	0.7–5.0 mcg/kg PO q8h	None
Mitaban® (amitraz)	10.6 mL in 9 L water, dip q2 week for three treatments, let it dry on	None
Morphine	0.1–0.5 mg/kg IV q2–4h; 0.5–1 mg/kg IM, SC q2–6h; 0.05–0.5 mg/kg/h IV; 0.1–0.3 mg/kg epidurally q8–24h	0.05–0.2 mg/kg SC, IM q2–6h
Morphine sulfate (tablets and oral liquid)	1 mg/kg PO q4–6h	Not recommended
Morphine sulfate SR (sustained release)	2–5 mg/kg PO q12h	Not recommended
Mucomyst® (acetylcysteine)	Acetaminophen toxicity: 280 mg/kg PO, IV, then 140 mg/kg q4h for seven treatments	Acetaminophen toxicity: 140 mg/kg PO, IV, then 70 mg/kg q6h for seven treatments
	Ocular: with artificial tears, dilute to 2% and apply topically q2h for max. of 48 hours	Same
	Antioxidant: 50 mg/kg diluted at least 1:1 slow IV over 1 hour, repeated every 6 hours for 24 hours	Same
Mycophenolate mofetil	20–40 mg/kg PO q8–12h	
Nafcillin	10 mg/kg PO, IM q6h	
Nalorphine (Nalline®)	0.1 mg/kg IV, IM, SC; max. dose = 5 mg	Same; max. dose = 1 mg
Naloxone (Narcan®)	0.01–0.04 mg/kg IV, IM, SC; 0.04–0.1 mg/kg IT	Same
Nandrolone decanoate	1–5 mg/kg SC, IM q7–10d; max. 40 mg	2–4 mg/kg IM, SC q7–10d; max. 20 mg
Naproxen (Aleve®, Naprosyn®)	2–5 mg/kg PO once; then 1–2 mg/kg PO q48h	None
Narcan® (naloxone)	0.01–0.04 mg/kg IV, IM, SC	Same
Naxcel® (ceftiofur)	2.2–4.4 mg/kg SC q12–24h	Same

Drug name	Dog	Cat
Nemex® (pyrantel pamoate, Strongid T®)	5 mg/kg PO, repeat in 7–10 days	10–20 mg/kg PO, repeat in 7–10 days
Neomycin	2.5–10 mg/kg PO q6–12h	Same
Neosar® (Cytoxan®, cyclophosphamide)	200–300 mg/m^2 IV bolus once; 200 mg/m^2 PO divided over 4 days (50 mg/m^2), stop for 3 days, repeat CBC and re-evaluate; 50 mg/m^2 PO q48h for 7 days, stop 3 days, repeat CBC and re-evaluate	6.25–12.5 mg/cat q24h × 4d/wk
Neostigmine (Stiglyn®)	1–2 mg IM as needed	Same
Neo-Synephrine Infant® (phenylephrine)	0.15 mg/kg IV; 10% solution topically in eye or in nostrils	Same
Neptazane® (methazolamide)	2.5–5 mg/kg PO q8–12h	Same
Neupogen® (G-CSF)	5–10 mg/kg SC, IV q24h	
Nitroglycerine cream	0.6–5.1 cm on skin q4–6h	0.3–1.3 cm q6–8h for 48 h
Nitroprusside sodium	0.5–10 mg/kg per min CRI IV	0.25–10 mg/kg per min CRI IV
Nizatidine (Axid AR®)	2.5–5 mg/kg PO q12h	None
Nizoral® (ketoconazole)	5–20 mg/kg PO q12–24h with acid food	5–10 mg/kg PO q24–48h
Norepinephrine	0.05–2 µg/kg/min CRI IV	Same
Norfloxacin	3–22 mg/kg PO q12h	
Normosol®-R	40–60 mL/kg per day IV, SC, IO; shock dose = 90 mL/kg per hour IV	20–30 mL/kg per day IV, SC, IO; shock dose = 60 mL/kg per hour
Norvasc® (amlodipine)	0.1 mg/kg PO q24h	0.625–1.25 mg PO q24h
Numorphan® (oxymorphone)	Sedation: 0.2 mg/kg (1 mL/4.5 kg) with diazepam (0.02 mg/kg) IV Analgesia: 0.05–0.1 mg/kg; IV q2–4h 0.05–0.2 mg/kg; IM, SC q2–6h	Sedation: 0.02–1 mg/kg IV or 0.02–0.03 mg/kg IV, IM Analgesia: 0.02–0.05 mg/kg; IV q2–4h 0.05–0.1 mg/kg; IM, SC q2–6h
Nystatin	100 000 units PO q6h	Same
Octreotide (Sandostatin®)	5–40 mg SC q8h	Same
Omeprazole	0.5–1.5 mg/kg PO q24h	0.5–1 mg/kg PO q24h
Ondansetron (Zofran®)	0.1–0.2 mg/kg IV q6–12h; 0.1–0.15 mg/kg IV q6–12h; 0.1 – 1 mg/kg IV or PO q12–24h	Same
Orbifloxacin (Orbax®)	2.5–7.5 mg/kg q24h PO	
Organidin (guaifenesin)	0.05–0.1 mL/kg PO q6h	Same
Orgotein (Palosein®)	2.5–5 mg IM, SC q24h for 6 days, then q48h for 8 days	None
Ormetoprim sulfonamide (Primor®)	55 mg/kg PO first day, then 27.5 mg/kg PO q24h for 2 days after remission	
Orudis-KT® (ketoprofen, ketofen)	1–2 mg/kg IV initial dose, then 1 mg/kg IV, IM, SC, PO q24h for a maximum of 5 days	1–2 mg/kg SC, IV, IM, then 1 mg/kg PO, SC, IV, IM q24h for a maximum of 5 days

Continued

Drug name	Dog	Cat
	Antipyretic dose: 0.25–0.5 mg/kg IV, IM, SC, PO	Antipyretic dose: 0.25–0.5 mg/kg SC
Oxacillin	11–22 mg/kg IV, IM, PO, q6–8h	Same
Oxazepam		Appetite stimulant: 0.1–0.25 mg/kg PO (2.5 mg/cat PO)
Oxycodone	0.1–0.3 mg/kg PO q6–12h	Not recommended
Oxygen	22.7–40.7 mL/kg per minute 6 L/min maximum	Same
Oxyglobin (HBOC)	15–30 mL/kg IV	5–20 mL/kg IV, given in 5 mL/kg IV increments
Oxymetholone (Anadrol®)	1–3 mg/kg q24h or 1 mg/kg PO q12–24h	
Oxymorphone (Numorphan®)	Sedation: 0.2 mg/kg (1 mL/4.5 kg) with diazepam (0.02 mg/kg) IV	Sedation: 0.02–1 mg/kg IV; or 0.02–0.03 mg/kg IV or IM
	Analgesia: 0.05–0.1 mg/kg; IV q2–4h; 0.05–0.2 mg/kg; IM, SC q2–6h	Analgesia: 0.02–0.05 mg/kg; IV q2–4h; 0.05–0.1 mg/kg; IM, SC q2–6h
Oxytetracycline	22 mg/kg PO q8h; 7–12 mg/kg IV, IM q12h	15 mg/kg PO q8h; 7–12 mg/kg IV, IM, q12h
Oxytocin	0.25–2.0 U to 4 U IM, IV, repeat q30–45min	0.25–2.0 U IM, IV
Packed red blood cells	10 mL/kg IV	Same
Palosein (Orgotein®)	2.5–5 mg IM, SC q24h for 6 days, then q48h for 8 days	None
2-PAM ((2-pyridine aldoxime methyl chloride, pralidoxime, Protopam®)	10–50 mg/kg IM, SC, IV over 15 min, q8–12h as needed; 10–20 mg/kg per hour CRI IV	20 mg/kg in 5% solution IM
Panacur® (fenbendazole)	50 mg/kg per day for 3 days and repeat in 3 weeks	50 mg/kg PO once
Pantoprazole (Protonix®)	0.7–1 mg/kg IV q24h	Same
Paregoric	0.05–0.06 mg/kg PO q12h	Same
D-Penicillamine	10–15 mg/kg q12h PO on an empty stomach	Same
	Lead toxicity: 110 mg/kg/day PO divided q6–8h for 1–2 weeks; if vomiting, decrease to 33–55 mg/kg per day divided q6–8h	
Penicillin G (aqueous) (Na or K)	40 000–100 000 U/kg PO q8h; 20 000–100 000 U/kg IV, IM, SC, q4–6h; 20 000 U/kg IM, SC, q12–24h	Same
Penicillin G (benzathine)	40 000 U/kg IM q120h	Same
Penicillin G (procaine)	10 000–50 000 U/kg IM, SC, q12h	Same
Penicillin G (procaine + benzathine)	3000–30 000 U/kg IM, SC, q48h	Same
Pentazocine (Talwin®)	1–3 mg/kg IV, IM, SC q1–6h; 2–10 mg/kg PO q4–6h	2.2–3.3 mg/kg IV, IM, SC

Drug name	Dog	Cat
Pentobarbital	Sedation: 2–4 mg/kg IV; Status epilepticus: 2–15 mg/kg IV to effect; 3–10 mg/kg/h CRI IV; 0.5–5 mg/kg PO q12–24h	Same
Pentothal® (sodium thiopental)	4–20 mg/kg IV to effect, given in increments of 2–4 mg/kg IV; less in dogs if combined with lidocaine 2 mg/kg IV	Same
Pepcid® (famotidine)	0.3–1 mg/kg IV, IM, PO q12–24h; 0.5–5 mg/kg PO q12–24h	Same
Pepto Bismol® (bismuth subsalicylate)	0–30 mL PO; 0.25–2 mL/kg PO q6–12h	0.25–0.5 mL/kg PO q12h for a maximum of 3 days
Periactin® (cyproheptadine)		1–2 mg PO q12h
Peritone® (aminopropazine)	2 mg/kg PO	Same
Phenobarbital	Status epilepticus: 15–200 mg/animal IV to effect; 4–16 mg/kg IV initially then 1–8 mg/kg q12h IV, IM, PO Oral loading dose: 6–8 mg/kg O unless on phenobarbital, hen 2–4 mg/kg PO Idiopathic epilepsy: 1–2 mg/kg O q12h to 8 mg/kg PO q12h	2.5 mg IV boluses to effect, maximum 16 mg/kg 1.1–2.5 mg/kg IV, IM, PO q12h; start with 7.5 mg PO q12h 0.5–1 mg/kg per hour CRI IV combined with diazepam CRI IV
Phenoxybenzamine (Dibenzyline®)	0.25–0.5 mg/kg PO q8–12h	2.5–5 mg PO q12–24h, gradually increase to 10 mg
Phenylephrine (Neo-Synephrine®)	0.15 mg/kg IV; 10% solution topically in eye	Same
Phenylpropanolamine (Proin@)	1–1.5 mg/kg PO q8–12h	Same
Phenytoin (Dilantin®)	15–40 mg/kg PO q8h	None
Phosphate (sodium or potassium)	0.01–0.03 mmol/kg/h CRI IV	
Physostigmine (Antilirium®)		0.02–0.06 mg/kg slow IV q12h
Pilocarpine (2%)	1 drop q4–6h	
Pimobendan	0.25 mg/kg PO q12h (0.1–0.3 mg/kg PO q12h)	
Piperacillin	50–70 mg/kg IV, IM q4–8h	Same
Piroxicam (Feldene®)	0.3 mg/kg PO q24–48h	1 mg/cat PO q24h for max. 5 days
Plasma	For coagulopathy: 10–15 mL/kg IV For hypoalbuminemia: 40 mL/kg IV	Same
Platelet-rich plasma	10–20 mL/kg IV	Same
Plavix® (clopidogrel)	5 mg/kg PO q24h	
Polyflex® (ampicillin trihydrate)	6.5–10 mg/kg IM, SC q12h	Same
Polysulfated glycosaminoglycan (Adequan®)	2–5 mg/kg IM, SC, or intra-articular q3–6 days, up to eight injections	

Continued

Appendices

Drug name	Dog	Cat
Potassium bromide	Loading dose: 400 mg/kg per day divided q12h for 2–3 days Maintenance: 22–30 mg/kg per day with phenobarbital or 70–80 mg/kg per day as a single agent	Not recommended
Potassium chloride	1–3 g/day PO, IV; max. 10 mEq/h; 0.10–0.25 mL/kg PO q8h	0.2 g/day PO
Potassium citrate	40–75 mg/kg PO q12h	
Potassium iodide	50 mg/kg per day	20 mg/kg per day
Potassium phosphate	0.01–0.03 mmol/kg per hour IV (put 1.3 mL in 500 mL fluids) and administer the fluids at a maintenance rate	Same
Pralidoxime (2-PAM, Protopam®)	0–50 mg/kg IM, SC, IV over 60 min, q8–12h as needed; 10–20 mg/kg/h CRI IV	20 mg/kg in a 5% solution IM
Praziquantel (Droncit®)	<6.8 kg: 7.5 mg/kg PO; >6.8 kg: 5 mg/kg PO; 2.7–4.5 kg: 6.3 mg/kg SC, IM; >5 kg: 5 mg/kg SC, IM	<1.8 kg: 6.3 mg/kg PO, SC; >1.8 kg: 5 mg/kg PO, SC
Prazosin (Minipress®)	0.25–2 mg PO q8–12h To decrease urethral sphincter tone: 1 mg/15 kg PO q8 – 24h	0.25–1 mg PO q8–12h To decrease urethral sphincter tone: 1 mg/15 kg PO q8–24h
PRBC	10–15 mL/kg IV	Same
Prednisone	Allergy: 0.5 mg/kg PO, IM q12h Immune suppression: 2.0 mg/kg PO, IM, q12h Physiologic: 0.2–0.3 mg/kg/day	1.0 mg/kg PO, IM q12h 3.0 mg/kg PO, IM q12h Same
Prednisolone sodium succinate (Solu Delta Cortef®)	0.25–2 mg/kg IV q12h	1–3 mg/kg IV q12h
Pregabalin (Lyrica®)	2–4 mg/kg PO q8h	1–2 mg/kg PO q12h
Primacor® (milrinone)	0.5–1.0 mg/kg PO q12h; 1–10 mg/kg per min CRI IV	None
Primaxin® (imipenem-cilastatin)	5 mg/kg CRI IV in IV fluids over 20–30 min q6 hours or 10 mg/kg q8h IV	Same
Primidone (Mysoline®)	5–10 mg/kg PO q8–12h; may need to increase to maximum dose of 50 mg/kg per day	None
Primor® (sulfadimethoxine/ormetoprim)	55 mg/kg PO first day, then 27.5 mg/kg PO q24h for 2 days after remission	Same
Procainamide	6–8 mg/kg IV; 8–20 mg/kg IM, PO q4–6h; 2 mg/kg IV bolus then repeated up to 20 mg/kg cumulative maximum dose, then 10–40 mg/kg per minute; CRI IV (22–55 mg/kg per minute CRI IV)	5–10 mg/kg PO q6–8h
Procalamine®	40–45 mL/kg per day CRI IV	Same
Prochlorperazine (Compazine®)	0.1–0.5 mg/kg IM, SC q6–8h	Same
Proglycem® (diazoxide)	5–13 mg/kg PO q8h; max. 20 mg/kg q8h	Same

Drug name	Dog	Cat
Propantheline bromide	0.25–0.5 mg/kg PO q8–12h	Same
Propofol	2–6 mg/kg IV then 0.1–0.4 mg/kg per min; 25% IV q30s until intubated; boluses of 1 mg/kg IV; after acepromazine, xylazine, opioid etc., administer 3–4 mg/kg IV	Same
Propranolol (Inderal®)	0.02–0.06 mg/kg IV over 5–10 min q8h; 0.2–1.0 mg/kg PO q8h	0.01–0.03 mg/kg IV; 2.5–5 mg PO q8–12h
Propulsid® (cisapride)	0.1–0.5 mg/kg PO q8–12h PO	1 mg/kg q8h; 1.5 mg/kg q12h; 2.5–5 mg/cat PO q8–12h
Protamine sulfate	0.5–1 mg per 100 U heparin slow IV if within 1 hour of heparin administration; 0.25–0.5 mg per 100 U heparin slow IV if within 1–2 hours of heparin administration; 0.12–0.25 mg per 100 U heparin slow IV if >2 hours after heparin administration	Same
Protopam® (2-PAM, pralidoxime)	10–50 mg/kg IM, SC, IV over 60 min, q8–12h as needed; 10–20 mg/kg per hour CRI IV	20 mg/kg in 5% solution IM
Proventil® (albuterol)	0.02–0.05 mg/kg PO q6–12h; nebulization of 0.5% solution in 4 mL saline 0.1 mL/5 kg	0.02–0.05 mg/kg PO q8–24h
Prozac® (fluoxetine)	1–2 mg/kg PO q24h	None
Pyrimethamine (Daraprim®)	0.5–1.0 mg/kg PO q24h for 2 days, then 0.25 mg/kg PO q24h for 2 weeks	Same
Pyrantel pamoate (Nemex®, Strongid T®)	5 mg/kg PO, repeat in 7–10 days	10–20 mg/kg PO, repeat in 7–10 days
Quibron® (guaifenesin-theophylline)	1–3 capsules q8h PO; 0.33 mL/kg q8h PO	0.5 capsule q8h
Quinidine sulfate	6–16 mg/kg IM, PO q6–8h	4–11 mg/kg IM, PO q8h
Ranitidine (Zantac®)	0.5–2 mg/kg IV, 1–2 mg/kg; PO q8–12h	2.5 mg/kg IV q12h; 3.5 mg/kg PO q12h
RBC (packed)	10–15 mL/kg IV	Same
Reglan® (metoclopramide)	0.2–0.5 mg/kg PO, IV, IM, SC q6–8h; 1–2 mg/kg IV drip over 24 hours (0.01–0.02 mg/kg/h)	Same
Rifampin (Rifadin®)	10–20 mg/kg PO q8–12h	Same
Rimadyl® (carprofen)	4 mg/kg IV, IM, SC once; 0.5–2.2 mg/kg IV, IM, SC, PO q12h	4 mg/kg SC once
Robaxin® (methocarbamol)	44.4–222.2 mg/kg IV, PO; 44.4 mg/kg PO q8h first day, then 22.2–44.4 mg/kg PO q8h	44.4 mg/kg PO, IV, IM, then 22.2–44.4 mg/kg PO q8h
Robinul-V® (glycopyrrolate)	Preanesthetic: 0.011 mg/kg IV, IM, SC; 0.01–0.02 mg/kg IM, Bradycardia: 0.005–0.01 mg/kg V, IM 0.01–0.02 mg/kg SC q8–12h	0.011 mg/kg IM 0.005–0.01 mg/kg SC q8–12h

Continued

Drug name	Dog	Cat
Robitussin Pediatric® cough syrup (1.5 mg/mL dextromethorphan)	1–2 mg/kg PO q6–8h	2 mg/kg PO q8h
Rocaltrol (calcitriol, 1,25-dihydroxyvitamin D)	1.5–60 ng/kg per day PO (0.0025–0.06 mg/kg per day PO)	Same
Rocephin® (ceftriaxone)	15–50 mg/kg q24h IV, IM	
Rompum® (xylazine)	1.1 mg/kg IV; 2.2 mg/kg IM	Emetic: 0.4–0.5 mg/kg IV; 1.1 mg/kg IM
7.5% saline (NaCl) (hypertonic saline	4–5 mL/kg IV over 2–5 min	2–3 mL/kg IV over 2–5 min
SAM-e	17–22 mg/kg PO q24h	Same
Sandostatin (octreotide)	5–40 mg SC q8h	Same
Scorpion antivenom	1 vial dilute in 50 mL slow IV over 15–30 min, may repeat	Same
Septiserum	4.4 mL/kg IV, diluted to at least 50% with IV crystalloid administered CRI IV over 1 hour	
Sildenafil citrate (Viagra®)	2.08–5.56 mg/kg/day PO; 3.13 mg/kg PO q24h	Same
Silymarin (milk thistle)	20–50 mg/kg PO q24h	Same
Simplicef® (cefpodoxime proxetil)	5–10 mg/kg q24h PO for 5–28 days	5 mg/kg PO q12h or 10 mg/kg PO q24h
Sodium bicarbonate	0.5 mEq/kg IV, IO	Same
Sodium nitroprusside	0.5–10 mg/kg per min IV CRI	0.25–10 mg/kg per min IV CRI
Sodium pentobarbital	Sedation: 2–4 mg/kg IV Status epilepticus: 2–15 mg/kg IV to effect, 3–10 mg/kg per hour CRI IV; 0.5–5 mg/kg PO q12–24h	Same
Sodium phosphate	0.01–0.03 mmol/kg/h IV (put 1.3 mL in 500 mL fluids)	Same
Sodium sulfate	1 g/kg PO; Cathartic: 10–25 g PO	2–4 g PO
Sodium thiopental (Pentothal®)	4–20 mg/kg IV to effect, given in increments of 2–4 mg/kg IV, less in dogs if combined with lidocaine 2 mg/kg IV	Same
Sodium thiosulfate	40–50 mg/kg IV (20% soln) q8–12h for 2–3 days or 0.5–3.0 g PO	None
Solu Medrol® (methyl-prednisolone sodium succinate)	Spinal trauma: initial dose of 20–30 mg/kg IV, followed by 10–12.5 mg/kg IV 2–3 h later, then 10–12.5 mg/kg IV 2–3 h later (4–6 h after presentation), then 6–9h after presentation start a continuous IV infusion of 2.5 mg/kg per hour for 24 h	Same
Solu Delta Cortef® (prednisolone sodium succinate)	5–20 mg/kg IV q4–6h	1–3 mg/kg IV q4–6h
Sorbitol (70%)	4 g/kg (3 mL/kg) PO	Same
Sotalol (Betapace®)	1–5 mg/kg PO q12h	1–2 mg/kg PO q12h
Spectinomycin	5–12 mg/kg IM q12h; 20 mg/kg PO q12h	Same Same
Spironolactone (Aldactone®)		0.25–2 mg/kg PO q12–24h

Drug name	Dog	Cat
Sporanox® (itraconazole)	5.0–10.0 mg/kg PO q12–24h; 2.5 mg/kg PO q12h; 5 mg/kg PO q24h	5 mg/kg PO q12h
Stanozol (Winstrol-V®)	0.5–2 tablets q12h PO; 25–50 mg IM weekly; 1–4 mg PO q12–24h	0.5–2 mg/cat PO q12h; 10–25 mg IM, PO weekly
Stiglyn® (neostigmine)	1–2 mg IM as needed	Same
Streptokinase (Streptase®)		90 000 IU CRI IV over 30 min then 45 000 IU/h CRI IV for up to 6 hours or until arterial pulses return
Streptomycin	7.5–20 mg/kg IM, SC q12h; 20 mg/kg PO q12h	5–20 mg/kg IM, SC q12h
Strongid T® (Nemex®, pyrantel pamoate)	5 mg/kg PO, repeat in 7–10 days	10–20 mg/kg PO, repeat 7–10 days
Succimer (Chemet®, DMSA, meso-dimercaptosuccinic acid)	10 mg/kg PO q8h × 10d	None
Sucralfate (Carafate®)	0.5–1 g PO q6–8h (34 mg/kg) Loading dose of 3–6 g PO if severe GI hemorrhage	0.25 g/cat PO q8h
Sulfadiazine-trimethoprim	15–30 mg/kg PO, SC q12–24h	30 mg/kg PO, SC q12–24h
Sulfadimethoxine (Albon®)	25–55 mg/kg PO, IV, IM q24h 55 mg/kg PO first day, then 27.5 mg/kg PO q24h for 14–20 days	Same
Sulfadimethoxine/ ormetoprim (Primor®)	55 mg/kg PO first day, then 27.5 mg/kg PO q24h for 2 days after remission	Same
Sulfasalazine (Azulfidine®)	15–50 mg/kg PO divided q8h (max. 4 g/day)	20–25 mg/kg PO q24h (max. 7 days)
Suprax® (cefixime)	10 mg/kg PO q12h; 5 mg/kg PO q12h for urinary tract infections	Same
Surital® (thiamylal sodium)	(2% soln) 8–20 mg/kg IV given to effect	Same
Tagamet® (cimetidine)	5–10 mg/kg PO, IV, IM, q6–8h	Same
Talwin® (pentazocine)	1–3 mg/kg IV, IM, SC, q1–6h; 2–10 mg/kg PO q4–6h	2.2–3.3 mg/kg IV, IM, SC
Taurine	500 mg/kg PO q12h	250–500 mg PO q12h
Tavist-D® (clemastine fumarate)	0.05 mg/kg PO q12h	0.1 mg/kg PO q12h
Tazicef® (Tazidine®, ceftazidime)	4.4 mg/kg IV loading dose, then 4.0 mg/kg/h IV CRI	
Tegaserod (Zelnorm®)	0.05–1 mg/kg PO, IV q12h	Same
Tegison® (etretinate)	0.75–1 mg/kg PO q24h	2 mg/kg PO q24h
Telazol® (tiletamine-zolazepam)	5–7 mg/kg IV, IM	Same
Telmintic® (mebendazole)	22 mg/kg PO q24h for 3 days, with food	Same
Tenormin® (atenolol)	6.25–25 mg PO q12h or 0.5 mg/kg PO q12h	6.25–12.5 mg PO q24h
Tensilon® (edrophonium chloride)	0.11–0.22 mg/kg IV	2.5 mg/cat IV

Continued

Appendices

Drug name	Dog	Cat
Tepoxalin (Zubrin®)	10–20 mg/kg PO day 1, then 10 mg/kg PO q24h	
Terbutaline	Small dog: 0.625–1.25 mg PO q12h	0.312–0.625 mg/cat
	Medium dog: 1.25–2.5 mg PO q12h	PO q8–12h
	Large dog: 2.5–5 mg PO q12h	
	0.01 mg/kg SC, IV, IM q4–6h	0.01 mg/kg SC, IV, IM
	Bradycardia: 2.5 mg PO q8h	q4h
Testosterone enanthate	50–150 mg IM every 1–4 weeks	
Testosterone propionate	10–15 mg/day IM	
Tetanus toxoid	100–500 U/kg (max. 20 000 U)	Same
Tetracycline	15–30 mg/kg PO q6–8h; 7–11 mg/kg IV, IM q8–12h	10–25 mg/kg PO q8–12h
Theophylline	9 mg/kg q6–8h PO	4 mg/kg q8–12h PO
	Bradycardia: 10–20 mg/kg PO q8h	
Theophylline extended release (Theo-Dur®)	10–25 mg/kg PO q12h	25 mg/kg PO q24h at night
Thiacetarsamide sodium	2.2 mg/kg IV q12h × 2 days	Not recommended
Thiamine	10–100 mg/day PO	100 mg PO, IM then 5–50 mg PO q12h
Thiamylal sodium (Surital®) (2% solution)	8–20 mg/kg IV given to effect	Same
Thiopental (Pentothal®)	4–20 mg/kg IV to effect, given in increments of 2–4 mg/kg IV, less in dogs if combined with lidocaine 2 mg/kg IV	Same
Thorazine® (chlorpromazine)	Antiemetic dose: 0.05–0.10 mg/kg IV q4–6h or 0.20–0.50 mg/kg SC, IM q6–8h or 1 mg/kg diluted in 1 mL 0.9% NaCl administered per rectum q8h	0.01–0.025 mg/kg IV q4h
	Tranquilization: 0.8–2.2 mg/kg PO q8–12h	0.5 mg/kg IM
L-Thyroxine	22 mg/kg PO q12h	20–30 mg/kg per day PO or divided q12h
Ticarcillin (Ticar®)	40–80 mg/kg IV, IM q6–8h	Same
Ticarcillin-clavulanate (Timentin®)	30–50 mg/kg IV, q6–8h	Same
Tigan® (trimethobenzamide)	3 mg/kg IM q8–12h	None
Tiletamine-zolazepam (Telazol®)	5–7 mg/kg IV, IM	Same
Tissue plasminogen activator (t-PA, Activase®)		0.25–1 mg/kg/h IV up to 1–10 mg/kg IV (4.2–16.5 mg/kg per min CRI IV)
Tobramycin	1.0–4 mg/kg SC IV, IM q8h	Same
Tocainide	10–20 mg/kg PO q8–12h	
Toradol® (ketorolac)	0.3–0.5 mg/kg IV, IM PO q12h for 1–2 doses; 5–10 mg/dog PO for no more than 3 days (10 mg for dogs >30 kg)	0.25 mg/kg IM q12h for 1–2 doses
Torbugesic® (Torbutrol®, butorphanol)	0.1–0.5 mg/kg IV q1–4h; 0.2–0.8 mg/kg SC, IM, PO q1–6h; or 0.55–1.1 mg/kg PO q6–12h; 0.1 mg/kg per hour CRI IV	0.1–0.8 mg/kg IV, IM, SC q1–6h; 0.5–2 mg/kg PO q4–8h

Drug name	Dog	Cat
	Cough suppressant: 0.05–0.12 mg/kg SC q6–12h; or 0.5–1 mg/kg PO q8–12h	
Torecan® (triethylperazine)	0.13–0.25 mg/kg IM q8–12h; 0.5 mg/kg rectal q8h	0.125 mg/kg IM q8–12h
Tracrium® (atracurium besylate)	0.2 mg/kg IV, then 3–8 mg/kg per minute CRI IV	Same
Tramadol®	2–8 mg/kg PO q6–12h	2-5 mg/kg PO q12h
Tresaderm®	Topically, q12h maximum of 7 days treatment	Same
Triethylperazine (Torecan®)	0.13–0.25 mg/kg IM q8–12h; 0.5 mg/kg rectal q8h	0.125 mg/kg IM q8–12h
Trimethobenzamide (Tigan®)	3 mg/kg IM q8–12h	None
Trimethoprim-sulfadiazine	15–30 mg/kg PO, SC q12–24h	30 mg/kg PO, SC q12–24h
Tussigon® (Hycodan®, hydrocodone)	0.25–0.5 mg/kg PO q6–12h	2.5–5 mg/cat PO q8–12h
Tylenol 4® (acetaminophen with codeine)	300 mg acetaminophen, with 60 mg codeine; give 0.5–2 mg/kg of codeine PO q6–8h	Not recommended
Tylosin (Tylan®)	5–25 mg/kg IV, IM, PO, q6–12h	5–15 mg/kg IV, IM, PO, q6–12h
Unasyn® (ampicillin-sulbactam)	20–50 mg/kg IV, IM q6–8h	Same
Urecholine® (bethanechol)	5–15 mg PO q8h	1.25–5 mg PO q8h
Ursodeoxycholic acid (Actigal®, Ursodiol®)	5–15 mg/kg PO q24h or divided q12h	10 mg/kg/day PO
Valium® (diazepam)	Status epilepticus: 0.5–3 mg/kg IV or 2.5–20 mg	Same
	Intratracheal: 0.1–0.5 mg/kg per hour CRI IV	
	Preanesthetic: 0.1 mg/kg IV	Same
	Restraint: 0.2–0.6 mg/kg IV	
	Per rectum or intranasal: 0.5–1 mg/kg	Same
	Behavior modification: 0.5–2.2 mg/kg PO PRN	1–2 mg PO q12h
		Appetite stimulation: 0.05–0.15 mg/kg IV q24–48h or 1.0 mg PO q24h
Valproic acid (Depakene®)	6–90 mg/kg per day PO	
Vancomycin (Vancocin®)	10–20 mg/kg IV q6–12h; 5–12 mg/kg PO q6h	Same
Vasopressin	0.2–0.8 U/kg IV, IO; 0.4–1.2 U/kg IT; 0.5–2 mU/kg/min IV CRI	Same
Vasotec® (Enacard®, enalapril)	0.25–3 mg/kg PO q12–24h	0.25–0.5 mg/kg PO q24–48h
Vasoxyl® (methoxamine)	1–2 mg IV or 0.01 mg/kg slow IV	None
Velosef ® (cephradine)	10–25 mg/kg PO, IV, IM q6–8h	Same
Verapamil	0.05–0.15 mg/kg IV q8h; 1–5 mg/kg PO q8–12h	Same
Versed® (midazolam)	0.1–0.25 mg/kg IV, IM; or 0.1–0.3 mg/kg per hour CRI IV	Same

Continued

Drug name	Dog	Cat
Vetamox® (Diamox®, acetazolamide)	Glaucoma: 2–10 mg/kg IV, PO q8–12h	50 mg/kg IV once; 7 mg/kg PO q8–12h
Viagra® (sildenafil citrate)	2.08–5.56 mg/kg/day PO; 3.13 mg/kg PO q24h	Same
Vicks Formula 44® (2 mg/mL, dextromethorphan)	1–2 mg/kg PO q6–8h	2 mg/kg PO q8h
Vincristine	0.5–0.75 mg/m^2 IV, repeat in 3 days, repeat again in 7 days if needed	Same
Vitamin B complex	0.5–2.0 mL IV, IM, SC q24h	0.5–1.0 mL IV, IM, SC
Vitamin B$_6$	2 mg/kg/day	
Vitamin C (ascorbic acid)	100–500 mg/day PO (maintenance); or 100–500 mg PO q8h (urinary acidifier) Acetaminophen toxicosis: 30 mg/kg PO, SC q6h or 20–30 mg/kg in IV fluids q6h	125 mg/cat PO, IV q6h
Vitamin D (Rocaltrol®, 1,25-dihydroxy-vitamin D, Calcitriol®)	1.5–60 ng/kg/day PO (0.0025–0.06 mg/kg per day PO)	Same
Vitamin D$_3$	500–2000 U/kg per day PO	Same
Vitamin K$_1$	2.5–5 mg/kg SC loading dose; 0.25–2.5 mg/kg SC, PO q12h (give with a fatty meal)	Same
Vivonex T.E.N.®	50% solution; 40–45 mL/kg per day PO divided q1–2h; give $\frac{1}{3}$ or 33% dose the first day, $\frac{2}{3}$ or 66% dose the second day and the full dose thereafter	Same
Warfarin	0.2 mg/kg PO once then 0.05–0.1 mg/kg PO q24h	0.25–0.5 mg/cat PO q24h
Whole blood	20–25 mL/kg IV	
Winstrol-V® (stanozolol)	0.5–2 tablets PO q12h; 25–50 mg IM weekly; 1–4 mg PO q12–24h	0.5–2 mg/cat PO q24h; 10–25 mg IM, PO weekly
Yohimbine	0.1 mg/kg IV	0.1–0.5 mg/kg IV
Xylazine (Rompum®)	1.1 mg/kg IV; 2.2 mg/kg IM	Emetic: 0.4–0.5 mg/kg IV; 1.1 mg/kg IM
Xylocaine Viscous® (lidocaine hydrochloride solution)	2–10 mL PO before feeding	
Zantac® (ranitidine)	0.5–2 mg/kg IV, 1–2 mg/kg; PO q8–12h	2.5 mg/kg IV q12h; 3.5 mg/kg PO q12h
Zefazone® (cefmetazole)	15 mg/kg IV, IM, SC	Same
Zelnorm® (Tegaserod)	0.05–1 mg/kg PO, IV q12h	Same
Zithromax® (azithromycin)	5–10 mg/kg PO q24h for 5 days	5 mg/kg PO q24–48h for 5 days
Zofran® (ondansetron)	0.1–0.2 mg/kg IV q6–12h; 0.1–1 mg/kg IV or PO q12–24h	0.1–0.15 mg/kg IV q6–12h; same
Zosyn® (piperacillin-tazobactam)	50 mg/kg IV, IM q4–6h	50 mg/kg IV, IM q4–6h
Zubrin® (tepoxalin)	10–20 mg/kg PO day 1 then 10 mg/kg PO q24h	Not recommended

I ANALGESICS

Boothe, D.M., (guest ed), 1998. The Veterinary Clinics of North America, Small Animal Practice. Clinical Pharmacology and Therapeutics 28 (2), 366–374.

Eeg, P.H., the Veterinary Medical Forum, 1998. New Advances in Control of Pain and Inflammation. Veterinary Learning Systems, Pfizer Animal Health, Trenton NJ, pp. 48, 51–52, 75.

Hansen, B., 2008. Analgesia for the critically ill dog or cat: an update. In: Mathews, K.A. (guest ed), The Veterinary Clinics of North America, Small Animal Practice 38 (6), 1353–1363.

Hellyer, P., Rodan, I., Brunt, J., et al., 2007. (AAHA/AAFP Pain Management Guidelines Task Force Members), AAHA/AAFP Pain Management Guidelines for Dogs and Cats. Journal of the American Animal Hospital Association 43, 235–248.

Ko, J.C., Freeman, L.J., Barletta, M., et al., 2011. Efficacy of oral transmucosal and intravenous administration of buprenorphine before surgery for postoperative analgesia in dogs undergoing ovariohysterectomy. Journal of the American Veterinary Medical Association 238, 318–328.

Lamont, L.A., 2008. Adjunctive analgesic therapy in veterinary medicine. In: Mathews, K.A. (Ed.), The Veterinary Clinics of North America, Small Animal Practice 38 (6), 1187–1203.

Looney, A.L., 2009. Acute pain management. In: Bonagura, J.D., Twedt, D.C. (Eds.), Kirk's Current Veterinary Therapy XIV. Saunders Elsevier, St Louis, pp. 9–17.

Mathews, K.A., 2006. Veterinary Emergency and Critical Care Manual, second ed. Lifelearn Inc., Guelph.

Quandt, J., Lee, J.A., 2006. Analgesia and constant rate infusions. In: Silverstein, D.C., Hopper, K. (Eds.), Small Animal Critical Care Medicine. Saunders Elsevier, St Louis, pp. 710–715.

Sparkes, A.H., Heiene, R., Lascelles, B.D.X., et al., 2010. ISFM and AAFP Consensus Guidelines, Long-term use of NSAIDs in cats. Journal of Feline Medicine and Surgery 12, 521–538.

Tranquilli, W.J., Fikes, L.L., Raffe, M.R., 1989. Selecting the right analgesics: indications and dosage requirements. Veterinary Medicine 84 (7), 692–697.

II BLOOD CROSS MATCHING

Giger, U., Stieger, K., Palos, H., 2005. Comparison of various canine blood-typing methods. American Journal of Veterinary Research 66, 1386–1392.

Giger, U., 2009. Blood typing and crossmatching. In: Bonagura, J.D., Twedt, D.C. (Eds.), Kirk's Current Veterinary Therapy XIV. Saunders Elsevier, St Louis, pp. 260–265.

Hohenhaus, A.E., 2011. Blood transfusion and blood substitutes. In: DiBartola, S.P. (Ed.), Fluid, Electrolyte, and Acid-Base Disorders in Small Animal Practice, fourth ed. Elsevier Saunders, St Louis, pp. 598–599.

Stieger, K., Palos, H., Giger, U., 2005. Comparison of various blood-typing methods for the feline AB blood group system. American Journal of Veterinary Research 66, 1393–1399.

III BLOOD COMPONENT INDICATIONS

Cotter, S.M. (Ed.), 1991. Advances in Veterinary Science, Comparative Medicine, Comparative Transfusion Medicine, vol 36. Academic Press, London.

Giger, U., 2006. Transfusion medicine. In: Silverstein, D.C., Hopper, K. (Eds.), Small Animal Critical Care Medicine. Saunders Elsevior, St Louis, pp. 281–287.

Hohenhaus, A.E., (guest ed), 1992. Problems in Veterinary Medicine. Transfusion Medicine 4 (4).

Hohenhaus, A.E., 2011. Blood transfusion and blood substitutes. In: DiBartola, S.P. (Ed.), Fluid, Electrolyte, and Acid-Base Disorders in Small Animal Practice, fourth ed. Elsevier Saunders, St Louis, pp. 585–604.

Kirby, R., Stamp, G.L., (guest eds), 1989. The Veterinary Clinics of North America, Small Animal Practice. Critical Care 19 (6), 1112–1113.

Kristensen, A.T., Feldman, B.F., (guest eds), 1995. The Veterinary Clinics of North America, Small Animal Practice. Canine and Feline Transfusion Medicine 25 (6).

Appendices

Schaer, M., (guest ed), 1989. The Veterinary Clinics of North America, Small Animal Practice. Fluid and Electrolyte Disorders 19 (2), 362–363.

IV FLUID THERAPY

DiBartola, S.P., 2011. Fluid, Electrolyte, and Acid-Base Disorders in Small Animal Practice, fourth ed. Elsevier Saunders, St Louis.

Kirk, R.W. (Ed.), 1983. Current Veterinary Therapy VIII. W B Saunders, Philadelphia, pp. 408–411.

National Research Council, 1985. Nutritional Requirements of the Dog. Bethesda, MD.

National Research Council, 1987. Nutritional Requirements of the Cat. Bethesda, MD.

Schaer, M., (guest ed), 1989. The Veterinary Clinics of North America, Small Animal Practice. Fluid and Electrolyte Disorders 19 (2), 205, 361–377.

Silverstein, D.C., Hopper, K., 2006. Small Animal Critical Care Medicine. Saunders Elsevier, St Louis.

V GUIDELINES FOR POTASSIUM SUPPLEMENTATION

DiBartola, S.P., 2011. Fluid, Electrolyte, and Acid-Base Disorders in Small Animal Practice, fourth ed. Elsevier Saunders, St Louis, pp. 107–108.

Feldman, E.C., Nelson, R.W., 2004. Table 13-10, Guidelines for potassium supplementation in intravenous fluids. Canine and Feline Endocrinology and Reproduction, third ed. Saunders Elsevier, St. Louis.

Mathews, K.A., 2006. Veterinary Emergency and Critical Care Manual, second ed. Lifelearn Inc., Guelph, pp. 395.

VI INSULIN PREPARATIONS AVAILABLE

Feldman, E.C., Nelson, R.W., 2004. Canine and Feline Endocrinology and Reproduction, third ed. Saunders Elsevier, St Louis.

Kirk, R.W., Bistner, S.I., Ford, R.B. (Eds.), 1989. Handbook of Veterinary Procedures and Emergency Treatment, fourth ed. W B Saunders, Philadelphia, pp. 113.

Nelson, R.W., Henley, K., Cole, C., the PZIR Clinical Study Group, 2009. Field safety and efficacy of protamine zinc recombinant human insulin for treatment of diabetes mellitus in cats.

Journal of Veterinary Internal Medicine 23, 787–793.

Plumb, D.C., 2011. Plumb's Veterinary Drug Handbook, seventh ed. Wiley-Blackwell, Ames.

Rucinsky, R., Cook, A., Haley, S., 2010. AAHA Diabetes Management Guidelines for Dogs and Cats. Journal of the American Animal Hospital Association 46, 215–224.

VIII POISONOUS PLANTS

Atkinson, K.J., Fine, D.M., Evans, T.J., et al., 2008. Suspected lily-of-the-valley (Convallaria majalis) toxicosis in a dog. Journal of Veterinary Emergency and Critical Care 18 (4), 399–403.

Knight, A.P., 2006. A Guide of Poisonous House and Garden Plants. Teton New Media, Jackson.

Langston, C.E., 2002. Acute renal failure caused by lily ingestion in six cats. Journal of the American Veterinary Medical Association 220 (1), 49–52.

Milewski, L.M., Khan, S.A., 2006. An overview of potentially life-threatening poisonous plants in dogs and cats. Journal of Veterinary Emergency and Critical Care 16 (1), 25–33.

Osweiler, G.D., Hovda, L.R., Brutlag, A.G., et al., 2011. Blackwell's Five-Minute Veterinary Consult Clinical Companion Small Animal Toxicology. Wiley-Blackwell, Ames.

Rumbeiha, W.K., Francis, J.A., Fitzgerald, S.D., et al., 2004. A comprehensive study of Easter lily poisoning in cats. Journal of Veterinary Diagnosis and Investigation 16, 527–541.

Saxon-Buri, S., 2004. Daffodil toxicosis in an adult cat. Canadian Veterinary Journal 45, 248–250.

Scanlan, S., Eagles, D., Vacher, N., et al., 2006. Duranta erecta poisoning in nine dogs and a cat. Australian Veterinary Journal 84, 367–370.

Tefft, K.M., 2004. Lily nephrotoxicity in cats. Compendium on Continuing Education for the Practicing Veterinarian 26 (2), 149–157.

IX RELATIVELY NONTOXIC INGESTIONS

Kirk, R.W., Bistner, S.I., Ford, R.B. (Eds.), 1990. Handbook of Veterinary Procedures and Emergency Treatment, fifth ed. W B Saunders, Philadelphia, pp. 166.

X DRUGS WITH POTENTIAL ADVERSE AFFECTS DURING PREGNANCY

Johnson, C.A., (guest ed), 1986. The Veterinary Clinics of North America: Small Animal Practice. Reproduction and periparturient care 16 (3), 531–533.

Plumb, D.C., 2011. Plumb's Veterinary Drug Handbook, seventh ed. Wiley-Blackwell, Ames.

XI DRUGS SAFE FOR USE DURING PREGNANCY

Johnson, C.A., (guest ed), 1986. The Veterinary Clinics of North America: Small Animal Practice. Reproduction and periparturient care 16 (3), 531–533.

Plumb, D.C., 2011. Plumb's Veterinary Drug Handbook, seventh ed. Wiley-Blackwell, Ames.

XII DRUGS TO AVOID IN SEVERE RENAL FAILURE

Kirk, R.W. (Ed.), 1983. Current Veterinary Therapy VIII. W B Saunders, Philadelphia, pp. 1038.

Plumb, D.C., 2011. Plumb's Veterinary Drug Handbook, seventh ed. Wiley-Blackwell, Ames.

XIII DRUGS REQUIRING DOSE REDUCTION IN PATIENTS WITH RENAL FAILURE

Plumb, D.C., 2011. Plumb's Veterinary Drug Handbook, seventh ed. Wiley-Blackwell, Ames.

XIV COMMONLY USED FORMULAE

Willard, M.D., Tvedten, H., Turnwald, G.H., 1989. Small Animal Clinical Diagnosis by Laboratory Methods. W B Saunders, Philadelphia.

XV CONSTANT RATE INFUSION FORMULAE

Bonagura, J.D., Kirk, R.W. (Eds.), 1995. Current Veterinary Therapy XII. W B Saunders, Philadelphia, pp. 186.

Silverstein, D.C., Hopper, K., 2006. Small Animal Critical Care Medicine. Saunders Elsevier, St Louis.

XVI DRUGS COMMONLY ADMINISTERED BY CRI

Mathews, K.A., 2006. Veterinary Emergency and Critical Care Manual, second ed. Lifelearn Inc., Guelph, pp. 229–262.

Silverstein, D.C., Hopper, K., 2006. Small Animal Critical Care Medicine. Saunders Elsevier, St Louis.

XVII METRIC CONVERSIONS CHART (APPROXIMATIONS)

Bonagura, J.D., Kirk, R.W. (Eds.), 1995. Current Veterinary Therapy XII. W B Saunders, Philadelphia, pp. 1417.

Plumb, D.C., 2011. Plumb's Veterinary Drug Handbook, seventh ed. Wiley-Blackwell, Ames, pp. 1157.

Rice, L., 1989. Lead poisoning in cats. Feline Health Topics, vol 4, no 2. Cornell Feline Health Center, Cornell University College of Veterinary Medicine, Ithaca, pp. 525.

XVIII BODY SURFACE AREA TABLES

Ettinger, S.J., 1975. Textbook of Veterinary Internal Medicine, Diseases of the Dog and Cat, second ed. W B Saunders, Philadelphia, pp. 146.

Plumb, D.C., 2011. Plumb's Veterinary Drug Handbook, seventh ed. Wiley-Blackwell, Ames, pp. 1154.

XIX COMMONLY USED EMERGENCY DRUGS (APPROXIMATE DOSAGES)

Bonagura, J.D., Twedt, D.C., 2009. Kirk's Current Veterinary Therapy XIV. Saunders Elsevier, St Louis.

Greene, C.E., 2006. Infectious Diseases of the Dog and Cat, third ed. Saunders Elsevier, Philadelphia.

Plumb, D.C., 2011. Plumb's Veterinary Drug Handbook, seventh ed. Wiley-Blackwell, Ames.

Silverstein, D.C., Hopper, K., 2006. Small Animal Critical Care Medicine. Saunders Elsevier, St Louis.

Index

Page numbers followed by 'f' indicate figures, 't' indicate tables, and 'b' indicate boxes.

INDEX

INDEX

Index

887

INDEX